Nova IVI Textbook of Infertility and Assisted Reproductive Technology

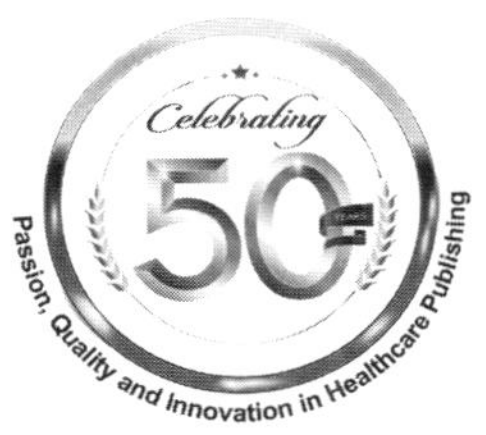

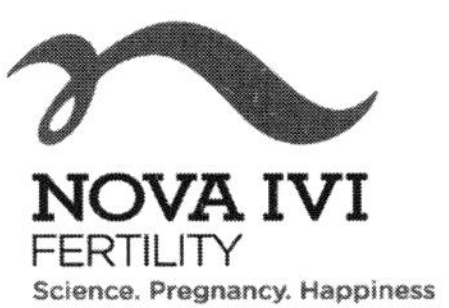

Nova IVI Textbook of Infertility and Assisted Reproductive Technology

Editor

Manish Banker MD
Medical Director
Nova IVI Fertility, India
Director
Pulse Women's Hospital
Ahmedabad, Gujarat, India
Past President
Indian Society for Assisted Reproduction (ISAR)

Co-Editors

Richa Jagtap
MD (Obs and Gyne) DGO Fellowship Reproductive Medicine, Singapore
Certificate Course in Fertility, Andrologist and Quality Management, Germany
Clinical Director and Consultant Reproductive Medicine
Nova IVI Fertility
Mumbai, Maharashtra, India
Founding Member
Fertility Preservation Society (India)

Ritu Hinduja
MD Masters Certificate Reproductive Medicine and IVF, UK
Diploma in Reproductive Medicine, Germany
Fellowship in Reproductive Medicine (India, Spain, Israel)
Certificate in Genetic Counselling
Consultant Reproductive Medicine
Nova IVI Fertility
Mumbai, Maharashtra, India

Sneha Sathe
MS Masters Certificate Reproductive Medicine and IVF, UK
Consultant Reproductive Medicine
Nova IVI Fertility
Mumbai, Maharashtra, India

Sulbha Arora
MD DNB Fellowship in Reproductive Medicine, Israel
Clinical Director and Senior
Consultant Reproductive Medicine
Nova IVI Fertility
Mumbai, Maharashtra, India

Foreword

Juan A Garcia-Velasco, José Remohi, Antonio Pellicer

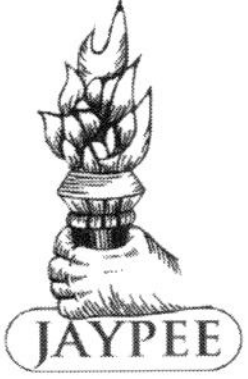

JAYPEE BROTHERS MEDICAL PUBLISHERS
The Health Sciences Publisher
New Delhi | London | Panama

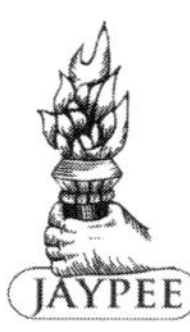

Jaypee Brothers Medical Publishers (P) Ltd

Headquarters

Jaypee Brothers Medical Publishers (P) Ltd
4838/24, Ansari Road, Daryaganj
New Delhi 110 002, India
Phone: +91-11-43574357
Fax: +91-11-43574314
Email: jaypee@jaypeebrothers.com

Overseas Offices

J.P. Medical Ltd
83 Victoria Street, London
SW1H 0HW (UK)
Phone: +44 20 3170 8910
Fax: +44 (0)20 3008 6180
Email: info@jpmedpub.com

Jaypee-Highlights Medical Publishers Inc
City of Knowledge, Bld. 235, 2nd Floor
Clayton, Panama City, Panama
Phone: +1 507-301-0496
Fax: +1 507-301-0499
Email: cservice@jphmedical.com

Jaypee Brothers Medical Publishers (P) Ltd
Bhotahity, Kathmandu, Nepal
Phone: +977-9741283608
Email: kathmandu@jaypeebrothers.com

Website: www.jaypeebrothers.com
Website: www.jaypeedigital.com

Inquiries for bulk sales may be solicited at: jaypee@jaypeebrothers.com

Nova IVI Textbook of Infertility and Assisted Reproductive Technology

First Edition: **2019**

ISBN 978-93-88958-84-4

Printed at Rajkamal Electric Press, Plot No. 2, Phase-IV, Kundli, Haryana.

Dedicated to

Dr Pravin Patel

Brother, Friend, Philosopher and Guide

Contributors

Aanchal Garg
Consultant
Nova IVI Fertility
Lucknow, Uttar Pradesh, India

Aarthi Maini MBBS MS
Fellow in Reproductive Medicine
NOVA IVI Fertility
New Delhi, India

Abha Bhat
MBBS DGO MRCOG PGDCE (PG Diploma in Clinical Embryology)
Clinical Director
Milann—The Fertility Center
Mumbai, Maharashtra, India

Aditi Kotdawala MSc
Clinical Embryologist and Lab Manager
Nova IVI Fertility
Ahmedabad, Gujarat, India

A Fabris MD
Gynecologist
Unit of Reproductive Medicine in IVIRMA-Madrid
Madrid, Spain

Aila Coello MSc
Embryologist
IVI Valencia
Valencia, Spain

Akanksha Allahbadia Gupta MS (Obstetrics & Gynecology)
Consultant Fertility Specialist
Indira IVF
New Delhi, India

Akila B MBBS MS
Assistant Gynecologist
Paul's Hospital
Centre for Advanced Endoscopy and Infertility
Kochi, Kerala, India

Alberto Pacheco Castro PhD
Director-Andrology Laboratory
IVI-Madrid, Spain
Associate Professor
Alfonso X "El Sabio" University, Madrid, Spain

Alberto Tejera PhD
Embryologist
IVI Valencia
Valencia, Spain

Alessandro Conforti MD
Professor of Obstetrics and Gynecology
Department of Neurosciences
Reproductive Sciences and
Odontostomatology
University of Naples Federico II
Naples, Italy

Alfredo Guillén MD
Gynecologist
Vice Director
IVI Madrid, Madrid, Spain

Ana Cobo PhD
Director
Cryopreservation Laboratory
IVI Valencia, Valencia
Associate Professor
Rey Juan Carlos University
Madrid, Spain

Anil Gudi MD MRCOG
Medical Director
Homerton Fertility Center
London, UK

Anisha Uberoi MSc
Clinical Embryologist and Lab Manager
Nova IVI Fertility
Chembur, Mumbai, India

Antonia Tocino Diaz MD
Reproductive Gynecology
IVI Seville, Avenida República, Argenita

Antonio Pellicer MD
Adjunct Professor
Department of Obstetrics and Gynecology
Yale University, USA
IVIRMA President
IVI Foundation President
Professor of Obstetrics and Gynecology
University Medical School, Valencia
Past Dean University Medical School, Valencia
Doctor honoris causa, Polytechnic University
Valencia
Co-Editor-in-Chief, Fertility and Sterility

Arati Gupte Shah MS
Associate Consultant
Nova IVI Fertility Clinics and
Pulse Women's Hospital
Ahmedabad, Gujarat, India

Arindam Rath MD
Consultant
Nova IVI Fertility
Kolkata, West Bengal, India

Ashvini Deshmukh MBBS MS (Obs & Gyn)
Assistant Gynecologist
Nova IVI Fertility
Mumbai, Maharashtra, India

Avantika Vaze (Parab)
MS (Obs & Gyne) Fellowship in Infertility and Reproductive Medicine
Assistant Gynecologist
Nova IVI Fertility
Mumbai, Maharashtra, India

Avinash Kumar BTech (IIT Kanpur) MBA (IIM Bengaluru)
Founder Director
Families of Joy Foundation
New Delhi, India

Aviva Pinto Rodrigues MBBS MD (Obs & Gyne)
Kasturba Medical College
Mangaluru University
Mangaluru, Karnataka, India
Clinical Director
Nova IVI Fertility
Bengaluru Karnataka, India

Azadeh Patel MS (Obs & Gyne)
Fellow
Reproductive Medicine and Endocrinology
IVI Madrid
Madrid, Spain
Assistant Consultant
Nova IVI Fertility
Ahmedabad, Gujarat, India

Barbara Lawrenz MD PhD
Consultant
IVI Middle East Fertility Clinic
Abu Dhabi, UAE

Belén Aparicio MSc
Embryologist
IVI Valencia
Valencia, Spain

Carlo Alviggi MD PhD
Assistant Professor
University of Naples
Federico II
Naples, Italy

Carlos Balmori MD FECMS
Consultant
Men's Health and Sexual Medicine
IVI-Madrid
Madrid, Spain

Carlos Dosouto Capel MD
Physician/Doctor
Hospital Universitario Dexeus
Reproductive Medicine Service
Barcelona, Spain

Carlos Iglesias Sánchez MD
Gynecologist (Reproductive Medicine)
Av del Talgo, IVI Madrid, Madrid, Spain

Carlos Marin MSc
Biologist, Igenomix
Valencia, Spain

Carlos Simon MD PhD
Professor (Obstetrics and Gynecology)
University of Valencia, Valencia, Spain
Scientific Director, Igenomix
Adjunct Clinical Professor
Department of Obstetrics and Gynecology
Stanford University School of Medicine, California, USA
Adjunct Professor
Department of Obstetrics and Gynecology
Baylor College of Medicine
Texas, USA

Carmela Albert PhD
IVF Laboratory Supervisor
IVI Valencia
Valencia, Spain

Carmen Rubio Llues PhD
Lab Director
Molecular Cytogenetics
Igenomix, Spain

Carmen Vidal MD PhD (Obs & Gyne)
Senior Consultant
Reproductive Medicine Unit
IVI Valencia
Valencia, Spain

Carol Rubina D'Souza MSc
Clinical Embryologist
Nova IVI Fertility
Bengaluru, Karnataka, India

Cinzia Caligara MD
Gynecologist
IVI Sevilla Clinic
Sevilla, Spain

Cristina González Ravina PhD
Director-Andrology Laboratory
IVI Sevilla, Spain
Associate Professor
Seville University, Spain

Deven Patel MSc
Clinical Embryologist and Regional Manager
Nova IVI Fertility
Ahmedabad, Gujarat, India

Devika Gunasheela
MBBS MRCOG (Lon) Fellow in Reproductive Medicine (RGUHS)
Director
Gunasheela Surgical and Maternity Hospital
Bengaluru, Karnataka, India

Diana Alecsandru MD PhD
Consultant Clinical Immunologist
Physician for Reproductive Immunology
Reproductive Immunology Unit
IVIRMA Madrid
Madrid, Spain

Diana Collado Muñoz MD PhD
Oocyte Donation Program
Gynecologist
IVI Madrid, Madrid, Spain

Diana Divya Crasta
Masters in Social Work with Medical and Psychiatric Specialization
Chief Psychological Counselor
Nova IVI Fertility
Bengaluru, Karnataka, India

Diksha Goswami Sharma
MD DNB MRCOG FNB (Reproductive Medicine)
IVF Consultant
Rainbow IVF
Agra, Uttar Pradesh, India

Esther Santamaría López MSc
Embryologist
IVI Sevilla Clinic
Sevilla, Spain

Gautam Nand Allahbadia
MD DNB FNAMS DGO DFP FICOG FCPS FICMU
Consultant Reproductive Endocrinology and IVF
Consultant Obstetrics and Gynecology
Orchid Fertility Centre, Dubai Health Care City, Dubai, UAE
Metropolitan Medical Center, Dubai, UAE

Geetha R MBBS MS
Assistant Gynecologist
Paul's Hospital
Centre for Advanced Endoscopy and Infertility
Kochi, Kerala, India

George Paul MBBS MS
Assistant Gynecologist
Paul's Hospital
Centre for Advanced Endoscopy and Infertility
Kochi, Kerala, India

Giuseppe De Placido MD
Professor
Department of Neurosciences, Reproductive Sciences and
Odontostomatology
University of Naples Federico II
Naples, Italy

Graciela Kohls Ilgner MD
Gynecologist
Specialized in Reproductive Medicine
IVI-Madrid
Madrid, Spain

Guillermo Martínez-Canillas MD
Department of Reproductive Endocrinology and Infertility
IVIRMA-Madrid
Madrid, Spain

Haahr T MD PhD
Clinical Assistant
Department of Clinical Medicine
The Fertility Clinic Skive
Skive Regional Hospital and Skive
Aarhus University, Aarhus, Denmark

Hetal Shukla MSc
Chief Andrologist
Nova IVI Fertility
Ahmedabad, Gujarat, India

Himani Agnihotri MSc
Lab Manager
Nova IVI Fertility
Coimbatore, Tamil Nadu, India

Human M Fatemi MD PhD
Director
Middle-East Operations
IVI Middle-East Fertility Clinic
Abu Dhabi, UAE

Irene Rubio Palacios PhD
Medical Affairs Department
IVIRMA Madrid

Israel Ortega Sanchez MD
Gynecologist
IVI Madrid, Madrid, Spain

Jaideep Malhotra
MD FICOG FICMCH FICS FRCOG FMAS
Managing Director ART
Rainbow IVF Hospital
Agra, Uttar Pradesh, India
Professor, Dubrovnik International University, Croatia
President Elect, ISPAT Editor-in-Chief, SAFOMS and SAFOG
Member, FIGO, RDEH
Regional Director of South Asia Ian Donald School of Ultrasound
Vice President, ISAR

Javier Herrero MSc
Medical Affairs Department
IVIRMA Madrid

Javier Martínez-Salazar Romero MD
Reproductive Unit
IVI-Madrid
Madrid, Spain

Jayesh Patel MS (Obs & Gyne)
Assistant Consultant
Nova IVI Fertility
Ahmedabad, Gujarat, India
Fellow, Reproductive Medicine and Endocrinology
IVI Madrid, Madrid, Spain

Jayesh Shinde
Master's Degree (Biotechnology of Human Assisted Reproduction Embryology)
Regional Manager and Clinical Embryologist
Embryology
Nova IVI Fertility
New Delhi, India

JM Puente MD
Specialist in Reproductive Ultrasound
H 12 de Octubre and IVIRMA-Madrid
Madrid, Spain

Jose Miravet-Valenciano MSc
Biologist, Igenomix
Valencia, Spain

José Remohí MD
IVIRMA President
Professor of Obstetrics and Gynecology
School of Medicine, University of Valencia, Spain

José V Medrano PhD
Health Research Institute La Fe
Valencia, Spain

Juan A García-Velasco MD PhD
Director
IVI Madrid, Madrid, Spain
IVI Director
Nova IVI Fertility India and GCC
Abu Dhabi, UAE
Professor of Obstetrics and Gynecology
Rey Juan Carlos University
Madrid, Spain

Juan Giles MD
Unit of Human Reproduction
Valencian Infertility Institute
University of Valencia
Valencia, Spain

Juan José Espinós-Gómez MD
Department of Obstetrics and Gynecology
Hospital de la Santa Creu I Sant Pau.
Fertty Barcelona
Universitat Autònoma de Barcelona
Barcelona, Spain

Julia K Bosdou MD MSc PhD
Obstetrics and Gynecology Resident
Unit for Home Reproduction
First Department of Obstetrics and Gynecology
Papageorgiou Hospital
Aristotle University of Thessaloniki Medical School
Thessaloniki, Greece

Kalyani Shrimali DNB MNAMS DRM (Germany)
Consultant
Nova IVI Fertility
Indore, Madhya Pradesh
Fellowship in Reproductive
Medicine
Indian College of Obstetricians and Gynaecologists
(ICOG)
Mumbai, Maharashtra, India

Kamini A Rao
DGO MRCOG DORCP DCh FRCOG (UK) MCh (UK) FICOG PGDMLE (Law) FNAMS
Medical Director (Obstetrics and Gynecology)
Milann (A Unit of BACC Health care Private Limited)
Bengaluru, Karnataka, India

Korula George MD MRACOG
Professor and Head
Reproductive Medicine Unit
Bangalore Baptist Hospital
Bengaluru, Karnataka, India

Krithika Devi J MBBS MD (Obs & Gyne)
Consultant
Fellowship in Andrology and
Reproductive Medicine
Nova IVI Fertility
Chennai, Tamil Nadu, India

Lakshmi Chirumamilla
MD (Obs & Gyne) MRCOG DFSRH
Clinical Director and Consultant Fertility Specialist
Nova IVI Fertility Clinic
Hyderabad, Telangana, India

Lovy Arora MBBS DGO
Fellow in Reproductive Medicine
Nova IVI Fertility
New Delhi, India

Manish Banker MD
Medical Director
Nova IVI Fertility, India
Director
Pulse Women's Hospital
Ahmedabad, Gujarat, India
Past President
Indian Society for Assisted Reproduction (ISAR)

Manjushri Kothekar MS (Obs & Gyne)
Assistant Gynecologist and Fellow
Department of Reproductive Medicine
Nova IVI Fertility
Mumbai, Maharashtra, India

Manuel Fernández-Sánchez PhD
Director IVI Seville
Av República Argentina
Seville, Spain

Marcos Meseguer PhD
IVF Scientific Supervisor
IVI Valencia, Valencia
Associate Professor
Valencia University
Valencia, Spain

Maria J de los Santos PhD
Director
IVF Laboratory
IVI Valencia, Valencia
IVI-INCLIVA Foundation
Valencia, Spain

Maria Ruiz-Alonso MSc
Biologist, Igenomix
Valencia, Spain

Mauro Cozzolino MD
IVIRMA Madrid-IVI Foundation
PhD Program in Universidad Rey Juan Carlos
Madrid, Spain

M Cerrillo MD
Specialist in Reproductive Medicine
Unit of Reproductive Medicine in IVIRMA-Madrid
Madrid, Spain

Megha Malik Aneja MBBS MS
Fellow in Reproductive Medicine
Nova IVI Fertility
New Delhi, India

Mirudhubashini Govindarajan MBBS FRCS (C)
Clinical Director and Consultant in Reproductive Medicine
Women's Center and Hospitals
Coimbatore, Tamil Nadu, India

Mohan S Kamath
MS DNB PGDMLS Fellow (Reproductive Medicine)
Professor
Reproductive Medicine Unit
Christian Medical College
Vellore, Tamil Nadu, India
Commonwealth Fellow (Reproductive Medicine), UK

Mona Shroff
Clinical Director and Consultant
Nova IVI Fertility
Seven Square Doctor House
Surat, Gujarat, India

Nalini Mahajan MD (Obs & Gyne) MMedSci (ART) (UK) FICOG
Director
Ferticity, New Delhi
President
Fertility Preservation Society (India)
Secretary
Asian Society for Fertility Preservation

Nameeta Mokashi Bhalerao
MBBS MS (Obs & Gyn) DNB FNB (Infertility) PGDMLE
Consultant Reproductive Medicine
Nova IVI Fertility
Pune, Maharashtra, India

Narendra Malhotra
MD FICOG FICMCH FRCOG FICS FMAS AFIAP
Professor
Dubrovnik International University
VP WAPM (World Association of Prenatal Medicine)
President, ISPAT (2017–2019)
Managing Director
Global Rainbow Healthcare
Agra, Uttar Pradesh, India

N Ashwini MBBS DNB Fellow in Reproductive Medicine (RGUHS)
Senior Consultant
Department of Obstetrics, Gynecology and Infertility
Gunasheela Surgical and Maternity Hospital
Bengaluru, Karnataka, India

Natalia Basile MSc PhD
Embryologist
IVI Madrid, Madrid, Spain

Naval Navin Shah
MSc Zoology (Endocrinology) Adv Dip Biotechnology
Regional Manager Embryology
Avhya ART Specialists Pvt Ltd
New Delhi, India

Navin Desai MSc
Clinical Embryologist
NIF, Mumbai, Maharashtra, India

Neharika Bora MD (Obs & Gyne) FICMCH FMAS
Infertility Consultant
Rainbow IVF Hospital
Agra, Uttar Pradesh, India
Assistant Professor
Bharati Vidyapeeth Medical College
Consultant, Malhotra Hospitals
Jr Consultant and Fellow, Reproductive Medicine,
Patankar Hospital
Pune, Maharashtra, India

Nicolás Prados Dodd
Embryologist and Laboratory Coordinator
IVI-RMA Headquarters Spain
Sevilla, TL

Nikita Banerjee MS (Obs & Gyne) DNB
Former Senior Resident
Maulana Azad Medical College and Lok Nayak Hospital
Fellow Reproductive Medicine
NOVA IVI, Mumbai, Maharashtra, India

Nisha Thakre MBBS MS (Obs & Gyne)
Clinical Research Fellow in fertility
Homerton Fertility Centre,
Homerton University Hospital
London, UK

Nozer Sheriar MD DNBE FICOG FCPS DGO
Consultant Obstetrics and Gynecology
Breach Candy, Hinduja Healthcare Surgical and Holy
Family Hospitals, Mumbai
Aviva Clinic for Women
Mumbai, Maharashtra, India
Past Secretary General and Chair
MTP Committee, Federation of Obstetric and
Gynecological Societies of India
Past President, Mumbai Obstetric and Gynecological
Society

Pallavi Menon MSc
Clinical Embryologist and Lab Manager
NIF Sadashivanagar
Bengaluru, Karnataka, India

Pallavi Prasad MBBS MD FNB
Consultant Gynecologist
Nova IVI Fertility
Bengaluru, Karnataka, India

Parnita Sardana
Fellow National Board
Nova IVI Fertility
Ahmedabad, Gujarat, India

Parul Katiyar MS (Obs & Gyne)
Senior Consultant
Infertility and Reproductive Medicine
Nova IVI Fertility
New Delhi, India

Paula Celada MD
Unit of Human Reproduction
Reproductive Medicine Unit
IVI Valencia
Valencia, Spain

Pere Mir Pardo PhD
Laboratory Manager
Igenomix Headquarters
Valencia, Spain

Peter Humaidan DMSc
Professor
Skive Regional Hospital and Faculty of Health
Aarhus University, Aarhus, Denmark

PG Paul MBBS DGO
Consultant Gynecologist and Endoscopic Surgeon
Paul's Hospital
Centre for Advanced Endoscopy and Infertility
Kochi, Kerala, India

Pilar Alamá Faubel MD PhD
Gynecologist
Oocyte Donation Program
Coordinator, Instituto Valenciano de
Infertilidad (IVI)
Valencia, Spain

Pilar Gámiz PhD
IVF Laboratory Supervisor
IVI Valencia
Valencia, Spain

PM Gopinath MD DGO FMMC FICS FICOG MBA
Director and Senior Consultant
Department of Obstetrics and
Gynecology and IVF
SIMS Hospitals
Chennai, Tamil Nadu, India

Pooja Dhir Bhayana
MBBS MD (Obs & Gyne) Fellowship in Reproductive Medicine
Consultant Reproductive Medicine
Nova IVI Fertility
Hisar, Haryana, India

Pravin Patel MD DGO
Director
Nova IVI Fertility Clinics and
Pulse Women's Hospital
Ahmedabad, Gujarat, India

Preeti Shah MSc
Clinical Embryologist and Regional Manager
Nova IVI Fertility
Ahmedabad, Gujarat, India

Puneet Rana Arora
MBBS MS MRCOF MSc (Reproduction and Development)
Senior Consultant and Reproductive Medicine Specialist
Infertility/Oncofertility
New Delhi, India

Rajneet Bhatia DGO
Clinical Associate
Obstetrics and Gynecology
Hinduja Healthcare Surgical Hospital
Mumbai, Maharashtra, India
Aviva Clinic for Women
Mumbai, Maharashtra, India

Rajni Khajuria PhD (Human Genetics)
Lab Manager
Igenomix
New Delhi, India

Ramya Jayaram MS (Obs & Gyne)
Fellowship in Reproductive Medicine Fellowship in Endogyne
Consultant
Women's Center and Hospitals
Coimbatore, Tamil Nadu, India

Reena Gupta MBBS MS FNB
Consultant
Nova IVI Fertility
New Delhi, India

Richa Jagtap
MD (Obs and Gyne) DGO, Fellowship Reproductive Medicine, Singapore, Certificate Course in Fertility, Andrologist and Quality Management, Germany
Clinical Director and Consultant Reproductive Medicine
Nova IVI Fertility
Mumbai, Maharashtra, India
Founding Member
Fertility Preservation Society (India)

Rishabh Bora MBBS MD (Radiology)
Radiology Consultant
Global Rainbow Hospital
Agra, Uttar Pradesh, India
Formerly, Senior Resident (Radiology)
Deen Dayal Upadhyay Hospital
New Delhi, India

Rishina Bansal MSc
Clinical Embryologist and Lab Manager
NIF, Mumbai, Maharashtra, India

Ritu Hinduja
MD Masters Certificate Reproductive Medicine and IVF, UK, Diploma in Reproductive Medicine, Germany, Fellowship in Reproductive Medicine (India, Spain, Israel) Certificate in Genetic Counselling
Consultant Reproductive Medicine
Nova IVI Fertility
Mumbai, Maharashtra, India

Rohit Gutgutia MBBS DGO
Clinical Director
Motherhood IVF
Kolkata, West Bengal, India

Rupin Shah MS MCh (Urology)
Consultant (Andrologist and Microsurgeon)
Department of Urology
Lilavati Hospital and Research Centre
Mumbai, Maharashtra, India

Sandeep Shah MBBS MD (Obstetrics and Gynecology)
Consultant Infertility
Nova IVI Fertility
Ahmedabad, Gujarat, India

Sandro C Esteves PhD MD
Medical and Scientific Director
Androfert
Andrology and Human
Reproduction Clinic
Center for Male Reproduction
Sao Paulo, Brazil

Saroja Koppala MRCOG RCOG
Consultant
Nova IVI Fertility
Hyderabad, Telangana, India

Sayali Palnitkar MSc (Microbiology) MS (Clinical Embryology)
Junior Embryologist
Nova IVI Fertility
Pune, Maharashtra, India

Shalu Gupta MS (Obs & Gyne) DNB MNAMS FNB (Rep Med)
Infertility Consultant
Nova IVI Fertility, New Delhi, India

Shashank Joshi
MD DM FRCP (Lon, Edin, Glasg) FACE (USA) FACP (USA) FICP
Consultant Endocrinologist
Joshi Clinic, Lilavati and Bhatia Hospitals
Mumbai, Maharashtra, India

Shridutt Gaitonde BSc
Clinical Embryologist
NIF, Mumbai, Maharashtra, India

Sneha Sathe
MS Masters Certificate Reproductive Medicine and IVF, UK
Consultant Reproductive Medicine
Nova IVI Fertility
Mumbai, Maharashtra, India

Stratis Kolibianakis MD MSc PhD
Associate Professor
Obstetrics, Gynecology and
Assisted Reproduction Unit for
Human Reproduction
Medical School
Aristotle University, Thessaloniki, Greece

Sujal Munshi MD DNB MICOG
Consultant Endoscopic Surgeon
National Innovation Foundation, Ahmedabad, Gujarat, India
Diploma in Advanced Gynec Endoscopic Surgeries
Kiel, Germany
CICE, France

Sulbha Arora
MD DNB Fellowship in Reproductive Medicine, Israel
Clinical Director and Senior
Consultant Reproductive Medicine
Nova IVI Fertility
Mumbai, Maharashtra, India

Sumeetkaur Mehta MBBS DNB FRM
Assistant Gynecologist
Paul's Hospital
Centre for Advanced Endoscopy and Infertility
Kochi, Kerala, India

Supreet Pal Singh MSc (Clinical Embryology)
Clinical Embryologist
Embryology
Nova IVI Fertility
Jalandhar, Punjab, India

Taswin Kaur DGO FRM
Consultant Reproductive Medicine
Department of Obstetrics and Gynaecology
Chandra Superspeacilty Hospital
Anantapur, Andhra Pradesh, India

Ujwala Rao BSc MBBS Master of Medicine
Reproductive Medicine and
Genetics University of Sydney
Sydney, Australia

Vineet Malhotra MBBS MS DNB (Urology)
Consultant Urologist and Andrologist
Nova IVI Fertility, Rockland Hospital
New Delhi, India

Yolanda Minguez PhD
IVF, Andrology and PDG Laboratory Coordinator
Vice Director
IVI Madrid, Madrid, Spain

Foreword

We have the pleasure to introduce this book edited by Dr Manish Banker which is a fantastic compendium of modern infertility management. He is one of the most recognized experts in infertility around the world and has made sure to include, as authors of the different chapters, many colleagues who have great expertise in the different topics that are covered herein.

The book begins by a thoughtful analysis of the current preconceptional evaluation and also evaluation of the infertile couple, making special emphasis on the ovarian reserve, which is a major problem in our daily practice.

There are a substantial number of chapters dedicated to male infertility. Contrary to what was thought in the past, male problems are found in approximately 50% of our couples. Modern techniques, especially intracytoplasmic sperm injection (ICSI), have completely changed the way we approach male infertility.

Polycystic ovarian syndrome (PCOS) is discussed in detail in a number of chapters, emphasizing its importance in many areas of the globe, including India. The way adolescent girls should be managed, the way PCOS women should be stimulated for assisted reproduction, the management of ovarian hyperstimulation syndrome, are all chapters that deserve careful reading.

Dr Manish Banker has also created two sections for problematic cases that include difficult ovaries or gynecological diseases such as the poor responder, the high responder, women with endometriosis, adenomyosis, or hydrosalpinx.

Another section of the book is dedicated to the modern ART laboratory. Although the contribution of the different stimulation protocols and introduction of ultrasound have been relevant, nothing compares to the advancement in the laboratories. Today, we generate much more better embryos with higher chances to implant due to the culture conditions and embryo selection methods. All these aspects are carefully analyzed in this book by world experts.

Last but not least, some chapters are dedicated to highlight the importance of Genetics and Ethics in our field; some medicolegal aspects; and also some new developments such as fertility preservation or management of recurrent pregnancy loss.

All in all, a complete and well-written manual to which we wish and predict a great success among our colleagues, medical students, and residents.

Juan A Garcia-Velasco
José Remohi
Antonio Pellicer

Preface

"Of all the rights of a woman, perhaps the greatest is to be a mother"!

—Lin Yutang

The field of infertility, though one of the most difficult and challenging, is at the same time the most satisfying! The hopes, dreams, and longings of the patient are pitched upon us and thus it becomes our great responsibility to leave no stone unturned in our diagnosis and treatment of these patients.

Many modern-day lifestyle issues have contributed to the rise in infertility and there has also been a rise in social pressure to beget a child!! Scientific knowledge is continuously evolving and reproductive medicine is certainly not immune to this phenomenon. However, there has been a lacuna in addressing these wide range of topics dealing with infertility.

This book was started as a series of handbooks on each topic related to reproductive medicine. However, seeing the need as well as demand for a handy, easy to read yet scientifically sound material, it has been compiled into a textbook. It covers a large range of topics from basic physiology and primary management of infertility to the very latest in implantation and embryo selection and screening. The chapters are authored by the acknowledged masters in their field. Sections on polycystic ovarian syndrome (PCOS), male infertility, laboratory procedures in ART have been added to make it a comprehensive and easy daily reference book for all of us attached to this field of medicine. The book ends with very thought provoking chapters dealing with Adoption, Counseling, Medicolegal and Ethical Aspects, Third Party and Cross Border Reproduction.

I hope this book will be helpful to the Postgraduate Students, Gynecologists, Embryologists, Infertility Counselors, and Fertility Specialists.

I want to acknowledge the debt I owe to my parents Dr Shyama and Dr Rajju Banker for inspiring me with their lifelong devotion to their patients in the field of Gynecology.

I thank all four co-editors for their enthusiasm and efforts.

"Babies are bits of star dust blown into our hands by God.
Lucky the woman who knows the pangs of birth for she has held a star!"

—Larry Barretto

Lucky are we indeed to have chosen this field of medicine as our profession. I hope this modest endeavor will be of use; for I will not have lived in vain if even one life is enriched by this book!

Manish Banker

Contents

Section 1: Investigating Infertility

Section 2: Practical Management of Male Infertility

Secttion 3: Intrauterine Insemination

Secton 4: Endocrinology in Infertility

Section 7: Abnormalities of Pelvis

Section 8: Miscellaneous

Section 1

Investigating Infertility

CHAPTER

1

Basics of Human Reproduction: As we Understand it Now

Azadeh Patel, Jayesh Patel, Manish Banker

INTRODUCTION

Reproduction as we understand happens when a sperm fertilizes the ovum to form a zygote which would further develop into an embryo, fetus, and deliver as a child in future. But the process of development and maturation of the gametes and fertilization is very complex. Understanding of biology of gametes and human reproduction has led to evolution of technologies and techniques to help the infertile couples, over the years. The techniques used, try to mimic the natural way of conception. Thus, it is very important to understand the anatomy of the reproductive tract and physiology of the conception to evaluate the cause of infertility and to provide proper necessary treatment.

The union of sperm and egg is one of the essentials of reproduction; however, the remote site of occurrence of this event and microscopic dynamic nature, made it difficult to study for many years. Greater understanding of sperm and egg development and union provides major benefits of the clinical application of the assisted reproductive technologies. This chapter includes understanding of gametogenesis, sperm and egg transport, fertilization, implantation with associated genetics and immunology.

HISTORY

In 1677, Anton van Leeuwenhoek of Delft, Holland, by Galileo's microscope described the "little animals of the sperm." After 198 years, Wilhelm August Oscar Hertwig, in Germany, demonstrated the union of sperm and egg, fertilization, in the sea urchin. In 1951, Min Chueh Chang and Colin Russell Austin made discovery of sperms spending some time in the female reproductive tract before acquiring ability to fertilize the egg was made in rat and rabbit respectively.[1,2]

MALE REPRODUCTIVE SYSTEM

Male reproductive system consists of scrotum and testes within it, epididymis, vas deferens, ejaculatory duct, urethra, penis and accessory glandular structure (SVs: seminal vesicles, bulbourethral glands, and prostate).

The testes contain two anatomical units:

1. A network of seminiferous tubules comprised of:
   - *Sertoli cells*: They contain follicle-stimulating hormone (FSH) receptors, and synthesize inhibin B, anti-Müllerian hormone (AMH) and androgen-binding protein.
   - *Germ cells*: This develops into sperm by spermatogenesis.
2. An interstitium containing Leydig cells that produce androgens (testosterone mainly) and peritubular myoid cells. Luteinizing hormone (LH) receptors are found on Leydig cells (Flowchart 1).

Tight junctions between the Sertoli cells separate the tissue into two functional compartments (basal and adluminal), which are distinct structure and have limited permeability for diffusion of macromolecules between them. The *basal* compartment consists of the outer layers of the seminiferous tubules containing the spermatogonia. The *adluminal* compartment contains the inner portion of the seminiferous tubules, including primary spermatocytes and more advanced stages of spermatogenesis.

Spermatogenesis (Flowchart 2)

The male gamete is called as spermatozoa or sperm. Spermatogenesis/spermiogenesis is a complex, multistep process involving the proliferation and differentiation of spermatogonia into mature sperm, taking place in testes.

Flowchart 1: Neuroendocrine control male.

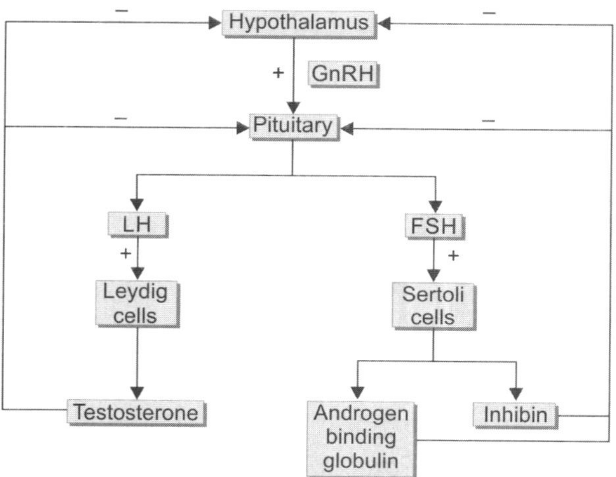

Flowchart 2: Spermatogenesis.

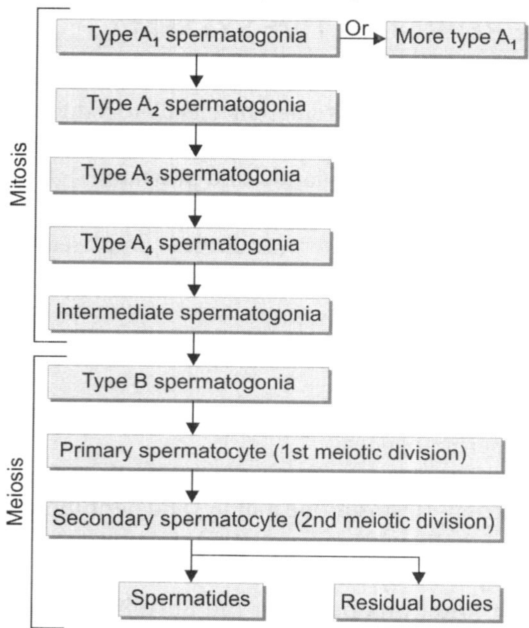

After the primary germ cells (PGCs) reaches the testes in the intrauterine life, they divide into Type A_1 spermatogonia, which has ovoid nucleus with chromatin and nuclear membrane. They are found near the basement membrane and are sperm stem cells. They are capable to divide into Type A_2 spermatogonia or self-renewal into Type A_1 spermatogonia. Type A_2 spermatogonia forms Type A_3 spermatogonia and successively Type A_4 spermatogonia. All these have capacity of self-renewal. If Type A_4 spermatogonia do not undergo self-renewal, it can undergo either cell death by apoptosis or differentiates into intermediate spermatogonium stage with the onset of puberty. Those who enter the process of spermatogenesis divide mitotically into Type B spermatogonia. From this, they divide mitotically to form Primary spermatocyte, which each undergo first meiotic division to form a pair of Secondary spermatocytes, which complete the second division of meiosis. The haploid cells thus formed are called spermatids. With the division from Type A_1 spermatogonium to spermatid, the cells move farther from the basement membrane toward the lumen. The spermatids located at the border of the lumen, loose their cytoplasmic connection and become sperm.[3] The seminiferous tubules empty into the network of tubules called as rete testes, through which sperm move to the epididymis.

Optimal spermatogenesis requires temperatures lower than body temperature, hence mammalian testis are located outside the body cavity.

Microscopic structure of sperm consists of:

- *Head*: Containing nucleus and acrosome
- *Mid-piece*: Containing mitochondria
- *Tail*: Containing axial filament and end piece.

Sperm Maturation and Transport

Sperm formation takes approximately 65 days from the spermatocyte stage,[3] and the transport of sperm through the epididymis to the ejaculatory ducts requires about 14 days. Maturation of sperm begins during their passage through the epididymis, as evidenced by enhancement of motility, but the final maturation (or capacitation) of sperm take place in the female genital tract after ejaculation. In epididymis, the sperm acquire surface glycoprotein (beta-defensin 126) that protects the sperm while they travel through the cervical mucus. The caudal epididymis stores sperm and make them available for ejaculation, thus providing repetitive fertile ejaculations. Adequate testosterone levels in circulation and maintenance of normal scrotal temperature is required for optimal sperm-function preservation and storage.[4] During ejaculation epididymal content is mixed with secretion from the prostate gland and seminal vesicle (SV).[5]

Otherwise the epididymis is believed to play only the storage role, as the sperm obtained by testicular biopsy is directly injected into an oocyte in intracytoplasmic sperm injection (ICSI), and is very successful in achieving fertilization and pregnancy.[6]

Semen forms a gel almost immediately following ejaculation but then liquefies in 20–30 minutes by prostatic enzymes. The alkaline pH of semen provides temporary protection for the sperm from the acidic environment of the vagina, but most sperm left in the vagina are immobilized within 2 hours. The most motile and fortunate sperms gain entrance into cervical mucus and then enter into the uterus. This entry is rapid, and sperm have been found in mucus within 90 seconds of ejaculation.[7] Contractions of the female reproductive tract occur during coitus and male forces (the flagellar activity of the sperm) are responsible for successful transport. The sperm swim and migrate through pores in the cervical mucus that are smaller than the sperm head; therefore, the sperm must actively push their way through the mucus. Those sperm incapable in motility are held at the level of cervical mucus.

FEMALE REPRODUCTIVE SYSTEM

- It comprises of two ovaries (female gonads) on each side of the body, two fallopian tubes, uterus, cervix and the vagina. Vagina is the female copulating organ and the sperms are deposited in the vagina after ejaculation.
- The function of the ovaries is to cyclically produce ovum for fertilization and of steroidogenesis by secreting cyclical estrogen and progesterone.

Oogenesis (Flowchart 3)

- Embryologically ovaries appear as early as 5th intrauterine week, and the PGCs start dividing by mitosis as early as 6–8th intrauterine week, reaching to 6–7 million oogonias by 16–20th intrauterine week. This represents the maximum ovarian capacity for the germ cells, mitosis does not occur after that.
- With the commencement of meiosis I by 7–8th intrauterine week the oogonia get arrested at the diplotene stage of prophase and they are now called as primary oocytes. The oogonia not undergoing meiosis are degenerated by apoptosis. So at the time of birth ovaries are left with only 2 million, and then 300,000 primary oocytes till puberty, out of which approximately only 400 will ovulate in reproductive years.
- Onset of puberty is marked by activation of HPO axis, and a cohort of oocytes is recruited by nonhormonal followed by hormonal selection for development and maturation by ovarian cycle every month. The oocyte of the dominant follicle undergoes resumption and completion of meiosis I with the onset of LH surge and the first polar body (containing 23X chromosomes and small amount of oocyte cytoplasm, in the perivitelline space) is released; now it is called as secondary oocyte. Just before the ovulation, it gets arrested at metaphase stage of second meiotic division, which is completed after sperm penetration.
- Thus, the ovum available for fertilization has 23X, and the rest 23 (X or Y) chromosomes come from sperm

Flowchart 3: Oogenesis.

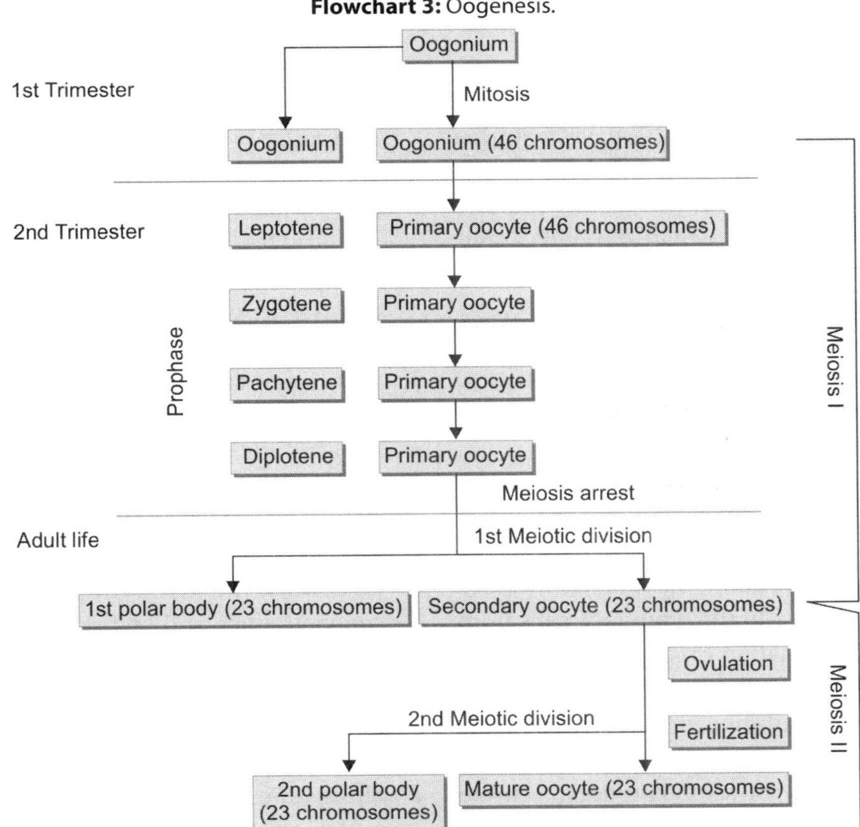

after fertilization. The second polar body containing 23X chromosomes from the oocyte with cytoplasm is released in the perivitelline space. Nowadays polar body biopsy from the metaphase II ovum, for patients undergoing IVF is possible to detect chromosomal abnormality of the ovum in case of high maternal age.[8]

- There is continuous loss of the oogonias and the oocytes by apoptosis from the intrauterine life to 45–50 years after birth. When the ovarian reserve gets exhausted it leads to menopause. The amount of the ovarian reserve can be measured by a marker AMH that is secreted by the preantral and small antral follicles in the ovarian cycle.[9] It suggests the number of the primordial follicles recruited from the primary pool of ovary. It is believed to be constant marker throughout the cycle.[10]

Physiology of Menstruation

The studies and ideas, over the past few decades have made a scientific progress in understanding the nature of the normal menstrual cycle and role of higher center and gonadal hormones in it. The normal cycle can be divided into:

- Follicular phase
- Ovulation
- Luteal phase.

Follicular Phase

This phase occurs over a period of 10–14 days, featuring action of hormones and local autocrine-paracrine peptides, leading to growth of the cohort of primordial follicles containing the follicle destined to ovulate through various stages of development.

The primordial follicle:

- The primordial follicle is resting stage of follicle containing oocyte, arrested in the diplotene stage of prophase of meiosis I, surrounded by single layer of spindled-shaped granulosa cells.
- The recruitment is nonhormonal and the selection of a cohort probably depends on residual pool of primordial follicles.
- Onset of follicular maturation is marked by increase in the oocyte size, change in the granulosa cells from spindle to cuboidal, formation of small gap junctions in between granulosa cells and oocyte which acts as pathway for exchange of nutrition, metabolite and signal interchange.
- Oocyte depends on the glycolysis end product, pyruvate for energy source from granulosa cells.[11]
- Activin and BMP are promoters and inhibin and AMH are inhibitors of primordial follicular development and growth.[12]

The preantral follicle:

- With the increasing follicular growth, the oocyte enlarges and is surrounded by a membrane called as *zona pellucida*, and the granulosa cells undergo multilayer proliferation and the theca cells form the surrounding stroma.
- Once the granulosa cells become 3–6 layered, they are separated from the stromal cells by *basement lamina*. The stromal cells close to the basement lamina are called as *theca interna cells*, and those in the outer region are called as *theca externa cells*.
- This growth of follicle is gonadotropin dependent.
- Follicle-stimulating hormone receptor number rise quickly till 1,500 receptors per granulosa cells in the preantral stage.[13]
- Role of androgens, in early follicular development is very complex. In low androgen concentration, by FSH stimulation, androgens are converted to estrogen by the process of *aromatization*, but higher concentration stimulates the 5α-reductase activity that reduces androgen to more potent 5 α -androgens. These further inhibits conversion to estrogen and also inhibits FSH-induced LH receptors formation[14-16] (Flowchart 4).

The antral follicle:

- Under synergistic influence of estradiol and FSH, there is increase in follicular fluid in the intracellular spaces of the granulosa cells, eventually coalescing to form a cavity, called as *antrum*, and the follicle is now called as *antral follicle*.
- The granulosa cells surrounding the oocyte are now called as *cumulus oophorus*.
- The antrum is rich in hormones mainly estrogen, growth factors and cytokines, and provides environment and nutrition for development and maturation of oocyte.
- The follicle with greatest rate of granulosa cells proliferation; produce highest estradiol concentration acquires dominance amongst them and is believed to yield a healthy oocyte.
- In contrary, those follicles with least estrogenic concentrations and higher androgenic levels, inhibits granulosa cell proliferation and undergo atresia and degeneration of oocyte.
- In case of premature LH rise, leads to excess androgen production that favors degeneration.
- The synthesis of the steroid hormones in a follicle, is explained by two-cell, two-gonadotropin system.

Flowchart 4: Aromatization.

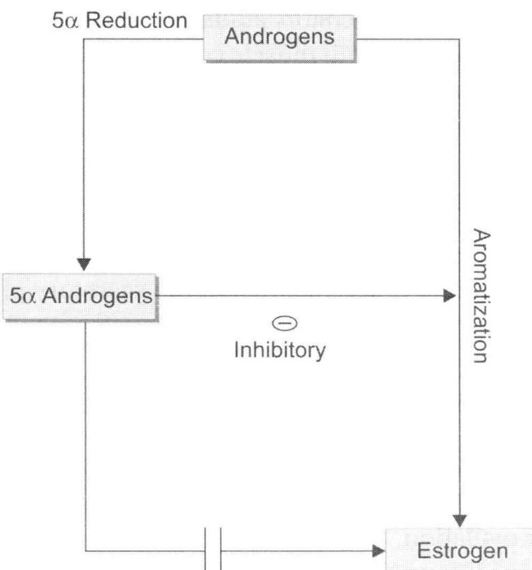

Two-cell, two-gonadotropin system (Flowchart 5):

- In preantral and antral follicles, the FSH receptors are located only on granulosa cells, and LH receptors on the theca interstitial cells located in the theca interna cells.
- The LH acts on the theca cells and facilitates conversion of low-density lipoprotein (LDL) cholesterol to androgens and these androgens are transported to granulosa cells and acts as a substrate to get converted into estrogens under the influence of FSH. This conversion depends upon follicular sensitivity to FSH, brought about by the action of FSH and estrogen.
- Thus, in the final stages of follicular maturation, LH is important for increasing amount of androgens, which are the substrate for estrogen production and promoting growth of the dominant follicle, with the regression of the smaller ones.

Selection of the dominant follicle:

- With the increasing concentration of estrogen, it exerts a negative feedback on the HPO axis and withdraws the release of FSH. This leads to regression of the all follicles by apoptosis, except the dominant follicle.
- The dominant follicle is selected by 5–7th day of the cycle and escapes the suppression, because of previous higher sensitivity and longer exposure to FSH. It has its own estrogen production and continues to grow.
- Also, the vascularity of theca cells of the dominant follicle increases as compared to others, thus delivering more gonadotropins to it than other.
- FSH now changes its action of estrogen production and starts up-regulation of LH receptors on granulosa cells. Once stimulated, LH can form its own receptors on FSH primed granulosa cells.[17,18]

Flowchart 5: Two-cell two-gonadotropin theory.

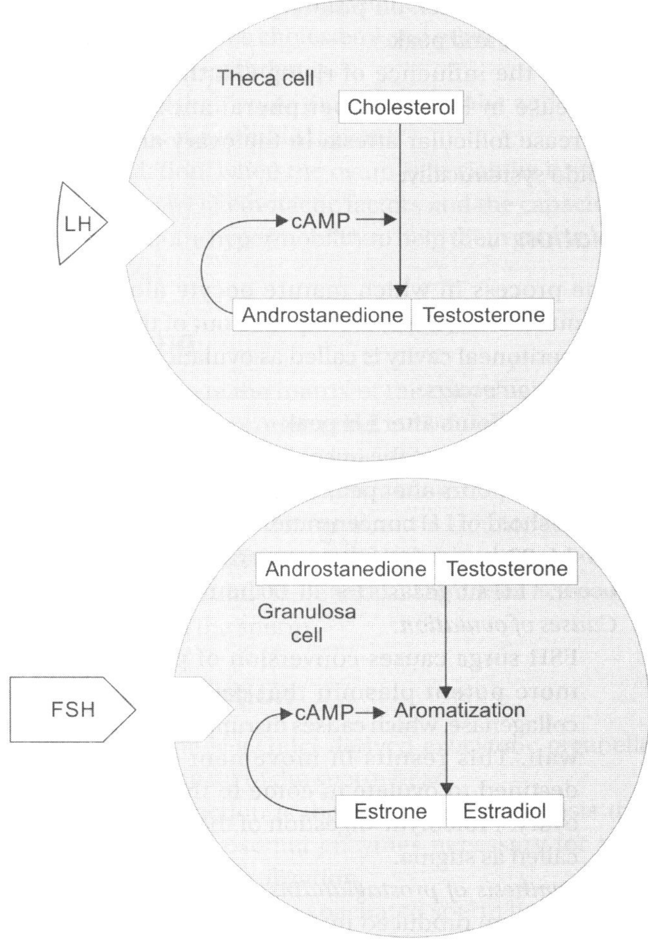

- With the decreasing concentration of FSH, and mid-follicular estrogen rise, exerts a positive feedback on HPO axis and influences LH release. LH levels rises steadily over the late follicular phase, stimulating more androgen production in the theca cells.

The preovulatory follicle:

- The granulosa cells of the preovulatory follicle enlarge and acquire lipid inclusions and the theca cells becomes vacuolated and vascular.
- The oocyte now proceeds with meiosis I.
- Estrogen rises slowly at first, and then rapidly, marking its peak 24–36 hours prior to the ovulation. Peak estradiol level stimulates the onset of LH surge.
- In preovulatory follicle, LH inhibits further growth of the follicle and promotes luteinization of the granulosa cells that results in progesterone production[19] and stimulates progesterone receptor expression on the granulosa cells, unlike traditionally believed it to be expressed mediated by estrogen.[20]

UTERUS, ENDOMETRIUM, AND IMPLANTATION

The uterus is an important female reproductive organ, which holds feto-placental unit during pregnancy. Endometrium is the dynamic inner mucosal lining of the uterus, which responds to the hormonal changes of ovarian cycle and sheds cyclically as well as provides favorable physiological environment for embryo implantation, thus it is considered essential for reproduction.

Layers of Endometrium

- *Functionalis layer (upper two-thirds)*: Consists of epithelial cells and glands. Its main purpose is to provide receptive environment for embryo (blastocyst) implantation.
- *Basalis layer (lower one-third)*: Consists of endometrial stem cells and basal cells, to regenerate functional endometrium following menstrual loss.[31]

Endometrial Changes during an Ovulatory Menstrual Cycle

Cyclical sequence of changes is essential to prepare receptive endometrium approximately every month for implantation, failing which the endometrium breaks down and sheds in the form of menses.

These changes occur in three main phases:

1. The menstrual phase
2. The proliferative phase
3. The secretory phase.

Menstrual Phase

- It is a transitional phase marked by exfoliation of endometrium till onset of endometrial proliferative phase of the next cycle.
- In histology, epithelial reparative changes along with remnants of menstrual shedding are seen.
- The epithelial repair is fast; by day 4 of the cycle, more than two-thirds of the cavity is covered with new epithelium.[32] By day 5–6, the entire cavity is re-epithelialized and stromal growth begins.
- *Ultrasound findings*: The endometrium is relatively indistinct during menses with menstrual blood collection seen sometimes and then becomes a thin hyperechoic line after cessation of menses.

Proliferative Phase

- It coincides with ovarian follicular phase and increased estrogen secretion by growing follicles. This estrogen is responsible for reconstruction, growth, and proliferation of the endometrium. Estrogen also induces progesterone receptors on endometrium.
- In histology, all of the tissue components (glands, stromal cells, and endothelial cells) demonstrate proliferation, which peaks on days 8–10 of the cycle, reflecting rising estradiol levels in the circulation and maximal estrogen receptor concentration in the endometrium.[33,34] Depending on the advancement of these histological changes, this phase is divided into early and late proliferative phase.
- *Ultrasound findings*: Endometrium becomes thicker, grows from approximately 1 mm to 7–10 mm and develops in "triple line" pattern.

Secretory Phase

- It is associated with the luteal phase of ovarian cycle after ovulation and it is a constant phase of 14 days; the endometrium now demonstrates a combined effect of estrogen and progesterone activity.
- Endometrial height is fixed now at its preovulatory extent (approximately 7–10 mm) despite continuous availability of estrogen.
- Progesterone secreted by corpus luteal cells is responsible for cessation of proliferative changes and it induces secretory changes in endometrial glands.
- The first histologic sign that ovulation has occurred is the appearance of subnuclear intracytoplasmic glycogen vacuoles in the glandular epithelium on cycle day 17–18.
- The glands acquire tortuosity and creates "cork-screw pattern" while spiral vessels become more coiled.
- The peak secretory changes are seen approximately 7 days after LH surge and it generally coincide with blastocyst implantation.
- *Ultrasound findings*: Endometrium loses its "triple line" image and becomes more uniformly hyperechoic.

Fate of Endometrium after Secretory Phase (Flowchart 7)

- In the absence of fertilization and implantation, corpus luteum regresses which causes hormonal support withdrawal.
- Estrogen and mainly progesterone withdrawal is responsible for various events which leads to endometrial breakdown and shedding.
- Endometrial tissue breakdown also involves a family of enzymes, matrix metalloproteinase, that degrade components (including collagens, gelatins, fibronectin, and laminin) of the extracellular matrix and basement membrane.[35,36]

Flowchart 7: Fate of endometrium after secretory phase.

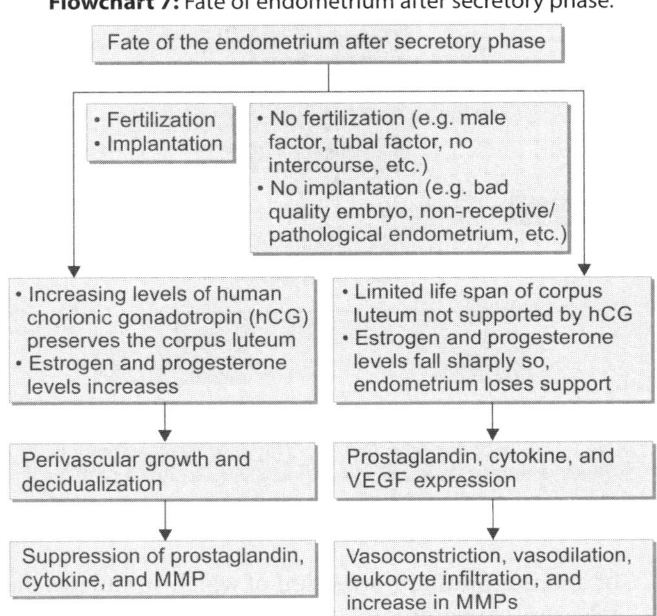

Source: Modified from Fritz MA, Leon Speroff L. Clinical Gynecologic Endocrinology and Infertility, 8th edition. Lippincott William and Wilkins; 2010. p. 134.

- Matrix metalloproteinase is activated under influence of increasing VEGF concentration (in response to progesterone withdrawal), which causes vasoconstriction and hypoxia in the endometrial layers to be shed.
- Also tumor necrosis factor (TNFα)-inhibits endometrial proliferation and induces apoptosis.
- Vasoconstriction and myometrial contractions associated with the menstrual events are believed to be significantly mediated by prostaglandins ($PGF_{2\alpha}$ and PGE_2).
- The basalis endometrium remains as it is during menses, and repair takes place from this layer.

Endometrial Preparation for Implantation

From the 7th to 13th day postovulation, with thickness of 7–10 mm, the endometrium is differentiated into three distinct zones, which after implantation forms the decidua of the pregnancy:

1. *Stratum basalis* (less than one-fourth of the tissue) is the unchanged basalis fed by its straight vessels and surrounded by indifferent spindle-shaped stroma.
2. *Stratum spongiosum* (mid-portion, approximately 50% of the total) is lace-like, composed of loose edematous stroma with tightly coiled spiral vessels and glands.
3. *Stratum compactum* (superficial one-fourth) containing all the components but tightly compacted.
   - The change from proliferative to secretory endometrium and preparing it for the arriving blastocyst is a very well synchronized process.
   - This process involves temporary expression of many biochemical and molecular events in the endometrium for a time being called implantation window.
   - *The endometrial receptivity array* consists of a customized array containing 238 differentially expressed genes in endometrial samples that are within the window of implantation regardless of their histologic appearance, is a recent diagnostic tool to predict receptive behavior of endometrium to blastocyst.[37]

Implantation

Implantation is defined as the process by which an embryo attaches to the endometrial lining and penetrates first the epithelium and then the circulatory system of the mother to form the placenta.

- Implantation begins with the loss of the ZP (hatching) about 2–3 days after, morula enters the uterine cavity.[38] Thus, implantation occurs 5–7 days after fertilization (at the 32–256 cells-blastocyst stage).
- Successful implantation requires invasion of healthy and genetically normal blastocyst and secretory receptive endometrium simultaneously. But there are various hormonal and immunological factors affecting implantation.

Implantation takes place in three stages:

1. Apposition
2. Adhesion
3. Invasion (and placentation).

Apposition and adhesion:

- Apposition begins at blastocyst stage as development of inner cell mass and trophectoderm are essential for initiating implantation.
- A prerequisite step for apposition to endometrial lining is hatching of blastocyst from ZP which occurs in vitro by contraction and expansion of blastocyst while in vivo by the presence of lytic enzymes in uterine fluid dissolve ZP.
- The polar trophoblast cells besides the inner cell mass are primarily involved in adhesion with endometrial epithelial cells.
- Various cytokines (CSF-1, LIF, and IL-1) and adhesion molecules (including integrins, selectins, and trophinin) play their role in the process of adhesion by increasing capillary permeability near implanting blastocyst and providing extracellular matrix support.

Invasion and placentation:

- Trophoblastic (called extravillous trophoblastic cells) invasion begins after the second week of ovulation and is completed after 10th or 11th day.

- The purpose of invasion (migration) is to remodel uterine vasculature by replacing maternal endothelium and converting high resistance, low flow vasculature in to high flow, low resistance vascular system in order to provide high blood flow interchange system between mother and fetus.
- Deep endometrial stromal invasion by human embryo is called interstitial implantation.
- The early embryo secretes a variety of enzymes (e.g. collagenase and plasminogen activators), that are important for digesting the intercellular matrix that holds the epithelial cells together.
- By invading endometrial stromal cells and basement membrane, blastocyst then erodes the endothelium of maternal capillaries to make sinusoidal sacs lined with endovascular trophoblast, thus providing connection with maternal blood.
- Further invasion is limited by various inflammatory cytokines secreted from the infiltrated lymphocytes in the endometrial cells and immunological factors like endometrial NK cells.

The first hormonal evidence of implantation (the appearance of hCG) occurs on 8, 9, or 10 days after ovulation; the earliest was 6 days and the latest 12 days.[39]

NEUROENDOCRINOLOGY

The HPO axis (Flowchart 8) plays a very important role by interplay of hormones. The direction signals sent by hypothalamus, and the operating signals given by anterior pituitary causes production of steroid hormones and ovulation. Depending upon, the amount of the hormone production, the lower centers send the positive or negative feedback signals in order to produce or reduce the signal for its hormone production respectively. This axis can be disturbed by various factors including increase in prolactin and TSH levels.

There are three types of feedback mechanisms:

1. *Long feedback mechanism*: From the ovary to pituitary and hypothalamus depending upon steroid hormone production.
2. *Short feedback mechanism*: From pituitary to hypothalamus depending upon gonadotropin secretion.
3. *Ultrashort feedback mechanism*: From pituitary or hypothalamus for their autoregulation.

Neurohormone/Gonadotropin-releasing Hormone

- It is a decapeptyl hormone, released from the arcuate nucleus of the hypothalamus into the portal circulation of anterior pituitary, secretion of which stimulates the release of gonadotropins (FSH and LH) from the anterior pituitary.

Flowchart 8: Neuroendocrine control in female.

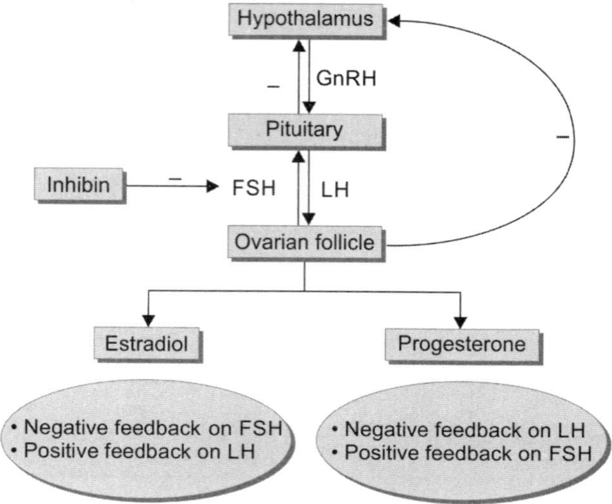

- It is released in pulsatile manner (also called as LH pulse), and changes its amplitude and frequency depending upon the cycle day and requirement of the gonadotropin (Table 1).
- Lower GnRH pulse frequencies and less amplitude favor FSH secretion, higher GnRH pulse frequency with higher amplitude favors LH secretion. Functions of GnRH on anterior pituitary:
  1. It causes synthesis and storage of gonadotropins.
  2. *Activation:* Movement of the gonadotropins from the storage site to the pool for direct secretion; a self-priming action.
  3. Direct secretion of gonadotropins.
- Also, GnRH stimulates synthesis of activin, inhibin and follistatin. Activin enhances GnRH response on pituitary by forming its receptors on pituitary.[40,41] Inhibin and follistatin suppresses the activity of activin.[42]
- Catecholaminergic system has direct effect on release of GnRH. Norepinephrine stimulates the release while dopaminergic pathway inhibits the release of GnRH.
- *GnRH antagonist* injections are now available by multiple amino acid substitution. They suppress gonadotropin secretion immediately by blocking the receptor site of GnRH on pituitary and thus making it unavailable for it. Nowadays, this is widely used as short protocol for COH in cases of patients undergoing IVF, in precocious puberty, endometriosis and prostate cancer. They degrade rapidly if given oral.
- GnRH agonists are also widely used in COH by long protocol, for down regulation before starting IVF cycle and for treatment of endometriosis.

Table 1: Gonadotropin-releasing hormone (GnRH) pulses.

Phase time	*GnRH pulse amplitude*	*GnRH pulse frequency*
Early follicular phase	6.5 IU/L	90 minutes
Mid-follicular phase	5.0 IU/L	-
Late follicular phase	7.2 IU/L	60–70 minutes
Early luteal phase	15.0 IU/L	100 minutes
Mid-luteal phase	12.2 IU/L	-
Late luteal phase	8.0 IU/L	200 minutes

Source: Clinical Gynecologic Endocrinology and Infertility, 8th edn. Lippincott Williams & Wilkins; 2011

Gonadotropin (FSH and LH)

- They are water-soluble glycoproteins of higher molecular weight.
- They are secreted by the beta cells of the anterior pituitary.
- They have two subunits α and β. The amino acid composition of α subunit of FSH, LH, and hCG is the same; they differ in their β-subunits.
- We have already understood the functions of FSH and LH in ovarian cycle.
- Injectable gonadotropins are widely used for COH in treatment of infertility.

Prolactin

- It is a polypeptide.
- Its use in reproductive physiology is not clearly understood.
- It is secreted by the alpha cells of anterior pituitary.
- Its secretion remains under chronic inhibition by the dopaminergic pathway.
- But if the prolactin levels increases in the blood, it stimulates hypothalamic-dopaminergic pathways, thus suppressing prolactin secretion but also GnRH secretion.
- That results into hypogonadotrophic hypogonadism.
- Mild hyperprolactinemia (20–50 ng/mL) causes poor preovulatory follicular growth and thus short luteal phase.[43,44] Moderate hyperprolactinemia (50–100 ng/mL) causes anovulation, oligomenorrhea, or amenorrhea. Severe hyperprolactinemia (> 100 ng/mL) causes hypogonadism and estrogen deficiency and related consequences.[45,46]

Thyroid Hormone

- Thyroid stimulating hormone (TSH) is released from the beta cells of the anterior pituitary.
- Higher TSH causes disturbed folliculogenesis and defective spermatogenesis and embryogenesis. Hypothyroidism can affect fertility due to anovulatory cycles, luteal phase defects, hyperprolactinemia, and sex hormone imbalance.[47]

We have already studied about estrogen and progesterone in ovarian cycle in this chapter.

GENETICS IN REPRODUCTION

Genetic abnormality is often one of the causes of infertility, failure of infertility treatment, miscarriage, congenital abnormalities in child and some of the comorbidity. Genetics contributes to reproduction by influencing varieties of physiological process including gametogenesis, quality of gametes and hormonal homeostasis.

Reproduction genetic is a branch which deals with the relationship between genotype and reproduction. It includes studying the transmission of the genetic material and its epigenetic modification from one generation to next and also the effects of abnormalities in the genetic material on reproduction.

Genetic Tests of Infertile Couple

Availability of genetic tests from basic to advance to diagnose any genetic abnormalities in infertile couples/patients helps selecting further treatment plans like ICSI with preimplantation genetic diagnosis (PGD) or donor gametes/zygote. Basic genetic evaluation includes:

- Karyotyping
  - In infertile female
  - In infertile male
  - In recurrent implantation failure
  - In recurrent miscarriage
- Cystic fibrosis gene mutation
- Fragile-X mental retardation gene mutation
- Y-chromosome microdeletion test.

Karyotyping

Karyotyping in infertile female:

- The prevalence of chromosomal abnormalities in women with regular ovulation, as reflected by a regular menstrual cycle, is reported to be 0.58%.[48]
- Chromosomal abnormalities are higher in women with primary amenorrhea, premature ovarian failure and in cases of recurrent miscarriage (RM).

- Women carrying extra X-chromosomes are at risk of reduced ovarian reserve and premature ovarian insufficiency (POI).
- Assessment of ovarian reserve is essential whenever numerical chromosomal translocations are involved.
- Women lacking an X-chromosome (Turner syndrome, 45XO) are known to be infertile with streak ovaries.

Karyotyping in infertile male:

- Chromosomal abnormalities account for approximately 5% of causes of infertility in males, and the prevalence increases to 15% in the population of azoospermic males.[49]
- Aneuploidy is the most common abnormality seen in infertile male, specifically of sex chromosome.
- Klinefelter's syndrome (nonmosaic, 47, XXY; and mosaic, 47, XXY/46, XY), is the most common chromosomal abnormality caused by aneuploidy with 5% prevalence in severe oligospermic men and 10% in azoospermic men.[50] The syndrome causes arrest of spermatogenesis at primary spermatocyte level. The affected men are sterile but sperm can be seen in the ejaculate of some men with nonmosaic pattern.
- Chromosomal translocation is another source of aneuploidy. Robertsonian translocations are more common in oligozoospermic and azoospermic men, with rates of 1.6% and 0.09%, respectively.[51,52] Carriers of Robertsonian translocations may exhibit a normal phenotype but could be infertile because of a lack of gamete production.

Karyotyping in recurrent implantation failure:

In couples presenting with RIF the prevalence of chromosomal abnormalities on karyotyping is 2.11%, more specifically 2.73% in women with RIF compared to 1.89% in male partners of women suffering from RIF.[53]

Karyotyping in recurrent miscarriage:

The prevalence of structural balanced chromosomal translocation in either partner of a couple experiencing RM increases according to the number of miscarriages; 2.2% after one miscarriage; 4.8% after two miscarriages; and 5.2% after three miscarriages.[54] However, the frequency of numerical chromosomal abnormalities in miscarriages with advancing age is also high.

Y-chromosome Microdeletion Test

- Y-chromosome microdeletions, in the AZF region, have been observed in between 3% and 15% of men with severe oligozoospermia and non-obstructive azoospermia.[55]
- Proper genetic counseling should be done, as this can be transmitted to the male offspring.

Cystic Fibrosis Gene Mutation

- Cystic fibrosis is the most common autosomal recessive condition in northern Europeans with a carrier rate of 1 in 25 Caucasians.
- Cystic fibrosis transmembrane regulator gene mutations are associated with reproductive tract abnormalities such as congenital absence of the vas deferens and congenital epididymal obstruction.[56-58]
- In contrast to patients with AZF deletions, these patients typically have normal spermatogenesis with normal testicular size and consistency, normal FSH, absence of the vas deferens, and/or an indurated epididymis.
- However, there has been no study to date showing that these genetic conditions are mutually exclusive. Therefore, the possibility exists that a single patient can genetically demonstrate both conditions.

Fragile X Mental Retardation 1 Gene Mutation

Fragile X syndrome has a prevalence of 1 in 4,000 males and 1 in 6,000 females and is the most common cause of mental retardation in men.[59] This syndrome is caused by mutation in fragile X mental retardation 1 (FMR-1) gene, which codes for fragile X mental retardation protein (FMRP), it might be associated with poor ovarian response during ovarian stimulation.

Couples with high maternal age or with RM and RIF can be offered IVF/ICSI with PGS. This involves taking a biopsy of a single blastomere from day 3 embryo or trophectoderm biopsy from a blastocyst and checking for any aneuploidy.[60,61] In this case there is a choice of transferring only euploid embryo. In case of couples with single gene disorders, IVF/ICSI along with PGD can be offered, which tests the single cell biopsied from the embryo for that specific genetic abnormality. The embryo, which is free from the disorder, can be transferred.[62]

IMMUNOLOGY IN REPRODUCTION

- *Autoimmunity influence reproduction by:*
  - Affecting the reproductive life and fertility of both sexes, and
  - Affecting implantation of the embryo by either failure of implantation or rejection of implantation resulting in abortion.
- Autoimmune disorders involve an immune response directed against a specific part of host or self, like systemic lupus erythematosus (SLE) and antiphospholipid antibody syndrome (APLA) syndrome.
- Alloimmune disorders involve an abnormal maternal immune response, to fetal or placental antigens, e.g.

maternal cytotoxic antibodies, absent maternal blocking antibodies, and disturbance of NK cell function and distribution.

- *Mechanisms involved in autoimmune disorders:*
  - Direct action of antibodies (antiphospholipid, antithyroid, antinuclear antibodies) without any clinical disorder.
  - By affecting process of spermatogenesis, oogenesis, implantation and pregnancy loss.
  - By causing vasculitis, impairing the blood circulation.

The major immunological disorders affecting fertility are:

- Antisperm antibodies (ASAs)
- APLA
- Human leukocyte antigen-killer cell immunoglobulin-like receptor (HLA-KIR)

Antisperm antibody: The presence of ASAs in serum and in the secretions of the reproductive system is seen in some infertile patients. Its role, however, in reproduction remains debatable as many authors have revealed ASA in a relatively high percentage of both infertile as well as fertile couples. Thus, ASA test is not an essential workup in the evaluation of infertile patients.

The role of ASAs is in various mechanisms have been proposed affecting male fertility: sperm agglutination and impaired cervical mucus penetration, complement-mediated sperm injury through the female genital tract, and interference with gametes interaction.[63]

Various tests for qualitative detection (like agglutination tests, MAR, complement-mediated sperm immobilization or cytotoxicity assays, anti-human antibody-coated immunobeads, IFA and immunogold assay) and for quantitative detection (like ELISA, radiolabeled antiglobulin assays, radioisotopes and enzymes are quantitative probes and FCM) and tests for identification of specific bond (like immunoblotting and affinity chromatography) have been evolved but have so far not been used in the routine laboratory investigation of the subfertile couple.

APLA syndrome or APS: APS is a systemic autoimmune inflammatory thrombotic disorder, characterized by the presence of antiphospholipid (aPL) antibodies in the serum of the patient and associated with an array of obstetric complication with or without vascular thromboembolic events.

The diagnostic criteria for APS are mentioned in Table 2.[64]

Antiphospholipid antibodies are directed against various phospholipid-binding proteins. The most important of these proteins is β-2 glycoprotein but some less frequent targets include prothrombin, thrombin, tPA, annexin-2, etc.

The exact mechanism through which these antibodies mediate the prothrombotic state is not clear but proposed mechanisms of action include:

- Activation of cellular elements (platelets, endothelial cells, and monocytes)
- Inhibition of the fibrinolytic system
- Activation of the coagulation cascade, and
- Activation of the complement system.

Anticoagulation and antiplatelet medications have been the mainstay of the treatment of this disease.

Human leucocyte antigens-killer immunoglobulin-like receptor: Blastocyst adheres and implants into the decidualized endometrial cell lining. HLA-KIR is an antigen antibody interaction, which if favorable results into successful correct implantation and placentation and if incorrect results into implantation failure or incorrect placentation leading to abortion, or pregnancy complications like preeclampsia, prematurity, etc.

HLA system is the locus of genes, which encodes for the proteins on the surface of the cells associated with the regulation of the immune system. EVT cells of the blastocyst express a large repertoire of class I HLA-C and nonclassical HLA-G and HLA-E antigens, whereas the class I antigens

Table 2: Diagnostic criteria for antiphospholipid syndrome (APS)[64] (the updated international preliminary classification criteria for APS).

Clinical criteria	*Laboratory criteria*
Vascular thrombosis (arterial/venous/microvascular)	
One or more clinical episodes of arterial, venous, or small vessel thrombosis, in any tissue or organ	Lupus anticoagulant present in plasma on two or more occasions at least 12 weeks apart, detected according to the guidelines of the International Society on Thrombosis and Hemostasis
Obstetric morbidity	
One or more premature birth of normal neonate before 34 weeks of gestation	Anticardiolipin antibody (IgG and/or IgM iso-type), in serum or plasma, present in medium or high titers on two or more occasions at least 12 weeks apart, measured by a standardized ELISA
One or more unexplained death of a normal fetus at or beyond 10 weeks of gestation	
Three or more unexplained spontaneous abortions before 10 weeks' gestation	Anti-β2 glycoprotein I antibody (IgG and/or IgM isotype) in serum or plasma, present on two occasions at least 12 weeks apart, measured by a standardized ELISA

HLA-A and HLA-B and class II antigens are absent.[65,66] HLA-C genotypes are the main one and could be HLA-C1 or HLA-C2.[67] Of the two, C2 is a stronger ligand than C1. HLA genes are inherited one from mother and one from father in each cell. So, EVT cell would express HLA C1C1, HLA C1C2, or HLA C2C2. HLA C1C1 is the most compatible, where as HLA C2C2 is the least.

Uterine NK cells express receptor KIR for ligand HLA of the EVT cells. The maternal KIR genotype could be haplotype AA (no activating KIRs), AB, or BB (1–10 activating KIRs).[67]

Interaction and compatibility between KIR and its HLA (ligand) facilitates migration followed by invasion of EVTs into maternal vasculature. Thus, maternal immune system is not going to reject the semiallogenic fetus. The recognition of HLA-C expressing trophoblasts by maternal KIR positive NK cells during pregnancy is important for successful placentation.[68-71]

Noncompatibility of expression of genotypes of HLA and KIR results in failure of trophoblastic invasion which might be correlated with an increased risk of RM, preeclampsia and fetal growth retardation.[70,71]

CONCLUSION

It is essential to understand reproductive biology, physiology and reproductive endocrinology to help in making differential diagnosis from various causes of infertility in evaluation of both the partners. Reproductive Genetics and immunology play a very important role in case of understanding reason for failure of infertility treatment, and thus helps to provide a treatment suitable to the conditions.

REFERENCES

1. Chang MC. Fertilizing capacity of spermatozoa deposited into the fallopian tubes. Nature. 1951;168(4277):697-8.
2. Austin CR. Observations on the penetration of the sperm in the mammalian egg. Aust J Sci Res B. 1951;4(4):581-96.
3. Dym M. Spermatogonial stem cells of the testis. Proc Natl Acad Sci USA. 1994;91:11287-9.
4. Foldesy RG, Bedford JM. Biology of the scrotum. I. Temperature and androgens as determinants of the sperm storage capacity of the rat cauda epididymis. Biol Reprod. 1982;26:673-82.
5. Cornwall GA. New insights into epididymal biology and function. Hum Reprod Update. 2009;15:213-27.
6. Devroey P, Liu J, Nagy Z, et al. Normal fertilization of human oocytes after testicular sperm extraction and intracytoplasmic sperm injection. Fertil Steril. 1994;62:639-41.
7. Sobrero AJ, MacLeod J. The immediate postcoital test. Fertil Steril. 1962;13:184-9.
8. Montag M, Köster M, Strowitzk T, et al. Polar body biopsy. Fertil Steril. 2013;100:603-7.
9. Visser JA, de Jong FH, Laven JS, et al. Anti-Müllerian hormone—a new marker for ovarian function. Reproduction. 2006;131(1):1-9.
10. van Disseldorp J, Lambalk CB, Kwee J, et al. Comparison of inter- and intra-cycle variability of anti-Müllerian hormone and antral follicle counts. Hum Reprod. 2010;25(1):221-7.
11. Su YQ, Sugiura K, Eppig JJ. Mouse oocyte control of granulosa cell development and function: paracrine regulation of cumulus cell metabolism. Seminars Reprod Med. 2009;27:32-42.
12. Trombly DJ, Woodruff TK, Mayo KE. Roles for transforming growth factor beta superfamily proteins in early folliculogenesis. Semin Reprod Med. 2009;27:14-23.
13. Erickson GF. An analysis of follicle development and ovum maturation. Semin Reprod Endocrinol. 1986;4:233.
14. McNatty KP, Makris A, Reinhold VN, et al. Metabolism of androstenedione by human ovarian tissues in vitro with particular reference to reductase and aromatase activity. Steroids. 1979;34:429-43.
15. Hillier SG, Van Den Boogard AM, Reichert LE, et al. Intraovarian sex steroid hormone interactions and the regulation of follicular maturation: aromatization of androgens by human granulosa cells in vitro. J Clin Endocrinol Metab. 1980;50:640-7.
16. Jia X-C, Kessel B, Welsh TH, et al. Androgen inhibition of follicle-stimulating hormone—stimulated luteinizing hormone receptor formation in cultured rat granulosa cells. Endocrinology. 1985;117:13-22.
17. Jia X-C, Hsueh AJ. Homologous regulation of hormone receptors: luteinizing hormone increases its own receptors in cultured rat granulosa cells. Endocrinology. 1984;115:2433-9.
18. Kessel B, Liu YX, Jia X-C, et al. Autocrine role of estrogens in the augmentation of luteinizing hormone receptor formation in cultured rat granulosa cells. Biol Reprod. 1985;32:1038-50.
19. Yong EL, Baird DT, Yates R, et al. Hormonal regulation of the growth and steroidogenic function of human granulosa cells. J Clin Endocrinol Metab. 1992;74:842-9.
20. Chandrasekher AY, Brenner RM, Molskness TA, et al. Titrating luteinizing hormone surge requirements for ovulatory changes in primate follicles. II. Progesterone receptor expression in luteinizing granulosa cells. J Clin Endocrinol Metab. 1991;73:584.
21. Zelinski-Wooten MB, Hutchison JS, Chandrasekher YA, et al. Administration of human luteinizing hormone (hLH) to Macaques after follicular development: further titration of LH surge requirements for ovulatory changes in primate follicles. J Clin Endocrinol Metab. 1992;75:502-7.
22. Hoff JD, Quigley ME, Yen SS. Hormonal dynamics at midcycle: a reevaluation. J Clin Endocrinol Metab. 1983;57:792-6.
23. Gougeon A. Regulation of ovarian follicular development in primates: facts and hypotheses. Endocr Rev. 1996;17:121-55.
24. Christenson LK, Stouffer RL. Follicle-stimulating hormone and luteinizing hormone/chorionic gonadotropin stimulation of vascular endothelial factor production by macaque granulosa cells from pre and periovulatory follicles. J Clin Endocrinol Metab. 1997;82:2135-42.
25. Anasti JN, Kalantaridou SN, Kimzey LM, et al. Human follicle fluid vascular endothelial growth factor concentrations are correlated with luteinization in spontaneously developing follicles. Hum Reprod. 1998;13:1144-7.

26. Dickson SE, Fraser HM. Inhibition of early luteal angiogenesis by gonadotropin-releasing hormone antagonist treatment in the primate. J Clin Endocrinol Metab. 2000;85:2339-44.
27. Bedford JM. Puzzles of mammalian fertilization—and beyond. Int J Dev Biol. 2008;52:415-26.
28. Zaneveld LJ, Polakoski KL, Williams WL. Properties of a proteolytic enzyme from rabbit sperm acrosomes. Biol Reprod. 1972;6:30-9.
29. Jones R. Identification and functions of mammalian spermegg recognition molecules during fertilization. J Reprod Fertil. 1990;42(Suppl):89-105.
30. Sathananthan AH, Trounson AO. Ultrastructure of cortical granule release and zona interaction in monospermic and polyspermic human ova fertilized in vitro. Gamete Res. 1982;6:225.
31. Chan RW, Schwab KE, Gargett CE. Clonogenicity of human endometrial epithelial and stromal cells. Biol Reprod. 2004;70:1738-50.
32. Ludwig H, Spornitz UM. Microarchitecture of the human endometrium by scanning electron microscopy: menstrual desquamation and remodeling, In: Bulletti C, Gurpide E (Eds). The Primate Endometrium. New York: The New York Academy of Sciences, New York; 1991. p. 28.
33. Bergeron C, Ferenczy A, Shyamala G. Distribution of estrogen receptors in various cell types of normal, hyperplastic, and neoplastic human endometrial tissues. Lab Invest. 1988;58:338-45.
34. Tabibzadeh SS. Proliferative activity of lymphoid cells in human endometrium throughout the menstrual cycle. J Clin Endocrinol Metab. 1990;70:437-43.
35. Fata J, Ho ATV, Leco KJ, et al. Cellular turnover and extra-cellular matrix remodelling in female reproductive tissues: functions of metal-loproteinases and their inhibitors. Cell Mol Life Sci. 2000;57:77-95.
36. Zhang J, Salamonsen LA. In vivo evidence for active matrix metalloproteinases in human endometrium supports their role in tissue breakdown at menstruation. J Clin Endocrinol Metab. 2002;87:2346-51.
37. Díaz-Gimeno P, Horcajadas JA, Martínez-Conejero JA, et al. A genomic diagnostic tool for human endometrial receptivity based on the transcriptomic signature. Fertil Steril. 2011;95:50-60.
38. Navot D, Scott RT, Droesch K, et al. The window of embryo transfer and the efficiency of human conception in vitro. Fertil Steril. 1991;55:114-8.
39. Wilcox AJ, Baird DD, Weinberg CR. Time of implantation of the conceptus and loss of pregnancy. New Engl J Med. 1999;340:1796-9.
40. Kaiser UB, Conn PM, Chin WW. Studies of gonadotropin-releasing hormone (GnRH) action using GnRH receptor-expressing pituitary cell lines. Endocr Rev. 1997;18:46-70.
41. Norwitz ER, Xu S, Jeong KH, et al. Activin A augments GnRH-mediated transcriptional activation of the mouse GnRH receptor gene. Endocrinology. 2002;143:985-97.
42. Bilezikjian LM, Corrigan AZ, Blount AL, et al. Pituitary follistatin and inhibin subunit messenger ribonucleic acid levels are differentially regulated by local and hormonal factors. Endocrinology. 1996;137:4277-84.
43. Seppala M, Ranta T, Hirvonen E. Hyperprolactinaemia and luteal insufficiency. Lancet. 1976;1:229-30.
44. Corenblum B, Pairaudeau N, Shewchuk AB. Prolactin hypersecretion and short luteal phase defects. Obstet Gynecol. 1976;47:486-8.
45. Biller BM, Baum HB, Rosenthal DI, et al. Progressive trabecular osteopenia in women with hyperprolactinemic amenorrhea, J Clin Endocrinol Metab. 1992;75:692-7.
46. Schlechte J, Walkner L, Kathol M. A longitudinal analysis of premenopausal bone loss in healthy women and women with hyperprolactinemia. J Clin Endocrinol Metab. 1992;75:698-703.
47. Verma I, Sood R, Juneja S, et al. Prevalence of hypothyroidism in infertile women and evaluation of response of treatment for hypothyroidism on infertility. Int J Appl Basic Med Res. 2012;2(1):17-9.
48. Papanikolaou EG, Vernaeve V, Kolibianakis E, et al. Is chromosome analysis mandatory in the initial investigation of normoovulatory women seeking infertility treatment? Hum Reprod. 2005;20:2899-903.
49. Ferlin A, Raicu F, Gatta V, et al. Male infertility: role of genetic background. Reprod Biomed Online. 2007;14:734-45.
50. Foresta C, Garolla A, Bartoloni L, et al. Genetic abnormalities among severely oligospermic men who are candidates for intracytoplasmic sperm injection. J Clin Endocrinol Metab. 2005;90:152-6.
51. Johnson MD. Genetic risks of intracytoplasmic sperm injection in the treatment of male infertility: recommendations for genetic counseling and screening. Fertil Steril. 1998;70:397-411.
52. Meschede D, Lemcke B, Exeler JR, et al. Chromosome abnormalities in 447 couples undergoing intracytoplasmic sperm injection—prevalence, types, sex distribution and reproductive relevance. Hum Reprod. 1998;13:576-82.
53. De Sutter P, Stadhouders R, Dutré M, et al. Prevalence of chromosomal abnormalities and timing of karyotype analysis in patients with recurrent implantation failure (RIF) following assisted reproduction. Facts Views Vis Ob Gyn. 2012;4:59-65.
54. Hook EB, Healy NP, Willey AM. How much difference does chromosome banding make? Adjustments in prevalence and mutation rates of human structural cytogenetic abnormalities. Ann Hum Genet. 1989;53:237-42.
55. Girardi SK, Mielnik A, Schlegel PN. Submicroscopic deletions in the Y chromosome of infertile men. Hum Reprod. 1997;12:1635-41.
56. Anguiano A, Oates RD, Amos JA, et al. Congenital bilateral absence of the vas deferens (A primarily genital form of cystic fibrosis). JAMA. 1992;267:1794-7.
57. Kaplan E, Shwachman H, Perlmutter AD, et al. Reproductive failure in males with cystic fibrosis. N Engl J Med. 1968;279:65-9.
58. Mak V, Zielenski J, Tsui LC, et al. Proportion of cystic fibrosis gene mutations not detected by routine testing in men with obstructive azoospermia. JAMA. 1999;281:2217-24.
59. Crawford DC, Acuña JM, Sherman SL. FMR1 and the fragile X syndrome: human genome epidemiology review. Genet Med. 2001;3(5):359-71.
60. Milán M, Cobo AC, Rodrigo L, et al. Redefining advanced maternal age as an indication for preimplantation genetic screening. Reprod Biomed Online. 2010;21:649-57.

61. Schoolcraft WB, Fragouli E, Stevens J, et al. Clinical application of comprehensive chromosomal screening at the blastocyst stage. Fertil Steril. 2010;94(5):1700-6.
62. Magli MC, Gianaroli L, Ferraretti AP. Chromosomal abnormalities in embryos. Mol Cell Endocrinol. 2001;183: S29-34.
63. Francavilla F, Santucci R, Barbonetti A, et al. Naturally-occurring anti-sperm antibodies in men: interference with fertility and clinical implications. An update. Front Biosci. 2007;12:2890-911.
64. Miyakis S, Lockshin MD, Atsumi T, et al. International consensus statement on an update of the classification criteria for definite antiphospholipid syndrome (APS). J Thromb Haemost. 2006;4:295-306.
65. King A, Allan DS, Bowen M, et al. HLA-E is expressed on trophoblast and interacts with CD94/NKG2 receptors on decidual NK cells. Eur J Immunol. 2000;30:1623-31.
66. Apps R, Murphy SP, Fernando R, et al. Human leucocyte antigen (HLA) expression of primary trophoblast cells and placental cell lines, determined using single antigen beads to characterize allotype specificities of anti-HLA antibodies. Immunology. 2009;127:26-39.
67. Uhrberg M, Valiante NM, Shum BP, et al. Human diversity in killer cell inhibitory receptor genes. Immunity. 1997;7:753-63.
68. Hiby SE, Walker JJ, O'shaughnessy KM, et al. Combinations of maternal KIR and fetal HLA-C genes influence the risk of preeclampsia and reproductive success. J Exp Med. 2004;200:957-65.
69. Hiby SE, Regan L, Lo W, et al. Association of maternal killer-cell immunoglobulin-like receptors and parental HLA-C genotypes with recurrent miscarriage. Hum Repro. 2008;23:972-6.
70. Hiby SE, Ashrafian-Bonab M, Farrell L, et al. Distribution of killer cell immunoglobulin-like receptors (KIR) and their HLA-C ligands in two Iranian populations. Immunogenetics. 2010;62:65-73.
71. Hiby SE, Apps R, Sharkey AM, et al. Maternal activating KIRs protect against human reproductive failure mediated by fetal HLA-C2. J Clin Invest. 2010b;120:4102-10.

CHAPTER

2

Role of History Taking and Clinical Examination in an Infertile Couple

Arindam Rath

Infertility is defined as a lack of pregnancy after 12 months of unprotected sexual intercourse with the same partner.[1] This condition may be affecting one in six couples worldwide. Reasons for such prevalence involve the decline in natural fertility with female age, an increased incidence of sexually transmitted infections, higher exposure to environmental toxins, and lifestyle factors such as smoking and obesity.[2]

It is estimated that 75% of infertile couples will achieve conception after evaluation and treatment for infertility. The success of therapeutic interventions depends on proper history taking, clinical examination and proper diagnostic evaluation of the couple.

In this chapter, we look at the role of history taking and clinical examination of the couple to achieve a working diagnosis.

BEFORE WE START HISTORY TAKING OF THE INFERTILE COUPLE

Even before history taking is commenced, a discussion of the process of reproduction and conception will help the infertile couple understand the basis for diagnostic testing and future treatment. It always makes sense to explain separately ovarian function, pelvic anatomy and the male factor including the role of coitus to put the couple at ease so that they can volunteer information accordingly. It is also good to point out that in at least one-third of couples, more than one potential cause for the infertility will be detected. This way we can cover other relevant fertility factors even when one particular factor seems obvious. Again, in 20–25% couples initial evaluation may not reveal any abnormality in which case a working diagnosis of unexplained infertility needs to be made. During history taking, there is ample opportunity for the clinician to discuss myths and facts regarding reproduction and dispel a few misconceptions gathered from friends and media.

Infertile couples often need the opportunity to express their concerns, frustrations, and fears, and support groups can help to meet that need.[3] Group meetings can help couples to realize that their problem is not unique and to learn how others cope with similar problems. Whereas severe anxieties can have adverse effects on ovulatory function and coital frequency, there is no substantial evidence that the usual anxieties of couples trying to conceive cause or contribute to their infertility.

We can also take this meeting as a chance to explain the various ART procedures so that they can realize the role of such procedures and find their suitability in their personal case.

So, we feel that the initial history taking session is a very important interface which shall determine the future course of the couples interaction with the clinician based on the interaction.

HISTORY TAKING AND CLINICAL EXAMINATION OF THE MALE

General Information

Age and other background information considered to be relevant to male fertility such as occupation, ethnic group, religion, and so on, should be recorded.

Fertility History

Determining whether infertility is primary or secondary is the first step in the fertility history. This is accomplished by asking the patient about previous marriages and outcomes.[4]

Primary male infertility is the case when the man has never impregnated a woman. Secondary male infertility applies when the man has at some time impregnated a woman, even if the woman is the partner in the presenting couple. In the case of secondary infertility, one should determine the time elapsed since impregnation. Whether a case of primary or secondary infertility, one should estimate the duration of infertility of the present couple. Inquiring about previous work-ups and/or treatment for infertility is important and should be discussed in detail.

Family History

The patient should be asked about the existence of a family history of infertility, spontaneous abortion, still birth, and congenital disease. Diethylstilbestrol (DES) exposure in utero may be a cause of male infertility.[5]

General History

Diseases can influence fertility either directly or indirectly. Diabetes mellitus affects fertility through vascular, neurological and metabolic alteration. Tuberculosis may destroy the urogenital tract. Fever exceeding 38°C can affect spermatogenesis for the succeeding 6 months. Hypogonadism, gynecomastia and testicular atrophy are commonly observed in men with hepatic cirrhosis.[6] Chronic renal failure is associated with hypogonadism and hyperprolactinemia.[6] Spermatogenic arrest has been observed in adrenogenital syndrome. Cystic fibrosis is a known factor in male infertility. Bronchiectasis may be a part of the immotile cilia syndrome or Young's syndrome. Neurological diseases such as paraplegia, spina bifida, neuropathies, and congenital abnormalities of autonomic innervation may affect sexual activity. Irradiation of the genital area is a risk factor and is dose-dependent: permanent sterility is observed for single dose field with 600 to 800 rads.[7] Cimetidine, spironolactone, nitrofurantoin, sulfasalazine, and cytotoxic drugs depress sperm density and quality.[5] Tranquillizers, depressant drugs and some antihypertensive drugs may cause impotence.

Urogenital History

Age at puberty (normal, precocious or delayed) should be registered. Any pathology that possibly causes testicular damage should be inquired about, with details concerning the site, the treatment given, complications due to treatment, and evolution of the pathology. A history of cryptorchidism may lead to testicular atrophy. Testicular injury may initiate antisperm antibody formation or testicular damage especially if it is accompanied by scrotal bleeding or hematuria. Testicular torsion leads to testicular damage if not treated within six hours. Mumps orchitis may be the cause of testicular atrophy. Varicocele can impair testicular function.[6]

History of Sexually Transmitted Diseases (STD)

A positive history of STD is suggestive of damage and/or obstruction of the genital tract. Data should be collected about the number of episodes, the time passed since the most recent episode, and treatment during the most recent episode. One should also inquire about the causative organism.

Surgical History Related to Infertility

Testicular and scrotal operations, e.g. orchiectomy, orchiopexy, testicular detorsion, repair of inguinal hernias, varicocelectomy and hydrocelectomy may be followed by decreased fertility. Operations of the epididymis and vas deferens such as epididymovasostomy and vasovasostomy may lead to antisperm antibody formation or genital tract obstruction. Prostatectomy is followed by impotence of variable degree and retrograde ejaculation. Urinary cystectomy, bladder neck operations, repair of urethral strictures and repair of a hypospadias can all affect fertility.

Habits

The subject should be questioned about environmental and/or occupational exposure to hazardous factors, such as radiation, chemicals, drugs, heat and traumas. Some personal habits can seriously affect men's fertility, such as wearing tight pants, taking excessively hot baths and sauna.[7] Cigarette smoking alters sperm motility and count. Alcohol consumption depresses sperm motility and count and, if used in high concentration, leads to impotence.[8]

Sexual History

Daily or more frequent intercourse may depress the sperm count below normal levels. Abstinence for seven days or more may decrease motility due to increased proportions of older sperms.[5] For most couples, coitus every 36 hours around the time of ovulation will give the optimal chance for pregnancy. Intercourse is considered adequate if it occurs more than twice per month, but if the frequency is twice or less per month it is considered inadequate and may be an etiologic factor of infertility and a possible sign of sexual dysfunction.[5]

Absence of libido or decreased libido is not only a cause of decreased coital frequency, but may also be a sign of an endocrine or a psychological disease. Dyspareunia may underlie either an organic or a psychological problem.

Impotence is defined as the inability to achieve or sustain an erection for a sufficient duration to have coitus and achieve an orgasm.[6] If coital erection is inadequate, inquiry about early morning erection and masturbatory erection should be made. If both occur normally, the diagnosis of primary impotence is excluded and coital impotence is attributed in most cases to a psychological factor. In primary impotence, erection cannot be achieved in any circumstance. It may be due to hypogonadism with androgen failure, pelvic vascular disease, or due to a systemic disease, such as diabetic neuropathy, anemia, tuberculosis and cancers. Secondary impotence is due to psychological factors in 90% of cases, and is characterized by failure of erection in the case of coitus only. Sometimes the man is impotent only when he consumes alcohol or with the use of some antihypertensive drugs or central nervous system (CNS) depressants.[8]

Ejaculation is considered adequate if it occurs intravaginally with emission of semen from the external urethral meatus. It is considered inadequate in the following conditions: (1) extravaginal ejaculation that may be due to ejaculation praecox or extreme hypospadias; (2) retrograde ejaculation into the bladder; and (3) anejaculation, i.e. failure of emission that may be of organic or psychological origin.[9] In the last case, if nocturnal and/or masturbatory ejaculation occurs normally, this indicates a psychological factor. Previous experience of painful ejaculation may also be a factor behind anejaculation.

Physical Examination

General Examination

Height, arm span, and the upper to lower body ratio should be measured to exclude eunuchoidism. Gait should be looked at, as it may indicate the presence of a neurological disease. Body weight, blood pressure and a general physical examination help assess the general health, and will disclose any chronic debilitating disease. If there is a history of neuropathy, endocrinopathy, cardiovascular, respiratory, renal or hepatic disease, or a clinical suspicion is aroused during the physical examination, the suspected disorder should be investigated thoroughly. Secondary sexual characteristics including hair distribution, body configuration, pubertal stage, and evidence of gynecomastia should be looked for carefully.

Urogenital Examination

The penis should be examined for size, circumcision, the presence of surgical or traumatic scars and induration plaques of Peyronie's disease that may cause deformation of the erect penis, thus hindering vaginal intercourse. If hypospadias is present, one should look for whether the urethral meatus is near the corona of the glans, or on the proximal part of the penile shaft. Delivery of semen could still occur intravaginally if the opening is in the distal part of the shaft. Semen will be delivered outside the vagina if the opening is proximal or lies in the perineal region. Any discharge from the urethra should be cultured. Nontender induration of the urethra suggests a stricture. Tenderness and induration may indicate periurethritis.[10]

Each scrotum should be examined individually for presence of the testis, its size, the presence of a hydrocele, masses, nodules, and tenderness. The average size of the adult testis is 5 × 3 cm, equivalent to a volume of 25 mL. The lower size limit for a mature testis is about 4 × 2.5 cm, corresponding to a volume of approximately 15 mL. Smaller than normal or very soft testes in an adult indicate impaired germinal tissue mass, due either to primary testicular failure or to hypothalamic-pituitary insufficiency. When determining the size of the testis, the patient should be examined in the recumbent position to avoid the risk of syncope. The scrotal skin is stretched over the testicle, the contours of which are isolated from the epididymis. The testis is palpated between the thumb and first two fingers. The volume of each testicle is compared with the corresponding ovoid of the Prader orchidometer.[9]

A varicocele can only be detected with the patient standing; if present it should be graded according to the following criteria: Grade III: if the distended venous plexus visibly bulges through the scrotal skin; Grade II: if there is intrascrotal venous distension which is easily palpable but not visible; and Grade I: distension is only palpable while the patient is performing a Valsalva maneuver. Subclinical varicocele should be recorded if no distension can be detected, but there is any abnormal finding during scrotal thermography and/or Doppler echography.

The epididymis should be examined while the patient is standing. The epididymis is examined between the thumb and forefinger along its entire course. A normal one is difficult to palpate, however if the epididymis is palpable it should have a regular outline, a soft consistency, and should not be tender. Nodular induration may suggest tuberculosis. Any swelling and tenderness may indicate epididymitis.

The vas deferens should be palpated along its entire course below the inguinal canal. A normal one should be palpable, but not thickened.[9,10]

Inguinal examination can be performed while the patient is standing, or in recumbent position. Any palpable or visible abnormalities should be recorded in detail. If the testes are not palpable in the scrotum, an attempt to palpate them in the inguinal region should be made.[9,10]

Rectal examination is carried out with the patient in the knee-elbow position. Palpation should be performed from the cranial to the caudal part and from lateral to medial. The prostate is normally soft, regular and not tender upon slight pressure. The central groove should be easily identified in a normal prostate. The seminal vesicles are not palpable, if normal.

After completion of the history and physical exam, some patients can be diagnosed directly as having sexual and/or ejaculatory dysfunction. Sexual dysfunction applies to those patients with inadequate erection and/or inadequate frequency of intercourse. Ejaculatory dysfunction applies when there is normal intercourse, but followed either by an ejaculation or ejaculation occurring outside the vagina. Retrograde ejaculation is suspected in patients with normal intercourse and orgasm, but no emission of semen. To be sure of the diagnosis, a postorgasm urine sample should be analyzed for the presence of spermatozoa.

Table 1 shows the summary of relevant history and physical examination findings for determining male factors in the infertile couple.

Table 1: Summary of relevant history and physical examination findings for determining male factors in the infertile couple.

History	*Physical examination*
• A history of poor fertility	• Examination of the penis, noting the location of the urethral meatus
• Coital frequency and timing	• Palpation and measurement of the testes
• Duration of infertility and prior fertility	• Presence and consistency of both the vasa and epididymides
• Childhood illness	• Presence or absence of a varicocele
• Developmental history	• Body habitus
• Systemic medical illness (e.g. diabetes, mellitus and upper respiratory disease)	• Hair distribution
• Previous surgery	• Breast development
• Medication	
• Sexual history (including sexually transmitted infections)	
• Exposures to gonadal toxins (including environmental and chemical toxins and heat)	

Source: Adapted from Practice Committee of the American Society for Reproductive Medicine.

HISTORY TAKING AND CLINICAL EXAMINATION OF THE FEMALE

Present History

The current problem/complaint, age, occupation, recent cervical smear findings, breast changes such as milk-like discharges, excessive hair growth with or without acne on face and chest, hot flushes, eating disorders, any current associated medical illness as diabetes and/or hypertension, drug intake prescribed as nonsteroidal antiinflammatory drugs (NSAIDs), sex steroids and cytotoxic drugs or recreational as marijuana and cocaine, smoking, alcohol, and caffeine consumption.[6]

Menstrual History[11]

Menstrual history alone often is sufficient to establish a diagnosis of anovulation. Menses in normally ovulating women generally are regular, predictable, consistent in volume and duration, and typically accompanied by a recognizable pattern of premenstrual and menstrual symptoms. Conversely, those in anovulatory women generally are irregular, unpredictable or infrequent, vary in flow characteristics, and exhibit no consistent pattern of molimina. Women with regular menses are almost always ovulatory. Women with irregular or infrequent menses may ovulate, but not consistently, and do not require specific diagnostic tests to prove what is already obvious. We need to check for the age of menarche, mid cycle symptoms, primary or secondary amenorrhea. All of these specific histories shall guide toward relevant investigations.

Obstetric History

Previous pregnancies, *if any*, and its outcome, recurrent pregnancy loss, induced abortion, postabortive infection or puerperal sepsis needs to be asked for.

Contraceptive History

Previous use of any contraceptive method, particularly intrauterine system, and any associated problems. If there is use of IU system then, we need to be proceed accordingly.

Sexual History

Coital frequency, timing in relation to the cycle, use of vaginal lubricant before, or vaginal douching after, coitus, loss of libido, as well as, any associated problems as difficult or painful coitus.

Past History

Medical or surgical as pelvic infection, tuberculosis, bilharziasis, ovarian cyst, appendicectomy, laparotomy, cesarean sections, and cervical conization. Immunization status especially regarding Rubella needs to be ascertained.

Family History

Similar problem among the female members, consanguinity, diabetes mellitus, hypertension, twins delivery, breast cancer in first degree relatives need to be asked.

Table 2: Summary of relevant history and physical examination findings for determining female factors in the infertile couple.

History	*Physical examination*
• Duration of infertility	• Weight, body mass index, blood pressure, and pulse
• Menstrual history	• Thyroid enlargement and presence of any nodules or tenderness
• Pregnancy history	• Breast secretions and their character
• Previous methods of contraception	• Signs of androgenexcess
• Coital frequency and sexual dysfunction	• Vaginal or cervical abnormality or discharge
• Past surgery (procedures, indications)	• Pelvic or abdominal tenderness, organ size, or masses
• Hospitalizations (illnesses or injuries)	• Uterine size, shape, position, and mobility
• Pelvic inflammatory disease (sexually transmitted diseases)	• Adnexal masses or tenderness
• Thyroid disease, galactorrhea, hirsutism	• Cul-de-sac masses, tenderness, or modularity
• Abnormal pap smears or cervical surgeries	
• Current medications and allergies	
• Family reproductive history	
• Exposure environmental hazards	
• Use of tobacco, alcohol, or illicit drugs	

Source: Adapted from Practice Committee of the American Society for Reproductive Medicine.

General Examination[11]

Vital signs (especially blood pressure), body height and weight (BMI = ratio between weight in kilograms and height in square meters) for over or under weights, secondary sexual characters, any excessive hairs with/without acne on face or chest, and acanthosis nigricans. Abnormal skin depigmentation as vitiligo may suggest an autoimmune systemic disease. Examination should include also the thyroid gland.

Breast examination: To evaluate its development and to exclude any pathology or presence of occult galactorrhea.

Chest examination: For lungs and heart.

Abdominal examination: For any abdominal mass, organomegaly, ascites, abdominal striae, and surgical scars.

Genital examination: Type of circumcision, size and shape of clitoris, hymen, vaginal introitus, site, size, shape, surface, consistency, mobility and direction of uterus, any palpable adnexal mass, vaginal discharge, tenderness, uterosacral ligament thickening, and nodules in the cul-de-sac denoting either endometriosis or tuberculosis by pervaginal (PV) examination. A perspeculum examination is also helpful to rule out certain conditions.

Table 2 shows summary of relevant history and physical examination findings for determining female factors in the infertile couple

CONCLUSION

To conclude, adequate history taking and examination would definitely help the clinician in decision making regarding investigations and the therapeutic options. This is very important in a multifactorial condition such as infertility where we could have myriad of investigations for both partners.

But more importantly, the quality of interaction during this session shall be of immense help to the infertile couple in understanding their situation, the solutions available and above all in reassuring them.

REFERENCES

1. Revised Glossary on ART Terminology, 2009. Journal article: Fertility and Sterility. 2009;92(5).
2. PLoS Med. 2012 Dec; 9(12): e1001356.
   Published online 2012 Dec 18. doi: 10.1371/journal.pmed.1001356
   National, Regional, and Global Trends in Infertility Prevalence Since 1990: A Systematic Analysis of 277 Health Surveys
   Maya N. Mascarenhas, Seth R. Flaxman, Ties Boerma, Sheryl Vanderpoel, and Gretchen A. Stevens.
3. Cousineau TM, Domar AD. Psychological impact of infertility. Best Pract Res Clin Obstet Gynaecol. 2007;21:293.

4. Urologic Nursing Examining Male Infertility Susanne Quallich Urol Nurs. 2006;26(4):277-88.
5. Speroff L, Glass RH, Kase NG (eds). Clinical Gynecologic Endocrinology and Infertility, 4th edition. Williams & Wilkins, Baltimore. 1989.
6. Yen SC, Jaffe RB (Eds). Reproductive Endocrinology, 3rd edition. W.B. Saunders Company, Philadelphia. 1991.
7. Martin-du Pan R, Campana A. Physiopathology of spermatogenic arrest. Fertil. Steril. 1993;60:937-46.
8. Labby DH: In: Benson RC (Ed), Current Obstetric & Gynaecologic Diagnosis & Treatment, 4th edition. Lang, California. 1982. pp. 486-501.
9. Rowe PJ, Comhaire FH, Hargreave TB, Mellows HJ (Eds). WHO manual for the standardized investigation and diagnosis of the infertile couple. Cambridge University Press, Cambridge. 1993.
10. Hammond MG. Evaluation of the infertile couple. Obstet. Gynecol. Clin. North Am. 1987;14:821-30.
11. Fertil Steril 2015;103:e4450. 2015 by American Society for Reproductive Medicine.

CHAPTER

3

Preconceptional Evaluation of a Couple

Lakshmi Chirumamilla

INTRODUCTION

From the earliest recorded time, women have been advised to increase their level of wellness and to avoid hazardous substances before becoming pregnant. Plutarch wrote that the ancient Spartans: "...ordered the maidens to exercise themselves with wrestling, running, throwing the quote and casting the dart, to the end that the fruit they conceived might, in strong and healthy bodies, take firmer root and find better growth."[1] In the Old Testament, the following passage appears: "And the angel of the Lord appeared unto the woman, and said unto her, 'Behold now thou art barren, and barest not: but thou shalt conceive and bear a son. Now, therefore beware, I pray thee, and drink not wine and strong drink, and eat not any unclean thing.' "[2]

As the modern practice of obstetrics evolved, it became a specialty that separated women's prepregnancy wellness from prenatal care, but in the last quarter century this has begun to change. The dominant model of prenatal care as the main perinatal prevention strategy has been re-examined, and recognition of the importance of the prepregnancy period has emerged. Today the general public and health-care professionals could easily be overwhelmed by the amount of information available which promotes prepregnancy or preconceptional health.[3]

"Interconception" care has come to represent efforts to address health status between pregnancies, birth spacing and intendedness of subsequent conceptions.[4] "Preconception" generally refers to the woman's health status and risks before the first pregnancy and her health status shortly before any conception. "Periconception" usually refers to the time immediately before conception through the period of organogenesis. It is important to note that this nomenclature is inconsistently applied and not universally accepted. In England, for instance, "preconception" is referred to as "preconceptual."

By 1985, the concept of preconceptional care and its potential advantages began to gain momentum. In that year, the Institute of Medicine published *Preventing Low Birth weight* and noted that numerous opportunities exist before pregnancy to reduce the incidence of low birth weight, but that they are too often overlooked in favor of interventions during pregnancy. The Committee emphasized the importance of prepregnancy risk identification, counseling and risk reduction; health education related to pregnancy outcome in general, and to low birth weight, in particular.

Preconception evaluation is part of preconception care.[6] The goal of the preconception care process is to make sure that the woman is healthy as she attempts to become pregnant, and to promote her health and the health of her children throughout her reproductive lifespan. PCC is defined as "a set of interventions that aim to identify and modify biomedical, behavioral, and social risks to a woman's health or pregnancy outcome through prevention and management, emphasizing those factors that must be acted on or before conception or early in pregnancy to have maximal impact." Preconception evaluation forms part of preconception care. It is essential to evaluate both the male and female so that effective actions can be offered to improve obstetric outcomes.

It is believed that through preconception care we can improve the outcomes of pregnancy and reduce maternal and perinatal mortality. The first antenatal visit is too late to address any perinatal risk factors or to assess exposure to unwanted substances. PCC includes assessment of risk factors from the couple in view of genetic, environmental and behavioral as well.

EVIDENCE-BASED EFFECTIVENESS

There is evidence that many preconception interventions reduce the risks of adverse pregnancy outcomes that include birth defects, fetal loss, low birth weight, and preterm delivery. The challenge for health professionals is to reach women and men with these interventions at the time they will be most effective in reducing risks.
Such interventions include:

- Managing medical conditions (such as diabetes, obesity, phenylketonuria, sexually transmitted infections, hypothyroidism, seizure disorders, and HIV).
- Counseling women to avoid certain risks (such as alcohol consumption, smoking, prescription and over-the-counter teratogenic drug use, excess vitamin intake, under nutrition, and exposure to toxic substances).
- Counseling women to engage in healthy behaviors (such as reproductive life planning,[38] folic acid consumption, and proper nutrition).
- Counseling women about the availability of vaccines to protect their infants from the consequences of infections that affect the mother (such as rubella, varicella, and hepatitis B).
- Counseling men to avoid certain risks (such as tobacco use and exposure to toxic substances).
- Counseling men to engage in healthy behaviors (such as reproductive life planning, proper nutrition, and healthy weight maintenance).

PRECONCEPTION CARE: TIMING IS KEY

The fetus is vulnerable to developing certain problems 17–56 days after conception. Prenatal health care, which usually begins in weeks 11 or 12 of pregnancy, may be too late to prevent these problems. This is particularly true in the case of certain prescription drugs that are known to cause birth defects and hazardous substances in the workplace and home.

Preconceptional evaluation of the couple should start from history pertaining to the couple which includes mainly medical and surgical history to assess the risks the woman could face during pregnancy and also to assess any risks that can be a cause of infertility. The medications taken by both the partners should be looked at as these can be teratogenic. So assessing the medications and switching to drugs that are safe during pregnancy is very important. More over if the woman is suffering from any medical conditions like epilepsy or diabetes she should be advised to refrain from pregnancy till the underlying medical problem is well under control. Otherwise especially if the woman enters into pregnancy when she has frequent attacks of seizures it can affect the baby and be risky to her as well. History should also include the vaccination history of the women. Sexual habits should also be evaluated. Sexually transmitted diseases can impact the fertility. Untreated STD like syphilis can affect the unborn fetus causing congenital abnormalities.

Basic observations like BMI, blood pressure should be part of the evaluation process. It is proven in many studies that women and men who enter into pregnancy at a high BMI take longer to conceive and also have increased risk of congenital abnormalities and miscarriages.

The concept of preconception evaluation is prevailing for women with pre-existing medical ailments. But this should be applied to the general population who are planning to conceive. It should include both men and women. A Cochrane review in 2009 restricted to randomized controlled trials, no systematic review comprising observational studies has been conducted to address preconception lifestyle interventions for women. A systematic review including observational studies is deemed valuable as the majority and most prominent studies are observational because of the behavioral changes that are included in PCC. Changes in individual behavior, clinical practice, community programs, and public policies are recommended.

Offering preconception care and evaluation is not only the responsibility of obstetricians and gynecologists but is also the duty of all medical practitioners who come in contact with men and women of reproductive age. Primary care providers potentially could routinely and efficiently use the tools available to screen for smoking, alcohol abuse, genetic risks, and occupational hazards; endocrinologists, geneticists, and nutritionists could become an integral part of a preconception care strategy. Moreover, settings such as family planning or STD clinics must become part of an integrated approach in order to reach many women at high risk for adverse pregnancy outcomes.

Preconception care and interventions are designed to reduce perinatal risk factors and, for optimal effectiveness, must be successfully implemented before the start of pregnancy. The components of preconception care, including an array of interventions to address medical, psychosocial, and environmental risks associated with childbearing, augment routine well woman care.

At the same time, preconception care must be tailored to meet the needs of the individual woman. Given that preconception care is a process, not a visit; some recommendations will be more relevant to women at specific stages in their lives or those with varying levels of health risks. Health promotion efforts, risk screening, and interventions would be different for a young woman who has never experienced pregnancy than for a 35-year-old woman who has had three children. Women with chronic diseases, prior pregnancy complications, or behavioral risk factors may need more intensive interventions. At the clinical level, it is especially important that individual interventions be tailored to the specific needs of the woman. Such variations in interventions also place constraints on how interventions can and should be bundled or pre-packaged.

A multigenerational medical family history graphically recorded as a pedigree or family tree is a cost-effective tool in preconception counseling to identify couples at risk to have offspring with inherited disorders and to identify if either partner has a personal risk for a disorder with a genetic etiology. Interpretation of a medical family history can provide risk assessment for reproductive planning and choices, inform a diagnosis to help identify a patient's medical screening needs and clinical management, and build rapport with the patient or couple. The use of standardized pedigree nomenclature is paramount to health-care delivery as electronic medical records become universal. The trend towards having patients prepare a medical family history in advance of the first clinic visit is a way to empower patients to take charge of their health, and also allow health professionals to spend more focused time in confirming and interpreting family history at the visit instead of constructing family history.

Preconceptional evaluation should encompass assessing the dietary habits of the couple also. Even in couple facing infertility it has been shown that certain types of diets like the Mediterranean diet, Dutch diet, or the high-protein diet improves the chances of conception in IVF cycles.

Recommendations that would advocate provider assistance for a woman and her partner in developing a reproductive life plan and in communicating her/their intentions through the implementation of that plan.

Male health and health care before conception has received little attention by many practitioners. It is also rare for a male patient to come to a clinic for preconception information. Only recently has the importance of preconception health for men been explored.

- The benefits of preconception care are important, including ensuring that all pregnancies are planned and wanted, improving the man's genetic and biologic contributions to the pregnancy, improving reproductive health and outcomes for female partners, improving the male's capacity and understanding of parenthood, and enhancing the man's overall health through access to primary care.
- Health-care professionals evaluating and advising men regarding their overall reproductive health need a comprehensive framework, which is outlined herein. Evaluation Reproduction Life Plan First, it is important to assess the goals and intentions of the male patient regarding reproduction goals. The Center for Disease and Control and Prevention recommends that all men, women, and couples to have a reproductive life plan. This is defined as a set of goals about having children or not having children based on personal values and resources and a plan to achieve these goals.
- Like women, the male patient should be questioned regarding any previous children, the desire to have any more children, whether there has ever been trouble conceiving, and what time frame the couple has for conception. A recent study noted that 10% of men can recall their primary care physician discussing preconception health care with them.
- If the couple is not currently interested in having children, it is important that the male patient be involved with contraception, and a discussion regarding proper methods should be addressed. Maximizing the health of the male patient to maximize outcomes, herein we aid in the assessment of the male patient who is considering having a child. If the patient has been trying to conceive without results for some time, a formal fertility evaluation is warranted for both the male patient (by a male infertility specialist) and his partner.
- *Medical and surgical history*: As with all patient encounters, a detailed medical and surgical history is important for the evaluation of a man's reproductive health. If these conditions exist, it is prudent to perform quantitative and qualitative analyses of semen. If abnormalities are found, referral to an infertility specialist is warranted (Tables 1 and 2).
- It is important to evaluate the patient's mental health as well. Although this may not directly impact the man's ability to father a child, there is evidence that the child of a father with depression may have behavioral and emotional developmental problems.
- *Medications*: The patient's medication history should be evaluated, including past and current prescription medications, nonprescription medications, herbal remedies.
- Medications may alter the hypothalamic-pituitary-gonadal axis, impair libido, affect erectile function, or have a direct toxic effect on the sperm. If the patient is

Table 1: Medical conditions associated with infertility.
Cryptorchidism, testicular torsion, and trauma[5]
Postpubertal mumps orchitis[7]
Congenital adrenal hyperplasia
Obesity[8]
Diabetes and poor glycemic control[9]
Erectile dysfunction[10,11]
Multiple sclerosis and spinal cord injury[12]
Hyper or hypothyroidism[13]
Varicocele[14]
Prostatitis, epididymitis, sexually transmitted diseases[15]
Malignancies (Hodgkin[16] and testicular cancer[17]) and any endocrine or metabolic effects of cancer[18]

Table 2: Surgical conditions associated with infertility.
Inguinal hernia repairs[19]
Scrotal or pelvic surgery
Retroperitoneal surgery in the setting of testicular cancer[20]
Incision of the bladder neck and transurethral resection of the prostate

Table 3: Medications that can affect fertility.

Medication	*Effect*
Exogenous testosterone	Decreased spermatogenesis
Androgen supplements	Impaired HPG axis
5-α reductase inhibition	ED, impaired sperm production[22]
α-blockers	Retrograde ejaculation
Cimetidine, spirinolactone, and ketoconazole	Direct inhibition of androgen production
Erythromycin, neomycin, tetracycline, nitrofurantoin, and gentamycin	Direct impairment of sperm production
Selective serotonin receptor inhibitors, monoamine oxidase inhibitors, lithium, and phenothiazines	Decreased libido, ED, and alteration of the HPG axis[23]
Chemotherapeutic agents	Direct impairment of spermatogenesis
Marijuana,[24] cocaine,[25] alcohol,[26] and tobacco[27]	May impair the HPG axis, spermatogenesis, and erectile function

(ED: ejaculatory dysfunction; HPG: hypothalamic-pituitary-gonadal).

taking medications that are known to impact fertility (Table 3), an alternative should be sought or the patient should be monitored appropriately.[29]

- *Family history and genetic risks* as part of the family history, a detailed genetic history should be obtained. Because sex-linked or autosomal disorders may skip generations, a three-generation history is important. Conditions to screen for include cystic fibrosis, which impairs infertility through a congenital absence of the vas deferens, and Klinefelter syndrome, which impairs fertility through sclerosis of the seminiferous tubules, resulting in azoospermia and small testicles. Families with intersex disorders should lead to the evaluation of the possibility of androgen receptor abnormalities. Social history, as noted earlier, the risks of tobacco, alcohol, and illicit drug use can directly affect spermatogenesis and impact erectile function.[30-33]
- However, a social history is also important to determine whether the patient is exposed to environmental hazards, including ionizing radiation, radiant heat, pollutants in the diet, lead, mercury, dichlorodiphenyltrichloroe thane, carbon disulfide, ethylene glycol ethers, dibromo-chloropropane, polycyclic aromatic hydrocarbons, polychlorinated biphenyls, dioxins, phlates, and acrylamide. A review of patient's hobbies should also be performed. Woodworking with oils used to finish furniture, painting, pottery with lead-based glazes, stained glass work, and gun cleaning and shooting may lead to toxic exposures to lead and other heavy metals that are harmful to sperm production.[36]
- *Physical examination*: A thorough physical examination should be performed as part of the preconception evaluation. This includes screening for hypertension and obesity through body mass index measurements. Overall body habitus should also be evaluated because it can offer clues about androgen abnormalities. Tall stature, gynecomastia, and decreased body hair could suggest Klinefelter syndrome. Hyperpigmentation may be a sign of underlying adrenal insufficiency; whereas abdominal striae, increased abdominal girth, and enlargement of the fat pad along the back of the neck and collar bone could be suggestive of Cushing syndrome. Excess sweating and essential tremor could be indicative of hyperthyroidism. An examination of visual fields should be performed; hemianopsia could indicate a pituitary adenoma. The thyroid gland should be evaluated because enlargement could be indicative of underlying hyper or hypothyroidism. Gynecomastia may be a sign of Klinefelter disease, excess estrogen, or androgen insensitivity, which may be associated with infertility. Underlying respiratory disease may be indicative of ciliary disease such as Kartagener syndrome, cystic fibrosis, or Young syndrome, which may inhibit fertilization through absence or obstruction of the vas deferens. A cardiovascular examination should be performed to identify any underlying arterial compromise, which may contribute to erectile

dysfunction. An abdominal examination should be performed to evaluate for any surgical scars, particularly in the lower abdomen or inguinal region, for any evidence of a previous operation that may have affected the patency of the vasa. Heptomegaly may indicate underlying hepatic dysfunction, which may impair the metabolism of sex steroids.

- A genital examination should be performed, beginning with the phallus. Penile lesions could indicate an underlying STD. Hypospadias, penile curvature, or chordee may impact the delivery of semen during intercourse. The scrotal skin and contents should be evaluated. The presence of scars could indicate previous scrotal surgery, which may impact patency of the vas deferens. Small testicles could indicate testicular failure, either primarily as is seen in Klinefelter syndrome,[35] or secondarily as seen with use of exogenous testosterone. Normal testicular size is 43 cm or a 20-mL volume.[28] Undescended testicles or absent testicles should also be noted.[37] Testicular masses may indicate an underlying neoplasm. Epididymal tenderness may be indicative of untreated epididymitis, which can affect sperm delivery. The presence of the vas deferens should be evaluated to rule out congenital absence of the vas deferens. Vasal nodularity or thickening could indicate a prior infection such as tuberculosis, whereas thickening may be indicative of obstruction. Finally, the patient should be examined in the supine and standing positions to determine the presence of a varicocele. Varicoceles are seen in 15% of normal men and are present in 19–41% of men with primary infertility and up to 81% of those with secondary infertility.
- Laboratory Testing Basic screening, as recommended by the US Preventive Service Task Force, should be offered to all male patients. This includes screening for lipid disorders beginning at age 35 (and for men ages 20–35 if they have diabetes, a family history of coronary artery disease or familial hyperlipidemia, or multiple risk factors for coronary heart disease) and screening for diabetes.[21] Targeted laboratory evaluation can be directed toward specific clinical signs and symptoms. Prolactin levels may be checked if there is any evidence of bitemoporal hemianospia. Thyroid function tests should be ordered if there are signs and symptoms of hyper- or hypothyroidism. Adrenal function tests may be necessary with any signs of Addison or Cushing syndrome. Liver function testing should be completed if there is evidence of hepatomegaly. Testosterone, estrogen, follicle-stimulating hormone, and luteinizing hormone should be evaluated if there are small testicles, gynecomastia, enuchoid body habitus, or signs of androgen resistance.

Recommendations for Health Promotion Achieving and maintaining a healthy weight is the starting point for discussion of health promotion.

Obesity has a number of detrimental health effects. In fact, every 20 lb overweight can lead to a 10% increase in the odds of infertility.[8] As part of the preconception evaluation, overweight and obese men should be counseled on the health and fertility benefits of weight loss; they should set goals and be offered the resources to achieve those goals. This may include referral to a nutritionist, a structured weight loss program, and promoting regular exercise. Stress reduction is also important to emphasize in male patients.[39,40] Although the mechanisms are not fully understood, there is a clear impact of stress on sperm morphology and concentration and decreasing testosterone.[41] The reason for these changes is believed to be mediated by impacts on the hypothalamic-pituitary-gonadal axis secondary to increased release of epinephrine and corticotrophin-releasing hormone, which impacts the natural pulsatility of luteinizing hormone.[43]

Approaches to stress reduction include regular exercise, proper sleep habits, and proper nutrition. The benefits of avoidance of tobacco, alcohol, and recreational drugs have been noted. Providers should also encourage those patients with a profession with hazardous environmental exposures to take appropriate precautions to minimize risk. This includes the use of leaded aprons for those with regular exposure to X-rays and proper use of gloves and masks when exposed to harmful toxins. Nutritional recommendations are not only an important part of helping a patient maintain a healthy weight and reducing stress,[42] but certain nutrients actually have been shown to affect the viability of sperm; zinc sulfate and folic acid have shown a positive effect on sperm production.[44]

Additional considerations men with findings during a physical exami nation that suggest hormonal or testicular abnormalities should be referred to an infertility expert.[46] In addition, the couple who has been attempting unsuccessfully to conceive should undergo an infertility evaluation. It is vital that male patients be included in such an infertility evaluation.[45]

Male patients should also be counseled regarding the growing evidence of increased risks associated with advanced paternal age.[49] The risk of a child with schizophrenia is twice as likely if the father is 45 or older compared with those in their 20s and 3 times more likely after the paternal age of 50.[47] Autism is 5.75 times more likely if the father is aged 40 or older compared with those men who father a child when they are younger than 40.[48] Autosomal dominant disorders also have been associated with advanced paternal age, including achondroplasia, Marfan syndrome, and osteogenesis imperfecta.

Improving preconception health requires changes in the knowledge, attitudes, and behaviors of individuals, families, communities, and institutions (e.g. government, health-care settings). The purpose is to improve the health of each woman before any pregnancy and to thereby affect the future health of the woman, her child, and her family. "If you raise the level of health of women in a society, you have raised the level of health of families and the community at the same time."[4] The successful implementation of the preconceptional care will help achieve the vision for preconception health and pregnancy outcomes where:

- All women and men of childbearing age have high reproductive awareness (e.g. understand risk factors related to childbearing)
- All women have a reproductive life plan (e.g. whether or when they wish to have children, how they will maintain their reproductive health)
- All pregnancies are intended and planned
- All women of childbearing age have health-care coverage
- All women of childbearing age are screened prior to pregnancy for risks related to the outcomes of pregnancy
- Women with a prior pregnancy loss (e.g. infant death due to very low birth weight or preterm birth) have access to intensive interconception care aimed at reducing their risks.

Conclude preconception care and planning is important for improving pregnancy outcomes, ensuring all pregnancies are planned and wanted, and enhancing the health of female partners and, particular to this review, of the male patient. The preconception examination is an excellent window to promote not only reproductive health but also to discuss overall health issues with the male patient. This includes promotion of proper nutrition and regular exercise, treatment and prevention of diseases, stress reduction, and avoidance of dangerous behaviors.

REFERENCES

1. Plutarch. Lycurgus 14 (trans. John Dryden). New York: Random House; 1932. pp. 59-60.
2. Old Testament (Judges 13:3–4).
3. Whitworth M, Dowswell T. Routine pre-pregnancy health promotion for improving pregnancy outcomes. Cochrane Database Syst Rev. 2009;4:CD007536.
4. Atrash H, Adams M, Cordero J, Johnson K, Howse J. Time to act on missed opportunities to improve perinatal outcomes: preconception care. Mat Child Health J. 2006;5(Suppl):S3-11.
5. Posner SF, Johnson K, Parker C, Atrash H, Biermann J. The national summit on preconception care: a summary of concepts and recommendations. Matern Child Health J. 2006;10(5 Suppl):S197-205.
6. Frey KA. Preconception care by the nonobstetric provider. Mayo Clin Proc. 2002;77:469-73.
7. Mirsa DP, Grason H, Weisman C. An intersection of women's and perinatal health: the role of chronic conditions. Women's Health Issues. 2000;10:256-67.
8. Brundage SC. Preconception Health Care. Washington, DC: American Academy of Family Physicians; 2002.
9. Korenbrot CC, Steinberg A, Bender C, Newberry S. Preconception care: a systematic review. Mat Child Health J. 2002;6(2):75-88.
10. Bennett RL. The family medical history as a tool in preconception consultation. J Community Genet. 2012;3(3):175-83.
11. Shindel AW, Nelson CJ, Naughton CK, Ohebshalom M, Mulhall JP. Sexual function and quality of life in the male partner of infertile couples: prevalence and correlates of dysfunction. The Journal of Urology. 2008;179(3):1056-9.
12. Twigt JM, Bolhuis ME, Steegers EA, Hammiche F, van Inzen WG, Laven JS, Steegers-Theunissen RP. The preconception diet is associated with the chance of ongoing pregnancy in women undergoing IVF/ICSI treatment. Hum Reprod. 2012 Aug;27(8):2526-31. doi: 10.1093/humrep/des157. Epub 2012 May 15.
13. Frey KA. Male reproductive health and infertility. Prim Care. 2010;37:643-52.
14. Frey KA, Navarro SM, Kotelchuck M, Lu MC. The clinical content of preconception care: preconception care for men. Am J Obstet Gynecol. 2008;199(6 Suppl 2):S389-95.
15. Johnson K, Posner SF, Biermann J, Cordero JF, Atrash HK, Parker CS, et al. CDC/ ATSDR Preconception Care Work Group; Select Panel on Preconception Care. Recommendations to improve preconception health and health care—United States. A report of the CDC/ATSDR Preconception Care Work Group and the Select Panel on Preconception Care. MMWR Recomm Rep. 2006;55(RR-6):1-23.
16. Files JA, Frey KA, David PS, Hunt KS, Noble BN, Mayer AP. Developing a reproductive life plan. J Midwifery Womens Health. 2011;56:468-74.
17. Frey KA, Engle R, Noble BB. Preconception healthcare: what do men know and believe? J Mens Health. 2012;9:25-35.
18. Puri P, Barton D, O'Donnell B. Prepubertal testicular torsion: subsequent fer-tility. J Pediatr Surg. 1985;20:598-601.
19. Werner CA. Mumps orchitis and testicular atrophy; a factor in male sterility. Ann Intern Med. 1950;32:1075-86.
20. Sallmen M, Sandler DP, Hoppin JA, Blair A, Baird DD. Reduced fertility among overweight and obese men. Epidemiology. 2006;17:520-3.
21. Padron RS, Dambay A, Suarez R, Mas J. Semen analyses in adolescent diabetic patients. Acta Diabetol Lat. 1984;21:115-21.
22. McCulloch DK, Campbell IW, Wu FC, Prescott RJ, Clarke BF. The prevalence of diabetic impotence. Diabetologia. 1980;18:279-83.
23. Sexton WJ, Jarow JP. Effect of diabetes mellitus upon male reproductive function. Urology. 1997;49:508-13.

24. Sonksen J, Biering-Sorensen F. Fertility in men with spinal cord or cauda equina lesions. Semin Neurol. 1992;12:106-14.
25. Velazquez EM, Bellabarba Arata G. Effects of thyroid status on pituitary gonadotropin and testicular reserve in men. Arch Androl. 1997;38:85-92.
26. Agarwal A, Deepinder F, Cocuzza M, et al. Efficacy of varicocelectomy in improving semen parameters: new meta-analytical approach. Urology. 2007;70:532-8.
27. Aitken RJ, De Iuliis GN. Value of DNA integrity assays for fertility evaluation. Soc Reprod Fertil Suppl. 2007;65:81-92.
28. Shin D, Lipshultz LI, Goldstein M, et al. Herniorrhaphy with polypropylene mesh causing inguinal vasal obstruction: a preventable cause of obstructive azoospermia. Ann Surg. 2005;241:553-8.
29. Nudell DM, Monoski MM, Lipshultz LI. Common medications and drugs: how they affect male fertility. Urol Clin North Am. 2002;29:965-73.
30. Close CE, Roberts PL, Berger RE. Cigarettes, alcohol and marijuana are related to pyospermia in infertile men. J Urol. 1990;144:900-3.
31. Hurd WW, Kelly MS, Ohl DA, Gauvin JM, Smith AJ, Cummins CA. The effect of cocaine on sperm motility characteristics and bovine cervical mucus penetration. Fertil Steril. 1992;57:178-82.
32. Muthusami KR, Chinnaswamy P. Effect of chronic alcoholism on male fertility hormones and semen quality. Fertil Steril. 2005;84:919-24.
33. Vine MF, Tse CK, Hu P, Truong KY. Cigarette smoking and semen quality. Fertil Steril. 1996;65:835-42.
34. Anguiano A, Oates RD, Amos JA, Dean M, Gerrard B, Stewart C, et al. Congenital bilateral absence of the vas deferens. A primarily genital form of cystic fibrosis. JAMA. 1992;267:1794-7.
35. Lanfranco F, Kamischke A, Zitzmann M, Nieschlag E. Klinefelter's syndrome. Lancet. 2004;364:273-83.
36. Bonde JP. Male reproductive organs are at risk from environmental hazards. Asian J Androl. 2010;12:152-6.
37. Charny CW. The spermatogenic potential of the undescended testis before and after treatment. J Urol. 1960;83:697-705.
38. Guide to Clinical Preventive Services, 2nd edition. Rockville, MD: Agency for Healthcare Research and Quality; 2010. [online] Available from: www.odphp. osophs. dhhs.gov/pubs/guidecps/ [Accessed January, 2013].
39. Giblin PT, Poland ML, Moghissi KS, Ager JW, Olson JM. Effects of stress and characteristic adaptability on semen quality in healthy men. Fertil Steril. 1988;49:127-32.
40. Zorn B, Auger J, Velikonja V, Kolbezen M, Meden-Vrtovec H. Psychological factors in male partners of infertile couples: relationship with semen quality and early miscarriage. Int J Androl. 2008;31:557-64.
41. Nilsson PM, Moller L, Solstad K. Adverse effects of psychosocial stress on gonadal function and insulin levels in middle-aged males. J Intern Med. 1995;237:479-86.
42. McGrady AV. Effects of psychological stress on male reproduction: a review. Arch Androl. 1984;13:1-7.
43. Schweiger U, Deuschle M, Weber B, Körner A, Lammers CH, Schmider J, et al. Testosterone, gonadotropin, and cortisol secretion in male patients with major depression. Psychosom Med. 1999;61:292-6.
44. Wong WY, Merkus HM, Thomas CM, Menkveld R, Zielhuis GA, Steegers-Theunissen RP. Effects of folic acid and zinc sulfate on male factor subfertility: a double-blind, randomized, placebo-controlled trial. Fertil Steril. 2002;77:491-8.
45. Jose-Miller AB, Boyden JW, Frey KA. Infertility. Am Fam Physician. 2007;75:849-56.
46. Kolettis PN. Evaluation of the subfertile man. Am Fam Physician. 2003;67:2165-72.
47. Malaspina D, Harlap S, Fennig S, et al. Advancing paternal age and the risk of schizophrenia. Arch Gen Psychiatry 2001;58:361-7.
48. Reichenberg A, Gross R, Weiser M, et al. Advancing paternal age and autism. Arch Gen Psychiatry. 2006;63:1026-32.
49. Stewart AF, Kim ED. Fertility concerns for the aging male. Urology. 2011;78:496-9.

CHAPTER

4

Assessing Ovulatory Function and Ovarian Reserve

Puneet Rana Arora, Shalu Gupta, Nalini Mahajan

INTRODUCTION

Ovulation is defined as growth, maturation, and rupture of an oocyte. It is a complex interplay and delicate balance between the hypothalamus, pituitary, ovary and endometrium. The hypothalamus produces GnRH in a pulsatile fashion and this in turn stimulates production of the gonadotrophins FSH and LH from the pituitary. The end result of this complex process is release of a mature oocyte from the ovary. It helps to indicate a fertile window which if timed with intercourse can lead to conception. The knowledge of fertile window has been used by some to avoid conception. If conception does not happen, it leads to the menstrual cycle. The number and quality of oocytes is assessed by ovarian reserve.

In approximately 15% of all infertile couples, ovulatory dysfunction will be identified and it accounts for up to 40% of infertility in women.[1] Hence prediction and timing of ovulation becomes important in evaluation of such couples. Ovulatory dysfunction is very commonly associated with irregularity in the menstrual cycle. The common causes of ovulatory dysfunction include polycystic ovaries (PCOS), obesity, weight gain, weight loss, strenuous exercise, thyroid dysfunction and prolactin disorder.

Unlike other species, there are no behavioral or obvious physical signs of impending ovulation in humans, although there may be hormonally induced changes in mood and behavior throughout the ovarian cycle.

NORMAL PHYSIOLOGY

Development of the ovarian follicle occurs in response to stimulation to these hormones from the pituitary gland. The ovary has two major roles: the first is its role in the formation of mature oocyte (gametogenesis) leading to the release of the oocyte (ovulation). Its second role is production of estrogen and progesterone, which in turn prepares the endometrium for the fertilized ovum to be implanted and achieving conception. Hence assessment of ovulatory function is very important as it helps the couple for timed intercourse and also provides guidance for procedures like intrauterine insemination.

A number of methods and tests are available to evaluate ovarian and ovulatory function. Each of the available tests has a varying degree of accuracy and no single test has been described as the gold standard for ovulation.

The first step in assessing ovarian health in the form of ovulatory function is a detailed medical history including menstrual history, sexual and contraceptive history, any previous pelvic surgery, weight gain or loss, any recent stressful events, level of exercise. This is followed by a complete physical and pelvic examination as well as assessment of adrenal, thyroid and pituitary glands. This guides as to the ovulatory or non-ovulatory status of the cycle.

The various tests used to assess the ovulatory status of the ovaries can be classified as definite, direct or presumptive methods. Even though direct methods give direct evidence of ovulation, these methods are invasive and assessing each month by invasive procedure is not only inconvenient to the women but also expensive.

Presumptive methods of assessment of ovulation:

- Menstrual cycle charting
- Basal body temperature
- Changes in the reproductive tract including cervix, endometrium, and vagina
- Steroid or gonadotropic hormone assays in the blood or urine.

Direct methods:

- Observation of corpus luteum with the presence of a stigma by laparoscopy or laparotomy
- Collapse of the ovulatory follicle and the appearance of fluid in the pouch of Douglas by high resolution transvaginal ultrasound.[2,3]

Definite methods:

- Establishment of pregnancy
- Recovery of an ovum from the fallopian tubes.

Menstrual Cycle Charting

The simplest and least expensive method is menstrual cycle charting. This involves recording the days of onset and cessation of menses for several months in succession. Menstrual cycles between 21 and 35 days are generally ovulatory. Variations in the cycle reflect ovulatory status and some variation is also seen with advancing age. Longer and shorter cycles may indicate anovulation. Shorter cycles may also occur due to a shortening of the follicular phase, as occurs in ovarian aging, or with a short (inadequate) luteal phase, which means that the endometrium is not appropriately prepared to receive a fertilized embryo.

Basal Body Temperature (BBT) Monitoring

Monitoring of BBT is one of the simplest means of predicting ovulation. Progesterone released from the corpus luteum after ovulation has potent effects on the hypothalamus, resulting in increase of body temperature. An approximately 0.5°F rise in body temperature can be detected in the luteal phase of the menstrual cycle compared with the follicular phase. In a normal cycle, the temperature rise begins 1 or 2 days after the LH surge and persists for at least 10 days. The fall in BBT can be used as an indicator of the imminent onset of menses. The temperature record shows a typical biphasic pattern during ovulatory cycles; in anovulatory cycles it remains monophasic. A preovulatory dip (possibly coinciding with estrogen peak) is usually, but not invariably, observed.

In practice, women are instructed to take their oral temperatures with a basal thermometer in the morning before starting any activity of the day including eating and drinking. Even though simple, it is cumbersome and stressful for some women. Other issues with BBT monitoring are that as the rise is so minimal, it can be missed and hence not always useful to time ovulatory function. Moreover, not every woman will show a biphasic pattern of BBT.

Changes in Cervical Mucus and its Testing

Secretion of cervical mucus is regulated by ovarian hormones. Under their influence, both the cervix and cervical mucus (their physical and chemical properties) undergo changes.

In the follicular phase—estrogen stimulates the production of large amounts of thin, watery, alkaline, acellular cervical mucus with intense ferning, spinnbarkeit, viscosity, and sperm receptivity. In the luteal phase, progesterone inhibits the secretory activity of cervical epithelia and produces scanty, viscous, cellular mucus with low spinnbarkeit and absence of ferning, which is impenetrable by spermatozoa.[2]

This method is a simple assessment of the ovulatory function as it does not require any hospital visits and no intervention. Its sensitivity and specificity is, however, low as it is a partly subjective assessment of the ovulatory function.

Changes in Endometrium and Endometrial Biopsy

Endometrial secretory activity during the luteal phase is usually indicative of ovulation and corpus luteum formation. Assessing ovulation through endometrial biopsy involves taking biopsy in the luteal phase of the cycle. Endometrial pattern indicating secretory activity is due to progesterone release from corpus luteum postovulation. Even though it is one of the reliable means of assessing ovulation, it is not frequently used these days due to being invasive. Also, as the results indicate when the ovulation has already happened, its role is limited.

Changes in Vagina and Vaginal Cytology

Papanicolaou described the variation in human vaginal smears during the menstrual cycle. A correlation between vaginal smear changes and the BBT curve and cyclic hormonal changes during the menstrual cycle has been established. Studies correlating have shown that the karyopyknotic index of vaginal cells increases gradually to mid-cycle and peaks on the day after the LH surge.[3] Thereafter, there is a steady decline of the index to the end of the menstrual cycle, when it reaches levels below those in the early proliferative phase. The mean peak of the index is reached 2 days after the total estrogen peak. This lag period is probably required before the vaginal epithelium responds to increased estrogenic stimulation. Because the peak of urinary estrogens precedes the LH surge by one day[3,4] and ovulation is presumed to occur within 24 h after the surge,[5] it follows that the peak of the index of the vaginal cells coincides with ovulation. Being invasive, it is inconvenient for the women each month to have this test done to detect ovulation. With the development of noninvasive methods of ovulation detection such as urinary LH testing, this method has lost its appeal.

Hormonal Assays

Measurement of levels of LH, estradiol (E2) and progesterone in the serum, urine and saliva has been used to assess ovulation. The temporal relation between ovulation and defined changes in the concentration of plasma E2, LH, FSH, and progesterone is well established.

Serum or Urinary LH

Laboratory assays of LH are used to detect LH surge and hence ovulation timing. Assays of LH can be done in serum or urine. Serial serum assay of LH is obviously cumbersome and unacceptable to most patients. The preovulatory LH rise appears to have a circadian cycle, occurring in the early morning in most women. Excretion of LH in urine is 6–7 hours later than serum and hence, results correlate best when LH surge testing is performed in late afternoon or early evening.

Urinary assay of LH is simpler and easy to perform. Several dipstick kits for rapid assay of urinary LH are available, known as ovulation predictor kits (OPK)/LH kits. These are based on enzyme immunoassay technique (monoclonal antibody technology). The patient at home can use them once or twice per day (morning and evening), beginning approximately 4 days before suspected ovulation.

It is claimed that these rapid enzyme immunoassays have an accuracy of more than 90% for detecting the LH surge. Several studies have compared urinary LH kits for ovulation prediction to ultrasonographic changes of follicular collapse to establish their reliability. Miller et al. after using a rapid colorimetric enzyme immunoassay test once every evening, found positive predictive values for follicular collapse within 24 or 48 hours after positive urine LH testing to be 73% and 92%, respectively.[6] In another report, sonographic evidence of ovulation was detected by the first day after the LH surge (day 1) in 35% of 269 cycles studied and not until day 2 in an additional 61% of cycles.[7]

Thus, urinary LH kits, if used properly, are one of the reliable methods of ovulation prediction for home use. Ovulation occurs within 14–24 hours after LH surge detection and almost always within 48 hours. Hence the most fertile period is the following 2 days post-LH surge. These kits are now widely used by patients and are recommended by physicians involved in the care of infertile couples for timing of coitus, artificial insemination, postcoital tests, and the like. However, their efficacy relative to improvement of fecundity remains to be established.[8] It is patient-friendly and can be done conveniently at home.

It is not of much use in clinical conditions such as premature ovarian insufficiency, early menopause, perimenopause and cases of polycystic ovarian syndrome where LH level may already be elevated. The urinary LH kit may provide a false-positive result and may not be reliable in predicting LH surge.

Urinary FSH

The preovulatory peak of FSH coinciding with that of LH is well established. In practice, first void morning sample is analyzed by an enzyme immunoassay method, and indexed by the concentration of creatinine in the same sample. In a study comparing the measurement of serum and urinary hormones with ovarian ultrasonography, the urinary FSH peak was found to be closer to the day of follicular collapse (–0.85 day) and follicle collapsed within 24 hours in 97% of cycles studied.[9] It is not widely used as a method for detection of ovulation.

Estrogen Assays

Serum E2 demonstrates a characteristic peak approximately one day before the LH surge and 37 hour before ovulation. Serial determinations of serum E2 at midcycle thus can detect the time of ovulation with a fair amount of accuracy. Rapid assays for serum E2 are available but require a specialized laboratory are time-consuming and expensive. Urinary estrogen assays have been used for detection and timing of ovulation. The preovulatory peak of urinary estrogens ranges from 40 to 100 µg per 24 hour. The mean interval between the first observable rise and the estrogen peak is 5.5 days. The day after estrogen peak (day of LH surge) is believed to be the day of maximal fertility. Direct assays of urinary metabolites of estrogens have been developed, and kits for self-detection of these metabolites are available. These tests have the potential to both predict ovulation and identify the limits of the fertile period in healthy women with regular menstrual periods. Three immunochemical tests have been developed, and their potential efficiency has been compared with results of other methods.

1. The first test involves the measurement of estrone-3 glucuronide (E3G) in daily samples of early morning urine. The day of a defined rise in the concentration is used to indicate the start of the probable fertile period, and the peak day plus four is used to indicate the last day of potential fertility or the start of the infertile (postovulatory) period.
2. The second test involves determining the ratio of E3G to pregnanediol-3α-glucuronide in a daily sample of early morning urine. Similar to the previous test, the day of a defined rise is used to identify the last day of potential

fertility or the start of the infertile period. Additional studies have suggested that the use of pregnanediol-3α-glucuronide alone or in combination with urinary LH or mucus testing may provide additional accuracy. After the first day of positive LH test or the end of fertile mucus, three consecutive days of pregnanediol-3α-glucuronide (PDG) testing over a threshold of 5 μg/mL indicated a 100% specificity for ovulation confirmation.[10]

3. The third test is designed to measure E3G and LH simultaneously. These kits measures changes in LH and E3G levels in urine using antibodies specific to these hormones. It stores information on hormone level changes gathered over the last six cycles to take into account cycle variations among individual women.[11] These assays have been field-tested by a task force of WHO. The results indicate that the E3G test can predict ovulation and define the fertile period in 78% of menstrual cycles. The ratio test can predict this fertile period in 74% of cycles.[11]

Progesterone Assays

A serum progesterone level is one of the simplest and most commonly used methods to document ovulation, as long as it is properly timed. Automated chemiluminescent assays available for serum progesterone, have considerably improved the accuracy and ease of documentation of ovulation. Serum progesterone levels are usually less than 1 ng/mL during the follicular phase. Coincident with the LH rise, serum progesterone begins to rise, and reaches a peak of greater than 10 ng/mL approximately 8 days after the LH peak or 7 days before menstruation starts. A progesterone level greater than 5 ng/mL is considered to be consistent with ovulatory cycles by most investigators.[12] Presumption of ovulation can be documented, therefore, by obtaining two blood samples on days 8 and 21 of a normal 28 days cycle. A rise of progesterone value from less than 1 ng/mL to greater than 5 ng/mL would be consistent with ovulation.

A progesterone concentration less than 3 ng/mL is considered anovulation except when withdrawn immediately postovulation or just before the onset of menses, when lower levels are naturally expected. The timing of testing of progesterone levels vary with cycle length and should be aimed a week before onset of menstruation, e.g. on day 18 in 25 day cycle or on day 28 in 35 day cycle.

Urinary assay of pregnanediol, a metabolite of progesterone, would also aid in ovulation detection. In the midluteal phase, pregnanediol levels reach 4–6 mg per 24 hour.[3] A urinary level of 2 mg or greater is thus consistent with ovulatory cycles. RIA or urinary pregnanediol-3α-glucuronide has demonstrated a significant rise of this metabolite in the urine 2 days after the LH peak.[13] As previously indicated, the peak of the ratio of E3G to pregnanediol-3α-glucuronide plus 5 signals the start of the postovulatory period.[11]

Other Assays

For couples with unexplained infertility the additional measurement of thyroid stimulating hormone and prolactin could be of importance.

Major problems with indirect methods include:

- The inability of indirect methods to detect luteinized unruptured follicle (there is an increased incidence of this syndrome in patients with chronic use of nonsteroidal anti-inflammatory drugs or in women treated with clomiphene citrate)
- The relatively high incidence of false negative results in methods depending on urine versus blood measurements
- The difficulty to time ovulation in women with prolonged follicular phases.

Transvaginal Ultrasound

Serial real-time pelvic ultrasonography has been described as a rapid, reliable method for monitoring follicular growth, rupture, and ovulation and formation of corpus luteum and regression. The introduction of transvaginal ultrasound has considerably improved the sensitivity of this technique for ovulation detection. Transverse and longitudinal scans are performed on both ovaries and the mean diameter of each follicle is calculated. Ovulation is deemed to have occurred if the follicle reached a mean diameter of 18–25 mm and subsequently changed in size, shape or sonographic density.

The changes in ultrasound image of the follicle that has ovulated are: (1) disappearance or sudden decrease in size of the follicle, (2) increased echogenicity, (3) irregularity of follicular wall, and (4) appearance of free fluid in the cul-de-sac or pouch of Douglas. Disappearance or sudden decrease in follicle size has been found to be the most frequent sign of ovulation.[14] Sensitivity and specificity of ultrasonography to document ovulation is 84% and 89%, respectively, and accuracy is about 85%.

The disadvantages include:

- Regression of an unruptured follicle documented as ovulation.
- The range of diameter of the dominant follicle before rupture is between 18 mm and 29 mm. This relatively large range makes it difficult to predict the day of ovulation prospectively.[15]

- A similar linear relation between follicle diameter and plasma E2 levels was reported by Bryce and coworkers,[16] but the variation within and between the two parameters was too large to predict ovulation to within less than 1.4 ± 1.2 days.
- Serial ultrasound determination is expensive.

Current practice is to use other methods of ovulation timing and to perform two or three ultrasonic measurements of follicular size close to the time of ovulation to confirm follicular maturation or collapse.[17]

OVARIAN RESERVE

Ovarian reserve is defined as the pool of ovarian follicles that can be stimulated to produce oocytes to achieve conception.

Ovarian Reserve Tests

Ovarian reserve assessment can be divided into clinical markers, dynamic tests, static tests. Previous failed cycle also is an important assessment for ovarian reserve.

- *Clinical markers*: Age, menstrual pattern, previous history of cancelled cycles
- *Endocrine static markers*: FSH, LH, E2, progesterone (P4), FSH:LH ratio, P4:E2 ratio, AMH, testosterone, vascular endothelial growth factors, insulin growth factor-1
- *Endocrine dynamic tests*: CCST, GAST, EFORT
- *Ultrasound markers*: AFC, ovarian volume, ovarian blood flow, ovarian follicular vascularity
- *Histology*: Ovarian biopsy.

Age

It is one of the important markers of the ovarian reserve. Natural fecundity and pregnancy rate decreases as age of women advances.[18] This is mainly due to decrease in quality and quantity of ovarian follicles, which in turn relates to efficiency and frequency of ovulation. Fecundability starts declining after the age of 30 years and is more significant after the age of 35 years. The prevalence of infertility increases after the age of 35 and 99% of women are infertile after the age of 45.

Menstrual Age

Menstrual cycle's length is primarily dependant on duration of follicular phase, which in turn is determined by rate and quality of follicular growth. Shortening in cycle length (especially follicular phase) can be associated with decrease ovarian reserve. The mechanism behind it is decrease in production of inhibin-B by small antral follicles, which lead to increase in FSH.

Duration of menstrual cycle has not only been related to ovarian reserve but in some studies has been found to be related to response to ovarian stimulation to gonadotrophin and quality of embryos in assisted reproductive techniques (ART) cycles with pregnancy rates higher with cycle duration of more than 34 days than less than 26 day cycle.

Previous Failed Cycle

It has been shown that in a standard stimulation protocol, history of poor follicular growth and cancellation of cycle is linked to cancellation in subsequent treatment cycles. This is more commonly associated with increasing age and high endocrine static markers.

Follicle-stimulating Hormone

It is the most commonly used endocrine test used to assess the ovarian reserve. Decrease in ovarian reserve is associated with increasing FSH levels. High FSH levels are related to poor response to gonadotrophin stimulation in ART cycles. Some authors observed reduced chances for spontaneous pregnancy when the levels exceeded 8 IU/L in women under 40 years[19] and others found FSH levels more than 15 IU/L as indicator of poor ovarian response and higher chances of ART cycle cancellation.[20] It has certain limitations, as it is associated with variability in its level within and between menstrual cycles, disparity between assays and being affected by external factors as smoking. But due to its low cost and easy accessibility, it is still used in some centers as means for assessing the ovarian reserve.

Luteinizing Hormone

Basal LH has not been related much to ovarian reserve and ovarian response in ART cycles, though it has been found that mean LH, LH amplitude and LH response to GnRH were higher in women with imminent ovarian failure (women with irregular menstrual cycles and high FSH levels).[21]

FSH:LH Ratio

An increase in basal FSH:LH ratio, even with normal FSH is a sign of decrease ovarian reserve[22] and poor response to COH.[23] Hence, the FSH:LH ratio appears to be clinically useful as it is considered as first sign of decreasing ovarian reserve. It increases before changes in serum FSH are observed.[24]

Estradiol

Basal E2 levels assists in predicting ovarian reserve when combined with FSH and age. On its own it has been found to have low predictive accuracy and lacks high sensitivity and specific cut off levels. Early elevations of E2 have been associated with advanced follicular recruitment and early development of ovarian follicle as observed in women with advancing age. It has been suggested that measurement of basal E2 in addition to FSH might improve prediction of fertility potential compared with basal FSH and chronological age alone.[25] Measurement of both FSH and E2 on cycle day 3 help to diminish the incidence of false-negative tests based on measurement of FSH alone; when both markers are precociously elevated, poor ovarian response is likely to occur.[26]

Decrease in estradiol levels with increasing FSH levels is a more certain sign of decreasing ovarian reserve. Evidence suggests that elevated early follicular E2 levels are associated with poorer prognosis.[27] Higher rates of cancelled ART cycles have been demonstrated with E2 levels less than 20 pg/mL or greater than or equal to 80 pg basal/mL.[28]

Inhibin A and B

Inhibins are glycoproteins from the superfamily of TGF-β. They are secreted by granulosa and theca cells of the ovarian follicle.[29] It has both paracrine and autocrine effect. It is known to inhibit pituitary FSH secretion and by its paracrine action, acts on the developing follicles. The systemic review by Broekmans et al. observed significant intercycle variability in inhibin B concentrations and also high rate of false positives in routine determination of basal inhibin levels.

Anti-Müllerian Hormone

Anti-Müllerian Hormone (AMH), also known as Müllerian inhibiting substance, is a member of the TGF-β super family. It is produced by the granulosa cells of growing preantral and small antral ovarian follicles as soon as they are recruited prior to their responsiveness to FSH.[30] Follicles secrete AMH till they are about the size of approximately 6 mm.[31] Serum AMH levels may be used as a marker of ovarian reserve, representing the quantity and quality of the ovarian follicle pool.[32] It may also estimate the quantity and quality of retrievable follicles in early stages of maturation and hence acts as a better predictor of ovarian response and reproductive potential.

Compared to other endocrine static hormones, AMH has the advantage of reduced variability of serum concentration along the menstrual cycle and also lower variations in serum levels between consecutive cycles. Overall, AMH is an important clinical marker in the assessment of female infertility. At present, poor response can be associated with AMH serum levels less than 1 ng/mL, normal response with levels from 1 ng/mL to 4 ng/mL, and high response with levels greater than 4 ng/mL.[33]

Endocrine Dynamic Tests

Clomiphene Citrate Challenge Test (CCCT)

This test involves administering 100 mg clomiphene citrate from days 5–9 of the menstrual cycle. FSH levels are measured on day 3 and day 10 of the cycle. Diminished ovarian reserve was determined by day 10 FSH more than day 3 FSH. An elevated serum progesterone level (>1.1 ng/mL) on menstrual cycle day 10 of a CCCT is also predictive of decrease ovarian reserve.[34] Due to the absence of standardized abnormal test definitions, CCCT is not being used commonly as a prognostic tool for testing ovarian reserve.

Gonadotropin Analogue Stimulating Test

GAST involves subcutaneous administration of the gonadotropin analogue, leuprolide acetate on day 2 and looking at change in FSH, LH, inhibin-B, E2 concentrations from day 2 to day 3.[35] Due to lack of standardization of GnRH analogue doses and administration timing, this has not been used routinely to test ovarian reserve.[36]

Exogenous FSH Ovarian Reserve Test

EFORT involves administration of 300 IU recombinant FSH at day 3 of the menstrual cycle. FSH, E2 and inhibin B levels are measured prior to FSH administration and 24 hours after FSH administration. The basal FSH levels and increase in E2 can be used to predict a woman's response in a later IVF cycle.[37]

ULTRASOUND

Antral Follicular Count

AFC is measured as follicles measuring between 2 mm and 10 mm between day 2 and day 5 of menstrual cycle. It has been shown to be predictor of ovarian stimulation. It was on its own also found superior to other different combination markers such as clinical, biochemical, and other ultrasonographic markers in predicting ovarian reserve and response.[38] Studies also demonstrated significant correlations between AFC and other commonly used serum ovarian reserve tests,[39] especially between

AFC and AMH.[30] Low numbers of antral follicles are a sign of ovarian ageing, and are observable earlier than arise in FSH serum level.[40]

AFC should be included in assessing the ovarian reserve as a tool for counseling the probability of achieving pregnancy and to individualize treatment protocols in IVF cycles. As with other endocrinology tests, it can also have intercycle variation and interobserver variation.[41]

Ovarian Volume

Sonographic measurements of ovarian volume have been shown to be important predictors of success in the treatment of infertility as well as early and specific indicators of normal ovarian aging.[42] Previously, significant correlations had been found between reduced ovarian measures, increased age and elevated serum FSH.[43] However, the review of ten well-designed studies concluded that OV presented little applicability in the prediction of poor response or pregnancy.[44] Hence its routine use should be used with caution in predicting ovarian reserve and response to stimulation. The reliability of measurement of OV using 2D ultrasound is also an issue.

Ovarian Blood Flow

Both ovarian stromal PSV and preovulatory follicular blood flow have been extensively assessed using transvaginal pulsed Doppler ultrasound. A recent meta-analysis assessing OBF as a predictor of IVF outcomes, found its clinical value unclear because of different flow-derived predictors used in literature.[45] Hence, ovarian blood flow may not be used to determine management of infertile couples in ART programs or predict ART outcome.[45]

Others

Previous Cancelled Cycles

Recent studies have shown that a history of cancelled cycles due to poor follicular response in a standard stimulation protocol is a better predictor of cancellation in subsequent treatment cycles than age or FSH.[46]

Ovarian Biopsy

The number of follicles per unit volume of cortical ovarian tissue can be calculated and defined as follicular density.[47] As is an invasive procedure it is no longer recommended to assess ovarian reserve.

REFERENCES

1. Mosher WD, Pratt WF. Fecundity and infertility in the United States: incidence and trends. Fertil Steril. 1991;56:192-3.
2. Moghissi K, Puscheck E, et al., Glob. libr. women's med. 2015. DOI 10.3843/ GLOWM.10325 (ISSN: 1756-2228).
3. Moghissi KS, Syner FN, Evans TN. A composite picture of the menstrual cycle. Am J Obstet Gynecol. 1972;114:405.
4. Abraham GE, Odell WD, Swerdloff RS, Hopper K. Simultaneous radioimmunoassay of plasma FSH, LH, progesterone, 17-hydroxyprogesterone and estradiol-17b during the menstrual cycle. J Clin Endocrinol Metab. 1972;34:312-8.
5. Yen SC, Vela P, Ramkin J, Littel AS. Hormonal relationship during the menstrual cycle. JAMA. 1970;211:1513-7.
6. Miller PB, Soules MR. The usefulness of a urinary LH kit for ovulation prediction during menstrual cycle of normal women. Obstet Gynecol. 1996;87:13-7.
7. Pearlstone AC, Surrey ES. The temporal relation between the urine LH surge and sonographic evidence of ovulation: determinant and clinical significance. Obstet Gynecol. 1994;83:184-8.
8. Guida M, Tommaselli GA, Palomba S, et al. Efficacy of methods for determining ovulation in natural family planning program. Feril Steril. 1999;72:900-4.
9. Li H, Chen J, Overstreet JW, Nakajima ST, Lasley BL. Urinary follicle-stimulating hormone peak as a biomarker for estimating the day of ovulation. Fertil Steril. 2002;77:961-6.
10. Ecochard R, Leiva R, Bouchard T, Boehringer H, Direito A, Mariani A, et al. Use of urinary pregnanediol 3-glucuronide to confirm ovulation. Steroids. 2013;78(10):1035-40.
11. Collins WP. Biochemical approaches to ovulation prediction and detection and the location of the fertile period in women. In: Jeffcoate SL (Ed). Ovulation: Methods for Its Prediction and Detection. New York: John Wiley & Sons; 1983. p. 49.
12. Ross GT, Cargille CM, Lipsett MB, Rayford PL, Marshall JR, Strott CA, et al. Pituitary and gonadal hormones in women during spontaneous and induced ovulatory cycles. Recent Prog Horm Res. 1970;26:1-62.
13. Samarajeewa P, Cooley G, Kellie AE. The radioimmunoassay of pregnanediol-3 alpha-glucuronide. J Steroid Biochem. 1979;11:1165-71.
14. Ecochard R, Marret H, Rabilloud M, Bradaï R, Boehringer H, Girotto S, et al. Sensitivity and specificity of ultrasound indices of ovulation in spontaneous cycles. Eur J Obstet Gynecol Reprod Biol. 2000;91:59-64.
15. Kerin J. Ovulation detection in the human. Clin Reprod Fertil. 1982;1(1):27-54.
16. Bryce RL, Shutter B, Sinosich MJ, Stiel JN, Picker RH, Saunders DM, et al. The value of ultrasound, gonadotropin and estradiol measurements for precise ovulation prediction. Fertil Steril. 1982;37:42-5.
17. Wilcox AJ, Weinberg ER, Baird DD. Timing of sexual intercourse in relation to ovulation: effects on the probability of conception, survival of pregnancy and sex of the baby. N Engl J Med. 1995;333:1517-21.
18. te Velde ER, Pearson PL. The variability of female reproductive aging. Hum Reprod Update. 2002;8:141-54.
19. van der Steeg JW, Steures P, Eijkemans MJ, et al. Predictive value and clinical impact of basal follicle stimulating hormone in subfertile, ovulatory women. J Clin Endocrinol Metab. 2007;92:2163-8.
20. Ashrafi M, Madani T, Tehranian AS, Malekzadeh F. Follicle stimulating hormone as a predictor of ovarian response in women undergoing controlled ovarian hyperstimulation for IVF. Int J Gynaecol Obstet. 2005;91:53-7.

21. de Koning CH, Popp-Snijders C, Schoemaker J, Lambalk CB. Elevated FSH concentrations in imminent ovarian failure are associated with higher FSH and LH pulse amplitude and response to GnRH. Hum Reprod. 2000;15:1452-6.
22. Barroso G, Oehninger S, Monzó A, Kolm P, Gibbons WE, Muasher SJ. High FSH:LH ratio and low LH levels in basal cycle day 3: impact on follicular development and IVF outcome. J Assist Reprod Genet. 2001;18:499-505.
23. Mukherjee T, Copperman AB, Lapinski R, Sandler B, Bustillo M, Grunfeld L. An elevated day three follicle-stimulating hormones: luteinizing hormone ratio (FSH:LH) in the presence of a normal day 3 FSH predicts a poor response to controlled ovarian hyperstimulation. Fertil Steril. 1996;65:588-93.
24. Kligman I, Rosenwaks Z. Differentiating clinical profiles: predicting good responders, poor responders, and hyperresponders. Fertil Steril. 2001;76:1185-90.
25. Licciardi FL, Liu HC, Rosenwaks Z. Day 3 estradiol serum concentrations as prognosticators of ovarian stimulation response and pregnancy outcome in patients undergoing in vitro fertilization. Fertil Steril. 1995;64:991-4.
26. Speroff L, Fritz MA. Female infertility. In: Speroff L, Fritz MA (Eds). Clinical Gynecologic Endocrinology and infertility. 7th edition. Philadelphia, Pa, USA: Lippincott Williams & Wilkins; 2005. pp. 1015-22.
27. Smotrich DB, Widra EA, Gindoff PR, Levy MJ, Hall JL, Stillman RJ. Prognostic value of day 3 estradiol on in vitro fertilization outcome. Fertil Steril. 1995;64:1136-40.
28. Frattarelli JL, Bergh PA, Drews MR, Sharara FI, Scott RT. Evaluation of basal estradiol levels in assisted reproductive technology cycles. Fertil Steril. 2000;74:518-24.
29. Hayes FJ, Hall JE, Boepple PA, Crowley WF. Differential control of gonadotropin secretion in the human: endocrine role of inhibin. J Clin Endocrinol Metab. 1998;83:1835-41.
30. Fanchin R, Schonäuer LM, Righini C, Guibourdenche J, Frydman R, Taieb J. Serum anti-Müllerian hormone is more strongly related to ovarian follicular status than serum inhibin B, estradiol, FSH and LH on day 3. Human Reprod. 2003;18:323-7.
31. Weenen C, Laven JSE, von Bergh AR, Cranfield M, Groome NP, Visser JA, et al. Anti-Müllerian hormone expression pattern in the human ovary: potential implications for initial and cyclic follicle recruitment. Mol Hum Reprod. 2004;10:77-83.
32. van Rooij IA, Broekmans FJ, te Velde ER, Fauser BC, Bancsi LF, de Jong FH, et al. Serum anti-Mullerian hormone levels: a novel measure of ovarian reserve. Hum Reprod. 2002;17:3065-71.
33. Muttukrishna S, McGarrigle H, Wakim R, Khadum I, Ranieri DM, Serhal P. Antral follicle count, antimullerian hormone and inhibin B: predictors of ovarian response in assisted reproductive technology? BJOG. 2005;112:1384-90.
34. Hofmann GE, Scott RT, Horowitz GM, Thie J, Navot D. Evaluation of the reproductive performance of women with elevated day 10 progesterone levels during ovarian reserve screening. Fertil Steril. 1995;63:979-83.
35. Winslow KL, Toner JP, Brzyski RG, Oehninger SC, Acosta AA, Muasher SJ. The gonadotropin-releasing hormone agonist stimulation test—a sensitive predictor of performance in the flare-up in vitro fertilization cycle. Fertil Steril. 1991;56:711-7.
36. Ramalho de Carvalho B1, Gomes Sobrinho DB, Vieira AD, Resende MP, Barbosa AC, Silva AA, et al. Ovarian Reserve Assessment for Infertility Investigation. ISRN Obstet Gynecol. 2012;2012:576385.
37. Fanchin R, de Ziegler D, Olivennes F, Taieb J, Dzik A, Frydman R. Exogenous follicle stimulating hormone ovarian reserve test (EFORT): a simple and reliable screening test for detecting 'poor responders' in in-vitro fertilization. Hum Reprod. 1994;9:1607-11.
38. Scheffer GF, Broekmans FJ, Looman CW, Blankenstein M, Fauser BC, teJong FH, et al. The number of antral follicles in normal women with proven fertility is the best reflection of reproductive age. Human Reprod. 2003;18;700-6.
39. Haadsma ML, Bukman A, Groen H, Roeloffzen EM, Groenewoud ER, Heineman MJ, et al. The number of small antral follicles (2–6 mm) determines the outcome of endocrine ovarian reserve tests in a subfertile population. Hum Reprod. 2007;22:1925-31.
40. Scheffer GJ, Broekmans FJ, Dorland M, Habbema JD, Looman CW, te Velde ER. Antral follicle counts by transvaginal ultrasonography are related to age in women with proven natural fertility. Fertil Steril. 1999;72:845-51.
41. Nahum R, Shifren JL, Chang Y, Leykin L, Isaacson K, Toth TL. Antral follicle assessment as a tool for predicting outcome in IVF—is it a better predictor than age and FSH? J Assist Reprod Genet. 2001;18:151-5.
42. de Boer EJ, den Tonkelaar I, te Velde ER, Burger CW, Klip H, van Leeuwen FE, et al. A low number of retrieved oocytes at in vitro fertilization treatment is predictive of early menopause. Fertil Steril. 2002;77:978-85.
43. Bowen S, Norian J, Santoro N, Pal L. Simple tools for assessment of ovarian reserve (OR): individual ovarian dimensions are reliable predictors of OR. Fertil Steril. 2007;88:390-5.
44. Hendriks DJ, Kwee J, Mol BW, te Velde ER, Broekmans FJ. Ultrasonography as a tool for the prediction of outcome in IVF patients: a comparative meta-analysis of ovarian volume and antral follicle count. Fertil Steril. 2007;87:764-75.
45. Gibreel A, Maheshwari A, Bhattacharya S, Johnson NP. Ultrasound tests of ovarian reserve; a systematic review of accuracy in predicting fertility outcomes. Hum Fertil. 2009;12:95-106.
46. Peñarrubia J, Fábregues F, Manau D, Creus M, Carmona F, Casamitjana R, et al. Previous cycle cancellation due to poor follicular development as a predictor of ovarian response in cycles stimulated with gonadotrophin-releasing hormone agonist-gonadotrophin treatment. Hum Reprod. 2005;20:622-8.
47. Lass A, Silye R, Abrams DC, Krausz T, Hovatta O, Margara R, et al. Follicular density in ovarian biopsy of infertile women: a novel method to assess ovarian reserve. Hum Reprod. 1997;12:1028-31.

CHAPTER

5

Tubal Evaluation: An Eternal Dilemma

Richa Jagtap, Manjushri Kothekar

INTRODUCTION

Fallopian tubes play an important role in female fertility. It gives the passage for spermatozoa to find the ovum, is the site for natural fertilization, and helps the developing embryo find its way toward uterine cavity for implantation. The fallopian tubes need not just be patent anatomically but they should be functional physiologically also. Tubal infertility is a major reason of infertility. The reported incidence varies from 15% to 20%.[1]

ANATOMY AND PHYSIOLOGY

Fallopian tubes are derived from Müllerian ducts in fetal life. There are two ducts which fuse with each other in the distal part. The proximal part of each tube forms the fallopian tubes and uterus is derived from the fused distal parts. Abnormalities in this fusion can lead to various congenital anomalies of uterus and tubes.[2]

Each tube has got four parts, starting from its proximal end, interstitial part, isthmus, ampulla, and infundibulum along with fimbria.[2] The fimbria have flower like petals which remain glued together. The tube has its inner mucosal layer which is lined by ciliated epithelium and outer serosal layer with intervening lamina propria. When the ovulation happens, the fimbria open and the released ovum are captured by them. The ciliary activity of the tubal epithelium is dependent on the gonadal steroidogenesis, being maximum near the ovulation, favoring egg transport.[3] The fertilization of sperm and ovum happens in the ampullary part usually and the embryo traverses the tube to enter the uterine cavity.

Which Patients will Need Evaluation of Tubes?

Patients who fail to achieve pregnancy after 1 year of unprotected intercourse, or 6 months if age of the female partner is more than 35 years will need tubal testing as a part of a thorough infertility evaluation.

In patients with anovulatory infertility, this evaluation can be deferred till three cycles of successful ovulation induction. For patients who will need in vitro fertilization (IVF) as a treatment modality due to severe male factor, etc. also will not need evaluation for tubal patency. That is why it is advisable that before subjecting a woman for tubal patency check, few important things, viz. husband's semen analysis and ovarian reserve assessment should be checked. If either of these tests shows that pregnancy is not possible naturally or even with intrauterine insemination (IUI), then the tubal patency checking can be bypassed in favor of IVF.

What is the Ideal Time to Test?

Ideal time for any tubal evaluation test is within day 5 to day 10 of menstrual cycle. Most of the patients stop bleeding by that time, also there is very less risk of disturbing any pregnancy.

Tubal Evaluation

Few clinical details for example, history of ectopic pregnancy, recurrent pelvic inflammatory disease (PID), etc. warrant a detailed evaluation of tube. History may not be able to diagnose the exact status; however, it will

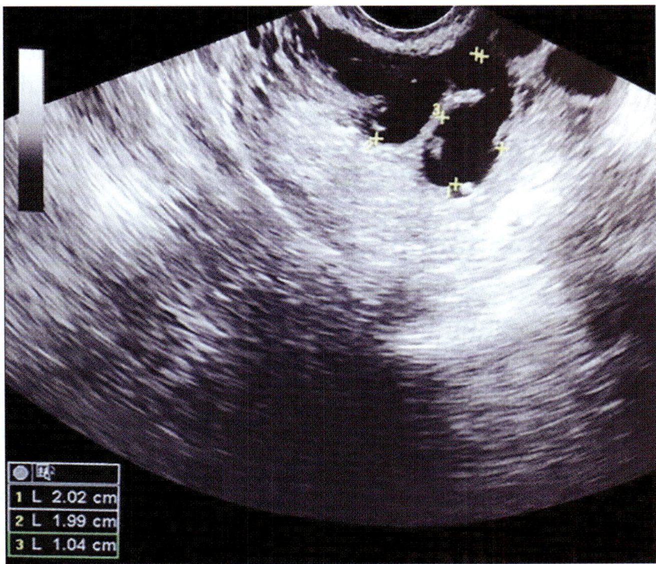

Fig. 1: Hydrosalpinx as seen on transvaginal examination.

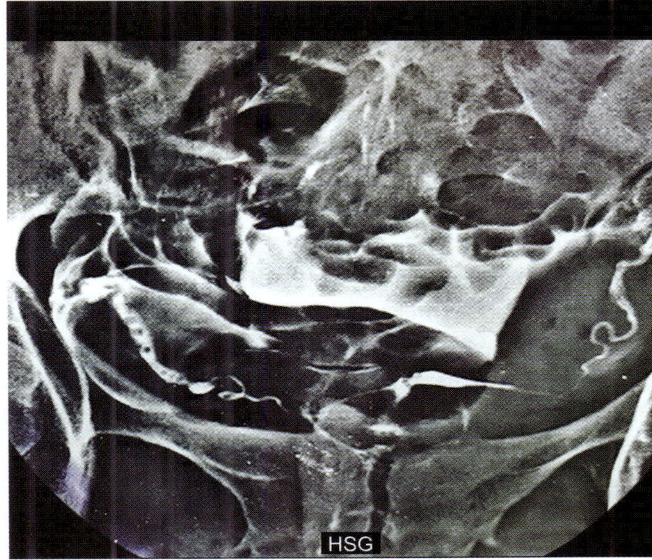

Fig. 2: Normal hysterosalpingography (HSG) showing bilateral spill.

definitely guide us regarding which is the best method to evaluate the tubal status in that patient.

Ultrasound examination is the cornerstone of infertility consultation. Ultrasonography (USG) is something what a stethoscope is for a general physician. A normal tube should not be visible on ultrasound and when seen, is always pathological. This would happen only if the tube is distended or edematous. A hydrosalpinx or a hematosalpinx is seen as a tubular structure in the adnexa. It could be uniloculated, but mostly it appears like a multiloculated adnexal structure (Fig. 1).

A routine transvaginal ultrasound examination will not help to assess tubal patency. Moreover, a patent tube which is dilated and or has lost its elasticity and mucosal characteristics, due to past infection will not be useful for fertility. Tubal evaluation ideally should include evaluation of the tubal patency along with its function. However, till date, we do not have any test which can definitively asses tubal function. Salpingoscopy, detailed later, is a step toward the same. Tubal patency can be checked by several ways which we will see one by one in details.

Hysterosalpingography

Hysterosalpingography (HSG) is an X-ray of uterus and patent tubes, taken after injecting radiocontrast dye inside uterus. It is the most simple and basic investigation for tubal patency. It is usually done without any anesthesia, but short general anesthesia can be offered to the patients if requested. In lithotomy position after emptying the bladder, cervix is gently visualized using a speculum under all aseptic precautions and the HSG cannula is attached to the cervix. Traditionally metallic HSG cannula was used, but nowadays disposable plastic HSG cannulas are also available which are little thinner and self-retaining. The cannula is fitted by small rotatory movements and radiocontrast dye is pushed through it.

Radiocontrast dye is available as oil-based as well as water-based preparations. Both were used historically, and much was studied regarding which type of contrast dye gives better results. But usually both the types are equal in terms of their usability in diagnosing tubal patency.[4] Some studies have found a serious lipogranulomatous type of allergic reaction to the oil-based contrast. The water soluble contrast is broadly used in current practice.

First a baseline image is captured before injecting the contrast and then 2–3 images are again captured immediately and 5 minutes after pushing the dye. Patent tubes will be outlined well from the cornual till fimbrial end, culminating in the pelvic spill documented by timely captured films (Fig. 2).

Sometimes late or delayed spillage is seen which is evident only in last image. Tubes will be seen distended without any spillage from fimbrial end in case of hydrosalpinx. In bilateral cornual block, both the tubes would not be opacified. Whenever there are peritubal adhesions, spillage will be loculated. Beading of the tube is seen in infectious pathology (Fig. 3).

Advantage of HSG is that it is a simple and least expensive test for tubal patency. It also lays down predictive direction for an upcoming laparoscopy if required and the operative intervention anticipated therein. In one study,

HSG has 83% concordance with laparoscopy.[5] Overall when compared with laparoscopy—the gold standard, HSG has 65% sensitivity and 85% specificity in diagnosing tubal pathology.[6]

Disadvantages of HSG include pain that originates from cervical cannulation and uterine inflation with dye. In best hand also the procedure will cause pain so as to make a permanent impact in a patient's mind. Other possible disadvantages include slight bleeding and infection. To avoid infection stringent aseptic precautions should be followed. It was reported that infection risk with HSG is 1%, but in high-risk population it can go up to 3%.[7] HSG causes radiation exposure, but the exposure is minimal and is considered to be safe.[8]

Another disadvantage is that of significant intraobserver and interobserver variations. Generally these variations are more when distal tube block is suspected, while proximal occlusion is easily diagnosed.[9,10]

Hysterosalpingography will cause some amount of flushing of the tubes with the media which may also have therapeutic effect on proximal tubal block. It was observed by some authors that tubal flushing with oil-soluble contrast media may increase the chance of pregnancy and live birth compared to no intervention.[11]

Hysterosalpingography is not conclusive in diagnosing peritubal pathology like adhesions, etc. False-positive diagnosis of bilateral cornual block can happen due to cornual spasm.

There are some contraindications for the procedure which include active pelvic infection and history of hypersensitivity to the radiocontrast dye.

So one can conclude that HSG can be offered as a baseline test to a couple for tubal patency assessment. If the report shows both tubes as patent, one can go ahead with simple treatment like ovulation induction with or without IUI. But if the report is suggestive of tubal block, then the findings should be confirmed by laparoscopy. In such a scenario, the possibility of need of operative correction in the same sitting should be taken in consideration.

Sonosalpingography

Sonosalpingography (SSG), also called as saline infusion sonography (SIS), is a procedure wherein normal saline (instead of the radiocontrast dye) is injected inside the uterine cavity using a pediatric Foley's catheter or special self-retaining catheter and spillage of the saline is assessed on sonography. It is a blend of HSG and USG.

Sonosalpingography can be attempted as an OPD procedure. No anesthesia is required. Patient lies in lithotomy position. Under all aseptic precautions a Cusco's speculum is introduced inside and cervix is visualized. An 8 No. pediatric Foley's catheter is introduced inside the uterus. After confirming its position in uterus, the bulb is inflated with 1–2 cc normal saline. Then slowly the speculum is removed and transvaginal sonography (TVS) ultrasound probe is inserted. Normal saline is pushed slowly through the catheter and spillage of the fluid in adnexa is visualized using the transvaginal ultrasound probe. The probe should be directed in each adnexa along the utero-ovarian axis while pushing saline. Not more than 10–15 cc normal saline needs to be pushed to diagnose the spill. One can also use the option of color flow which can detect the sudden gush of fluid (Fig. 4).

If free fluid is noted in the pouch of Douglas postprocedure, it surely indicates either of the tubes is patent.

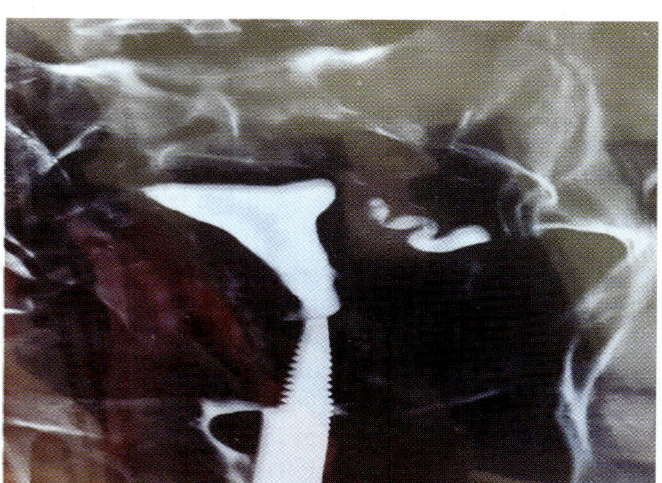

Fig. 3: Hysterosalpingography showing hydrosalpinx.

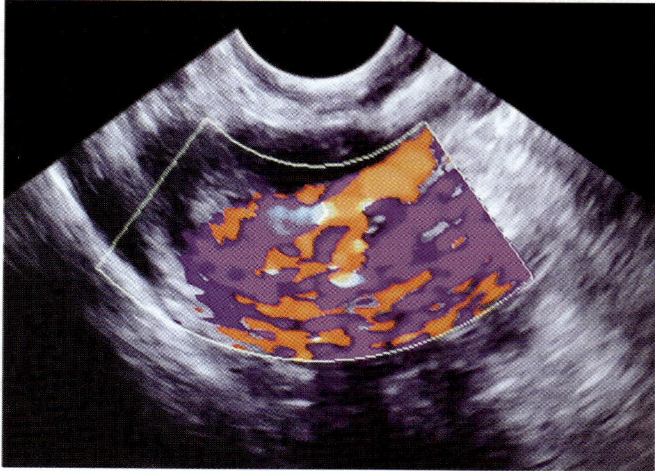

Fig. 4: Sudden gush of fluid noted in adnexa suggestive of patent tube.

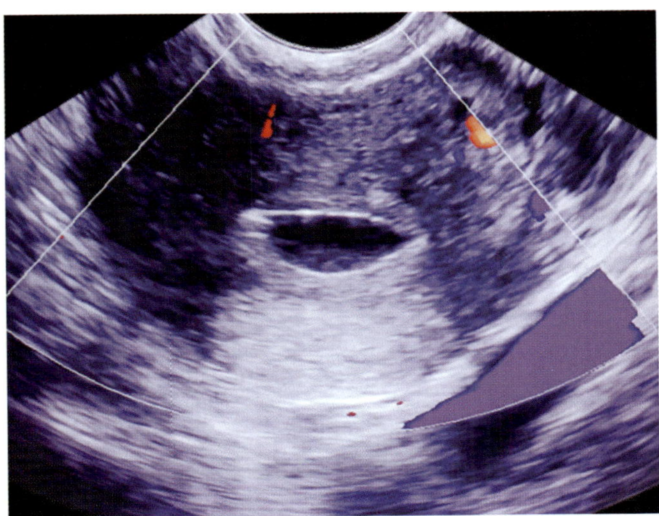

Fig. 5: Distended cavity postdeflation of catheter bulb.

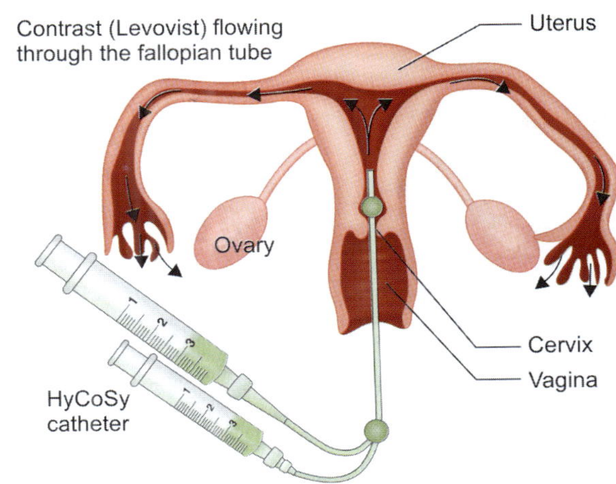

Fig. 6: Hysterosalpingo-contrast-sonography (HyCoSy) procedure.

In case of a blocked tube, the uterine cavity will get unduly distended due to the saline (Fig. 5).

Advantage of SSG over HSG is mainly its simplicity. SSG can be done in a normal gyne OPD wherein an ultrasound machine is available. Assessment of uterus along with ovaries is possible at the same time. It also helps to assess the uterine cavity and any intrauterine polyp; submucosal polyp can be well-delineated due to the distended cavity and fluid interface.

One study has found SSG to have 97% sensitivity and 92% specificity as compared to laparoscopy for assessing tubal patency.[12.]

The main disadvantage of SSG is that it is very subjective test wherein there can be a lot of interobserver disagreement. In case of SSG, as it is just plain normal saline which is not radioopaque, tubes are not delineated. Only the spill, which is seen as a sudden gush of fluid defines tubal patency. Furthermore if the tubes are blocked, level of the blockade cannot be ascertained as in HSG. The ultrasound evaluation is difficult in obese patients and in patients with difficultly placed ovaries.

Possible complications include pain, which is significantly lesser than HSG mainly due to the cannula used and the smaller amount of fluid distension used. Introduction of infection, vasovagal spasms, etc. are the other documented complication as of any other intervention.

Hysterosalpingo-Contrast-Sonography

It is a procedure which is in principle similar to SIS (sonosalpingography). The only difference being instead of normal saline a radiocontrast dye is instilled inside the uterine cavity. It is also an office procedure. The patient lies in lithotomy position. Under all aseptic precautions, cervix is visualized and a pediatric Foley's catheter is introduced in the uterine cavity and its bulb is inflated inside with normal saline. After that the radiocontrast dye is introduced inside through the catheter. Initially Echovist, which is a combination of 20% D-galactose carrier along with D-galactose microparticles, was used. As it was not approved by the Food and Drug Administration (FDA) in USA, some investigators have used saline with air as a contrast media (Fig. 6).[13]

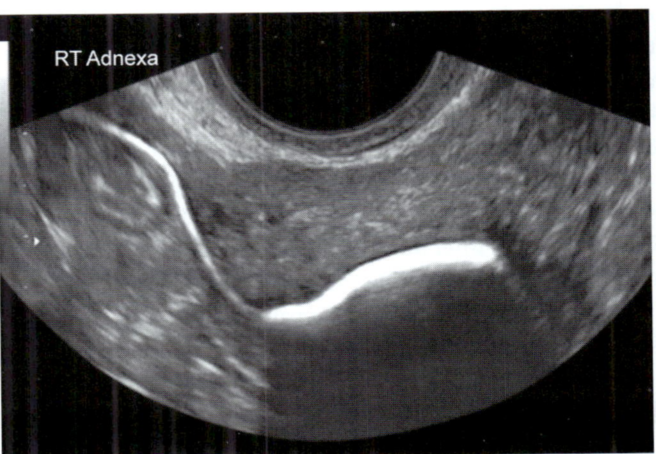

Fig. 7: Tubal outline seen after contrast injection.

The uterus along with tubes will be delineated clearly due to the radiocontrast and spillage of the contrast can be seen on transvaginal or sometimes transabdominal ultrasound (Fig. 7).

Advantage of hysterosalpingo-contrast-sonography (HyCoSy) over other procedures is that here there is no

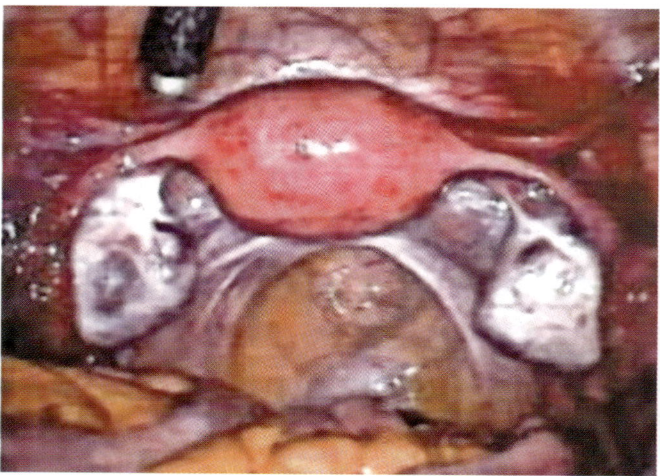

Fig. 8: Panoramic view on laparoscopy.

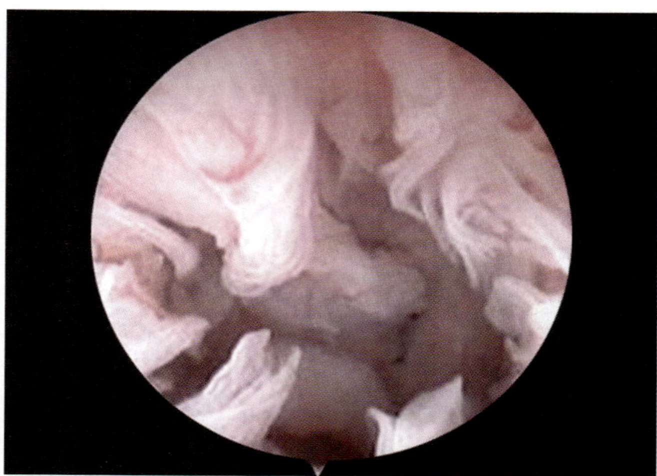

Fig. 9: Normal intraluminal folds.
Courtesy: Dr Sanjay Patel, Dr Haresh Vaghasia.

radiation exposure, but still the tubes are clearly delineated. HyCoSy results were found to be concordant with the HSG results in 83–89% cases. Its concordance with laparoscopy was found to be 86%.[14,15] In one study the investigators have found HyCoSy to have a sensitivity of 97% and specificity of 82% as compared to laparoscopy.[16]

The common complications include abdominal and sometimes shoulder pain.[14] Other complications include introduction of infection, vasovagal spasm, etc. The overall complication rate was 5%.

But when HyCoSy was compared with HSG, no significant difference was found in patient tolerance.[17]

Laparoscopy

It is by and large considered as the gold standard in evaluation of fallopian tubes. Laparoscopy gives the opportunity to examine the tubes thoroughly along with the surrounding structures. For laparoscopy, patient is given general anesthesia after completing the preoperative formalities. Usually for diagnostic laparoscopy two ports are sufficient, but if some operative correction is required then a third port also needs to be introduced. Fallopian tubes are identified; they are attached to the uterine cornua in between round ligament and ovarian ligament. The tubes are inspected from cornual end till fimbrial end. Presence of adhesions, tubercles, etc. if any is noted. If required biopsy can be taken from the suspicious sites and sample can be sent for histopathological examination. Spill is checked by instilling methylene blue inside the uterus though a cannula inserted from the vaginal end (Fig. 8).

Laparoscopy can be combined together with salpingoscopy for a more detailed examination. Salpingoscope is basically a microendoscope which can be introduced from the fimbrial end within the tubal lumen. One can see the endosalpingeal folds or cilia lining the tube. The findings help to assess the prognosis. If they appear agglutinated or so then it is pathological. It is found that the extent of intraluminal adhesions does not always correlate with the peritubal adhesions (Fig. 9).[18]

There are some classification systems based on the salpingoscopy findings which help to predict the tubal function (Figs. 10A and B).

The main advantage of laparoscopy is that it allows correction of the problem apart from diagnosing in same sitting. Laparoscopy also gives the opportunity to study the peritubal structures.

Main disadvantage includes its operative nature, need of anesthesia, and cost. The operative complications are injury to major vessels, injury to bowels, hemorrhage, and infection and anesthetic hazards. Overall 0.2–10% complication rate was observed in laparoscopies all over the world.[19]

Apart from these modalities few other modes are also published in literature.

Selective Salpingography and Tubal Catheterization

Selective salpingography means direct injection of the radioopaque dye into the tubal ostium with the help of a catheter introduced transcervically under fluoroscopic control. It rules out false-positive results due to tubal spasm or debris. It also allows to measure tubal perfusion pressure which has supposed to have a prognostic value.[20,21]

This procedure can be combined with tubal catheterization to treat proximal tubal block. The reported successful catheterization rates are high in the form of

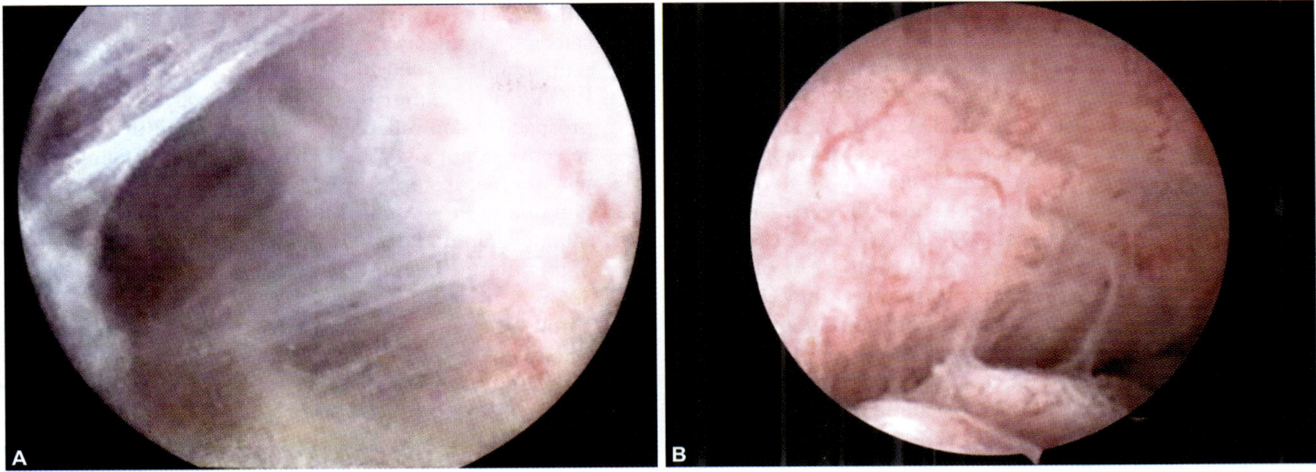

Figs. 10A and B: Intraluminal adhesions in different grades of severity.
Courtesy: Dr Sanjay Patel, Dr Haresh Vaghasia

62–90%. But the pregnancy rates after it are low—30%, the possible reasons could be reocclusion of the tubes or presence of coexisting tubal inflammatory pathology. The disadvantage of this procedure is that it requires skill and it also increases the radiation exposure time. There is 2% risk of tubal perforation and ectopic pregnancy.[22]

Office Hysteroscopy with Selective Tubal Perfusion

Selective pertubation with office hysteroscopy is also proposed as a method for evaluation of tubal patency. The flushing effect as evident by HSG is also seen in this. The flushing effect observed in it is found to be noninferior to HSG. Hysteroscopic tubal assessment is quoted to have a positive predictive value of 87.5%, and a negative predictive value of 76.7%.[23,24]

We can conclude by saying that HSG can be offered as a simple baseline investigation to assess the tubal patency. When the option of HyCoSy is available it can replace HSG. When either of these tests shows a tubal pathology, or whenever a pathology like endometriosis or pelvic inflammatory disorder is suspected, then laparoscopy should be offered.

REFERENCES

1. Hoffman L, Chan K, Smith B, et al. The value of saline salpingography as a surrogate test of tubal patency in low resource setting. Int J Fertil Womens Med. 2005;50(3):135-9.
2. Verco CJ. Fallopian tube anatomy, microanatomy, microcirculation and counter-current exchange. Fallopian Tube. 1993; pp.3-15.
3. Hunter RHF. The Fallopian Tubes: Their Role in Fertility and Infertility. Springer Science & Business Media. 2012
4. Lindequist S, Justesen P, Larsen C, et al. Diagnostic quality and complications of hysterosalpingography: Oil-versus water-soluble contrast media—a randomized prospective study. Radiology. 1991;179:69-74.
5. Strandell A, Bourne T, Bergh C, et al. The assessment of endometrial pathology and tubal patency: A comparison between the use of ultrasonography and X-ray hysterosalpingography for the investigation of infertility patients. Ultrasound Obstet Gynecol. 1999;14:200.
6. Swart P, Mol BW, van der Veen F, et al. The accuracy of hysterosalpingography in the diagnosis of tubal pathology: a meta-analysis. Fertil Steril. 1995;64:486-91.
7. Stumpf PG, March CM. Febrile morbidity following hysterosalpingography: Identification of risk factors and recommendations for prophylaxis. Fertil Steril. 1980;33:487-92.
8. Karande VC, Pratt DE, Balin MS, et al. What is the radiation exposure to patients during a gynecoradiologic procedure? Fertil Steril. 1997;67:401-3.
9. Mol BW, Swart P, Bossuyt PM, et al. Reproducibility of the interpretation of hysterosalpingography in the diagnosis of tubal pathology. Hum Reprod. 1996;11:1204-8.
10. Glatstein IZ, Sleeper LA, Lavy Y, et al. Observer variability in the diagnosis and management of the hysterosalpingogram. Fertil Steril. 1997;67:233-7.
11. Mohiyiddeen L, Hardiman A, Fitzgerald C, et al. Tubal flushing for subfertility. Cochrane Database Syst Rev. 2015;(5):CD003718.
12. Seal SL, Ghosh D, Saha D, et al. Comparative evaluation of sonosalpingography hysterosalpingography, and laparoscopy for determination of tubal patency. J Obstet Gynecol India. 2007;57(2):158-61.
13. Volpi E, Zuccaro G, Patriarca A, et al. Transvaginal sonographic tubal patency testing using air and saline solution as contrast media in a routine infertility clinic setting. Ultrasound Obstet Gynecol. 1996;7:43-8.
14. Holz K, Becker R, Schurmann R. Ultrasound in the investigation of tubal patency. A meta-analysis of three comparative studies of Echovist-200 including 1007 women. Zentralbl Gynakol. 1997;119:366-73.

15. Exacoustos C, Zupi E, Carusotti C, et al. Hysterosalpingo-contrast sonography compared with hysterosalpingography and laparoscopic dye pertubation to evaluate tubal patency. J Am Assoc Gynecol Laparosc. 2003;10(3):367-72.
16. Luciano DE, Exacoustos C, Johns DA, et al. Can hysterosalpingocontrast sonography replace hysterosalpingography in confirming tubal blockage after hysteroscopic sterilization and in the evaluation of the uterus and tubes in infertile patients? Am J Obstet Gynecol. 2011;204(1):79.e1-79.e5.
17. Ayida G, Kennedy S, Barlow D, et al. A comparison of patient tolerance of hysterosalpingocontrast sonography (HyCoSy) with Echovist-200 and X-ray hysterosalpingography for outpatient investigation of infertile women. Ultrasound Obstet Gynecol. 1996;7:201-4.
18. Marana R, Catalano GF, Muzii L. Salpingoscopy. Curr Opin Obstet Gynecol. 2003;15(4):333-6.
19. Magrina JF. Complications of laparoscopic surgery. Clin Obstet Gynecol. 2002;45:469-80.
20. Thurmond AS, Machan LS, Maubon AJ, et al. A review of selective salpingography and fallopian tube catheterization. Radiographics. 2000;20:1759-68.
21. Woolcott R, Fisher S, Thomas J, et al. A randomized, prospective, controlled study of laparoscopic dye studies and selective salpingography as diagnostic tests of fallopian tube patency. Fertil Steril. 1999;72:879-84.
22. Papaioannou S, Afnan M, Sharif K. The role of selective salpingography and tubal catheterization in the management of the infertile couple. Curr Opin Obstet Gynecol. 2004;16:325-9.
23. Török P, Major T. Accuracy of assessment of tubal patency with selective perturbation at office hysteroscopy compared with laparoscopy in infertile women. J Minim Invasive Gynecol. 2012;19(5):627-30.
24. Török P, Lőrincz J, Dobrai M, et al. Tubal flushing effect of hysteroscopic patency test. Middle East Fert Soc J. 2017;22(4):273-4.

CHAPTER

6

Mechanical Issues in Fertility: How do we evaluate?

Jayesh Patel, Azadeh Patel, Juan A García-Velasco

INTRODUCTION

Infertility is one of the most prevalent rising health problems in young adults. It is a medical condition that involves a couple, rather than a single individual. It is a disease defined by the failure to achieve a successful pregnancy after 12 months or more of appropriate, timed unprotected intercourse.[1] Earlier evaluation and treatment may be justified based on medical history and physical findings. It is warranted after 6 months for women over age of 35 years.

Some clinicians use the term subfertility to describe this failure to conceive unless the couple has been proven to be sterile, which is in fact more appropriate unless absolute factors—azoospermia, bilateral tubal blockage, premature ovarian failure (POF), congenital absence or surgical removal of uterus and/or ovaries—are diagnosed.

After normal ovulation, for fertilization and implantation we need normal patent and functional fallopian tubes, normal uterine cavity and normal male reproductive tract. Any obstruction or distortion will hamper passage of the gametes or embryo and contributes to mechanical hindrance to pregnancy.

EPIDEMIOLOGY

Distribution of causes of infertility is population based and varies accordingly. In a study by WHO involving 8500 infertile couples belonging to developed countries, female factor infertility was reported in 37%, male factor in 8% and combined factor infertility in 35%.[2] Common causes of female infertility are:

- *Ovulatory disorders*: 25%
- *Tubal blockage*: 11%
- *Other tubal abnormalities*: 11%
- *Endometriosis*: 15%
- *Pelvic adhesions*: 12%
- *Uterine causes*: 1–2%
- *Cervical causes*: 3–4%

Mechanical Causes of Infertility

- Female factors
  - *Tubal factor*: It is the most common site of obstruction. It would be covered in detail in separate chapter
  - *Cervical factor*: It includes stenosis and anatomical distortion of the cervix
  - *Vaginal factor*: Vaginismus
  - *Uterine factor*: Space occupying lesions such as fibroids, polyps, and Asherman's syndrome
  - Endometriosis
  - *Pelvic adhesions*: Due to pelvic infection or previous surgery.
- Male factors
  - Obstructive azoospermia (OA)
  - Ejaculatory dysfunction
  - Coital and deposition problem.

MECHANICAL CAUSES IN FEMALE INFERTILITY

Cervical Stenosis

Cervix is a narrow lumen, located at the neck of the uterus, between vagina and the uterus. Cervical stenosis is either congenital or acquired. It is usually caused by scar tissue contraction, agglutination of raw surfaces within the endocervical canal or obliteration of the endocervical canal by polyp or tumor (e.g. endometrial or cervical cancer).

It may sometime lead to distortion of cervical canal. It is said to be stenosed when the diameter becomes less than 2.5 mm.[3]

Causes

1. Congenital cervical stenosis
2. Acquired causes:
   - Any surgical cervical or uterine procedure, colposcopy, conization of cervix, cryosurgery on cervix for dysplasia, dilatation and curettage
   - Trauma to the cervix
   - Asherman's syndrome
   - Cervical cancer
   - Radiotherapy for any pelvic or endometrial cancer
   - *Chronic cervicitis:* Long-standing leading to hypertrophied cervix
   - Cervical fibroid or polyp
   - Postmenopausal: due to cervical atrophy

Symptoms

Before menopause it can lead to:
- Dysmenorrhea
- Oligo/amenorrhea
- Infertility as it hinders with the sperm transport to the uterus
- Hematometra/Pyometra and its consequences
- Endometriosis in long-standing and ignored cases
- Irregular bleeding, contact bleeding in case of cervical cancer.

In postmenopausal women it can lead to hydrometra/pyometra in long-standing cases.

Location

- *Internal os stenosis*: Internal os is the junction of the cervix and the uterus, and its stenosis with patent canal.
- *Anywhere below the internal os*: Localized or throughout the canal length.

Impact on Infertility

- Cervical stenosis can lead to infertility by preventing the transport of the sperms from the vagina to uterus.
- It can lead to difficult passage of intrauterine catheter for artificial insemination or embryo transfer in IVF due to distorted cervical canal and mechanical obstruction during treatment.

Evaluation

- *History*: Specific history of any previous cervical procedure/surgery, oligo/amenorrhea in previously normorrhagic women, dysmenorrhea, previous cervical dystocia during labor, lower abdominal bulge, infertility, weight loss.
- *Examination*:
  - Diagnosis can be done by passing a sterile catheter (used for IUI or IVF) after proper visualization of external os in per speculum examination, if it does not give way easily then the procedure should be performed guided with transabdominal ultrasound.
  - In suspected cervical cancer, diagnosis can be made by cervical cytology, colposcopy, and cervical biopsy for primary diagnosis.
- *Hysteroscopic evaluation*: Diagnostic hysteroscopy can be performed.

Treatment

Simple cervical dilation under general anesthesia using cervical dilators, or hysteroscopic resection by scissors can be performed under ultrasound guidance.

Vaginismus

It is defined as involuntary contraction of vaginal and pelvic muscles before sexual intercourse, making it painful, difficult or impossible. It is mostly psychological and is linked with past experience of sexual abuse/trauma, painful intercourse and emotions. It can be:
1. *Primary vaginismus*: When sexual penetration has never been achieved.
2. *Secondary vaginismus*: When penetration is not possible after gynecological surgery or radiation therapy.

It can lead to infertility by preventing intercourse and thus proper ejaculation in the vagina. Diagnosis can be made by digital or per speculum vaginal examination. Treatment is by proper psychological counseling and education by an expert, use of vaginal dilators and Kiegel's exercises.

Fibroid/Leiomyoma/Myoma

Introduction

Fibroids are benign tumors of uterus composed of smooth muscles cells, fibrous tissue and collagen. They are estrogen-dependent tumors. Incidence of fibroid is 20–40% of the women of reproductive age group. Uterine factor contributes to 1–2 % of the female infertility causes.[4]

Fibroid may affect fertility by:

- *Causing distortion of the uterus and uterine cavity (in large fibroids):* Causing mechanical obstruction interfering with transport of gametes and embryo.
- Causes endometrial vascular changes and affecting the embryo implantation.
- Space occupying nature (especially submucous fibroid) interfering with implantation.

Types of fibroids (depending on location):

1. Uterine fibroids.
2. *Cervical fibroids*: It is located within the cervix facing anterior/posterior/laterals and isthmic region.
3. *Broad ligament*: It is located between two sleeves of broad ligament.

Classification of Uterine Fibroids

1. *Submucous*: It is located beneath the endometrial cavity and it grows generally into uterine cavity and may become pedunculated. It is classified by ESGE classification[5] (Table 1).
2. *Intramural/intramyometrial:* It is located within myometrium of uterus.
3. *Subserous*: It is located beneath the uterine serosa and growth occurs outward in the pelvic cavity; they may become pedunculated. Generally it does not contribute to infertility.

The location of a fibroid, and not its size, is the key factor regarding fertility.[6] Fibroids that distort the uterine cavity (submucosal or intramural with an intracavitary component) result in difficulty in conceiving and have an increased risk of miscarriage.[6,7] In contrast, subserosal fibroids do not impact fertility. The role of intramural fibroids in infertility is controversial still today.[6,7] Women with submucosal or intramural with intracavitary component fibroids were less likely to become pregnant (RR 0.36, 95% CI 0.18–0.74) and more likely to have a spontaneous abortion (RR 1.7, 95% CI 1.4–2.1).[6] Women with submucosal fibroid who did versus did not undergo myomectomy had a significant increase in conception rate (RR 2.03, 95% CI 1.08–3.83). But, there was no significant decrease in the risk of spontaneous abortion in women who did versus did not undergo myomectomy (38.5 vs 50%; RR 0.77, 95% CI 0.36–1.66); however, this result was based on a single RCT study of 52 women and lacks adequate statistical power.[6,8]

Table 1: ESGE classification of submucous myoma.

Type	*Presentation of submucous myoma*
Type 0	• Entirely within endometrial cavity • No myometrial extension (pedunculated)
Type I	• < 50% myometrial extension (sessile) • < 90 degree angle of myoma surface to uterine wall
Type II	• ≥ 50% myometrial extension (sessile) • ≥ 90 degree angle of myoma surface to uterine wall

Source: Modified from reference 5.

Intramural fibroids that are not affecting the endometrial cavity have effect on alteration of expression of some endometrial genes but do not affect the genes involved in implantation and so do not affect the endometrial receptivity.[9] While in patients with submucous myomas have generalized decreased expression of *HOX* gene in endometrium, thus affecting endometrial receptivity for implantation.[10]

Symptoms

- *Menstrual abnormality*: It causes excessive and irregular menstruation, but only in submucous fibroids, the rest locations are mainly asymptomatic. In long-term it may lead to chronic iron deficiency anemia.
- *Pelvic pain*: It is not very common-pain with or without menstruation, varying from mild discomfort to debilitating pain, depending upon size, location of fibroid in relation to pelvic structures.
- *Compressive symptoms*: If the fibroid is large in size, it can cause compression of the urinary bladder anteriorly and cause urinary retention, difficult urination leading to hydroureter and hydronephrosis. Posterior compression on the rectum can cause tenesmus and bowel obstruction (very rare).
- *Subfertility/infertility*: Only in fibroids pressing on or distorting the cavity [submucus] or interfering with tubal function.
- *History of repeated abortions*: Only in submucous fibroids.

Diagnosis

Precise fibroid mapping (localization, measurement, characteristics) is important because both the modalities of treatment (medical and surgical) are available and are equally effective. The decision whether to treat the fibroid or not, and to operate the patient or give medical therapy is important for infertility patients.

Ultrasound: Most of the fibroids are asymptomatic and so is a chance finding on a routine ultrasound. Ultrasound is frequently used, relatively cost-effective, easily available and with an experienced skilled operator can detect fibroid of as small as of 5 mm size. It being operator dependent it is

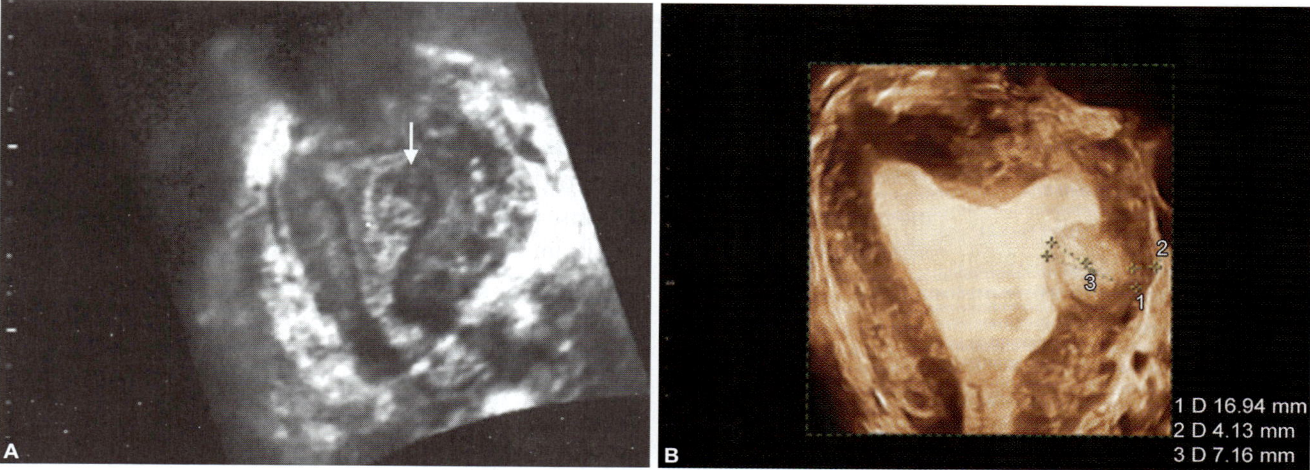

Figs. 1A and B: Ultrasound images of fibroid. (A) Showing lateral wall submucous fibroid (mixed echogenic globular area marked by arrow) distorting endometrial cavity (ESGE class: Type II submucous fibroid); (B) Showing 3D view of that submucous fibroid measuring 16.94 x 4.13 x 7.16 mm.
Source: Dr Jose Manuel Puente, IVI Madrid, Spain.

considered of having inferior reproducibility to magnetic resonance imaging (MRI).[11]

Transabdominal and transvaginal route are used, TVS being the preferred route, as it has better sensitivity to smaller fibroids. Transabdominal scans are difficult to perform in obese patient.

Ultrasound findings (Figs. 1A and B):

- Uterus may be normal sized or bulky and can be displaced from its normal position.
- Fibroids appear well-defined, solid whorled like with echogenicity same as myometrium or hypoechoic to them.
- In patients with infertility, uterine cavity distorting fibroids causing distortion or displacement of the endometrium are important ones. For example, 1.5 cm submucous fibroid is far more important for removal than 5 cm subserous or intramural fibroid away from the cavity.

Saline-infusion sonohysterography (SIS) (Fig. 2): By infusion of saline in the uterine cavity with TVS guidance can be used to delineate submucous fibroid, which has same echogenicity as that of myometrium in hypoechoic fluid. It is difficult to distinguish between submucous fibroid, endometrial polyp and blood clot.

It has limitation of quality and accuracy of the image obtained which depends upon the amount of the saline injected, and tolerance of the patients. So this test has a limited role in diagnosis now a day, where better well-tolerated tests are available.

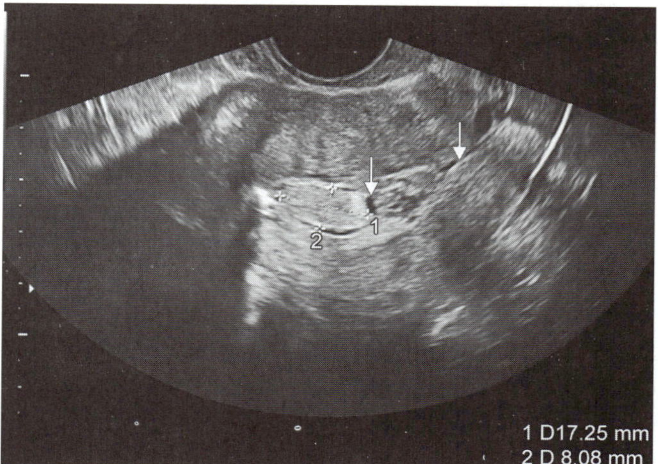

Fig. 2: Saline infusion sonohysterography (SIS). After saline infusion through cervix by small catheter, fluid (hypoechoic area marked by arrow) with endometrial polyp measuring 17.25 × 8.08 mm (echogenicity same as myometrium) seen inside the uterine cavity.
Source: Dr Jose Manuel Puente, IVI Madrid, Spain.

Magnetic resonance imaging (Figs. 3A and B): It is more costly and the most sensitive test available for diagnosis of the fibroid. It can detect the smallest possible fibroid with its sensitivity of 88–93% and specificity of 66–91%.[12,13] It can differentiate adenomyosis from fibroid. Submucosal fibroid, intramural fibroid and subserous fibroid can easily be differentiated with MRI. It can be used to detect fibroids of smaller than 5 mm size and that in unusual location.[14]

Leiomyomas are low signal intensity to the myometrium on T2W images and isointense to the surrounding myometrium on T1W images.[15,16] They produce different signal intensities depending upon their calcification and necrosis. MRI can also diagnose comorbidity due to large fibroid.

MRI along with patient's clinical findings can prevent unnecessary laparoscopy or exploratory laparotomy.[17]

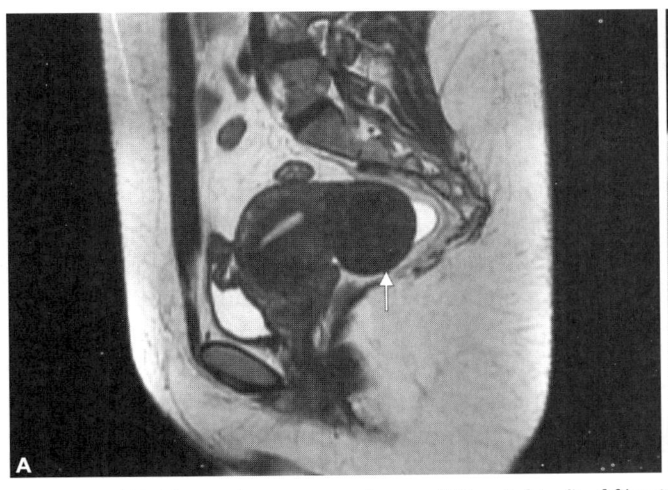

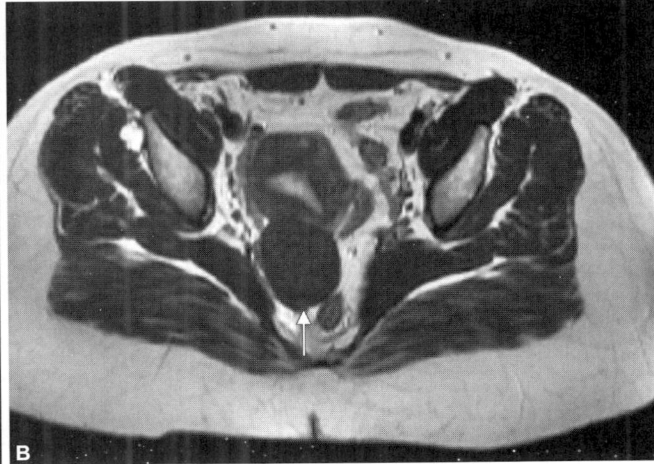

Figs. 3A and B: Magnetic resonance image (T2-weighted) of fibroid. (A) Sagittal view showing subserous fundal fibroid (low intensity globular area marked by arrow) has made uterus retroverted; (B) Axial view of that subserous fibroid (marked by arrow).
Source: Dr Rishi Patel, Infocus Diagnostic Center, Ahmedabad.

However, with high-resolution transvaginal scanners today there is no need to request an MRI to a patient being investigated for infertility, as we will be able to diagnose almost every fibroid the patient may have. 3D ultrasound or color Doppler does not add to the diagnostic accuracy.

Hysteroscopy: It can be used to confirm the diagnosis of submucous fibroids already done by transvaginal scans.

Endometrial polyps: They do not cause infertility by mechanical obstruction unless very large in size or causing proximal tubal blockage. They affect the endometrial receptivity and implantation; thus are mandatory for transcervical hysteroscopic resection in patients of infertility.[18] They can be confirmed by TVS in the proliferative phase and by hysteroscopy.

Asherman's Syndrome

Intrauterine adhesions usually occur due to trauma to the basal layer of the endometrium following mechanical curettage, postpartum hemorrhage, and elective abortion.[19] Cesarean sections, endometrial ablation, septum resection and submucous fibroid removal are less common causes. It can lead to partial or complete uterine cavity obliteration by fibrous bridges between the two uterine walls.[20] It causes amenorrhea or hypomenorrhea, infertility and recurrent pregnancy loss.

It causes infertility mainly by affecting the endometrial growth and its space-occupying characteristic. But it can affect transportation of the gametes when adhesions cause cervical stenosis and proximal or distal tubal block.

Diagnosis can be made by:

- TVS (obliteration of the cavity, very thin nondefined endometrium, hyperechoic bands within the cavity)
- Hysteroscopy
- It can be suspected when there is no endometrial growth with exogenous estradiol therapy.

Treatment is by hysteroscopic resection of the fibrous bands with scissors followed by cyclic estrogen-progesterone.

Endometriosis

It is defined as ectopic endometrial implants, where the functional endometrium grows outside the endometrial cavity. It usually affects the pelvis but can occur outside it. More common sites are ovaries, posterior vaginal wall, anterior and posterior cul-de-sacs, uterosacral ligaments, etc.

It can lead to infertility by causing deep dyspareunia, decreasing the oocyte quality, mechanical obstruction by causing pelvic adhesions by inflammation and thus affecting the normal anatomy of fallopian tubes, tubo-ovarian relationship, uterus and tubal blockage.

Pelvic Adhesions

Pelvic adhesions can be caused by pelvic inflammatory diseases and pelvic tuberculosis, history of any previous pelvic surgeries, radiotherapy, and other pelvic pathologies. It distorts the normal pelvic anatomy, like endometriosis and imparts mechanical obstruction to the normal transport of gametes.

MECHANICAL CAUSES IN MALE INFERTILITY (TABLE 2)

Mechanical causes (sperm transport disorders) are responsible for 10–20% of male factor infertility and mainly divided into:

Table 2: Mechanical factors in male infertility.	
Obstructive azoospermia (OA)[28]	• Congenital bilateral absence of the vas deferens (CBAVD) (relating to CFTR mutations) • Vasectomy • Infections causing obstruction of the vas deferens (e.g. gonorrhea, chlamydia, tuberculosis) • Iatrogenic injury • Ejaculatory duct obstruction • Young syndrome (OA with chronic sinopulmonary infection)
Ejaculatory dysfunction	• Anejaculation – Failure of antegrade ejaculation (spinal cord injury, psychological) – Retrograde ejaculation (diabetes, drugs) • Premature ejaculation
Penile (coital and deposition problem)	• Erectile dysfunction (ED) • Hypospadiasis

- Obstructive azoospermia (OA)
- Ejaculatory disorders
- Coital (erectile dysfunction) and deposition problems.

Obstructive Azoospermia (Obstructions in the Ductal System)

It is known that sperm maturation occurs outside the testes in the epididymis where they are stored. Motility and the ability to fertilize are acquired gradually as the sperm pass into the epididymis. The vas deferens then transports sperm from the epididymis to the urethra, where secretions from the seminal vesicles and prostate dilute them. Abnormalities at any of these sites, particularly the epididymis and vas deferens, can cause infertility. Finally, semen must be ejaculated properly and deposited in vaginal fornix.

Azoospermia is defined as complete absence of sperm from the ejaculate. It is present in less than 1% of all men and in 10–15% of infertile men. Although there are many causes of azoospermia, obstruction of the ductal system is responsible for approximately 40% of cases.[21] IVF/ICSI with the sperms retrieved through epididymis or testicular biopsy is better treatment of choice if we see success rate and time interval to get pregnancy.[22]

Causes

Male infertility can result from congenital or acquired abnormalities of the ductal system (epididymis, vas deferens, ejaculatory ducts, etc.)

- *Congenital bilateral absence of the vas deferens*: Approximately 1–2% of infertile men have CBAVD, which can be detected in routine examination by the andrologist. It is almost always related to mutations in the CFTR gene.[23] The respiratory and pancreatic disease manifestations of cystic fibrosis are not commonly associated with this mutation.
- *Vasectomy*: Voluntary ligation of the vas deferens is a medically induced cause of infertility. It may be reversible, but IVF/ICSI with percutaneous epididymal sperm aspiration (PESA) is recommended.
- *Infections*: Epididymitis is most common sexually transmitted genitourinary infection in men. Previously it was responsible for obstructive azoospermia 8–46% of infection after vasal reconstruction surgery.[24] It is caused by *Gonorrhea, Chlamydia, Trichomonas, Brucellosis, Mycobacterium Tuberculosis, Ureaplasma, Mycoplasma,* coliforms bacteria, adenovirus, and enterovirus. Infection leads to intense inflammation, and secondary scarring of the epididymis. Thus it leading to its obstruction and enlargement. On examination enlarged epididymis is found. Tuber-culosis can lead to enlarged and nodular vas deferens. IVF/ICSI with sperm retrieval biopsy for azoospermic men is recommended after treatment of tuberculosis.[25]
- *Iatrogenic injury*: Trauma is a rare cause of vasal obstruction. It is responsible for obstruction in 8–19% of patients after vasoepididymostomy.[24] Vasal injury is attributed to inguinal, scrotal and pelvic surgeries; like herniorrhaphy, hydrocelectomy, appendicectomy, and renal transplant.
- *Young syndrome*: It is a genetic disease consisting of a triad of bronchiectasis, chronic rhinosinusitis and infertility due to vas deferens obstruction, in which case cystic fibrosis (CF) and primary ciliary dyskinesia are excluded. One assumed etiology is mercury exposure during childhood.[25] There is rising evidence that modern day Young syndrome may be genetic variant of Kartagener's syndrome,[27] or cystic fibrosis transmembrane conductance regulator (CFTR) gene mutation.[26]
- *Ejaculatory duct obstruction*: It is a rare cause of OA, approximately 1% of men presenting with infertility.[28] Occasionally it causes pain during ejaculation. Traditionally transurethral resection of ejaculatory duct (TURED) was the treatment. But now vesiculoscopy with ejaculatory duct dilation is also a treatment option.[29] It is presented with severe oligospermia or azoospermia, palpable vasa and low-volume ejaculate with normal testis volume, particularly when the semen is acidic and contains little or no fructose.

Ejaculatory Disorders

It includes:

- *Anejaculation* is either due to
  - Failure of antegrade ejaculation is consequence of spinal cord disease or trauma, sympathectomy, autonomic disease (e.g. diabetes mellitus), psychological anejaculation or
  - Retrograde ejaculation backwards in to urinary bladder is due to sphincter damage during prostate surgery, diabetes or drug induced (e.g. tamsulosin, fluoxetine).
- *Premature ejaculation* becomes a fertility problem when ejaculation occurs before full penetration. It is a great cause of stress for the couple but can be adequately treated with psychological counseling.

Coital and Deposition Problems

Problem with proper erection and improper deposition of semen also contribute in male infertility.

- *Erectile dysfunction*: It is the inability to achieve or maintain an erection that is sufficiently rigid for achieving satisfying sexual intercourse.[30] Its causes include:
  - *Surgery/trauma*: Mainly seen after radical rectal surgery, and retroperitoneal surgeries
  - Diabetes (mainly due to Type I)
  - Congenital spinal abnormalities
  - Multiple sclerosis
  - *Spinal cord injury*: Lumbar region
  - *Drug induced*: Cimetidine, spironolactone, antidepressants, etc.
  - *Endocrine disorders*: Testosterone deficiency
- *Hypospadias*: It is very common congenital anomaly, in which external urethral meatus opens on the ventral surface of the penis. It causes ventral curvature of the erect penis which is called as chordee, and it is responsible for defective penis size and so improper sexual satisfaction and ejaculatory disorders.[31] Otherwise it does not cause infertility.

Evaluation of Mechanical Issues in Male Infertility

The components of the evaluation of the man include:

- History
- Semen analysis
- Physical examination
- Endocrine evaluation
- Ultrasound
- Testicular biopsy
- Genetic tests.

History

A thorough history of the infertile couple at the time of the initial consultation will frequently reveal conditions that could affect semen quality. Some of the important factors to consider are as follows:

- Reproductive history, including previous pregnancies with this and other partners.
- Sexual history, including libido, timing and frequency of intercourse, and previous fertility assessments of the man and his partner as well as the duration of their infertility.
- *Past medical and surgical history*: Regarding any childhood illness, diabetes, sexually transmitted diseases, prostatitis, or epididymitis, as well as scrotal trauma or surgery—including varicocele repair, vasectomy, inguinal herniorrhaphy, and vasovasostomy.
- Exposure to medication, drugs, toxins and adverse environmental conditions such as temperature extremes in occupational and leisure activities, either in the past or in the present.

Semen Analysis

The hallmark of the evaluation of the male remains the semen analysis. Semen parameters in particular man is dependent on days of abstinence, container, collection, interval between collection and analysis, recent history of any acute medical disease.

In 2010, the WHO published revised lower reference limits for semen analyses, which represent the fifth centile in a population of over 1,900 men from eight countries on three continents whose partners conceived within 12 months[32] (Table 3).

Table 3: Semen analysis reference values in fertile men.*

Semen parameters	*Reference value (95%; CI)*
Volume	1.5 (1.4–1.7) mL
Sperm concentration	15 (12–16) million/mL
Total sperm number	39 (33–46) million/ejaculate
Total motility	40 (38–42)%
Progressive motility	32 (31–34)%
Normal morphology	4 (3–4)%
Vitality	58 (55–63)%

*World Health Organization. WHO Laboratory Manual for the Examination of Human Semen. 5th edition. Geneva, Switzerland: WHO Press, 2010. pp. 223-5.

Mechanical issue in male infertility particularly obstruction in sperm transport presents with azoospermia in semen analysis but this has to be differentiated from the azoospermia due to primary testicular failure due to defective spermatogenesis (more common cause of azoospermia). Azoospermia defined as the absence of sperm on standard microscopic examination. The semen specimen should be centrifuged at high speed (3,000X *g* for 15 minutes) and the pellet is examined with high magnification (400X); the absence of sperm should be documented on at least two separate occasions to establish the diagnosis.[33]

Oligospermia is defined by a sperm concentration of less than 15 million/mL and is considered severe when it is below 5 million/mL. Endocrine and genetic evaluation is indicated for men with severe oligospermia or azoospermia (discussed below).

Poor sperm motility (< 32% motility, asthenospermia) suggests testicular or epididymal dysfunction.

Postejaculatory Urine Analysis

It should be considered when the ejaculate volume is less than 1 mL with no or low semen volume and azoospermia, and observed for presence of any sperm suggesting retrograde ejaculation.

Physical Examination

Examination should be performed by an andrologist in case of grossly abnormal semen parameters:

- Examination of the penis and localization of the urethral meatus.
- Palpation of the testes and measurement of their size. Small testes suggest testicular failure.
- The presence and consistency of both the vasa and epididymis. Epididymal fullness suggests ductal obstruction or epididymitis. Bilateral absence of palpation of vas in CBAVD, but it requires confirmation by testicular sonography.
- Presence of any varicocele.
- Secondary sexual characteristics, including body habitus, hair distribution, and breast development.
- Digital rectal examination to diagnose prostate, seminal vesicles and ejaculatory duct abnormalities. Presence of dilated seminal vesicles suggest ejaculatory duct obstruction.

Endocrine Evaluation

Indications:

- Abnormal semen analysis (particularly a sperm concentration less than 10 million/mL).
- Sexual dysfunction (decreased libido, impotence), and other clinical symptoms or findings that suggest a specific endocrinopathy.[34]

A basic endocrine evaluation of the infertile male involves (Table 4).

Ultrasound

- Transscrotal ultrasonography helps to clarify uncertain physical findings or to confirm the presence of mass.
- Transrectal ultrasonography is indicated to confirm diagnosis of ejaculatory duct obstruction.[35]

Testicular Biopsy

It is diagnostic and therapeutic in azoospermic men. Very low probability of sperm retrieval is there in patients with high FSH (> 10 IU/mL) suggesting secretory (nonobstructive) azoospermia; however, FSH below 10 IU/mL are indicative of obstruction and sperm can be found in most of these biopsies.

Table 4: Basal hormonal levels in various clinical states.

Clinical condition	*Follicle-stimulating hormone*	*Luteinizing hormone*	*Testosterone*	*Prolactin*
Normal spermatogenesis	Normal	Normal	Normal	Normal
Hypogonadotrophic hypogonadism	Low	Low	Low	Normal
Abnormal spermatogenesis*	High/Normal	Normal	Normal	Normal
Complete testicular failure/ Hypergonadotrophic hypogonadism	High	High	Normal/ Low	Normal
Prolactin (PRL) secreting pituitary tumor	Normal/Low	Normal/Low	Low	High

*Many men with abnormal spermatogenesis have normal serum FSH, but a marked elevation of serum FSH is clearly indicative of an abnormality in spermatogenesis.

Source: Modified from Practice Committee. Evaluation of the infertile male. Fertil Steril. 2015.

Genetic Evaluation

Genetic abnormality can affect infertility by affecting sperm production or transport. When indicated, efforts to identify genetic problems have impact on the choice and outcome of treatment. It can be evaluated by:

- *CFTR gene mutation*: At least two-thirds of men with CBAVD have a demonstrable CFTR gene mutation and almost all men with cystic fibrosis have CBAVD.[36,37] Prevalence is high in some part of the world (Mediterranean population).
- *Karyotyping*: Karyotyping should be offered to men with nonobstructive azoospermia or severe oligospermia (less than 5 million/mL) before their sperm are used for IVF with ICSI.[34] It is recommended always if sperm concentration is less than 1 million/mL. The overall prevalence of chromosomal anomalies in infertile men is approximately 7% and inversely related to sperm concentration; the prevalence is highest in azoospermic men (10–15%), lower in oligospermic men (approximately 5 %) and very low in men with normal semen quality (less than 1%).[38,39] By far, the most common chromosomal anomaly in infertile men is Klinefelter syndrome (47, XXY or mosaic 46, XY/47, XXY), which accounts for about two-thirds of chromosomal abnormalities in infertile men.[40]
- *Y-chromosome microdeletion*: Approximately 7% of infertile men harbor a Y-chromosome microdeletion that cannot be detected with a standard karyotype or cytogenetics, but can be identified using more sophisticated molecular biological techniques like polymerase chain reaction.[41] The incidence increases to 16% in azoospermic and severely oligospermic men.[41] There are three locations of deletion (AZF) along with the long arm of Y-chromosome (Yq11) which affect spermatogenesis accordingly: AZFa (proximal), AZFb (central), and AZFc (distal). If the AZFc region is deleted there is sufficient sperm production, and the sperm would appear in ejaculate (in reduced number) in oligospermic men, and sperm can be retrieved with testicular biopsy in azoospermic men.[42] But men with deletion in AZFa or AZFb region have a very poor prognosis for sperm retrieval even with extensive testicular biopsy.[43,44] Sons of the men with Y-chromosome microdeletion will inherit the microdeletion and may consequently become infertile.[45] Treatment with ICSI may lead to vertical transmission, expansion, and *de novo* Y-chromosome microdeletion in male fetuses.[46] Thus, screening for Y-chromosome microdeletion should be offered to all men with nonobstructive azoospermia or severe oligospermia (less than 5 million/mL) who are candidates for IVF with ICSI.[34]

CONCLUSION

Most of the mechanical issues, which are affecting fertility, cause infertility by preventing gamete interaction. Diagnosing mechanical obstruction in the gamete pathway is necessary to select better treatment plan, either by removing those obstruction and waiting for natural conception or enhancing it with IUI, or bypassing treatment for the obstruction and accepting IVF/ICSI, which is more effective and most advanced method of artificial reproductive techniques (ART).

REFERENCES

1. Practice Committee of the American Society for Reproductive Medicine. Definitions of infertility and recurrent pregnancy loss: a committee opinion. Fertil Steril. 2013;99:63.
2. WHO Technical Report Series. Recent Advances in Medically Assisted Conception Number 820, 1992. pp. 1-111.
3. Baldauf JJ, Dreyfus M, Ritter J, Meyer P. Risk of cervical stenosis after large loop excision or laser conization. Philippe Obstet Gynecol. 1996;88(6):933-8.
4. Buttram VC, Reiter RC. Uterine leiomyomata: etiology, symptomatology and management. Fertil Steril. 1981;36:433-45.
5. Wamsteker K, Emanuel MH, de Kruif JH. Transcervical hysteroscopic resection of submucous fibroids for abnormal uterine bleeding: results regarding the degree of intramural extension. Obstet Gynecol. 1993;82:736-40.
6. Pritts EA, Parker WH, Olive DL. Fibroids and infertility: an updated systemic review of the evidence. Fertil Steril. 2009;91:1215-23.
7. Klatsky PC, Tran ND, Caughey AB, Fujimoto VY. Fibroids and reproductive outcomes: a systematic literature review from conception to delivery. Am J Obstet Gynecol. 2008;198:357-66.
8. Casini ML, Rossi F, Agostini R, Unfer V. Effects of the position of fibroids on fertility. Gynecol Endocrinol. 2006;22(2):106-9.
9. Horcajadas JA, Goyri E, Higón MA, Martínez-Conejero JA, Gambadauro P, García G, et al. Endometrial receptivity and implantation are not affected by the presence of uterine intramural leiomyomas: a clinical and functional genomics analysis. J Clin Endocrinol Metab. 2008;93:3490-8.
10. Rackow BW, Taylor HS. Submucosal uterine leiomyomas have a global effect on molecular determinants of endometrial receptivity. Fertil Steril. 2010;93:2027-34.
11. Levens ED, Wesley R, Premkumar A, Blocker W, Nieman LK. Magnetic resonance imaging and transvaginal ultrasound for determining fibroid burden: implications for research and clinical care. Am J Obstet Genecol. 2009;200(5):537.e1-7.
12. Byun JY, Kim SE, Choi BG, et al. Diffuse and focal adenomyosis: MR imaging findings. Radiographics. 1999;19(Spec No):S161-70.
13. Ascher SM, Arnold LL, Patt RH, Schruefer JJ, Bagley AS, Semelka RC, et al. Adenomyosis: Prospective comparison of MR imaging and transvaginal sonography. Radiology. 1994;190:803-6.

14. Wilde S, Scott-Barrett S. Radiological appearances of uterine fibroids. Indian J Radiol Imaging. 2009;19(3):222-31.
15. Brosens JJ, de Souza NM, Barker FG. Uterine junctional zone: function and disease. Lancet. 1995;346:558-60.
16. Ueda H, Togashi K, Konishi I, Kataoka ML, Koyama T, Fujiwara T, et al. Unusual appearances of uterine leiomyomas: MR imaging findings and their histopathologic backgrounds. Radiographics. 1999;19(Suppl 1):s131-45.
17. Livermore JA, Adusumilli S. MRI of benign uterine conditions. Appl Radiol. 2007;36(9):8-18.
18. Rackow BW, Jorgensen E, Taylor HS. Endometrial polyps affect uterine receptivity. Fertil Steril. 2011;95:2690-2.
19. Robinson JK, Swedarsky Colimon LM, Isaacson KB. Postoperative adhesiolysis theapy for intrauterine adhesions (Asherman's syndrome). Fertil Steril. 2008;90(2):409-14.
20. March CM. Management of Asherman's syndrome. Reproductive BioMedicine Online. 2011;23(1):63-76.
21. Jarow JP, Espeland MA, Lipshultz LI. Evaluation of the azoospermic patient. J Urol. 1989;142:162-5.
22. Belker AM, Thomas AJ, Fuchs EF, Konnak JW, Sharlip ID. Results of 1,469 microsurgical vasectomy reversals by the vasovasostomy study group. J Urol. 1991;145:505-11.
23. Patrizio P, Asch RH, Handelin B, Silber SJ. Aetiology of congenital absence of vas deferens: genetic study of three generations. Hum Reprod. 1993;8:215-20.
24. Chan PT, Brandell RA, Goldstein M. Prospective analysis of outcomes after microsurgical intussusception vasoepididymostomy. BJU Int. 2005;96(4): 598-601.
25. Paick J, Kim SH, Kim SW. Ejaculatory duct obstruction in infertile men. BJU Int. 2000;85(6):720-4.
26. Goeminne PC, Dupont LJ. The sinusitis-infertility syndrome: Young's saint, old devil. Eur Respir J. 2010;35(3):698.
27. Ichioka K, Kohei N, Okubo K, Nishiyama H, Terai A. Obstructive azoospermia associated with chronic sinopulmonary infection and situs inversus totalis. Urology. 2006;68:204.e5-7.
28. Baker K, Sabanegh E. Obstructive azoospermia: reconstructive techniques and results. Clinics (Sao Paulo). 2013;68(Suppl 1):61-73.
29. Wang H, Ye H, Xu C, Liu Z, Gao X, Hou J, et al. Transurethral seminal vesiculoscopy using a 6F vesiculoscope for ejaculatory duct obstruction. J Androl. 2012;33(4):637-43.
30. NIH Consensus Conference Impotence. NIH consensus development panel on impotence. JAMA. 1993;270:83-90.
31. Mieusset R, Soulié M. Hypospadias: psychosocial, sexual and reproductive consequences in adult life. J Androl. 2005;26:163-8.
32. Cooper TG, Noonan E, von Eckardstein S, Auger J, Baker HW, Behre HM, et al. World Health Organization reference values for human semen characteristics, Hum Reprod Update. 2010;16:231-45.
33. World Health Organization, Laboratory Manual for the Examination of Human Semen and Sperm-Cervical Mucus Interaction. 4th edition. Cambridge University. 1999.
34. Sharlip ID, Jarow JP, Belker AM, Lipshultz LI, Sigman M, Thomas AJ, et al. Best practice policies for male infertility. Fertil Steril. 2002;77:873-82.
35. Carter SS, Shinohara K, Lipshultz LI. Transrectal ultrasonography in disorders of the seminal vesicles and ejaculatory ducts. Urol Clin North Am. 1989;16: 773-90.
36. Anguiano A, Oates RD, Amos JA, Dean M, Gerrard B, Stewart C, et al. Congenital bilateral absence of the vas deferens. A primarily genital form of cystic fibrosis. JAMA. 1992;267:1794-7.
37. Oates RD, Amos JA. The genetic basis of congenital bilateral absence of the vas deferens and cystic fibrosis. J Androl. 1994;15:1-8.
38. Foresta C, Garolla A, Bartoloni L, Bettella A, Ferlin A. Genetic abnormalities among severely oligospermic men who are candidates for intracytoplasmic sperm injection. J Clin Endocrinol Metab. 2005;90:152-6.
39. Ravel C, Berthaut I, Bresson JL, Siffroi JP. Prevalence of chromosomal abnormalities in phenotypically normal and fertile adult males: large-scale survey of over 10,000 sperm donor karyotypes. Hum Reprod. 2006;21:1484-9.
40. De Braekeleer M, Dao TN. Cytogenetic studies in male infertility: a review. Hum Reprod. 1991;6:245-50.
41. Pryor JL, Kent-First M, Muallem A, Van Bergen AH, Nolten WE, Meisner L, et al. Microdeletions in the Y chromosome of infertile men. New Engl J Med. 1997;336:534-9.
42. Oates RD, Silber S, Brown LG, Page DC. Clinical characterization of 42 oligospermic or azoospermic men with microdeletion of the AZFc region of the Y chromosome, and of 18 children conceived via ICSI. Hum Reprod. 2002; 17:2813-24.
43. Brandell RA, Mielnik A, Liotta D, Ye Z, Veeck LL, Palermo GD, et al. AZFb deletions predict the absence of spermatozoa with testicular sperm extraction: preliminary report of a prognostic genetic test. Hum Reprod. 1998;13:2812-5.
44. Krausz C, Quintana-Murci L, McElreavey K. Prognostic value of Y deletion analysis. What is the clinical prognostic value of Y chromosome microdeletion analysis? Hum Reprod. 2000;15:1431-4.
45. Kent-First MG, Kol S, Muallem A, et al. The incidence and possible relevance of Y-linked microdeletions in babies born after intracytoplasmic sperm injection and their infertile fathers. Mol Hum Reprod. 1996;2:943-50.
46. Lee SH, Ahn SY, Lee KW, Kwack K, Jun HS, Cha KY. Intracytoplasmic sperm injection may lead to vertical transmission, expansion, and de novo occurrence of Y-chromosome microdeletions in male fetuses. Fertil Steril. 2006;85:1512-5.

CHAPTER

7

How to Assess the Receptivity of the Human Endometrium

Jose Miravet-Valenciano, Carlos Marin, Maria Ruiz-Alonso, Carlos Simon

ENDOMETRIAL FACTOR AND ITS IMPORTANCE IN ASSISTED REPRODUCTIVE TECHNIQUES

A 2012 World Health Organization (WHO) study[1] indicates that female infertility affects an estimated 48 million women worldwide, with the highest prevalence in South Asia, Sub-Saharan & North Africa, Middle East, Central Eastern Europe and Central Asia. The study, based on women from 190 countries, shows that the overall burden of infertility has remained similar in estimated levels and trends from 1990 to 2010. Infertility is caused by many different factors, both male and female in origin. Describing the endometrial factor and how to assess it is the main objective in this chapter.

The human endometrium is a dynamic organ that undergoes cyclic physiological and morphological changes in response to ovarian steroid hormones (estrogen and progesterone), cytokines, prostaglandins (PGs), growth factors, chemokines, and other factors.[2,3] These factors induce the principal biological processes according to endometrial gene expression (Fig. 1).

An embryo seeks to attach and invade the endometrium to gain access to essential nutrients for growth and development. During this complex process, the semiallogenic embryo needs to be accepted by the endometrium. Successful implantation depends on appropriate embryo development to a viable blastocyst stage, the proper preparation of the endometrium to become receptive to the embryo, and an efficient cross-talk between them mediated by a set of complex molecules that will be discussed later.

For most of the menstrual cycle, the endometrium is not adhesive for embryo implantation, and it only becomes receptive for a short, self-limited period of time. During this brief time, the attachment of the blastocyst to the endometrial epithelium, and later invasion of the decidualized stroma, can occur. This process is the result of the interaction between paracrine signals and ovarian hormones, growth factors, lipid mediators, cytokines, integrins, PGs, and transcription factors.[4] The concept of receptivity was suggested in the 1950s and was later strengthened by Wilcox, who showed that implantation occurred between 8 days and 10 days after ovulation.[5] This state of receptivity occurs in the mid-secretory phase and is known as the window of implantation (WOI), a term coined by Harper in 1992.[6] By default, the WOI opens for 2 days after 5 days of exposure to exogenous or endogenous progesterone.[7] A successful dialog between the embryo and the endometrium during the WOI will allow the apposition of the embryo, its adhesion, and invasion of the decidualized stroma.[8] The most studied factor in human implantation has been the embryo itself; however, the endometrial factor has also been extensively studied since the 50s, when the first "gold standard" for evaluating the endometrial status—the histological criteria of Noyes—was published.[9]

Despite the interest in understanding the regulation of endometrial receptivity, the role of the endometrium in implantation remains a challenge. Using the single-molecule approach, many putative biochemical markers to be discussed later have been proposed as predictors of endometrial receptivity, but none of them have achieved the status of a diagnostic or predictive clinical tool.[10] Currently, the implementation of "omic" technologies such as transcriptomics and proteomics has enabled new

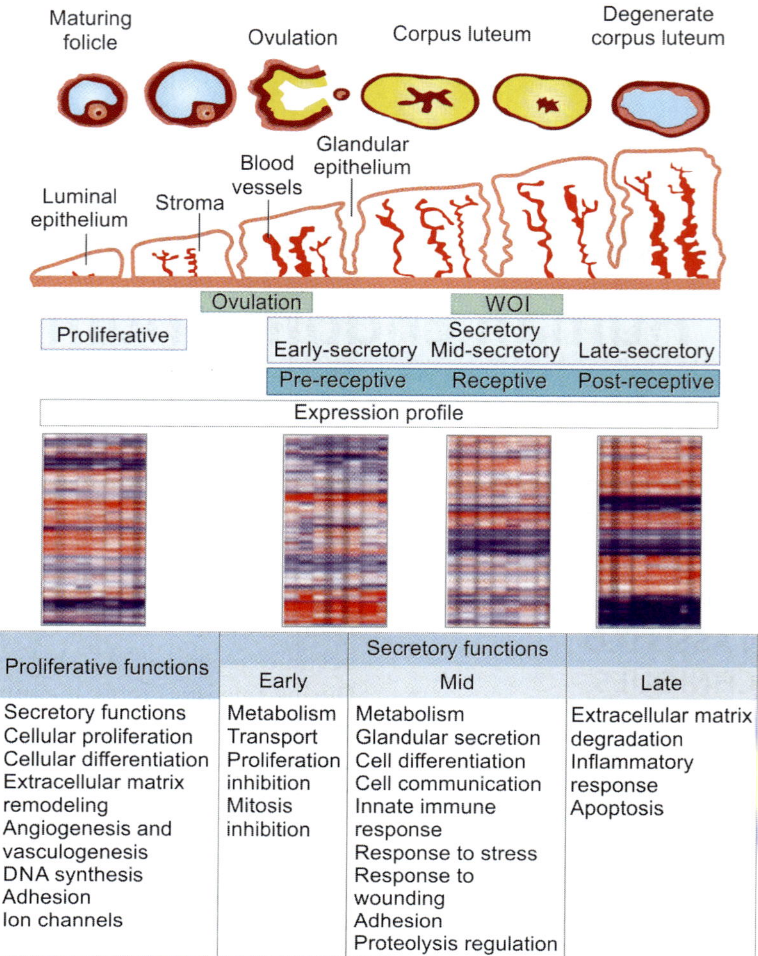

Proliferative functions	Secretory functions		
	Early	Mid	Late
Secretory functions Cellular proliferation Cellular differentiation Extracellular matrix remodeling Angiogenesis and vasculogenesis DNA synthesis Adhesion Ion channels	Metabolism Transport Proliferation inhibition Mitosis inhibition	Metabolism Glandular secretion Cell differentiation Cell communication Innate immune response Response to stress Response to wounding Adhesion Proteolysis regulation	Extracellular matrix degradation Inflammatory response Apoptosis

Fig. 1: Evolution of the endometrium along the menstrual cycle related to the gene expression and biological processes implied in each endometrial stage. (WOI: window of implantation)

approaches to improve our knowledge about the process of receptivity and implantation. Such studies have produced a large amount of information that, when combined with bioinformatics techniques, will lead to a better understanding of endometrial physiology and the clinical translation of biomarkers for receptivity. Recent studies have also found promising results analyzing the relation between an altered uterine microbiome and impaired reproductive clinical outcome.

DIAGNOSIS OF ENDOMETRIAL RECEPTIVITY

Despite the transfer of good-quality embryos (identified by standard embryological techniques) in assisted reproductive techniques (ART), most of them fail to implant. This phenomenon makes the assessment of endometrial receptivity an essential component of ART. The scientific and medical community is aware of the importance of deepening the understanding of endometrial receptivity to increase pregnancy rates and to achieve successful outcomes for in vitro fertilization (IVF) treatments.

In this part of the chapter we will describe the current diagnostic techniques used to assess the endometrium. The review begins with Noyes criteria and will be followed by a view of ultrasound techniques and luteinizing hormone (LH) surge as a reference. After that, we will take a look into morphological and biochemical markers, concluding with the latest discoveries in molecular biomarkers.

Histological Criteria and Their Use in Reproductive Medicine

In the late 1930s, the idea of endometrial receptivity came into its own with the work of Rock and Bartlett.[11] They later formalized a method of endometrial dating, published in 1950 in the inaugural issue of *Fertility and Sterility* with Noyes as the first author.[9] In this article, the group described a novel method for endometrial dating based on histological characteristics and morphological changes of the endometrium caused by the temporal responses to estrogens and progesterone, known as the Noyes histological criteria.

Noyes and colleagues examined the histological features of endometrial biopsies obtained during 8,000 natural cycles in 300 sterile women.[9,12] Correlating basal body temperature with histological changes, they were able to relate different histological patterns with specific days of the luteal phase. These criteria consider eight basic histological characteristics of the endometrium: degree of glandular mitosis, pseudostratification of nuclei, basal vacuolation, secretion, stromal edema, pseudodecidual reaction, stromal mitosis, and leukocytic infiltration.

The classic work of Noyes marked a milestone for endometrial dating. This methodology was considered the "gold standard" for over 50 years. However, the accuracy and functional relevance of Noyes criteria depend on multiple factors, including the method of determining the day of ovulation when the biopsy needs to be performed, the state of the biopsy, fixation techniques, interobserver variability, and intercycle variations. These criteria have been questioned in retrospective,[13,14] prospective,[15,16] and randomized[17,18] clinical trials. The limitations of these criteria include:

- The dating should be performed only on a functional endometrium, without injury and devoid of all elements of the basal layer and the lower uterine segment.
- Polyps, endometritis, or hormone therapy make it impossible to correctly apply the classic criteria of Noyes.
- Ovarian stimulation, commonly used in ART, produces changes in endometrial maturation compared to natural cycles, so it is not possible to date an endometrium in a controlled stimulated cycle using the histological methodology.[19]
- These criteria fail to discriminate between fertile and infertile women.[18]
- The histological normality of the endometrium does not necessarily imply a functional normality.
- *Subjectivity*: There is an interobserver, intraobserver, and intercycle variability that alters the consistency of the results obtained.[17]

These limitations, together with the incorporation of molecular techniques and the need to answer specific questions about the WOI posed by ART programs, suggest that the traditional criteria are not precise and indicate the need for new and updated methods to functionally assess the endometrium. In fact, Noyes' purpose was not to date the endometrium but describe the morphological changes occurring under the influence of ovarian hormones.

Diagnosis of the Menstrual Cycle

Menstrual cycle parameters have been used throughout history as reference points for predicting ovulation and therefore achieving pregnancy. These parameters include:

- Basal body temperature shift
- Start of menstrual flow
- Determination of cervical mucus levels and its characterization
- Changes in saliva composition
- Ultrasonographic features (ovulation and endometrial thickness); and
- Luteinizing hormone surge.

Since recent studies have contributed to our knowledge of female fertility, most of the parameters mentioned are today obsolete for use in IVF techniques.[13,20,21] Thus, we will focus on ultrasound and LH surge.

Ultrasound

Ultrasound has emerged as a critical tool in ART, not only for follicular monitoring, but also for evaluation of the endometrium. Furthermore, it is a noninvasive method and relatively inexpensive.

Various sonographic markers have been proposed to evaluate endometrial receptivity, such as endometrial thickness and pattern. With the advent of Doppler ultrasound, studying endometrial blood flow has emerged as an important means of evaluating endometrial receptivity. Markers related to endometrial perfusion have been studied at different levels of the uterine vascular tree such as uterine arteries, radial and spiral arteries, endometrial and subendometrial mapping with Doppler color and power Doppler, and more recently, the study of the endometrial vascularization as a whole by three-dimensional power Doppler ultrasound.[22]

A triple-layered pattern and an endometrial thickness greater than 7 mm have been proposed as markers for endometrial receptivity. Although some authors have found a relationship between endometrial thickness and pregnancy rate in patients undergoing IVF,[23-26] others have found no such association.[27-29] Moreover, Soares et al. in a large study analyzing 3,089 cycles, found no statistical difference between endometrial thickness and pregnancy rate.[30]

A good blood supply to the endometrium is generally considered necessary for implantation, but due to the suggestion that the increase in vascularization within the endometrium coincides with the opening of the WOI, it has been studied in rare cases. Furthermore, ovarian or abdominal abnormalities could interfere with adequate ultrasound investigation.[31] Although all of these metrics, including thickness and volume of the endometrium, have been debated for use as prognostic parameters in ART gestation,[32,33] we consider an acceptable endometrium as between 6 mm and 12 mm, being considered 5 mm or less as atrophic and 12 mm or more as hyperplastic.

Luteinizing Hormone Surge

Around the 13th day of the menstrual cycle, the LH surge occurs; 36 hours later ovulation follows. The day of LH surge is termed day LH+0, and the receptive endometrium, corresponding to the WOI, is between LH + 6 and LH + 8 (days 19–21 of the menstrual cycle).

Ovulation detection is fundamental in the diagnostic work-up of infertile women, for optimal artificial insemination timing, and for successful embryo transfers (ET), and can be measured in urine and in blood serum. The effectiveness of measurement of urinary LH levels for the purpose of monitoring ovarian activity and detecting ovulation is well-documented.[34,35] However, Kawano et al.[36] suggested that urine LH determination is good for predicting ovulation in spontaneous cycles, but it is also necessary to monitor follicle sizes by ultrasonography for ovulation in induced cycles. The most accurate method to predict ovulation is measuring the LH surge in blood serum. However, repeated measurement of circulating LH is invasive and expensive compared to methods used to detect the LH surge in urine; urine measurements, though, have a higher incidence of false-negative results.

Importantly, the LH surge does not occur in the same way in all women.[37] In fact, although the LH surge is classically described as a single peak, it may also be a double peak or even a plateau; furthermore, the duration of the surge may vary from 3 days to 11 days. Direito et al.[38] described the relationship between the characteristics of the LH surge and other characteristics of the menstrual cycle, affirming that multiple-peak LH surges are associated with smaller preovulatory follicles (follicular insufficiency), and prolonged LH surges for more than 3 days after ovulation are associated with delayed luteinization (luteal insufficiency). These conclusions, together with the fact that the menstrual cycle in the same woman can vary from one cycle to another, confirm the existence of multitude of variables that can affect the endometrial evaluation by this method.

Morphological Markers: Pinopodes

Martel et al.[39] and Nikas et al.[40] using scanning electron microscopy (SEM) on the uterine luminal epithelium, demonstrated the presence of specialized cell-surface formations called pinopodes. Pinopodes seem to be induced by endocytosis of endometrial fluid[41] and appear to act in modulating the volume of the uterine cavity that becomes virtual at the time of embryonic adhesion.

During natural cycles, pinopodes appear on days 19, 20, and 21 of a 28-day cycle. In contrast, in stimulated cycles, the endometrium shows advancement in the development of pinopodes compared with the spontaneous cycle, and they can be observed on days 16, 17, and 18.[42]

These structures were initially proposed as morphological markers of endometrial receptivity because they coincide with WOI. However, their utility in assessing endometrial receptivity has some drawbacks:

- SEM is needed to detect pinopodes, making it an invasive and expensive method.
- Pinopodes persist in the post-receptive endometrium, therefore their presence is not specific to the receptivity phase.[43]

Biochemical Markers

Although a fair number of biomarkers have been described in the literature, in this part of the chapter we will focus on proteins and lipids.

Proteins

Proteomic approaches, which identify differential levels of detectable proteins, closely reflect cellular functions. Thus, these are considered the next step in the study of biological systems,[44] despite the relative lack of sensitivity of such technology, which has slowed its incorporation into the field of reproductive research. However, new developments in mass spectrometry have increased the number of studies related to the profile of proteins expressed in both the endometrial tissue and endometrial fluid and have been very useful to improve the knowledge about the underlying biological processes.

In the 1990s, the Lessey group published several papers related to the role of integrins in uterine receptivity. In 1994, they discovered an association between the lack of the beta-3 integrin subunit and the diagnosis of endometriosis.[45] One year later they reported that alpha-1, alpha-4, and beta-3 integrin subunits are abnormally expressed in women with unexplained infertility, using immunohistochemical staining in endometrial biopsies obtained during days

20–24 of the menstrual cycle.[46] These discoveries led them to develop a clinical test to assess endometrial receptivity based on the evaluation of the beta-3 integrin subunit in an endometrial biopsy and complementary endometrial dating by the classical histological criteria, known as the E-tegrity test. Three different patterns could be diagnosed with this test: a normal pattern (beta-3 integrin positive with an "in-phase" endometrium from cycle days LH + 7 to LH + 11), patients with luteal phase defect (beta-3 integrin negative with an "out-of-phase" endometrium), and patients with unexplained infertility, minimal or mild endometriosis, or hydrosalpinx (beta-3 integrin negative in a patient with a normal "in phase" endometrium). But attention is required to address the proper use of biomarkers to assess endometrial receptivity, especially when studying endometriosis; not all women with endometriosis are infertile and not all lack expression of individual biomarkers, and, further, not all endometriosis cases are verifiable by the pathologist.[47] In addition to this, some studies have found that integrins are not useful biomarkers,[16,48-50] and we have already discussed the drawbacks concerning the histologic criteria.

An initial attempt to identify differential protein markers between the proliferative and secretory endometrium was published in 2005 by the DeSouza group.[51] The authors described a quantitative proteomics approach using the isotopic method repertoire of isotope-coded affinity tags (ICAT), affinity purification, and liquid chromatography coupled with mass spectrometry (LC-MS) to compare proliferative and secretory endometrium. Five proteins with significant differential expression were found, being of particular interest the frequently rearranged in advanced T-cell lymphomas 1 protein (FRAT1) and the subunit zeta-1 precursor of the N-methyl-D-aspartate (NMDA) glutamate receptor. However, the utility of these proteins for endometrial assessment remains unknown.

In a study published in 2009[52] proteins with differential expression throughout the menstrual cycle and in uterine fluid were identified. The analysis revealed upregulation of calreticulin, isozyme 5 of adenylate kinase, and transferrin in the proliferative endometrium; and annexin A5, alpha 1 antitrypsin, creatine kinase, and peroxiredoxin 6 in the mid-secretory phase. The bidimensional map of middle secretory phase endometrium and endometrial fluid was also compared. This analysis showed the presence of thermal stress protein 27, transferrin, and alpha-1 antitrypsin precursor both in the endometrium and endometrial fluid.

Our group studied endometrial receptivity by comparing the human proteome in a prereceptive (LH + 2) versus a receptive (LH + 7) endometrium.[53] For this purpose, endometrial biopsies were obtained from a group of fertile women ($n = 6$) in the same menstrual cycle. 35 differentially expressed proteins were detected in receptive endometrium compared to the prereceptive one, with 12 proteins upregulated and 23 downregulated. Notably, two proteins showed consistently differential expression: annexin A2 and stathmin 1. These proteins, associated with the cytoskeleton, show a consistently opposite adjustment in the prereceptive endometrium compared to the receptive. This is not surprising since the phenotype of the receptive endometrium is associated with the remodeling of the epithelial phenotype, primarily as a result of the disruption of the cytoskeleton in response to an external stimulus.[54] These proteins were functionally analyzed on a refractory endometrium model induced by the insertion of an intrauterine device. The analysis indicated that the labeling pattern for these proteins was similar to that present in the prereceptive endometrium, suggesting that annexin A2 and stathmin 1 are functionally involved in endometrial receptivity. Therefore, both molecules may be important in predicting the state of receptivity and could serve as targets for interception.[53]

Two recent studies analyzed protein expression patterns in prereceptive and receptive endometrial tissues. In the first publication,[55] a total of 31 proteins with differential expression (17 upregulated and 14 downregulated) between LH + 2 and LH + 7 endometrium were identified. In the second publication,[56] 57 differentially expressed proteins were identified. Among these structural proteins were molecular chaperones, signaling proteins, metabolic proteins, immune-related proteins, and ribonucleic acid (RNA) and protein biosynthesis molecules.

Garrido-Gómez et al.[57] performed proteomics of endometrial receptivity using the endometrial receptivity array (ERA) test (discussed later in this chapter). Receptive and nonreceptive endometrial samples were compared, revealing 24 proteins that were differentially expressed between phases. These included progesterone receptor membrane component 1 (PGRMC1), a nonclassical progesterone receptor, which was detected at a significantly lower level during the receptive phase; this finding was validated by Western blot and immunohistochemistry.

Proteomic techniques have also been applied to analyze the endometrial fluid in studies of endometrial receptivity. This viscous liquid, a complex biological fluid secreted by the glands, provides nutrients that enable the survival of the blastocyst and constitutes the microenvironment where the endometrial-blastocyst dialog occurs before implantation.[58] The advantage of working with endometrial fluid is that it can easily be aspirated, so it is considered a minimally invasive and painless procedure.[59] Furthermore, uterine secretions are less complex than endometrial tissues at the protein level, and can serve as a biomarker pool for endometrial function research.

The composition of the endometrial secretion varies during the menstrual cycle as a result of changes in concentrations of ovarian steroids.[60] Two studies[60,61] revealed three different protein patterns that are equivalent to the respective phases of the menstrual cycle: intermediate, proliferative, and secretory phases. These results show "families" of protein bands corresponding to 63 proteins, some of which were identified by their molecular weight.[62]

The endometrial fluid can be obtained by transcervical aspiration and analyzed immediately before ET without reducing the implantation rate.[63] However, although aspiration of endometrial fluid is a safe method, sometimes the material is not sufficient for analysis or is diluted through washing, making the results difficult to interpret.[64] Further, most of the identified proteins correspond to serum proteins, masking the identification of proteins present in lower concentrations.

Lipids

Lipidomics can be defined as the large-scale study of different lipids and the relationships among them. The objective of this study is full characterization, identification, and quantification of molecular lipid species and their biological roles according to the expression of proteins involved in the metabolism and function of lipids, including gene regulation.[65] Lipidomics are currently possible thanks to the implementation and further development of protocols and bioinformatics tools.[66]

Studies in animal models have shown the importance of lipids at the time of embryo implantation, with the identification and characterization of different lipids during the receptive stage. Lipid molecules such as endocannabinoids, lysophosphatidic acid, and PGs have been described as some of the most studied in embryo implantation lipids, meaning that endometrium can be assessed by a specific pattern of lipids.

Recently, defective endometrial prostaglandin synthesis has been linked to repetitive implantation failure in assisted reproduction patients,[67] indicating the importance of lipids as mediators in early gestational development. Most of these studies have focused on the role of PGs, which produce an increase in vascularization and decidualization of the endometrium.[68] PGs have also been suggested as important in endometrial maturation and implantation.[69-72]

In 2013, our group demonstrated that the lipidomic signature of PGs prostaglandin E2 (PGE2) and prostaglandin F2α (PGF2α) in endometrial fluid offers a noninvasive biomarker of endometrial receptivity.[73] These results are significant for three reasons: first, they prove that the endometrial fluid is suitable for lipid analysis in humans, a possibility never investigated before; second, they illustrate how the lipid profile changes in endometrial fluid throughout the menstrual cycle and open the possibility of developing noninvasive methods to determine endometrial receptivity; and finally, the information can be immediately generated, providing the possibility of ET within 24 hours after the test is performed.[74]

Immunological Studies

A successful pregnancy involves adaptation of the immune response to the semiallogenic developing embryo. In contrast to its classical role in protecting the organism from invading foreign antigens, the endometrial immune system supports invasion and maintenance of the fetal semiallograft[75] and has been thought to play a role in reproductive problems such as recurrent miscarriage, infertility, and implantation failure.

Leukocytes in human endometrium comprise of different subpopulations, including uterine natural killer (uNK) cells, macrophages, and dendritic cells.[76] Natural killer (NK) cells represent 5–12% of all lymphocytes[77] and are classified as $CD16^+$ $CD56^{dim}$ NK cells or $CD16^-$ $CD56^{bright}$ NK cells by their surface markers.[78] NK cells are the most abundant immune cells infiltrating the uterine implantation site.[79] In the peripheral blood, the main population of NK cells consists of $CD16^+$ $CD56^{dim}$ NK cells; in the endometrium, $CD16^-$ $CD56^{bright}$ NK cells are the main population.[79,80] Peripheral NK cells have been demonstrated to show significant cytotoxic activity with well-established antiviral and antineoplastic functions. uNK cells have little cytotoxic activity but are a rich source of growth factors and cytokines, particularly angiogenic ones, with possible roles in regulation of trophoblast invasion and angiogenesis.[80-82]

The uNK cells represent 40% of the total leukocyte population during the proliferative phase, which increases to 60% by mid-secretory phase and up to 75% in early pregnancy.[83] Dysregulation of uNK number and/or cell function (cytotoxicity, receptor expression, cytokine secretion, or gene expression) has been associated with reproductive disorders such as unexplained infertility (UI), unexplained recurrent pregnancy loss (uRPL), and endometriosis.[84] The assessment of peripheral blood NK cells in women with recurrent implantation failure (RIF) was popularized by Beer et al.[85] who claimed that elevated numbers of peripheral blood NK cells or higher levels of natural killer activity were predictors of pregnancy loss.

Giuliani et al.[84] investigated the expression of CD16 and NKp46 (natural cytotoxicity receptor of uNK). The percentage of CD16$^+$ cells was higher in women with uRPL and UI, even when these conditions were associated with endometriosis compared with fertile patients. Likewise, the ratio of NKp46$^+$/CD56$^+$ cells was higher in women with uRPL and UI even when these conditions were associated with endometriosis compared with fertile patients. They concluded that women who have larger populations of cytotoxic CD16$^+$ uNK cells may be at greater risk of infertility disorders resulting from an inflammatory environment occurring during implantation or later during decidualization.

With the main objective of evaluating the peripheral blood NK cells in women who have experienced RIF, Sacks et al.[86] analyzed the concentration of the CD56^{dim} and NK cell number. This study has demonstrated that women with RIF have altered peripheral blood NK cell parameters compared with normal fertile controls. The results of peripheral blood NK cell activity and concentration of the CD56^{dim} were significantly higher in women with RIF. Similarly, Karami et al.[87] investigated the implication of CD56^{dim} in recurrent spontaneous abortion (RSA) and RIF. They saw that the percentage of CD56^{dim} cells and the level of peripheral blood NK cell cytotoxicity in RSA patients and women with IVF failure were also significantly higher than those in controls. These findings suggest that increase in the percentage of CD56^{dim} cells and NK cytotoxicity in peripheral blood may be important contributing factors for both RSA and RIF.

Such studies alluded that testing NK cells (uNK and pNK) might be useful in women with RIF and RSA during the mid-secretory and late-secretory phase; however, there are also conflicting reports.[88] Furthermore, there are a series of case-control studies reporting an association between pNK cell numbers and recurrent miscarriage (RM), as well as some studies that have shown no difference in pNK cell parameters between RM and controls.[89-91] There is also inconsistency in the association of pNK cells[92] and uNK cells with infertility.[93]

In a recent study, Liu et al.[94] found that the prognostic value of uNK cell count is significantly increased when the result is combined with histological dating, but limitations of this classical approach have already been discussed in this chapter.

Additionally, it has been difficult to associate NK cells with reproductive failure in women or to develop them as clinical targets, so the prognostic value of measuring pNK or uNK cell parameters remains uncertain. More studies are needed to confirm or refute the role of NK cell assessments as a predictive test for screening women who may benefit from immunotherapy.

ENDOMETRIAL TRANSCRIPTOMICS

Gene expression is the most fundamental level at which the genotype gives rise to the phenotype. The transcriptome reflects the genes that are being actively expressed at any given time in a specific cell population.[95] Transcriptomics, or expression profiling, also allows gene expression characterization at the messenger RNA (mRNA) level of a population, leading to a sample-specific molecular profile. This fact led to a new concept of biomarker and thus represents new opportunities to characterize function or disease phenotypes.[96,97]

Gene expression in different endometrial cell types is regulated by ovarian steroids and paracrine-secreted molecules from neighboring cells.[98] The study of endometrial transcriptomics examines the mRNAs in the endometrium throughout the menstrual cycle. These studies have revealed hundreds of simultaneously up- and downregulated genes involved in the acquisition of endometrial receptivity and embryo implantation. The advances in gene expression profiling, first based on microarray technology,[97,99] and nowadays facilitated by the development of next-generation sequencing (NGS) techniques, make it possible to deepen the investigation of the endometrial receptivity process from a global genomic perspective. The main objective of transcriptomic studies is to identify the genes differentially expressed among predefined classes of samples to develop a mathematical function based on the expression profiles that can accurately predict the biologic group, diagnostic category, or prognostic stage.[98]

In the last decade, the development of microarray and NGS technology has prompted research to reveal the existence of specific expression profiles for different menstrual cycle phases. These findings initiated the possibility of classifying the molecular status of the endometrium according to its transcriptomic profile.[100,101] The most commonly used strategy to search for the human endometrial receptivity signature has been to compare expression profiles during the WOI versus other stages of the menstrual cycle.[102-105]

Despite the differences among all the studies performed, all agreed on the existence of a specific transcriptomic profile during the WOI. This characteristic profile suggested that a unique transcriptional process occurs to achieve a receptive phenotype, with the gatekeeper being the activation of the

Table 1: Concordance between endometrial receptivity array (ERA) and Noyes criteria.

	Pathologist 1 (P1)	*Pathologist 2 (P2)*	*P1 vs P2*	*ERA*
Kappa value	0.618 (0.446–0.791)	0.685 (0.545–0.824)	0.622 (0.435–0.839)	0.922 (0.815–1.000)

progesterone receptor.[98,102,104,106] The different regulation of genes (up or down) includes those involved in the processes of metabolism, glandular secretion, cell differentiation, cell communication, innate immune response, response to stress, response to wounding, cell adhesion, and proteolysis regulation.[102,104,107] Further, of all of the endometrial stages, the most interesting is the mid-secretory phase. During this phase, the endometrium acquires the receptive phenotype and most of the genes are upregulated compared to their expression in the prereceptive phase.[95,98,102]

Based on earlier studies, our group[86] defined a list of 25 target genes for endometrial receptivity, and Tseng et al.[105] found 128 genes for the diagnosis of endometrial disorders. Subsequently, Díaz-Gimeno et al. identified a set of 238 genes that are differentially expressed in the transition from the prereceptive to the receptive state, creating a diagnostic tool named the ERA.[102]

The ERA, first based on microarray data, is now performed using NGS coupled to a computational predictor. ERA facilitates the assessment of the endometrial receptivity state by defining the transcriptomic profile of the endometrium during the WOI.[102] The original predictor was created and trained with the transcriptomics profiles of each endometrial stage. The endometrial samples used (n = 79) to train the predictor were obtained from fertile women during their menstrual cycle, and were classified as proliferative (days 8–12 of the menstrual cycle), prereceptive (LH + 1 to LH + 5), receptive (LH + 7), and postreceptive (LH + 11 to LH + 13).[18] This analysis has a sensitivity of 0.99758 and specificity of 0.8857, and its effectiveness and consistency have recently been demonstrated.[102] Following the accumulation of data after 6 years, algorithms have been developed to provide a new computational predictor based on NGS technology. The new ERA predictor defines a shorter, optimal WOI frame. To define this receptivity signature, the training of the new predictor was performed by selecting well-defined and curated endometrial profiles. This technique has been refined and improved such that the predictor potency provides more detailed insights into the use of gene signature profiles for patient stratification.

As has already been discussed, histological criteria have been used since the 1950s to date the endometrium,[9,12] despite the major limitations for predicting endometrial receptivity, as shown in randomized studies.[17,18] The accuracy of both the ERA and the histological methods were evaluated to determine which method is more reliable. To do so, a dating set comprising 49 endometrial biopsies was analyzed by the ERA microarray and by two independent pathologists who followed the Noyes criteria. The concordance between each method was statistically analyzed by the quadratic weighted Kappa index;[108] the result is shown in Table 1.

The most important contribution of the ERA test has been the objective diagnosis of the WOI, leading to the creation of the concept of personalized embryo transfer (pET). The basis of the test implies that pET must be performed after a "receptive" result in a subsequent cycle (or even several cycles later) under the same conditions (day and type of cycle) as the original endometrial biopsy.

The reproducibility and consistency of the ERA were tested by analyzing a second biopsy obtained from the same patient several months later (29–40 months). The reproducibility set comprised four endometrial samples obtained at LH + 7 (Receptive, n = 4), and three samples outside the WOI (Proliferative, n = 2/Postreceptive, n = 1).[108] The intercycle variation observed in the patients studied showed a full consistency in the ERA test diagnosis between the first and second analysis in the same patient with the same diagnostic probability.[108] Paired-sample gene expression analysis by principal components analysis and clustering showed the reproducibility of the tool and demonstrated that the transcriptomic profile did not substantially change between cycles or over relatively long periods of the women's reproductive life. Therefore, the ERA is a highly reproducible method, even up to 40 months after diagnosing the receptivity status of the endometrium for the first time.[108,109] In conclusion, the accuracy, reproducibility, and consistency of the ERA test for assessing endometrial receptivity is superior to classical histology methods.[108] The diagnostic and clinical value of the ERA test has also been analyzed in patients with RIF in a prospective interventional, multicenter, clinical trial.[110] An RIF study group included 85 patients with failed ovum donation cycles (≤51 years old) and IVF patients (≤40 years old) with at least three previous failed cycles. Patients with one or no failed ART cycles served as the control group. Endometrial biopsies were obtained on day LH + 7 in a natural cycle or on day P + 5 in a hormone replacement therapy (HRT) cycle. In the control group, the ERA test result was "receptive" (R) in 22 out of 25 patients (88.0%) and "nonreceptive" (NR) in only 3 patients (12.0%). Interestingly, in RIF patients, the percentage of R results was 74.1% (63 out of 85 patients) and the percentage of NR results 25.9% (22 patients). The clinical outcome showed a pregnancy rate (PR) and an implantation rate (IR) of 81.8% and 59.1%, respectively in the comparison group versus 51.7% and 33.9% in the RIF group.

The clinical value of pET has been proven in locating the WOI in RIF patients with a previously nonreceptive endometrium. After pET, patients achieved a 50.0% pregnancy rate and a 38.5% implantation rate, as shown in Table 2. This is very close to that of patients who had a receptive result at their first biopsy.

The value and clinical potential of the ERA test is in detecting the personalized WOI in patients with repetitive implantation failure and guiding their pET. A pilot study included 17 patients undergoing oocyte donation who

Table 2: Summary of the diagnostic and clinical outcomes of repeated implantation failure (RIF) and comparison group patients following the endometrial receptivity array (ERA) test. Clinical outcome of nonreceptive RIF and comparison group patients that underwent pET. The endometrial biopsy was obtained on day LH + 7 in a natural cycle or on day P + 5 in an HRT.

	RIF vs. control		*No-receptive RIF vs. pET*	
No. of patients	85	25		
Age (year)	38.4–4.7	39.9–5.1		
No. of receptive ERA/Total analyzed (%)	63/85 (74.1)	22/25 (88.0)	No. of receptive ERA/Total analyzed	25/85
No. of previous failed cycle	4.8–2.1	0.5–0.5	No. of previous failed cycle RIF patients	5.0–0.6
Total patients with pET after receptive ERA	29	11	No. of previous failed cycle control patients	0.3–0.6
Implantation rate after 1st pET (%)	19/56 (33.9)	11/20 (59.1)	ERA prediction	
Pregnancy rate after 1st pET (%)	15/29 (51.7)	9/11 (81.8)	Prereceptive	21/25 (84.0)
Biochemical pregnancies (%)	3/15 (20)	2/9 (22.2)	Postreceptive	4/25 (16.0)
Clinical abortions (%)	0/15 (0.0)	0/9 (0.0)	2nd ERA at the specific day (P+4;+6;+7; LH+9)	18
Ovum donation patients/Total (%)	22/63 (34.9)	13/22 (59.1)	Months between 1st and 2nd ERA	2.6–2.8
Patients with pET after receptive ERA	16	8	2nd ERA receptive at specified day	15
Implantation rate after 1st pET (%)	12/33 (36.4)	7/15 (46.7)	Patients with pET after 2nd receptive ERA	8
Pregnancy rate after 1st pET (%)	9/16 (56.2)	6/8 (75.0)	Months between 2nd receptive ERA and pET	1.8–0.7
Biochemical pregnancies (%)	2/9 (22.2)	1/6 (16.7)	Implantation rate using pET (%)	5/13 (38.5)
Clinical abortions (%)	0/9 (0.0)	0/6 (0.0)	Pregnancy rate using pET (%)	4/8 (50.0)
IVF/ICSI patients/Total (%)	41/63 (65.1)	9/22 (40.9)	Biochemical pregnancies (%)	0/4 (0.0)
Patients with pET after receptive ERA	13	3	Clinical abortions (%)	0/4 (0.0)
Implantation rate after 1st pET (%)	7/23 (30.4)	4/5 (80.0)		
Pregnancy rate after 1st pET (%)	6/13 (46.2)	3/3 (100.0)		
Biochemical pregnancies (%)	1/6 (16.7)	1/3 (33.3)		
Clinical abortions (%)	0/6 (0.0)	0/3 (0.0)		
No. of nonreceptive ERA/Total analyzed (%)	22/85 (25.9)	3/25 (12.0)		
No. of previous cycles	5.0–1.8	0.3–0.6		
Ovum donation patients/Total (%)	11/22 (50.0)	2/3 (66.6)		
IVF/ICSI patients/ Total (%)	11/22 (50.0)	1/3 (33.3)		

(HRT: hormone replacement therapy; ICSI: intracytoplasmic sperm injection; IVF: in vitro fertilization; pET: personalized embryo transfer.)
Source: Ruiz-Alonso et al. (2013).[110]

suffered failed implantations with the routine embryo transfer and underwent pET after the personalized diagnosis of their WOI.[111] All the patients with RIF had the implantation window displaced (16 prereceptive and 1 postreceptive). The ET before the ERA test showed 11% and 19% of IR and PR, respectively; after pET, the results present 40% of IR and 60% of PR. Therefore, the clinical potential of the ERA has been demonstrated for detecting the personalized WOI in patients with repetitive implantation failure and guiding their pET as a novel therapeutic strategy.

The differences among endometrial transcriptomics under diverse IVF treatments,[107,108] among healthy patients and patients with endometriosis,[112] and in endometrial cancer have also been studied.[113] Hence, for the first time, a molecular tool based on the expression of a cluster of endometrial genes has been clinically used in reproductive medicine to assess the endometrial factor with proven accuracy and consistency.[100,114] We now have the ability to diagnose a displacement of the WOI in RIF patients and to schedule a pET, helping to improve clinical success from the endometrial perspective using the ERA test. This highlights the need to synchronize embryonic development and endometrial receptivity, personalizing the timing of ET.

ENDOMETRIAL MICROBIOME

As our body contains 10 more times the number of bacteria than cells, a main question regarding their potential relationship with reproduction has recently been answered in a study published by Moreno et al.[115] In this study, the species-specific sequences of the variable regions of the 16S rRNA gene were analyzed by NGS to evaluate the relative abundances of each microorganism present in the microbial population.

The first part of the study included a comparison between the microbiota of paired samples of endometrial fluid and vaginal aspirates from 13 healthy and fertile subjects in prereceptive (LH + 2) and receptive phase (LH + 7) in natural cycles. From all the samples, nine were colonized only by *Lactobacillus* spp., while the rest showed a combination of different operational taxonomic units (OTUs) in addition to *Lactobacillus*. In 24 out of 26 pairs of samples, there were found slight differences between endometrial and vaginal microbiota, but in 6 of them the bacterial communities were completely different with a high proportion of potential pathogens in the endometrium or in the vagina; the same bacterial OTUs were present in only 2 pairs of samples. The conclusion was that the uterine cavity is not sterile and endometrial and vaginal microbiomes are different in asymptomatic women.

The second part of the study consisted of investigating the hormonal regulation of the endometrial microbiota. For this purpose, the endometrial fluid from 22 healthy and fertile women was taken on LH + 2 and LH + 7 in the same natural cycle. The bacterial communities found were clustered according to the different bacterial OTUs identified and their abundances. The resulting heat map showed two sets of samples classified depending on the percentage of *Lactobacillus* OTUs identified. The first set of samples included those with a high abundance of *Lactobacillus* (over 90%) and very low or nonexistent other OTUs. The second set of samples was formed by lower *Lactobacillus* abundances that coexisted with bacteria represented by other OTUs. Clustering of individual samples showed two groups depending on the abundance of *Lactobacillus* OTUs. This part of the study concluded that endometrial microbiome is not regulated by hormones during the acquisition of endometrial receptivity.

Finally, the functional impact of the endometrial microbiota composition on reproductive outcome in patients undergoing IVF was studied, concluding that low abundance of *Lactobacillus* in endometrial microbiota is associated with poor reproductive outcomes in IVF patients. In fact, subjects with a non-*Lactobacillus* dominant microbiota had significantly lower implantation (60.7% vs. 23.1%, $p = 0.02$), pregnancy (70.6% vs. 33.3%, $p = 0.03$), ongoing pregnancy (58.8% vs. 13.3%, $p = 0.02$), and live birth (58.8% vs. 6.7%, $p = 0.002$) rates, as well as higher miscarriage rates (16.7% vs. 60%, $p = 0.007$), although this was not statistically significant, compared to those with a *Lactobacillus*-dominant microbiota.

In conclusion, the uterine cavity is not sterile. A human endometrial microbiota exists, and it is different from the vaginal microbiomes in asymptomatic women. Furthermore, the endometrial microbiome is not hormonally regulated during the acquisition of endometrial receptivity and the existence of non-*Lactobacillus* bacteria is related to negative impacts in reproduction.

The molecular microbiology method has also been used to identify culturable and nonculturable endometrial pathogens associated with chronic endometritis such as *Enterobacteriaceae*, *Enterococcus*, *Streptococcus*, *Staphylococcus*, *Mycoplasma*, and *Ureaplasma*.[116]

Chronic endometritis is a persistent inflammation of the endometrial mucosa that can be asymptomatic, but it is found in up to 40% of infertile patients and is responsible for repeated implantation failure and recurrent miscarriage.

With this aim, the classical methods used for diagnosis of chronic endometritis (hysteroscopy of the uterine cavity, endometrial biopsy with plasma cells being identified histologically, and microbial culture) were compared to the molecular method by evaluating 113 endometrial samples from patients assessed for chronic endometritis by real-time PCR. The results were lately confirmed by the microbiome assessed by next-generation sequencing. In the endometrial samples with concordant results in the three classic methods, the molecular microbiology diagnosis demonstrates 75% sensitivity, 100% specificity, 100% positive and 25% negative predictive values, and 0% false-positive and 25% false-negative rates, concluding that the molecular microbiology method is a fast and inexpensive diagnostic tool that allows for the identification of culturable and nonculturable endometrial pathogens associated with chronic endometritis.

Thus, the microbiological level as well as the morphological and molecular viewpoints should be considered to perform an endometrial receptivity assessment.

IMPROVING ENDOMETRIAL RECEPTIVITY ASSESSMENT THROUGH PERSONALIZED MEDICINE

Histological, biological, and physiological characteristics of the endometrium during the implantation window are the result of changes occurring at the level of gene transcription attached to post-transcriptional modification and epigenetic changes. Currently, the "omic" techniques allow us to accelerate the endometrial assessment. However, there remain limitations in the techniques that prevent the unification of the results. Transcriptomics, proteomics, secretomics, and lipidomics are complementary approaches that provide different but comparable perspectives that will improve our understanding of the complexity of this process and the identification of new biomarkers that determine endometrial receptivity, different causes of infertility, the development of a noninvasive diagnostic tool for endometrial receptivity that allows clinicians to obtain a quick result and, finally, to investigate potential interception targets to prevent or stimulate implantation. The use of sequencing technologies and the integration of this information into systematic biological models is nowadays helping to achieve a global understanding of endometrial receptivity.

The idea behind personalized medicine is to tailor health care to a person's unique genetic profile. It is moving us closer to more precise, predictable, and powerful individually customized medicine. Genetic analyses of patients dealing with different types of cancer[117-120] are driving treatment advantages that can usher in new perspectives in reproductive medicine.

Going further and moving endometrial assessment into personalized medicine, ART will evolve by shifting the emphasis from reaction to detection, prescribing customized fertility treatments, eliminating trial-and-error inefficiencies that inflate health care costs and demotivate patients, and reducing the time enabling pET, which therefore gives faster outcome feedback to aspiring mothers. Currently, the ERA test is the most reliable technique for bringing ART one step closer to personalized medicine, through identification of WOI displacements and introduction of the concept of pET.

REFERENCES

1. Mascarenhas M, Flaxman S, Boerma T, et al. National, regional, and global trends in infertility prevalence since 1990: A systematic analysis of 277 health surveys. PLoS Med. 2012;9:e1001356.
2. Diedrich K, Fauser BC, Devroey P, et al. Evian annual reproduction (EVAR) workshop group, the role of the endometrium and embryo in human implantation. Hum Reprod Update. 2007;13:365-77.
3. Hawkins SM, Matzuk MM. The menstrual cycle: Basic biology. Ann NY Acad Sci. 2008;1135:10-8.
4. Cha J, Vilella F, Dey SK, et al. Molecular interplay in successful implantation. Ten Critical Topics in Reproductive Medicine. S. Senders. 2013 (Ed). 44-8.
5. Wilcox AJ, Baird DD, Weinberg CR. Time of implantation of the conceptus and loss of pregnancy. N Engl J Med. 1999;340:1796-9.
6. Harper MJ. The implantation window. Baillieres Clin Obstet Gynaecol. 1992;6:351-71.
7. Finn CL, Martin L. The control of implantation. J Reprod Fertil. 1974;39:195-206.
8. Garrido-Gómez T, Dominguez F, Quiñonero A, et al. Annexin A2 is critical for embryo adhesiveness to the human endometrium by RhoA activation through F-actin regulation. FASEB J. 2012;26(9):3715-27.
9. Noyes RW, Hertig AT, Rock J. Dating the endometrial biopsy. Am J Obstet Gynecol. 1975;122(2):262-3.
10. Aghajanova L, Simon C, Horcajadas JA. Are favourite molecules of endometrial receptivity still in favour? Expert Rev Obstet Gynecol. 2008;3:487-501.
11. Rock J, Bartlett MK. Biopsy studies of human endometrium: Criteria of dating and information about amenorrhea, menorrhagia and time of ovulation. J Am Med Assoc. 1937;108:2022-8.
12. Noyes RW, Hertig AT, Rock J. Dating the endometrial biopsy. Am J Obstet Gynecol. 1975;122(2):262-3.
13. Shoupe D, Mishell DR, Lacarra M, et al. Correlation of endometrial maturation with four methods of estimating day of ovulation. Obstet Gynecol. 1989;73:88-92.
14. Balasch J, Fábreques F, Creus M, et al. The usefulness of endometrial biopsy for luteal phase evaluation in infertility. Hum Reprod. 1992;7:973-7.
15. Creus M, Ordi J, Fábregues F, et al. Alpha v beta3 integrin expression and pinopod formation in normal and out-

of-phase endometria of fertile and infertile women. Hum Reprod. 2002;17:2279-86.

16. Ordi J, Creus M, Quintó L, et al. Within subject between-cycle variability of histological dating, alpha v beta 3 integrin expression, and pinopod formation in the human endometrium. J Clin Endocrinol Metabol. 2003;88:2119-25.
17. Murray MJ, Meyer WR, Zaino RJ, et al. A critical analysis of the accuracy, reproducibility, and clinical utility of histologic endometrial dating in fertile women. Fertil Steril. 2004;81:1333-43.
18. Coutifaris C, Myers ER, Guzick DS, et al. Histological dating of timed endometrial biopsy tissue is not related to fertility status. Fertil Steril. 2004;82:1264-72.
19. Papanikolaou EG, Tournaye H, Verpoest W, et al. Early and late ovarian hyperstimulation syndrome: Early pregnancy outcome and profile. Hum Reprod. 2005;20:636-41.
20. Barron ML, Fehring RJ. Basal body temperature assessment: is it useful to couples seeking pregnancy? MCN Am J Matern Child Nurs. 2005;30(5):290-6.
21. Lenton EA, Weston GA, Cooke ID. Problems in using basal body temperature recordings in an infertility clinic. Br Med J. 1977;1(6064):803-5.
22. Mercé LT, Barco MJ, Bau S, et al. Are endometrial parameters by three dimensional ultrasound and power Doppler angiography related to in vitro fertilization/embryo transfer outcome? Fertil Steril. 2008;89(1):111-7.
23. Oliveira JB, Baruffi RL, Mauri RL, et al. Endometrial ultrasonography as a predictor of pregnancy in an in-vitro fertilization programme after ovarian stimulation and gonadotrophin-releasing hormone and gonadotrophins. Hum Reprod. 1997;12(11):2515-8.
24. Raga F, Raga F, Bonilla-Musoles F, et al. Assessment of endometrial volume by three-dimensional ultrasound prior to embryo transfer: clues to endometrial receptivity. Hum Reprod. 1999;14(11):2851-4.
25. Zhang X, Chen CH, Confino E, et al. Increased endometrial thickness is associated with improved treatment outcome for selected patients undergoing in vitro fertilization–embryo transfer. Fertil Steril. 2005;83(2):336-40.
26. McWilliams GD, Frattarelli JL. Changes in measured endometrial thickness predict in vitro fertilization success. Fertil Steril. 2007;88(1):74-81.
27. Remohí J, Ardiles G, García-Velasco JA, et al. Endometrial thickness and serum oestradiol concentrations as predictors of outcome in oocyte donation. Hum. Reprod. 1997;12(10):2271-6.
28. Garcia-Velasco JA, Pellicer A. New concepts in the understanding of the ovarian hyperstimulation syndrome. Curr Opin Obstet Gynecol. 2003;15(3):251-6.
29. Puerto B, Creus M, Carmona F, et al. Ultrasonography as a predictor of embryo implantation after in vitro fertilization: A controlled study. Fertil Steril. 2003;79(4);1015-22.
30. Soares SR, Troncoso C, Bosch E, et al. Age and uterine receptiveness: Predicting the outcome of oocyte donation cycles. J Clin Endocrinol Metab. 2005;90(7):4399-404.
31. Guermandi E, Vegetti W, Bianchi MM, et al. Reliability of ovulation tests in infertile women. Obstet Gynecol. 2001;97(1):92-6.
32. Dickey RP, Olar TT, Curole DN, et al. Endometrial pattern and thickness associated with pregnancy outcome after assisted reproduction technologies. Hum Reprod. 1992;7(3):418-21.
33. Noyes N, Liu HC, Sultan K, et al. Implantation: Endometrial thickness appears to be a significant factor in embryo implantation in in-vitro fertilization. Hum Reprod. 1995;10(4):919-22.
34. Martinez AR, Bernardus RE, Vermeiden JP, et al. Reliability of home urinary LH tests for timing of insemination: a consumer's study. Hum Reprod. 1992;7:751-3.
35. Robinson JN, Lockwood GM, Dalton JD, et al. A randomized prospective study to assess the effect of the use of home urinary luteinizing hormone detection on the efficiency of donor insemination. Hum Reprod. 1992;7(1):63-5.
36. Kawano T, Matsuura K, Honda R, et al. Prediction of ovulation by urinary LH surge. Nihon Naibunpi Gakkai zasshi. 1992;68(11):1188-96.
37. Park SJ, Goldsmith LT, Skurnick JH, et al. Characteristics of the urinary luteinizing hormone surge in young ovulatory women. Fertil Steril. 2007;88(3):684-90.
38. Direito A, Bailly S, Mariani A, et al. Relationships between the luteinizing hormone surge and other characteristics of the menstrual cycle in normally ovulating women. Fertil Steril. 2013;99(1):279-85.
39. Martel D, Monier MN, Roche D, et al. Hormonal dependence of pinopode formation at the uterine luminal surface. Hum Reprod. 1991;6(4):597-603.
40. Nikas G, Drakakis P, Loutradis D, et al. Uterine pinopodes as markers of the 'nidation window' in cycling women receiving exogenous oestradiol and progesterone. Hum Reprod. 1995;10(5):1208-13.
41. Nikas G. Cell-surface morphological events relevant to human implantation. Hum Reprod. 1999;14:37-44.
42. Psychoyos A, Nikas G. Uterine pinopodes as markers of uterine receptivity. Assist Reprod Rev. 1994;4:26-32.
43. Quinn CE, Casper RF. Pinopodes: A questionable role in endometrial receptivity. Hum Reprod Update. 2009;15:229-36.
44. Shankar R, Cullinane F, Brennecke SP, et al. Applications of proteomics methodologies to human pregnancy research: A growing gestation approaching delivery? Proteomics. 2004;4:1909-17.
45. Lessey BA, Castlebaum AJ, Sawin SW, et al. Aberrant integrin expression in the endometrium of women with endometriosis. J Clin Endocrinol Metab. 1994;79:643-9.
46. Lessey BA, Castlebaum AJ, Sawin SW, et al. Integrins as markers of uterine receptivity in women with primary unexplained infertility. Fertil Steril. 1995;63:535-42.
47. Lessey BA. Assessment of endometrial receptivity. Fertil Steril. 2011;96:522-9.
48. Creus M, Ordi J, Fábregues F, et al. Integrin expression in normal and out-of-phase endometria. Hum Reprod. 1998;13(12):3460-8.
49. Hii LL, Rogers PA. Endometrial vascular and glandular expression of integrin alpha (v) beta3 in women with and without endometriosis. Hum Reprod. 1998;13(4):1030-5.
50. Surrey ES, Lietz AK, Gustofson RL, et al. Does endometrial integrin expression in endometriosis patients predict enhanced in vitro fertilization cycle outcomes after prolonged GnRH agonist therapy? Fertil Steril. 2010;93(2):646-51.

51. DeSouza L, Diehl G, Yang EC, et al. Proteomic analysis of the proliferative and secretory phases of the human endometrium: Protein identification and differential protein expression. Proteomics. 2005;5:270-81.
52. Parmar T, Gadkar-Sable S, Savardekar L, et al. Protein profiling of human endometrial tissues in the midsecretory and proliferative phases of the menstrual cycle. Fertil Steril. 2009;92:1091-103.
53. Dominguez F, Garrido-GÓmez T, Lopez JA, et al. Proteomic analysis of the human receptive versus non-receptive endometrium using differential in-gel electrophoresis and MALDI-MS unveils stathmin 1 and annexin A2 as differentially regulated. Hum Reprod. 2009;24:2607-17.
54. Martin JC, Jasper MJ, Valbuena D, et al. Increased adhesiveness in cultured endometrial-derived cells is related to the absence of moesin expression. Biol Reprod. 2000;63:1370-6.
55. Li J, Tan Z, Li M, et al. Proteomic analysis of endometrium in fertile women during the prereceptive and receptive phases after luteinizing hormone surge. Fertil Steril. 2011;95(3):1161-3.
56. Rai P, Kota V, Sundaram CS, et al. Proteome of human endometrium: Identification of differentially expressed proteins in proliferative and secretory phase endometrium. Proteomics Clin Appl. 2010;4(1):48-59.
57. Garrido-Gómez T, Quiñonero A, Antúnez O, et al. Deciphering the proteomic signature of human endometrial receptivity. Hum Reprod. 2014;29(9):1957-67.
58. Cheong Y, Boomsma C, Heijnen C, et al. Uterine secretomics: A window on the maternal-embryo interface. Fertil Steril. 2013;99(4):1093-9.
59. van der Gaast MH, Beier-Hellwig K, Fauser BC, et al. Endometrial secretion aspiration prior to embryo transfer does not reduce implantation rates. Reprod Biomed. 2003;7:105-9.
60. Carson DD, Lagow E, Thathiah A, et al. Changes in gene expression during the early to mid-luteal (receptive phase) transition in human endometrium detected by high-density microarray screening. Mol Hum Reprod. 2002;8:971-9.
61. Horcajadas JA, Pellicer A, Simón C. Wide genomic analysis of human endometrial receptivity: New times, new opportunities. Hum Reprod Update. 2007;13:77-86.
62. Lessey BA, Killam AP, Metzger DA, et al. Immunohistochemical analysis of human uterine estrogen and progesterone receptors throughout the menstrual cycle. J Clin Endocrinol Metab. 1988;67:334-40.
63. Kao LC, Germeyer A, Tulac S, et al. Expression profiling of endometrium from women with endometriosis reveals candidate genes for disease-based implantation failure and infertility. Endocrinology. 2003;144:2870-81.
64. Borthwick JM, Charnock-Jones DS, Tom BD, et al. Determination of the transcript profile of human endometrium. Mol Hum Reprod. 2003;9:19-33.
65. Quehenberger O, Armando AM, Brown AH, et al. Lipidomics reveals a remarkable diversity of lipids in human plasma. J Lipid Res. 2010;51(11):3299-305.
66. Gawrisch K, Eldho NV, Polozov IV. Novel NMR tools to study structure and dynamics of biomembranes. Chem Phys Lipids. 2002;116(1-2):135-51.
67. Mirkin S, Arslan M, Churikov D, et al. In search of candidate genes critically expressed in the human endometrium during the window of implantation. Hum Reprod. 2005;20:2104-7.
68. Wenk MR. The emerging field of lipidomics. Nat Rev Drug Discov. 2005;4:594-610.
69. Achache H, Tsafrir A, Prus D, et al. Defective endometrial prostaglandin synthesis identified in patients with repeated implantation failure undergoing in vitro fertilization. Fertil Steril. 2010;94:1271-8.
70. Ye X, Hama K, Contos JJ, et al. LPA3-mediated lysophosphatidic acid signalling in embryc implantation and spacing. Nature. 2005;435:104-8.
71. Durn JH, Marshall KM, Farrar D, et al. Lipidomic analysis reveals prostanoid profiles in human term pregnant myometrium. Prostaglandins Leukot Essent Fatty Acids. 2010;82:21-6.
72. Huang JC, Wun WS, Goldsby JS, et al. Stimulation of embryo hatching and implantation by prostacyclin and peroxisome proliferator-activated receptor delta activation: implication in IVF. Hum Reprod. 2007;22:807-14.
73. Vilella F, Ramirez L, Berlanga O, et al. PGE2 and PGF2 concentrations in human endometrial fluid as biomarkers for embryonic implantation. J Clin Endocrinol Metab. 2013;98(10):4123-32.
74. Miravet-Valenciano JA, Rincon-Bertolin A, Vilella F, et al. Understanding and improving endometrial receptivity. Curr Opin Obstet Gynecol. 2015;27(3):187-92.
75. Robertson SA. Control of the immunological environment of the uterus. Rev Reprod. 2000;5(3):164-74.
76. Gnainsky Y, Dekel N, Granot I. Implantation: mutual activity of sex steroid hormones and the immune system guarantee the maternal-embryo interaction. Semin Reprod Med. 2014;32(5):337-45.
77. Thum M, Bhaskaran S, Abdalla H, et al. An increase in the absolute count of CD56dim CD16+ CD69+ NK cells in the peripheral blood is associated with a poorer IVF treatment and pregnancy outcome. Hum Reprod. 2004;19:2395.
78. Saito S, Nakashima A, Myojo-Higuma S, et al. The balance between cytotoxic NK cells and regulatory NK cells in human pregnancy. J Reprod Immunol. 2008;77:14-22.
79. Moffett-King A. Natural killer cells and pregnancy. Nat Rev Immunol. 2002;2:656-63.
80. Dosiou C, Giudice LC. Natural killer cells in pregnancy and recurrent pregnancy loss: Endocrine and immunologic perspectives. Endocr Rev. 2005;26:44-62.
81. Bulmer JN, Lash GE. Human uterine natural killer cells: A reappraisal. Mol Immunol. 2005;42:511-21.
82. Vacca P, Moretta L, Moretta A, et al. Origin, phenotype and function of human natural killer cells in pregnancy. Trends Immunology. 2011;32:517-23.
83. Tang AW, Alfirevic Z, Quenby S. Natural killer cells and pregnancy outcomes in women with recurrent miscarriage and infertility: A systematic review. Hum Reprod. 2011;26:1971-80.
84. Giuliani E, Parkin KL, Lessey BA, et al. Characterization of uterine NK cells in women with infertility or recurrent pregnancy loss and associated endometriosis. Am J Reprod Immunol. 2014;72(3):262-9.
85. Beer AE, Kwak J, Ruiz J. Immunophenotypic profiles of peripheral blood lymphocytes in women with recurrent pregnancy losses and in infertile women with multiple failed in vitro fertilization cycles. Am J Reprod Immunol. 1996;35:376-82.

86. Sacks G, Yang Y, Gowen E, et al. Detailed analysis of peripheral blood natural killer cells in women with repeated IVF Failure. Am J Reprod Immunol. 2012;67(5):434-42.
87. Karami N, Boroujerdnia MG, Nikbakht R, et al. Enhancement of peripheral blood CD56 (dim) cell and NK cell cytotoxicity in women with recurrent spontaneous abortion or in vitro fertilization failure. J Reprod Immunol. 2012;95(1-2):87-92.
88. Tang AW, Alfirevic Z, Quenby S. Natural killer cells and pregnancy outcomes in women with recurrent miscarriage and infertility: A systematic review. Hum Reprod. 2011;26(8):1971-80.
89. Emmer PM, Nelen WL, Steegers EA, et al. Peripheral natural killer cytotoxicity and CD56 (pos) CD16 (pos) cells increase during early pregnancy in women with a history of recurrent spontaneous abortion. Hum Reprod. 2000;15:1163-9.
90. Souza SS, Ferriani RA, Santos CM, et al. Immunological evaluation of patients with recurrent abortion. J Reprod Immunol. 2002;56:111-21.
91. Wang Q, Li TC, Wu YP, et al. Reappraisal of peripheral NK cells in women with recurrent miscarriage. Reprod Biomed Online. 2008;17:814-9.
92. Vujisic S, Lepej SZ, Aksamija A, et al. Band T-cells in the follicular fluid and peripheral blood of patients undergoing IVF/ ET procedures. Am J Reprod Immunol. 2004;52:379-85.
93. Matteo MG, Greco P, Rosenberg P, et al. Normal percentage of CD56 bright natural killer cells in young patients with a history of repeated unexplained implantation failure after in vitro fertilization cycles. Fertil Steril. 2007;88:990-3.
94. Liu B, Mariee N, Laird S, et al. The prognostic value of uNK cell count and histological dating in the mid-luteal phase of women with reproductive failure. Eur J Obstet Gynecol Reprod Biol. 2014;181:171-5.
95. Garrido-Gomez T, Dominguez F, Ruiz M, et al. The analysis of endometrial receptivity. Textbook of Assisted Reproductive Techniques, 4th edition. Vol. 1. Laboratory Perspectives. USA: CRC Press; 2012. pp. 366-79.
96. Nevins JR, Potti A. Mining gene expression profiles: Expression signatures as cancer phenotypes. Nat Rev Genet. 2007;8(8):601-9.
97. Díaz-Gimeno P, Ruiz-Alonso M, Blesa D, et al. Transcriptomics of the human endometrium. Int J Dev Biol. 2013;58(2-4):127-37.
98. Ruiz-Alonso M, Blesa D, Simón C. The genomics of the human endometrium. Biochim Biophys Acta. 2012;1822:1931-42.
99. Altmae S, Esteban FJ, Stavreus-Evers A, et al. Guidelines for the design, analysis and interpretation of 'omics' data: Focus on human endometrium. Hum Reprod Update. 2013;20:12-28.
100. Ponnampalam AP, Weston GC, Trajstman AC, et al. Molecular classification of human endometrial cycle stages by transcriptional profiling. Mol Hum Reprod. 2004;10:879-93.
101. Talbi S, Hamilton AE, Vo KC, et al. Molecular phenotyping of human endometrium distinguishes menstrual cycle phases and underlying biological processes in normo-ovulatory women. Endocrinology. 2006;147:1097-121.
102. Díaz-Gimeno P, Horcajadas JA, Martínez-Conejero JA, et al. A genomic diagnostic tool for human endometrial receptivity based on the transcriptomic signature. Fertil Steril. 2011;95(1):50-60.
103. Carson DD, Lagow E, Thathiah A, et al. Changes in gene expression during the early to mid-luteal (receptive phase) transition in human endometrium detected by high-density microarray screening. Mol Hum Reprod. 2002;8:871-9.
104. Riesewijk A, Martin J, van Os R, et al. Gene expression profiling of human endometrial receptivity on days LH+2 versus LH+7 by microarray technology. Mol Hum Reprod. 2003;9:253-64.
105. Tseng LH, Chen I, Chen MY, et al. Genome-based expression profiling as a single standardized microarray platform for the diagnosis of endometrial disorder: An array of 126-gene model. Fertil Steril. 2010;94:114-9.
106. Borthwick JM, Charnock-Jones DS, Tom BD, et al. Determination of the transcript profile of human endometrium. Mol Hum Reprod. 2003;9:19-33.
107. Horcajadas JA, Minguez P, Dopazo J, et al. Controlled ovarian stimulation induces a functional genomic delay of the endometrium with potential clinical implications. J Clin Endocrinol Metab. 2008;93:4500-10.
108. Díaz-Gimeno P, Ruíz-Alonso M, Blesa D, et al. The accuracy and reproducibility of the endometrial receptivity array is superior to histology as a diagnostic method for endometrial receptivity. Fertil Steril. 2013;99:508-17.
109. Garrido-Gómez T, Ruiz-Alonso M, Blesa D, et al. Profiling the gene signature of endometrial receptivity: clinical results. Fertil Steril. 2010;99(4):1078-85.
110. Ruiz-Alonso M, Blesa D, Díaz-Gimeno P, et al. The endometrial receptivity array for diagnosis and personalized embryo transfer as a treatment for patients with repeated implantation failure. Fertil Steril. 2013;100(3):818-24.
111. Ruiz-Alonso M, Galindo N, Pellicer A, et al. What a difference two days make: "Personalized" embryo transfer (pET) paradigm: A case report and pilot study. Hum Reprod. 2014;29(6):1244-7.
112. Matsuzaki S. DNA microarray analysis in endometriosis for development of more effective targeted therapies. Front Biosci (Elite Ed). 2011;3:1139-53.
113. Doll A, Abal M, Rigau M, et al. Novel molecular profiles of endometrial cancer-new light through old windows. J Steroid Biochem Mol Biol. 2008;108:221-9.
114. Ruíz-Alonso M, Gómez E, Díaz-Gimeno P, et al. Clinical application of the endometrial receptivity array. Médecine de la Reproduction, Gynécologie et Endocrinologie. 2014;16:120-6.
115. Moreno I, Codoñer FM, Vilella F, et al. Evidence that the endometrial microbiota has an effect on implantation success or failure. Am J Obstet Gynecol. 2016;215(6):684-703.
116. Moreno I, Cicinelli E, Garcia-Grau I, et al. The diagnosis of chronic endometritis in infertile asymptomatic women: a comparative study of histology, microbial cultures, hysteroscopy, and molecular microbiology. Am J Obstet Gynecol. 2018;218(6):602.e1-602.e16.
117. van't Veer LJ, Bernards R. Enabling personalized cancer medicine through analysis of gene-expression patterns. Nature. 2008;452(7187):564-70.
118. Heinemann V, Douillard JY, Ducreux M, et al. Targeted therapy in metastatic colorectal cancer—an example of personalized medicine in action. Cancer Treat Rev. 2013;39(6):592-601.
119. Swanton C, Burrell RA, Futreal PA. Breast cancer genome heterogeneity: A challenge to personalized medicine. Breast Cancer Res. 2011;13(1):104.
120. Ross JS, Slodkowska EA, Symmans WF, et al. The HER-2 receptor and breast cancer: Ten years of targeted anti-HER-2 therapy and personalized medicine. Oncologist. 2009;14(4):320-68.

CHAPTER

8

Assessment of the Male

Rupin Shah

INTRODUCTION

The male partner of an infertile couple should be evaluated to assess the following:

- Male fertility potential
- The presence of correctable gonadotoxic factors that may be impairing fertility
- History of illnesses in the past that may have permanently damaged the testes and would hence influence current decision-making
- Sexual dysfunction that may be contributing to the infertility or that may be resulting from the fertility treatment
- Difficulty in semen collection that may pose a problem during intrauterine insemination (IUI)/in vitro fertilization (IVF).

This will entail a specific history, examination, and investigations.

HISTORY

Textbooks provide a huge list of potential causes of impaired male fertility, and an equally long list of questions to be asked. Since most men would already have a semen test done it is more practical to tailor the history to the abnormality shown in the semen report.

Azoospermia

History of undescended testes, orchitis, testicular swelling followed by atrophy, testicular malignancy, chemotherapy or radiation would suggest primary testicular failure (PTF). Azoospermia in siblings should arouse the suspicion of PTF due to a genetic cause.

History of hernia or hydrocele surgery raises the possibility of iatrogenic obstructive azoospermia, though hernia surgery may also lead to atrophy.

History of testicular torsion with removal of one side and fixation of the other raises the possibility of iatrogenic obstruction on the fixed side. A nonpainful scrotal swelling and discharging sinus treated with long-term medication is usually indicative of genital tuberculosis with resultant obstruction. Previous urethral discharge or sexually transmitted diseases (STD) suggest infective obstruction of the epididymis.

If there has been delayed puberty and the need for a long course of injections (testosterone) to induce puberty then it would suggest hypogonadotropic hypogonadism, though some men with severe hypergonadotropic hypogonadism may also need testosterone to complete pubertal development. An increasing number of muscular men will admit to use of testosterone and anabolic steroids, which would cause azoospermia by suppressing the hypothalamopituitary axis.

Isolated Asthenozoospermia

Ask about recurrent respiratory tract infections—this would suggest a primary ciliary defect. Previous significant urinary infection would indicate the need to look for persistent accessory gland infection.

Oligoasthenoteratozoospermia

Enquire about various gonadotoxic factors—undescended testis, orchitis, heat or chemical exposure, gonadotoxic drugs or medications, excessive physical or mental stress, recurrent fever, and any major illness.

Sexual History

About 5% of infertility is primarily due to a sexual problem. Additionally, many couples develop sexual dysfunction due to the mechanization of sex that occurs during infertility treatment. Hence, it is important to enquire about the sexual history of all couples.

Ask about frequency of intercourse, adequacy of penetration, need for lubrication (many are spermicidal), difficulty in getting an erection at ovulation, and anejaculation. Also, enquire about premature ejaculation; this is not a cause of infertility unless it is so severe that there is ejaculation before penetration, but it is a common problem (usually untreated) and diagnosing and treating it can offer additional value to the couple.

It is important to ask the man if he is able to collect a semen sample by masturbation in the clinic. Situational anejaculation is common. Some men can ejaculate during intercourse but not by masturbation, others can ejaculate at home but not in the clinic, and some have a problem only when under pressure such as during a known fertile period. Detecting this problem in advance will allow for appropriate corrective measures.[1]

EXAMINATION

After a general examination for secondary sexual characters and any stigmata of a chronic illness, a careful examination of the genitalia should be performed.

Assess the following: scrotal skin (thickening due to chronic fungal infection can cause increase in local temperature); presence, size and consistency of testes; whether the epididymis is flabby or turgid, enlarged, irregular or adherent; presence or absence of the vas, and any thickening or nodularity of the vasa; thickening of the spermatic cord and presence and grade of any varicocele; any penile abnormality which may affect intercourse or deposition of semen.

It is a good practice to examine men with normal semen parameters to develop a feel for the normal, so that the abnormal can be detected with greater confidence. *An ultrasound study is not a substitute for a proper physical examination.*

INVESTIGATIONS

Semen Analysis

This is the first and most vital step in assessing male fertility potential. However, there are some very important points to bear in mind:

- Semen analysis is very operator dependent. The same sample may be reported very divergently. Hence, it is important to have a semen test done at a laboratory that has properly trained technicians. Most laboratories merely quote the World Health Organization parameters but do not follow the prescribed methodology.[2]
- Correct interpretation of the report is important. The latest norms have been revised but many clinicians and pathologists continue to refer to old norms resulting in a wrong diagnosis.
- Even a properly done and correctly interpreted, semen report is only a rough predictor of a man's fertility potential since eventually it is only one normal sperm that is required to produce a pregnancy, and often a young fertile wife can compensate for a subfertile male. On the other hand, seemingly normal semen may still be infertile due to subtle physiological defects that are not evident in the routine semen test. Thus, there is a significant overlap between the semen parameters of fertile and infertile men.[3]
- Hence, the semen report must be interpreted in conjunction with the "trying time." A couple who has been trying since only a short period of time still has a good chance of a natural conception despite a poor semen report, while a couple who has been trying since a long time probably have a sperm or egg defect despite seemingly normal reports and is likely to need assisted reproductive technology (ART).[4]

Hormone Tests

Not all infertile men need hormone testing, nor are all tests indicated. If the count is over 10 million/mL the hormone profile will be normal and testing is not required. If the count is less than 10 million/mL then an assay of total testosterone and follicle-stimulating hormone (FSH) should be asked for [guidelines of the American Urology Association (AUA)].[5] If testosterone is in the upper half, it indicates adequate testicular stimulation and no hormone therapy is indicated. If FSH is high it indicates testicular failure and one would not expect significant improvement in semen after treatment. Luteinizing hormone (LH) is relevant if testosterone is low. Unlike in women, elevated prolactin is usually not the cause of male infertility; its greater impact is on libido and erection; mild elevations are common, but are not of significance. Hence, routine prolactin assay is not indicated. Thyroid-stimulating hormone (TSH) can be assayed to screen for hypothyroidism, and recent reports suggest that detecting low levels of vitamin D3 may be relevant.[6]

Sonographic Evaluation

Scrotal sonography is *not* recommended as a test to be performed routinely in the evaluation of an infertile male. In most cases a good clinical examination will pick up all relevant findings. Sonography is then done only to confirm a clinical diagnosis of varicocele or some other relevant finding. The AUA *Practice Guidelines*[5] recommend scrotal sonograpahy only "in those patients in whom physical examination of the scrotum is difficult or inadequate or in whom a testicular mass is suspected."

Many gynecologists are not comfortable examining the male genitalia and rely on a scrotal ultrasound instead. This is not a good practice because:

- Some physical findings are not picked up on ultrasound.
- The relevance of many ultrasound findings has to be correlated with the clinical picture. For example, since treating a subclinical varicocele is not beneficial, an ultrasound-detected varicocele in the absence of a clinical varicocele is not relevant.

Transrectal ultrasound (TRUS) is indicated in cases of azoospermia or severe oligoasthenospermia (OAS) associated with low volume ejaculate (<1 mL) to look for ejaculatory duct obstruction which may be amenable to surgical correction.

Antisperm Antibody Testing

Antisperm antibodies (ASA) can affect sperm motility, cervical mucus penetration, acrosome reaction or fertilization. Despite this, testing for ASA is controversial. The National Institute for Health and Care Excellence *(NICE) guidelines* do not recommend ASA testing since "the significance of ASA is unclear and the effectiveness of systemic corticosteroids is uncertain."[7]

In practice, ASA testing has lost clinical relevance since most centers routinely proceed to IUI, and then intracytoplasmic sperm injection (ICSI), and ICSI results are unaffected by the presence of ASA. Further, the test routinely performed in most laboratories in India for detecting ASA is an enzyme-linked immunosorbent assay (ELISA) using the serum; this test is not relevant because it is only the antibodies attached to sperm that affect fertility, and serum titers do not correlate with seminal ASA. Further, the ELISA test detects many antigens which are not on the sperm surface, and hence are not relevant.

The recommended test for ASA is the IBT (Immunobead test) or the MAR (mixed agglutination reaction) test, both of which directly identify antibodies attached to the sperm.

Sperm DNA Integrity Testing

Damaged sperm DNA is common in men with infertility and high levels can cause impaired fertilization as well as increased pregnancy loss.[8] Hence testing for sperm DNA fragmentation is often advised for couples with idiopathic infertility, poor or failed fertilization or recurrent IVF failure. It may also help decide about the need for surgery in men with large varicoceles but normal conventional semen parameters.

A variety of tests are available and results do not always correlate between tests.[9] Also, the routine use of sperm DNA testing is still controversial. Thus, the British Fertility Society guidelines state that there is "no consensus on the best testing procedures, clinical reference values, and how patients with an adverse result should be managed."[10]

Genetic Tests

An increasing number of genetic causes of male infertility are being continuously identified and in future a complete genetic profile, combined with proteonomic profiling may revolutionize our evaluation of the infertile male. Currently, however, only a few genetic studies are recommended in clinical practice.[11] Men with nonobstructive azoospermia should undergo karyotyping for chromosomal numerical disorders and polymerase chain reaction (PCR) to detect microdeletions on the long arm of the Y chromosome (Yq micro-deletions). Men with vas aplasia need to be assessed for cystic fibrosis transmembrane conductance regulator (CFTR) gene mutations that are related to cystic fibrosis. In cases of recurrent pregnancy loss, karyotyping to look for chromosomal translocations may be helpful.

Other Specialized Tests

These include a variety of sperm function tests, computer-assisted semen analysis (CASA), and measurement of reactive oxygen species (ROS) in the semen. While these are useful research tools, they do not add to the clinical management of the infertile male and, hence, the American Society for Reproductive Medicine (ASRM) guidelines do not recommend these as part of routine evaluation.[12]

CONCLUSION

Whenever a woman presents for assessment of her fertility it is important to simultaneously assess the male partner. All too often the woman is investigated in great detail before a semen test is asked for, only to then discover that the male is azoospermic! Basic evaluation of the male should include a medical and sexual history, a clinical examination, and a semen analysis. Further evaluation through specific investigations should be individualized to each case. Use of a battery of investigations in every case through a "male infertility panel" is frequently a waste of resources.

REFERENCES

1. Shah R. Ejaculatory Failure. In: Rao KA, Carp H, Fischer R (Eds). Principles & Practice of Assisted Reproductive Technology. Vol. 2. New Delhi: Jaypee Brothers; 2014. pp. 911-4.
2. World Health Organization. (2010). WHO Laboratory Manual for the Examination and Processing of Human Semen (5th edition). [online] WHO website. Available from http://www.who.int/reproductivehealth/publications/infertility/9789241547789/en/ [Accessed October 2018].
3. Guzick DS, Overstreet JW, Factor-Litvak P, et al. Sperm morphology, motility, and concentration in fertile and infertile men. N Engl J Med. 2001;345(19):1388-93.
4. Hargreave TB, Elton RA. Is conventional sperm analysis of any use? Br J Urol. 1983;55:774-9.
5. AUA Male Infertility Panel. (2011). The optimal evaluation of the infertile male: Best practice statement reviewed and validity confirmed 2011. [online] AUA website. Available from https://www.auanet.org/guidelines/male-infertility-optimal-evaluation-(reviewed-and-validity-confirmed-2011) [Accessed October 2018].
6. Dabrowski FA, Grzechocinska B, Wielgos M. The role of vitamin D in reproductive health: A Trojan Horse or the Golden Fleece? Nutrients. 2015;7(6):4139-53.
7. National Institute for Health and Care Excellence (2013). Fertility problems: assessment and treatment. (NICE Clinical Guideline No. 156). Retrieved from https://www.nice.org.uk/guidance/cg156/chapter/recommendations#investigation-of-fertility-problems-and-management-strategies.
8. Zini A, Boman JM, Belzile E, et al. Sperm DNA damage is associated with an increased risk of pregnancy loss after IVF and ICSI: Systematic review and meta-analysis. Hum Reprod. 2008;23:2663-8.
9. Cissen M, Wely MV, Scholten I, et al. Measuring sperm DNA fragmentation and clinical outcomes of medically assisted reproduction: A systematic review and meta-analysis. PLoS One. 2016;11(11):e0165125.
10. Tomlinson M, Lewis S, Morroll D, et al. Sperm quality and its relationship to natural and assisted conception: British Fertility Society guidelines for practice. Hum Fertil (Camb). 2013;16:175-93.
11. Hotaling J, Carrell DT. Clinical genetic testing for male factor infertility: Current applications and future directions. Andrology. 2014;2:339-50.
12. Practice Committee of the American Society for Reproductive Medicine. (2014). Diagnostic evaluation of the infertile male: A committee opinion. Available from https://www.asrm.org/globalassets/asrm/asrm-content/news-and-publications/practice-guidelines/for-non-members/diagnostic_evaluation_of_the_infertile_male_a_committee_opinion-noprint.pdf [Assessed on October 2018].

CHAPTER

9

Role of Semen Analysis in Understanding Fertility Potential

Sayali Palnitkar, Irene Rubio Palacios, Javier Herrero

HISTORY/BACKGROUND

Semen analysis basically has a long history. In the 19th century, presence or absence of spermatozoa was only identified in cervical mucus samples from postcoital tests. By 1929, a recognizable predecessor of semen analysis was reported as a quantitative test in a medical journal.[1]

In 1965, World Health Organization (WHO) developed a human reproduction unit. In 1980 development and research in human reproduction (HRP) published the 1st edition of WHO Semen Manual with the intention not only to facilitate male contraceptive studies, but also to improve and standardize male infertility investigations.

The manual also defines standards to exclude influences such as the health of the patient over the previous spermatogenic cycle; duration of sexual abstinence, and temperature. The manual has been periodically updated since then (1992, 1999, and 2010).[2]

A basic semen analysis is still the most important test in male infertility investigation, as per the current criteria set by WHO in last two decades.[3]

SEMEN ANALYSIS

Evaluation of Male Fertility by Semen Analysis

Semen is mainly composed of spermatozoa and secretion from testis and epididymis (seminal fluid). Sperm (Fig. 1) consists of head, where genetic material is covered by the acrosome, the mid piece, with mitochondria, and tail (flagellum and principle piece) with microtubules forming the axoneme enclosed by a fibrous sheath, which helps in the progressive motion of the sperm.[4]

Seminal fluid is not essential for fertility as sperm taken from the vas deferens can also fertilize the oocyte. However, the fluid plays an important role in transportation and acts as a source of energy in their journey. Similarly, the seminal fluid helps to buffer the pH against the acidity of the vaginal fluid and also contains reducing agents which prevent the formation of toxic-free oxide radicals (Table 1). Seminal plasma transports sperms and also white blood cells, infective agents too (e.g., HIV, Hepatitis B).[5]

The variable morphology of human spermatozoa makes its assessment difficult but observations on spermatozoa recovered from the female reproductive tract, especially in postcoital endocervical mucus and also from the surface of the zona pellucida, have helped to define the

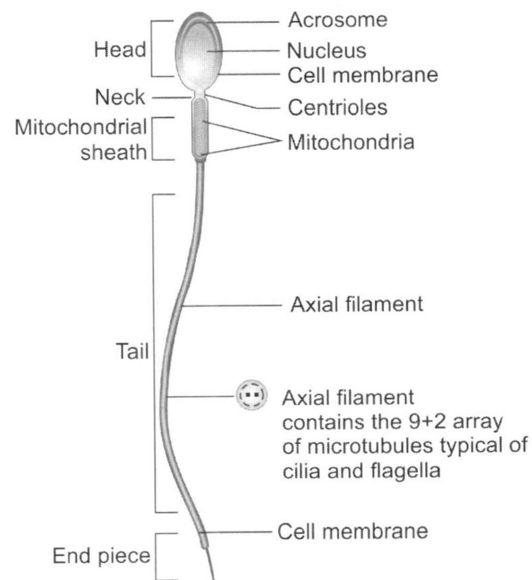

Fig. 1: Structure of sperm.

Table 1: Composition of semen.[5]

Parameters	*Reference range*
Volume	2–6 mL
Sperm concentration ($x10^6$)	50–150
Sodium (mM)	43–112
Potassium (mM)	14–28
Calcium (mM)	5–7
Chlorine (mM)	28–56
Fructose (mM)	2–33
Glucose (mM)	0.4
Inositol (mM)	3–3.5
Citric acid	5.2–7.3
Glycerophosphocholine (mM)	2–3.3
Phosphocholine (mM)	14–21
Acid phosphatase (mM)	2470

appearance of potentially fertilizing (morphologically normal) spermatozoa. To this day, controversy persists as to what constitutes the "normal" spermatozoa in semen, as normal and "pathologic" forms coexist in the semen samples.[6] However, it seems clear that factors such us obesity or lifestyle impact semen quality and fertility potential negatively.

By the strict application of certain criteria of sperm morphology, relationship between the percentage of normal forms and various fertility endpoints [time-to-pregnancy (TTP), pregnancy rates in vivo and in vitro] have been established, which may be useful for the prognosis of fertility.

Sperm velocity assessment often presents a high grade of subjectivity. There has been a time trend toward the simplification of the assessment paying more attention to the proportion of progressively motile sperm rather than the type of motility making it also more objective.[7]

Routine Semen Analysis

Routine semen examination composed of an analysis of physical characteristics as well as macroscopic and microscopic parameters. Prior to the analysis, the sample has to be collected and then liquefied as described below.

Collection of the Sample

Sample should be collected in sterile container after a minimum of 2 days and a maximum of 7 days of sexual abstinence. If additional samples are required, the number of days of sexual abstinence should be as constant as possible at each visit.

Liquefaction

Immediately after collection, semen is a semisolid coagulated mass. As liquefaction progresses it becomes more homogeneous and watery. It may take 15–60 minutes for a sample to liquefy completely. Sample may contain jelly-like bodies (gelatinous bodies) which will not liquefy and they do not have any clinical significance on the analysis.

Macroscopic Parameters[8]

Viscosity

It can be measured by gently aspirating it in wide-bored (1.5 mm diameter) plastic disposable pipettes. Semen should be dropped by gravity and the thread length observed. If the thread length is more than 2 mm, semen is marked as an abnormal sample.

Semen volume: Lower reference limit for normal semen sample is 1.5 mL.

pH: Normal semen sample should have a PH of 6–10 after liquefaction.

Microscopic Parameters

While the aforementioned variables are easily measured, the microscopic parameters present a certain level of subjectivity associated to the observer. The microscopic attributes of the seminal fluid include sperm concentration, motility, and morphology.[3]

Sperm Concentration

Sperm concentration is defined as the total number of spermatozoa per milliliter of sample in the ejaculate. The consistency in the measurement of sperm concentration and semen volume will give precision in calculating sperm output. It is considered as a biomarker for male infertility. Due to the considerable variation described in human semen ejaculates, it is advisable to analyze more than one sample before giving a diagnosis. Interestingly, there have been described geographic differences in the sperm concentration across different countries.[9]

Motility

Sperm motility can be defined as the concentration of progressively motile sperm in the ejaculate. Sperm motility within semen should be assessed as soon as possible after liquefaction of the sample but in any case after 1 hour following ejaculation, to limit the deleterious effects of dehydration, pH, or changes in temperature on motility.

Most of the systems for grading motility are based on the distinction between progressively or non-progressively motile spermatozoa from those that are immotile:

- *Progressive motility (PR)*: Spermatozoa moving actively, either linearly or in a large circle, regardless of speed.
- *Non-progressive motility (NP)*: All other patterns of motility with an absence of progression, e.g. swimming in small circles, the flagellar force hardly displacing the head, or when only a flagellar beat can be observed.
- *Immotility (IM):* No movement.

Motility is directly related to the fertilizing ability of the sample.

Methodology for Sperm Concentration and Motility

Different procedures can be used to get precision in counting and also in morphology prediction. Motility is calculated on visual basis under the microscope and quantified as a:

- Percentage motile
- Progressively motile
- Spermatozoa with no motility

Motility can be calculated using different counting chambers. Some chambers such as the *Makler chamber* is the most preferred which can count sperm concentration and their motility simultaneously but on the *Neubauer chamber*, only the sperm concentration can be calculated (Table 2).

Makler Chamber

Sample is analyzed after liquefaction, viscosity should be broken so that it will not interfere with the count and motility judgment.

This is done by placing the last drop contained in the syringe in the center of the disc area of the *Makler chamber*, otherwise a Pasteur pipette can be also used. Grasp the cover glass with your fingers opposite the black dots and immediately place the cover glass on the four pins. Press gently, looking again for the appearance of the color fringes. The drop will get spread on the entire area of the disc into a thickness of 10 microns; depth of the *Makler chamber* is 0.010 mm. Some surplus volume does not interfere with proper analysis as long as the tips are not flooded.

Evaluation is done using ×20 objective. The ×10 objective is not recommended because sperm will be seen too small. Never use a ×40 objective with the *Makler chamber*, the cover glass may get damaged while trying to focus. Even while using the proper ×20 objective, take care not to press on the cover glass. The image is usually seen clear when the tip of the objective is about 1 mm above the surface (Fig. 2).

After the sperms are brought into focus, adjust the chamber so that the grid lines will appear in vertical and horizontal position. If during the search of the sperm, sample is not spread uniformly or there is some blurring in the same focal plane, the loading procedure has to be repeated from the beginning.

Neubauer Chamber

Analysis of low count samples is challenging and should be handled carefully. To reduce human error in the analysis it is advisable to use a different counting chamber (*Neubauer chamber*), (Fig. 2) especially designed for low concentration cell samples (WHO). The sample needs to be diluted due to which motility cannot be assessed and the dilution factor has to be considered for the final calculation of the concentration.

Table 2: Comparison of counting chambers.[8]

Criteria	Neubauer hemocytometer	Makler chamber
Use	Count sperm concentration	Count and motility of sperm
Depth	100 µL	10 µL
Grid pattern	3 mm × 3 mm pattern of gridlines etched on the glass surface. Each counting area is divided into 1 mm × 1 mm grids	The grid is subdivided into 100 squares each of 0.1 × 0.1 mm.
Accuracy	Less accurate because motility and count is done separately	More accurate motility and count done simultaneously
Image	(Ref. www.mtg-de.com)	(Ref. www.micropticsl.com)

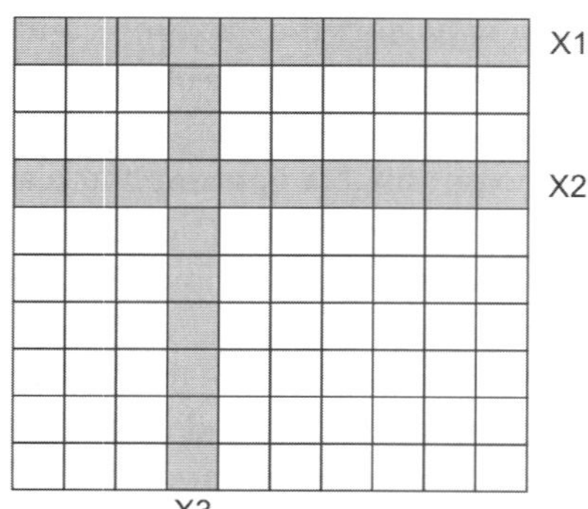

Fig. 2: Makler chamber grid.

Determination of the Concentration and Motility by Using the Makler Chamber

The concentration can be calculated by counting the sperm contained within a strip of 10 squares of the grid (Fig. 2). This number represents their concentration in millions per mL. The count should be repeated in another strip or two so that the count is representative even if the distribution of the sample in the counting chamber were uneven. In the case of oligospermic samples, it is suggested to count sperm in the entire grid area.

Likewise, the motility can be determined in the same way. By counting all motile sperm (progressively motile) contained within a strip of 10 squares of the grid, the percentage that the motile sperm represents from the total number contained in the same strip/s can be estimated. Again, the counting should be repeated in another strip or two to determine the average and for low count samples the entire grid area should be considered.

Morphology

Morphology refers to the analysis of the appearance of the different parts of the sperm: Head, neck, and tail.

Morphology is usually observed after staining a smear of ejaculate under microscope oil immersion lens. Preferably, two or more smears should be made from the fresh semen sample so that the assessment is performed in replicate since there may be significant slide variation in sperm morphology. Details are covered in the section below (Fig. 3).

Head Defects

The main head-related defects are large or small, tapered, pyriform, round, amorphous, vacuolated (more than two vacuoles or >20% of the head area occupied by unstained vacuolar areas), vacuoles in the postacrosomal region, small or large acrosomal areas (<40% or >70% of the head area), and double heads.

Neck and Midpiece Defects

Asymmetrical insertion of the midpiece into the head, thick or irregular, sharply bent, and abnormally thin neck are the most common defects affecting this structure.

Principal Tail Defects

Tail defects include short, multiple, broken, smooth hairpin bends, sharply angulated bends, irregular width and coiled tails.

Excess Residual Cytoplasm (ERC)

This is associated with abnormal spermatozoa produced from a defective spermatogenic process. Spermatozoa characterized by large amounts of irregularly stained cytoplasm, one third or more of the sperm head size, often associated with defective midpieces are abnormal.[10]

Different kinds of sperm malformations are observed in the semen sample, mostly due to defective spermiogenesis and some epididymal pathologies. Usually abnormal sperm lowers the fertilization potential; it is also observed that the increase in DNA fragmentation is associated with morphological defects. Normal spermatozoa can be defined as sperm without any morphological defects, present in the ejaculate (Fig. 4).

Cut-off Reference Values and Classification of Semen Samples

All the aforementioned microscopic parameters have a lower reference value for the sample to be considered as normal. These values are referred to as cut-off values. As shown in Table 3, WHO has periodically updated the cut-off values, incorporating a significantly general decrease over the years.

Taking into account the parameters described above and the set cut-off values, the WHO has also established a diagnostic classification of semen samples (Table 4).

Limitation of Semen Analysis

By early 1980s, Mortimer and his colleagues were apprehensive about the relationship between different variables in semen analysis and concept of quality control in semen analysis.[12] Both practical experience and theoretical knowledge is helpful in raising the skills of laboratory personnel in relation to semen analysis.[12] In most of the places, semen analysis is used as a biomarker to predict male fertility potential. Semen analysis is not a test of fertility since it provides no information regarding functionality of the spermatozoa to fertilize an ovum due to which it

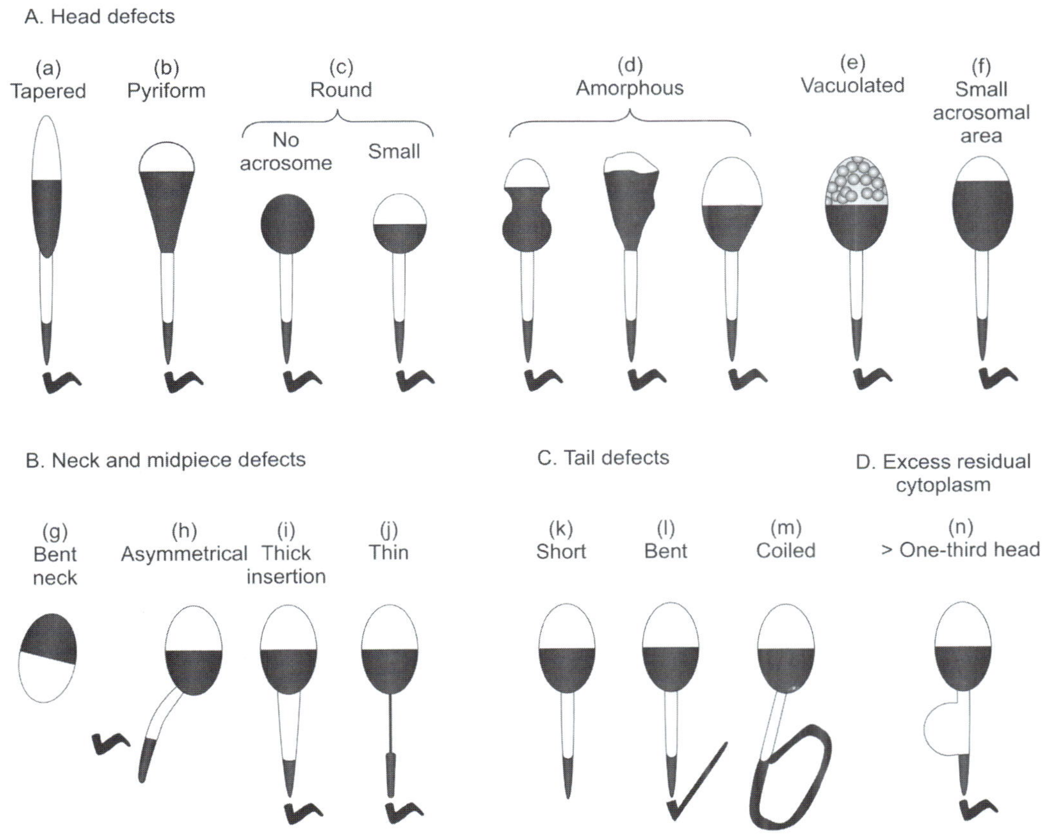

Fig. 3: Abnormal forms of human spermatozoa.[8]

cannot be considered as a direct measure of fertility.[11] There are some IVF techniques designed to select normal sperm like physiological intracytoplasmic sperm injection (PICSI) which is based on the binding of mature sperm to hyaluronic acid or magnetic activated cell sorting (MACS), based on the binding of apoptotic sperm to certain proteins.

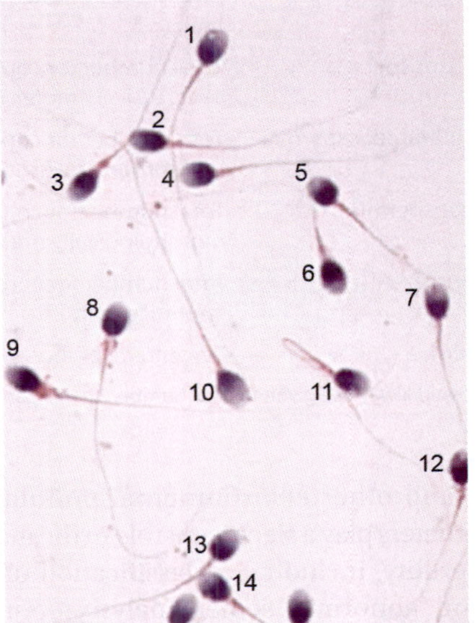

Fig. 4: Normal sperm.[8]

Controversies

There is a complex relationship between semen analysis and pregnancy outcome. In order to help in calculating the relative male fertility, WHO has established evidence-based thresholds as a reference. However, clinicians still depend on the semen analysis report to decide treatment for the patient. Interestingly, for the first time WHO 2010 has indicated reference values for semen analysis, are inclusive of analysis of healthy fertile men with known TTP (time to pregnancy); where earlier manual had values from fertile males but unknown TTP. TTP is defined as months (or cycles) from stopping contraception to achieving pregnancy, which is analyzed.[7,8]

It is worth mentioning that the adoption of the new WHO reference values[8] may lead more men to be classified as "fertile" as compared with the 1999 WHO reference values, which raises the question mark on how 2010 WHO reference threshold would affect current infertility practices. Some authors claim that those lower reference thresholds result from declining sperm counts caused by endocrine

Table 3: Cut-off reference values for semen characteristics as published in consecutive World Health Organization (WHO) manuals.[11]

Semen characteristics	*WHO 1980*	*WHO 1987*	*WHO 1992*	*WHO 1999*	*WHO 2010*
Volume (mL)	-	≥2	≥2	≥2	1.5
Sperm count (x 10^6/mL)	20–200	≥20	≥20	≥20	15
Total sperm count (10^6)	-	≥40	≥40	≥40	39
Sperm motility (% motile)	≥60	≥50	≥50	≥50	40
Progressively motile	≥2	≥25	≥25	≥25	32
Vitality (% alive)	-	≥50	≥75	≥75	58
Morphology (% normal forms)	80.5	≥50	≥30	14^5	4^8
Leukocyte (10^6/mL)	≤4.7	≤1.0	≤1.0	≤1.0	≤1.0

Table 4: Classification of semen samples.

Aspermia	No semen (no or retrograde ejaculation)
Asthenozoospermia	Percentage of progressively motile (PR) spermatozoa below the lower reference limit
Asthenoteratozoospermia	Percentages of both progressively motile (PR) and morphologically normal spermatozoa below the lower reference limits
Azoospermia	No spermatozoa in the ejaculate (given as the limit of quantification for the assessment method employed)
Cryptozoospermia	Spermatozoa absent from fresh preparations but observed in a centrifuged pellet
Hemospermia (hematospermia)	Presence of erythrocytes in the ejaculate
Leukospermia (leukocytospermia, pyospermia	Presence of leukocytes in the ejaculate above the threshold value
Necrozoospermia	Low percentage of live, and high percentage of immotile, spermatozoa in the ejaculate
Normozoospermia	Total number (or concentration, depending on outcome reported)* of spermatozoa, and percentages of progressively motile (PR) and morphologically normal spermatozoa, equal to or above the lower reference limits
Oligoasthenozoospermia	Total number (or concentration, depending on outcome reported)* of spermatozoa, and percentage of progressively motile (PR) spermatozoa, below the lower reference limits
Oligoasthenoteratozoospermia	Total number (or concentration, depending on outcome reported)* of spermatozoa, and percentages of both progressively motile (PR) and morphologically normal spermatozoa, below the lower reference limits
Oligoteratozoospermia	Total number (or concentration, depending on outcome reported)* of spermatozoa, and percentage of morphologically normal spermatoza, below the lower reference limits
Oligozoospermia	Total number (or concentration, depending on outcome reported)* of spermatozoa below the lower reference limit
Teratozoospermia	Percentage of morphologically normal spermatozoa below the lower reference limit

*Preference should always be given to total number, as this parameter takes precedence over concentration.

disruption and other environmental pollutants. Thus, semen parameters play a significant role in the management of male infertility, including reclassification of patient in "normal" and "abnormal" semen analysis reports.

Implication of WHO Criteria

- *Declining male infertility:* As the values for semen parameters are lower in WHO 2010 than the values in previous manuals, it suggests a declining trend in male fertility.[7] These lower values indicate that either because of environmental factor male infertility is globally reduced or there is methodological bias created by different ways of data generation.
- *Referral for assessment of male partner decreases:* With application of new WHO Manual earlier classified abnormal male has become normal. There has to be an association of male and female age, to reproductive outcome so, male infertility counting should go beyond semen analysis, supplemented with clinical examination.

What Routine Semen Analysis Cannot Assess?

The standardized semen analysis allows comparison across laboratories, where they follow reference values which are set by studies on fertile males. Semen has three types of abnormalities.

1. Low sperm count
2. Low motility
3. Abnormal sperm morphology

Any one of this is a sign of male infertility but their normalcy does not guarantee a fertile sperm sample.[9]

Spermatozoa undergo many changes before they can fertilize an oocyte. In IVF, sperm mitochondria are important for calcium homeostasis and for control of reactive oxygen species. This is important for sperm to function normally. The process of capacitation involves generation of adenyl cyclase which activates protein kinase A. This results into phosphorylation of sperm protein tyrosin, enabling spermatozoa to acquire fertilization capacity.[9]

Spermatozoa penetrate cumulus without undergoing acrosome reaction. It must be coated with the sperm protein ADAM3 to allow passage through cumulus to bind to zona. For fertilization, it is important to have IZUM0 on sperm and CD9 on the oocytes.[13] The acquisition of sperm surface proteins which are required for zona binding cannot assessed by routine semen analysis. Thus, we cannot identify sperm which has an ability to fertilize an oocyte.

Sperm Functional Tests

Sperm function tests are not done regularly. If required then genetical testing can be done. There are some studies which demonstrated that sperm DNA damage and chromatin damage are associated with male infertility. Integrity of sperm is correlated with motility and sperm membrane characteristics.[14]

Sperm vitality test: The test assesses membrane integrity of sperm. It can be used for the routine samples, and is especially advised for samples with motility less than 40%. Test is assessed after complete liquefaction of the sample; this will help to avoid effect of dehydration and effect of temperature change on sperms. The stain used is Eosin-Nigrosin. There is advantage of Eosin-Nigrosin stain that contrast created in staining makes the assessment very easy. Observation is done with oil immersion lens. If limited part of head is stained then it is called as "leaky neck membrane." The lower reference limit for vitality (membrane-intact spermatozoa) is 58% (5th centile, 95% CI 55–63) (Fig. 5).[8]

Hypo-osmotic swelling: Normal spermatozoa swell within 5 minutes in hypo-osmotic solution and flagellar shapes are stabilized after 30 minutes. Swelling solutions contain sodium citrate dehydrate and fructose. The lower reference limit for vitality (membrane-intact spermatozoa) is 58% (5th centile, 95% CI 55–63).[8] This test is preferred when staining is not done, e.g. while selecting sperm for ICSI (Fig. 6).

Antisperm antibody assay: IgG and IgA are two antibodies that may be found in semen; they can be detected on sperm cells. There is indirect detection and direct detection of antibodies.

Tests for Antibodies on Spermatozoa (Direct Tests)

There are two direct tests. The mixed antiglobulin reaction (MAR) test and the immunobead (IB) test. The MAR test is performed on a fresh semen sample while the IB test uses washed spermatozoa. Polyacrylamide beads are used in the IB test, and in the MAR test, latex particles with a

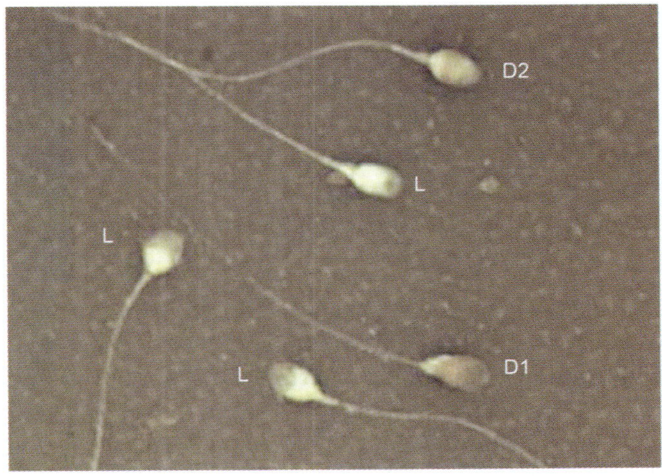

Fig. 5: Sperm vitality test: Staining of spermatozoa.[8] Spermatozoa with red (D1) or dark pink (D2) heads are considered dead (membrane-damaged), whereas spermatozoa with white heads (L) or light pink heads are considered alive (membrane-intact).

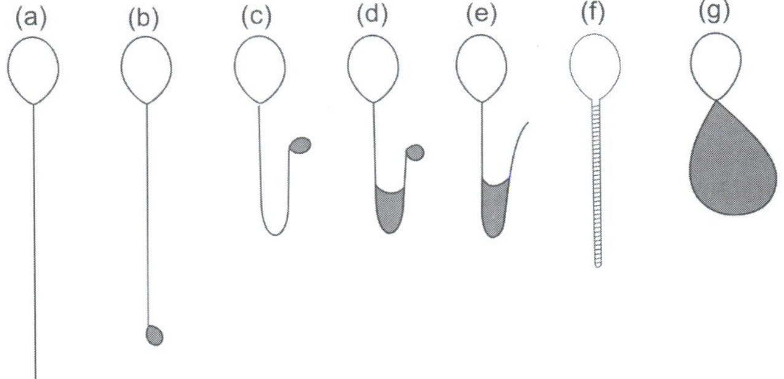

Fig. 6: Pictorial representation of human spermatozoa in the hypo-osmotic solution.[8] (a) No change. (b)-(g) various types of tail changes. Swelling in tail is indicated by the grey area.

uniform diameter of 2 μm are used. In the MAR test for immunoglobulin IgG, the particles are coated with IgG, and they do attach to the region of the spermatozoa where the antisperm antibodies are located. This attachment is obtained by adding strong and highly specific anti-IgG to the mixture of fresh, untreated spermatozoa, and latex beads. There are also sperm MAR tests for IgA and IgM.[15]

The MAR test using latex particles does not require preliminary separation of the spermatozoa, whereas the IB test requires washing the spermatozoa free of seminal plasma. As a result, the MAR test is easier and faster, and it requires less volume of ejaculate (10–12 μL). It can also be applied in semen samples with a lower motile sperm concentration than the IB test. While comparing both tests MAR test is more accurate than IB test. Also, the sperm MAR test for IgA detects only secretory IgA in semen, whereas the IB test sometimes reacts with nonsecretory IgA present in serum.[15]

The experimental protocols for the IB and MAR tests vary, but for both the sperm bead preparation is examined with a microscope. The beads adhere to the motile and immotile spermatozoa that have surface-bound antibodies; the percentage of motile spermatozoa with bound beads is recorded.[15]

Tests for Antisperm Antibodies in Sperm-free Fluids ("Indirect" Test)

In these tests, the diluted, heat-inactivated fluid suspected of containing antisperm antibodies (ASAs) is incubated with antibody-free donor spermatozoa that have been washed free of seminal fluid. Any ASAs in the suspect fluid will bind specifically to the donor spermatozoa, which are then assessed in a direct test, as above.[8]

Sperm Chromatin Integrated Assay

Limitation of semen analysis led to the investigation of sperm DNA damage as one of the markers for male subfertility. In recent studies, sperm DNA damage testing has shown its association with decreased fertilization, slow early embryonic development, reduced implantation, and miscarriages.[16,17] In somatic cells, DNA is associated with histones in organizational units called nucleosomes, whereas in sperm these histones are replaced by protamines. Fully protaminated sperm DNA is highly stable and resistant to damage, but deficiencies in protamination results in poorly compacted DNA, prone to damage.[18]

Variety of different tests is available to measure sperm DNA damage, where each tests analyses slightly different aspects of DNA damage (*see* Table 1).

- Indirect tests:
  - Sperm chromatin dispersion (SCD/Halo)[19]
  - Sperm chromatin structure assay (SCSA).[20]
- Direct tests:
  - The Comet assay[21]
  - The TUNEL assay.[22]

Benefits of Sperm DNA Testing

Incorporation of new tests into clinical care can help to avoid loss of biological time along with cost of failed cycles. There is significant increase in miscarriages in the patient with high DNA fragmentation observed, if compared with patient with low DNA fragmentation.[23]

Limitation of Sperm DNA Testing

The prime limitation for DNA testing assays is, the "tested sperm" becomes unacceptable for clinical use. To overcome this problem some noninvasive tests are established and their correlation with DNA damage is assessed (Table 5).[16]

Reactive Oxygen Species

Oxidative stress (OS) occurs when reactive oxygen species (ROS) offset the concentration of antioxidants in human serum. Physiologically ROS are important for sperm maturation as they undergo capacitation, hyper-activation, acrosome reaction and oocyte fusion.[24] WHO has recognized OS as vital parameter in male infertility.[8]

Reactive oxygen species are oxygen-based chemical reactive molecules that are kept at an equilibration with antioxidant in the system called a redox system.[25,26] When excessive amounts of ROS are produced or when antioxidant activity fails, this redox system is disrupted, resulting in a state of OS, which can result in lipid peroxidation, DNA damage and aggravated apoptosis.[27]

Measurement of Oxidation-Reduction Potential (ORP)

Galvanostat-based technology is used to measure ORP. A 30 μL sample suspension is loaded on the sample port of the sensor. The test starts when the sample fills the reference electrode, thereby completing the electrochemical circuit. After a short period, the sORP values, in millivolts (mV), are displayed on the screen. A higher sORP level indicates an imbalance in the activity of all available oxidants relative to all available antioxidants in the seminal ejaculate—a state of OS (Table 6).[28]

Table 5: Tests to measure DNA damage.

Assay	*Method of detection*	*Advantages*	*Disadvantages*
Sperm chromatin dispersion (SCD)/Halo[19]	Sperm loaded in agarose, denatured in acid solution, stained and observed with fluorescence microscopy for chromatin dispersion/halos. Sperm with non-dispersed chromatin (i.e. small halos) have fragmented DNA. Interpreted as percentage of sperm with non-dispersed chromatin.	Commercial assay available Interpretation does not depend on fluorescence or flow cytometry.	Indirect assay only detects ssDNA breaks. Involves acid denaturation.
Sperm chromatin structure assay (SCSA)[20]	Acid denaturation, then staining with acridine orange and measurement with flow cytometer. Green-staining sperm have intact DNA while red-staining sperm have denatured DNA. Interpreted as percentage of red-staining sperm (denatured sperm).	Has extensive body of literature and established clinical thresholds. Can be performed in fresh or frozen samples.	Proprietary protocol with no commercial assay available. Indirect assay only detects ssDNA breaks. Involves acid denaturation.
Comet Assay[21]	With gel electrophoresis, fragmented DNA forms tail while intact DNA stays in head. Can be performed in alkaline or neutral conditions. Tail size correlates to amount of DNA fragmentation within individual spermatozoon. Interpreted as mean amount of DNA damage per individual spermatozoon.	Requires small number of sperm cells. Direct assay can examine damage at level of individual spermatozoon. Can detect multiple types of DNA fragmentation.	No established standardized protocol. Time and labor intensive. Requires fresh semen sample.
TUNEL Assay[22]	Labeled nucleotide added to sites of DNA fragmentation with subsequent fluorescence measured by flow cytometry or fluorescence microscopy. Fluorescent sperm have fragmented DNA. Interpreted as percentage of fluorescent sperm.	Direct assay. Commercial assay available. Can be performed in fresh or frozen samples. Detects ssDNA and dsDNA breaks.	No established standardized protocol. Variable clinical thresholds in literature.

Table 6: List of some key findings on ORP and male infertility in clinical studies.

Study	*Findings*
Agarwal et al. (2016)[28]	ORP can be measured in semen and seminal plasma ORP measurements are stable up to 120 minutes Negative correlation between ORP and semen concentration/total sperm count regardless of fertility status
Agarwal et al. (2017)[29]	Elevated levels of ORP in infertile patients compared to those of controls Negative correlation between ORP and semen parameters (concentration, total sperm count, motility, and morphology) in all subjects ORP value of 1.3^6 mV/106 sperm/mL to distinguish fertile from infertile men Low intraobserver and interobserver variability
Agarwal et al. (2017)[30]	Elevated levels of ORP in abnormal semen parameters (of infertile patients) Sperm concentration and motility improves as ORP decreases ORP value of 2.59 mV/10^6 sperm/mL best predicts oligozoospermia A combination of ORP and at least 1 other abnormal semen parameter (especially concentration) is more robust in identifying OS than ORP alone
Agarwal et al. (2017)[31]	ORP is highly predictive of OZ and AZ samples regardless of fertility status. There is a weaker predictive value for TZ and OAT samples ORP is best at predicting OZ samples Elevated levels of ORP in all subgroups when compared to NZ samples A combination of ORP and two other abnormal semen parameters is more robust in identifying OS than ORP alone

Contd...

Contd...

(Agarwal et al. (2017)[25]	Collectively and individually between the Cleveland Clinic and Doha, Qatar, there were poorer semen parameters and higher ORP values present in infertile semen samples when compared to those of healthy controls. No significant differences between infertile groups in both data sets except progressive motility and morphology No significant differences between control groups in both data sets except morphology Elevated levels of ORP in abnormal semen groups ORP value of 1.42 mV/10^6 sperm/mL to distinguish fertile from infertile men
Arafa et al. (2018)[32]	ORP value of 1.38 mV/10^6 sperm/mL to distinguish normal from abnormal semen samples ORP value of 1.41 mV/10^6 sperm/mL to distinguish fertile from infertile men

(ORP: oxidation-reduction potential; OZ: oligozoospermic; AZ: asthenozoospermic; TZ: teratozoospermic; OAT: oligoasthenoteratozoospermic; NZ: normozoospermic)

FUTURE OF ANDROLOGY LABORATORY

Epidemiological data shows that 1:7 couples are reported as a subfertile couple and sperm dysfunction is a common cause of infertility that affects 1:15 men.[13]

Sperm functional tests show association with fertilization in vitro but none of the tests can predict consistently better TTP than sperm concentration and sperm morphology. The clinicians who are treating infertility patients can find out the type and severity of the problem with the male partner by means of semen analysis.[9,13]

However, the future of sperm functional tests will be to predict the success of fertilization in vitro and whether progeny will be normal. This may include epigenetics and deep sequencing studies. Sperms have small noncoding RNA defects and other subtle genetic abnormalities that may affect fertilization and outcome progeny.[9,13]

Further development in proteome will be able to identify proteins associated with the specific events in sperm function, even specific signaling complexes.[13]

Computer-assisted sperm analysis (CASA) is the upcoming technique used by some laboratories but unfortunately it is not standardized, and inadequate data is available to support its routine use. In CASA, sperm concentration between 2×10^6 per mL and 50×10^6 per mL can be measured. Samples with a sperm concentration higher than 50×10^6 per mL will need to be diluted.

CONCLUSION

Semen analysis plays a vital role in diagnosing infertility. The World Health Organization periodically releases manuals with guidelines to analyze semen and the multinational studies which predict globally changing fertility potential in males. The latest manual was published in 2010. Semen parameters within the reference values do not guarantee fertility nor do values outside limit imply infertility.

As the studies in epigenetics, proteomics and sequencing will develop, our understanding of sperm fertility will increase. This will help us to standardize procedures and parameters along with the reference values in the semen analysis.

With more powerful screening tools we will be able to design new tests which will enhance sperm function and can avoid unnecessary ART treatment.

SUMMARY

The chapter covers the importance of semen analysis in infertility treatment. Taking an overview of WHO manuals, and their changes in the reference values as time progresses, indicates decline in fertility potential globally. WHO manual also includes different functional tests and their use in understanding fertility potential of sperm. Development in epigenetics and proteomics will portrait powerful screening tools for sperm functioning and will define most suitable sperm with highest fertility potential.

REFERENCES

1. Handelsman DJ, Cooper TG. Foreword to Semen Analysis in 21st Century Medicine special issue in Asian Journal of Andrology. Asian J Androl. 2010;12:7-10.
2. Lewis SE. Is sperm evaluation useful in predicting human fertility? Reproduction. 2007;134:31-40.
3. Said TM, Agarwal A. Interpretation of basic semen analysis and advanced semen testing. Current Clinical Urology: Male Infertility: Problems and Solutions. Springer; 2011. pp. 15-22.
4. Wang C. How does semen analysis assist in understanding the reproductive status of the male? Handbook of Andrology, 2nd edition. USA: American Society of Andrology.
5. Fleming S, Cooke S. Textbook of Assisted Reproduction for Scientist in Reproductive Technology. Fertility Society of Australia. Australia: Vivid Publishing; 2008.
6. Nallella KP, Sharma RK, Aziz N, et al. Significance of sperm characteristics in the evaluation of male infertility. Fertil Steril. 2006;85:629-34.
7. Esteves SC, Agarwal A. Impact of the new WHO guidelines on diagnosis and practice of male infertility. Open Reprod Sci J. 2011;3:7-15.
8. WHO 2010. WHO Laboratory Manual for the Examination and Processing of Human Semen, 5th edition. Geneva: WHO; 2010.

9. Wang C, Swerdloff RS. Limitation of semen analysis as a test of male fertility and anticipated needs from newer tests. Fertil Steril. 2014;102(6):1502-7.
10. Mortimer D, Menkveld R. Sperm morphology assessment—historical perspectives and current opinions. J Androl. 2001;22:192-205.
11. Esteves SC. Clinical relevance of routine semen analysis and contraversies surrounding the 2010 World Health Organnisation criteria for semen examination. IBJU. 2014;40:443-53.
12. Jequier AM. Is quality assuarance in semen analysis still realy necessary? A clinician's view point. Hum Reprod. 2005;20:2039-42.
13. Lefièvre L, Bedu-Addo K, Conner SJ, et al. Counting sperm does not add up more: Time for a new euquation? Reproduction. 2007;133:675-84.
14. Zini A, Jamal W, Cowan L, et al. Is sperm DNA damage associated with IVF embryo quality? A systematic review. J Assist Reprod Genet. 2011;28(5):391-7.
15. Mahmoud A, Comhaire F. 2000. Debate: Antisperm antobodies, use of mixed aggultination reaction test using latex beads. Hum Reprod. 2000;15(2):231-3.
16. Sharif K, Lewis SEM. Sperm DNA fragmentation testing: To do or not to do? Middle East Fertil Soc J. 2013;18:78-83.
17. Lewis SE, John Aitken R, Conner SJ, et al. The impact of sperm DNA damage in assisted conception and beyond: Recent advances in diagnosis and treatment. Reprod Biomed Online. 2013;27(4):325-37.
18. Aitken RJ, De Iullis GN, McLachlan RI. 2009. Biological and clinical significance of DNA damage in the male germ line. Int J Androl. 2009;32:46-56.
19. Fernández JL, Muriel L, Goyanes V, et al. Simple determination of human sperm DNA fragmentation with an improved sperm chromatin dispersion test. Fertil Steril. 2005;84(4):833-42.
20. Evenson DP. Sperm chromatin structure assay (SCSA®) Methods Mol Biol. 2013;927:147-64.
21. Olive PL, Banáth JP. The comet assay: A method to measure DNA damage in individual cells. Nat Protoc. 2006;1(1):23-9.
22. Sharma R, Masaki J, Agarwal A. Sperm DNA fragmentation analysis using the TUNEL assay. Methods Mol Biol. 2013;927:121-36.
23. Robinson L, Gallos ID, Conner SJ, et al. The effect of sperm DNA fragmentation on miscarriage rates :a systematic review and meta-analysis. Hum Reprod. 2012;27(10):2908-17.
24. Aitken RJ. Reactive oxygen species as mediators of sperm capacitation and pathological damage. Mol Reprod Dev. 2017;84:1039-52.
25. Agarwal A, Arafa M, Chandrakumar R, et al. 2017a. A multicenter study to evaluate oxidative stress by oxidation-reduction potential, a reliable and reproducible method. Andrology. 2017a;5:939-45.
26. Agarwal A, Hamada A, Esteves SC. Insight into oxidative stress in varicocele-associated male infertility: Part 1. Nat Rev Urol.2012;9:678-90.
27. Agarwal A, Roychoudhury S, Sharma R, et al. Diagnostic application of oxidation-reduction potential assay for measurement of oxidative stress: Clinical utility in male factor infertility. Reprod Biomed Online. 2017;34(1):48-57.
28. Agarwal A, Sharma R, Roychoudhury S, et al. MiOXSYS: A novel method of measuring oxidation reduction potential in semen and seminal plasma. Fertil Steril. 2016;106:566-73.
29. Agarwal A, Roychoudhury S, Sharma R, et al. Diagnostic application of oxidation-reduction potential assay for measurement of oxidative stress: clinical utility in male factor infertility. Reprod Biomed Online. 2017;34:48-57.
30. Agarwal A, Wang SM. Clinical relevance of oxidation-reduction potential in the evaluation of male infertility. Urology. 2017;104:84-9.
31. Agarwal A, Henkel R, Sharma R, et al. Determination of seminal oxidation-reduction potential (ORP) as an easy and cost-effective clinical marker of male infertility. Andrologia. 2018;50(3).
32. Arafa M, Agarwal A, Al Said S, et al. Semen quality and infertility status can be identified through measures of oxidation-reduction potential. Andrologia. 2018;50(2).

CHAPTER

10

Role of Endoscopy in Infertility

PG Paul, Geetha R, Sumeetkaur Mehta, George Paul, Akila B

INTRODUCTION

Reproductive surgery involves procedures for correction of anatomical disorders of the reproductive tract to improve reproductive function. It made remarkable progress in the 1980s with refinements in the technique of laparoscopic surgery. In the 1990s, there was a dramatic improvement in the pregnancy rates in assisted reproductive technologies (ART) and this challenged the role of reproductive surgery. Since then several studies have tried to redefine the role of reproductive surgery in current practice. Reproductive surgery could be a primary treatment for infertility or, can be carried out to enhance ART outcome. Most commonly, reproductive surgeries are done for tubal disorders and endometriosis.

TUBAL SURGERIES

Tubal disease is responsible for 25–35% of female infertility and more than half of these are due to salpingitis.[1] In a study of 413 patients, Desai et al. found that 39% of damaged tubes in women with tubal infertility were caused by genital Koch's.[2]

Proximal Tubal Occlusion

Proximal tubal obstruction and occlusion account for 10–25% of tubal factor.[1] Proximal tubal occlusion diagnosed by hysterosalpingogram has high false positive rate up to 50% mostly due to spasm of uterotubal ostium.[3] True occlusions are relatively less common and are caused by fibrosis due to salpingitis isthmic nodosa (SIN), pelvic inflammatory disease (PID), or endometriosis.

Hysteroscopic tubal cannulation is a relatively simple treatment for functional proximal tubal occlusion. It offers a number of advantages over fluoroscopic-guided cannulation. It is performed under direct vision and any distal tubal disease can also be diagnosed as it is done along with laparoscopy. Commercially available hysteroscopic cannulation set like Modified Novy cornual cannulation set (Cook medical, Brisbane, Australia) is commonly used for cannulation. Hysteroscopy is performed with continuous flow hysteroscope with a 5/7 Fr operating channel and tubal ostia are identified. The transparent outer catheter, stabilized with a stiffening obturator is introduced through the operating channel. The obturator is removed, and an inner catheter with wire guide is passed till the soft tip is visible beyond the tip of the outer catheter. The outer catheter is now directed toward the ostium and the tip of the catheter is wedged into the tubal ostium. The inner catheter alone is now pushed into the ostium for 2–3 cm to negotiate the uterotubal junction and the isthmus of the tube (Fig. 1). A slight rotation or forward movement of the outer catheter helps in the cannulation process. Simultaneous laparoscopic observation and

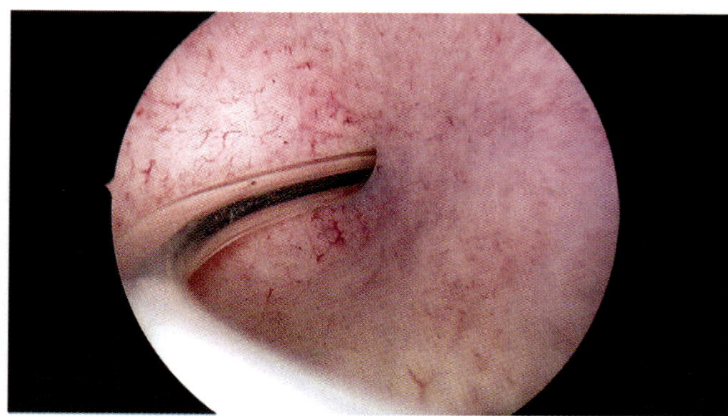

Fig. 1: Tubal cannulation with Novy's outer catheter and Terumo guidewire on the left side.

straightening of the tube with a laparoscopic grasper can help the cannulation. The wire guide is removed, and chromopertubation is done with dilute methylene blue dye. If spillage is observed, tubal patency is confirmed. We perform tubal cannulation with Novy's outer catheter and radifocus guidewire M (0.64 mm, Terumo Corporation, Japan) which is simpler and cost-effective. Tubal patency is confirmed by chromopertubation, after removing the hysteroscope (Fig. 2).

We had reported our experience of hysteroscopic cannulation in 31 cases (58 tubes) of proximal tubal obstruction.[4] At least one tube could be cannulated in 26 cases (83.9%). The associated distal tubal disease was present in three cases. Nine patients conceived after hysteroscopic cannulation. Five of these patients had associated pathologies. There were no ectopic pregnancies.

Considering the simplicity of the procedure, hysteroscopic cannulation should be tried as the first-line procedure for the proximal tubal block. If the procedure is not successful or pregnancy is not achieved, ART is recommended. Microsurgical tubocornual anastomosis is rarely performed in modern practice.

Tubal Anastomosis

Female sterilization is a prevalent method of birth control worldwide.[5] However, 2–13% of women develop poststerilization regret, and 1–3% seek tubal reanastomosis.[6] The treatment options available to these couples are either reversal procedures or ART. These patients are usually otherwise fertile and have good success with both procedures. Reversal of tubal ligation is achieved by opening the occluded ends of proximal and distal segments and anastomosing them with fine sutures using magnification and microsurgical techniques. Traditionally, tubal anastomosis has been done by open microsurgical techniques. A review on tubal anastomosis has shown that laparoscopic tubal anastomosis is equally effective as microsurgical procedures by laparotomy.[7]

Surgical Technique

The surgical procedure involves transection of the tubal stumps and removal of scar tissue, approximation of the mesosalpinx, anastomosis of the muscle and mucosa, and approximation of the serosal layer.

A 10 mm primary trocar is inserted through the umbilicus after creating pneumoperitoneum. Two ancillary 3 mm trocars lateral to the right and left epigastric vessels and a 5 mm median suprapubic trocar are inserted. The site of sterilization is identified and held with a fine grasper. Dilute vasopressin is injected into the mesosalpinx to reduce bleeding. A circular incision is made on the proximal segment about half a centimeter from the probable site of transection. The proximal segment is transected with scissors 5 mm distal to the serosal incision (Fig. 3). Any scarred portion is excised as it may lead to poor healing. Chromopertubation is done through the cervix to check the patency of the proximal segment (Fig. 4). The distal segment is also prepared in two layers similarly. The patency of the distal segment is also checked by chromopertubation from

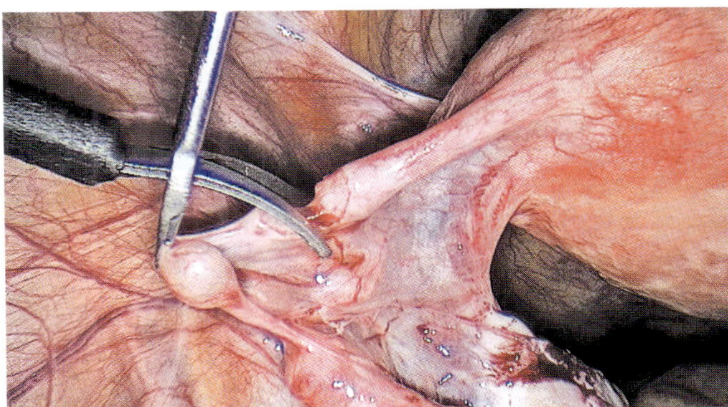

Fig. 3: Preparation of proximal segment of the tube in two layers with scissors.

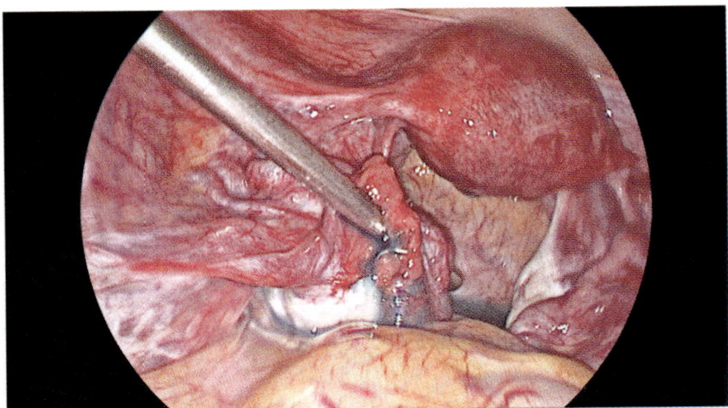

Fig. 2: Chromopertubation shows spill of dye at laparoscopy.

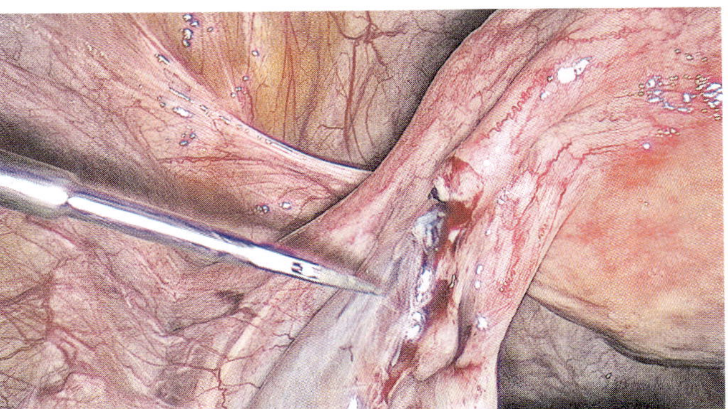

Fig. 4: Spill of dye from the transected proximal stump.

the proximal end with a chromopertubator ('KohUltramicro Series'™ Karl Storz, Tuttlingen, Germany). The anastomosis is then done by four 6-0 prolene sutures. The first suture is at 6 O'clock position (Fig. 5). The sutures are taken through the lumen ignoring the mucosa. 9 O'clock suture is then taken and tied as this is the most difficult to access location. 3 O'clock and then 12 O'clock sutures are taken and tied (Fig. 6). The serosa and mesosalpinx are then approximated with three or four interrupted 6-0 sutures and chromopertubation done to check integrity and patency (Figs. 7 and 8).

We have tried to simplify this suturing technique by using barbed sutures as they do not require knotting. Two separate 5-0 Quill barbed sutures (Angiotech Puerto Rico Inc, Aguadilla, Puerto Rico) are used in this technique. The first suture is used for taking 6 and 3 O' clock stitches. The second suture is used for taking 9 and 12 O'clock stitches. With this technique, the purse-string effect on the tubal lumen is reduced. This technique of laparoscopic tubal reanastomosis using barbed sutures is a simpler alternative to conventional suturing.[8]

Laparoscopic tubal anastomosis gives an intrauterine pregnancy rate of 60–80% and very low ectopic pregnancy rate of 1–6%.[9] Success rate mainly depends on the woman's age and the type of sterilization; Falope rings and clips give a higher success rate than Pomeroy's and other techniques. Two other prognostic factors associated with success of the procedure were tubal length and type of anastomosis.[10] Tubal anastomosis should not be considered if final tubal length is less than 4 cm, there are significant tuboovarian adhesions or stage 3–4 endometriosis, and/or more than a mild male factor.

It is difficult to compare ART with tubal surgery since the probability of an in vitro fertilization (IVF) pregnancy is limited by the number of cycles performed. It allows women to conceive naturally and is, therefore, an option for couples with ethical and religious concerns. More than one pregnancy is also possible with tubal surgery. ART is much costlier than tubal surgery, and many patients cannot afford this treatment. Risks of tubal surgery are very low. So, laparoscopic tubal anastomosis should be offered for younger patients with good prognostic factors.

Salpingo-ovariolysis

Pelvic adhesions involving tubes and ovaries can impair ovum pickup mechanism. Laparoscopic salpingo-ovariolysis is preferred for mild to moderate pelvic

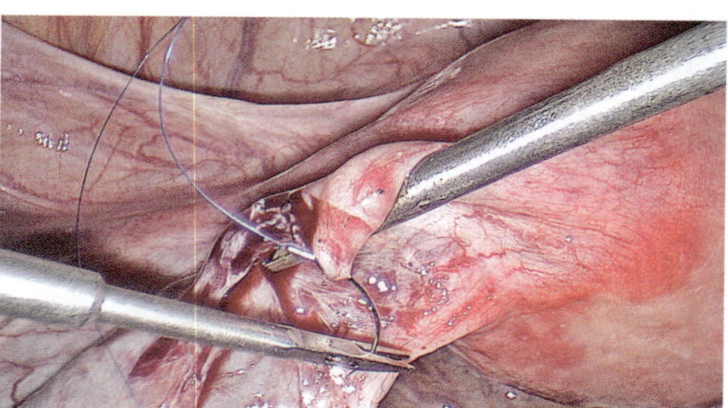

Fig. 5: Six O' clock suture.

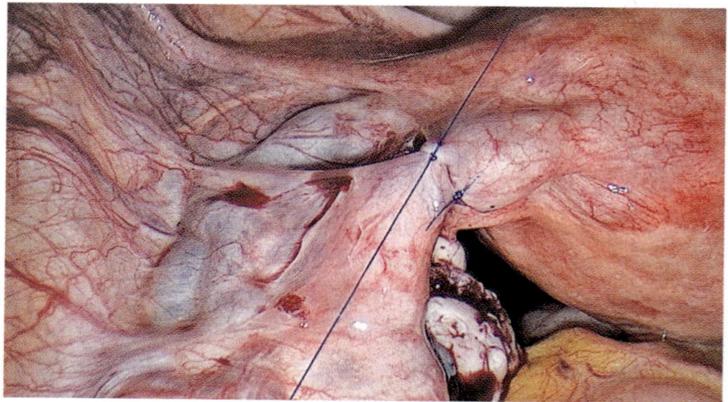

Fig. 7: Seromuscular sutures.

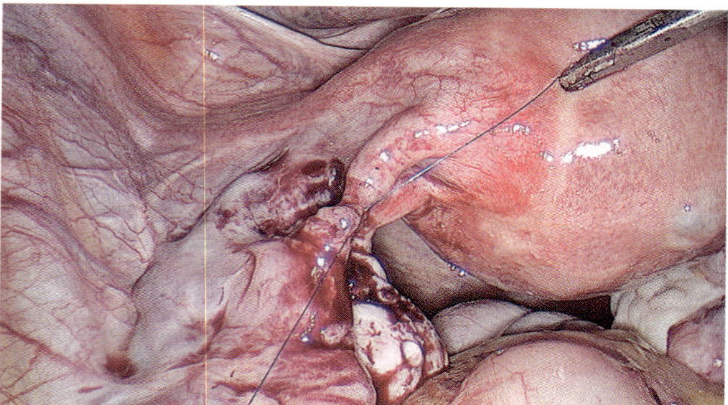

Fig. 6: Tying of 3 O' clock suture

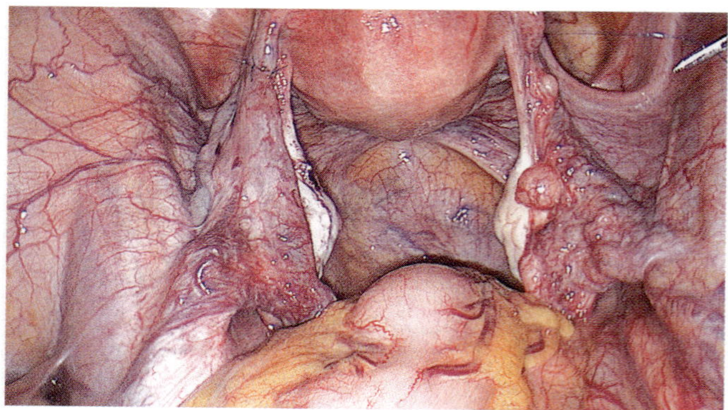

Fig. 8: Completed anastomosis on the left side.

adhesions and can achieve a pregnancy rate up to 60%.[11] In severe adhesions the chance of reformation of adhesions is high and hence the pregnancy rate is lower in these groups. The decision to operate on cases with severe pelvic adhesions should be based on the extent of tubal damage and patient's wishes. ART may be a better option in severe pelvic adhesions with tubal damage.

Hydrosalpinx

Tubal disease is responsible for 25–35% of female infertility and more than half of these are due to salpingitis.[1] Hydrosalpinx due to distal tubal occlusion is the most common tubal disease and usually treated by salpingostomy or salpingoneostomy which can be performed by laparoscopy. The pregnancy and ectopic pregnancy rate after laparoscopic salpingostomy are 41.6% and 3.9%, respectively.[12] Pregnancy rate may depend on the severity of mucosal damage. When fimbriae are agglutinated due to adhesions, tubal anatomy can be restored with fimbrioplasty which gives better pregnancy outcome than salpinogostomy.[13] In cases with severe mucosal damage, pregnancy rates are very poor and ART may be preferred.

Hydrosalpinx and Assisted Reproductive Technology

Assisted reproductive technology pregnancy rates are reduced by 50% when associated with bilateral hydrosalpinx diagnosed by ultrasonography.[14] This can be due to the toxic fluid affecting implantation or direct toxic effect on the embryo. Several measures like laparoscopic salpingectomy, proximal tubal occlusion, or hysteroscopic tubal occlusion are suggested to prevent entry of hydrosalpinx fluid into the uterine cavity. A Cochrane review has suggested salpingectomy in all women with hydrosalpinx before IVF treatment.[15] However, there is a concern over the reduction in ovarian function due to the compromise on ovarian vascularity following salpingectomy, but there is no consensus in literature regarding this. It is important to excise the hydrosalpinx close to the tube with minimal damage to the surrounding vessels. In severe tuboovarian adhesions, care must be taken to avoid damage to the infundibulopelvic ligament. It is a good technique to start dividing from cornual end and proceed toward the fimbrial end. Proximal tubal occlusion similar to sterilization is an alternative to salpingectomy in severe pelvic adhesions and has shown to give pregnancy rates similar to those following salpingectomy.

ENDOMETRIOSIS

Traditionally, surgery is considered the first line of treatment in patients with endometriosis-associated infertility. Diagnostic laparoscopy followed by surgical correction was the most common management option offered, as it serves simultaneous diagnosis and treatment. However, with the advent of improved imaging modalities especially transvaginal sonography (TVS), diagnosis can be made with sufficient accuracy, and diagnostic laparoscopy is not warranted. With the advances in ART, there is an ongoing debate on whether these patients should be offered ART directly, or, surgery with or without ART.

Conservative Surgery

Conservative surgery involves adhesiolysis for the restoration of anatomy, destruction of endometrial implants, and surgery for endometriomas.

Minimal and Mild Endometriosis

Patients with minimal and mild endometriosis have lower monthly fecundity rate compared with women with unexplained infertility.[16] A recent Cochrane review of two randomized controlled trials (RCTs) suggested an overall absolute difference of 8.6% in favor of surgical treatment compared with no treatment for minimal and mild endometriosis.[17] We prefer to do a laparoscopy when endometriosis is clinically suspected and perform excision or ablation for stage I and II endometriosis. To excise the implants, the margin of the lesions identified, and an outline is marked around with the cutting instrument. If vital organs are close by, a relaxing incision is made between the organ and the lesion to avoid inadvertent injury to a vital organ. The implant is now held with a grasper and separated from the underlying tissues with scissors or energy source (Fig. 9). The difficulty of the procedure depends on the

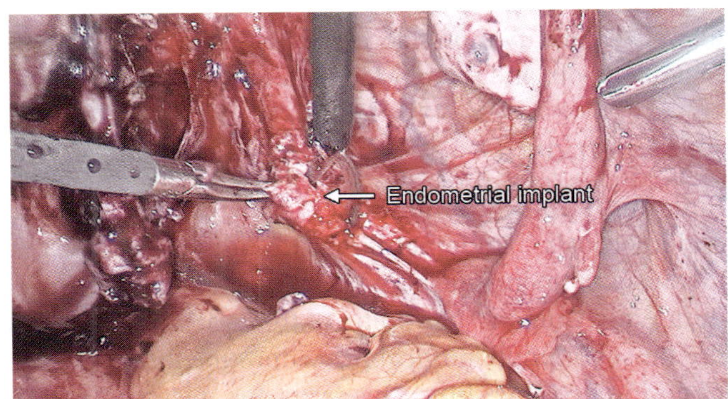

Fig. 9: Excision of the endometrial implant with scissors.

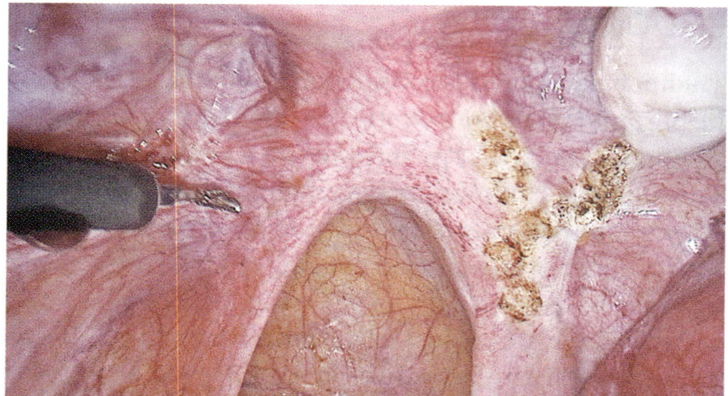

Fig. 10: Ablation of endometrial implants using monopolar electrode.

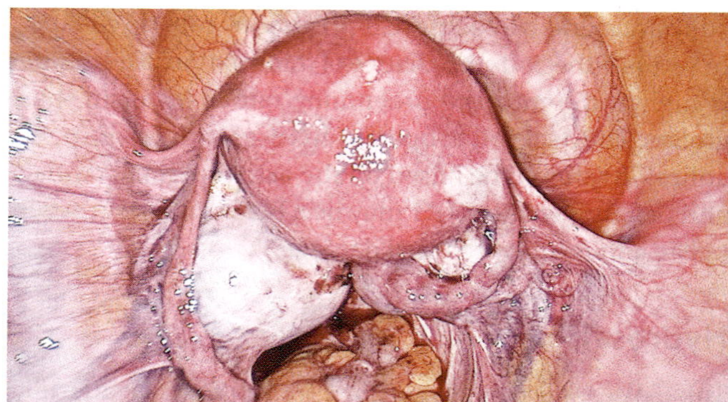

Fig. 11: Bilateral endometriomas with adhesions.

location, thickness, and size of the implant. Very small implants can be ablated by sparking with a monopolar electrode (Fig. 10). There are many reports of using plasma energy for ablation.[18] Superficial implants can be coagulated with a bipolar forceps also. This technique is less precise but easier for beginners. Advantages of excision are complete removal of the lesion and specimen is available for histopathological examination. Disadvantages are risk of injury to adjacent vital organs and requirement for advanced skill. There are two randomized controlled studies that compared ablation with excision and did not show any difference in pain scores at 12 months for mild endometriosis.[19,20] Follow-up of one study at 5 years showed that the excision group had lower rates of dyspareunia and were less likely to need medical treatment.[21]

Moderate and Severe Endometriosis

There are no RCTs available on whether surgical excision of moderate to severe endometriosis enhances pregnancy rates. But most of these women have either endometrioma or pelvic pain requiring surgery. We offer laparoscopic surgery as the first line of treatment for moderate and severe endometriosis, since laparoscopic surgery alone can give approximately 50% pregnancy rate.[22] Laparoscopic view allows visualization of inaccessible areas in pelvis, image magnification, and thereby facilitates precise surgery.

Endometrioma

Endometriomas are found in 17–44% of patients with endometriosis.[23] Endometriomas do not respond well to medical treatment, and surgical management is preferred in infertile women.[24] Stripping of the ovarian cyst wall is the most common surgical procedure for the treatment of endometrioma, but it leads to decrease in ovarian reserve and risk of premature ovarian failure.[25] Presence of endometrioma itself also causes a decrease in the ovarian reserve leading to infertility.[26]

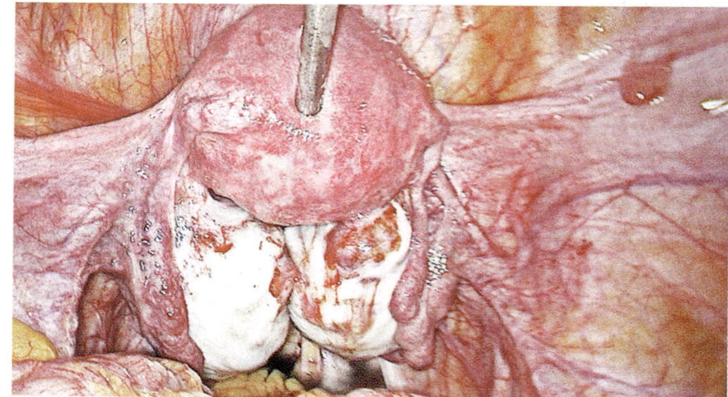

Fig. 12A: Injecting dilute vasopressin into the uterus.

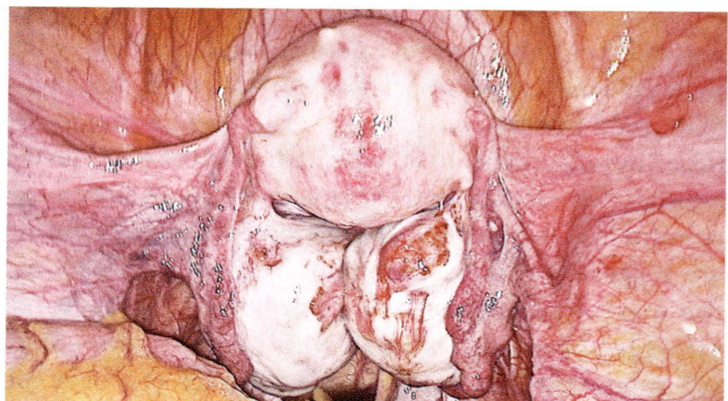

Fig. 12B: Blanching of the uterus after vasopressin injection.

We offer laparoscopic ovarian cyst enucleation for endometrioma more than 4 cm size (Fig. 11). We use the following surgical technique for endometrioma management. Dilute vasopressin (20 IU in 200 mL of normal saline) is injected into the myometrium till the uterus is blanched which helps in achieving initial hemostatic dissection of the adnexa and rectosigmoid (Figs. 12A and B). After anteverting the uterus with a Spackman's cannula,

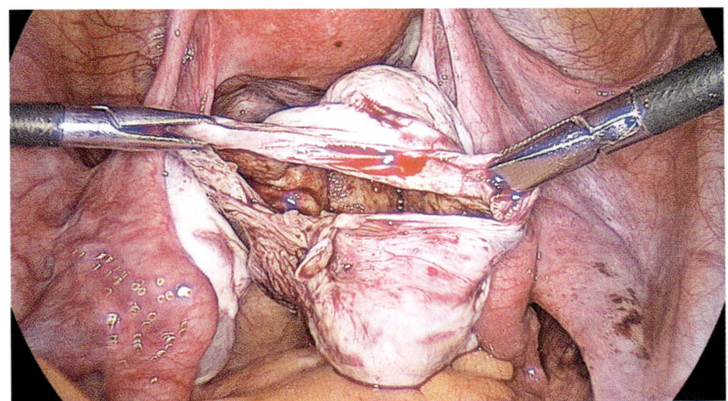

Fig. 13: Traction on the cyst wall with two graspers.

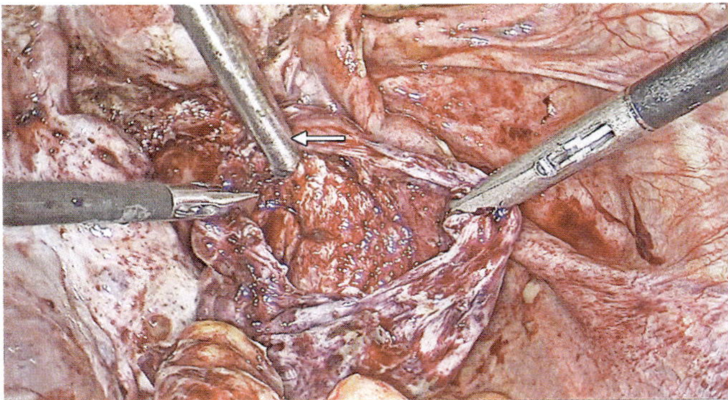

Fig. 15A: Injecting dilute vasopressin below the cyst wall.

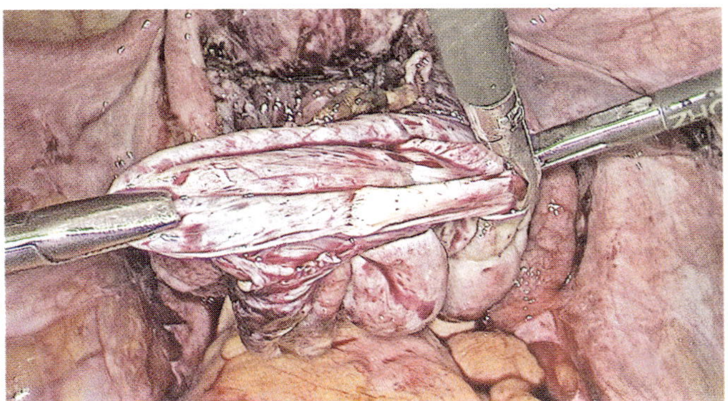

Fig. 14: Enucleation of the cyst wall.

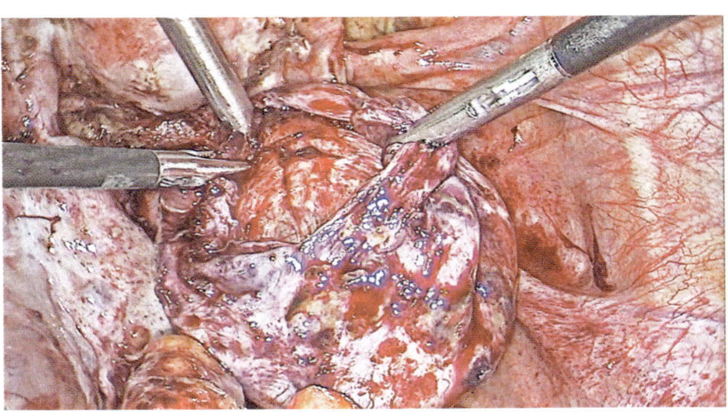

Fig. 15B: Bulging of the cyst wall.

salpingo-ovariolysis is done with sharp dissection. All fleshy adhesions from the uterus and pouch of Douglas are excised. All superficial endometriosis implants are coagulated, and deep ones are excised. The ovary with small endometrioma is mobilized from the pelvic ovarian fossa, and when the chocolate material invariably leaks out, the leaked out contents are aspirated, followed by complete irrigation and aspiration of the cyst. For large endometriomas, we puncture the cyst with a trocar and aspirate the chocolate material. Cyst wall opening is now enlarged to allow complete inspection of the inside of the cyst (Fig. 13). Any solid excrescence and number of loculi are now inspected. A controlled tear of 1 cm is made on the edge of the cyst by traction with two graspers, rather than using sharp cutting. This step separates the cyst wall from the ovarian tissue. After identification of the cleavage plane, the cyst wall is enucleated through traction exerted in opposite directions with two grasping forceps (Fig. 14). The cyst wall is held with a toothed grasper, and ovarian tissue is held with an atraumatic grasper. Traction and counter traction is done to separate the cyst from the ovarian tissue. Complete removal of the cyst wall is done. Enucleation is done gently near the ovarian ligament and hilum to avoid bleeding and injury. For smaller and multiloculated endometriomas, injection of dilute vasopressin below the cyst wall is useful to reduce the loss of ovarian tissue (Figs. 15A and B). Any residual endometriosis on the edges of the ovary is excised. At the end of the procedure, only the active bleeding vessels are controlled with bipolar coagulation. No sutures are used for approximation of the ovarian edges. The ovarian edges are held together to reconstruct the ovary and then held with a bowel grasper for 5 minutes for hemostasis and approximation (Figs. 16A and B).

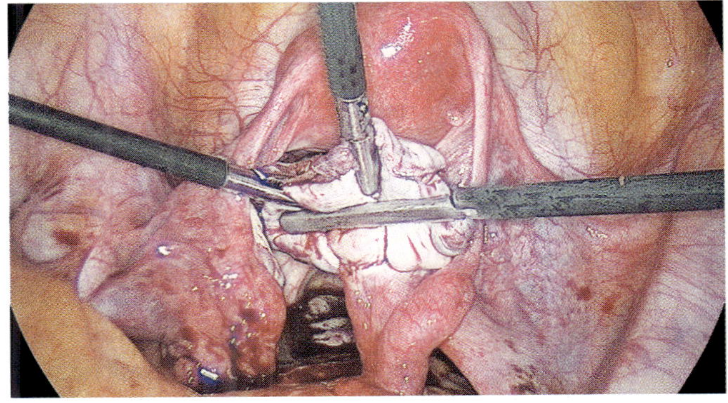

Fig. 16A: Reconstruction of right ovary.

Another alternative for cystectomy or excision is drainage of cyst and ablation, with bipolar coagulation, CO_2

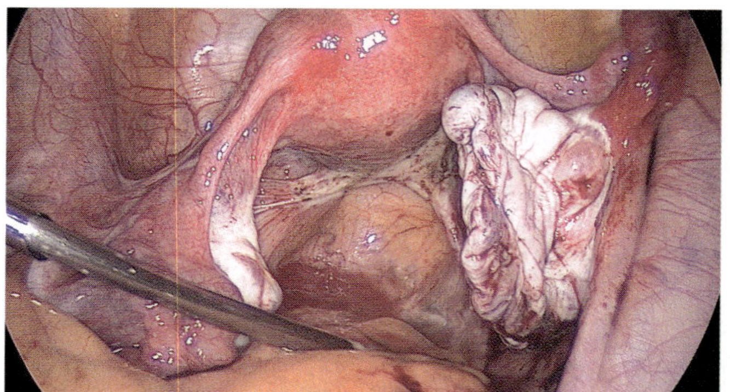

Fig. 16B: Right ovary after reconstruction.

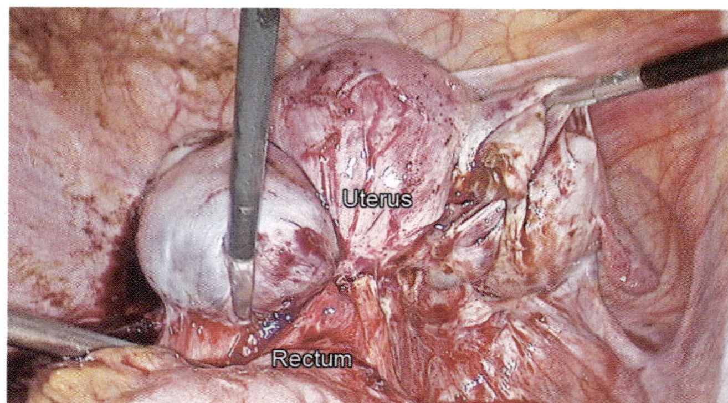

Fig. 17: Obliteration of pouch of Douglas due to rectal adhesions to the uterus.

laser or plasma energy, but studies have shown excision is superior because of high recurrence with the latter.[27]

Surgery for bilateral endometrioma appears to have a more deleterious effect on ovarian reserve than unilateral endometrioma. The factors which affect the ovarian reserve are age, size of cyst, and type of cyst. Advanced aged, smaller cyst, and fibroblastic type of cyst reduce the ovarian reserve. So, surgical techniques for endometrioma enucleation have to be performed with the utmost care to reduce the loss of ovarian tissue.

Deep Infiltrating Endometriosis (DIE)

Deep infiltrating endometriosis (DIE) is different from peritoneal and ovarian endometriosis and is characterized by infiltration of more than 5 mm below the peritoneum. Most common locations are uterosacral ligaments, rectovaginal septum, and rectum and vesicouterine pouch. DIE is present in 20% of women with endometriosis. Pelvic pain is the most common symptom, but some women may also have associated infertility. Laparoscopic excision of DIE can relieve the pelvic pain and also improve fertility in these women.[28] However, surgery for deep endometriosis needs more expertise, and is associated with complications.

Rectovaginal endometriosis typically refers to an infiltrative disease involving the cervix, vagina, rectovaginal septum, and rectum. It can occur in isolation or extend to other pelvic structures causing complete obliteration of the pouch of Douglas (Fig. 17). DIE is more common in the posterior compartment with a predisposition for left hemipelvis and predominantly affecting uterosacral ligaments. Isolated uterosacral lesions are present in 83%, but in 16.8% of cases, the involvement of vagina, bowel, and bladder may coexist.[29] Surgical excision of isolated uterosacral ligaments is done after identifying the ureters as they may be more medial due to the fibrotic nature of the disease. If the ureters are not clearly visualized, ureterolysis is done, and any endometriotic nodule on the uterosacral ligaments are excised safely (Figs. 18 and 19). In cases of bilateral disease with or without vaginal nodule, ureterolysis is done bilaterally. When a vaginal nodule is present, it may be adherent to the rectum and needs to be released from it before excision (Fig. 20). Once released from the rectum, it can be excised along with the cervical and vaginal nodule en masse. Deep dissection of bilateral uterosacral disease can damage the inferior hypogastric plexus resulting in urinary retention and sexual dysfunction. So surgery is aimed at preservation of these nerve plexuses if possible.

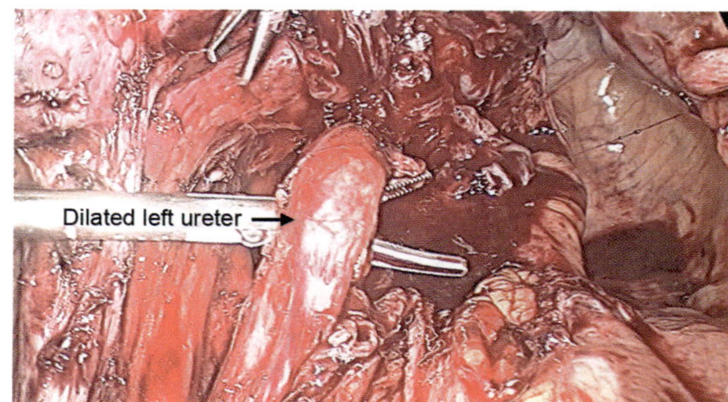

Fig. 18: Ureterolysis of left hydroureter.

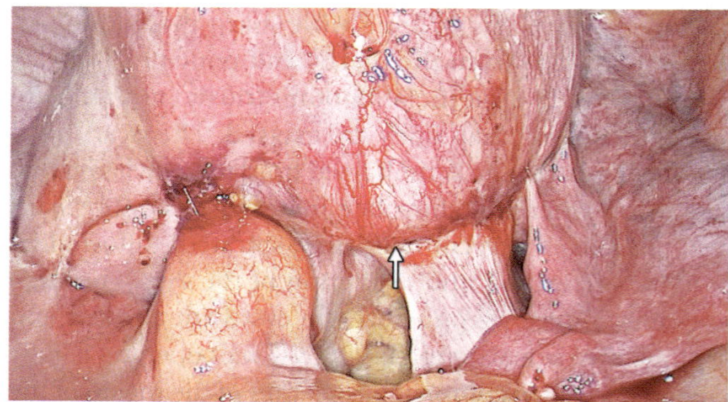

Fig. 19: Endometriosis involving uterosacral ligaments.

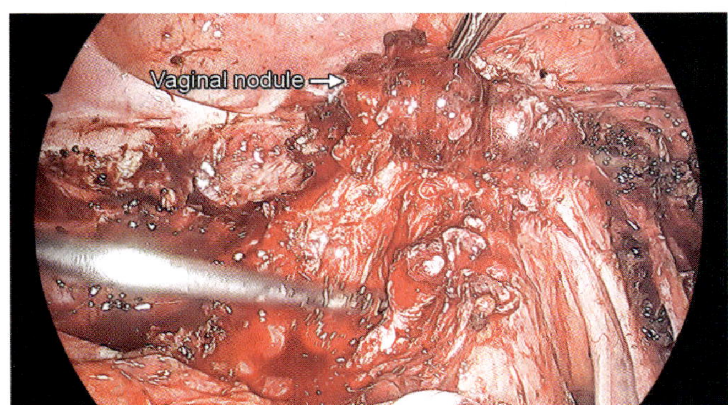

Fig. 20: Excision of vaginal nodule.

Deep infiltrating endometriosis needs surgical treatment when associated with pelvic pain and infertility, but should be done in experienced centers.

MYOMA

Uterine fibroids are the most common tumor in women and have a prevalence of 8–10% in women of 30–40 years.[30] Prevalence of fibroids is higher in women with infertility but if all other causes of infertility are excluded fibroids may be responsible only in 2–3% of the cases.[30]

There is no consensus on whether all types of fibroids affect the reproductive potential of women. A meta-analysis of 18 studies found that, fibroids in general, led to a statistically significant decrease in fertility, clinical pregnancy, and birth rates.[31] They found submucosal fibroids reduce clinical pregnancy rate up to 70%. An RCT found that removal of submucous fibroids led to a significant increase in pregnancy rate from 27.2% to 43.3% in 52 patients.[32] Subserous fibroids rarely cause infertility and do not need surgical removal.[31]

The role of intramural fibroids in causing infertility is not well established. A meta-analysis of 19 trials including 6,089 patients found that in women undergoing IVF, the fibroids not distorting endometrial cavity were associated with significantly lower clinical pregnancy and live birth rates. The size of intramural fibroids ranged from 0.7 cm to 5 cm.[33] There are few studies trying to find out the size and the number of intramural fibroids that interfere with the fertility potential. The fibroids that are more than 3–4 cm in size may interfere with fertility.[34]

Hysteroscopic resection is performed for all myomas less than 3 cm with more than 50% intracavitary component (Type 0, 1). Hysteroscopic surgery for myomas larger than 3 cm or type 2 myomas can be managed in two stage procedure depending on the skill of the surgeon. Laparoscopic myomectomy is considered the procedure of choice for myomas not amenable hysteroscopic resection.

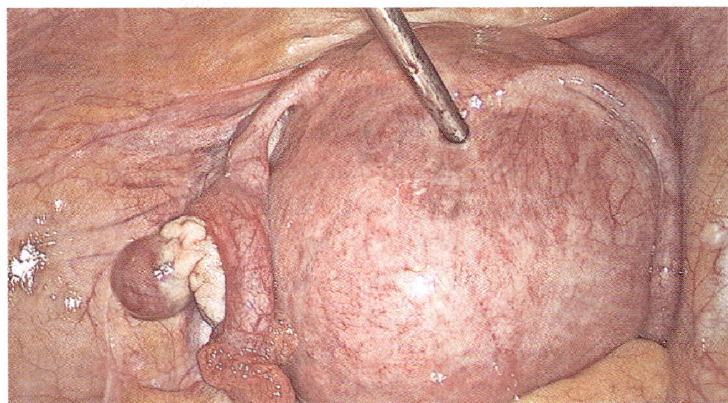

Fig. 21: Injection of vasopressin into the myometrium.

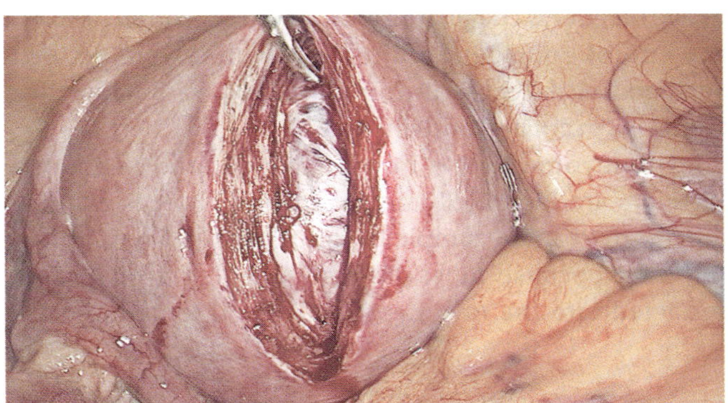

Fig. 22: Incision over myoma using ultrasonic scalpel.

Laparoscopic myomectomy for myomas more than 10 cm in size or more than four in number is challenging and depends on the skill of the surgeon. Laparotomy may be needed in very large myomas, especially when they are multiple.

Laparoscopic Myomectomy

The primary trocar is introduced above the umbilicus depending on the size of the uterus. Three 5 mm secondary trocars are now inserted under vision and may be placed at a higher level depending on the size of the myomas. Dilute vasopressin (Vasopressin 20 units in 200 cc normal saline) is injected into the myometrium over the proposed site of myomectomy (Fig. 21). Vasopressin injection is stopped when good blanching is achieved to avoid the potential side effects. A unipolar diathermy electrode or ultrasonic scalpel is used for making the incision over the most bulging portion of the myoma (Fig. 22). We make a transverse incision over anterior myomas and a vertical incision over posterior myomas to make the uterus in anteverted position after suturing, although both types of incisions cause comparable bleeding. Transverse incisions should not be extended too far laterally to avoid injuring uterine branches.

The incision is made deep to myoma cutting the capsule and exposing the myoma. This is necessary to get the correct plane of enucleation. The myoma is now firmly fixed with a myoma spiral and a 5 mm toothed grasper on the myometrium and the pseudocapsule for counter- traction (Fig. 23). The myoma is enucleated by traction on the myoma screw and counter traction with the 5 mm grasper. The ultrasonic scalpel from the suprapubic port helps in enucleation as well as achieving hemostasis (Fig. 24). The myoma spiral and 5 mm grasper are released and regrasped frequently so that traction and countertraction can be applied to attain enucleation in small steps with minimum injury to the vessels on the pseudocapsule. Any active bleeder is coagulated with an energy source. Toward the end of enucleation, the vessels that were actually surrounding the capsule are now seen as a vascular pedicle which is coagulated and divided.

The myoma bed is now inspected, and any active bleeders are identified and coagulated if necessary. The aim is not to attain complete hemostasis, which is difficult to attain because most of these bleeders have already retracted into the myometrium. A good technique is to attain hemostasis during enucleation itself. If there is poor visibility due to generalized oozing, a repeat dose of remaining vasopressin can be injected into the myometrium before suturing.

Closure of the uterine incision is done in two layers comparable to laparotomy technique. We use barbed knotless sutures more frequently and use the regular sutures only when there are multiple small incisions. The inner layers of the myometrial incision is approximated with deep bites approximately 1.5 cm apart in a continuous fashion to avoid dead space (Fig. 25). The same suture is continued for the second layer and is completed with base ball sutures to invert the edges (Fig. 26). When there is tension at suture line a grasper can help to maintain approximation of the edges till the suturing is completed. Two or three extra bites are taken before cutting the suture close to the tissues (Fig. 27).

Myoma specimen is usually removed by power morcellation. However, unexpected malignancies have been reported at surgery for presumed benign symptomatic fibroids.[35] A good preoperative screening with ultrasound imaging and Doppler velocimetry, lactate dehydrogenase

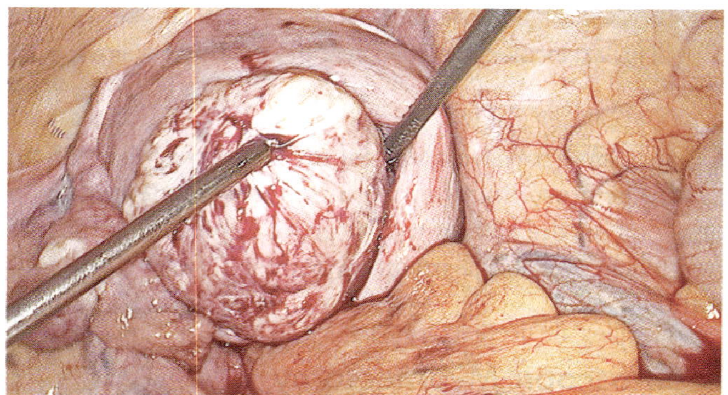

Fig. 23: Traction with myoma spiral and countertraction with grasper.

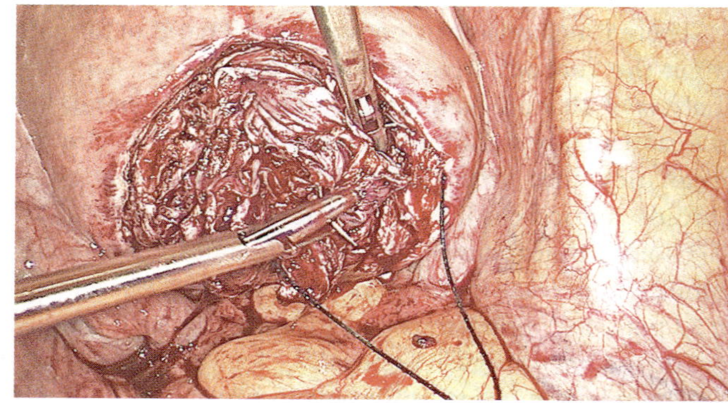

Fig. 25: First layer of continuous suturing.

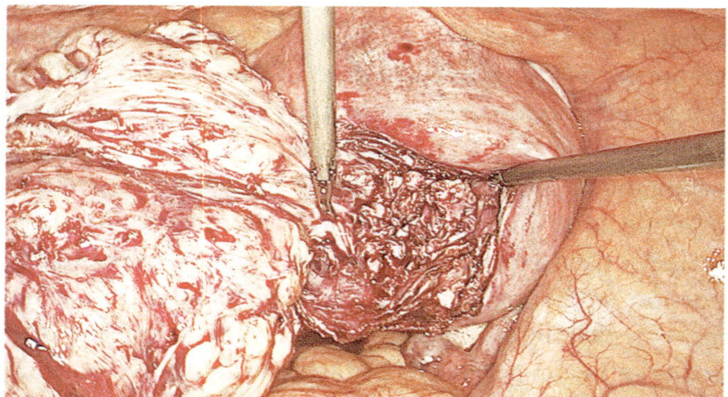

Fig. 24: Enucleation of myoma inside pseudocapsule with ultrasonic scalpel.

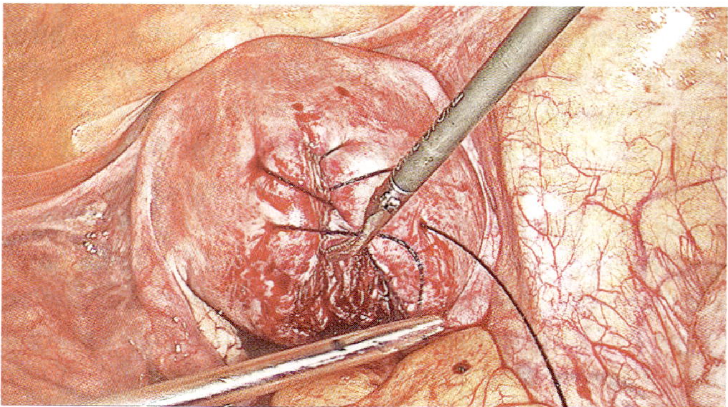

Fig. 26: Second layer of baseball suturing.

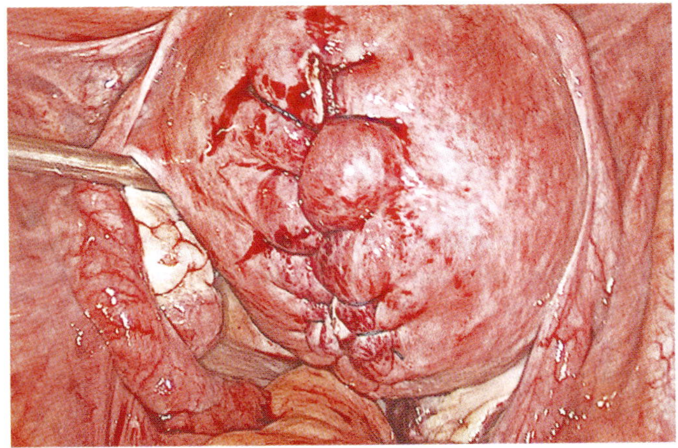

Fig. 27: Completed suturing with hemostasis.

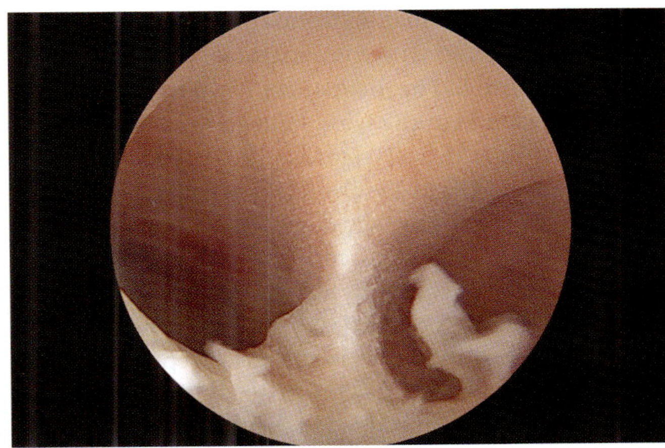

Fig. 28: Uterine septum.

(LDH) isoenzyme three assays, endometrial biopsy for patients with abnormal uterine bleeding especially older women and diffusion-weighted magnetic resonance imaging (MRI) may be performed in high-risk cases.[36] We use an in-bag morcellation technique for doubtful cases.[37]

We perform laparoscopic myomectomy for myomas up to 10–15 cm, but do a laparoscopic-assisted myomectomy with a 4 cm abdominal incision to avoid prolonged surgery and also to reduce blood loss in selected cases of multiple myomas.

LAPAROSCOPIC OVARIAN DRILLING

Polycystic ovarian syndrome (PCOS) is a predominant cause of anovulatory infertility with a prevalence of 4–8% in reproductive age women.[38] Clomiphene citrate (CC) is still the first line of treatment with a reported ovulation rate of 75–80% per woman.[39] Clomiphene-resistant patients can be treated with gonadotrophins or laparoscopic ovarian drilling (LOD). A recent Cochrane review found LOD resulted in a pregnancy rate of 39.7% without increased risk of multiple pregnancies or ovarian hyperstimulation syndrome.[40]

Laparoscopic ovarian drilling is performed using monopolar needle electrode. Armar et al. described a technique with only four punctures per ovary, each with 4 seconds at a power setting of 40 watts.[41] The punctures are made with an electrode of 2 mm diameter to a depth of 8 mm. If the volume of the ovary is more than 10 cc, we make few extra punctures.

Based on current evidence, LOD gives better reproductive outcome in women with CC-resistant polycystic ovarian syndrome (PCOS) when infertility is of less than 3 years duration, body mass index (BMI) less than 25 kg/cm^2, luteinizing hormone (LH) levels less than 10 IU/L, testosterone levels less than 1.3 ng/mL, and basal anti-Müllerian hormone (AMH) less than 7.7 ng/mL.[42]

We prefer to perform a diagnostic laparoscopy and ovarian drilling in clomiphene-resistant patients after counseling.

UTERINE SEPTUM

The uterine septum has been associated with pregnancy wastage rates as high as 90% (Fig. 28) but the association of septum and infertility is less clear.[43] A comparative study of two groups of women with unexplained fertility, one group with septate uteri who underwent hysteroscopic metroplasty and a control group without septate uteri showed a live birth rate of 38.6% vs. 20.4%, respectively.[44] In another study of women with septum length of more than 2.5 cm when compared with women with septum of less than 2.5 cm, pregnancy rate was 66.7% in those with septum length more than 2.5 cm and 42.8% in those with less than 2.5 cm, respectively.[45]

The role of septum incision in women undergoing IVF/ICSI was also studied in a large group. Live birth rate was 2.7% before surgery and 15.6% after surgery.[46] Hysteroscopic metroplasty not only increases the live birth rate but also allows spontaneous conception in unexplained infertility.

Hysteroscopic Metroplasty

A uterine septum is usually diagnosed with TVS and can be confirmed with 3D TVS, and MRI is rarely needed. A laparoscopy is usually performed during hysteroscopic septum incision which allows evaluation of the adnexae and pelvic cavity for possible pelvic adhesions, tubal or ovarian distortions, and endometriosis that could be treated during the same session. If a laparoscopy had been already performed, hysteroscopic septum incision could be monitored with intraoperative transabdominal ultrasonography. The best time for performance of septum incision is in the early follicular phase when the endometrium is thin. Hysteroscopic metroplasty can be accomplished with the use of mechanical scissors or electrosurgery with specially designed electrodes fitted to the hysteroscope or resectoscope.

We use 5 mm operating hysteroscope with 5Fr semirigid scissors for the division of thin septa. The monopolar or bipolar electrode can also be used. Thicker septa are divided with smaller resectoscopes (16/21Fr) with an L-shaped electrode. The septum is divided systematically from side to side at the midpoint of the septum. It is continued until both uterotubal openings can be seen and the cavity is near normal and over correction is avoided. A panoramic view from internal os is useful for making this decision. The intrauterine pressure of the distending fluid can be decreased before completing the procedure; if arterial bleeding occurs, selective coagulation can be performed. The final goal is to produce a satisfactory uterine cavity.

INTRAUTERINE ADHESIONS

Intrauterine adhesions are associated with infertility, recurrent miscarriage, preterm labor, and abnormal placentation. Intrauterine adhesions can cause infertility by complete or partial occlusion of the tubal ostia, uterine cavity or the cervical canal, preventing the migration of sperm or the implantation of the embryo.[47] Intrauterine adhesions are caused by trauma to the basal layer endometrium due to surgical or infectious damage (Fig. 29). The severity of adhesions is classified as mild (<25% uterine cavity with thin filmy adhesions), moderate (25–75% of the cavity containing adhesions causing partial occlusion of the ostium and upper fundus), and severe (>75% of the cavity with agglutination of the wall or thick bands).[48]

Hysteroscopic Adhesiolysis

The semirigid hysteroscopic scissors are used to divide adhesions at midpoint allowing the cut edges to retract. Thick vascular and dense adhesions are incised using resectoscopes utilizing the thin electro surgery (Collin's) knife or bipolar electrodes.

Postoperative balloon catheter or plastic intrauterine contraceptive devices can be used in case of severe adhesions to avoid apposition of uterine walls. Estrogen is usually prescribed for 1–3 months to stimulate the endometrial growth.

An observational study has shown that conception rate after hysteroscopic lysis was 58% for mild adhesions, 30% for moderate adhesions, and 33.3% for severe adhesions.[49]

ENDOMETRIAL POLYPS

Polyps may cause infertility due to irregular endometrial bleeding, endometrial inflammatory changes, and mechanical obstruction to sperms and embryos (Fig. 30).[50]

Hysteroscopic Polypectomy

Hysteroscopic polypectomy can be done using an operative hysteroscope with removal of the polyp using grasping forceps inserted through the operative channel. The grasping forceps should be directed at the base of the polyp and moved in and out to detach the polyp. The polyp is held with the grasper and removed along with the hysteroscope itself. Several attempts may be required to remove the polyp in its entirety or it may be removed in piece meal if the size of polyp is bigger. When there are multiple small polyps, a

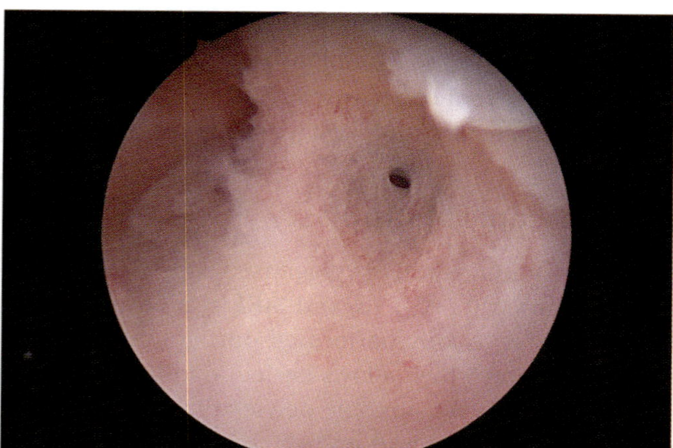

Fig. 29: Intrauterine adhesions.

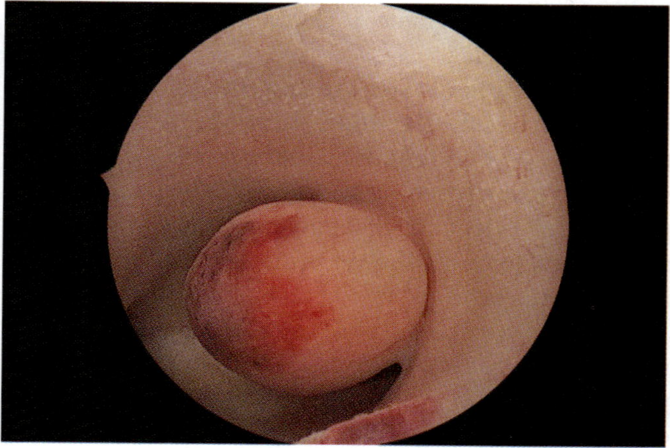

Fig. 30: Endometrial polyp.

suction evacuation can be done and check hysteroscopy is done to remove any residual polyps. Another technique involves the use of a hysteroscopic morcellator.

A randomized trial of 215 patients with polyps undergoing intrauterine insemination with and without polypectomy had a pregnancy rate of 51.4% and 25.4%, respectively.[51] A retrospective study of 230 women to determine the significance of the location of endometrial polyp found that uterotubal polypectomy was associated with a 50–60% pregnancy rate.[52]

SUMMARY

Reproductive surgery has a definite role in the diagnosis and treatment of a wide variety of conditions in selected infertile patients.

- Diagnostic laparoscopy has a limited role but should be considered in women younger than 35 years, short duration of infertility, and normal male factor with clinical suspicion of endometriosis, pelvic adhesions or tubal disease.
- Hysteroscopic cannulation should be tried as the first line of treatment for proximal tubal block.
- Laparoscopic tubal anastomosis gives good pregnancy rate for reversal of sterilization in experienced hands.
- Laparoscopic salpingoovariolysis is preferred for mild to moderate pelvic adhesions. Laparoscopic salpingoneostomy or fimbrioplasty for hydrosalpinx is reserved for cases with mild mucosal damage and in young women with short duration of infertility. Laparoscopic salpingectomy is performed for severe tubal damage to improve the results of ART.
- Laparoscopic ablation or excision of mild endometriosis marginally improves pregnancy rate.
- We prefer laparoscopic conservative surgery for moderate and severe endometriosis as the first line of treatment.
- Laparoscopic enucleation of endometriomas should be performed with minimum damage to the ovarian tissue. Repeat surgeries are avoided as a treatment for infertility alone.
- Submucous myomas can affect reproductive potential and are treated by hysteroscopic myomectomy.
- Laparoscopic myomectomy is performed for intramural myomas distorting the endometrial cavity or when more than 4 cm in size.
- Laparoscopic ovarian drilling is done for clomiphene-resistant PCOS with good prognostic factors.
- Hysteroscopic incision of uterine septum is an acceptable treatment option in unexplained infertility and before ART.
- Hysteroscopic adhesiolysis and polypectomy are indicated for intrauterine adhesions and polyps, respectively.

REFERENCES

1. Honore GM, Holden AEC, Schenken RS. Pathophysiology and management of proximal tubal blockage. Fertil Steril. 1999;5:785-95.
2. Desai SK, Desai S, et al. Genital tuberculosis and infertility. In: Desai S, Allahbadia G (Eds). Infertility and Transvaginal Sonography: Current Concepts. New Delhi: Jaypee Brothers Medical Publishers (P) Ltd; 1995.
3. Novy M, Thurmond AS, Patton P, et al. Diagnosis of cornual obstruction by transcervical fallopian tube cannulation. Fertil Steril. 1988;50:434-40.
4. Paul PG, Jeevanraj, Rani JS. Hysteroscopic cannulation for proximal tubal obstruction. J Obstet Gynaecol India. 1998;48:65-67.
5. United Nations, Department of Economic and Social Affairs, Population Division. World Contraceptive Use; 2009.
6. Liskin L, Rinehart W, Blackburn R, et al. Minilaparotomy and laparoscopy: Safe, effective, and widely used. Popul Rep C. 1985;9:C125-67.
7. La Grange J, Kruger TF, Steyn DW, et al. Fallopian tube reanastomosis by laparotomy versus laparoscopy: A meta-analysis. Gynecol Obstet Invest. 2012;74:28-34.
8. Paul PG, Khurd AS, Garg R, et al. Laparoscopic tubal reanastomosis using barbed sutures. J Minim Invasive Gynecol. 2017;24(1):11.
9. Yoon TK, Sung HR, Kang HG, et al. Laparoscopic tubal anastomosis: Fertility outcome in 202 cases. Fertil Steril. 1999;72:1121-6.
10. Paul PG, Bhosale SA, Khan S, et al. Fertility outcome in laparoscopic single tube reanastomosis. J Reprod Med. 2015;60(1-2):30-6.
11. Gomel V, McComb PF. Microsurgery for tubal infertility. J Reprod Med. 2006;51:177-84.
12. Mossa B, Patella A, Ebano V, et al. Microsurgery versus laparoscopy in distal tubal obstruction hysterosalpingographically or laparoscopically investigated. Clin Exp Obstet Gynecol. 2005;32:169-71.
13. Saleh WA, Dlugi AM. Pregnancy outcome after laparoscopic fimbrioplasty in nonocclusive distal tubal disease. Fertil Steril. 1997;67:474-80.
14. Practice Committee of American Society for Reproductive Medicine in collaboration with Society of Reproductive Surgeons. Salpingectomy for hydrosalpinx prior to in vitro fertilization. Fertil Steril. 2008;90:S66-8.
15. Johnson N, van Voorst S, Sowter MC, et al. Surgical treatment for tubal disease in women due to undergo in vitro fertilisation. Cochrane Database Syst Rev. 2010;(1).
16. Berube S, Marcoux S, Langevin M, et al. Fecundity of infertile women with minimal or mild endometriosis and women with unexplained infertility. The Canadian Collaborative Group on Endometriosis. Fertil Steril. 1998;69(6):1034-41.
17. Jacobson TZ, Duffy JMN, Barlow DH, et al. Laparoscopic surgery for subfertility associated with endometriosis. Cochrane Database Syst Rev. 2010;(1).

18. Roman H. Deep rectal shaving using plasma energy for endometriosis causing rectal stenosis - a video vignette. Colorectal Dis. 2014;16:834-6.
19. Wright J, Lotfallah H, Jones K, et al. A randomized trial of excision versus ablation for mild endometriosis. Fertil Steril. 2005;83:1830.
20. Healey M, Ang WC, Cheng C. Surgical treatment of endometriosis: A prospective randomized double-blinded trial comparing excision and ablation. Fertil Steril. 2010;94:2536.
21. Healy M, Cheng C, Kaur H. To excise or ablate endometriosis? A prospective randomized double-blinded trial after 5-year follow-up. J Minim Invasive Gynecol. 2014;21:999-1004.
22. Vercellini P, Somigliana E, Viganò P, et al. Surgery for endometriosis-associated infertility: A pragmatic approach. Hum Reprod. 2009;24(2):254-698.
23. Alborzi S, Keramati P, Younesi M, et al. The impact of laparoscopic cystectomy on ovarian reserve in patients with unilateral and bilateral endometriomas. Fertil Steril. 2014;101(2):427-34.
24. Ruiz-Flores FJ, Garcia-Velasco JA. Is there a benefit for surgery in endometrioma-associated infertility? Curr Opin Obstet Gynecol. 2012;24(3):136-40.
25. Benaglia L, Somigliana E, Vighi V, et al. Rate of severe ovarian damage following surgery for endometriomas. Hum Reprod. 2010;25:678-82.
26. Gupta S, Agarwal A, Agarwal R, et al. Impact of ovarian endometrioma on assisted reproduction outcomes. Reprod Biomed Online. 2006;13(3):349-60.
27. Chapron C, Vercellini P, Barakat H, et al. Management of ovarian endometriomas. Hum Reprod Update. 2002;8(6): 591-7.
28. Chapron C, Fritel X, Dubuisson JB. Fertility after laparoscopic management of deep endometriosis infiltrating the uterosacral ligaments. Hum Reprod. 1999;14:329-32.
29. Chapron C, Fauconnier A, Dubuisson JB, et al. Deep infiltrating endometriosis: The relation between severity of dysmenorrhoea and extent of disease. Hum Reprod. 2003;4:760-6.
30. Bulun SE. Uterine fibroids. N Engl J Med. 2013;369:1344-55.
31. Pritts EA, Parker WH, OliveDL. Fibroids and infertility: An updated systematic review of evidence. Fertil Steril. 2009;91:1215-23.
32. Casini ML, Rossi F, Agostini R, et al. Effects of the position of fibroids on fertility. Gynecol Endocrinol. 2006;22:106-9.
33. Sunkara SK, Khairy M, El-Toukhy T, et al. The effect of intramural fibroids without uterine cavity involvement on the outcome of IVF treatment: A systematic review and meta-analysis. Hum Reprod. 2010;25:418-29.
34. Yan L, Ding L, Li C, et al. Effect of fibroids not distorting endometrial cavity on the outcome of IVF treatment: A retrospective cohort study. Fertil Steril. 2014;10(1):716-21.
35. Paul PG, Rengaraj V, Das T, et al. Uterine sarcomas in patients undergoing surgery for presumed leiomyomas: 10 years' experience. J Minim Invasive Gynecol. 2016;23(3):384-9.
36. Seki K, Yoshihara T, Nagata I. Leiomyosarcoma of the uterus: Ultrasonography and serum lactate dehydrogenase level. Gynecol Obstet Invest. 1992;33(2):114-8.
37. Paul PG, Thomas M, Das , et al. Contained morcellation for laparoscopic myomectomy within a specially designed bag. J Minim Invasive Gynecol. 2016;23(2):257-60.
38. Overbeek A, Lambalk CB. Phenotypic and pharmacogenetic aspects of ovulation induction in WHO II anovulatory women. Gynecol Endocrinol. 2009;25(4):222-34.
39. Messinis IE. Ovulation induction: A mini review. Hum Reprod. 2005;20(10):2688-97.
40. Farquhar C, Brown J, Marjoribanks J. Laparoscopic drilling by diathermy or laser for ovulation induction in anovulatory polycystic ovary syndrome. Cochrane Database Syst Rev. 2012;(6).
41. Armar NA, McGarrigle HHG, Honour J, et al. Laparoscopic ovarian diathermy in the management of anovulatory infertility in women with polycystic ovaries: Endocrine changes and clinical outcome. Fertil Steril. 1990;53:45-9.
42. Abu Hashim H. Predictors of success of laparoscopic ovarian drilling in women with polycystic ovary syndrome: an evidence-based approach. Arch Gynecol Obstet. 2015;291: 11-8.
43. Kormanyos Z, Molnar BG, Pal A. Removal of a residual portion of a uterine septum in women of advanced reproductive age: Obstetric outcome. Hum Reprod. 2006;21:1047-51.
44. Mollo A, De Franciscis P, Colacuci N, et al. Hysteroscopic resection of the septum improves the pregnancy rate of women with unexplained infertility: A prospective controlled trial. Fertil Steril. 2009;91:2628-31.
45. Shokeir T, Abdelshaheed M, El-Shafie M, et al. Determinants of fertility and reproductive success after hysteroscopic septoplasty for women with unexplained primary infertility: A prospective analysis of 88 cases. Eur J Obstet Gynecol Reprod Biol. 2011;155:54-7.
46. Tomazevic T, Ban-Frangež H, Virant-Klun I, et al. Septate, subseptate, and arcuate uterus decrease pregnancy and live birth rates in IVF/ICSI. Reprod BioMed Online. 2010;21(5):700-5.
47. Bosteels J, Weyers S, Puttemans P, et al. The effectiveness of hysteroscopy in improving pregnancy rates in subfertile women without other gynecological symptoms: A systematic review. Hum Reprod Update. 2010;16:1-11.
48. March C. Hysteroscopy for infertility. In: Baggish M (Ed). Diagnostic and Operative Hysteroscopy. Chicago: Year Book Medical; 1989. pp. 136-44.
49. Roy KK, Baruah J, Sharma JB, et al. Reproductive outcome following hysteroscopic adhesiolysis in patients with infertility due to Asherman's syndrome. Arch Gynecol Obstet. 2010;281:355-61.
50. Richlin SS, Ramachandran S, Shanti A, et al. Glycodelin levels in uterine flushings and in plasma of patients with leiomyomas and polyps: Implications for implantation. Hum Reprod. 2002;17:2742-7.
51. Perez-Medina T, Bajo-Arenas J, Salazar F, et al. Endometrial polyps and their implication in the pregnancy rates of patients undergoing intrauterine insemination: A prospective, randomized study. Hum Reprod. 2005;20:163-5.
52. Yahaihara A, Yorimitsu T, Motoyama H, et al. Location of endometrial polyp and pregnancy rate in infertility patients. Fertil Steril. 2008;90:180-2.

CHAPTER 11

Ultrasound and Color Doppler in Fertility

Narendra Malhotra, Neharika Bora, Jaideep Malhotra, Rishab Bora

INTRODUCTION

Ultrasound is one of the most indispensable investigations as far as an infertile couple is concerned. A comprehensive ultrasound examination can replace the multiple diagnostic tests needed in an infertile female, often at different sites and over multiple visits. Two-dimensional (2D) ultrasound is a primary tool to evaluate the pelvis and can be combined with a three-dimensional (3D) scan to enable volume reconstruction. Color Doppler adds valuable information for the diagnosis and treatment of the infertile female. Dynamic changes of the menstrual cycle in a reproductively active female are picked up very well by transvaginal color Doppler and definite conclusions can be drawn regarding the diagnosis, prognosis and treatment of infertile patients.

ROLE OF ULTRASOUND AND DOPPLER IN INFERTILE COUPLE

- For understanding the anatomy and physiology and to rule out major pelvic pathologies
- Prediction of fertility potential before starting infertility treatment by means of antral follicle count (AFC) to determine the ovarian reserve
- Monitoring intrauterine insemination (IUI) and in-vitro fertilization (IVF) cycles, decide dose and type of drugs
- To predict of the response to ovarian stimulation in assisted conception, assessment of oocyte quality based on perifollicular flow and parameters influencing implantation following embryo transfer using Doppler
- Prevention of complications in assisted reproductive technology (ART) like hyperstimulation or poor response to stimulation.

BASELINE SCAN IN INFERTILITY

Baseline scan is a performed between day 3–7 of the cycle. It is known as a baseline scan because at this time of the cycle, endometrium is thin like a single line as it has shed off during menstruation and this is an absolute baseline status of the ovaries. It should comprise of a systematic approach in which first transabdominal scanning should be done, following which, after emptying the bladder transvaginal scanning for cervix, uterus and bilateral ovaries. All the findings should be documented and saved electronically. The proposed sequence of examination is to evaluate the uterus first using both 2D ultrasound and 3D ultrasound to determine the appearance and symmetry of the endometrium, myometrium, and junctional zone, rule out the presence of congenital or acquired anatomic abnormalities. The adnexa should be evaluated next for any tubal or ovarian pathology and for evidence of polycystic ovaries. The sonohysterogram can be combined with hysterosalpingo-contrast-sonography (HycoSY) between D6-8 of the cycle to test for tubal patency.

Technical Aspects of Transvaginal Sonography

Transvaginal sonography probe consists of a head, shaft and handle (grip). It may be straight or bend type. Straight probes are better for examination, bent probes may be better for TVS guided interventional procedures. An ideal set up should have privacy, a female attendant should be present and there should be a comfortable gynecological chair.

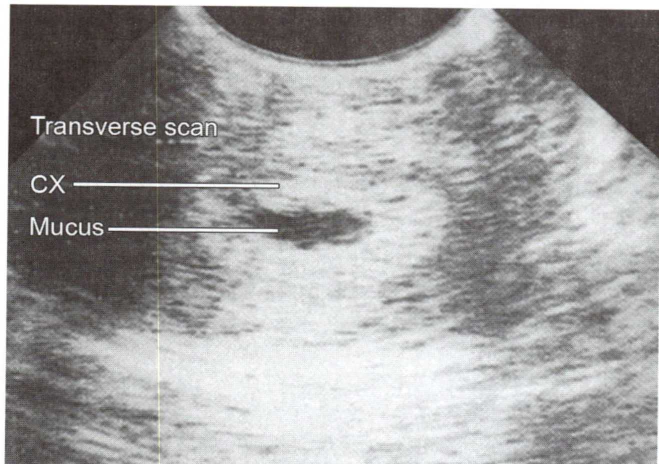

Fig. 1: Cervical mucus.

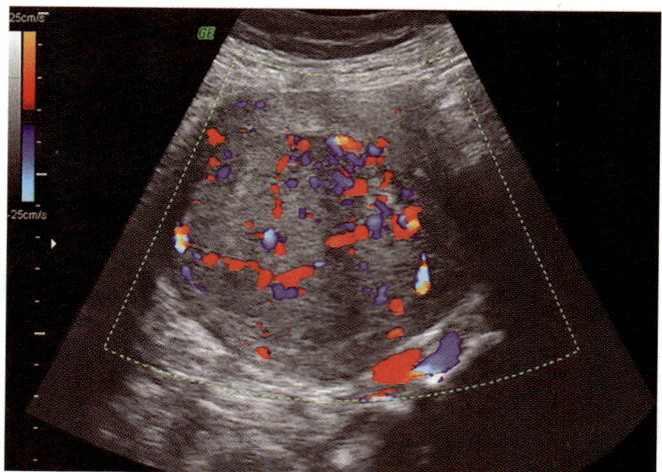

Fig. 3: Penetrating vessels in adenomyosis.

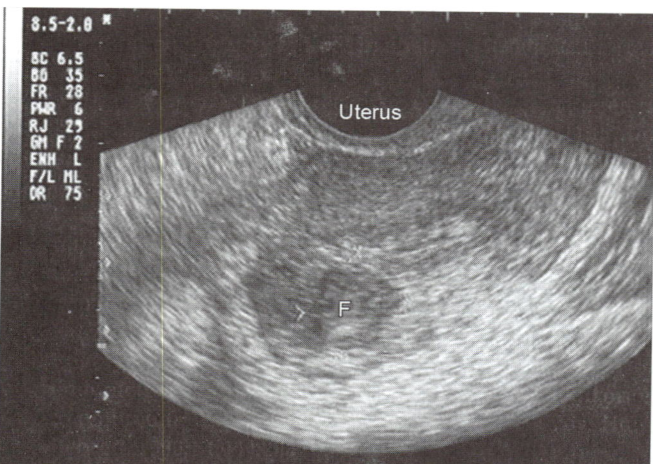

Fig. 2: Fibroid.

Table 1: Distinguishing features between fibroid and adenomyoma.

Fibroid/Adenomyoma	
Fibroid	*Adenomyoma*
• Iso-Hypoechoic • Cavity distorting • Distal acoustic shadowing • Doppler-peripheral draping vessel	• Hyperechoic • Cavity displacing • Pencil line/streaky shadows • Doppler-penetrating vessel

- *Cervix:* Cervix is evaluated for echotexture, cervicitis, nabothian cysts and cervical mucus (Fig. 1).
- *Uterus:* Transvaginal ultrasound is done to rule out any myometrial, endometrial abnormalities or uterine anomalies. The uterus should be scanned completely in transverse and sagittal planes. Imaging of the uterus helps in identifying pathologies like fibroids, adenomyosis, polyps and congenital malformations. Fibroids appear as hypoechoic, well-defined, discrete masses with distal acoustic shadowing on 2D scan with peripheral blood flow (Fig. 2).[1] The sonographic features of adenomyosis include, globular uterus, poor definition of the endometrial—myometrial junction, asymmetrical thickening of the anterior or posterior wall (Fig. 3), anechoic lacunae or cysts of poorly circumscribed areas within the myometrium 1–7 mm diameter, subendometrial echogenic linear striations and heterogeneous myometrium.[2] Table 1 enumerates the distinguising features between fibroid and adenomyoma.[3] Polyps usually appear as echogenic structures within the endometrium, often containing a feeder vessel easily demonstrated with color Doppler imaging.
- *Endometrium:* The endometrial cavity should be visualizable as a separate entity within the uterus in virtually all menstruating patients. It is generally centrally located in the uterus. Endometrium might be difficult to visualize in axially positioned uteri or in case of uterine rotation due to endometriosis or previous surgery-related adhesions. Endometrial thickness is measured in the sagittal plane at maximum thickness including both endometrial layers, placing the calipers at two opposite endometrial-myometrial interfaces (Fig. 4).[4] In case of fluid, thickness of both single layers is measured and is added. Assessment of the endometrial morphology should include endometrial echogenicity (Figs. 5A to D), endometrial midline (Figs. 6A to D) and endometrial-myometrial interface.[4]

The cyclic histologic changes and changes in the thickening of the endometrium with hormonal stimulation can be imaged using transvaginal ultrasound during the different phases of the menstrual cycle. Sakamoto described the characteristic sonographic image noted during the menstrual cycle in 1985.[5] The proliferative endometrium is characterized by:

- The presence of a well-defined three line sign
- A hypoechogenic functional layer
- A minimal or absent posterior acoustic enhancement

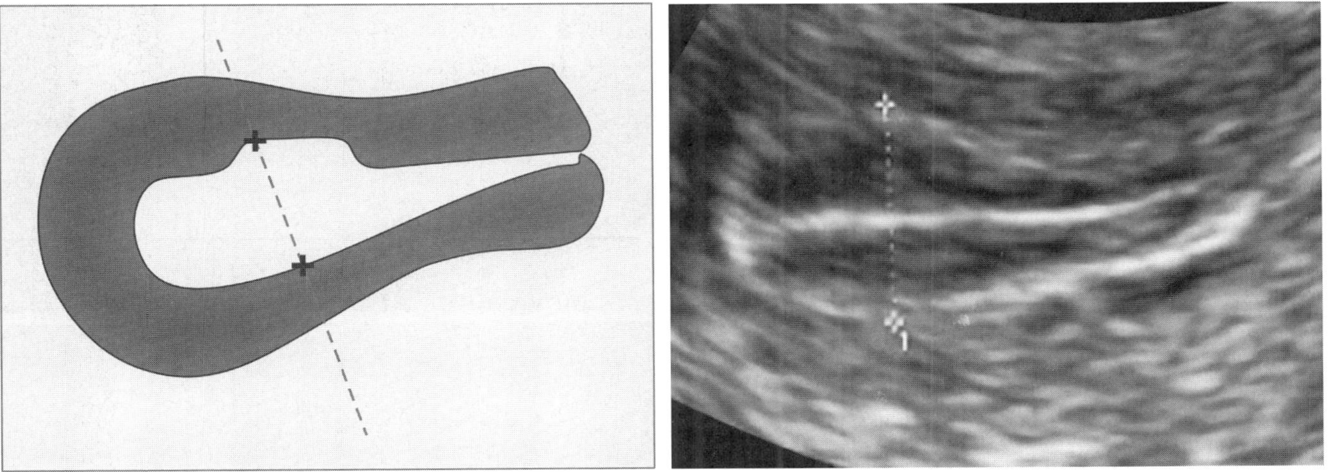

Fig 4: Measurement of endometrial thickness.

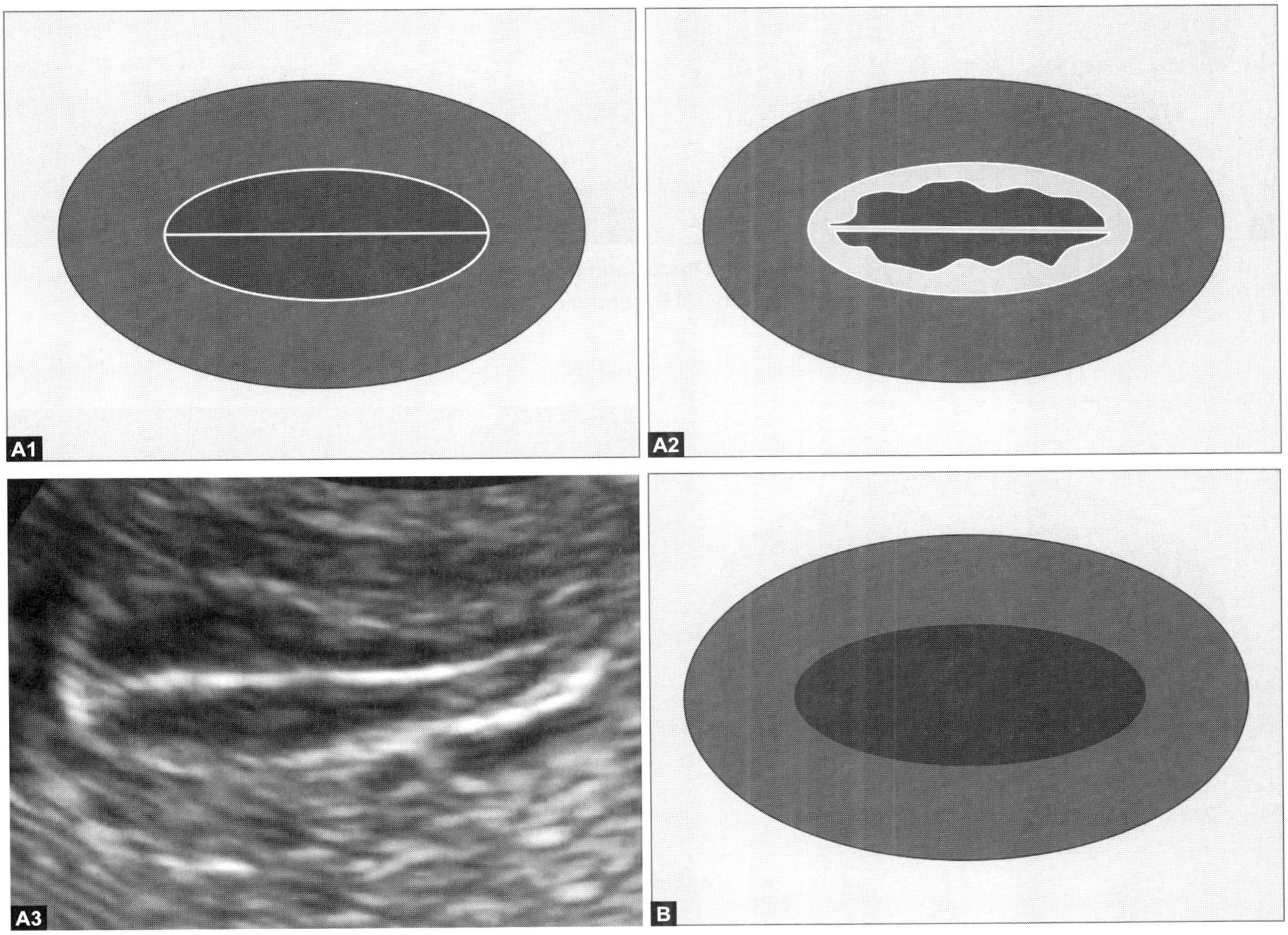

A1

A2

A3

B

Figs. 5A and B

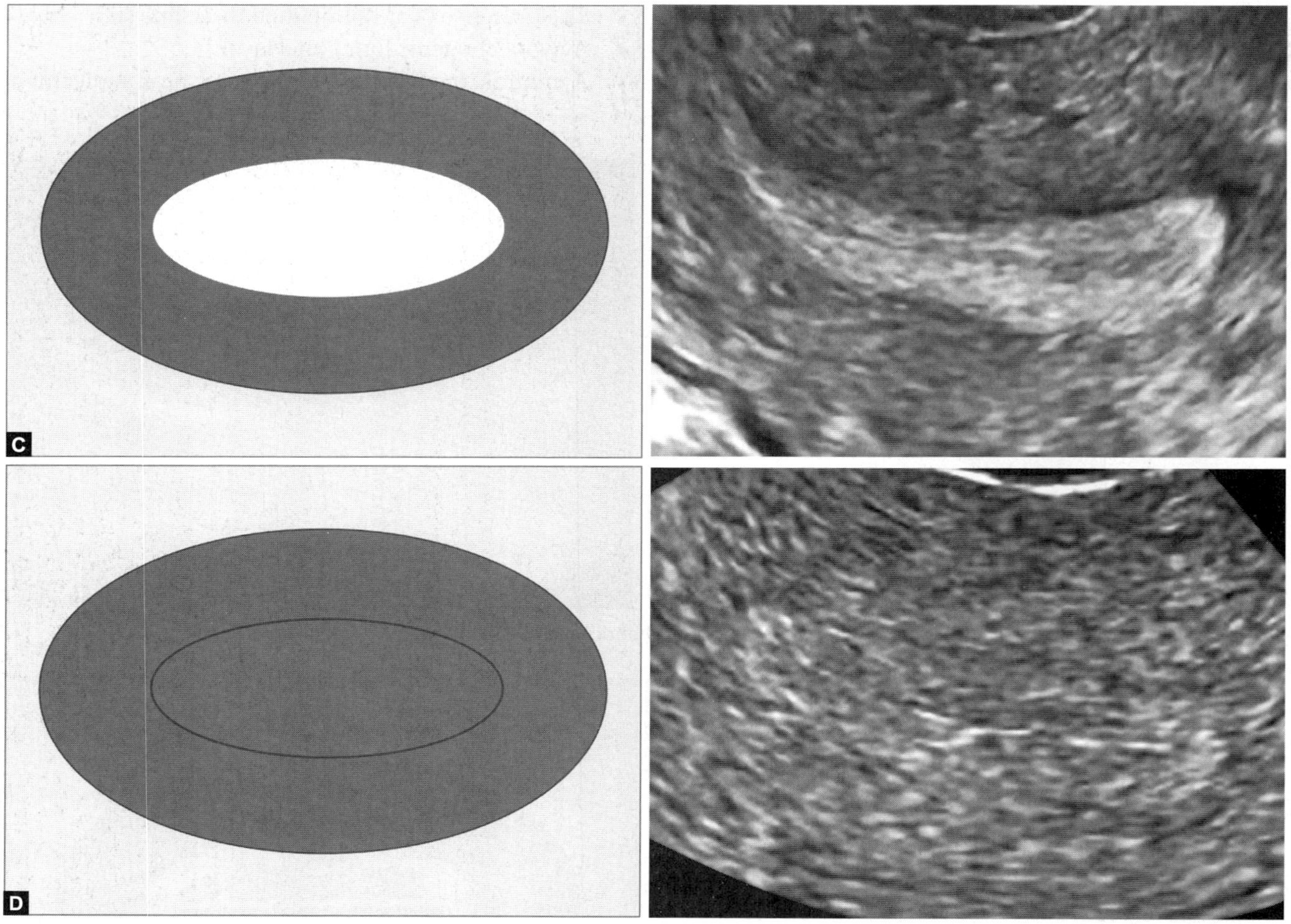

Figs. 5C and D

Figs. 5A to D: Endometrial echogenicity. (A) Hypoechoic, (B) iso-, (C) hyperechoic, (D) Isoechoic

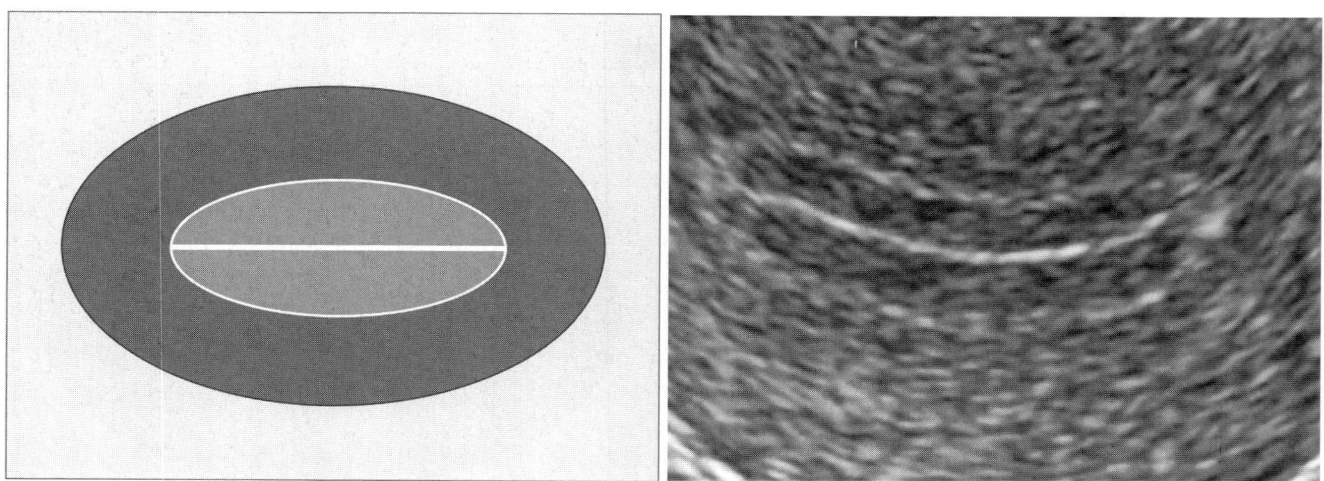

Figs. 6A

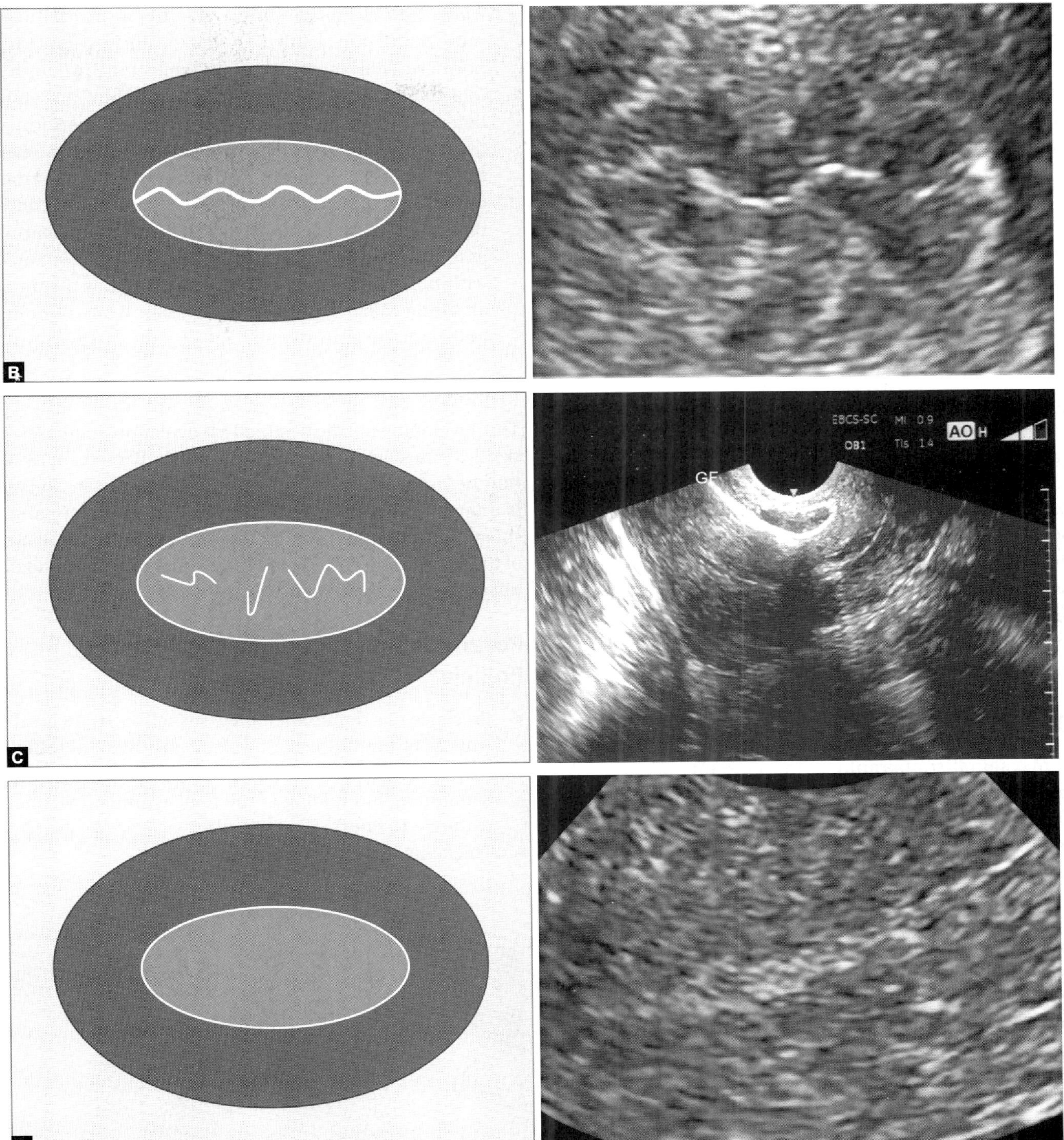

Figs. 6A to D: Endometrial midline; linear (A) non-linear, (B) irregular, (C) and not defined, (D)

The three line sign is formed by the central hyperechoic reflection representing the endometrial cavity and the additional hyperechoic reflection representing the thin developing layer of endometrium. There is also a surrounding hypoechoic halo.[4]

Luteal phase endometrium is:

- Hyperechoic
- Posterior enhancement is present
- Three line sign and halo are absent

Various studies have compared endometrial thickness in predicting pregnancy outcome in ART cycles with varied results. Although an appropriate conclusion has not been made, it is accepted that a very thin endometrium below 7 mm negatively impacts implantation rates.

Tubes

Fallopian tubes are isoechoic and cannot be normally seen on ultrasound unless pathological or fluid surrounds the tubes. Three-dimensional ultrasound is the key to differentiating a tubal from an ovarian mass because the entire tube can be displayed within the volume. On two-dimensional scan hydrosalpinx usually appears as a fusiform cystic lesion, cogwheel sign, adnexal cyst with incomplete septae and has a thickened cyst wall in all acute inflammations (Fig. 7).

Ovary

Transvaginal sonography is the modality of choice for imaging of the ovaries and detects common pathologies. The ovaries are placed medial to the internal iliac vessels on either side of the uterus. TVS can accurately track follicular development, predict and confirm ovulation.

- *Antral follicle count (AFC):* Healthy antral follicles more than 2 mm usually respond to follicle-stimulating hormone (FSH) stimulation and reflect the primordial follicle pool, being described as "selectable." A scan to determine the antral follicle count should be performed in the early follicular phase of the menstrual cycle when there are less chances of including coexisting ovarian cysts or the corpus luteum in the AFC. It is recommended that all antral follicles 2–10 mm in diameter, appearing as round or oval transonic structures should be counted within the entire ovary. AFC is obtained as a sum of all antral follicles in both the ovaries, while omitting follicles more than 10 mm.[6]

Follicular Development

The developing follicle destined for ovulation, increases in size 2–3 mm/day and reaches a maximum diameter of 16–33 mm before ovulation. Selection of the dominant follicle is thought to occur by cycle days 5–7 but is not apparent sonographically until cycle days 8 to 12. Other antral follicles of the developing cohort generally undergo atresia and do not exceed 14 mm in diameter.

Potential Signs Seen in a Preovulatory Follicle[7]

- Presence of a dominant follicle (usually > 16–18 mm)
- Anechoic area, double contour, around the follicle (possible ovulation within 24 hours)
- Separation and folding of the follicle lining (ovulation within 6–10 hours) (Figs. 8 and 9)
- Thickened proliferative endometrium

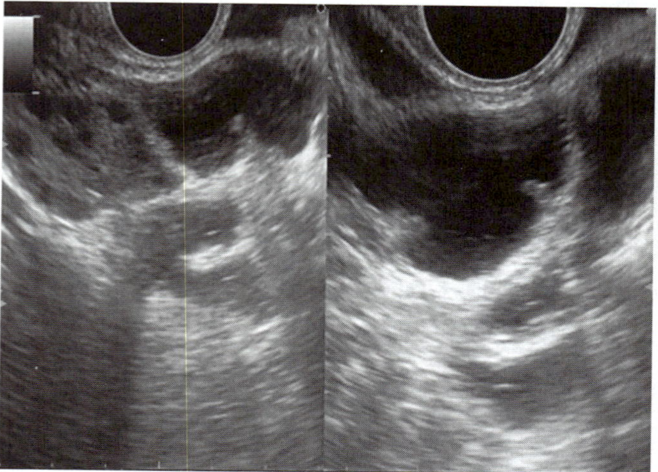

Fig. 7: Hydrosalpinx.

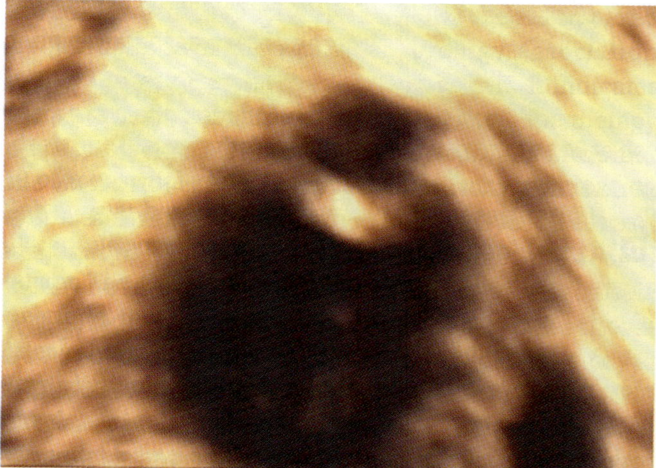

Fig. 8: Cumulus oophorus.

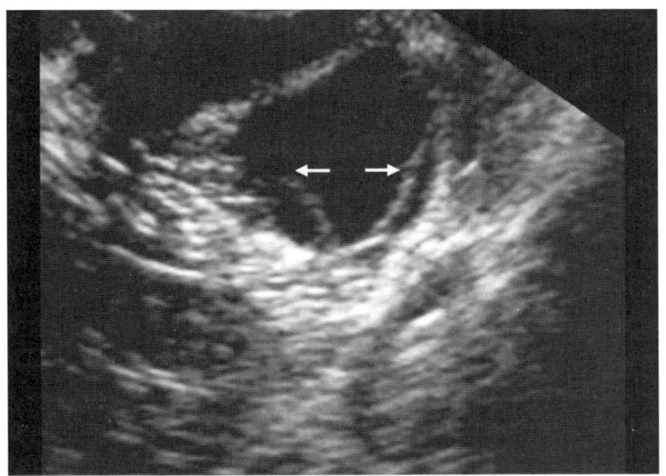

Fig. 9: Infolding of the follicle lining.

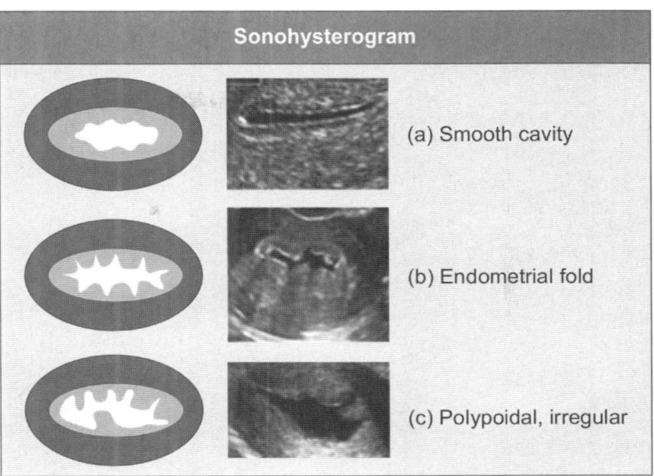

Fig. 10: Figure showing sonohysterogram (SHG) nomenclature.

Confirmation of Ovulation[8]

- Disappearance of the follicle (91% cases)
- Decrease in follicle size (9% cases)
- Fluid in cul de sac when not present in a previous scan
- Development of intrafollicular echoes suggesting the formation of a hemorrhagic corpus luteum

Common Ovarian Pathologies

Ultrasound diagnosis of polycystic ovarian morphology according to Rotterdam criteria is presence of more than or equal to 12 follicles in each ovary of 2–9 mm in size or ovarian volume more than 10 mL in at least one of the ovaries. Distribution may be peripheral or scattered in dense stroma along with stromal hypertrophy or echogenicity. New criteria proposed by the Androgen Excess Society include increasing the follicle number per ovary (FNPO) to 25, for establishing diagnosis of PCOS.

A good 2D ultrasound can help differentiate between common pathologies of the ovary.[7] Dermoid cysts are usually unilocular cysts with mixed echogenicity due to varying composition of fat, bone and fluid. Rokitansky nodule which appears as a distinct hyperechoic mural nodule is pathognomic of dermoid cyst and represents areas of floating hair. Endometriotic cysts are commonly unilocular with diffuse low level echoes-ground glass appearance in 82–95% and low-level blood flow in the wall. Atypical endometriomas can have papillary projections and malignancy should be ruled out.

USG EVALUATION OF TUBAL PATENCY

Sonosalpingography also known as "SION TEST" is a test to assess the tubal patency using ultrasound and Doppler. Sion test is a noninvasive, cheap outdoor screening procedure for tubal testing but cannot replace hysterosalpingogram (HSG) or laparoscopy as it cannot determine the site of block or intratubal pathology.

Method—the patient is asked to evacuate the bladder and base line vaginal scan is performed. Then a no. 8 Foleys catheter is introduced into the uterus and bulb is inflated with 2 mL distilled water. 20–60 mL of solution containing diploes, hyalase and dexamethasone is taken in 50 mL syringe and pushed via Foley's catheter; spill is confirmed as turbulence from the fimbrial end or presence of periovarian fluid or fluid in pouch of Douglas.

Table 2: Distinguishing features between polyps and fibroid on sonohysterography (SHG). (Fig. 11)

Intracavitary lesion	
Polyp	*Fibroid*
• Echogenicity—similar to endometrium	• Echogenicity—similar to myometrium
• Epicenter—endometrial based	• Epicenter—myometrial based
• Vascularity—feeder vessel at pedicle	• Vascularity—peripheral draping vessel

UTERINE CAVITY EVALUATION (FIG. 10)

Sonosalpingography (SSG) can be combined with sonohysterography (SHG) for a complete infertility workup. It can very accurately delineate the cavity and pick up pathologies like irregular endometrium, polyps, Asherman syndrome, submucous fibroids, septum, unicornuate and T-shaped uterus. Saline infusion sonohysterography can establish the location of the fibroid with respect to the endometrial lining. Table 2 enumerates the distinguishing features between polyps and fibroid on SHG.

Sonohysterography is done in the proliferative phase by introducing a No.8 Foley's catheter or an infant feeding

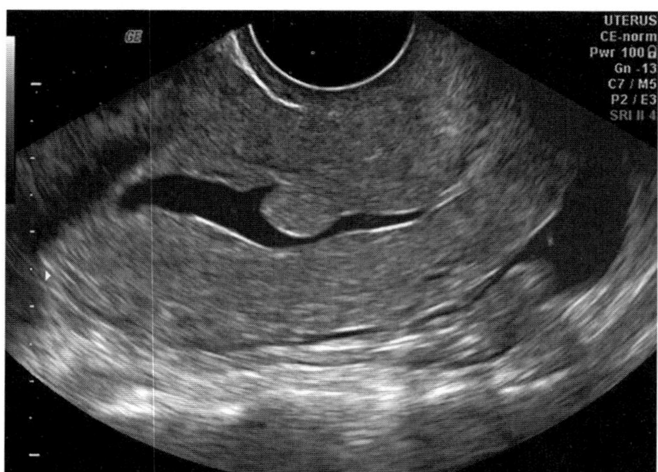

Fig. 11: Cavity lesion on sonohysterogram (SHG).

tube into the uterine cavity and injecting a sterile fluid media under ultrasound visualization (normal saline, hydrotubation fluid or commercially available echocontrast media: ECHOVIST).

ROLE OF USG MONITORING IN STIMULATED CYCLES

Follicular monitoring is important to assess the follicular response to stimulation in IUI or IVF cycles. This scan should be done on the day 5/6 of stimulation for an assessment of both number and size of follicles and helps to adjust the dosage of gonadotropins along with estradiol estimation. Hackeloer et al. (1979) reported a good correlation between follicular diameter and plasma estradiol levels in women in spontaneous menstrual cycles. The follicular diameters must be measured in the transverse and longitudinal planes to get the average diameter.

Follicular sizes also help to decide timing of human chorionic gonadotropin (hCG) trigger which is usually 20 mm in clomiphene cycle and 17–18 mm in gonadotropin cycles. In IVF cycles trigger is given when at least 2–3 lead follicles are more than 18 mm and majority are more than 14 mm. Total number of follicles on day of trigger also helps to assess the risk of *ovarian hyperstimulation syndrome* (OHSS) so that preventive measures can be initiated.

ULTRASOUND-GUIDED PROCEDURES

Ultrasound is an integral part of key IVF procedures like oocyte retrieval and embryo transfer.

Role of 3D Scan in Infertility

Müllerian duct anomalies are estimated to occur in 3% to 4% of all women, 7% of infertile women, 5–10% of patients with recurrent early miscarriages and more than 25% of women who present with recurrent late miscarriages and preterm deliveries.[9] Three-dimensional sonography has a sensitivity and specificity of 100% for diagnosing müllerian abnormalities. In comparison hysterosalpingography has a sensitivity of 78% and accuracy of 86% as there is nonvisualization of the fundal contour and it is diffcult to distinguish between bicornuate and septate uterus on HSG.[10] 3D ultrasound provides an accurate picture of the uterine cavity, serosal surface, and the myometrium in between. 3D ultrasound is also of paramount importance in detecting polyps and pinpointing the location of fibroids. Scoring systems like STEPW or LASMAR score have been devised which help decide feasibility of hysteroscopic surgery for submucous fibroids (Table 3).[11]

SonoAVC (Sonography-based Automated Volume Count) (Fig. 12)

This software automatically calculates the volume and mean diameter of all hypoechoic regions and depicts

Table 3: STEPW or LASMAR score.

	Size (cm)	*Topography*	*Extension of the base*	*Penetration*	*Lateral wall*	*Total*
0	< 2	Low	< 1/3	0		
1	> 2 a5	Middle	> 1/3 – 2/3	< 50%	+1	
2	> 5	Upper	> 2/3	> 50%		
Score	+	+	+	+	+	
Score	*Group*	*Complexity and therapeutic options*				
0 to 4	I	Low complexity hysteroscopic myomectomy.				
5 to 6	II	High complexity hysteroscopic myomectomy. Consider GnRH use? Consider two-step hysteroscopic myomectomy.				
7 to 9	III	Consider alternatives to the hysteroscopic technique				

(GnRH: Gonadotropin releasing hormone)

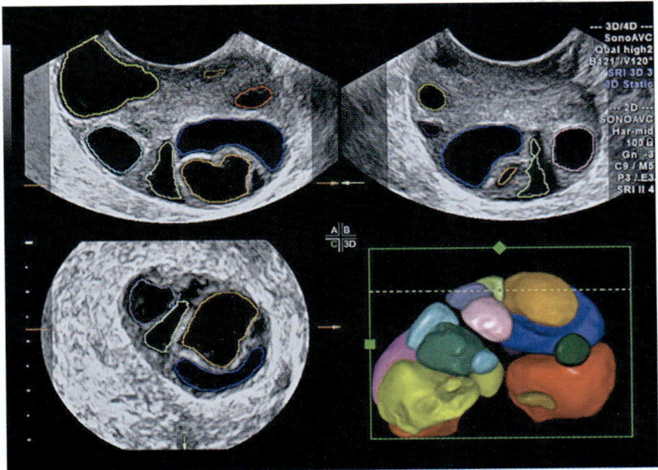

Fig. 12: SonoAVC (Sonography-based automated volume count).

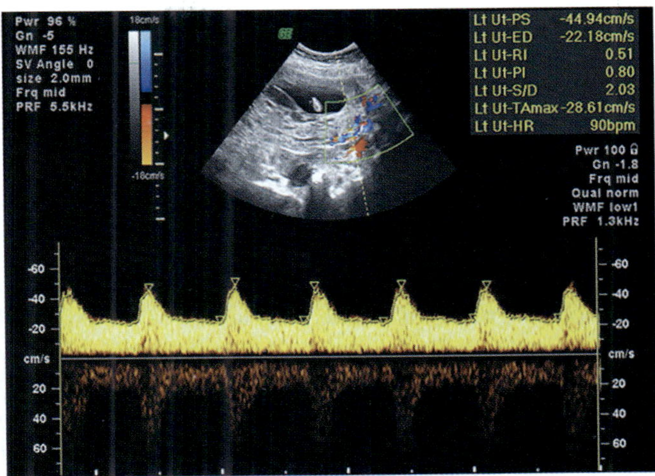

Fig. 13: Uterine artery waveform.

them pictorially in different colors to help study follicular development in the ovary. It is found to be highly accurate and reproducible in assessing individual antral follicles and exact follicular size saving time but needs post processing and was not found to improve the clinical outcomes.[12]

ROLE OF COLOR DOPPLER IN INFERTILITY

Addition of color to a two-dimensional TVS while evaluating infertility is an important tool to study the whole of the menstrual cycle. Color Doppler provides vital information about follicular dynamics like blood flow to the growing follicle, the vascular supply of the endometrium and corpus luteum vascularization which are very important for a successful outcome in terms of pregnancy.

Changes in the Ovary

The blood supply to ovary is by the ovarian artery via the infundibulopelvic ligament and ovarian branch of the uterine artery. Dominant follicle within the ovary can be identified by Doppler usually on day 8–10 by its increased perifollicular flow appearance due to neovascularization. These vessels become more abundant and prominent as the follicle grows in size. In general the Doppler index values are high in the early part of menstrual cycle and fall as ovulation approaches. According to Kurjak et al. the perifollicular resistance index (RI) in the early proliferative phase is 0.54 +/- 0.04 and falls the day before ovulation (LH Peak) when it is about 0.44 +/- 0.04.[13]

This is the best time for administration of surrogate HCG. Impending ovulation is heralded by an increase in peak systolic velocity with a relatively constant RI. The lowest RI values were obtained during the mid-luteal phase (RI 0.42 ± 0.06) with a return to higher vascular resistance (0.50 ± 0.04) during the late luteal phase. If the ovary having corpus luteum shows high RI (>0.50) it is associated with nonviable outcome.

Uterine Perfusion (Fig. 13)

Uterus receives its blood supply by the uterine artery via the arcuate arteries located in the outer one-third of the myometrium. These arcuate vessels branch into radial arteries at the endomyometrial border and further into basal arteries and the spiral arteries.

Usually uterine artery RI remains around 0.88 ± 0.04 in the follicular phase, with an increase in uterine artery impedance 3 days after the luteinizing hormone (LH) peak (day 16). This is due to the compression of vessels traversing the uterine wall, which decrease their diameter and consequently cause higher resistance to flow. The uterine artery impedance again declines to its lowest in the mid-luteal phase (RI = 0.84 ± 0.04) favoring implantation.

Similarly, blood flow changes in the spiral arteries can be used to predict implantation more precisely than uterine artery waveforms. Blood flow velocity wave form changes in the spiral arteries during normal ovulatory cycles are characterized by lower velocity and lower impedance to blood flow than in the uterine arteries.

Changes in the Endometrium

Michael Applebaum in his study with transvaginal color Doppler divided the endometrium and periendometrial areas into 4 zones. In the study conducted by him no pregnancy was reported in IVF patients unless vascularity was demonstrated in Zone III or with in Zone III or IV prior to transfer.

Zone 1: 2 mm thick area surrounding the hyperechoic outer layer of the endometrium
Zone 2: The hyperechoic outer layer of the endometrium
Zone 3: The hypoechoic inner layer of the endometrium
Zone 4: The endometrial cavity

Luteinized Unruptured Follicle (LUF)

This condition is recognized by serial ultrasonography to monitor the growth of follicle, with failure to see expected changes at the time of ovulation. LUF can be identified by means of color Doppler. Rising PSV (peak systolic velocity) with steady low RI suggests that follicle is close to rupture while steady or declining PSV with rising RI is indicative of follicle proceeding to LUF.

Luteal Phase Defect

This is due to decreased vascularization of corpus luteum. In the LPD group, no difference was obtained in terms of intraovarian RI during the follicular phase. The mean RI throughout the luteal phase (0.56 ± 0.04) was significantly higher compared to that in the normal women. Furthermore it did not show any difference between the early, middle and late luteal phase. In the LPD group no difference occurred in terms of intraovarian RI between the sides.

Color Doppler in In-vitro Fertilization

Color Doppler could prove valuable in the prediction of the response of patients to ovarian stimulation in assisted conception, assessment of oocyte quality based on perifollicular flow and parameters influencing implantation following embryo transfer.

- *Prediction of patient response to ovulation stimulation:* It is seen that women with greater ovarian stromal peak systolic blood flow velocity have increased intraovarian perfusion and need less amount of gonadotropins.
- *Follicular characteristics assessment in predicting oocyte quality (Fig. 14):* Nargund et al.[14] showed that oocytes obtained from highly vascularized follicle were of higher quality and were more likely to fertilize and result in pregnancy. From the available data, it appears that assessment of perifollicular vascular perfusion could lead to a better selection of oocytes and ultimately a higher pregnancy rate.
- *Implantation:* Friedler et al.[15] showed that the uterine artery impendence was different in the mid-luteal phase in women with subinfertility compared with those with normal fertility. They grouped the patients according to whether the PI was low (1–1.99), medium (2–2.99) or high (> 3.0). There were no pregnancies in high PI group and the PI was significantly lower in women who become pregnant as compared with those who did not.

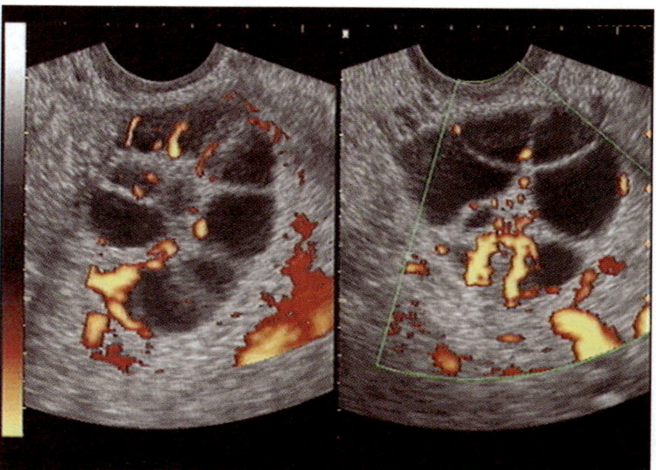

Fig. 14: Perifollicular blood flow.

The ability to predict implantation before the administration of hCG allows the clinician the option to delay giving hCG until the uterine artery PI improves.

CONCLUSION

Ultrasonography offers a reproducible method of comprehensive complete infertility evaluation of the female patient which can replace a multitude of other diagnostic tests and give information about the entire pelvis. Addition of color gives us more information about organ perfusion and addition of 3D has opened a new dimension to diagnosis of pelvic pathologies.

REFERENCES

1. Caoili EM, Hertzberg BS, Kliewer MA, et al. Refractory Shadowing from Leiomyoma. Am J Radiol. 2000:174(1):97-101
2. Fedele et al. Sonographic differentiation of Adenomyoma and Leiomyoma. Am J Obstet Gynecol. 1992:167(3):603-6
3. Botsis D, Kassanos D, Antoniou G, et al. Imaging characteristics of Adenomyoma and Leiomyoma. J Clin Ultrasound. 1998;26(1):21-5.
4. Leone FP, Timmerman D, Valentin L, et al. Terms, definitions and measurements to describe the sonographic features of the endometrium and intrauterine lesions: a consensus opinion from the International Endometrial Tumor Analysis (IETA) group. Ultrasound Obstet Gynecol. 2010;35(1):103-12.
5. Sakamoto C. Sonographic criteria of phasic changes in human endometrial tissue. Int J Gynecol Obstet. 1985;23(1):7-12.
6. Broekmans FJ, de Ziegler D, Howles CM, et al The antral follicle count: practical recommendations for better standardization. Fertil Steril. 2010;94(3):1044-51.

7. Picker RH, Smith DH, Tucker MH, et al. Ultrasonic signs of imminent ovulation J Clin Ultrasound. 1983;11(1):1-2.
8. Jaffe R, Ben Aderet N. Ultrasonic screening in predicting the time of ovulation. Gynecol obstet Invest.1984;18(6):303-5.
9. Chan YY, Jayaprakasan K, Zamora J, et al. The prevalence of congenital uterine anomalies in unselected and high-risk populations: a systematic review. Hum Reprod Update. 2011;17(6):761-71.
10. Saravelos SH, Cocksedge KA, Li TC. Prevalence and diagnosis of congenital uterine anomalies in women with reproductive failure: a critical appraisal. Hum Reprod Update. 2008;14(5)415-29.
11. Lasmar RB, XInmei Z, Indman PD, et al. Feasibility of a new system of classification of submucous myomas: a multicenter study. Fertil Steril. 2011;95(6):2073-7.
12. Raine-Fenning N, Jayaprakasan K, Deb S, et al. Automated follicle tracking improves measurement reliability in patients undergoing ovarian stimulation. Reprod Biomed Online. 2009;18(5):658-63.
13. Kujak A, Kupesic S. Transvaginal color Doppler and pelvic tumor vascularity: lessons learned and future challenges. Ultrasound Obstet Gynecol. 1995;6(2):145-9.
14. Nargund G, Doyle PE, Bourne TH, et al. Ultrasound derived indices of follicular blood flow before HCG administration and prediction of oocyte recovery and preimplantation embryo quality. Hum Reprod. 1996;11(11):2512-7.
15. Freidler S, Schenker JG, Herman A, et al. The role of ultrasonography in the evaluation of endometrial receptivity following assisted reproductive treatments: a critical review. Hum Reprod Update. 1996;2(4):323-35.

CHAPTER

12

When to Stop Investigating and Start Treating?

Rohit Gutgutia

INTRODUCTION

As the chapters in this treatise by various illustrious authors have demonstrated, investigating a couple desirous of a child is not a child's play. We need to be methodical as well as rational when asking for investigations. The aim is always to treat and not *merely* to investigate.

Which is why, there exists an entity called unexplained infertility. In fact, 15–30% couples shall be diagnosed as unexplained infertility after their diagnostic work-up.[1] In today's era, this should not be so. There are investigative tools which can diagnose the cause of infertility but beyond a point investigations are not carried out and instead a working diagnosis of unexplained infertility is made and treatment initiated.

This brings us to the moot point: when is it time to stop investigating and start treating the couple for their inability to conceive. There are, as would be expected in medicine, no clear answers to this question. We attempt in this chapter to understand the implications of delaying treatment in favor of further investigation to arrive at a firm diagnosis.

The Practice Committee of the American Society for Reproductive Medicine (ASRM) has published guidelines for a standard infertility evaluation.[2] It includes a semen analysis, assessment of ovulation, a hysterosalpingogram, and, if indicated, tests for ovarian reserve and laparoscopy. When these tests are inconclusive, a provisional diagnosis of unexplained infertility is made.[1] There is approximately 15–30% chance that these reports shall come out normal. So, there is a large group of couples who do not have working diagnosis prior to starting treatment. The practicing clinician can choose to further investigate the couple or go ahead with treatment based on the available information.

ROLE OF FURTHER INVESTIGATIONS

As we have been made aware by other authors in this treatise, there exists an array of specialized tests for further evaluation of both male and female factors.

Male Factor Investigations

Conventional semen analysis is a critical first step in the evaluation of male fertility, but provides limited information about sperm function.[3] In a subset of patients, specialized semen tests will be needed to elucidate the etiology of subfertility.[4] These tests are useful for determining specific defects of human sperm physiology. Newer sperm function tests may eventually be useful clinically, but more information is needed to determine if these tests will truly predict fertility potential.

Female Factor Investigations

Assessment of Ovulation and Ovarian Reserve Tests

Beyond assessing for ovulation, various ovarian reserve tests have recently become popular with practitioners due to the noninvasive nature of such tests collectively known as ovarian reserve tests. These tests have been proposed to derive a predictive model of sorts for the efficacy of the treatment procedures. However, such attempts have not been very successful, even with multiple markers. Despite the multitude of ovarian reserve tests available, age remains the best predictor of pregnancy.[5]

Assessment of Uterus and Tubes

Assessing the uterine contour and the patency of fallopian tubes remains an integral part of initial investigations.

Beyond hysterosalpingography (HSG), there are other options as mentioned elsewhere. In fact, the concordance of HSG with laparoscopic dye perturbation is estimated as close to 90%.[6] However, patent fallopian tubes on HSG do not confirm that ovum pickup will occur. For example, women with severe endometriosis may have adherent ovaries in the cul-de-sac with normal fallopian tubes.

So the general consensus is that while some advanced tests may have some role in identifying the cause of infertility and thus allow more targeted approach, by and large such tests do not help much in the treatment planning for majority of couples. It makes more sense to treat such couples.

TREATMENT OPTIONS

The treatment for unexplained infertility is therefore, by definition, empiric because it does not address a specific defect or functional impairment. The principal treatments for unexplained infertility include expectant observation with timed intercourse and lifestyle changes, clomiphene citrate and intrauterine insemination (IUI), controlled ovarian hyperstimulation (COH) with IUI and in-vitro fertilization (IVF).

Expectant Management and Lifestyle Changes

Epidemiological studies indicate cigarette smoking, abnormal body mass index (BMI), and excessive caffeine and alcohol consumption reduce fertility in the female partner. The female partner should be counseled to achieve a normal BMI, reduce caffeine intake to no more than 250 mg daily (2 cups of coffee), and reduce alcohol intake to no more than four standardized drinks per week.[7]

Although expectant management is associated with the lowest cost, it results in the lowest cycle fecundity rates, and is therefore inferior to the commonly available reproductive techniques outlined below. It may provide an option for a couple with unexplained infertility in whom the female partner is young and the problem of oocyte depletion is not an immediate concern.

Laparoscopy as a Treatment

A Cochrane review on the topic published in 2002 concluded that laparoscopic surgery in the treatment of minimal and mild endometriosis may improve pregnancy success rates, but that the "relevant trials have some methodological problems and further research in this area is needed."[8] If laparoscopy is performed in a patient with unexplained infertility and minimal/mild endometriosis is identified, we recommend ablation of endometriosis.[9] However, the current literature does not support performing a diagnostic laparoscopy in all patients with unexplained infertility.

Intrauterine Insemination (IUI) as a Treatment

IUI involves the placement of washed sperm into the uterine cavity around the time of ovulation. It can be performed in conjunction with natural ovulation timed with lutienizing hormone (LH) kit, ovulation induction using clomiphene citrate, or injectable gonadotropins. Few data exist on the use of IUI without COH.

The theoretical rationale for COH in women with a normal ovulatory assessment is that subtle ovulatory defects missed by standard testing may be overcome, and that an increased number of eggs available for fertilization may increase the likelihood of pregnancy. In a similar fashion, introducing washed sperm into the uterine cavity using IUI may increase the density of motile sperm available to ovulated oocytes, which should maximize the chance of fertilization.[10]

In-vitro Fertilization (IVF) or Intracytoplasmic Sperm Injection (ICSI) as a Treatment

The most expensive, but also most successful treatment of unexplained infertility consists of the spectrum of assisted reproductive technology including IVF, with or without ICSI. IVF is the treatment of choice for unexplained infertility when the less costly, but also less successful treatment modalities outlined above have not worked. In some IVF programs ICSI is performed in all couples with unexplained infertility for an undetected but suspected fertilization problem.

CONCLUSION

A thorough but time-efficient investigation of the infertile couple is required prior to a diagnosis of unexplained infertility. Couples should undergo a semen analysis, ovulation testing, assessment of ovarian reserve, and imaging to assess for tubal and uterine factors. This work up can ideally be completed in one menstrual cycle.

There is not much sense in doing further investigations solely to establish a diagnosis while delaying treatment. Instead a working diagnosis of unexplained infertility can be made and prompt treatment instituted on that basis. A smaller group of couples may benefit from further investigations based on their individual considerations but the advanced tests are by and large not applicable to the general population.

The treatment options that are available are expectant management with lifestyle changes, IUI with COH and IVF/ICSI. While a comparative analysis of all these treatment options has never been performed, the European Society of Human Reproduction and Embryology (ESHRE) Multicentre Trial reported in 1991 that pregnancy rates per cycle were 15.2% in gonadotropin-only cycles, 27.4% in gonadotropin and IUI cycles, and 25.7% in IVF cycles.[11] The pregnancy rate for IVF cycles has since increased with availability of improved and sequential media, embryo micromanipulation, and extended embryo culture. The ASRM Practice Committee published an analysis on the appropriate roles and the cost- effectiveness of the various procedures in the management of unexplained infertility by analysis of previously published data.[12] There is limited information on the costeffectiveness of various treatments; however, it appears that there is a correlation between the cost of a treatment modality and its pregnancy rates. Therefore, depending on the individual couple and their particular clinical situation, COH with IUI may be attempted first, with transition to IVF/ICSI if pregnancy is not achieved in a timely manner.

The optimal treatment strategy needs to be based on individual patient characteristics such as age, treatment efficacy, side-effects profile such as multiple pregnancies, and cost consideration.

REFERENCES

1. The Practice Committee of the American Society for Reproductive Medicine, authors. Effectiveness and treatment for unexplained infertility. Fertil Steril. 2006; 86(5 suppl):S111–4.
2. The Practice Committee of the American Society for Reproductive Medicine, authors. Optimal evaluation of the infertile female. Fertil Steril. 2006;86(5 suppl): S264–7.
3. World Health Organization. Laboratory manual of the WHO for the examination of human semen and sperm-cervical mucus interaction. Ann Ist Super Sanita. 2001;38(1):I-XII, 1-123.
4. Guzick DS, Overstreet JW, Factor-Litvak P, et al. Sperm morphology, motility, and concentration in fertile and infertile men. N Engl J Med. 2001;345:1388–93.
5. Eijkemans MJ, Lintsen AM, Hunault CC, et al. Pregnancy chances on an IVF/ICSI waiting list: a national prospective cohort study. Hum Reprod. 2008;23:1627–32.
6. Exacoustos C, Zupi E, Carusotti C, et al. Hysterosalpingo-contrast sonography compared with hysterosalpingography and laparoscopic dye pertubation to evaluate tubal patency. J Am Assoc Gynecol Laparosc. 2003;10:367–72.
7. Barbieri RL. The initial fertility consultation: recommendations concerning cigarette smoking, body mass index, and alcohol and caffeine consumption. Am J Obstet Gynecol. 2001;185:1168–73.
8. Jacobson TZ, Barlow DH, Koninckx PR, et al. Laparoscopic surgery for subfertility associated with endometriosis. Cochrane Database Syst Rev. 2010;1: CD001398.
9. Marcoux S, Maheux R, Berube S. Laparoscopic surgery in infertile women with minimal or mild endometriosis. Canadian Collaborative Group on Endometriosis. N Engl J Med. 1997;337:217–22.
10. Verhulst SM, Cohlen BJ, Hughes E, et al. Intra-uterine insemination for unexplained subfertility. Cochrane Database Syst Rev. 2006;4:CD001838.
11. Crosignani PG, Walters DE, Soliani A. The ESHRE multicentre trial on the treatment of unexplained infertility: a preliminary report. European Society of Human Reproduction and Embryology. Hum Reprod. 1991;6:953–8.
12. Guzick DS, Sullivan MW, Adamson GD, et al. Efficacy of treatment for unexplained infertility. Fertil Steril. 1998;70:207–13.

Section 2

Practical Management of Male Infertility

CHAPTER

13

Understanding the New WHO 2010 Semen Parameters

Cristina González Ravina, Alberto Pacheco Castro

INTRODUCTION

As it is well known, the first *Laboratory Manual for the Analysis of Human Semen and Its Interaction with the Cervical Mucus* was published in 1980. This was as a response to the high necessity of standardizing the protocols to carry out this analysis.[1] This manual has subsequently been reviewed three times. In 2010, the fifth edition of the *Laboratory Manual for the Examination and Processing of Human Semen* was published. In this edition, the latest so far, the reference values, the algorithms for diagnosis, the clinical interpretation of diagnosis, and other relevant aspects have been reviewed. Until last year, every andrology or assisted reproduction laboratory worked according to the guidelines recommended in the latest manuals published by the WHO.[1-3]

After making a revision of these manuals and the reference values that existed up to the year 2010, it can be observed that they were useful when established in 1999, but nowadays an update of these was necessary. It should be remembered that the studies performed to establish the reference values in 1999 were based in the analysis of two semen samples from a not-very-high number of males in different laboratories where the work method had not yet been standardized nor the pertinent quality systems had yet been introduced.

THE PREVIOUS WHO MANUAL

In the manual published in 1999, spermatozoa were classified in four categories regarding their motility: type a [rapid progressive motility (PM)], type b (slow PM), type c [nonprogressive motility (NP)], and type d [immotility (IM)]. One of the main restrictions from this classification is the acknowledgment that sperm PM (types a + b) studies and morphology studies were not only subjective but also they did not follow any standard protocol in the laboratories.[4-6] However, the values obtained regarding sperm concentration and total motility (a + b + c) were considered acceptable. This is because they could be measured in a reproducible way in most centers. For this reason, it was recommended that each laboratory established their own limit values of normality for these variables, and they were also advised to include the appropriate internal and external quality assurances. These quality assurances are fully developed in the new manual of 2010.

In spite of this, reference ranges for the main seminal parameters were defined through a statistics analysis by comparing the sperm characteristics of a group of males. These reference ranges distinguished two different populations studied (fertile vs. subfertile or subfertile vs. infertile).[7,8]

The reference values established in 1999 are shown in Table 1. Regarding morphology, the WHO manual discusses the start of a multicenter study for the analysis of seminal parameters. The edition of 1999 specifies that the data obtained in centers with assisted reproduction programs suggest a connection between morphology values less than 15% and a decrease in IVF (in vitro fertilization) rate.[9]

Regarding the nomenclature, these are the terms used to express seminogram values lower than the reference values:

- *Asthenozoospermia*: PM less than 50% types a + b or less than 25% type a
- *Oligozoospermia*: Concentration less than 20 million/mL
- *Teratozoospermia*: Morphology less than 15% normal shapes

Table 1: The reference values established in the WHO Laboratory Manual of 1999.

Seminal parameter	*Lower reference value*
Volume	2.0 mL
pH	7.2
Concentration	20 million spermatozoa per milliliter
Total number of spermatozoa	40 million spermatozoa per ejaculation
Motility	50% type a + b spermatozoa per ejaculation 25% type a spermatozoa per ejaculation
Vitality	75% spermatozoa alive per ejaculation
Morphology	15% normal shape

- *Necrozoospermia*: Vitality less than 75%
- *Cryptozoospermia*: Absence of spermatozoa in the first analysis of the ejaculation sample and presence of spermatozoa after centrifugation
- *Azoospermia*: Absence of spermatozoa in the first analysis of the ejaculation sample and absence of spermatozoa after centrifugation; concentration = 0
- *Aspermia*: Absence of ejaculation; volume = 0

Based on the male's seminal classification, his medical history and his physical exploration, as well as any other additional information, a diagnosis of the male could be given through a diagram based on different sperm concentration ranging from azoospermia, cryptozoospermia, and oligozoospermia samples.[1-3] It should be emphasized that in the manual of 1999, a subclassification for the different seminal alterations (oligo-, asteno-, terato-, and necrozoospermia) is used, with a range from mild to moderate to severe.

CHANGES IN THE NEW 2010 WHO MANUAL

Eleven years after the edition of 1999, a review and update of the reference values and the established work protocols became more and more necessary. Therefore, the new online edition of the WHO manual of 2010 presents much more detail regarding seminal analysis: work solutions, procedures, calculations, and results interpretation. Furthermore, it recommends using a specific method in those cases in which there is more than one possible analysis technique.

Considering this, the main changes in the fifth edition include the following:

- A new work protocol to determine sperm concentration. The recommended semen dilutions and the counting chamber areas necessary to establish the number of spermatozoa (concentration) in order to count 200 spermatozoa by replicate have been modified. The goal of reducing sampling errors has been intensified, giving more importance to the sample volume, which was not so relevant before. This sample volume must be measured with precision and using the method recommended by the WHO manual (by weighing the sample in the vessel in which it is collected).
- Regarding azoospermia, there is a change in the work protocols to be followed on this type of samples, in which there are no spermatozoa in the ejaculate. It differentiates the necessity to obtain a concentration value and/or an accurate motility value from centrifuging the sample to increase the chances of finding spermatozoa after washing.
- There are significant changes in the sperm motility classification. From now on, spermatozoa should be only differentiated according to three categories: PM—combining former types a + b, NP—former type c, and IM—former type d.
- The morphology analysis is dealt with in more detail in this edition. It includes pictures of spermatozoa considered normal and spermatozoa with one or several morphological anomalies, as well as accurate explanations to improve the technician's training regarding the study of this seminal parameter.
- On the other hand, the manual includes an improved chapter on semen cryopreservation, with a well-described section on sperm preparation.

It also dedicates a full chapter to quality assurance that, apart from being the novelty, involves a recommendation from the WHO to have quality assurance in our laboratories. This includes both the external and the internal quality assurance.

Therefore, the fifth edition of the Manual is divided into three parts:

- Semen analysis (Chapters 2–4)
  i. Standard procedures
  ii. Optional procedures
  iii. Research procedures
- Sperm preparation (Chapters 5 and 6)
- Quality assurance (Chapter 7)

METHODOLOGY AND INCLUSION CRITERIA

For this study, semen samples from 4,500 males from 14 countries and four continents were analyzed. They were divided into three wide groups: fertile males, males with unknown fertility, and normozoospermic males according to the manual of 1999. The group of males whose partner had become pregnant in a time period less than or equal to 12 months was selected as the control group to establish the reference values of seminal parameters (1,953 males, five studies in eight countries from three continents).

All the laboratories participating in this study obtained their data by using the standard methods of semen analysis.[1-2] Each laboratory was taken into account at the moment of assessing the results because this manual offers different methods to determine volume, sperm concentration, and morphological stain. Moreover, many laboratories implemented with delay the internal and external quality assurances. For this reason, the data were reviewed to calculate the reference distribution considering that fact.[10]

For this study, only one ejaculated semen sample per male, which was gathered with a sexual abstinence period of 2–7 days, was used. Concentration was measured in most cases with the improved Neubauer hemocytometer. Motility data were gathered on total motility (WHO 1999: a + b + c) and PM (WHO 1999: a + b).[11] Morphology data were taken into account only in those centers using Tygerberg's strict criteria.[1-3] Finally, vitality, analyzed by eosin-nigrosin staining, got a significantly lower number of samples studied than the other seminal parameters, only two centers provided data. The advantage of having standard work protocols is that the analytic error has been minimized and the values presented are considered representative of the seminal characteristics of a fertile male.

NEW REFERENCE VALUES AND DIAGNOSIS

This edition reviews old reference values and establishes new ones with which we have to work nowadays (Table 2).

Table 2: Distribution of values, lower reference limits, and their 95% confidence interval (CI) for semen parameters from fertile men those partners had a time-to-time pregnancy of 12 months or less.

Seminal parameter	*95% CI*
Volume	1.5 milliliter
pH	7.2
Concentration	15 million spermatozoa per milliliter
Total number of spermatozoa	39 million spermatozoa per ejaculation
Motility	40% total motility (progressive + nonprogressive) 32% progressive motility
Vitality	58% spermatozoa alive per ejaculation
Morphology	4% normal shape

These are available in a free access article published in May 2010 in *Human Reproduction Update*[12] offering, with more clarity, lower reference limits of the fifth percentile of the values for a fertile male reference population.

This is accompanied by some changes in the samples diagnosis. Therefore, despite maintaining the nomenclature, there are some changes:

- *Teratozoospermia*: Normal shape by strict criteria (Tygerberg) less than 4%
- *Asthenozoospermia*: PM less than 32% does not take into account total motility (% PR + NP) even if under the reference value.
- *Oligozoospermia*: Total number of spermatozoa less than 39 million. The WHO prefers this parameter to sample concentration, which was the selectable parameter in the Manual of 1999.
- *Necrozoospermia*: Vitality less than 58% and very high IM percentage. The second criterion is arbitrary since the WHO does not specify a number, but it does talk about much IM. This way, fake necrozoospermia, which can alarm unjustifiably, is avoided.
- *Cryptozoospermia/azoospermia*: There are no changes from 1999.

PROBLEMS AND IMPROVEMENTS OF THE NEW WHO CLASSIFICATION

As it occurs in every change or review, we have found not only significant improvements but also some issues that we will need to solve as we get familiarized with the modifications. Some of these issues were as follows:

- *New concept of oligozoospermia:* In 1999, the WHO assigned this diagnosis to those samples with concentration under the reference value of this parameter (20 million/mL). However, it has become clear that this concentration depends on the final volume of the sample. That is the reason why the manual of 2010 links preferably the oligozoospermia diagnosis to the total number of spermatozoa, provided that it is under 39 million. This is an improvement in the assessment of this parameter.
- *New categories of sperm motility:* The old category "a" from the manual of 1999 was difficult to justify without a computerized system to count motility in the sample. It was actually observed that the relevant information from this parameter was in the total number of PM (a + b). For these two reasons, sperm motility categories were modified. Now, it is recommended to differentiate spermatozoa in three categories or types: PM, NP, and IM. Some centers consider the new classification as an advantage.

- *Decrease of the percentage of normal shapes in morphology analysis:* It is well known that this is not only the most subjective parameter of the semen analysis but also the one which creates the most controversy when choosing one treatment type or another in assisted reproduction clinics. Numerous articles have been published for and against the importance of morphology in many key aspects of these treatments: pregnancy rate, implantation rate, fertilization success, etc.[13-17] Anyway, it has always been debated not only in andrology and IVF laboratories but also between these departments and the clinical departments. This is due to the fact that, apart from extreme morphology cases with many anomalies, it is difficult to unify morphological assessment criteria to evaluate the samples, even when performing the appropriate internal and external quality assurances.
- *Sperm vitality and necrozoospermia:* It looks like this parameter, not included in the WHO as a "compulsory study" in the seminogram but as something very advisable, is gaining importance in this new edition. Because this parameter is linked to the percentage of sperm IM but there is not an exact fixed value from which necrozoospermia can be diagnosed, each group can decide that value individually depending on the methodology employed in their center and the information expected from the diagnosis. It is well-known that the vitality study is essential in those cases with a percentage of sperm IM over 50%. It is not the same to have a high percentage of immotile spermatozoa that are alive after the stain test, which would guide toward possible structural flaws in the tail,[18] than a high percentage of immotile spermatozoa which are also dead, more related to an epididymis pathology.[19,20]
- The disappearance of the "adjectives" mild, moderate, and severe results in diagnosis of the samples being incomplete and obliges to take into account numerical values of volume, concentration, motility, and morphology to get a real idea of the state of the sample. Depending on the number of millions of progressive motile spermatozoa, each center or laboratory, can decide the type of treatment for a couple.
- Finally, the most remarkable aspect is probably the different male seminogram reference values and parameters in 1999 and 2010. In Table 3, a comparison of the two possible situations is described.

Table 3: Different male seminogram reference values and parameters in 1999 and 2010.

Seminal parameter	*Semen 1999*	*Semen 2010*
Volume	2.0 milliliter	1.5 milliliter
Concentration	20×10^6 spermatozoa per milliliter	15×10^6 spermatozoa per milliliter 39×10^6 total spermatozoa
Progressive motility	50%	32%
Morphology	15% normal shape	4% normal shape
Millions of progressive motile	20	7.2 12

As it can be observed, the number of millions of progressive motile spermatozoa is reduced by 64%—or 40% if we use the total spermatozoa criterion that is now advised—to the number obtained for a semen sample of a male according to the reference values of 1999. The change of this aspect could cause more problems at clinical consultation level, since males now diagnosed as normal may still receive the recommendation to be submitted to an intrauterine insemination (IUI) or even an IVF cycle. Obviously, each center should decide whether they change their criteria or they explain to every patient that with the current reference values there is the possibility that, even being "normal", they could have subfertility that would need a specific assisted reproduction treatment.

DEBATE

First of all, it is important to remember that the seminogram does not have diagnosis capacity per se—sensitivity and specificity—to indicate male infertility. Seminogram diagnosis is better understood merely as a sample description to check that they "are similar" to the values of a fertile population. Nonetheless, they could be useful in the clinical diagnosis to detect cryptozoospermia or azoospermia.

On the other hand, for people who work in assisted reproduction, it is important to differentiate between the male seminal diagnosis and the "real" use of the sample in an infertility treatment. We know that WHO establishes clearly that being under the reference values or having a sample not "normozoospermic" does not necessarily mean male infertility but it shows that seminal parameter is under the fifth percentile in a reference population of fertile males, i.e. it means that this value is under 95% of the values presented by these fertile males. Theoretically, it is likely that the reference values keep on updating as population studies get widened, especially due to the way those values were obtained—statistics of parameters in 2,000 fertile male. Apart from its utility for the diagnosis of an infertile couple, the seminogram is, together with the other tests and examinations, a useful tool to make therapeutic decisions. Its main goal is to evaluate if the sample, once prepared, allows obtaining the minimum number of millions of progressive motile spermatozoa to follow one reproduction treatment or another: artificial insemination or IUI, in vitro fertilization or IVF, or intracytoplasmic sperm injection (ICSI). We could think that for standard IVF the new reference values should not modify the internal values established by every laboratory according to their insemination protocols. However, we should be careful with normozoospermic samples containing values under the lower limits of the different parameters, as aforementioned. Finally, morphology determination is still a parameter with doubtful clinical utility to recommend a patient directly to IVF or ICSI treatment, and therefore should be considered with caution. In fact, a recent article from 2017 reports that males with 0% of normal forms have a capacity to conceive spontaneously of 29.2%, which reinforces the fact that sperm morphology alone should not be used as a factor prognosis of pregnancy, implantation or live newborn,[21] nor be direct indication in these males of assisted reproduction techniques when it is an isolated factor.[22]

REFERENCES

1. World Health Organization. WHO Laboratory Manual for the Examination of Human Semen and Sperm-Cervical Mucus Interaction, 4th edition. Cambridge: Cambridge University Press; 1999. pp. 128.
2. World Health Organization. Sperm Collection and Processing Methods. Cambridge: Cambridge University Press; 1999.
3. World Health Organization. WHO Manual for the Standardized Investigation and Diagnosis of the Infertile Male. Cambridge: Cambridge University Press; 1999.
4. Cooper TG, Neuwinger J, Bahrs S, et al. Internal quality control of semen analysis. Fertil Steril. 1992;58:172-8.
5. Dunphy BC, Kay R, Barratt CL, et al. Quality control during the conventional analysis of semen, an essential exercise. J Androl. 1989;10:378-85.
6. Neuwinger J, Behre HM, Nieschlag E. External quality control in the andrology laboratory: An experimental multicenter trial. Fertil Steril. 1990;54:308-14.
7. Comhaire FH, Vermeulen L, Schoonjans F. Reassessment of the accuracy of traditional sperm characteristics and adenosine triphosphate (ATP) in estimating the fertilizing potential of human semen in vivo. Int J Androl. 1987;10:653-62.
8. Ombelet W, Bosmans E, Janssen M, et al. Semen parameters in a fertile versus subfertile population: A need for change in the interpretation of semen testing. Hum Reprod. 1997;12:987-93.
9. Ombelet W, Wouters E, Bolees L, et al. Sperm morphology assessment: Diagnostic potential and comparative analysis of strict or WHO criteria in a fertile and subfertile population. Int J Androl. 1997;20:367-72.
10. Castilla JA, Alvarez C, Aguilar J, et al. Influence of analytical and biological variation on the clinical interpretation of seminal parameters. Hum Reprod. 2006;21:847-51.
11. Cooper TG, Yeung CH. Computer-aided evaluation of assessment of "grade a" spermatozoa by experienced technicians. Fertil Steril. 2006;85:220-4.
12. Cooper TG, Noonan E, von Eckardstein S, et al. World Health Organization reference values for human semen characteristics. Hum Reprod Update. 2010;16(3):231-45.
13. Kruger TF, Menkveld R, Stander FS, et al. Sperm morphologic features as a prognostic factor in vitro fertilization. Fertil Steril. 1986;46:1118-23.
14. Kruger TF, Acosta AA, Simmons KF, et al. Predictive value of abnormal sperm morphology in vitro fertilization. Fertil Steril. 1988;49:112-7.
15. Menkveld R, Stander FSH, Kotze TJ, et al. The evaluation of morphological characteristics of human spermatozoa according to stricter criteria. Hum Reprod. 1990;5(5):586-92.
16. Mortimer D, Menkveld R. Sperm morphology assessment. Historical perspectives and current opinions. J Androl. 2001;22:192-205.
17. Garrido N, Meseguer M, Martínez-Conejero JA, et al. Impacto de los criterios estrictos de morfología espermática en reproducción Asistida. Cuadernos de Medicina Reproductiva. 2005;11(1).
18. Chemes HE, Rawe VY. Sperm pathology: A step beyond descriptive morphology. Origin, characterization and fertility potential of abnormal sperm phenotypes in infertile men. Hum Reprod Update. 2003;9:405-28.
19. Wilton LJ, Temple-Smith PD, Baker HWG, et al. Human male infertility caused by degeneration and death of sperm in the epididymis. Fertil Steril. 1988;49:1052-8.
20. Correa-Pérez JR, Fernández-Pelegrina R, Aslanis P, et al. Clinical management of men producing ejaculates characterized by high levels of dead sperm and altered seminal plasma factors consistent with epididymal necrospermia. Fertil Steril. 2004;81(4):1148-50.
21. Kovac JR, Smith RP, Cajipe M, et al. Men with a complete absence of normal sperm morphology exhibit high rates of success without assisted Reproduction. Asian J Androl. 2017;19:39-42.
22. Shabtaie SA, Gerkowicz SA, Kohn TP, et al. Role of abnormal sperm morphology in predicting pregnancy outcomes. Curr Urol Rep. 2016;17:67.

CHAPTER

14

Investigating the Subfertile Male: Which Tests are Practically Relevant?

Alberto Pacheco Castro, Cristina González Ravina

INTRODUCTION

Male infertility is directly or indirectly responsible for 50% of the cases involving fertility-related failures in reproductive couples. Since intracytoplasmic sperm injection (ICSI) into oocytes was described, most of these cases have been treated with this procedure, especially when that failure is due to severe male factor infertility.[1,2] However, current success rates of this procedure remain suboptimal. The reason for this is that current diagnoses of male factor infertility are mainly based on sperm parameters of concentration, motility, viability, and morphology. Also, nowadays, selection of sperm during ICSI is mainly based on motility and morphology.[3] These criteria are clearly inadequate to detect abnormalities at a molecular level, which may have a negative impact on pregnancy rate. Invisible anomalies such as intracellular oxidative stress, externalization of plasma membrane phosphatidylserine, disruption of mitochondrial membrane potential and, more importantly, damaged chromatin are barely taken into account.[4]

In a large number of reproductive centers, male factor is only determined by an anamnesis and a semen profile. Indeed, male factor infertility is usually defined in terms of conventional semen analysis, where descriptive information is only given concerning the number of spermatozoa present in the ejaculate sample and the proportion of them which are motile or morphologically normal and related to "normal" threshold values established by World Health Organization.[5]

Thus, when conventional seminal study confirms a serious defect, especially at the level of sperm concentration (<5 million/mL), supplementary studies are required to improve the diagnosis, especially in order to determine genetic or chromosomal abnormalities. Among them, the most desirable (apart from karyotype analysis) are (1) study of chromosomal alterations by fluorescence in situ hybridization assay, (2) study of prevalent genetic mutations, e.g. cystic fibrosis, and (3) analysis of Y-chromosome microdeletions. Depending on the results, the clinician can evaluate the possibility of carrying out an assisted reproduction technique (ART) or performing a complementary technique (preimplantation genetic diagnosis). However, if the risk of transmitting genetic disorders to the offspring is high, or if the probabilities of a successful treatment are very low, the clinician should consider the suitability of a change of male gamete for the ART.

However, a high proportion of patients attending clinics present normal values or only moderate defects in sperm analysis. In most cases, no additional tests are performed in these subfertile or "normal" individuals. It is important to mention that normal reference values for semen parameters do not equate with the minimum values required for pregnancy. *Patients with semen variables outside the reference ranges may be fertile and, conversely, men with values within the reference range may still be infertile.* Clearly, in such cases, conventional semen analysis has been unable to identify the functional defects responsible for infertility,[6] indicating that if the only evaluation made on the patient is a semen analysis, then an underlying pathology can be missed.

In the past decade, several methods have been developed to improve diagnosis of male subfertility. Many of them have been shown to exhibit prognostic utility that eluded the conventional semen analysis. As a consequence, nowadays, we have new tools to investigate the functional capacity of sperm and, if necessary, to separate spermatozoa through other parameters different from the motility as used in conventional separation methods. In this chapter, several of them will be discussed, highlighting the laboratory methods available to assess these aspects of sperm structure and function and focusing on their clinical application.

SPERM DNA FRAGMENTATION

Deoxyribonucleic acid (DNA) integrity is one of the most important elements of sperm quality and it correlates not only with impaired pregnancy rates in vivo and in vitro but also with the health and well-being of the offspring.[7]

Deoxyribonucleic acid damage can be a consequence of many different factors: drugs, pollution, alcohol, smoking, increased testicular temperature, infections, varicocele, male age, or genetic lesions.

Although the main role of sperm DNA integrity is well known[8] and it is also established that abnormal DNA damage is more frequent in infertile patients,[9] there is considerable controversy about the possible diagnostic and/or prognostic value of the tests currently used to study sperm DNA fragmentation. This can be due to several factors:

- *Origin of DNA damage*: There are different mechanisms by which DNA can be damaged: defective sperm chromatin condensation during maturation, apoptosis,[10] oxidative stress,[11] and genetic lesions.[12] This damage may originate from intrinsic (changes in spermatogenesis, genetic causes) or extrinsic (genital infections) factors, and maybe interdependent between them.
- *Types of sperm DNA damage*: There are two types of DNA strand breaks: single- and double-stranded breaks. These breaks could develop from different clinical causes. Double-stranded breaks are less capable of being repaired by the oocyte than single-stranded breaks. They indicate more profound defects and clinical implications.
- *Sperm DNA fragmentation tests*: There are many different clinical tests (Table 1) used to analyze sperm DNA fragmentation, among which: (1) single-cell gel electrophoresis assay (COMET),[9] (2) sperm chromatin structure assay (SCSA),[13] (3) terminal deoxynucleotidyl transferase-mediated dUTP Nick end labeling (TUNEL),[14] and (4) alkaline gel electrophoresis,[15] or sperm chromatin decondensation (SCD) test. These tests have different cutoff values (20% for TUNEL assay, 30% for SCSA) and the results obtained from them do not exactly correlate in some cases, suggesting that all tests do not analyze the same level of DNA damage.

Clinical Applications of Sperm DNA Fragmentation

The study of sperm DNA fragmentation would be especially useful in (1) older patients (>45 years old), (2) patients with "normal" seminal parameters or slight alterations but long

Table 1: Main sperm DNA fragmentation tests.

Test	*Author/year*	*Mechanism analyzed*	*Pretreatment*	*Technique of analysis*
TUNEL	Gorczyca et al.[16] (1993)	Incorporation of fluorescent labeled dUTP by TdT enzyme	No	Fluorescence microscopy or cytometry
SCSA	Evenson et al.[17] (1995)	Metachromatic properties of acridine orange with single- and double-stranded DNA	Yes (acid)	Cytometry
COMET	Aitken et al.[18] (1998)	Differences of single- and double-stranded DNA migration in an electric field	No	Electrophoresis
SCD	Fernandez et al.[19] (2002)	Differences on release of DNA loops	Yes (acid)	Microscopy

(TUNEL: deoxynucleotidyl transferase-mediated dUTP nick end labeling assay; SCSA: sperm chromatin stability assay; COMET: single-cell electrophoresis assay; SCD: sperm chromatin decondensation assay; TdT: terminal deoxynucleotidyl transferase)

duration infertility (>3 years), and (3) patients with severe seminal alterations but no genetic anomalies.

Since there is a strong correlation between sperm DNA fragmentation and miscarriage,[20] other relevant candidates for this study are couples with previous failures using ART without known female factor and cases of recurrent miscarriages.

More importantly, this analysis of sperm DNA damage will enable us to obtain significant functional sperm quality data. However, it does not explain the origin of functional alteration. Thus, the best approach would be performing the DNA fragmentation test and other functional tests (such as H3 oxidative stress and H4 apoptosis) to help us determine the source of the damage and/or take a different clinical approach (reduction of sexual abstinence, antioxidant therapy, and selection of nonapoptotic spermatozoa).

OXIDATIVE STRESS

Sperm oxidative status is crucial to spermatozoa functionality.[21] Human spermatozoa are particularly sensitive to oxidative stress due to their high cellular content of polyunsaturated fatty acids, together with a defective natural antioxidant defense capacity.[22] Indeed, oxidative stress created by excessive generation of reactive oxygen species (ROS) and/or impairment of antioxidant protection within the male reproductive tract[7] can cause damage in the plasma membrane (lipid peroxidation) and in the mitochondrial function as well as a disruption of cell functionality. Finally, this triggers alterations in sperm DNA integrity and results in cell death by apoptotic processes. Under physiological conditions, these spermatozoa are retained in the female reproductive tract and never reach the oocyte. But when experts are working with the sample in the laboratory, this selection process does not occur correctly and, as a result, the spermatozoa with less functionality can be used for ART.

At present, there are several methods to analyze sperm oxidative stress, which have advantages and disadvantages. Historically, the most commonly used method has been the chemiluminescence analysis. But the main problem with this technique is that the measurement obtained may be contaminated by oxidative stress produced by leukocytes, cells with much greater power for ROS generation. Therefore, it is essential to eliminate the cells which may contain some magnetic particles having anti-CD45 (leukocyte cell-specific) antibodies. An alternative technique uses certain lipophilic fluorescent compounds that give us a direct measure of cellular oxidative status. Among them, the most used are DHE (dihydroethidium), DCFH (dichlorodihydrofluorescein), and 8-hydroxyguanosine. Nonetheless, in order to accomplish these steps, a flow cytometer is needed so that the results obtained are representative and consistent.

Oxidative stress can also be analyzed by determining the cellular lipid peroxidation.[23] In these cases, the most common tests are the ones that determine malondialdehyde by ELISA (enzyme-linked immunosorbent assay) and the analysis of lipid peroxidation by flow cytometry using BODIPY compound.[24] Finally, another commonly used analysis focuses on determining sperm DNA fragmentation through different techniques. This analysis is also a good procedure, somehow related indirectly to the oxidative status, therefore correlating oxidative status and sperm functional capacity.[8]

Clinical Application of Oxidative Stress Analysis: Antioxidant Therapy

Today, there are several products in the market with antioxidant properties to improve sperm oxidative status and, as a result, to improve the semen quality (increasing its concentration and improving sperm motility). Among them, the most commonly used are selenium, vitamin C, vitamin E, and zinc.[25] Not only do they improve semen parameters but also these compounds can help improve other functional characteristics (Table 2) of sperm and, thus, they help to increase pregnancy rates in infertile couples. Indeed, a recent Cochrane meta-analysis about the use of oral antioxidant in cases of male infertility found that these agents significantly improve pregnancy rates and live birth rates.[26] Interestingly, in this analysis, a significant decrease of sperm DNA damage was also found after 2–3 months of antioxidant therapy, but improvements in semen parameters were not evident, suggesting that these treatments improve functional capability of spermatozoa rather than testicular function. However, more studies are needed to confirm these promising results.

Table 2: Compounds commonly used as antioxidant properties in oral antioxidant therapy.

Compound	*Sperm functional properties*
Selenium	Reduces lipid peroxidation
Vitamin E	Improves cell and mitochondrial membrane integrity
Vitamin C	Scavenger of oxidative species molecules, reduces DNA fragmentation
Q10	Improves of cell membrane integrity, reduces DNA fragmentation coenzyme
Zinc	Reduces sperm oxidative stress and sperm DNA fragmentation
Lycopene	Reduces sperm DNA fragmentation

SPERM APOPTOSIS

It is well known that apoptosis plays an important role in the regulation of spermatogenesis. It implies the induction of a series of cellular and biochemical changes that lead the cell to commit suicide without eliciting an inflammatory response.[27] Apoptosis is based on a genetic mechanism, whose main objective is to control the overproduction of spermatozoa, restricting it to normal levels of proliferation. Tests show that germ cell apoptosis occurs during spermatogenesis, mainly in spermatogonia and the meiotic cell division. This generates excessive breakage of chromatin and increased DNA fragmentation. Indeed, multiple studies have established that in patients diagnosed with male infertility, the proportion of apoptotic sperm in ejaculated semen samples is higher.[28,29] Several studies have studied the relationship between seminal parameters and apoptosis in ejaculated semen. A significant negative correlation between the proportion of apoptotic cells and sperm viability and motility in ejaculated semen has been reported.[29-31]

Mature sperm cells have been reported to express distinct markers of apoptosis-related cell damage.[27,32,33] One of the earlier markers is the externalization of phosphatidylserine (EPS) residues to the sperm outer membrane leaflet. Nevertheless, it is not clear whether the apoptotic markers detected in spermatozoa are residues of an abortive apoptotic process started before ejaculation or whether they result from apoptosis initiated in the postejaculation period.[27,34,35]

In order to select nonapoptotic spermatozoa fraction and improve sperm preparation protocols for ICSI, a new sperm selection technique called MACS (magnetic-activated cell sorting) has been described. This technique is based on the EPS to the outer surface of the sperm membrane in apoptotic sperm. This allows its binding with annexin-V-conjugated paramagnetic microbeads, which could be used to label and separate apoptotic spermatozoa using an MACS system.[36] A heterogeneous sperm cell suspension is incubated with annexin-V-conjugated microbeads, which bind to only apoptotic sperm with EPS. Then, the bead or sperm mixture is allowed to run through the MACS column, which is placed inside a magnet. The magnetic force will cause the retention of the cells labeled with microbeads inside the column, while the nonlabeled cells will flow freely.

OTHER FUNCTIONAL TESTS

There are a series of functional tests that have been employed mainly in research studies, although some of them may be used for the diagnosis of male infertility in the near future. One of the more promising tests is the analysis of acrosome reaction of human sperm induced by different agents (calcium ionophore or progesterone). Also, the measurement of different biochemical markers such as sperm creatine kinase or Catsperm function may be of interest in the improvement of male diagnosis. But currently these tests have a limited role, because they have little proven clinical utility.

CONCLUSION

Determination of reliable and accurate methods to study the fertilizing potential of sperm is of vital importance to provide a definitive diagnosis of the underlying causes of idiopathic male fertility. Identifying the exact nature of the defect will help select the appropriate procedures, which in turn will improve natural and assisted reproduction success rates and help ensure healthy offspring. This may also help identify the group of men and their offspring that, through techniques such as ICSI, may propagate their genetic complement linked to male infertility.

REFERENCES

1. Sherins RJ, Thorsell LP, Dorfmann A, et al. Intracytoplasmic sperm injection facilitates fertilization even in the most severe forms of male infertility: pregnancy outcome correlates with maternal age and number of eggs available. Fert Ster. 1995;64:369-75.
2. Jain T, Gupta RS. Trends in the use of intracytoplasmic sperm injection in the United States. N Engl J Med. 2007;357:251-7.
3. Henkel RR, Schill WB. Sperm preparation for ART. Reprod Biol Endocrinol. 2003;1:108.
4. Zhang HB, Lu SM, Ma CY, et al. Early apoptotic changes in human spermatozoa and their relationships with conventional semen parameters and sperm DNA fragmentation. Asian J Androl. 2008;10:227-35.
5. World Health Organization. WHO Laboratory Manual for the Examination of Human Semen and Sperm-Cervical Mucus Interaction, 5th edition. Cambridge: Cambridge University Press; 2010.
6. Nallela KP, Sharma RK, Aziz N, et al. Significance of sperm characteristics in the evaluation of male infertility. Fert Ster. 2006;85(3):629-34.
7. Aitken RJ, Bennetts LE, Sawyer D, et al. Impact of radio frequency electromagnetic radiation on DNA integrity in the male germline. Int J Androl. 2005;28(3):171-9.
8. Lewis S, Aitken RJ. DNA damage to spermatozoa has impacts on fertilization and pregnancy. Cell Tissue Res. 2005;322:33-41.
9. Irvine DS, Twigg JP, Gordon EL, et al. DNA integrity in human spermatozoa: relationships with semen quality. J Androl. 2000;21:33-44.
10. Shen H, Ong C. Detection of oxidative DNA damage in human sperm and its association with sperm function and male infertility. Free Radic Biol Med. 2000;28:529-36.

11. Said TM, Aziz N, Sharma RK, et al. Novel association between sperm deformity index and oxidative stress-induced DNA damage in infertile male patients. Asian J Androl. 2005;7:121-6.
12. Sharma RK, Said T, Agarwal A. Sperm DNA damage and its clinical relevance in assessing reproductive outcome. Asian J Androl. 2004;6:139-48.
13. Evenson DP, Jost LK, Marshall D, et al. Utility of the sperm chromatin structure assay as a diagnostic and prognostic tool in the human fertility clinic. Hum Reprod. 1999;14(4):1039-49.
14. Sun JG, Jurisicova A, Casper RF. Detection of deoxyribonucleic acid fragmentation in human sperm: correlation with fertilization in vitro. Biol Reprod. 1997;56:602-7.
15. Sawyer DE, Mercer BG, Wiklendt AM, et al. Quantitative analysis of gene-specific DNA damage in human spermatozoa. Mutat Res. 2003;529(1):21-34.
16. Gorczyca W, Traganos F, Jesionowska H, et al. Presence of DNA strand breaks and increased sensitivity of DNA in situ to denaturation in abnormal human sperm cells: analogy to apoptosis of somatic cells. Exp Cell Res. 1993;207:202-5.
17. Evenson D, Jost L, Gandour D, et al. Comparative sperm chromatin structure assay measurements on epiillumination and orthogonal axes flow cytometers. Cytometry. 1995;19: 295-303.
18. Aitken RJ, Gordon E, Harkiss D. et al. Relative Impact of Oxidative Stress on the Functional Competence and Genomic Integrity of Human Spermatozoa. Biol Reprod. 1998;59:1037-46.
19. Fernández JL, Muriel L, Rivero MT, et al. The sperm chromatin dispersion test: a simple method for the determination of sperm DNA fragmentation. J Androl. 2003;24:59-66.
20. Robinson L, Gallos ID, Conner SJ, et al. The effect of sperm DNA fragmentation on miscarriage rates: a systematic review and meta-analysis. Hum Reprod. 2012;27(10):2908-17.
21. Henkel RR. Leukocytes and oxidative stress: dilemma for sperm function and male fertility. Asian J Androl. 2011;13(1):43-52.
22. Aitken RJ, Baker MA. Oxidative stress, sperm survival and fertility control. Mol Cell Endocrin. 2006;250(1):66-9.
23. Gomez E, Irvine DS, Aitken RJ. Evaluation of a spectrophotometric assay for the measurement of malondialdehyde and 4-hydroxyalkenals in human spermatozoa: relationships with semen quality and sperm function. Int J Androl. 1998;21:81-94.
24. Aitken RJ, Wingate J, de Iuliis GN, et al. Analysis of lipid peroxidation in human spermatozoa using BODIPY C11. Mol Hum Reprod. 2007;13:203-11.
25. Ross C, Morriss A, Khairy M, et al. A systematic review of the effect of oral antioxidants on male infertility. RBM Online. 2010;20(6):711-23.
26. Showell MG, Brown J, Yazdani A, et al. Antioxidants for male subfertility. Cochrane Database Syst Rev. 2011;(1):CD007411.
27. Grunewald S, Paasch U, Wuendrich K, et al. Sperm caspases become more activated in infertility patients than in healthy donors during cryopreservation. Syst Biol Reprod Med. 2005;51(6):449-60.
28. Sakkas D, Seli E, Bizzaro D, et al. Abnormal spermatozoa in the ejaculate: abortive apoptosis and faulty nuclear remodelling during spermatogenesis. RBM Online. 2003;7:428-32.
29. Taylor SL, Weng SL, Fox P, et al. Somatic cell apoptosis markers and pathways in human ejaculated sperm: potential utility as indicators of sperm quality. Mol Hum Reprod. 2004;10(11):825-34.
30. Marchetti C, Obert G, Deffosez A, et al. Study of mitochondrial membrane potential, reactive oxygen species, DNA fragmentation and cell viability by flow cytometry in human sperm. Hum Reprod. 2002;17:1257-65.
31. Said TM, Grunewald S, Paasch U, et al. Effects of magnetic-activated cell sorting on sperm motility and cryosurvival rates. Fert Ster. 2005;83:1442-6.
32. Muratori M, Piomboni P, Baldi E, et al. Functional and ultrastructural features of DNA-fragmented human sperm. J Androl. 2000;21(6):903-12.
33. Shen HM, Dai J, Chia SE, et al. Detection of apoptotic alterations in sperm in subfertile patients and their correlations with sperm quality. Hum Reprod. 2002;17(5):1266-73.
34. Tesarik J. Paternal effects on cell division in the preimplantation embryo. RBM Online. 2005;10(3):370-5.
35. Lachaud C, Tesarik J, Cañadas ML, et al. Apoptosis and necrosis in human ejaculated spermatozoa. Hum Reprod. 2004;19(3):607-10.
36. Lee TH, Liu CH, Shih YT, et al. Magnetic-activated cell sorting for sperm preparation reduces spermatozoa with apoptotic markers and improves the acrosome reaction in couples with unexplained infertility. Hum Reprod. 2010;25:839-46.

CHAPTER 15

Managing Ejaculation Failure

Rupin Shah

INTRODUCTION

Failure to ejaculate is a relatively uncommon, and therefore poorly understood, cause of infertility, and can prove be a major stumbling block during infertility treatment. In this chapter, we outline a practical approach to the diagnosis and management of this problem.

Failure to ejaculate may be situational or total. In *situational anejaculation*, the man is able to ejaculate under some circumstances but not in others. In *total anejaculation*, the man never ejaculates during intercourse or masturbation.

Situational anejaculation occurs due to psychological reasons. No investigations are needed. Therapy is focused on strategies to anticipate and prevent the problem, and to obtain a semen sample if the problem does occur.

Total anejaculation may occur because a man never reaches conscious orgasm and therefore does not ejaculate—*anorgasmic anejaculation*, or may occur despite a man reaching an orgasm—*orgasmic anejaculation*. Excluding men with spinal cord injury, anorgasmic anejaculation occurs due to psychological or physiological reasons, while orgasmic anejaculation is always due to a physical defect—usually anatomical or neurological.[1]

SITUATIONAL ANEJACULATION

There are various types of situational anejaculation. The diagnosis is obvious from history and no investigations are needed. The various types of situational anejaculation, and strategies for their prevention and management, are discussed below:

- *Unexpected failure of ejaculation*: This happens to a man who has had no problem giving a semen sample in the past but suddenly, unexpectedly, fails to give a sample on the day of intrauterine insemination (IUI) or ovum pickup (OPU) during an in vitro fertilization (IVF) cycle. This happens due to the stress of the infertility treatment and the pressure of having to give a sample under such conditions. This can happen to anyone and so the best preventive measure is to cryopreserve a sample in advance for all IVF couples. If that has not been done, a semen sample may be obtained by the use of a vibrator or electroejaculation, or sperm can be aspirated from the testis and used for intracytoplasmic sperm injection (ICSI).
- *Periovulatory anejaculation/on-demand anejaculation*: In this situation, the man has difficulty in collecting a semen sample at the time of ovulation, when he is under pressure to perform, though he is able to ejaculate easily at other times. Sometimes, the infertility specialist contributes to the problem by giving a specific time of ovulation so that the wife wakes up the husband at 4 AM to have sex at the right time!! This treatment-induced sexual dysfunction can be minimized by giving the couple a fertile period and emphasizing that they can have sex during this period as per their inclination and pleasure. Some men will benefit from the use of an erectogenic drug like sildenafil that can be given in a dose of 50 mg, one hour before intercourse, and is safe for conception. In refractory cases, a vibrator may be used to get a semen sample that can be used for IUI.
- *Clinic anejaculation*: A fair number of men, who can ejaculate easily at home, find it difficult to ejaculate in the clinic because they become self-conscious and feel under pressure. This problem can be avoided by ensuring that the semen collection room is discretely

placed, is clean, and has a bed so that the couple can be together, if required. Sometimes providing erotic material will help. If the problem has been identified during the sexual history at the initial interview (these questions should be part of standard fertility history) then the man can be allowed to bring the sample from home. Otherwise, most men with this problem can ejaculate in the clinic with the help of a vibrator.

- *Masturbation anejaculation*: Some men are unaccustomed to masturbation and are unable to give a sample by manipulation even though they ejaculate during intercourse. Therefore, when asking a man to produce a semen sample it is always important to check whether he will be able to produce a sample by masturbation in the clinic. If he expresses his inability to do so he can be asked to collect a sample at home by coitus interruptus.
- *Intercourse anejaculation*: In this condition, a man can ejaculate during masturbation but not by intercourse. The cause is usually psychogenic or technical (lack of adequate stimulation). Treatment is through sex therapy and counseling but is often difficult. Fertility can be easily achieved by IUI used the masturbatory sample.

ANORGASMIC ANEJACULATION

In this condition, the man does not ejaculate because he never reaches an orgasm, either during intercourse or during masturbation.

The etiology may be:

- *Psychological*: Due to early negative sexual experiences or strict, inhibitory religious upbringing.
- *Technical*: Inadequate stimulation during intercourse due to poor erections or improper intercourse.
- *Physiological*: Due to a high ejaculatory threshold (the opposite of premature ejaculation). This seems to be the most common cause in our experience.
- *Pharmacological*: Due to antipsychotics that can cause marked inhibition and delay of orgasm.
- *Neurological*: Spinal cord injury, or reduced glans sensation or dorsal nerve neuropathy.

Diagnosis is based on the history alone and usually does not need investigations. Classically, the man gives a history of prolonged intercourse without reaching an orgasm, and finally stopping because he is tired. However, a man who has never experienced orgasm is often unclear about whether he has reached an orgasm or not, and hence the history may be unclear. Many of these men will, however, state that they though do not ejaculate during intercourse they have spontaneous ejaculations at night. *A history of nocturnal emissions is very important because it rules out an organic cause of anejaculation.*

Treatment through psychosexual therapy may help in some cases but is time-consuming and frequently unfruitful. When the primary concern is fertility (rather than orgasm and sexual pleasure) then more active measures to obtain sperm by vibrator stimulation[2] or electroejaculation[3,4] should be tried right away.

ORGASMIC ANEJACULATION

These men reach an orgasm but do not ejaculate. The cause is always organic.

When a man reaches a climax the orgasm is usually accompanied by ejaculation that occurs in three phases:

- *Phase 1 (emission)*: Stimulation of the sympathetic fibers causes the seminal vesicles, prostate, vasa, and tails of the epididymides to contract and deposit seminal fluid into the posterior urethra.
- *Phase 2 (bladder neck closure)*: Simultaneously, again under sympathetic control, the bladder neck closes to prevent retrograde ejaculation.
- *Phase 3 (antegrade propulsion)*: Seminal fluid flows from the posterior into the bulbar urethra. Rhythmic contractions of the bulbocavernosus muscle propel the fluid out of the urethra with forceful squirts.

Any of these three phases can be affected by anatomical, neurogenic, or pharmacological factors resulting in orgasmic anejaculation. Some of the common causes are listed below:

- *Phase 1 disorder—failure of emission*:
  - Anatomical causes—ductal obstruction due to genitourinary tuberculosis
  - Neurogenic causes—spinal cord injury, lumbar sympathectomy, pelvic surgery, retroperitoneal lymph node dissection, diabetic neuropathy, and α-adrenergic blockers
  - Endocrine causes—severe hypogonadism (very low testosterone) due to primary or secondary testicular failure.
- *Phase 2 disorder—retrograde ejaculation:*
  - Anatomical causes—bladder neck disruption due to bladder neck trauma (fracture pelvis), bladder neck incision (iatrogenic), and congenitally wide bladder neck
  - Neurogenic causes—diabetic neuropathy and α-adrenergic blockers.
- *Phase 3 disorder—failure of antegrade propulsion:*
  - Anatomical causes—outflow obstruction due to stricture, diverticulum or urethral pouch, damage

to the bulbocavernosus muscle during urethral reconstruction

- Neurogenic cause—paralysis of the bulbocavernosus muscle.

Diagnosis is frequently possible from history alone. Retrograde ejaculation is diagnosed by examination of the post-orgasm urine for sperm.

Treatment depends on etiology. Neurogenic failure of emission or retrograde ejaculation due to neuropathy may respond to a 5-day course of a combination of a sympathomimetic (ephedrine 30 mg TDS; pseudoephedrine 60 mg TDS, phenylephrine 10 mg TDS) and an anticholinergic (imipramine 50 mg HS).[5] Other cases of neurogenic failure can be treated with vibrator stimulation or electroejaculation.[6] In men with spinal cord injury success will depend on the spinal level of the lesion.[7] Retroperitoneal lymph node dissection (RPLND) usually results in failure of ejaculation rather than retrograde ejaculation; semen can be obtained by electroejaculation.[8]

Anatomical obstruction causing failure of emission is usually too extensive to be corrected by endoscopic surgery and the only option is epididymal or testicular sperm aspiration and ICSI.

Retrograde ejaculation due to diabetic neuropathy may respond to medical therapy as above. Otherwise sperm can be retrieved from the bladder and used for IUI or ICSI depending on the quality. When sperm is being retrieved from the bladder, the urine must be made alkaline and dilute to improve sperm survival. Accordingly, the patient is given a urinary alkalizer (sodium bicarbonate or potassium citrate thrice a day) for 3 days. On the day of retrieval, he consumes three glasses of water with the alkalizer and then passes urine every 30 minutes. The urine pH is checked each time and when it is above 7.5, the man masturbates and then immediately voids urine. This is quickly centrifuged to separate the sperm; the sperm pellet is then rewashed with medium and used for IUI. If the motility of the recovered sperm is poor then an alternative method is to instill 30 mL of sperm washing medium in the bladder and then ask the man to masturbate.

When there is failure of antegrade propulsion, the semen will dribble out later. This can be collected and used for IUI or IVF. In all cases of orgasmic anejaculation, if other measures fail, sperm retrieval from the testes and ICSI is the final solution.

VIBRATOR THERAPY

This is extremely useful in treating situational anejaculation, anorgasmic anejaculation, and some cases of neurogenic orgasmic anejaculation.

The vibrator works by strongly stimulating the afferent pathways of the ejaculatory reflex. This overcomes inhibition due to situational, psychological, or neurogenic factors, thus resulting in orgasm and ejaculation.

The patient is prepared for the vibrator by counseling him that the ejaculation will happen automatically and that he should *not try* to ejaculate. This will allow him to be relaxed and will reduce cortical inhibition of ejaculation due to anxiety. It also helps avoid pseudoejaculation of urine that happens when a nonorgasmic man strains to ejaculate.

He then sits on a bed in a quiet room and self-stimulates and fantasizes to achieve some tumescence. A full erection is not mandatory and the patient is reassured that he would be able to ejaculate even if he does not have an erection. If the man is very anxious then an anxiolytic and phosphodiesterase type 5 (PDE5) inhibitor may be given. The vibrator is then positioned so that the undersurface of the glans penis rests upon the vibrating head. Gentle pressure is applied to the penis so that maximum vibration is felt. Simultaneously, he continues to fantasize; visual erotic materials may help.

The stimulation is continued till the man ejaculates, or till 30–60 minutes are over. Some men succeed only on the second or third attempt.

Success rates are 90% for situational anejaculation, 60% for anorgasmic anejaculation, and around 50% for neurogenic anejaculation (depending on the level and extent of the spinal lesion).

ELECTROEJACULATION

Electroejaculation involves direct electrical stimulation of the sympathetic nerves innervating the prostate, seminal vesicles, and terminal vas resulting in their contraction and ejaculation.[9]

It is performed using the Seager electroejaculator that delivers an alternating current at an intensity ranging from 0 volts to 50 volts, corresponding to 0 to 1 amperes of current. The procedure is painful and requires a short general anesthesia unless the patient has spinal cord injury with loss of sensation.

The patient is positioned in the lithotomy or left lateral position and a rectal examination and proctoscopy are performed to rule out any rectal pathology. The electrode is lubricated copiously with jelly and then introduced per rectum with the electrode's stimulation strips facing anteriorly. The electrode is pushed against the prostate and seminal vesicles and the stimulation is started.

The standard technique involves stimulation in one second bursts, starting at 5 V. The current is turned up to 5 volts, held for a second and then turned back to zero. For the next stimulus the current is turned up to 7 volts, held for a second and then lowered to zero. The stimulus is progressively increased by a couple of volts each time till ejaculation occurs. Two to three stimulations are delivered at this level and then increased again to see if any further ejaculate can be obtained.

If there is no antegrade ejaculation, the bladder is catheterized and the urine is checked for retrograde ejaculation.

This author has modified the technique and directly stimulates at 50 volts. This usually results in an ejaculate in 1 or 2 stimulations, and the entire procedure is over in 10 stimulations. In this technique, it is essential that the patients have complete muscle relaxation since there can be violent muscle contractions.

Electroejaculation is successful in most cases of situational anejaculation and anorgasmic anejaculation and those cases of neurogenic anejaculation where the thoracolumbar outflow is intact. However, the quality of semen is unpredictable and sometimes, inexplicably, count or motility may be poor.[10] Depending on the semen quality, IUI or ICSI can be done with the sample.[11]

SUMMARY

Failure to ejaculate can pose a frustrating problem. Classification of the problem as situational or total, and anorgasmic or orgasmic, provides a practical way of understanding the problem. Diagnosis is easy once the etiological factors are understood. Treatment varies depending on the etiology. The use of vibratory stimulation or electroejaculation is very useful in many of the cases.

REFERENCES

1. Shah R. Management of anejaculation. In: Pandian N (Ed). Handbook of Andrology. Chennai: T.R. Publishers; 1999. pp. 129-39.
2. Wheeler JS Jr, Walter JS, Culkin DJ, et al. Idiopathic anejaculation treated by vibrator stimulation. Fertil Steril. 1988;50:377-9.
3. Hovav Y, Shotland Y, Yaffe H, et al. Electro-ejaculation and assisted fertility in men with psychogenic anejaculation. Fertil Steril. 1996;66:620-3.
4. Soeterik TF, Veenboer PW, Lock TM. Electroejaculation in psychogenic anejaculation. Fertil Steril. 2014;101:1604-8.
5. Kamischke A, Nieschlag E. Treatment of retrograde ejaculation and anejaculation. Hum Reprod Update. 1999;5:448-74.
6. Nehra A, Werner MA, Bastuba M, et al. Vibratory stimulation and rectal probe electroejaculation as therapy for patients with spinal cord injury: Semen parameters and pregnancy rates. J Urol. 1996;155:554-9.
7. Chéhensse C, Bahrami S, Denys P, et al. The spinal control of ejaculation revisited: A systematic review and meta-analysis of anejaculation in spinal cord injured patients. Hum Reprod Update. 2013;19:507-26.
8. Hsiao W, Deveci S, Mulhall JP. Outcomes of the management of postchemotherapy retroperitoneal lymph node dissection-associated anejaculation. BJU Int. 2012;110:1196-200.
9. Bennett C, Seager S, Vasher E, et al. Sexual dysfunction and electroejaculation in men with spinal cord injury: Review. BJU. 1991;67:191-4.
10. Meng X, Fan L, Liu J, et al. Fresh semen quality in ejaculates produced by nocturnal emission in men with idiopathic anejaculation. Fertil Steril. 2013;100:1248-52.
11. Ohl DA, Wolf LJ, Menge AC, et al. Electroejaculation and assisted reproductive technologies in the treatment of anejaculatory infertility. Fertil Steril. 2001;76:1249-55.

CHAPTER

16

Management of Oligoasthenoteratozoospermia

PM Gopinath

INTRODUCTION

Approximately 10–15% of all couples of reproductive age groups seek fertility assessment. With an increasing population of working women and the associated delay in the ages of marriage and first childbearing, infertility services are being increasingly utilized.[1] With the advent of assisted reproductive techniques and with the increasing success achieved, the evaluation of the male partner and an attempt at curative treatment is often overlooked. Male factor is involved in about half of the infertility cases. Normal fertile couples of reproductive age have a conception rate of 20–25% per month, with more than 90% conceiving within 1 year. Male factor infertility is involved in approximately 50% of infertile couples and in 30% of the cases an abnormality is discovered solely in men. Hence, it is essential to identify the pathology and treat the male which may allow couples to improve their fertility potential and conceive through natural intercourse. Figure 1 illustrates the various etiologies of male factor and their impact on fertility.

The suboptimal semen condition where a man has a combination of a low sperm count (oligozoospermia), poor

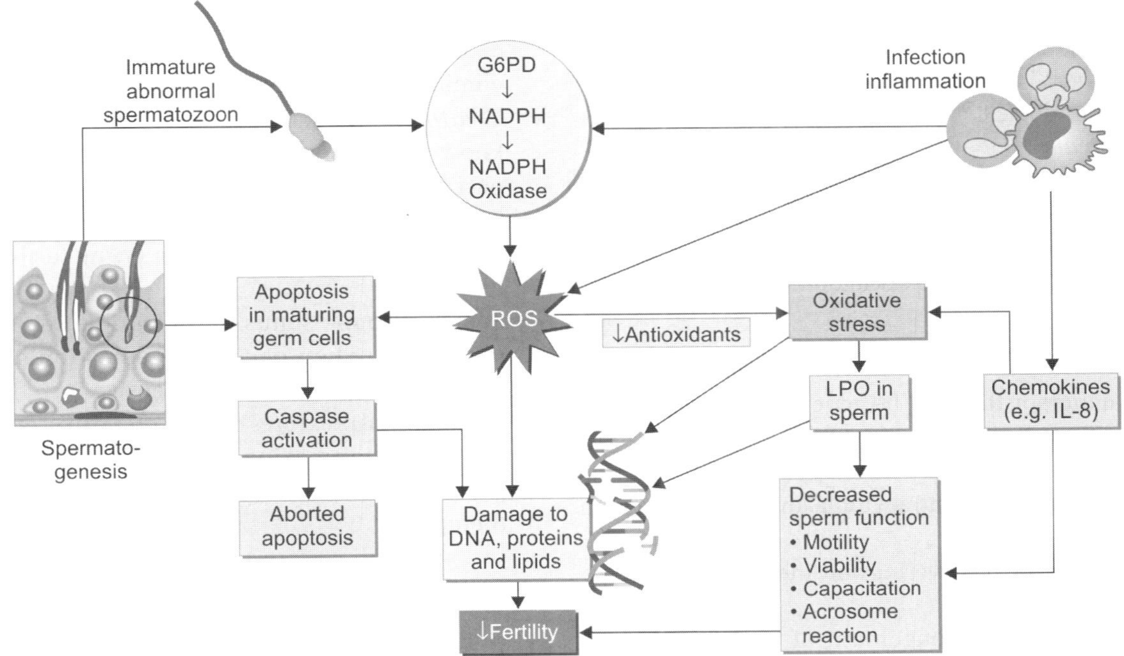

Fig. 1: Various etiology of ROS and its impact on fertility. (DNA: deoxyribonucleic acid; G6PD: glucose-6-phosphate dehydrogenase; IL: interleukin; LPO: lipid peroxidation; NADPH: nicotinamide adenine dinucleotide phosphate; ROS: reactive oxygen species).

sperm motility or movement (asthenozoospermia), and abnormal sperm shape or morphology (teratozoospermia) is termed as oligoasthenoteratozoospermia (OAT). A major problem in severe OAT is the reduced chance for sperm selection regarding morphology. Fertilization rates of spermatozoa with several morphological defects are lower regardless of their source. Injection of morphologically abnormal spermatozoa has been associated with a lower implantation rate. A correlation has been found between higher incidence of meiotic errors and lower sperm counts. Significantly higher aneuploidy rates of sex chromosomes are evident in patients with severe OAT (<5 M/mL) in comparison to less severe OAT patients.

The new World Health Organization (WHO) guidelines on semen analysis[2] are exciting and make one wonder whether we have over treated the male partners previously. Oligoasthenoteratozoospermia known as OAT syndrome is a commonly encountered problem in male infertility.

There are various causes of OAT and the medical treatment to be selected would be based on it. The causes are classified as follows:

- *Pretesticular*
  - *Endocrine*: Hypogonadotropic hypogonadism, hyperthyroidism, hyperprolactinemia, and diabetes.
  - *Coital disorders*: Erectile dysfunction and ejaculatory failure.
- *Testicular*
  - *Genetic*: Klinefelter syndrome, Y chromosome deletion, and immotile cilia syndrome.
  - *Congenital*: Cryptorchidism, infective, antispermatogenic agents, like heat, irradiation, and chemotherapy.
  - *Vascular*: Torsion and varicocele.
  - Immunological.
- *Post-testicular*
  - *Obstructive*: Epididymal (congenital and infective), vasal (genetic-cystic fibrosis, acquired-vasectomy ejaculatory duct obstruction, accessory gland infection, immunological, idiopathic post vasectomy).

TREATMENT OPTIONS IN OAT

- Medical therapy that may be general or specific.
- Surgical therapy.
- Assistance reproductive technology (ART): Intrauterine insemination (IUI) or intracytoplasmic sperm injection (ICSI).

In this article, we are covering only the medical management of OAT.

Specific medical management of OAT is based on identifying reversible causes of infertility and treating them with appropriate medications to achieve a pregnancy. Despite the advancements in diagnostic methodology, no identifiable cause can be found in majority of infertile males. This is referred to as idiopathic OAT. These patients are treated with nonspecific, empirical medications based on theoretical concepts, in an attempt to improve semen parameters and to improve fertility potential.

FACTORS INFLUENCING THE CHOICE OF MEDICAL THERAPY IN OAT

- *Age of the couple and duration of infertility*: A young couple with a short trying time should be given the option of medical therapy in order to buy time to achieve a natural pregnancy. On the other hand, an older couple with a much longer trying time should be counseled to move toward ART.
- *Severity of OAT and realistic chances of improvement expected*: Thus, a patient with severe OAT (<5 million/mL with very poor progressive motility) with no obvious reversible factors is better off being referred for ART.
- *Past illness causing irreversible damage*: For example, a patient who had postmumps orchitis and testicular atrophy, or who was operated for undescended testes. In such patients, it is unlikely that medical therapy will help.
- *Reversible, correctable gonadotoxic factors*: If there is occupational exposure to gonadotoxins (heat, chemical fumes), heavy smoking, recent febrile illness, accessory gland infections, etc. then such patients can be given supportive medical therapy to buy time for improvement of semen parameters once the gonadotoxic factors are eliminated or modified.
- *Treatment history is imperative*: It is important to know what drugs a patient has already tried in the past (whether they were effective or not) so that there is no repetition. If various drugs have already proved ineffective there is no point in giving further medical therapy.
- Socioeconomic status of the couple should also be considered when deciding medication since many empirical drugs are rather expensive.
- Psychosocial pressures on the couple play an important role in decision making. In a couple that is socially hard pressed for a baby, less time should be spent on medical therapy.

SPECIFIC MEDICAL THERAPY

With history, physical examination, and specific investigations, it is possible to diagnose and treat certain specific medical conditions that will contribute to OAT.

Chronic Scrotal Fungal Dermatitis

This can affect fertility by thickening the scrotal skin and thus increasing the local temperature. This is treated with topical, antifungal plus steroid creams.

Genital Tract Infection

The WHO defines leukocytospermia as seminal white blood cells (WBC) levels more than 1×10^6/mL (WHO 1999) with the prevalence among male infertility patients being about 10–20%. The clinician must ensure that the laboratory should clearly differentiate between leukocytes and immature germ cells using cytologic staining or immunohistochemical techniques. All men with elevated seminal WBC levels (>1×10^6/mL) should be evaluated for a genital tract infection or inflammation, and a semen culture should be performed. Common organisms responsible are *Streptococcus faecalis, Escherichia coli, Chlamydia trachomatis,*[3] and *Ureaplasma urealyticum*. Because of the difficulty of culturing *Chlamydia* or *Ureaplasma* we often give doxycycline 100 mg/day on an empirical basis for 15 days and then start antibiotics as per culture reports. Commonly used are fluoroquinolones 0.5–1 g/day, cotrimoxazole (sulfamethoxazole 800 mg, trimethoprim 160 mg), or erythromycin 1.5 g/day. These drugs are administered for 2–3 weeks along with advice of frequent ejaculation. It is also a better option to rotate the antibiotics. However, culture-negative patients with proven leukocytospermia should be treated with anti-inflammatory therapy and frequent ejaculation, because empiric antibiotic therapy generally provides no benefit in these cases and may be harmful. In cases of refractory leukocytospermia, sperm washing can be performed before IUI to remove the white cells.

Immunologic Infertility

Oral prednisolone is commonly used to suppress antibody production, but no double-blind, randomized large trial has confirmed the efficacy of this therapy. Small studies following different protocols report pregnancy rates between 0% and 44%. Studies in which treatment was continued for more than 3 months reported a significant increase in the number of pregnancies among those receiving prednisolone compared with placebo.[4]

Intracytoplasmic Sperm Injection

It is considered to be the treatment of choice for patients with severe sperm autoimmunity. Recently, higher fertilization rates during in vitro fertilization (IVF) were reported in patients with antisperm antibodies who received immunosuppressive therapy compared to IVF without immunosuppressive therapy. Therefore, treatment of antisperm antibodies using corticosteroids should not be prescribed routinely, but can be considered in patients with antisperm antibodies and earlier failed fertilization during IVF or ICSI. High doses of prednisolone should be avoided even on short-term due to the rare but catastrophic risk of avascular necrosis of femoral head. It is recommended to use tablet prednisolone 5 mg, thrice-a-day for 10 days, then twice-a-day for 10 days, then once-a-day for 10 days.

Chronic Epididymo-orchitis

Many subfertile men have clinical evidence of chronic filarial epididymo-orchitis—residence in an endemic area, enlarged adherent epididymis, thickened cord, lax hydrocoele, history of (h/o) hydrocoele surgery, h/o testicular swelling with fever, and occasionally ultrasound evidence of the "filarial dance". Such men sometimes show good improvement in semen parameters after a course of antifilaria therapy (diethylcarbamazine 100 mg thrice-a-day for 20 days in combination with doxycycline 100 mg twice-a-day for 10 days) followed by low-dose steroids as given above.

Adrenogenital Syndrome

It is a rare congenital cause of gonadotropin deficiency, in which an enzyme defect in the steroid pathway for synthesis of cortisol results in increased adrenocorticotropic hormone, with stimulation of the adrenals and overproduction of androgen. The excess androgen suppresses pituitary gonadotropin secretion and the testes are not stimulated. The diagnosis when testosterone (T) is in elevated levels and decreased follicle stimulating hormone (FSH) and luteinizing hormone (LH). Administration of glucocorticoids in slightly higher than physiologic doses suppresses adrenal androgen production by negative feedback on adrenocorticotropic hormone secretion and enables gonadotropin levels to rise. This would result in growth, spermatogenesis, and high rate of fertility.

NONSPECIFIC OR EMPIRICAL THERAPY

In patients with idiopathic OAT, a variety of empirical medical therapies[5] have been recommended. Although there are numerous reports that support a multitude of compounds, the vast majorities are nonrandomized studies and unfortunately no medical therapy has demonstrated consistent efficacy in multiple, rigorous, well-controlled, randomized, placebo-controlled trials. Because of isolated case reports and small series demonstrating efficacy of some agents, there is continued hope that they may be effective in select subpopulations of men with idiopathic reproductive dysfunction.

Nonspecific treatments[5] include the following:

- *Hormonal agents:* Androgens, antiestrogens, aromatase inhibitors (AIs), gonadotropins.
- *Antioxidants:* Glutathione, lycopene, and vitamin E.
- *Sperm vitalizers:* L-carnitine, coenzyme Q10.
- *Nutritional supplements:* Folic acid, zinc, multivitamins, and trace elements.
- *Miscellaneous:* Indomethacin, kallikrein, and low-dose corticosteroids.
- Elimination of gonadotoxic factors.

Hormonal Agents

Androgens

- *Rationale (direct therapy)*: Exogenous androgens, administered at a dose that will not influence the pituitary-gonadal axis, may have a direct stimulatory effect on spermatogenesis or influence sperm transport and maturation through an effect on the epididymis, vas deferens, and seminal vesicles.
- *Drugs used and dosage*: Mesterolone 25 mg thrice daily or T undecanoate[6] 40 mg two to four capsules daily.
- *Rationale (rebound therapy)*: High doses of exogenous androgens will suppress the hypothalamic-pituitary-testicular (HPT) axis and result in azoospermia. Subsequently, after cessation of androgens, the gonadotropin levels will rise again, during which period there may be a rebound increase in sperm counts above baseline. However, the spermatogenesis which rebounds after suppression did not increase the rates of fertility. Hence, rebound therapy has been given up because of uncertain results and risk of permanent azoospermia.

Antiestrogens[7]

- *Rationale*: Antiestrogens inhibit the negative feedback effect of estrogen by blocking estrogen receptors in the hypothalamus, which in turn increases endogenous gonadotropin secretion. In turn, the raised FSH and LH stimulate Sertoli and Leydig cells with a possible improvement in spermatogenesis. Another antiestrogen, testolactone, similarly promotes testicular function both centrally and directly by decreasing the influence of estradiol. However, it does not function by competition for the estrogen receptor but by directly decreasing the conversion of androgen to estradiol through aromatase inhibition.
- *Drugs used and dose*: Clomiphene citrate 25 mg daily or alternate days or tamoxifen citrate 10–20 mg daily. Tamoxifen 20 mg/day for 4–12 months daily.

Tamoxifen citrate is an antiestrogen that exhibits less estrogenic activity than clomiphene citrate and has been used in the treatment of male infertility. Uncontrolled studies have reported improvement in sperm density and pregnancy rates after clomiphene citrate treatment, whereas others failed to show benefit. It was also found that the administration of antiestrogens does not immediately provide higher sperm quality and number, but over time there is a gradual increase.[8]

Aromatase Inhibitors[9-12]

- *Rationale*: Estrogen has a potent negative feedback effect on gonadotropin secretion. The intent is to reduce the estrogenic effect on spermatogenesis. High estrogen levels in combination with low T levels have been shown to impair proper spermatogenesis. More importantly, elevated levels of estrogen will lead to feedback inhibition of the hypothalamic-pituitary-gonadal (HPG) axis, and the end result is a decrease in the LH necessary for the production of T, and FSH to optimize sperm production. The activity of aromatase inhibition regardless of patient body mass index (BMI) suggests that aromatase activity in the Leydig cells is responsible for the T to estradiol conversion and impaired semen parameters.
- *Drugs used and dose*: Letrozole 2.5 mg daily orally, or anastrozole 1 mg daily. The use of the AI letrozole in the treatment of men with oligospermia or azoospermia showed a marked improvement in the hormonal profile, and an improvement in the semen parameters including an increase in sperm concentration. 20% of treated oligospermic men achieved spontaneous pregnancy and 24% of azoospermic men had sperm identified in the ejaculate. Since most men with low sperm concentration appear to commonly have excess aromatase activity leading to diminished T/E ratio, AIs seem to be effective in restoring LH, FSH, and T levels, improving semen parameters, and re-establishing fertility. Men that benefited the most had the diagnosis of nonobstructive azoospermia or idiopathic oligoasthenospermia and low T and T/E less than 10:1 ratio. AI therapy is usually well-tolerated with rare side effects including nausea, decreased libido, and asymptomatic mild elevation

in the liver function tests. A very important side effect of AI is the possible decrease of bone mineral density and increase in the total body fat due to the decrease in availability of estrogen.

Gonadotropins[13-18]

- *Rationale*: Some patients with idiopathic infertility may have a subclinical endocrinopathy that results in abnormalities in the bioactivity, half-life, or pulsatility of gonadotropin secretion.[8] Such men may benefit from exogenous gonadotropins despite normal levels on immunoassay. Initially, human chorionic gonadotropin (hCG) is administrated alone. After several months of treatment, if no sperm is detected but adequate serum T levels are achieved, then treatment with FSH is introduced.
- *Drugs used and dose*: Human chorionic gonadotropin (1,500 IU IM three times per week), human menopausal gonadotropin (hMG; 37.5–75 IU IM three times per week).

Even though gonadotropin-releasing hormone (GnRH) and gonadotropins have proven their benefit and shown success in the induction of spermatogenesis, there is limited evidence for the use of gonadotropins in men with idiopathic infertility. Some of the randomized controlled studies which evaluated the use of hMG or FSH in combination with hCG for the treatment of normogonadotropic OAT did not show any benefits from treatment. However, some studies have shown that men with hypospermatogenesis on a fine needle aspiration will have improvement in the seminal parameters and pregnancy rates when treated with gonadotropins compared to other pathology on testicular tissue. Currently, there is a lack of consensus on the use of FSH or LH substitute for the treatment and since the majority of men with testicular failure have elevated FSH greater than 8.4 IU/L, the rationale to administer more gonadotropins is not completely justified. Therefore, these treatments should be considered empirical and more evidence from placebo-controlled trials is required.

Dopamine Agonist[19-21]

- *Rationale:* Elevated levels of prolactin inhibit the pulsatile secretion of GnRH, men will present with hypogonadism and infertility.

Study shows that treatment with cabergoline for 6 months is successful in normalizing serum prolactin (PRL) levels and in rapidly restoring gonadal function in men with prolactinoma, with an excellent tolerability. Thus, cabergoline could be successfully employed in the treatment of male hyperprolactinemic hypogonadism.

- *Drugs used and dose:* Cabergoline (0.125–1 mg twice weekly) is the preferred choice because it has the highest efficacy.

Antioxidants[22-30]

Increased rates of infertility have been found in men with seminal fluid containing high levels of reactive oxygen species (ROS). These ROS are associated with sperm dysfunction, germ cell DNA damage with the possibility of impaired fertility, but the exact mechanism is not completely understood. These associations have led clinicians to treat infertile men with antioxidant supplements. A variety of clinical trials have suggested that the use of antioxidant supplements have a slight benefit in improving sperm function and DNA integrity. However, most of these studies are not randomized controlled trials, and to date there are no convincing trials that have demonstrated a significantly higher unassisted pregnancy rate after treating men with antioxidant therapy. Moreover, the benefits of antioxidants might be limited to certain groups of patients that are not, as yet, clearly defined. The use of individual antioxidants is very common. These trends have led pharmaceutical companies to produce and market specific combinations of antioxidants and numerous studies have looked at the benefit of these combinations. Use of vitamin E and C in combination found no improvement in semen parameters but meaningful reduction in DNA fragmentation. A systematic review of 17 randomized trials, including 1,665 infertile men, was conducted to evaluate the effects of oral antioxidants (vitamins C and E, zinc, selenium, folate, carnitine and carotenoids) on sperm quality and pregnancy rates in infertile men. 14 of the 17 (82%) trials showed an improvement in either sperm quality or pregnancy rate after antioxidant therapy. Ten trials examined pregnancy rate and six showed a significant improvement after antioxidant therapy.[9]

- *Rationale*: Elevated seminal ROS levels have been recognized as an independent marker of male factor infertility, irrespective of whether patients have normal or abnormal semen parameters. Spermatozoa are particularly susceptible to oxidative stress induced damage. Antioxidants in seminal plasma are the most important form of protection available to spermatozoa against ROS. Many studies[9] have supported the use of exogenous antioxidants in the treatment of idiopathic infertility.

- *Drugs used and dose*: Glutathione 250 mg daily (50–600 mg/day), lycopene 4–8 g daily, and vitamin E 400–800 mg daily. L-carnitine and acetyl carnitine 1 g, thrice-a-day; coenzyme Q10 100–300 mg/day.

Other most commonly studied antioxidants were vitamin E, vitamin C, selenium, CoQ10, N-acetyl-cysteine, L-carnitine, and zinc and their favorable effect was confirmed. According to this review, favorable effects on idiopathic OAT have been determined with CoQ10, vitamin E, selenium, and also vitamin C and N-acetyl-cysteine treatments. In case of oligozoospermia vitamin E and CoQ10 were most often proved to be effective. Favorable effects on asthenozoospermia have most often been determined with vitamin E, CoQ10, and selenium treatments. In teratozoospermia selenium and CoQ10 treatments were most often proved to be effective. In addition, combination of vitamin C and E showed the biggest favorable effect on DNA fragmentation; similar effects were determined with zinc and selenium treatments.

Pentoxifylline[31,32]

- *Rationale*: When taken orally and secreted in the seminal fluid, pentoxifylline and its metabolites will appear in the semen. They inhibit phosphodiesterase and increase cyclic adenosine monophosphate (cAMP) concentrations in the ejaculated spermatozoa thereby improving their motility, hyperactivation and acrosome reaction.
- *Drugs used*: Pentoxifylline of 1,200 mg daily over 6 months.

Antiprostaglandins[33]

It has been suggested that antiprostaglandins improve spermatogenesis. In a controlled study by Barkay and coworkers, indomethacin (50–75 mg/day for 60 days) was found to improve significantly both semen parameters and pregnancy rates compared with no improvement in the placebo group. The best results (pregnancy rate of 36%) were obtained at the 75 mg dose. These results need to be confirmed by additional controlled studies.

Nutritional Supplements[34]

- *Rationale*: In our country, majority of the people from the lower socioeconomic strata are nutritionally depleted and therefore may not have the necessary levels of vitamins and trace elements to facilitate spermatogenesis.
- *Drugs used*: Multivitamin combinations with zinc (up to 50 mg/day), selenium (55–100 µg), folic acid (400 mg per day), and B12. Various combinations of nutraceuticals are available.[10]

Out of the available supplements it is found that zinc deficiency has been linked to low sperm counts and T levels. Exposure to stress, cigarette smoke, pollution, and alcohol can deplete zinc. Zinc supplements have been shown to improve sperm count, motility, form, function, quality, and fertilizing capacity.

Selenium supplementation has shown to improve sperm formation, quantity, structure, quality, motility and function. The epididymis, the tube through which sperm passes from the testicle through the penis, needs selenium to function properly. Selenium deficiency has been linked to male infertility, while selenium supplementation in men has been shown to improve pregnancy rates.

Other vitamins and minerals for treatment of male infertility:

- Vitamin A 5,000 IUs
- Vitamin B6 50 mg
- Vitamin B12 100 μg
- Copper 2 mg
- Iron 2 mg
- Magnesium 250–500 mg
- Manganese 1–2 mg

Miscellaneous

- *Rationale*: Some of these therapies have aimed at improving sperm quality by boosting the Kallikrein-Kinin system (kallikreins) or by interfering with the production of prostaglandins (phosphodiesterase inhibitors, nonsteroidal anti-inflammatory agents).
- *Drugs used*: Kallikreins 600 IU daily; indomethacin.

ART Techniques

Intrauterine Insemination

Artificial insemination with husband semen has been used to treat infertile couples for almost 200 years. It is an accepted form of treatment for men with severe hypospadias, retrograde ejaculation, neurologic impotence, and sexual dysfunction refractory to counseling. It also has been used in the presence of oligospermia, asthenozoospermia, low or high ejaculate volumes, and antisperm antibodies; however, the success rate in these settings is low and the utility is open to review. The technique also has been used in the presence of abnormal cervical mucus, stenotic cervical canal, or antisperm antibodies in the female. The desire to bypass poor cervical mucus or to assist sperm transit in male factor infertility has led to the technique of IUI. Abandoned because of serious allergic reactions, IUI with unprepared semen has been replaced with IUI with "washed sperm".[35] There are a variety of techniques designed to separate sperm from the other seminal fluids, remove antibodies or debris, and isolate a fraction of sperm with optimal motility and morphology. These include simple washing, where semen is diluted into a volume of culture medium and centrifuged, the supernatant decanted, and then the process repeated. The final product has the seminal fluid portion removed but all sperm and cellular components remain. The swim-up and Percoll techniques are designed to isolate a population of sperm with better motility and morphology and thus higher pregnancy rates.[36,37]

In the swim-up procedure, after washing and centrifugation, the specimen is incubated, allowing the most motile sperm to swim up from the pellet into the medium. The specimen for insemination is obtained from the supernatant, rather than the pellet. It contains fewer sperm, but the motility is enhanced. With the Percoll procedure, motile sperm are separated differentially by means of their ability to traverse progressively more dense layers of a viscous medium.

The number of sperm for insemination should not be less than 1 million, and pregnancy rates are not increased to greater than 15 million, although the multiple pregnancy rate is increased to more than 20 million. However, others have not been able to demonstrate increased pregnancy rates with IUI over timed intercourse in oligoasthenospermic infertility.[38]

Recently, IUI in conjunction with superovulation has become a popular treatment for male factor infertility, as well as unexplained infertility. The combination of IUI and superovulation with gonadotropins has the theoretical advantage of placing a greater number of motile and morphologically normal sperm in close proximity to multiple mature oocytes. Pregnancy rate or cycle was significantly greater for the combination of IUI and gonadotropin superovulation (26.4%) than for IUI alone (2.7%) or superovulation alone (6.1%).[39-42]

Donor Insemination

For couples who have failed to conceive despite therapy or those with extreme idiopathic oligospermia, donor insemination offers the couple an alternative to adoption. In the absence of contributing female-factor infertility, donor insemination is extremely successful (70% with 5–6 cycles). If donor insemination is unacceptable and adoption is not desired, the male who wants to pursue having his own genetic offspring can avail himself of the new reproductive technologies: IVF and micromanipulation.

Sperm Retrieval Techniques for IVF and Microassisted Fertilization[42-44]

There are a variety of techniques involved in the retrieval of spermatozoa for utilization in IVF and microassisted fertilization, such as ICSI. This includes masturbation, electroejaculation or vibratory stimulation, percutaneous epididymal sperm aspiration (PESA), microsurgical epididymal sperm aspiration (MESA), and testicular sperm extraction (TESE). Masturbation requires 2–3 days of abstinence before production of the sample, which subsequently undergoes sperm preparation before use. Electroejaculation or vibratory stimulation requires the use of a device and urinary alkalization in patients with ejaculatory dysfunction to produce an adequate sample. PESA and MESA are used in men with azoospermia secondary to obstructive and nonobstructive disorders. PESA involves local anesthesia and multiple blind passages with a 21 to 23-gauge needle through the epididymis, with the advantage of avoiding a skin incision. However, the disadvantage is the "blind" nature of the procedure, which may cause significant damage to the epididymis, making future attempts at conception difficult. Conversely, MESA provides retrieval of many sperm, with less epididymal damage, which then may be cryopreserved and used for future procedures. TESE involves an open surgical biopsy of the testicle when epididymal sperm retrieval is unable to occur and provides similar pregnancy rates when using microassisted fertilization.

In vitro fertilization[45]*:* In vitro fertilization and its micromanipulative innovations show promise of being an advance for male infertility on the level that traditional IVF has been for female tubal infertility. The concept of IVF originated with the desire to treat infertility caused by failed gamete union secondary to tubal obstruction. The first successful in vitro manipulation of gametes by conventional IVF occurred with the birth of Louise Brown in England in 1978. Although the methodology of processing and storing sperm had been available for many years, the ability to recruit, collect, and culture oocytes was required before the possibility of enhancing fertilization by the in vitro incubation of gametes became possible. Since the delivery of the first baby some 21 years ago, the technique has spread worldwide, and consistent results are now obtained. Moreover, the indications soon expanded to include unexplained infertility and male factor.

Although it was logical that inseminating oocytes in vitro would facilitate fertilization, the number of motile sperm originally used for insemination (2–6 million/oocyte) limited application of the technique in oligospermic infertility. With time and experience, the number of motile sperm used for insemination has declined (50,000–100,000/oocyte) with maintenance of fertilization rates and tolerable levels of polyspermic fertilization. This development opened the door for treatment of the oligospermic male using IVF. Additionally, controlled ovarian hyperstimulation with hMG allows the recruitment of multiple ovarian follicles and retrieval of multiple oocytes, which then can be inseminated using processed sperm from the male partner.

Conventional IVF and the Oligospermic Male[46-51]

Male factor infertility is the indication for approximately 25% of IVF cycles. Oligospermia, abnormal morphology, and motility adversely influence fertilization rates. However, once fertilization has occurred, the implantation rate per transfer is equal to that of other IVF patients. The national IVF registry has demonstrated consistently an increased chance of failed fertilization in male factor infertility (50%) compared with tubal infertility (15%). These low fertilization rates result in fewer embryos for transfer and a lower overall success rate (deliveries/retrieval).

Failure of fertilization at IVF is devastating to the infertile couple. The financial and emotional investment is of such magnitude that even when it is anticipated because of known severe andrological infertility, the disappointment is great. What can the patient be offered after failed fertilization, and what of the patient with such extreme semen abnormalities that even conventional IVF is not a consideration? Several new techniques have been developed to assist the fertilization process, some of which promise to make conceiving a pregnancy a reality for even the most severe oligospermic, asthenospermic, and teratospermic males. When there is failure of fertilization at IVF or when a male factor is anticipated or known, options include gamete intrafallopian transfer (GIFT), repeat conventional IVF, modification of sperm concentration, and microassisted fertilization. Although recommended by some, the use of a second sperm sample (husband/partner or donor) to reinseminate (rescue) oocytes that have failed to undergo fertilization has not proven efficacious.

Intrafallopian Transfer Procedures[52-56]

In nontubal infertility, intrafallopian transfer procedures have gained popularity because of modestly increased clinical pregnancy rates compared with IVF (25% vs. 10%). It is not clear whether these results are due to the benefits of the in vivo tubal environment or whether they only reflect differences in patient selection. The rationale for GIFT is that the oviduct, being the natural location for fertilization, offers the optimal environment. In nonmale-factor patients, the usual number of sperm placed with the oocytes in the oviduct is 100,000. In male-factor cases, some investigators suggest the use of increased sperm numbers (325,000 sperm/oviduct), whereas others report using reduced numbers (2,500/oviduct). It is likely in these cases that the criteria used to define a male factor are different. Indeed, in retrospect, a male factor may not even exist because functional sperm are clearly present. A drawback with GIFT is that in the absence of pregnancy, fertilization cannot be confirmed. Thus, some investigators perform fertilization in vitro and then transfer the zygote to the fallopian tube. In one study of planned zygote intrafallopian transfer (ZIFT) cycles, failure of fertilization was observed in 34 (43.6%). These results would not have been available if GIFT was the planned procedure, and perhaps 34 patients would have undergone unnecessary laparoscopy.

Although some retrospective studies have shown advantages of ZIFT over IVF, a prospective, randomized study comparing IVF and ZIFT found no advantage of ZIFT over IVF for the treatment of male factor infertility. Furthermore, with ZIFT, one-cell zygotes are transferred before determination of pronuclear stage arrest or cleavage failure, both of which are more common in male factor infertility; thus, not permitting embryo preselection, as has been shown advantageous in IVF. Both ZIFT and GIFT have the added disadvantage of requiring laparoscopy and general anesthesia for transfer with consequent increased cost. The possibility of transcervical-intrafallopian transfer of cleavage-stage embryos could impact the success and cost equation, but the efficacy of these procedures has yet to be determined.

Thus, conventional IVF provides advantages in cost and convenience when compared with GIFT or ZIFT, and success rates probably are not significantly different. If GIFT is considered, it should be limited to cases of mild to moderate male factor infertility, where fertilization potential is known or expected to be good.

Repeat Conventional In Vitro Insemination

Studies have noted that of male factor patients who had one IVF cycle with failed fertilization, 81% had achieved successful fertilization after another cycle. However, with the new microassisted fertilization techniques such as ICSI, with more effective fertilization and pregnancy rates yet slightly higher costs, many clinicians have recommended going directly to these procedures rather than IVF.[57]

Heavy Conventional Insemination

Although concentrations of 50,000–100,000 sperm/mL are customary for conventional IVF, much higher concentrations are appropriate for male factor infertility. Several groups recommend that in the presence of severe male-factor infertility or conventional IVF fertilization failures, patients undergo an IVF cycle with "heavy" conventional insemination. The effective sperm concentration can be as high as 1–5 million/Ml.[58] When oligospermia is severe and insufficient sperm are available, these concentrations frequently can be obtained using the microdrop technique. Sperm concentrations of 1 million/mL can be obtained by placing as few as 25,000 cells in 25 mL droplets of medium under oil. Another technique that can be employed when sperm numbers are limited is to inseminate multiple oocytes in a single dish. Fertilization can be enhanced further in male factor cases by inseminating with not only a high concentration of sperm but with a highly motile population as well. Special procedures (e.g. mini-Percoll), designed to separate a highly motile subpopulation of sperm have evolved for this purpose.[59,60]

Microassisted Fertilization

Although conventional IVF has been very helpful in treating couples with long-term andrological infertility, there are patients with severe male factor infertility (extreme oligospermia, absence of normal morphology, and motility), and fertilization failure patients with no currently detectable semen abnormalities, who are appropriately considered for treatment by more aggressive techniques. Philosophical extremes still exist in deciding which patients should be considered for micromanipulation: a last resort procedure or one appropriate for all suspected or diagnosed male factor infertility. These techniques involve the use of micromanipulators to mechanically assist the sperm–egg interaction process.

The Micromanipulation Technique

Under visualization on the stage of an inverted microscope, oocytes in culture medium droplets under oil are held and micromanipulated with specially prepared holding and injection pipettes. The oocyte is immobilized with gentle suction applied by the holding pipette, and the injection pipette is used to incise the zona pellucida (ZP), deposit several sperm in the perivitelline space, or inject a single sperm directly into the ooplasm. These techniques can be classified as zonal, subzonal, and intracytoplasmic procedures. Although known by many names such as zona drilling, subzonal insertion, and direct egg injection, the following terms are used in this chapter: partial zona dissection (PZD), subzonal injection (SUZI), and ICSI.

Partial Zona Dissection[61-66]

Before fertilization can occur, sperm must penetrate the ZP, traverse the perivitelline space, and fuse with the oolemma in the process of entering the ooplasm. The ZP, an acellular glycoprotein coat surrounding the oocyte, plays several roles in fertilization and early development, including the provision of a species-specific barrier to fertilization, a barrier to polyspermia, and a protective shell for the preimplantation embryo. Because ZP passage represents a prerequisite step for the fertilizing sperm, the creation of gaps or slits in the zona should facilitate this process.

Oocytes dissected in this manner are inseminated subsequently with standard concentrations of capacitated sperm. Chemical, mechanical, and laser techniques have been employed. The ZP was first opened using acidified Tyrode's solution delivered through a microneedle (zona drilling). This process was successful in mice but not when applied in human IVF because of induced oocyte damage.

To minimize damage to the oocyte during this process, limited shrinkage is induced by conducting the procedure in sucrose. The technique usually involves placing the micropipette through the ZP into the perivitelline space and then continuing out through the opposite side of the ZP without entering the ooplasm. Releasing the oocyte from the holding pipette, the ZP overlying the micropipette is rubbed against the side of the holding pipette until a slit is created in the ZP. Other investigators have advocated using laser for PZD because of its simplicity and precision.

However, the overall success of PZD has been limited. It is estimated that only 100–150 live births have resulted from the method. In a comparative study involving 130 male factor cycles, no differences were found between IVF and PZD with respect to fertilization (12% vs. 13%); the cleavage rate was higher for the IVF group (89% vs. 73%); and the pregnancy rate for IVF was 33% compared with 12% for PZD.99 The conclusion was drawn that PZD was no better than conventional IVF. Furthermore, PZD is complicated by excessive rates of polyspermia, variously reported at 30–47%. Although rates of polyspermia may be modulated by patient selection, gap size, and sperm concentration, results have been inconsistent. In most centers, the implantation capacity also is reduced, most likely because of oocyte damage during the procedure (2–30%), or improper culture conditions during the micromanipulation (temperature and pH). These problems and inconsistent results have led many investigators to abandon PZD.

Subzonal Injection

The second generation of micromanipulation techniques includes SUZI or the direct subzonal insertion of sperm through and under the ZP into the perivitelline space. Depending on their morphologic appearance, several sperms (3–6) are aspirated into a sharp, beveled microneedle and injected through the ZP. Because the ZP and its ZP3, the zona glycoprotein implicated in acrosome reaction induction, are bypassed in this process, strategies to prematurely induce the acrosome reaction have been conceived. Two methods designed for this purpose are washed sperm incubated for 24 hours in Tyrode's medium plus 50% follicular fluid, and electroporation plus incubation in 3.5 mmol/L pentoxifylline.[67] Although these procedures increase the acrosome-free sperm to as high as 54%, their efficacy remains unproven. Indeed, motile sperm in the perivitelline space still may be exposed to ZP3 present on the inner aspects of the zona. In theory, increasing the number of reacted sperm should allow the use of fewer sperm (3 vs. 6), thereby decreasing the risk of polyspermic fertilization.

Unfortunately, the clinical success with SUZI has been less than spectacular, with fertilization rates hovering around 20% and pregnancy rates around 10%.[68,69]

The drawbacks of SUZI are the same as those for PZD: polyspermic fertilization and impaired implantation. Because the oolemma cannot block multiple sperm fusion, SUZI is inherently complicated by polyspermic fertilization. The fertilization rate with SUZI can be increased by increasing the number of sperm placed in the perivitelline space, but the proportion of polyspermic embryos may become unacceptably high. However, polyspermia may be lower than with PZD and can be influenced by the number of sperm inserted. Implantation rates with SUZI embryos also may be better than for PZD. Likewise, the risk of blastomere or cytoplasm extrusion and contamination of the perivitelline space with medium is reduced with SUZI (smaller gap). However, this technique recently has been superseded by ICSI.

Intracytoplasmic Sperm Injection[70-84]

The next logical step was to use micromanipulation to inject a single sperm through the ZP and oolemma directly into the ooplasm. Although the most invasive technique, the inherent advantage to ICSI is avoidance of polyspermic fertilization because only one sperm is injected. Initial concerns with ICSI centered on whether the cytoskeleton would be disrupted, causing defective cell division (minimized by injecting distal to the meiotic spindle); whether fertilization would occur with genetically abnormal sperm; and whether oocyte activation (completion of the fertilization process, initiation of cleavage, and development), if triggered, would be normal.

In animals, the ICSI procedure has not always resulted in activation, and various treatment regimens have been developed to overcome this limitation. For instance, oocytes can be activated by exposure to ethanol, calcium ionophore, or electrical fields (electroporation). The common mediator with these methods is most likely elevation of intracellular calcium ion concentration, either by extracellular calcium influx or by intracytoplasmic mobilization of calcium stores. It has become apparent that injection of a single sperm into the cytoplasm is sufficient stimulus in humans to trigger activation. In addition, the increased intracellular calcium associated with the injection process does not, in and of itself, provoke egg activation, but rather, the release of a sperm factor appears to be required. Interestingly, an intact acrosome is not a deterrent to ICSI success.

Although preclinical trials of ICSI established that fertilization could be obtained, 106 clinical pregnancies were not reported until 1992. High fertilization and pregnancy rates with ICSI currently are routine in several centers around the world. The most extensive experience has been realized in a program in Brussels. In their ICSI technique, sperms either were incubated overnight, treated with pentoxifylline and deoxyadenosine, electroporation, or were exposed transiently to elevated calcium levels to increase the chance for fertilization. These recipes for success have been largely abandoned. Percoll-gradient processed sperm are dispersed in polyvinylpyrrolidone, a viscous solution that allows separation of motile sperm from immotile cells, specifically in conditions of severe oligoasthenozoospermia.

Subsequent immobilization of the spermatozoa by various techniques, such as crimping the tail of the spermatozoa at the tip, allows for delivery into the micropipette. Beveled, injection micropipettes (7 µm outer and 5 µm inner diameter) then are front-loaded tail first, with the resultant immobilized spermatozoa for injection into the ooplasm. In men with complete asthenozoospermia, there are no motile sperm and less than 50% of the sperm are viable. As a result, the hypo-osmotic swelling test was developed and used to enhance fertilization and pregnancy in these patients, as well as in previously cryopreserved sperm that usually have poor motility. When sperms are incubated in a hypo-osmolar medium, those that are viable and functional undergo swelling of the cytoplasmic space and the sperm tail fibers curl. These sperm in turn may be used in ICSI and provide a better outcome.

The indications for ICSI are the absence of fertilization, a failure to fertilize in a previous cycle of IVF, antisperm antibodies, teratozoospermia, sever oligoasthenozoospermia, obstructive azoospermia, such as with congenital bilateral absence of the vas deferens, nonobstructive azoospermia, and anejaculation.

In the early developmental phase of the ICSI procedure, a comparison of 750 cycles of ICSI and SUZI was conducted, and a fertilization rate of 55% for ICSI vs. 17% for SUZI was obtained. ICSI quickly was adopted as the standard assisted fertilization treatment for couples unable to benefit from conventional IVF.

Although concerns about disruption of chromosomal or cytoskeletal elements or the consequences of fertilization with genetically abnormal sperm continue, confidence is accumulating that clinical outcomes will be normal. In infertile men, approximately 7% have a major sex chromosome abnormality, half of which are accounted for by a mosaic Klinefelter condition. The incidence rises from 2% in men with normal sperm concentration to 20% in those with azoospermia. Despite these data and an apparently high risk for chromosome abnormalities in ICSI fetuses, it was found that the risk of chromosomal abnormalities to be approximately 1%, similar to the general newborn population.

Sperm employed for ICSI can be morphologically very abnormal; pregnancies have occurred with very low counts, 0% motility, 0% normal morphology, as well as with cryopreserved sperm. In fact, in situations of previously diagnosed primary testicular failure with FSH levels greater than 30 mIU/mL, nearly 50% of men had mature sperm on testicular biopsy suitable for ICSI. In addition, application of round spermatid nuclei injection (ROSNI) in humans is undergoing careful consideration, with fertilization rates of approximately 30%, two pregnancies, and resultant childbirth. Because ICSI allows fertilization by sperm, which under natural conditions are incapable of ZP penetration and oocyte-sperm fusion, concern also exists that germline mutations might be transmitted, resulting in heritable defects. The inheritance of susceptibility to infertility is another concern and would not be recognized until late in the next generation (the reproductive years). Once sexing of the spermatozoa becomes routinely available, prevention of sex-linked diseases may be preventable by selecting the healthier gender. Thus, careful evaluation, genetic consultation with the couples, and follow-up of the pregnancies resulting from ICSI are necessary.

Elimination of Gonadotoxic Factors

Elimination of chronic exposure to heat at the workplace (furnace, kitchen, etc.) or in leisure activities (sauna, steam bath), cessation of heavy smoking, avoidance of exposure to pesticides [dichlorodiphenyltrichloroethane (DDT) spray] or chemical fumes (aromatic amines), reduction of excessive stress, regularization of diet, and lifestyle can also help some men significantly.

CONCLUSION

- As physicians taking care of couples with OAT, it is our duty to give the patients a very clear road map of their course of therapy.
- Therapy must be individualized and it is mandatory that a treatment timeline and endpoints be established prior to initiation of medical therapy.
- When empiric pharmacologic therapy is going to be used, treatment should last at least 3 months to incorporate a full 74 day spermatogenic cycle, and should be followed by a semen analysis.
- If there is significant improvement then the medications should be continued and further improvement monitored monthly. If there is no improvement then the medication should be changed or the therapy may be escalated to ART.
- Patients must be counseled regarding the inconsistent response to medical therapy and to have realistic expectations from the same.
- Most importantly, we must not be guilty of wasting precious time and money over medical therapy when the circumstances call for assisted reproductive therapy.

REFERENCES

1. Petraglia F, Serour GI, Chapron C. The changing prevalence of infertility. Int J Gynecol Obstet. 2013;123(Suppl 2):S4-8.
2. World Health Organization. (2010). WHO Laboratory Manual for the Examination of and Processing of Human Semen, 5th edition.
3. Cai T, Mazzoli S, Mondaini N, et al. Chlamydia trachomatis infection: challenge for the urologist. Microbiol Res. 2011;2(2):e14.
4. Hendry WF, Hughes L, Scammell G, et al. Comparison of prednisolone and placebo in subfertile men with antibodies to spermatozoa. Lancet. 1990;335(8681):85-8.
5. Safarinejad MR, Safarinejad S, Shafiei N, et al. Effects of the reduced form of coenzyme Q10 (ubiquinol) on semen parameters in men with idiopathic infertility: a double-

blind, placebo controlled, randomized study. J Urol. 2012;188(2):526-31.

6. Samplaski MK, Loai Y, Lo K, et al. Testosterone use in the male infertility population: short and longer term effects on semen and hormonal parameters. J Urol. 2013:189(4):E779.
7. Chua ME, Escusa KG, Luna S, et al. Revisiting oestrogen antagonists (clomiphene or tamoxifen) as medical empiric therapy for male infertility: a meta-analysis. Andrology. 2013;1(5):749-57.
8. Farmakiotis D, Farmakis C, Rousso D, et al. The beneficial effects of toremifene administration on the hypothalamic-pituitary-testicular axis and sperm parameters in men with idiopathic oligozoospermia. Fertil Steril. 2007;88(4):847-53.
9. Saylam B, Efesoy O, Cayan S. The effect of aromatase inhibitor letrozole on body mass index, serum hormones, and sperm parameters in infertile men. Fertil Steril. 2011;95(2):809-11.
10. Roth MY, Amory JK, Page ST. Treatment of male infertility secondary to morbid obesity. Nat Clin Pract Endocrinol Metab. 2008;4(7):415-9.
11. Zumoff B, Miller LK, Strain GW. Reversal of the hypogonadotropic hypogonadism of obese men by administration of the aromatase inhibitor testolactone. Metabolism. 2003;52(9):1126-8.
12. Gregoriou O, Bakas P, Grigoriadis C, et al. Changes in hormonal profile and seminal parameters with use of aromatase inhibitors in management of infertile men with low testosterone to estradiol ratios. Fertil Steril. 2012;98(1):48-51.
13. Finkelstein JS, Lee H, Burnett-Bowie SA, et al. Gonadal steroids and body composition, strength, and sexual function in men. N Engl J Med. 2013;369(11):1011-22.
14. Knuth UA, Hönigl W, Bals-Pratsch M, et al. Treatment of severe oligospermia with human chorionic gonadotropin/human menopausal gonadotropin: a placebo-controlled, double blind trial. J Clin Endocrinol Metab. 1987;65(6):1081-7.
15. Kamischke A, Behre HM, Bergmann M, et al. Recombinant human follicle stimulating hormone for treatment of male idiopathic infertility: a randomized, double-blind, placebo-controlled, clinical trial. Hum Reprod. 1998;13(3):596-603.
16. Foresta C, Bettella A, Garolla A, et al. Treatment of male idiopathic infertility with recombinant human follicle-stimulating hormone: a prospective, controlled, randomized clinical study. Fertil Steril. 2005;84(3):654-61.
17. Sikaris K, McLachlan RI, Kazlauskas R, et al. Reproductive hormone reference intervals for healthy fertile young men: evaluation of automated platform assays. J Clin Endocrinol Metab. 2005;90(11):5928-36.
18. Gordetsky J, van Wijngaarden E, O'Brien J. Redefining abnormal follicle-stimulating hormone in the male infertility population. BJU Int. 2012;110(4):568-72.
19. Webster J, Piscitelli G, Polli A, et al. Dose-dependent suppression of serum prolactin by cabergoline in hyperprolactinaemia: a placebo controlled, double blind, multicentre study. European Multicentre Cabergoline Dose-finding Study Group. Clin Endocrinol (Oxf). 1992;37(6):534-41.
20. Verhelst J, Abs R, Maiter D, et al. Cabergoline in the treatment of hyperprolactinemia: a study in 455 patients. J Clin Endocrinol Metab. 1999;84(7):2518-22.
21. Melmed S, Casanueva FF, Hoffman AR, et al. Diagnosis and treatment of hyperprolactinemia: an Endocrine Society clinical practice guideline. J Clin Endocrinol Metab. 2011;96(2):273-88.
22. Nieschlag E, Lenzi A. The conventional management of male infertility. Int J Gynecol Obstet. 2013;123(Suppl 2):S31-5.
23. Sharma RK, Agarwal A. Role of reactive oxygen species in male infertility. Urology. 1996;48(6):835-50.
24. Saleh RA, Agarwal A. Oxidative stress and male infertility: from research bench to clinical practice. J Androl. 2002;23(6):737-52.
25. Rolf C, Cooper TG, Yeung CH, et al. Antioxidant treatment of patients with asthenozoospermia or moderate oligoasthenozoospermia with high-dose vitamin C and vitamin E: a randomized, placebo-controlled, double-blind study. Hum Reprod. 1999;14(4):1028-33.
26. Greco E, Iacobelli M, Rienzi L, et al. Reduction of the incidence of sperm DNA fragmentation by oral antioxidant treatment. J Androl. 2005;26(3):349-53.
27. Paradiso Galatioto G, Gravina GL, Angelozzi G, et al. May antioxidant therapy improve sperm parameters of men with persistent oligospermia after retrograde embolization for varicocele? World J Urol. 2008;26(1):97-102.
28. Ross C, Morriss A, Khairy M, et al. A systematic review of the effect of oral antioxidants on male infertility. Reprod Biomed Online. 2010;20(6):711-23.
29. Showell MG, Brown J, Yazdani A, et al. Antioxidants for male subfertility. Cochrane Database Syst Rev. 2011;(1):CD007411.
30. Agarwal A, Sekhon LH. Oxidative stress and antioxidants for oligoasthenoteratospermia: is it justified? Indian J Urol. 2011;27(1):74-85.
31. Merino G, Martinez Chequer JC, Barahona E, et al. Effects of pentoxifylline on sperm motility in normagonadotropic asthenozoospermic men. Arch Androl. 1997;39(1):65-9.
32. Tesarik J, Thebault A, Testart J. Effect of pentoxifylline on sperm movement characteristics in normozoospermic and asthenozoospermic specimens. Hum Reprod. 1992;7(9):1257-63.
33. Barkay J, Haysaz-Karpel S, Ben-Ezra, et al. The prostaglandin inhibitor effect of anti-inflammatory drugs in the therapy of male infertility. Fertil Steril. 1984;42(3):406-11.
34. Ko EY, Sabanegh ES. The role of over-the-counter supplements for the treatment of male infertility—fact or fiction? J Androl. 2012;33(3):292-308.
35. Carrell DT, Kuneck PH, Peterson CM, et al. A randomized, prospective analysis of five sperm preparation techniques before intrauterine insemination of husband sperm. Fertil Steril. 1998;69(1):122-6.
36. Berger T, Marrs RP, Moyer DL. Comparison of techniques for selection of motile human spermatozoa. Fertil Steril. 1985;43(2):268.
37. Kerin J, Byrd W. Supracervical placement of spermatozoa. In: Soules MR (Ed). Controversies in Reproductive Endocrinology and Infertility. Amsterdam: Elsevier; 1989.
38. Ho PC, Poon IML, Chan SYW, et al. Intrauterine insemination is not useful in oligoasthenospermia. Fertil Steril. 1989;51(4):682-4.
39. Kemmann E, Bohrer M, Shelden R, et al. Active ovulation management increases the monthly probability of pregnancy occurrence in ovulatory women who receive intrauterine insemination. Fertil Steril. 1987;48(6):16.

40. Serhal PF, Katz M, Little V, et al. Unexplained infertility—the value of Pergonal superovulation combined with intrauterine insemination. Fertil Steril. 1988;49(4):602.
41. Dodson WL, Haney AF. Controlled ovarian hyperstimulation and intrauterine insemination for treatment of infertility. Fertil Steril. 1991;55(3):457-67.
42. Ombelet W, Puttemans P, Bosmans E. Intrauterine insemination: a first-step procedure in the algorithm of male subfertility treatment. Hum Reprod. 1995;10(Suppl 1):90-102.
43. Kim ED, Lipshultz LI. Male subfertility: diagnostic and therapeutic advances. Br J Urol. 1997;80:633-41.
44. Ghazzawi IM, Sarraf MG, Taher MR, et al. Comparison of the fertilizing capability of spermatozoa from ejaculates, epididymal aspirates and testicular biopsies using intracytoplasmic sperm injection. Hum Reprod. 1998;13(2):348-52.
45. Wolf DP, Byrd W, Dandekar P, et al. Sperm concentration and the fertilization of human eggs in vitro. Biol Reprod. 1984;31(4):837-48.
46. Jeulin C, Feneux D, Serres C, et al. Sperm factors related to failure of human in vitro fertilization. J Reprod Fertil. 1986;76(2):735-44.
47. Matson PL, Blackledge DG, Richardson PA, et al. The role of gamete intrafallopian transfer (GIFT) in the treatment of oligospermia infertility. Fertil Steril. 1987;48(4):608-12.
48. Tournaye H, Devroey P, Camus M, et al. Comparison of in vitro fertilization in male and tubal infertility: a 3 year survey. Hum Reprod. 1992;7(2):218-22.
49. Cohen J, Edwards R, Fehilly C, et al. In vitro fertilization: a treatment for male infertility. Fertil Steril. 1985;43(3):422-32.
50. American Fertility Society/Society for Assisted Reproductive Technology. Assisted reproduction technology in the United States and Canada: 1992 results generated from the American Fertility Society/Society for Assisted Reproductive Technology Registry. Fertil Steril. 1994;62(6):1121-8.
51. Hughes EG, King C, Wood ED. A prospective study of prognostic factors in in vitro fertilization and embryo transfer. Fertil Steril. 1989;51(5):838-44.
52. Khan I, Camus M, Staessen CK, et al. Success rate in gamete intrafallopian transfer using low concentrations of washed spermatozoa. Fertil Steril. 1988;50(6):922-7.
53. Tournaye H, Devroey P, Camus M, et al. Zygote intrafallopian transfer or in vitro fertilization and embryo transfer for the treatment of male-factor infertility: A prospective randomized trial. Fertil Steril. 1992;58(2):344-50.
54. Tournaye H, Camus M, Khan I, et al. In vitro fertilization, gamete- or zygote intrafallopian transfer for the treatment of male infertility. Hum Reprod. 1991;6(2):263-6.
55. Puissant F, Van Rysselberge, Barlow P, et al. Embryo scoring as a prognostic tool in IVF treatment. Hum Reprod. 1987;2(8):705-8.
56. Bustillo M, Schulman JD. Transcervical ultrasound guided intrafallopian placement of gametes, zygotes and embryos. J In Vitro Fert Embryo Transf. 1989;6(6):321-4.
57. Ben-Shlomo I, Bider D, Dor J, et al. Failure of fertilization in couples with male factor infertility: what next? Fertil Steril. 1992;58(1):187-9.
58. Tucker MJ, Wiker SR, Massey J. Rational approach to assisted fertilization. Hum Reprod. 1993;8(11):1778.
59. Bayer SR, Lee MA, McInnes DR, et al. In vitro fertilization and male factor infertility: a critical review and update. Assisted Reprod Rev. 1993;3:244.
60. Ord T, Patrizio P, Marello E, et al. Mini-Percoll: a new method of semen preparation for IVF in severe male factor infertility. Hum Reprod. 1990;5(8):987-9.
61. Malter HE, Cohen J. Partial zona dissection of the human oocyte: a non-traumatic method using micromanipulation to assist zona pellucida penetration. Fertil Steril. 1989;51(1):139-48.
62. El-Danasouri I, Westphal LM, Neeve Y, et al. Zona opening with 308 nm XeC1 excimer laser improves fertilization by spermatozoa from long-term vasectomized mice. Hum Reprod. 1993;8:464.
63. Cohen J, Wiemer KE, Alikani M. Advanced laboratory techniques for assisted reproduction. Assisted Reprod Technol. 1993;4:733.
64. Calderon G, Veiga A, Penella J, et al. Two years of assisted fertilization by using partial zona dissection. Fertil Steril. 1993;60(1):105-9.
65. Tucker MJ, Bishop FM, Cohen J, et al. Routine application of partial zona dissection for male factor infertility. Hum Reprod. 1991;6(5):676-81.
66. Palermo G, Joris H. Devroey P, et al. Induction of acrosome reaction in human spermatozoa used for subzonal insemination. Hum Reprod. 1992;7(2):248-54.
67. Ng SC, Bongso TA, Liow SL, et al. Microinsemination sperm transfer (MIST) and its application to male subfertility: current strategies to improve results. Ann Acad Med Singapore. 1992;21(4):561-4.
68. Cohen J, Malter HE, Talansky BE, et al. Micromanipulation of Human Gametes and Embryos. New York: Raven Press; 1992. pp. 152.
69. Edward RG, Van Steirteghem AC. Intracytoplasmic sperm injections (ICSI) and human fertilization: Does calcium hold the key to success? Hum Reprod. 1993;8(7):988-9.
70. Tesarik J, Sousa M, Testart J. Human oocyte activation after intracytoplasmic sperm injection. Hum Reprod. 1994;9(3):511-8.
71. Lanzendorf SE, Slusser MS, Maloney MK, et al. A preclinical evaluation of pronuclear formation by microinjection of human spermatozoa into human oocytes. Fertil Steril. 1988;49(5):835-42.
72. Palermo G, Joris H, Devroey P, et al. Pregnancies after intracytoplasmic injection of single spermatozoon into an oocyte. Lancet. 1992;340(8810):17-8.
73. Van Steirteghem A, Liu J, Nagy Z, et al. Use of assisted fertilization. Hum Reprod. 1993;8(11):1784-5.
74. Fujii Y, Motoyama H, Hiraguchi K, et al. A simple method for recovering the motile spermatozoa from extremely low quality sperm samples. Hum Reprod. 1997;12(6):1218-21.
75. Chen SU, Ho HN, Chen HF, et al. Intracytoplasmic sperm injection (ICSI) for severe semen abnormalities: Dissecting the tail of spermatozoa at the tip. Hum Reprod. 1996;11(12):2640-4.
76. Casper RF, Meriano JS, Jarvi KA, et al. The hypo-osmotic swelling test for selection of viable sperm for intracytoplasmic sperm injection in men with complete asthenozoospermia. Fertil Steril. 1996;65(5):972-6.

77. Kim ED, Lamb DJ, Lipshultz LI. Intracytoplasmic sperm injection for treatment of the infertile male. Tex Med. 1997;93(7):50-6.
78. Palermo GD, Cohen J, Rosenwaks Z. Intracytoplasmic sperm injection: A powerful tool to overcome fertilization failure. Fertil Steril. 1996;65(5):899-908.
79. Ubaldi F, Nagy Z, Liu J, et al. A survey of four years of experience with intracytoplasmic sperm injection. Acta Europaea Fertilitatis. 1995;26(1):7-11.
80. Baker HW, Liu DY, Bourne H, et al. Diagnosis of sperm defects in selection of patients for assisted fertilization. Hum Reprod. 1993;8(11):1779-80.
81. Persson JW, Peters GB, Saunders DM. Is ICSI associated with risks of genetic disease? Implications for counseling, practice and research. Hum Reprod. 1996;11:921-32.
82. Bonduelle M, Legein J, Buysse A. Prospective follow-up study of 423 children born after intracytoplasmic sperm injection. Hum Reprod. 1996;11(7):1558.
83. Abuzeid MI, Sasy MA, Salem HH. Intracytoplasmic sperm injection for treatment of non-obstructive azoospermia. Gynecol Endocrinol. 1997;11(5):335-9.
84. De Jonge CJ, Pierce J. Intracytoplasmic sperm injection-What kind of reproduction is being assisted? Hum Reprod. 1995;10:2518-28.

CHAPTER 17

Varicocele Surgery: Does it Help?

Vineet Malhotra

INTRODUCTION

It is known that infertility affects 15% of couples of reproductive age. The infertile male has long been an ignored and untreated part of infertility. It has been found that the male factor maybe relevant in up to 50% of all cases of infertility. There has been a lot of interest and controversy regarding the various causes leading to male infertility and their appropriate treatment.[1,2]

Idiopathic infertility is the commonest cause of male factor infertility. Varicoceles (abnormally dilated veins in the pampiniform plexus) are the most common surgically correctable cause of male infertility and are found in 4.4–22.6% of men in the general population. They are present in 20–40% of men with primary infertility and in 75–81% men with secondary infertility. It was the Greek physician Celsus who, in first century AD, first described varicoceles as swollen and twisted veins over the testicle causing them to be smaller in size. There have been anecdotal reports of crude surgical maneuvers such as wiring of the scrotum to treat these dilated swollen veins.[3-6]

It was much later in the early 1950s that Tulloch reported his results of surgical repair of varicoceles and the resultant improvement in sperm parameters.[7]

There has been immense controversy regarding the standardization of diagnosis and classification of a varicocele. There is also lack of agreement over the need for treatment and the response to treatment.[8]

The predictive value of semen analysis as a marker of male fertility is limited and has been shown by various authors.[9]

Smith et al.[10] reported that up to 25% men with sperm densities below 12.5 million/mL could father a child through spontaneous conception. On the other hand, even with counts of up to 25 million/mL, which is normal by the WHO standards, 10% of men could not father a child with a fertile female.

A more effective outcome parameter would be pregnancy rates since pregnancy is the ultimate endpoint of therapy. When using pregnancy as the endpoint of treatment outcome, it is important to consider the spontaneous pregnancy rate in supposedly infertile couples on no therapy. The spontaneous pregnancy rate is about 1% per month, reaching cumulatively to 26% over 3 years. Obviously, any treatment option being used should improve upon this result. On the other hand, the benefit from an intervention like varicocelectomy may be neutralized by a concomitant untreated female factor.

Good clinical trials require a placebo-controlled, double-blind format. Such a trial, with sham surgery, is ethically impossible in humans. Moreover, randomization on a large scale for such surgeries is also difficult due to the intense social pressure and stress faced by infertile couples resulting in them seeking early intervention. During the course of a multicenter, prospective, randomized trial, in Germany, on radiological embolization of varicoceles, only 67 patients could be randomized in 3 years against a target of 460.[11] Further, follow-up is a major problem among individuals affected by infertility, since they are a young and mobile population. Varicocelectomy results are incremental and pregnancies may occur even 2 years after the surgery. Thus, in another study on surgically treated varicoceles, only 130 out of an original 480 patients remained in the study at the end of 1 year.[12] There is also inconsistency regarding the populations studied, initial grading of varicocele, age of patient and partner, duration of follow-up, and type of treatment applied. Certain nomograms have been created to predict changes in semen parameters in infertile men after varicocele repair.[13]

Based on current evidence, it is the practice guideline of both the American Urological Association (AUA) and the American Society for Reproductive Medicine (ASRM) that correction of a varicocele should be offered to infertile men with palpable lesions and one or more abnormal semen parameters.[14]

We have attempted to address the issue and provide our view on this debate regarding surgery for varicocele. We will attempt to outline the contentious issues with regards to classification/grading of a varicocele, the effect it may have on fertility, treatment types available, treatment of different grades, unilateral/bilateral varicoceles. We will also discuss the relevance of treating varicoceles with small testicular size, azoospermia, with isolated sperm defects and in adolescents. Finally, we will discuss surgery versus assisted reproductive techniques in the era of Assisted reproductive technology (ART).

DIAGNOSIS AND CLASSIFICATION

Varicoceles are usually diagnosed on clinical examination in an upright position and confirmed by scrotal ultrasound. There is significant examiner bias and variation in classification of varicoceles.[14] The classification of varicoceles on physical examination was described by Dubin[15] (Dubin grading system) into three grades, with grade 3 being visible while the patient is standing, grade 2 is palpable without Valsalva maneuver, and grade 1 is not able to be visualized and only palpable with Valsalva maneuver.

A clinical varicocele is one which is detected on physical examination, either visible or palpable. A nonpalpable enlargement of spermatic veins which is only identifiable by imaging techniques is referred to as a subclinical varicocele.

The imaging techniques used for grading varicoceles include scrotal ultrasound and color Doppler imaging. They have low accuracy and clinical utility as most data have shown a poor correlation between varicoceles detected only on imaging and response to surgery.

For those who utilize scrotal ultrasound as a diagnostic modality, criteria for diagnosing a subclinical varicocele by scrotal ultrasound requires at least the presence of dilated veins with diameter > 3.0 mm with concomitant reversal of flow after Valsalva.

Color Doppler Ultrasound Classification of Varicocele (Sarteschi)[16]

Grade Features

- Reflux in vessels in the inguinal channel is detected only during the Valsalva maneuver, while scrotal varicosity is not evident in the standard ultrasound study.
- Small posterior varicosities that extend to the superior pole of the testis. Their diameters increase and venous reflux is seen in the supratesticular region only during the Valsalva maneuver.
- Vessels appear enlarged at the inferior pole of the testis when the patient is evaluated in a standing position; no enlargement is detected if the patient is examined in a supine position. Reflux observed only during the Valsalva maneuver.
- Vessels appear enlarged even when the patient is studied in a supine position; the dilatation is more marked in the upright position and during the Valsalva maneuver. Testicular hypotrophy is common at this stage.
- Venous ectasia is evident even in the prone decubitus and supine positions. Reflux is observed at rest and does not increase during the Valsalva maneuver.

PATHOPHYSIOLOGY

Varicocele has been postulated to affect testicular function and spermatogenesis through various mechanisms that include elevation of testicular temperature and intratesticular pressure. Other factors such as reflux of toxic metabolites from adrenal glands and hormonal abnormalities have also been implicated. One theory suggests the reduction of blood flow leading to hypoxia and impaired spermatogenesis.

The malfunction of valves of the internal spermatic veins, cremasteric veins, and occasionally the external spermatic veins leads to a reflux and rise of intrascrotal temperatures. This may cause thermal damage to the spermatogenic cells and Leydig cells leading to impaired spermatogenesis.[17-22]

The low sperm concentration is attributed by some researchers to the high germ cell apoptosis usually observed in these men, while the low motility is attributed to the increased concentration of reactive oxygen species.

The exact mechanism by which the above factors contribute to the adverse effect of varicocele on spermatogenesis has not been fully clarified. It is speculated that the main mechanism is DNA damage in sperm heads due to oxidative stress. The latter is caused either by the presence of high levels of reactive oxygen species or by reduced antioxidant capacity. It is interesting to note that these results were confirmed in fertile as well as in infertile men with varicocele. Thus, it becomes obvious that oxidative stress is directly related to varicocele, independent of the fertility status.[23-26]

Nevertheless, oxidative stress is known to have adverse effects on sperm structure and function, such as membrane lipid alterations, disruption of sperm metabolism, reduction of its motility, DNA fragmentation, and reduced overall sperm quality.[27-30]

THE DEBATE

There are several early studies that showed benefit of intervention in cases of subclinical varicoceles. These found results of intervention to be independent of the grade of varicocele and were responsible for the widespread practice of treating all varicoceles by intervention.[31,32] Later, in the early 1990s, studies revealed that there was no significant difference in outcomes between patients with subclinical varicoceles in the observation versus intervention arm.[33,34]

It is now generally agreed that patients with subclinical varicoceles do not warrant any intervention as an isolated causative factor for male infertility.[35] Several studies have questioned the role of intervention in case of clinical varicoceles and that has been the basis of a Cochrane database review that did not offer conclusive support to intervention [an odds ratio of postoperative spontaneous pregnancy as 1.10 (95% CI: 0.73–1.68)] over expectant management in subfertile couples.[36-40] In a recent meta-analysis published by Kroese et al. the search methodology included the Cochrane Menstrual disorders and Subfertility Group Trials Register (September 12, 2003 to January 2012), the Cochrane Central Register of Controlled trials (Central) in the Cochrane library issue 1, 2012, Medline (January 1966 to January 2012), Embase (January 1985 to January 2012), PsycINFO (to Week 1, 2012), and reference list of articles.[40a] They have also checked cross-references, references from review articles, and contacted researchers in the field. The meta-analysis included 894 men (10 studies) and showed a combined fixed-effect odds ratio of 1.47 for the outcome of pregnancy (very low quality evidence) favoring intervention.

The study design, patient inclusion criteria, and analysis of these studies have been questioned, as they included patients with normal semen parameters, different methods of intervention, and significant patient dropout.

Madgar et al.[41] studied infertile men with clinical varicoceles and subjected them to intervention versus observation for a period of 12 months. If the patients in the observation group did not report a pregnancy, they were reassigned to the intervention arm. This study revealed a significantly higher pregnancy rate in the immediate (60% in the intervention vs 10% in observation arm) and delayed treatment (44% vs 10%) groups.

The conclusions of Evers and Collins in their systematic review spurred Ficarra et al.[42,43] and Marmar et al.[44] both to re-evaluate the existing data with meta-analyses as well. Ficarra et al. published a meta-analysis including only three of the randomized controlled trials and excluded those where subjects with normal semen analyses or subclinical varicoceles were included. The authors concluded that the heterogeneity of the data and poor quality of study design do not allow for formal analysis. At the same time, the authors used this same argument to refute the conclusions by Evers and Collins. Marmar et al. published a meta-analysis of five studies on surgical repair only on infertile men with clinical varicocele and abnormal semen analysis looking at spontaneous pregnancy rates. The authors included randomized controlled trials and also observational studies. While accepting that this is not standard for the meta-analysis format, the authors state that their inclusion and exclusion criteria allow for less heterogeneity in the population studied and intervention being studied. Odds ratio of spontaneous pregnancy after varicocelectomy was calculated to be 2.87 (95% CI: 1.33–6.20, $P = 0.007$). Pregnancy rates were also significantly higher in treated patients than in not treated (33% vs 15.5%, respectively).

Though varicoceles most commonly present on the left side, this swelling can occur on the right side as well, individually or in unison. *Bilateral* varicocele would seemingly be more detrimental than a unilateral defect. Several investigations have examined whether bilateral repair is similar or superior to one-sided repair. Kondoh et al. reported a small cases series of 27 men with bilateral varicoceles and 40 unilateral left-sided varicoceles and noted less improvements in sperm density in the group with bilateral when compared to the left-sided only group. Four subsequent reports all have demonstrated evidence to support the contrary.[45-47] Scherr et al.[48] prospectively studied 91 men with moderate-to-large left varicocele and small (grade 1) right varicocele and noted significant greater improvements in motile sperm concentrations in those with bilateral repair. Fujisawa et al. and Libman et al. observed significantly greater improvements in concentration and/or motility after bilateral surgical repair.[49,50] Furthermore, Libman et al. and Baazeem et al.[51] noted significantly higher spontaneous pregnancy rates in those with bilateral repair compared to unilateral repair. This evidence would support the notion that subfertility in men with abnormal semen analyses and bilateral palpable varicoceles is the result of an additive effect of both and would justify simultaneous repair, even if small.

Additional studies have examined impact of unilateral or bilateral repair of a clinical varicocele in the presence of a subclinical varicocele with conflicting results. However, grade of varicocele should not dictate treatment. Therefore, in these cases, bilateral repair is likely warranted.

There has been a lot of debate regarding relationship between varicocele and *azoospermia*. Historically, varicocele repair has been a primary treatment strategy of male infertility with the goal of improving spontaneous pregnancy rates. Severe *oligozoospermia* and nonobstructive *azoospermia* are both conditions that significantly reduce a couple's chances at spontaneous pregnancy. Early reports of varicocele repair demonstrate the potential, in some, to induce spermatogenesis and regain the potential for otherwise unassisted fertility. Additionally, the introduction of in vitro fertilization (IVF) and intracytoplasmic sperm injection (ICSI) has allowed for further research on the role of varicocele repair as an adjunct to ART. The presence of varicocele in an azoospermic patient may be causative or coexistent with primary testicular failure and this has led to a disparate management protocol especially with regards to surgical intervention.

It is important to understand the etiology of azoospermia and impaired histology in a patient with clinical varicocele. A small flabby testes with Maturation arrest or Sertoli cell only histology and azoospermia may represent a coexistent pathology or irreversible state and may not benefit from repair of varicocele.

These patients may not show significant benefit even to become candidates for sperm retrieval (TESE) followed by ICSI. Approximately 4–13% of men with a palpable varicocele will present with azoospermia or severe oligoasthenozoospermia. Matthews et al.[52] first published a study looking specifically at this population of men. The authors prospectively evaluated patients after microsurgical varicocelectomy and followed for improvements in semen parameters as well as pregnancies. The majority of the cohort was observed to have return of motile sperm to the ejaculate postoperatively, 55% (12/22) of azoospermic men and 69% (35/51) of those with severe oligoasthenospermia. Mean total motile sperm count increased from $0.08 \pm 0.02 \times 10^6$ to $7.2 \pm 2.3 \times 10^6$ illustrating the potential for men to conceive a subsequent spontaneous pregnancy. Twenty-four (31%) conceived pregnancies, fifteen of which were unassisted. Additionally, testicular atrophy on initial examination had no prognostic value. A subsequent study by Kim et al. noted return of motile sperm as well, but no spontaneous pregnancies.[53]

Varicocele repair led to spermatogenesis and presence of motile sperm in ejaculate of 33% azoospermic men in one study. Fifty-five percent of these men became progressively azoospermic within 1 year of the repair. The study design has been questioned due to lack of a control arm. In another study, 9.6% of men who underwent surgery had sperms which could be used for ICSI.

It is suggested that surgery maybe attempted in azoospermic men with normal-sized testes and large clinical varicoceles though results from different studies has been variable.

Based on the studies by Kim et al., Kadioglu et al., Esteves et al., and Lee et al., those with hypospermatogenesis and maturation arrest at later stages are more likely to see return of motile sperm and pregnancies postoperatively.[54-56]

Pasqualotto et al. and Lee et al. showed that patients are at risk for relapse to azoospermia in the follow-up period and recommend cryopreservation of postoperative samples containing motile sperm.

Pasqualotto et al.[57] reviewed the records of 15 azoospermic men who underwent testicular biopsy and microsurgical varicocelectomy for azoospermia. Forty-seven percent (7/15) men had return of sperm in their ejaculate following surgery with one establishing a spontaneous pregnancy. They noted that even a preoperative biopsy showing germ cell aplasia was not a contraindication to surgery. However, the benefit was not sustained, with five of the seven relapsing to azoospermia after 6 months.

In another retrospective review, Schelegel and Kaufmann reported return of sperm to the ejaculate of 22% of 31 men who underwent microsurgical varicocelectomy.[58] However, only three had adequate motile sperm in the ejaculate for ICSI, while the rest still required testicular sperm extraction (TESE). The authors concluded that such men rarely have adequate sperm in the ejaculate after varicocele repair and most still need TESE. Cakan and Altug reported 13 infertile patients who had complete azoospermia and clinical varicocele, and underwent inguinal varicocele repair. Induction of spermatogenesis was achieved in 3 (23%) patients.[59] None could father a child spontaneously; nor did their sperm result in a successful ICSI. Matthews et al. obtained motile sperm in the semen of 12 out of 22 azoospermic men following varicocele repair; there were three pregnancies (two unassisted and one following ICSI using ejaculated sperm). Only patients whose testicular biopsies showed hypospermatogenesis had motile sperm after surgery. This role of testicular biopsy in nonobstructive azoospermic men has been reaffirmed in a meta-analysis by Elzanaty.[60]

The role of varicocelectomy in *nonobstructive azoospermia* is unresolved. There are no well-defined predictors of success in this group of patients and while surgery may result in spontaneous conception, this eventuality is rare. Careful case selection (large varicocele, reasonable-sized testes and absence of other causes of infertility) with adequate preoperative counseling is mandatory before considering this option.

The management of children or *adolescents* with varicocele has remained a contentious issue.[61-67]

Current AUA guidelines recommend a conservative, nonsurgical approach for an adolescent with varicocele, as early intervention has not shown to be of any benefit.

The recommendations for early repair of varicoceles in children and adolescents have been listed as follows:

- Varicocele with a significantly small ipsilateral testis
- Additional testicular conditions affecting fertility
- Bilateral palpable varicoceles
- Pathological sperm quality (older adolescents)
- Supranormal response to GnRH stimulation test
- Symptomatic varicocele.

It is AUA best practice policy to follow adolescents annually with testicular volume estimation and semen analysis (when possible).

Infertile men with varicoceles have benefitted significantly by the use of *ART* methods to enable them to father children. Varicocele repair has been postulated to downstage and improve the results of ART. Cayan et al.[68] evaluated a cohort of 540 infertile men with clinical varicocele who underwent microsurgical varicocelectomy. The total motile sperm counts were evaluated for each patient preoperatively and postoperatively and the patients were divided into four groups according to the type of assisted reproductive technology for which they qualified: 0–1.5 million, ICSI; 1.5–5 million, IVF; 5–20 million, intrauterine insemination (IUI); 20 million or greater, possibility of spontaneous pregnancy. These men were followed > 1 year postoperatively for alterations in semen quality and conception. An overall spontaneous pregnancy rate of 36.6% was achieved after varicocelectomy with a mean time to conception of 7 months. Another 31% who preoperatively were assessed as suitable for IVF or ICSI improved enough to become candidates for IUI, while 42% of the IUI candidates gained the potential for spontaneous pregnancy.

Surgery may also help improve the results of assisted reproduction techniques. In a study of 58 patients with a varicocele, patients undergoing varicocelectomy prior to IUI had higher pregnancy rates than those who did not. The authors also noted that while there was no significant improvement in the semen parameters in the two groups, the improved pregnancy rate may be an indicator of improved sperm function, a parameter not evaluated on routine semen analysis.

Marmar et al. initially reported IUI as a possible treatment option for men with history of a varicocele and refractory infertility. Of the 71 couples who underwent 187 inseminations, only 6 achieved a pregnancy. Pregnancy rates were observed to be much higher in a subsequent analysis by Daitch et al. who studied whether varicocele repair improved chance of success with IUI. They studied 58 couples with varicocele-associated infertility, 34 who previously underwent inguinal or subinguinal microsurgical repair and 24 who chose not to undergo repair. Pregnancy rates per cycle were noted to be 6.3% in the untreated group compared to 11.8% in those who underwent surgical repair ($p = 0.04$). Odds of pregnancy were 4.4-fold higher in the surgically treated group favoring varicocelectomy as a strategy to improve chances of pregnancy with assisted means.[69,70]

Several studies have examined effect of varicocele repair on various semen analysis parameters in attempts to correlate varicocelectomy with improved fertility. Unfortunately, these endpoint measurements are limited and more functional endpoint measurements are difficult to assess.

A study by Ashkenazi et al.[71] utilized patients who previously failed to achieve pregnancy following IVF/ICSI, and attempted to attribute subsequent pregnancy success with IVF/ICSI following varicocele repair to the corrective surgery itself. However, it is impossible to attribute this success to the repair procedure and potential improved sperm quality without a more well-controlled study design. Additionally, other studies indicate varicocele repair has no impact on rates of pregnancy following IVF/ICSI, though it may decrease their pursuit of additional ART procedures. Whether this is attributed to improved fertility or simply due to cost, ethical concerns related to ART, or other factors is unknown.[72]

Three cost analyses have been published that both favor varicocele repair as a more cost-effective strategy. Schlegel et al. and Meng et al. reported decision analyses that favor varicocele repair over ART.[73,74] Schlegel estimated cost per live delivery after varicocelectomy and after ICSI to be $26, 268 and $89,091, respectively. However, a subsequent analysis including only men with nonobstructive azoospermia who would require microsurgical TESE favored microTESE as the more cost-effective strategy to varicocelectomy in this subpopulation.[75]

DISCUSSION

The Male Infertility Best Practice Policy Committee of the American Urological Society recommends that varicocele treatment should be offered to the male partner of a couple attempting to conceive when all of the following are present:

- A varicocele is palpable.
- The couple has documented infertility.

- The female has normal fertility or potentially correctable infertility.
- The male partner has one or more abnormal semen parameters or sperm function test results.

In addition, adult men who have a palpable varicocele and abnormal semen analyses findings but are not currently attempting to conceive should also be offered varicocele repair. The indications for repairing varicoceles in adolescents include the presence of significant testicular asymmetry (> 20%) demonstrated on serial examinations, testicular pain, and abnormal semen analysis results. Young men with varicoceles but normal ipsilateral testicular volume should be offered follow-up monitoring with annual objective measurements of testicular volume, semen analyses, or both.

Contrary to the opinion offered by the Cochrane Database review, a cost-analysis study by Schlegel showed the significant cost advantage of varicocele repair over ICSI. In addition, varicocele repair had the potential for improving the male factor, rather than using unknown sperm. ICSI also involves intervention in the female partner in the form of controlled ovarian hyperstimulation and surgical egg retrieval which carries some risks.

Cayan et al.[76] specifically evaluated rates of postoperative complications and spontaneous pregnancies and excluded studies involving subclinical varicoceles. After pooling the data from 4,473 men undergoing repair by various techniques, pregnancy rates were compared and significant differences were noted depending on the technique. The highest rates were seen with the microsurgical technique, followed by nonmicrosurgical approaches. This method was also noted to have the least documented recurrences, postoperative hydroceles, or other complications. Agarwal et al. conducted a meta-analysis that included both randomized controlled trials and observational studies in attempts to evaluate the data with more focused attention on men with documented infertility, abnormal semen analysis, and clinical varicoceles. While accepting their study was subject to bias from the variability of semen data in sequential analyses, the authors highlight the significant number of data that document a direct positive relationship between improvements in semen parameters over time and varicocele repair. Agarwal et al. illustrate significant improvements in concentration, motility and morphology in studies evaluating high ligation and microsurgery.[77,78]

CONCLUSION

How to treat an infertile male with varicocele is one of the most debated issues in the field of male infertility, specifically with regard to surgical intervention. It is agreed that the surgical repair of varicocele should include a very small group of infertile men. There are no fixed guidelines for selecting the candidates fit for surgery.

Varicoceles are relatively common in the adult male population in general and the infertile male population in particular. In many, but not all, of these infertile men it is can be the cause of their infertility. However, it is important to exercise restraint and clinical judgment before advocating surgery for these patients. Consensus guidelines advocate surgery only for infertile men with clinically obvious varicoceles and persistent seminal abnormalities. About 60% of the operated men will show good improvement in semen parameters. Surgery should also be recommended in adolescent boys with ipsilateral testicular atrophy so as to preserve future fertility. Among the various modes of therapy, microsurgical ligation is the gold standard and should be the procedure of choice. Since success is not guaranteed, and there are no clear predictors of success, it is important to counsel patients about possibility of no benefit after surgery, and discuss the alternative option of assisted reproductive techniques.

Varicocele repair is a reasonable consideration as the primary treatment option when a couple with documented infertility involves a male with a palpable varicocele and suboptimal semen quality and female partner has a normal evaluation. Bilateral repair is warranted when varicoceles are noted on both sides, regardless of grade. However, approach to varicocele treatment should be based on the physician's experience and the additional options available. Assisted reproductive technologies may serve as a viable adjunct or alternative to surgery to improve chances of pregnancy. With improvements in ART laboratory technology, future research efforts are warranted to delineate the benefit of varicocele repair in patients who will require subsequent IVF/ICSI.

Certain additional factors that must be considered before deciding the therapeutic approach of varicocele in infertile couples include:

- The advanced age of the wife (older than 35 years) and high serum FSH levels should drive the decision toward the ICSI solution rather than repair of varicocele.
- In case of chronic presence of varicocele and advanced male age, surgery should be avoided.
- Surgical repair of varicocele is recommended in case of secondary male infertility. On the other hand, if the patient has primary infertility, azoospermia, small testicular size, and high serum FSH levels, the presence of varicocele should be ignored and surgery should be avoided as it indicates a primary testicular failure.

- The diagnosis of Sertoli cell only or early maturation arrest denotes primary testicular failure. Thus, the presence of varicocele should be ignored. On the contrary, the presence of mild or moderate hypospermatogenesis can be attributed to varicocele in which case surgery can be a reasonable therapeutic approach.

REFERENCES

1. World Health Organisation. The influence of varicocele on parameters of fertility in a large group of men presenting to infertility clinics. Fertil Steril. 1992;57:1289-93.
2. World Health Organisation. Laboratory Manual for the Examination of Human Semen and Sperm–Cervical Mucus Interaction, 4th edition. New York: Cambridge University Press; 1999.
3. Greenberg SH. Varicocele and male infertility. Fertil Steril. 1977;28:699-706.
4. Esteves SC, Miyaoka R, Agarwal A. An update on the clinical assessment of the infertile male. Clinics. 2011;66(4):691-700.
5. Baker HW. Male infertility. Endocrinol Metab Clin North Am. 1994;23:783-93.
6. Saypol DC. Varicocele. J Androl. 1981;2:61.
7. Tulloch WS. Varicocele in subfertility: result of treatment. BMJ. 1955; 4935: 356-8
8. Gorelick JI, Goldstein M. Loss of fertility in men with varicocele. Fertil Steril. 1993;59(3):613–6
9. Mallidis C, Howard EJ, Baker HW. Variation of semen quality in normal men. Int J Androl. 1991;14:99-107.
10. Smith KD, Rodriguez-Rigau LJ, Steinberger E. Relation between indices of semen analysis and pregnancy rate in infertile couples. Fertil Steril. 1977;28:1314-9.
11. Krause W, Muller HH, Schafer H, et al. Does treatment of varicocele improve male fertility? Results of the "Deutsche Varikozelenstudie", a multicentre study of 14 collaborating centres. Andrologia. 2002;34:164-71.
12. Samplaski MK, Yu C, Kattan MW, et al. Nomograms for predicting changes in semen parameters in infertile men after varicocele repair. Fertil Steril. 2014;102(1):68-74.
13. Male Infertility Best Practice Policy Committee of the American Urological Association; Practice Committee of the American Society for Reproductive Medicine. Report on varicocele and infertility. Fertil Steril. 2004;82(Suppl 1): S142-5.
14. Stahl P, Schlegel PN. Standardization and documentation of variccocele evaluation. Curr Opin Urol. 2011;21(6):500-55.
15. Dubin L, Amelar RD. Varicocele size and results of varicocelectomy in selected subfertile men with varicocele. Fertil Steril. 1970;21:606-9.
16. Sarteschi LM. Lo studio del varicocele con eco-Doppler. G Ital Ultrasonologia. 1993;4:43-9.
17. Sharma RK, Agarwal A. Role of reactive oxygen species in male infertility. Urology. 1996;48:835-50.
18. Holland MK, Alvarez JG, Storey BT. Production of superoxide and activity of superoxide dismutase in rabbit epididymal spermatozoa. Biol Reprod. 1982; 27:1109-18.
19. de Lamirande E, Gagnon C. Impact of reactive oxygen species on spermatozoa: a balancing act between beneficial and detrimental effects. Hum Reprod. 1995;10:15-21.
20. Aitken RJ. The Amoroso lecture. The human spermatozoon—a cell in crisis? J Reprod Fertil. 1999;115:1-7.
21. Zini A, de Lamirande E, Gagnon C. Reactive oxygen species in semen of infertile patients: levels of superoxide dismutaseand catalase-like activities in seminal plasma and spermatozoa. Int J Androl. 1993;16:183-8.
22. Allamaneni SS, Agarwal A, Nallella KP, et al. Characterization of oxidative stress status by evaluation of reactive oxygen species levels in whole semen and isolated spermatozoa. Fertil Steril. 2005;83:800-3.
23. Ozdamar AS, Soylu AG, Culha M, et al. Testicular oxidative stress. Effects of experimental varicocele in adolescent rats. Urol Int. 2004;73:343-7.
24. Hendin BN, Kolettis PN, Sharma RK, et al. Varicocele is associated with elevated spermatozoal reactive oxygen species production and diminished seminal plasma antioxidant capacity. J Urol. 1999;161:1831-4.
25. Saleh RA, Agarwal A, Sharma RK, et al. Evaluation of nuclear DNA damage in spermatozoa from infertile men with varicocele. Fertil Steril. 2003;80:1431-6.
26. Mostafa T, Anis TH, El-Nashar A, et al. Varicocelectomy reduces reactive oxygen species levels and increases antioxidant activity of seminal plasma from infertile men with varicocele. Int J Androl. 2001;24:261-5.
27. Cam K, Simsek F, Yuksel M, et al. The role of reactive oxygen species and apoptosis in the pathogenesis of varicocele in a rat model and efficiency of vitamin E treatment. Int J Androl. 2004;27:228-33.
28. Barqawi A, Caruso A, Meacham RB. Experimental varicocele induces testicular germ cell apoptosis in the rat. J Urol. 2004;171:501-3.
29. Onur R, Semercioz A, Orhan I, et al. The effects of melatonin and the antioxidant defence system on apoptosis regulator proteins (Bax and Bcl-2) in experimentally induced varicocele. Urol Res. 2004;32:204-8.
30. Trigo RV, Bergada I, Rey R, et al. Altered serum profile of inhibin B, Pro-alphaC and anti-Mullerian hormone in prepubertal and pubertal boys with varicocele. Clin Endocrinol (Oxf). 2004;60:758-64.
31. Dubin L, Amelar RD. Varicocelectomy: 986 cases in a twelve year study. Urology. 1977;10:446-8.
32. Jarow JP, Ogle SR, Eskew LA. Seminal improvement following repair of ultrasound detected subclinical varicoceles. J Urol. 1996;155:1287-90.
33. Marsman JW, Schats R. The subclinical varicocele debate. Hum Reprod. 1994;9:1-8.
34. Yamamoto M, Hibi H, Hirata Y, et al. Effect of varicocelectomy on sperm parameters and pregnancy rate in patients with subclinical varicocele: a randomized prospective controlled study. J Urol. 1996;155:1636-8.
35. Unal D, Yeni E, Verit A, et al. Clomiphene citrate versus varicocelectomy in treatment of subclinical varicocele: a prospective randomized study. Int J Urol. 2001;8:227-30.
36. Nieschlag E, Hertle L, Fischedick A, et al. Update on treatment of varicocele: counselling as effective as occlusion of the vena spermatica. Hum Reprod. 1998;13(8):2147-50.

37. Nieschlag E, Hertle L, Fischedick A, et al. Update on treatment of varicocele: counselling as effective as occlusion of the vena spermatica. Hum Reprod. 1998;13:2147-50.
38. Evers JL, Collins JA, Vandekerckhove P. Surgery or embolisation for varicocele in subfertile men. Cochrane Database Syst Rev. 2001;(1):CD000479.
39. Evers JL, Collins JA. Assessment of efficacy of varicocele repair for male subfertility: a systematic review. Lancet. 2003;361(9372):1849-52.
40. Evers JL, Collins JA. Surgery or embolisation for varicocele in subfertile men. Cochrane Database Syst Rev. 2004;(3):CD000479.

40a. Kroese AC, de Lange NM, Evers JL, et al. Surgery or embolisation for varicocele in subfertile men. Cochrane Database Syst Rev. 2012;10:CD000479.

41. Madgar I, Weissenberg R, Lunenfeld B, et al. Controlled trial of high spermatic vein ligation for varicocele in infertile men. Fertil Steril. 1995;63(1):120–4
42. Ficarra V, Cerruto MA, Liguori G, et al. Treatment of varicocele in subfertile men: the Cochrane Review—a contrary opinion. Eur Urol. 2006;49(2):258-63.
43. Ficarra V, Crestani A, Novara G, et al. varicocele repair for infertility: what is the evidence? Eur Urol. 2011;60(4):795-808.
44. Marmar JL, Kim Y. Subinguinal microsurgical varicocelectomy: a technical critique and statistical analysis of semen and pregnancy data. J Urol. 1994; 152:1127-32.
45. Zheng YQ, Gao X, Li ZJ, et al. Efficacy of bilateral and left varicocelectomy in infertile men with left clinical and right subclinical varicoceles: a comparative study. J Urol. 2009;73(6):1236-40.
46. Elbendary MA, Elbadry AM. Right subclinical varicocele: how to manage in infertile patients with clinical left varicocele? Fertil Steril. 2009;92(6):2050-53.
47. Kondoh N, Koh E, Matsui T, et al. Improvement of semen characteristics after surgical repair of bilateral testicular varicocele as compared to unilateral varicocele patients. Arch Androl. 1990;24(1):61-7.
48. Scherr D, Goldstein M. Comparison of bilateral versus unilateral varicocelectomy in men with palpable bilateral varicoceles. J Urol. 1999;162(1):85-8.
49. Fujisawa M, Ishikawa T, Takenaka A. The efficacy of bilateral varicocelectomy in patients with palpable bilateral varicoceles: comparative study with unilateral varicocele. Urol Res. 2003;31(6):407-9.
50. Libman J, Jarvi K, Lo K, et al. Beneficial effect of microsurgical varicocelectomy is superior for men with bilateral versus unilateral repair. J Urol. 2006;176 (6 Pt 1):2602-5.
51. Baazeem A, Boman JM, Libman J, et al. Microsurgical varicocelectomy for infertile men with oligospermia: differential effect of bilateral and unilateral varicocele on pregnancy outcomes. BJU Int. 2009;104(4):524-8.
52. Matthews GJ, Matthews ED, Goldstein M. Induction of spermatogenesis and achievement of pregnancy after microsurgical varicocelectomy in men with azoospermia and severe oligoasthenospermia. Fertil Steril. 1998;70(1):71-5.
53. Kim KH, Lee JY, Kang DH, et al. Impact of surgical varicocele repair on pregnancy rate in subfertile men with clinical varicocele and impaired semen quality: a meta-analysis of randomized clinical trials. Korean J Urol. 2013;54(10):703-9.
54. Kadioglu A, Tefekli A, Cayan S, et al. Microsurgical inguinal varicocele repair in azoospermic men. Urology. 2001;57(2):328-33.
55. Esteves SC, Glina S. Recovery of spermatogenesis after microsurgical subinguinal varicocele repair in azoospermic men based on testicular histology. Int Braz J Urol. 2005;31(6):541-8.
56. Lee JS, Park HJ, Seo JT. What is the indication of varicocelectomy in men with nonobstructive azoospermia? Urology. 2007;69(2):352-5.
57. Pasqualotto FF, Sobreiro BP, Hallak J, et al. Induction of spermatogenesis in azoospermic men after varicocelectomy repair: an update. Fertil Steril. 2006; 85(3):635-9.
58. Schlegel PN, Kaufmann J. Role of varicocelectomy in men with nonobstructive azoospermia. Fertil Steril. 2004;81(6):1585-8.
59. Cakan M, Bakirtas H, Aldemir M, et al. Results of varicocelectomy in patients with isolated teratozoospermia. Urol Int. 2008;80(2):172-6.
60. Elzanaty S. Varicocele repair in non-obstructive azoospermic men: diagnostic value of testicular biopsy—a meta-analysis. Scan J Urol. 2014;8:1-5.
61. Cayan S, Akbay E, Bozlu M, et al. The effect of varicocele repair on testicular volume in children and adolescents with varicocele. J Urol. 2002;168:731-4.
62. Thomas JC, Elder JS. Testicular growth arrest and adolescent varicocele: does varicocele size make a difference? J Urol. 2002;168:1689-91.
63. Lund L, Tang YC, Roebuck D, et al. Testicular catch-up growth after varicocele correction in adolescents. Pediatr Surg Int. 1999;15:234-7.
64. Rivilla F, Casillas JG. Testicular size following embolization therapy for paediatric left varicocele. Scand J Urol Nephrol. 1997;31:63-5.
65. Haddad NG, Houk CP, Lee PA. varicocele: a dilemma in adolescent males. Pediatr Endocrinol Rev. 2014;11(Suppl 2):274-83.
66. Pinto KJ, Kroovand RL, Jarow JP. Varicocele related testicular atrophy and its predictive effect upon fertility. J Urol. 1994;152:788-90.
67. Ku JH, Son H, Kwak C, et al. Impact of varicocele on testicular volume in young men: significance of compensatory hypertrophy of contralateral testis. J Urol. 2002;168:1541-4.
68. Cayan S, Shavakhabov S, Kadio lu A. Treatment of palpable varicocele in infertile men: a meta-analysis to define the best technique. J Androl. 2009;30(1):33-40.
69. Marmar JL, Agarwal A, Prabakaran S, et al. Reassessing the value of varicocelectomy as a treatment for male subfertility with a new meta-analysis. Fertil Steril. 2007;88(3):639-48.
70. Daitch JA, Bedaiwy MA, Pasqualotto EB, et al. Varicocelectomy improves intrauterine insemination success rates in men with varicocele. J Urol. 2001;165(5): 1510-13.
71. Ashkenazi J, Dicker D, Feldberg D, et al. The impact of spermatic vein ligation on the male factor in in vitro fertilization-embryo transfer and its relation to testosterone levels before and after operation. Fertil Steril. 1989;51(3):471-4.
72. Evers JH, Collins J, Clarke J. Surgery or embolisation for varicocele in subfertile men. Cochrane Database Syst Rev. 2009;(1):CD000479.

73. Schlegel P. Is assisted reproduction the optimal treatment for varicoceleassociated male infertility? A cost effective analysis. Urology. 1997;49(1):83-90.
74. Meng MV, Greene KL, Turek PJ. Surgery or assisted reproduction? A decision analysis of treatment costs in male infertility. J Urol. 2005;174(5):1926-31.
75. Lee R, Li PS, Goldstein M, et al. A decision analysis of treatments for nonobstructive azoospermia associated with varicocele. Fertil Steril. 2009;92(1):188-96.
76. Cayan S, Erdemir F, Ozbey I, et al. Can varicocelectomy significantly change the way couples use assisted reproductive technologies? J Urol. 2002;167(4):1749-52.
77. Gabriele R, Conte M, Egidi F, et al. Results of surgical treatment of varicocele in male infertility. Curr Opin Urol. 2012;22(6):489-94.
78. Agarwal A, Deepinder F, Cocuzza M, et al. Efficacy of varicocelectomy in improving semen parameters: new meta-analytical approach. Urology. 2007; 70(3):532-8.

CHAPTER

18

Evaluation and Management of Azoospermia

Carlos Balmori

DEFINITION, DIAGNOSIS, AND EPIDEMIOLOGY

Azoospermia is defined as the complete absence of sperm in the ejaculate. The presence of even a small number of spermatozoa is defined as cryptozoospermia. Aspermia is distinct from azoospermia and is defined by the complete absence of seminal fluid emission at time of orgasm.

The diagnosis of azoospermia must be confirmed by centrifugation of the semen specimen at 3,000 g for 15 minutes at room temperature and a high-powered microscopic examination of the pellet. The presence of any mature sperm in the semen excludes the possibility of complete absence of spermatogenesis.

The semen analysis should be performed according to the 2010 World Health Organization guidelines, and at least two semen samples obtained > 2 weeks apart should be examined.[1] Azoospermia is found in approximately 1% of all men and 10–15% of infertile males.[2]

ETIOLOGICAL CLASSIFICATION

Traditionally azoospermia is classified into obstructive azoospermia (OA) and *nonobstructive* azoospermia (NOA).[3] In obstructive cases spermatogenesis is normal but there is obstruction in the seminal ducts, while in nonobstructive cases there is deficient, or absent spermatogenesis. Obstructive azoospermia and nonobstructive azoospermia can be further divided into congenital, acquired, or iatrogenic according to their etiology (Table 1). Azoospermia due to ejaculatory duct dysfunction and hypogonadotrophism are rare, accounting for about 2% of azoospermia.[4]

Table 1: Etiology of OA and NOA.

	Type of azoospermia	
Etiology	*Obstructive azoospermia (OA)*	*Nonobstructive azoospermia (NOA)*
Congenital	• Congenital bilateral absence of the vas deferens (CBAVD) • Young syndrome • Prostatic cysts (Müllerian cysts) • Idiopathic epididymal obstruction	• Cryptorchidism • Sertoli only syndrome • Steiner's syndrome • Reifenstein's syndrome • Kallmann's syndrome • Noonan syndrome • Klinefelter's syndrome • Prader-Willi's syndrome • Y-chromosome microdeletions • Androgen insensitivity syndrome • Meiotic and meiosis abnormalities during spermatogenesis
Acquired	• Vasectomy • Prostatitis, epididymitis • Testicular trauma	• Orchitis • Testicular neoplasm • Testicular injury (trauma, torsion) • Pituitary tumor • Varicocele
Iatrogenic	• Postsurgical (hernia, scrotum)	• Radiation • Medication (cytotoxic, antiandrogens, cimetidine, ketoconazole, spironolactone, testosterone) • Postsurgical (bladder neck, retroperitoneal)

Another clinical classification[5] is *pretesticular* (due to deficient hormonal stimulation of the testis), *testicular* (due to testicular dysfunction), and *post-testicular* (due to seminal ductal obstruction or dysfunction) (Table 2).

Table 2: Classification of azoospermia based upon the area problem.

Area problem	*Etiology*	
Pretesticular	Hypogonadotrophic hypogonadism	• Idiopathic • Kallmann's syndrome • Pituitary tumors
Testicular	• Idiopathic • Cryptorchidism • Cytotoxic therapy • Irradiation • Testicular neoplasm • Systemic illness (Cirrhosis, renal failure) • Viral or inflammatory orchitis • Drugs • Vascular injury • Varicocele • Testicular torsion • Genetic disorders • Y-chromosome microdeletions	
Post-testicular	Seminal ducts obstruction	• Vasectomy • Postsurgical (hernia, scrotum) • Postinfective (epididymitis, orchitis, prostatitis) • Congenital bilateral absence of the vas deferens (CBAVD) • Idiopathic epididymal obstruction • Prostatic cysts (Müllerian cysts) • Young's syndrome
	Ejaculatory ducts dysfunction	• Retrograde ejaculation • Anejaculation • Spinal cord injury • Neurological illness • Diabetes mellitus • Erectile dysfunction • Postsurgery (retroperitoneal lymphadenectomy, bladder neck)

Whereas the pretesticular and post-testicular causes of azoospermia frequently are correctable, the testicular causes of azoospermia are not.

EVALUATION OF AZOOSPERMIC PATIENTS

Aims

- To determinate the cause and any treatment options that may be effective.
- To recognize that azoospermia may be the initial manifestation of a severe medical condition.
- To estimate the probability of recovering sperm in patients with NOA.
- To assess the risks of genetic abnormalities in these males.

Clinical Assessment

The initial evaluation of the azoospermic male patient should be rapid, noninvasive, and cost-effective. A great number of conditions causing azoospermia in men can be diagnosed by history, physical examination, semen analysis, and hormonal and genetic tests. Further evaluation can then be done as necessary. A rational approach is necessary to perform the appropriate workup and to choose the best treatment options for the couple.

History

A detailed history must include information about not only medical and surgical problems, but also developmental issues, occupational and social habits, and exposures.

- *Childhood illnesses*: This includes questions related to cryptorchidism, mumps, hypospadias, gynecomastia, herniorrhaphy or scrotal surgery, and the onset of pubertal changes. Precocious or delayed puberty may be the sign of a serious underlying endocrinologic disorder. Hormonally active tumors from the testicle, adrenal gland, or pituitary, along with adrenal hyperplasia, primary testicular insufficiency, or end-organ androgen insensitivity, may alter the onset of puberty. Testicular torsion and trauma may result in testicular atrophy and the production of antisperm antibodies.
- *Adult illnesses*: A history of anosmia in combination with azoospermia or severe oligospermia and low gonadotropins suggests Kallmann's syndrome. Bronchiectasis, sinusitis, and OA can be observed in Young's syndrome or cystic fibrosis. Smallpox, postpubertal mumps, prostatitis, orchitis, seminal vesiculitis, and urethritis may lead to azoospermia. Liver and renal diseases lead to hypogonadism and feminization because of primary testicular failure and increased estrogen levels. Obesity causes an increased peripheral conversion of testosterone to estrogen and decreased LH pulse amplitude. Ejaculatory dysfunction may be secondary to diabetes mellitus. Patients should be questioned about recent fevers and systemic illness, because spermatogenesis may be adversely affected for 2–3 months, and semen analysis must be repeated at timely intervals up to 6 months after such episodes. Spinal cord injury can cause infertility through epididymal, testicular, prostatic, seminal vesicular, or ejaculatory dysfunction.

- *Medical or surgical treatments*: Many therapeutic drugs are associated with decreased sperm production and sperm quality: anabolic steroids, Dilantin, manganese, colchicine, methadone, methotrexate, phenytoin, Thioridazine, calcium channel blockers, spironolactone, cyproterone, ketoconazole, cimetidine, tetracycline, nitrofurantoin, valproic acid, or sulfasalazine. History of cancer and related chemotherapy or radiation must be sought, not only for the potential effects on spermatogenesis, but also for determination of a time interval after which retrieved sperm can be safely used after such therapies.
- *Sexual history*: Anejaculation may masquerade as azoospermia when the man collects urethral secretions or urine in lieu of semen.
- *Environmental or occupational assaults*: Overexposure to these assaults can cause azoospermia, either by direct suppression of sperm production or by affecting hormone secretion. Some chemicals that affect sperm production are as follows: free oxygen radicals, pesticidal chemicals (DDT, aldrin, dieldrin, PCPs, dioxins, and furans) with estrogen-like effects, plastic softening chemical like phthalates, and hydrocarbons (ethylbenzene, benzene, toluene, and xylene). Chronic exposure to heavy metals such as lead, cadmium, or arsenic may affect the hypothalamic pituitary axis and cause azoospermia in otherwise healthy men.
- *Social habits and exposures*: Emotional stress or excessive heat exposure may cause a temporary decrease in sperm production but rarely azoospermia. The same applies to tobacco and alcohol. The relationship of tobacco with sperm concentration is shown in several studies.[6] Meanwhile, it seems to be difficult to relate alcohol consumption with an impairment of sperm counts as a single factor.[7]

Physical Examination

Signs of endocrinopathy or genetic alterations as a cause of azoospermia should be sought. The amount and distribution of body hair, including beard growth, axillary hair, and pubic hair should be noted. The ethnic origin of the patient should be considered in this assessment. Any decrease in body hair or decrease in beard growth should also be noted. The presence and degree of gynecomastia should be recorded. The presence of galactorrhea would suggest pronounced hyperprolactinemia, usually associated with some degree of hyperestrogenism.[8] Eunuchoid stature, subvirilization, and disproportionately long extremities can be associated with genetic disorders such as Klinefelter's syndrome (KS) characterized by testosterone deficiency.[9]

The genital examination should include palpation of the spermatic cord, the aspect and symmetry of the scrotum, and testicular mobility and consistency. Length and width of the testes, or its volume, should be measured by using calipers, a Prader orchidometer, or ultrasound. Some testicular disorders may selectively affect production of sperm without influencing production of testosterone. Because approximately 85% of testicular mass consists of germinal tissue, a reduced germinal cell mass would be associated with a reduced testicular size and a soft consistency.

Testicular consistency should be noted. If the germinal epithelium was damaged before puberty, the testes are generally small and firm. If postpubertal damage occurred, the testes are usually small and soft.

A through palpation of the epididymis—its caput, corpus, and cauda— is of importance. Epididymal enlargement, induration, and cysts are indicative of OA.

The presence of the vas deferens should be ascertained while palpating the spermatic cord. The complete absence bilaterally of the vasa is observed in men with mutations in one or both copies of the *CF* gene. Sometimes these men may have only a partial defect in the vas. Surgical scars in the inguinal or scrotal area may indicate possible injuries to the testicular blood supply and/or vas deferens.

Abnormal shapes of the penis or wrong opening of the urethral meatus are not a cause of azoospermia.

A complete physical examination of males with azoospermia must include a rectal examination to exclude ejaculatory duct obstruction. Midline prostatic cysts, such as Müllerian duct cysts, and dilated seminal vesicles can be palpated; a definite diagnosis can be confirmed by transrectal ultrasound scanning and deferentovesiculography.[10] Prostatic induration or tenderness supports a diagnosis of prostatitis.

One study has investigated whether anogenital distance (AGD) could distinguish men with OA from those with NOA. Anogenital distance is a marker for endocrine disruption in animal studies in which decreased male AGD has been associated with testicular dysfunction.[11]

Semen Analysis

Once azoospermia has been established, semen analysis can provide additional valuable information about the likely origin of azoospermia. It allows assessment of accessory glands' function, and detection of immunological, inflammatory, or infectious problems.

A low ejaculate volume indicates absence of seminal vesicular fluid. This is commonly due to absence of the seminal vesicles in association with vas aplasia, but may also occur if there is ejaculatory duct obstruction. Occasionally, this may be due to incomplete ejaculation or partial retrograde ejaculation, or severe hypogonadism resulting in failure of accessory gland secretions. Large volumes are sometimes found in association with infection of the genital tract or after long periods of sexual abstinence.

The pH is determined by acidic secretions of the prostate and alkaline secretions of the seminal vesicles. If the pH exceeds 8.0, infection should be suspected with decreased secretion of acidic products by the prostate, such as citric acid. Abnormal pH may also be recorded in cases of incomplete ejaculation. Acidic pH (< 6.5) is found in cases of agenesis or obstruction of the seminal vesicles.

The presence of agglutination is suggestive of, but not sufficient evidence to prove, the existence of an immunological factor.[12]

The biochemical analysis of semen enables us to detect disturbances for each organ involved in seminal fluid production. The fructose level for seminal vesicular function, citrate or acid phosphatase for the prostate gland, and free carnitine as an index of epididymal function.[13]

Hormonal Analysis

According to the American Urological Association (AUA) Infertility Best Practice Statement,[14] the minimum initial hormonal evaluation should consist of measurements of serum follicle-stimulating hormone (FSH) and serum testosterone levels. If the testosterone level is low, a repeat measurement of total and free testosterone (or bioavailable testosterone) as well as determination of serum luteinizing hormone (LH) and prolactin (PRL) levels should be obtained.

LH and FSH are synthesized in the pituitary gland, released into the systemic blood circulation, and carried to the target end organs—the gonads. The pituitary also secretes PRL. In the testis, LH stimulates testosterone secretion and FSH is important in the initiation and maintenance of spermatogenesis. The secreted testicular androgens—testosterone and its activated form dihydrotestosterone (DHT)—act on numerous target end organs causing the development of male secondary sexual characteristics and inhibiting the pituitary secretion of LH and FSH. Spermatogenesis is dependent on pituitary FSH and on intratesticular testosterone. FSH and androgens seem to have different preferential sites of action during spermatogenesis.

In the presence of normal spermatogenesis, FSH secretion is regulated by negative inhibition from inhibin. With primary testicular failure, inadequate Leydig and Sertoli cell functions result in elevated gonadotropin levels with normal or low testosterone levels. Hypothalamic or pituitary dysfunction resulting in inadequate levels of gonadotropins causes low peripheral levels of testosterone and an absence of spermatogenesis. Men who have selective injury to the germinal epithelium (seminiferous tubules) have elevated serum FSH, but normal LH and testosterone levels. In OA, FSH levels are normal, but normal levels do not exclude a testicular cause of azoospermia—FSH is normal in 40% of men with primary spermatogenic failure. Inhibin B seems to have a higher predictive value for normal spermatogenesis[15] (Table 3).

Table 3: Hormonal status and clinical diagnosis of azoospermia.

Clinical Status	*FSH*	*Inhibin B*	*LH*	*Testosterone*
• Normal	Normal	Normal	Normal	Normal
• Spermatogenic arrest	Normal	Normal	Normal	Normal
• Aplasia germinal	High	Low	Normal	Normal
• Hypergonadotropic hypogonadism (testicular failure)	High	Low	High	Normal or low
• Hypogonadotropic hypogonadism	Low		Low	Low

Elevated FSH levels have been associated with a low probability for the retrieval of spermatozoa in men and lower pregnancy rates in their female partners using random biopsy testicular sperm extraction (TESE) techniques. Although FSH reflects the predominant pattern of spermatogenesis, it may not reflect isolated areas of spermatogenesis within the testis. Thus, micro-TESE has been shown to be more successful in sperm retrieval than a single biopsy or multiple random biopsies.[16]

Genetic Analysis

Genetic factors explain 21–29% of azoospermia, and another 12–41% of azoospermic cases are idiopathic and most likely related to unknown genetic factors.[17] Some researchers believe that approximately 75% or more cases of infertility have a genetic basis, but our current ability to diagnose these defects remains limited.[2] A particular difficulty is the huge number of candidate genes to be studied; there are > 2,300 genes expressed in the testis alone, and hundreds of those genes influence reproductive function in humans and could contribute to male infertility.

Cytogenetic analysis of patients with azoospermia and severe oligozoospermia is mandatory before infertility treatment with assisted reproduction technologies. We must research the main genetic factors related to azoospermia: chromosomal abnormalities, cystic fibrosis gene mutations, and Y-chromosome microdeletions.

Chromosomal abnormalities can be identified by karyotype of peripheral leukocytes in approximately 7% of infertile men. The prevalence of such abnormalities relates inversely to the sperm concentration,[18] being 10–15% in azoospermic men, 5–12.8% in oligospermic men, and < 1–1.1% in patients with normozoospermia.[19,20] The most common chromosomal aberrations that are associated with severe spermatogenic defects are sex chromosome aneuploidies and chromosomal translocations. Among the various cytogenetic abnormalities, KS is the major cytogenetic/sex chromosome/numerical anomaly that is detected in infertile men.[17]

Klinefelter's syndrome is the most prevalent chromosomal disorder in humans, with an estimated frequency of 1:500 to 1:1,000 men.[21] It is also the most frequent genetic cause of azoospermia.[22] Men with KS have an extra paternal X chromosome in nearly half of all cases. In nonmosaic KS of both paternal and maternal origin, the extra X chromosome is the result of meiotic nondisjunction or possibly of premature separation of sister chromatids.[23,24]

Approximately 8% of adult men with KS have sperm present, with sperm concentrations $< 1 \times 10^6$/mL, and impairment in sperm motility and morphology.[25] In those patients with azoospermia and Sertoli cell-only pattern on pretreatment testicular histology, sperm retrieval using microdissection TESE was successful in 70% of the cases.[26] Given the potential for increased chromosomal abnormalities in the offspring of men with KS, preimplantation genetic diagnosis of embryos obtained using TESE-ICSI has been recommended.[27]

Patients with congenital bilateral absence of vas deferens (CBAVD) or unexplained OA and low-semen volume should be tested for abnormalities of the cystic fibrosis transmembrane conductance regulator *(CFTR)* gene. The *CFTR* gene is located on chromosome 7 q31.2 and has been implicated in the formation of excurrent seminal ducts.[28] Patients with congenital bilateral absence of vas deferens accounts for ~1–2% of the population of infertile, but otherwise healthy, males and up to 25% of those with OA. Imaging studies and surgical exploration generally are unnecessary for diagnosis but may help to identify other abnormalities associated with vasal agenesis. Patients with congenital bilateral absence of vas deferens, having detectable CFTR mutations in most of them, are able to father their children with help of assisted reproductive technologies, so CFTR mutations may be artificially transmitted to the offspring as a consequence. Therefore, genetic testing should be offered to these CBAVD patients before undergoing assisted reproduction, which allows for better evaluation of the genetic risk for the offspring.[29] Many mutations of the CFTR are undetectable using commercial kits and hence it should be assumed that the male is a carrier, even when testing negative, and testing should be offered to his female partner to exclude the possibility that she too may be a carrier.[19]

Yq microdeletion is another recognized cause of spermatogenic failure, causing azoospermia or severe oligozoospermia. Yq microdeletions involve loss of one or more of three discreet loci on the q arm of Y chromosome.[30]

The prevalence of Yq microdeletions is ~7.4%. In an azoospermic population, the prevalence is higher (9.7%), while in oligozoospermic men, the prevalence is 6.0%. The Yq contains three "azoospermia factor (AZF)" regions: AZFa, AZFb, and AZFc. Deletions of the complete AZFc region are most frequently detected (69%), followed by deletions of the AZFb region (14%) and deletions of the AZFa region (6%).[31] Yq microdeletions contribute only marginally to the totality of human male infertility, but when present, the use of ICSI may allow for the transmission of such mutations to the next generation. Couples should be offered this information, as they must understand that their male offspring will almost certainly be subfertile and require reproductive care.[32]

The occurrence and type of microdeletion correlates with testicular phenotype and is a good predictor of sperm retrieval during microdissection TESE. Sperm retrieval is not successful in those patients with AZFa, AZFb, AZFb+c, and complete Yq deletions; however, patients with AZFc have better prognosis, and sperm retrieval is possible.[33] Also, oligozoospermic men with microdeletions have been reported to progress to azoospermia over time, and higher incidence of poor-quality embryos has been observed in couples where the male partner has microdeletions.[34]

TREATMENT OF AZOOSPERMIA

Some men can be managed with surgical or medical treatment. In other cases, operative spermatic recovery techniques will be necessary.

Medical Management

Less than 3% of NOA men have a primary hormonal etiology[35] like hypogonadotropic hypogonadism.

Among men with NOA, gonadotropin therapy for hypogonadotropic hypogonadism is the only specific indication that has universally shown an improvement in semen analysis and pregnancy rates. Gonadotropins (hCG and rFSH in combination) are the standard therapy, while GnRH therapy is reserved for nonresponders. Avoiding the use of drugs that inhibit the hypothalamic axis, such as tranquilizers or steroids can be useful in some cases. The medical management of other forms of NOA, such as patients who have primary Leydig cell damage, remains empirical. Drug therapy with aromatase inhibitors and gonadotropins shows potential promise in improving outcomes in men requiring surgical sperm retrieval, but there is lack of level I clinical evidence for this indication.[36]

Surgical Management

Microsurgical reconstruction may be possible when OA has resulted from previous vasectomy, or epididymal obstruction. The main surgical techniques are the vasovasostomy and the vasoepididymostomy. Occasionally, transurethral resection of obstructed ejaculatory ducts can be curative. Some men with large varicoceles may have reappearance of sperm in the ejaculate after varicocelectomy.

Vasovasostomy

About 2–6% men who undergo vasectomy will desire reversal of their vasectomy at a later time.[37] Vasectomy reversal can be performed in a variety of ways. Variability exists in the size and number of sutures used as well as in the number of layers anastomosed. Microsurgical vasovasostomy, as described by Owen[38] and Silber,[39] is the gold standard with overall patency and pregnancy rates reported by the vasovasostomy Study Group of 86% and 52%, respectively.[40] While a two-layer technique has been advocated, it is often tedious and time-consuming, and no difference has been demonstrated compared to a microsurgical one-layer closure. Fibrin glue vasovasostomy is potentially less time-consuming than standard microsurgical vasovasostomy.[41]

Vasoepididymostomy

The need to perform vasoepididymostomy has been reported to be as high as 62% in patients undergoing reversal 15 or more years after vasectomy.[42] Patients with epididymal obstruction from other causes (congenital or infection) are also candidates for vasoepididymostomy. Nonmicrosurgical epididymovasostomy, based upon the creation of a fistula between several openings in the epididymal tubule and the lumen of the vas, was first described by Martin.[43] Dubin and Amelar[44] suggested the use of loupes.

Later microsurgical techniques were developed. End-to-end and end-to-side anastomoses (Schlegel and Goldstein[45]) and longitudinal and triangulation intussusception (Schiff[46]) are currently favored techniques. With epididymovasostomy restoration of patency can be achieved in 65% of cases with a 38% natural pregnancy rate.[47]

In men undergoing vasostomy or vasoepididymostomy, sperm retrieval and cryopreservation during the operation is recommended for surgical and pregnancy failure.[48]

SPERM RETRIEVAL TECHNIQUES

Unreconstructable OA and NOA have historically been relatively untreatable conditions that required the use of donor spermatozoa. ICSI has transformed treatment for this type of severe male factor infertility. Sperm retrieval with IVF/ICSI is also preferred to surgical treatment when the female partner is advanced in age or there is female infertility requiring IVF. Depending on the type of azoospermia, sperm can be retrieved either from the epididymis or the testes.

The sperm retrieval methods can be either open surgery or percutaneous acquisition. Both of them can be performed by macro- or microsurgical techniques (Table 4; Figs. 1A to C). Historical prognostic factors for sperm recovery in NOA are related to the clinical, laboratory, and surgical technique, the testicular tissue processing method in the gamete laboratory; and the histological pattern of

Table 4: Sperm retrieval techniques.

Type of surgery	*Open surgery*	*Percutaneous acquisition*
Nonmicrosurgical	• Open epididymal fine-needle aspiration • Testicular sperm extraction (TESE) • Single seminiferous tubule biopsy	• Percutaneous epididymal sperm aspiration (PESA) • Percutaneous testicular sperm aspiration (TESA) • Percutaneous testicular fine-needle aspiration (TEFNA)
Microsurgical	• Microsurgical epididymal sperm aspiration (MESA) • Microsurgical testicular sperm extraction (Micro-TESE)	

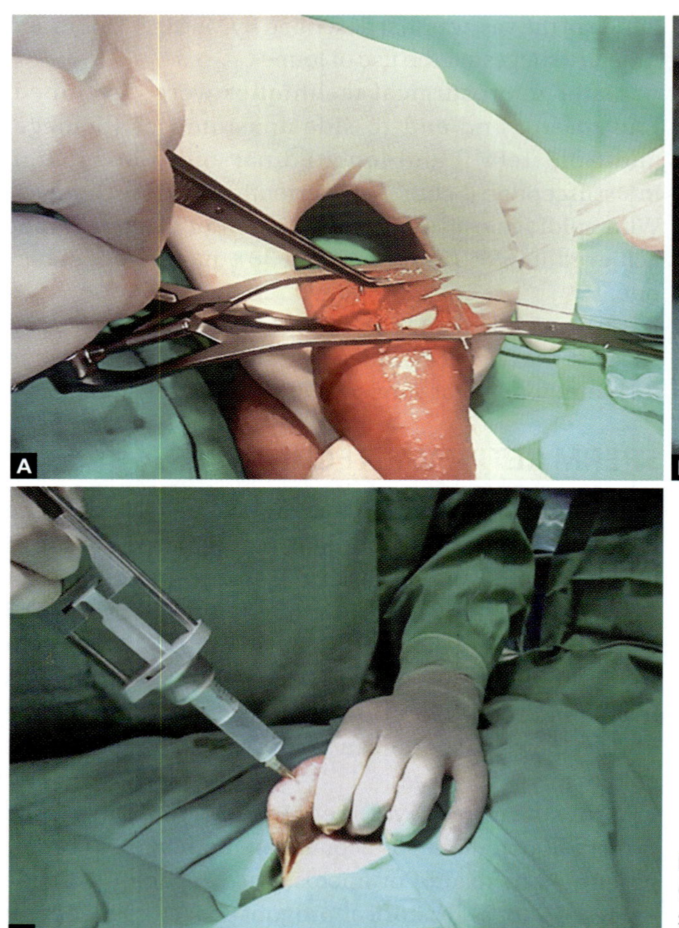

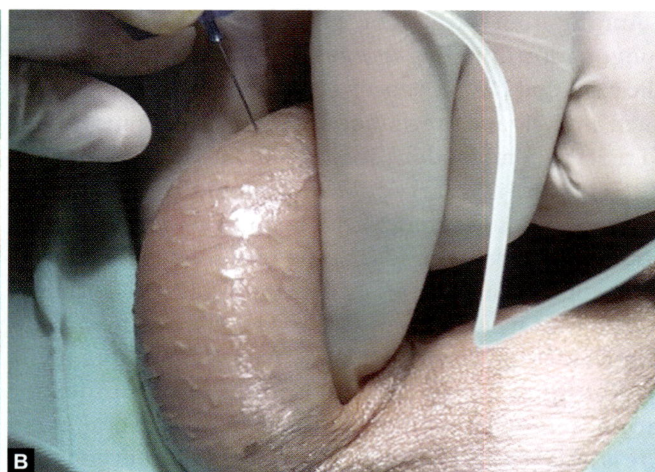

Figs. 1A to C: Nonmicrosurgical sperm retrieval techniques. (A) Testicular sperm extraction (TESE). (B) Percutaneous epididymal sperm aspiration (PESA). (C) Percutaneous testicular sperm aspiration (TESA).

the testis. Nonobstructive azoospermia remains the most challenging diagnosis for andrologists, and there are no positive prognostic factors that guarantee sperm recovery for these patients. The only reliably negative prognostic factor is the presence of AZFa and AZFb microdeletions.[49]

REFERENCES

1. WHO. WHO Laboratory Manual for the Examination and Processing of Human Semen, 5th edition. Geneva: WHO Press; 2010.
2. Cocuzza M, Alvarenga C, Pagani R. The epidemiology and etiology of azoospermia. Clinics. 2013;68(S1):15-26.
3. Ezeh UI. Beyond the clinical classification of azoospermia. Hum Reprod. 2000;15(11): 2356-9.
4. Hull MGR, Glazener CMA, Kelly NJ, et al. Population study of causes, treatment and outcome of infertility. Brit Med J. 1985;291:1693-7.
5. Sharif K. Reclassification of azoospermia: the time has come? Hum Reprod. 2000;15(2): 237-8.
6. Ramlau-Hansen C, Thulstrup AM, Aggerholm AS, et al. Is smoking a risk factor for decreased semen quality? A cross-sectional analysis. Hum Reprod. 2007;22:188-96.
7. Martini AC, Molina RI, Estofán D, et al. Effects of alcohol and cigarette consumption on human seminal quality. Fertil Steril. 2004;82:374-7.
8. Petak SM. AACE Hypogonadism Guidelines. Endocr Pract. 2002;8(6):440-56.
9. Gudeloglu A, Parekattil SJ. Update in the evaluation of the azoospermic male. Clinics. 2013;68(S1):27-34.
10. Shebel HM, Farg HM, Kolokythas O, et al. Cysts of the lower male genitourinary tract: embryologic and anatomic considerations and differential diagnosis. Radiographics. 2013;33(4):1125-43.
11. Eisenberg ML, Shy M, Walters RC, et al. The relationship between anogenital distance and azoospermia in adult men. Int J Androl. 2012;35(5):726-30.
12. Hoover P, Naz RK. Do men with prostate abnormalities (prostatitis/benign prostatic hyperplasia/prostate cancer) develop immunity to spermatozoa or seminal plasma? Int J Androl. 2012;35(4):608-15.
13. Wetterauer U. Recommended biochemical parameters for routine semen analysis. Urol Res. 1986;14(5):241-6.
14. Jarow J, Sigman M, Kolettis PN, et al. 2010. The evaluation of the azoospermic male: AUA best practice statement, reviewed and revised 2011. American Urological Association Education and Research, Inc. http://www.auanet.org/ common/pdf/

education/clinical-guidance/Male-Infertility-b.pdf.Accessed Feb.2014
15. Jungwirth A, Giwercman A, Toumaye H, et al. European Association of Urology Guidelines on Male Infertility: The 2012 Update. Eur Urol. 2012;62(2):324-32.
16. Ramasamy R, Lin K, Gosden LV, et al. High serum FSH levels in men with nonobstructive azoospermia does not affect success of microdissection testicular sperm extraction. Fertil Steril. 2009;92(2):590-93.
17. Hamada AJ, Esteves SC, Agarwal A. A comprehensive review of genetics and genetic testing in azoospermia. Clinics. 2013;68(S1):39-60.
18. Clementini E, Palka C, Iezzi I, et al. Prevalence of chromosomal abnormalities in 2078 infertile couples referred for assisted reproductive techniques. Hum Reprod. 2005;20:437-42.
19. ASRM Practice Committee. Evaluation of the azoospermic male. Fertil Steril. 2008;90:S74-7.
20. Pylyp LY, Spinenko LO, Verhoglyad NV, et al. Chromosomal abnormalities in patients with oligozoospermia and non-obstructive azoospermia. J Assist Reprod Genet. 2013;30: 729-32.
21. Bojesen A, Juul S, Gravholt CH. Prenatal and postnatal prevalence of Klinefelter syndrome: a national registry study. J Clin Endocrinol Metab. 2003;88:622-6.
22. Tuttelmann F, Werny F, Cooper TG, et al. Clinical experience with azoospermia: aetiology and chances for spermatozoa detection upon biopsy. Int J Androl. 2011;34:291-8.
23. Hassold T, Hunt P. To err (meiotically) is human: the genesis of human aneuploidy. Nat Rev Genet. 2001;2:280-91.
24. Thomas NS, Hassold TJ. Aberrant recombination and the origin of Klinefelter syndrome. Hum Reprod Update. 2003;9:309-17.
25. Selice R, Di Mambro A, Garolla A, et al. Spermatogenesis in Klinefelter syndrome. J Endocrinol Invest. 2010;33:789-93.
26. Schlegel PN. Nonobstructive azoospermia: a revolutionary surgical approach and results. Semin Reprod Med. 2009;27:165-70.
27. Mehta A, Paduch DA. Klinefelter syndrome: an argument for early aggressive hormonal and fertility management. Fertl Steril. 2012;98(2):274-83.
28. Rommens JM, Iannuzzi MC, Kerem B, et al. Identification of the cystic fibrosis gene: chromosome walking and jumping. Science. 1989;245(4922):1059-65
29. Yu J, Chen Z, Ni Y, Li Z. CFTR mutations in men with congenital bilateral absence of the vas deferens (CBAVD): a systemic review and meta-analysis. Human Reprod. 2012;27(1):23-35.
30. Foresta C, Moro E, Ferlin A. Y chromosome microdeletions and alterations of spermatogenesis. Endocr Rev. 2001;22:226-39.
31. Massart A, Lissens W, Tournaye H, et al. Genetic causes of spermatogenic failure. Asian J Androl. 2012;14:40-48.
32. Sagnak L, Ersoy H, Ozok U, et al. The significance of Y chromosome microdeletion analysis in subfertile men with clinical variocele. Arch Med Sci. 2010;6(3):382-7.
33. Stahl PJ, Masson P, Mielnik A, et al. A decade of experience emphasizes that testing for Y microdeletions is essential in American men with azoospermia and severe oligozoospermia. Fertil Steril. 2010;94(5):1753-6.
34. Sen S, Pasi AR, Dada R, et al. Y chromosome microdeletions in infertile men: prevalence, phenotypes and screening markers for the Indian population. J Assist Reprod Genet. 2013;30:413-22.
35. Sigman M, Jarow JP. Endocrine evaluation of infertile men. Urology. 1997;50: 659-64.
36. Kumar R. Medical management of non-obstructive azoospermia. Clinics. 2013;68(S1):75-9.
37. Potts JM, Pasqualotto FF, Nelson D, et al. Patient characteristics associated with vasectomy reversal. J Urol. 1999;161:1835-9.
38. Owen ER. Microsurgical vasovasostomy: a reliable vasectomy reversal. Aust NZJ Surg. 1977;47:305.
39. Silber SJ. Microscopic vasectomy reversal. Fertil Steril. 1977;28:1191.
40. Belker AM, Thomas AJ, Fuchs EF, et al. Results of 1,469 microsurgical vasectomy reversals by the Vasovasostomy Study Group. J Urol. 1991;145:505.
41. Ho Kl, Witte MN, Bird ET, et al. Fibrin glue assisted 3-suture vasovasostomy. J Urol. 2005;174(4Pt1):1360-63.
42. Fuchs EF, Burt RA. Vasectomy reversal performed 15 years or more after vasectomy: correlation of pregnancy outcome with partner age and with pregnancy results of in vitro fertilization with intracytoplasmic sperm injection. Fertil Steril. 2002;77:516-19.
43. Martin E, Carnett, JB, Levi JV, et al. The surgical treatment of sterility due to obstruction at the epididymis. Together with a study of the morphology of human spermatozoa. Univ Pa Med Bull. 1902;15:2-15.
44. Dubin L, Amelar RD. Magnified surgery for epididymovasostomy. Urology. 1984;23:525-8.
45. Schlegel PN, Goldstein M. Microsurgical vasoepididymostomy: refinements and results. J Urol. 1993;150:1165-8.
46. Schiff J, Chan P, Li PS, et al. Outcome and late failures compared in 4 techniques of microsurgical vasoepididymostomy in 153 consecutive men. J Urol. 2005;174:651-5.
47. Smrkolj T, Virant-Klun I, Sinkovec J, et al. Epididymovasostomy as the firstline treatment of obstructive azoospermia in young couples with normal spermatogenesis. Reprod Biomed Online. 2010;20(5):594-601.
48. Lee HS, Seo JT. Advances in surgical treatment of male infertility. World J Mens Health. 2012;30(2):108-13.
49. Glina S, Vieira M. Prognostic factors for sperm retrieval in non-obstructive azoospermia. Clinics. 2013;68(S1):121-4.

CHAPTER 19

Surgical Management of Azoospermia

Rupin Shah

INTRODUCTION

Many men with azoospermia can now father their own genetic children with the help of microsurgical reconstructive techniques to correct obstructive azoospermia (OA), or by the use of intracytoplasmic sperm injection (ICSI) to achieve fertilization using sperm retrieved from the epididymis or testis. The use of the correct surgical procedure is important in obtaining the best outcome. Since the techniques of microsurgical reconstruction for OA, and for operative sperm retrieval have been extensively described,[1-3] in this chapter we will focus on the pros and cons of each procedure, and discuss the optimal approach to sperm retrieval.

Operative procedures for azoospermia may be divided into:

- *Reconstructive procedures (for OA)*
  - Vaso-epididymal anastomosis (VEA)
  - Vaso-vasal anastomosis (VVA)
  - Transurethral resection of ejaculatory duct (TURED)
- *Sperm retrieval procedures: Epididymal*
  - Percutaneous epididymal sperm aspiration (PESA)
  - Microsurgical epididymal sperm aspiration (MESA)
- *Sperm retrieval procedures: Testicular*
  - Testicular sperm aspiration (TESA)
  - Needle testicular sperm extraction/needle aspiration biopsy (nTESE/NAB)
  - Tru-cut needle biopsy
  - Conventional open biopsy (cTESE)
  - Testicular mapping by single seminiferous tubule (SST) biopsy technique
  - Microdissection TESE (mdTESE).

RECONSTRUCTIVE SURGERY

Vaso-epididymal Anastomosis

Vaso-epididymal anastomosis is performed for men with OA due to a block in the epididymis. Diagnosis is based on:

- Physical findings of a turgid epididymis and palpable normal vas.
- Absence of inguinal or pelvic surgery (to rule out vas obstruction).
- Presence of fructose with normal semen volume (to rule out ejaculatory duct block).
- Normal spermatogenesis on testicular biopsy.

Several techniques have been described.[4] The older, conventional nonmicrosurgical VEA, which relied on the creation of a fistula, has been given up due to poor success rates. The currently preferred technique is a direct microsurgical anastomosis between a side hole created in the epididymal ductule and the mucosa of the vas using double-armed 10-0 nylon to intussuscept the epididymal ductule into the vas lumen. Patency rates average 50% and vary depending on the extent of epididymal damage and the etiology of the block. Half of those with a patent anastomosis will achieve a natural pregnancy.

ICSI versus VEA

Is a patient with epididymal obstruction better off with VEA or sperm aspiration and ICSI?

- *Advantages of VEA:*
  - Allows a natural pregnancy.
  - Second pregnancy possible without treatment.
  - Corrects the primary problem.
  - Saves the wife from unnecessary treatment.

- *Disadvantages of VEA:*
  - Needs special expertise in microsurgery.
  - Can take 1 year for sperm to appear and even longer for pregnancy to occur.
  - High failure rate if there is extensive epididymal damage.
- *Advantages of ICSI:*
  - Avoids need for a long and difficult surgical procedure.
  - Much quicker results.
  - Can be done when VEA has failed or has poor prognosis.
  - More readily available than microsurgery.
- *Disadvantages of ICSI:*
  - Places burden of therapy on normal female partner, with attendant risks of hormonal stimulation and the in vitro fertilization (IVF) procedure.
  - Needs to be repeated for every pregnancy.
  - More expensive than microsurgery.
  - Not "natural".

Hence, VEA can be recommended when the couple is young and not in a hurry, or if they are insistent on a natural pregnancy, or if cost is a factor. ICSI is recommended if the couple is aging and there is no time to waste, or if the couple is in a hurry due to social reasons, or they are not interested in surgery, or if surgery has failed.

Vaso-vasal Anastomosis

The most common reason for VVA is reversal of vasectomy.[5] In such cases, success depends on whether there is a secondary epididymal block due to back pressure from the vasectomy site. The longer the duration since vasectomy, the greater is the likelihood of a secondary epididymal block.

If there is no epididymal block the technical success of microsurgical VVA[6] is over 90%. Hence, if the female partner is relatively young then VVA is more cost-effective than ICSI. If female fertility is compromised then ICSI with sperm aspirated from the epididymis is a better option.

Transurethral Resection of Ejaculatory Duct

Transurethral resection of ejaculatory duct is indicated when there is ejaculatory duct obstruction (EDO) with dilatation of the ejaculatory ducts. When this is due to a congenital intraprostatic cyst compressing the ejaculatory ducts then the urologist can introduce a resectoscope and easily deroof the cyst by cutting the floor of the urethra near the veru. Occasionally, the block may be due to infection and the ejaculatory ducts are individually dilated. In such a case surgery is more difficult since deroofing has to be more precise and there is a greater chance of restenosis.

However, often the blockage that follows an infection is fibrous (especially after tuberculosis). In such cases, the ejaculatory ducts and seminal vesicles do not dilate; TUR is not possible, and sperm aspiration with ICSI is required.

This important distinction between cystic and fibrous EDO is made on the basis of a transrectal ultrasound (TRUS). In a man with azoospermia, low volume of ejaculate, absent fructose, and palpable vasa, if TRUS shows dilated seminal vesicles with intraprostatic dilatation of the ejaculatory ducts or an intraprostatic cyst then this is a cystic obstruction amenable to TURED. If TRUS shows nondilated ejaculatory ducts and seminal vesicles then this is indicative of a fibrous, nonoperable type of block.

SPERM RETRIEVAL PROCEDURES

Percutaneous Epididymal Sperm Aspiration

Sperm can be retrieved from the epididymis only in cases of OA. It is not indicated in men with nonobstructive azoospermia (NOA).

Percutaneous epididymal sperm aspiration is a simple procedure that involves percutaneous puncture of the epididymis with a fine needle and aspiration of epididymal fluid.[7] One may use a 24-gauge scalp vein connected to a syringe, or a tuberculin syringe with a 26-gauge needle (author's preference). The aspiration must be performed from the proximal epididymis (caput region) since in an obstructed system the distal sperm are old and degenerating and the best sperm are the most recent ones that are found in the caput.

Since the procedure is blind, several punctures at different locations on the head may be required to get adequate numbers of motile sperm. Only motile epididymal sperm are used for ICSI since immotile epididymal sperm may be dead sperm.

Percutaneous epididymal sperm aspiration is easy and inexpensive, with no major complications, and can be repeated.[8] Hence, it has generally replaced the more complex MESA.

Microsurgical Epididymal Sperm Aspiration

Microsurgical epididymal sperm aspiration is the original technique described for sperm retrieval from the epididymis.[9] It involves open surgical exposure of the epididymis and mobilization of a loop of epididymal ductule under magnification. The ductule is incised and the outpouring fluid is aspirated and checked for sperm.

Multiple ductules can be opened at different locations so as to retrieve a large number of sperm.

While MESA allows for retrieval of a large number of sperm, adequate for many cycles of ICSI, it seems unnecessarily complex compared to PESA that can provide enough sperm in most cases.

Testicular Sperm Aspiration

Testicular sperm aspiration is like fine needle aspiration cytology (FNAC) of the testis. A 24-gauge needle is attached to a syringe and suction is applied while making several passes through the testis. The aspirate is examined for sperm. FNAC of the testis has been used extensively both for diagnosis (to distinguish between OA and NOA) and for therapy as a method of sperm retrieval. However, on both counts, it falls short.

Diagnostically, FNAC can be misleading because a few sperm may be seen in the aspirate even in cases of NOA with focal spermatogenesis. Thus, relying on FNAC to diagnose obstruction can lead to false explorations for corrective microsurgery.

Therapeutically, the opposite is also true for FNAC. It may fail to retrieve sperm in cases where there is only focal spermatogenesis. Several studies have compared sperm retrieval by FNAC vs. tissue biopsy and have found fewer positive retrievals, and also fewer number of sperm retrieved.[10,11]

Hence, FNAC is better replaced by a needle biopsy that is equally noninvasive but more useful as described below.

Needle Aspiration Biopsy of the Testis

Needle aspiration biopsy differs from FNAC in that a larger bore scalp vein needle (18 gauge) is used. Suction is applied with a 10 mL or 20 mL syringe and the needle is passed in and out only in one direction, so that what is aspirated is not just fluid but a large chunk of testicular tissue containing many seminiferous tubules.[12] In fact, often the amount of tissue that is recovered by NAB may be more than traditionally removed by an open biopsy.

Diagnostically, NAB is equivalent to an open conventional biopsy because it can provide enough tissue for histopathological examination.

Therapeutically, NAB is far more efficient than FNAC in retrieving sperm since large amounts of tissue are available for processing. In fact, even in men with NOA we are often able to retrieve enough sperm by NAB alone and avoid the need for the more invasive, open microsurgical sperm retrieval procedures.

Tru-Cut Needle Biopsy of the Testis

Commercial needle biopsy systems may also be used to obtain testicular biopsy percutaneously,[13] but their cutting action makes them more traumatic than the NAB procedure with a scalp vein needle.

Conventional Open Biopsy

This is the traditional method of obtaining a testicular biopsy through a small incision in the skin and tunica. Performed correctly, it is a simple and safe method of obtaining one or two diagnostic or therapeutic biopsies. However, in most cases the same amount of tissue can usually be obtained by the NAB procedure that is less invasive. Hence, the author reserves diagnostic open biopsy for those cases where NAB fails due to fibrosis.

The conventional open biopsy has limited use for therapeutic sperm retrieval in men with testicular failure since, in these cases, often multiple biopsies are needed to find sperm. Each open biopsy can cause some degree of permanent testicular devascularization.[14,15] If sperm are retrieved within a couple of biopsies then no harm is done, but for a more extensive search the microsurgical techniques described below are more efficient and less harmful than multiple conventional open biopsies.

Single Seminiferous Tubule Biopsy Technique for Therapeutic Testicular Mapping

This is an open microsurgical procedure that allows extensive sampling of the testis without the need for an incision in the tunica and with no risk of devascularization of testicular tissue.[16]

After exposure of the testis, an avascular area of the tunica is punctured with a fine needle. The opening is widened with the prong of a microforceps till a loop of seminiferous tubule pops out. This is grasped and pulled out and inspected under the operating microscope. If it appears promising then more tubule is extracted. If not, then another puncture is made a centimeter away and the procedure repeated. In this manner, the entire testicular surface can be mapped with 15–30 seminiferous tubule biopsies All the microbiopsies are sent to the IVF laboratory where they are processed for sperm retrieval. The small punctures do not need any suturing and since no vessels are cut there is no damage to the testis. The SST technique is useful for sperm retrieval in men with testicular failure since it allows for extensive sampling while being less traumatic than mdTESE.

It may not be possible to use this technique in very small or fibrotic testis in which no tissue protrudes through the puncture. In such cases, mdTESE is more useful.

Microdissection TESE

The testis is exposed and the tunica is incised along the circumference resulting in bivalving of the testis. The parenchyma is dissected and inspected under an operating microscope, looking for larger tubules that are more likely to contain sperm; these are biopsied. Thus, the entire testis is explored and a large number of microbiopsies can be taken while removing only a small amount of tissue in total.[17,18]

Microdissection TESE offers the most thorough method for finding rare sperm in a case of testicular failure.[19] However, it is invasive and needs special training. There is risk of hematoma, infection and, rarely, atrophy if care is not taken to preserve vascularity.

Choice of Sperm Retrieval Technique

The technique to be used will depend on whether the man has OA or NOA.

In men in whom the distinction between OA and NOA is not clinically obvious, a diagnostic biopsy will be required. This should not only differentiate between OA and NOA, but also, in cases of NOA, identify whether focal spermatogenesis is present, and obtain sperm for cryopreservation. Hence, for diagnosis, the single, conventional biopsy should be replaced by a four quadrant NAB from both sides. One specimen is sent for histopathology, while the rest go to the IVF laboratory for sperm retrieval, and cryopreservation if sperm are found. If no sperm are found in any of the eight biopsies then the patient can be counseled that the chances of finding sperm by mdTESE are less than 10%.

For sperm retrieval in men with obstructive azoospermia, PESA is the technique of choice, offering a simple, painless method for retrieving a good number of motile sperm. When PESA is unsuccessful then MESA can be done, or sperm can be retrieved percutaneously from the testis by NAB. In men with OA, pregnancy rates are the same whether epididymal or testicular sperm are used.

In men with clinically obvious testicular failure, the author recommends a staged approach in one session. This is based on the finding that in the some cases of testicular failure, sperm can be found by doing just a few biopsies,[20] while other cases will require extensive exploration and a large number of biopsies. Thus we start with four quadrant NAB. If sperm are retrieved then further invasive procedures are not required. If no sperms are retrieved then the testis is exposed and mapped by SST biopsies. If still no sperm are found then the procedure is extended into a mdTESE. If no sperms are found then the procedure is repeated on the opposite side.

With such a staged approach it will be possible to avoid the more aggressive, open techniques in many men in whom sperm are found by a simple needle biopsy.[21] And if sperms are not found by simpler methods then the patient immediately gets the benefit of the more invasive methods of sperm retrieval. The best chance of finding sperm is at the first attempt, and the use of fresh sperm is associated with higher embryo transfer rates.[22,23] Hence, it is best to be prepared with all methods of sperm retrieval at the first session.

CONCLUSION

There have been many advances in the surgery for azoospermia, both in reconstructive procedures and in sperm retrieval techniques. Microsurgery plays an important role in optimizing results in reconstructive surgery. Many techniques are available for operative sperm retrieval. The optimal technique for a given patient will vary depending on his clinical picture and the surgeon should have a variety of techniques available in his repertoire for best results.

REFERENCES

1. Marmar JL. Techniques for microsurgical reconstruction of obstructive azoospermia. Indian J Urol. 2011;27(1):86-91.
2. Donoso P, Tournaye H, Devroey P. Which is the best sperm retrieval technique for non-obstructive azoospermia? A systematic review. Hum Reprod Update. 2007;13(6):539-49.
3. Shah R. Surgical sperm retrieval: techniques and their indications. Indian J Urology. 2011;27(1):102-9.
4. Chan PT. The evolution and refinement of vasoepididymostomy techniques. Asian J Androl. 2013;15(1):49-55.
5. Ramasamy R, Schlegel PN. Vasectomy and vasectomy reversal: an update. Indian J Urol. 2011;27(1):92-7.
6. Herrel L, Hsiao W. Microsurgical vasovasostomy. Asian J Androl. 2013;15(1):44-8.
7. Shrivastav P, Nadkarni P, Wensvoort S, et al. Percutaneous epididymal sperm aspiration for obstructive azoospermia. Hum Reprod. 1994;9(11):2058-61.
8. Rosenlund B, Westlander G, Wood M, et al. Sperm retrieval and fertilization in repeated percutaneous epididymal sperm aspiration. Hum Reprod. 1998;13(10):2805-7.
9. Patrizio P, Silber S, Ord T, et al. Two births after microsurgical sperm aspiration in congenital absence of vas deferens. Lancet. 1988;2(8624):1364.
10. Friedler S, Raziel A, Strassburger D, et al. Testicular sperm retrieval by percutaneous fine needle aspiration compared with testicular sperm extraction by open biopsy in men with NOA. Hum Reprod. 1997;12(7):1488-93.
11. Houwen J, Lundin K, Söderlund B, et al. Efficacy of percutaneous needle aspiration and open biopsy for sperm

retrieval in men with non-obstructive azoospermia. Acta Obstet Gynecol Scand. 2008;87(10):1033-8.
12. Shah RS. Surgical and nonsurgical methods of sperm retrieval. In: Hansotia M, Desai S, Parihar M (Eds). Advanced Infertility Management. New Delhi: Jaypee Brothers Medical Publishers (P) Ltd; 2002. pp. 253-8.
13. Morey AF, Deshon GE Jr, Rosanski TA, et al. Technique of biopty gun testis needle biopsy. Urology. 1993;42(3): 325-6.
14. Schlegel PN, Su LM. Physiological consequences of testicular sperm extraction. Hum Reprod. 1997;12(8):1688-92.
15. Ron-El R, Strauss S, Friedler S, et al. Serial sonography and colour flow Doppler imaging following testicular and epididymal sperm extraction. Hum Reprod. 1998;13(12): 3390-3.
16. Shah RS. Operative sperm retrieval for ART. In: Goenka ML, Goenka D (Eds). Recent Advances in Infertility Management. Guwahati: Goenka; 2001. pp. 179-83.
17. Schlegel PN, Li PS. Microdissection TESE: sperm retrieval in non-obstructive azoospermia. Hum Reprod Update. 1998;4(4):439.
18. Schlegel PN. Testicular sperm extraction: microdissection improves sperm yield with minimal tissue excision. Hum Reprod. 1999;14(1):131-5.
19. Schlegel PN. Nonobstructive azoospermia: a revolutionary surgical approach and results. Semin Reprod Med. 2009;27(2):165-70.
20. Altay B, Hekimgil M, Cikili N, et al. Histopathological mapping of open testicular biopsies in patients with unobstructed azoospermia. BJU Int. 2001;87(9):834-7.
21. Colpi GM, Colpi EM, Piediferro G, et al. Microsurgical TESE versus conventional TESE for ICSI in non-obstructive azoospermia: a randomized controlled study. Reprod Biomed Online. 2009;18(3):315-9.
22. Verheyen G, Vernaeve V, Van Landuyt L, et al. Should diagnostic testicular sperm retrieval followed by cryopreservation for later ICSI be the procedure of choice for all patients with non-obstructive azoospermia? Hum Reprod. 2004;19(12):2822-30.
23. Craft I, Tsirigotis M. Simplified recovery, preparation and cryopreservation of testicular sperm. Hum Reprod. 1995;10(7):1623-6.

Section 3

Intrauterine Insemination

CHAPTER 20

An Overview of Intrauterine Insemination

Sneha Sathe, Avantika Vaze

INTRODUCTION

Intrauterine insemination (IUI) is the process of placing washed spermatozoa transcervically into the uterine cavity for the treatment of infertility. Compared with in vitro fertilization (IVF) and intracytoplasmic sperm injection (ICSI), IUI is a simple and inexpensive technique which is easy to learn and can be performed without expensive infrastructure. It is a relatively safe procedure with minimal risks when appropriately monitored and is more acceptable to patients.

Intrauterine insemination can be performed using the husband's sperm or with sperm from a donor. It may involve timed insemination of sperm into the uterus in natural (unstimulated) cycles or insemination following stimulation of the ovaries using oral ovulogens or gonadotropins.[1,2]

Intrauterine insemination with or without ovarian stimulation (OS) is one of the most popular methods of assisted reproductive technology (ART) worldwide and is often the first-line treatment option for many infertile couples. There is extensive literature on the subject of IUI using husband's sperm, however, its effectiveness particularly in relation to IVF or ICSI is still controversial.[3-7]

There are wide variations in the indications of IUI, OS protocols, semen preparation techniques, timing, number and technique of insemination, and number of treatment cycles. This chapter gives a brief overview of the evidence based data available on the subject of IUI.

INDICATIONS

Intrauterine insemination using husband's sperm can be offered for a wide range of indications; these are summarized in Box 1. The indications for IUI using donor sperm are summarized in Box 2.

Box 1: Indications for IUI with husband's or partner's sperms.

Male subfertility
- Mild oligo/asthenozoospermia

Unexplained infertility
Cervical factor
Minimal to mild endometriosis
Sexual dysfunction
- Vaginismus
- Erectile dysfunction
- Ejaculation problems

Oligo/Anovulation
Other
- To reduce risk of transmission to wife/female partner in case of HIV/HBsAg/HCV positive husband/male partner.
- Use of cryopreserved semen due to nonavailability of husband/partner because of work or other reasons and in case of cancer patients who have undergone semen freezing prior to radio/chemotherapy.

(HIV: human immunodeficiency virus; HBsAg: hepatitis B virus surface antigen; HCV: hepatitis C virus; IUI: intrauterine insemination)

Box 2: Indications for IUI with donor's sperms.

Azoospermia
- Nonobstructive
- Obstructive

Severe oligoasthenospermia when not willing for IVF/ICSI
Inheritable genetic disease in husband/male partner
Severe rhesus isoimmunization
Lesbian couples
Single women

(ICSI: intracytoplasmic sperm injection; IUI: intrauterine insemination; IVF: in vitro fertilization)

Mild Male Factor Infertility

Male factor infertility is the only cause of infertility in approximately 30% of couples and a contributing factor in another 20–30%.[8] It is usually defined by abnormal results on semen analysis. However, even if results of semen analysis are normal, other male factors may be present. The category of "male subfertility" includes couples that are heterogeneous for the type and degree of semen abnormality as well as for the female fertility potential.

There is no shared minimal cut-off of semen parameters for IUI indication. Two Cochrane reviews found insufficient evidence to conclude whether IUI is effective or not in moderate and mild male infertility.[5,9] However, based on evidence from older studies, it is suggested that IUI may be offered to couples with male factor infertility, in a low technology setting.[1]

A couple with severe male factor infertility is not a candidate for IUI but for ICSI.[10]

Unexplained Infertility

Up to 30% of couples who are unable to conceive are determined to have unexplained infertility.[2] Traditionally diagnosis is made only when basic infertility workup fails to reveal any obvious abnormality. Basic workup should provide evidence of ovulation, normal semen parameters, and patency of tubes.

The treatment options for unexplained infertility include expectant observation with timed intercourse (TI), IUI with clomiphene citrate (CC) or gonadotropins for controlled OS (COS), and IVF or ICSI.

The chance of spontaneous pregnancy in untreated couples varies from 30% to 70% within 2 years.[11] A recent Cochrane systematic review[12] which included 14 trials with 1,867 women concluded that there was no difference in live birth rates between IUI and TI, both in natural or stimulated cycles. However, there was an increase in live birth rate in stimulated cycle IUI in comparison to natural cycle IUI without an increase in multiple pregnancy rate.

In the Fast Track and Standard Treatment (FASTT) Trial,[13] patients were randomized to receive either a conventional treatment regimen of three cycles of CC or IUI, three cycles of follicle stimulating hormone (FSH) or IUI, and up to six cycles of IVF or to receive an accelerated treatment course of three cycles of CC or IUI and then up to six cycles of IVF. An increased pregnancy rate was observed in the accelerated arm compared with the conventional arm. Median time to pregnancy was 8 and 11 months in the accelerated and conventional arms, respectively.

Endometriosis

Classical studies suggest that 25–50% of infertile women have endometriosis and that 30–50% of women with endometriosis are infertile.[14] The European Society of Human Reproduction and Embryology (ESHRE) guideline[15] on the management of women with endometriosis recommends IUI with COS instead of expectant management and instead natural cycle IUI as it increases live birth rates and pregnancy rates, respectively. However, these are grade C recommendations of moderate quality.

Factors such as the woman's age, duration of infertility, ability to undergo IVF, family history, and pelvic pain must be taken into consideration before deciding the course of treatment.

The National Institute for Health and Care Excellence (NICE) guidelines[16] recommend that for couples with unexplained infertility, male factor infertility, and mild endometriosis, failed expectant management for up to 2 years should be followed directly by IVF, suggesting the limited role of IUI for these indications. The ESHRE Capri Workshop[6] on IUI concluded that IUI requires OS to achieve modest results, but the associated high multiple pregnancy rates make it a poor substitute for IVF.

However, since then, a few trials have been published supporting the value of IUI[17,18] and more randomized controlled trials (RCTs) are needed on IUI with mild stimulation protocols and on the order of IUI and other treatments.

Polycystic Ovarian Syndrome

Ovulatory dysfunction, per se, is not an indication for IUI and the primary treatment for women with polycystic ovarian syndrome (PCOS) is ovulation induction (with TI). IUI can be considered if there is an associated male factor or in women who fail to conceive in spite of successful induction of ovulation.[19] The few studies available on the results of OS and IUI in women with PCOS report clinical pregnancy rates of 11–20% and multiple pregnancy rates ranging from 11% to 36%.[20-22] However, current recommendations suggest that IUI should not be the first-line therapy in anovulatory women.[23]

Cervical Factor Infertility

The average incidence of cervical factor infertility among infertile couples is 5%.[24] Previously, the postcoital test (PCT) for assessing sperm motility in a sample of postcoital cervical mucus was considered an integral part of the basic infertility evaluation, but today, the PCT has been largely abandoned and is not recommended as a component of the standard infertility investigation.[25] A recent Cochrane review concluded that there is no evidence to suggest that IUI is an effective treatment for cervical hostility.[26]

Ejaculatory Failure

Ejaculatory dysfunction is an uncommon cause of male infertility, accounting for approximately 2% of cases.[27] It is the major cause of infertility in patients with spinal cord injury (SCI).[28] Other causes of anejaculatory infertility include retroperitoneal lymph node dissection for testis cancer,[29] diabetic neuropathy,[30,31] multiple sclerosis[32] and psychogenic anejaculation.[33]

In most men with SCI, semen can easily be obtained by penile vibratory stimulation (PVS) or electroejaculation (EEJ) and IUI has successfully been used to achieve pregnancy.[34] Several studies, however, have shown that sperm obtained by EEJ is of poor quality and hence IVF or ICSI may be a more suitable option in these groups of patients.[35,36]

CONTROLLED OVARIAN STIMULATION

Intrauterine insemination can be performed in the natural cycle or can be combined with COS. The rationale of COS is to increase the number of oocytes available for fertilization and thereby increase the chance of conception. Stimulation also enhances steroid production, which may improve the chance of fertilization and implantation.[37]

There is a spectrum of OS protocols for IUI, varying from the use of clomiphene, tamoxifen or letrozole alone, or in combination with gonadotropins, and gonadotropins alone, or in combination with gonadotropin-releasing hormone (GnRH) agonists or antagonists.

A Cochrane systematic review[38] which included 43 trials involving 3,957 women, was conducted to evaluate COS protocols for IUI for all indications. It was concluded that when IUI is combined with COS, gonadotropins may be the most effective. When using gonadotropins, daily regimens and low-dose protocols are advised. There is no significant difference in pregnancy rates between the different types of gonadotropins and the addition of GnRH agonist or antagonist does not provide added benefit. There is no significant difference in pregnancy rates between antiestrogens and aromatase inhibitors.

When deciding whether or not to use COS for IUI and the choice of the drug and protocol; the benefit of a potential increase in success rates must be balanced against the increased cost of medication and monitoring, as well as potential complications like ovarian hyperstimulation syndrome (OHSS) and multiple pregnancy.

Strict ultrasound monitoring of each stimulated cycle is important. The aim should be two dominant follicles larger than 15 mm but all follicles larger than 10 mm should be measured and considered when defining cancellation criteria.[39] Although evidence-based data are lacking, it is recommended that secondary preventive measures to prevent multiple pregnancies are needed when four or more follicles more than or equal to 14 mm are present at the time of human chorionic gonadotropin (hCG) injection. These measures include cancellation of the cycle, the aspiration of supernumerary follicles, and/or escape IVF.[6]

NUMBER OF INSEMINATIONS

The IUI procedure is timed around ovulation and can be done once or twice. There is no evidence that double inseminations give rise to higher pregnancy rates as compared to single inseminations.[40-44]

SEMEN PREPARATION

The rationale behind sperm preparation for IUI is to remove prostaglandins, infectious agents and antigenic proteins, as well as to remove immotile spermatozoa, leukocytes, and immature germ cells. The ideal sperm preparation technique is the one which will achieve the largest number of morphologically normal motile spermatozoa in a small volume of culture media, free from seminal plasma, leukocytes, and bacteria.[45]

Simple sperm wash, swim-up, and density gradient centrifugation (DGC) are the most commonly used methods. Although DGC is superior to the swim-up and simple wash technique as far as semen parameters are concerned, there is insufficient evidence to recommend any specific technique when speaking about clinical outcome after IUI.[46]

Although there is no final consensus on the semen parameters which should qualify for ICSI rather than IUI, the recommended lower limits when considering IUI are:[47]

- Inseminating motile count (IMC): 1 million
- Sperm morphology using strict criteria: 4% normal
- Total motile sperm count (TMC) in native sample: 5–10 million
- Total motility (TM) in native sample: 30%.

TYPES OF CATHETER

Various types of IUI catheters are available commercially, such as soft or rigid, disposable or metal, with or without stylet. There is no evidence of significant difference in pregnancy or live birth rates with the type of catheter used.[48]

LUTEAL PHASE SUPPORT

Progesterone is essential for implantation and for the maintenance of an early pregnancy. However, the minimum amount of progesterone essential is unknown and successful pregnancies have been reported when the concentration of progesterone was never above 15 nmol/L for the first 14 days.[49]

An updated meta-analysis[50] which included 11 RCTs concluded that progesterone supplementation improves pregnancy and live birth rates in gonadotropin stimulated IUI cycles and has no benefit in clomiphene stimulated cycles. Regarding clomiphene or letrozole plus gonadotropin IUI cycles, the evidence was insufficient.

NUMBER OF CYCLES

Most authors recommend treatment with IUI for up to three to four cycles[51-55] and some advice to continue IUI even after six or more cycle.[56-58] 88% of the pregnancies are reported to occur in the first three cycles of IUI.[59] The NICE guidelines and a Cochrane systematic review support using IUI as treatment for up to 6 cycles.[2,19]

FACTORS INFLUENCING IUI OUTCOME

Success rates with IUI depend on the age of the female partner, duration of infertility, sperm quality and tubal patency.[60] The woman's age is the most important factor influencing the likelihood of pregnancy, whatever treatment is chosen (IUI or IVF).[53,61] The longer the duration of infertility, the lower the likelihood of success with IUI.[62-64]

Some studies report an association between the number of large follicles in the late follicular phase and pregnancy rates,[65-68] but there are others that do not.[69-71] However, it is important to note that all studies have confirmed a relationship between follicle number and multiple gestation. A cycle involving the development of many follicles carries the risk of higher-order multiple pregnancy and OHSS and should be cancelled.

Although the literature does not reveal level 1 evidence on the relationship between sperm quality and IUI success, the following cut-off values for semen parameters are suggested when considering IUI: IMC more than 1 million, sperm morphology using strict criteria more than 4%, TMCs of 5–10 million, and TM of more than 30%.[47]

COMPLICATIONS

The complications of IUI are few. Unsuccessful IUI or failure of treatment is the most frequent outcome since reported pregnancy rates range from 5% to 25%. A rare, but most serious complication with grave consequences is insemination of the wrong semen sample. Painful uterine contractions may occur during insemination. This can usually be minimized by inseminating slowly. Intrauterine infection and rarely anaphylaxis may occur particularly if neat semen which should never be used, is used. There is a risk ectopic pregnancy and of miscarriage but this is similar to that after other infertility treatments. The two most serious complications are multiple pregnancy and OHSS and the risk is related to the use of COS with IUI.

CONCLUSION

Intrauterine insemination is a simple, noninvasive, cost-effective first-line treatment option for certain diagnostic groups of infertile couples. Results are best in young women with short periods of infertility, patent fallopian tubes, no or mild ovulatory disorder, and no severe degree of male infertility in their partners. Thorough counseling about the procedure, its effectiveness, the cost involved, and the potential complications is important. Mild OS protocols with close monitoring of treatment cycles are essential. If there is no pregnancy within three to four cycles of IUI, it is better to move on to IVF or ICSI.

REFERENCES

1. Abdelkader AM, Yeh J. The potential use of intrauterine insemination as a basic option for infertility: a review for technology-limited medical settings. Obstet Gynecol Int. 2009;2009:584837.
2. National Institute for Health and Clinical Excellence: Guidance. Fertility: Assessment and Treatment for People with Fertility Problems. London: RCOG Press; 2004.
3. Cohlen BJ. Should we continue performing intrauterine inseminations in the year 2004? Gynecol Obstet Invest. 2005;59(1):3-13.
4. Ombelet W. IUI and evidence-based medicine: an urgent need for translation into our clinical practice. Gynecol Obstet Invest. 2005;59(1):1-2.
5. Bensdorp AJ, Cohlen BJ, Heineman MJ, et al. Intra-uterine insemination for male subfertility. Cochrane Database Syst Rev. 2007;(3):CD000360.
6. ESHRE Capri Workshop Group. Intrauterine insemination. Hum Reprod Update. 2009;15(3):265-77.
7. Pashayan N, Lyratzopoulos G, Mathur R. Cost-effectiveness of primary offer of IVF vs. primary offer of IUI followed by IVF (for IUI failures) in couples with unexplained or mild male factor subfertility. BMC Health Serv Res. 2006;6:80.
8. Kolettis PN. Evaluation of the subfertile man. Am Fam Physician. 2003;67(10):2165-72.
9. Cissen M, Bensdorp A, Cohlen BJ, et al. Assisted reproductive technologies for male subfertility. Cochrane Database Syst Rev. 2016;2:CD000360.
10. Van Voorhis BJ, Barnett M, Sparks AE, et al. Effect of the total motile sperm count on the efficacy and cost-effectiveness of intrauterine insemination and in vitro fertilization. Fertil Steril. 2001;75(4):661-8.

11. Smeenk JM, Braat DD, Stolwijk AM, et al. Pregnancy is predictable: a large-scale prospective external validation of the prediction of spontaneous pregnancy in subfertile couples. Hum Reprod. 2007;22(8):2344-5.
12. Veltman-Verhulst SM, Hughes E, Ayeleke RO, et al. Intrauterine insemination for unexplained subfertility. Cochrane Database Syst Rev. 2016;2:CD001838.
13. Reindollar RH, Regan MM, Neumann PJ, et al. A randomized clinical trial to evaluate optimal treatment for unexplained infertility: the fast track and standard treatment (FASTT) trial. Fertil Steril. 2010;94(3):888-99.
14. Missmer SA, Hankinson SE, Spiegelman D, et al. Incidence of laparoscopically confirmed endometriosis by demographic, anthropometric, and lifestyle factors. Am J Epidemiol. 2004;160(8):784-96.
15. Dunselman GA, Vermeulen N, Becker C, et al. ESHRE guideline: management of women with endometriosis. Hum Reprod. 2014;29(3):400-12.
16. National Institute for Health and Clinical Excellence: Guidance. Fertility problems: assessment and treatment. London: RCOG Press; 2013.
17. Bensdorp AJ, Tjon-Kon-Fat RI, Bossuyt PMM, et al. Prevention of multiple pregnancies in couples with unexplained or mild male subfertility: randomised controlled trial of in vitro fertilisation with single embryo transfer or in vitro fertilisation in modified natural cycle compared with intrauterine insemination. BMJ. 2015;350:g7771.
18. Farquhar CM, Liu E, Armstrong S, et al. Intrauterine insemination with ovarian stimulation versus expectant management for unexplained infertility (TUI): A pragmatic, open-label, randomised, controlled, two-centre trial. Lancet. 2018;391(10119):441-50.
19. Cohlen BJ, Vandekerckhove P, te Velde ER, et al. Timed intercourse versus intra-uterine insemination with or without ovarian hyperstimulation for subfertility in men. Cochrane Database Syst Rev. 2000;(2):CD000360.
20. Gerli S, Casini ML, Unfer V, et al. Recombinant versus urinary follicle-stimulating hormone in intrauterine insemination cycles: a prospective, randomized analysis of cost effectiveness. Fertil Steril. 2004;82(3):573-8.
21. Mitwally MF, Casper RF. Aromatase inhibition reduces the dose of gonadotropin required for controlled ovarian hyperstimulation. J Soc Gynecol Investig. 2004;11(6):406-15.
22. Palomba S, Falbo A, Orio F Jr, et al. A randomized controlled trial evaluating metformin pre-treatment and co-administration in non-obese insulin-resistant women with polycystic ovary syndrome treated with controlled ovarian stimulation plus timed intercourse or intrauterine insemination. Hum Reprod. 2005;20(10):2879-86.
23. Thessaloniki ESHRE/ASRM-Sponsored PCOS Consensus Workshop Group. Consensus on infertility treatment related to polycystic ovary syndrome. Hum Reprod. 2008;23(3):462-77.
24. Collins JA, Van Steirteghem A. Overall prognosis with current treatment of infertility. Hum Reprod Update. 2004;10(4):309-16.
25. Practice Committee of the American Society for Reproductive Medicine. Optimal evaluation of the infertile female. Fertil Steril. 2006;86(5 Suppl 1):S264-7.
26. Helmerhorst FM, Van Vliet HA, Gornas T, et al. Intrauterine insemination versus timed intercourse for cervical hostility in subfertile couples. Cochrane Database Syst Rev. 2005;(4):CD002809.
27. Dubin L, Amelar RD. Etiologic factors in 1294 consecutive cases of male infertility. Fertil Steril. 1971;22(8):469-74.
28. Sønksen J, Biering-Sørensen F. Fertility in men with spinal cord or cauda equina lesions. Semin Neurol. 1992;12(2):106-14.
29. Donohue JP, Foster RS, Rowland RG, et al. Nerve-sparing retroperitoneal lymphadenectomy with preservation of ejaculation. J Urol. 1990;144(2 Pt 1):287-91.
30. Sexton WJ, Jarow JP. Effect of diabetes mellitus upon male reproductive function. Urology. 1997;49(4):508-13.
31. Dunsmuir WD, Holmes SA. The aetiology and management of erectile, ejaculatory, and fertility problems in men with diabetes mellitus. Diabet Med. 1996;13(8):700-8.
32. Valleroy ML, Kraft GH. Sexual dysfunction in multiple sclerosis. Arch Phys Med Rehabil. 1984;65(3):125-8.
33. Stewart DE, Ohl DA. Idiopathic anejaculation treated by electroejaculation. Int J Psychiatry Med. 1989;19(3):263-8.
34. Ohl DA, Wolf LJ, Menge AC. Electroejaculation and assisted reproductive technologies in the treatment of anejaculatory infertility. Fertil Steril. 2001;76(6):1249-55.
35. Buch JP, Zorn BH. Evaluation and treatment of infertility in spinal cord injured men through rectal probe electroejaculation. J Urol. 1993;149(5 Pt 2):1350-4.
36. Chung PH, Yeko TR, Mayer JC, et al. Assisted fertility using electroejaculation in men with spinal cord injury-a review of literature. Fertil Steril. 1995;64(1):1-9.
37. Wallach EE. Gonadotropin treatment of the ovulatory patient: the pros and cons of empiric therapy for infertility. Fertil Steril. 1991;55(3):478-80.
38. Cantineau AE, Cohlen BJ, Heineman MJ. Ovarian stimulation protocols (anti-oestrogens, gonadotrophins with and without GnRH agonists/antagonists) for intrauterine insemination (IUI) in women with subfertility. Cochrane Database Syst Rev. 2007;(2):CD005356
39. Ombelet W. Evidence-based recommendations for IUI in daily practice. Middle East Fertil Soc J. 2013;18(2):74-7.
40. Alborzi S, Motazedian S, Parsanezhad ME, et al. Comparison of the effectiveness of single intrauterine insemination (IUI) versus double IUI per cycle in infertile patients. Fertil Steril. 2003;80(3):595-9.
41. Osuna C, Matorras R, Pijoan JI, et al. One versus two inseminations per cycle in intrauterine insemination with sperm from patients' husbands: a systematic review of the literature. Fertil Steril. 2004;82(1):17-24.
42. Cantineau AEP, Heineman MJ, Cohlen BJ. Single versus double intrauterine insemination (IUI) in stimulated cycles for subfertile couples. Cochrane Database of Sys Rev. 2003;(1):CD003854.
43. Polyzos NP. Double versus single intrauterine insemination for unexplained infertility: A meta-analysis of randomized trials. Fertil Steril. 2010;94(4):1261-6.
44. Zarek SM, Hill MJ, Richter KS, et al. Single-donor and double-donor sperm intrauterine insemination cycles: does double intrauterine insemination increase clinical pregnancy rates? Fertil Steril. 2014;102(3):739-43.

45. Pardo M, Bancells N. Artificial insemination with husbands' sperm (AIH): techniques for sperm selection. Arch Androl. 1989;22(1):15-27.
46. Boomsma CM, Heineman MJ, Cohlen BJ, et al. Semen preparation techniques for intrauterine insemination. Cochrane Database Syst Rev. 2007;(4):CD004507.
47. Ombelet W, Dhont N, Thijssen A, et al. Semen quality and prediction of IUI success in male subfertility: A systematic review. Reprod BioMed Online. 2014;28(3):300-9.
48. van der Poel N, Farquhar C, Abou-Setta AM, et al. Soft versus firm catheters for intrauterine insemination. Cochrane Database Syst Rev. 2010;(11):CD006225.
49. Csapo AI, Pulkkinen M. Indispensability of the human corpus luteum in the maintenance of early pregnancy. Luteectomy evidence. Obstet Gynecol Surv. 1978;33(2):69-81.
50. Green KA, Zolton JR, Schermerhorn SM, et al. Progesterone luteal support after ovulation induction and intrauterine insemination: An updated systematic review and meta-analysis. Fertil Steril. 2017;107(4):924-33.
51. Aboulghar MA, Mansour RT, Serour GI, et al. Ovarian superstimulation and intrauterine insemination for the treatment of unexplained infertility. Fertil Steril. 1993;60(2): 303-6.
52. Plosker SM, Jacobson W, Amato P. Predicting and optimizing success in an intra-uterine insemination programme. Hum Reprod. 1994;9(11):2014-21.
53. Yang JH, Wu MY, Chao KH, et al. Controlled ovarian hyperstimulation and intrauterine insemination in subfertility. How many treatment cycles are sufficient? J Reprod Med. 1998;43(10):903-8.
54. Nuojua-Huttunen S, Tomas C, Bloigu R, et al. Intrauterine insemination treatment in subfertility: an analysis of factors affecting outcome. Hum Reprod. 1999;14(3):698-703.
55. Sahakyan M, Harlow BL, Hornstein MD. Influence of age, diagnosis, and cycle number on pregnancy rates with gonadotropin-induced controlled ovarian hyperstimulation and intrauterine insemination. Fertil Steril. 1999;72(3): 500-4.
56. Campana A, Sakkas D, Stalberg A, et al. Intrauterine insemination: evaluation of the results according to the woman's age, sperm quality, total sperm count per insemination and life table analysis. Hum Reprod. 1996;11(4): 732-6.
57. Berg U, Brucker C, Berg FD. Effect of motile sperm count after swim-up on outcome of intrauterine insemination. Fertil Steril. 1997;67(4):747-50.
58. Custers IM, Steures P, Hompes P, et al. Intrauterine insemination: how many cycles should we perform? Hum Reprod. 2008:23(1):885-8.
59. Morshedi M, Duran HE, Taylor S, et al. Efficacy and pregnancy outcome of two methods of semen preparation for intrauterine insemination: a prospective randomized study. Fertil Steril. 2003;79(3):1625-32.
60. Steures P, van der Steeg JW, Mol BW, et al. Prediction of an ongoing pregnancy after intrauterine insemination. Fertil Steril. 2004;82(1):45-51.
61. Goverde AJ, McDonnell J, Vermeiden JP, et al. Intrauterine insemination or in-vitro fertilisation in idiopathic subfertility and male subfertility: a randomised trial and cost-effectiveness analysis. Lancet. 2000;355(9197):13-8.
62. Nulsen JC, Walsh S, Dumez S, et al. A randomized and longitudinal study of human menopausal gonadotropin with intrauterine insemination in the treatment of infertility. Obstet Gynecol. 1993;82(5):780-6.
63. Crosignani PG, Walters DE. Clinical pregnancy and male subfertility; the ESHRE multicenter trial on the treatment of male subfertility. Hum Reprod. 1994;9(6):1112-8.
64. Nuojua-Huttunen S, Tomas C, Bloigu R, et al. Intrauterine insemination treatment in subfertility: an analysis of factors affecting outcome. Hum Reprod. 1999;14(3):698-703.
65. Khalil MR, Rasmussen PE, Erb K, et al. Intrauterine insemination with donor semen. An evaluation of prognostic factors based on a review of 1131 cycles. Acta Obstet Gynecol Scand. 2001;80(4):342-8.
66. Dickey RP, Taylor SN, Lu PY, et al. Effect of diagnosis, age, sperm quality, and number of preovulatory follicles on the outcome of multiple cycles of clomiphene citrate-intrauterine insemination. Fertil Steril. 2002;78(5):1088-95.
67. Ibérico G, Vioque J, Ariza N, et al. Analysis of factors influencing pregnancy rates in homologous intrauterine insemination. Fertil Steril. 2004;81(5):1308-13.
68. Ghesquiere SL, Castelain EG, Spiessens C, et al. Relationship between follicle number and (multiple) live birth rate after controlled ovarian hyperstimulation and intrauterine insemination. Am J Obstet Gynecol. 2007;197(6):589.
69. Goverde AJ, Lambalk CB, McDonnell J, et al Further consideration on natural or mild hyperstimulation cycles for intrauterine insemination treatment: effects on pregnancy and multiple pregnancy rates. Hum Reprod. 2005;20(11):3141-6.
70. Gulumser C, Narvekar N, Conway G, et al. Limiting multiple pregnancies in 4,242 cycles of IUI: increase in follicle numbers increases multiple pregnancy but not clinical pregnancy rate! Hum Reprod. 2008;23(Suppl 1):i63.
71. van Rumste MM, Custers IM, van der Veen F, et al. The influence of the number of follicles on pregnancy rates in intrauterine insemination with ovarian hyperstimulation: a meta-analysis. Hum Reprod Update. 2008;14(6):563-70.

CHAPTER

21

Stimulation Protocols for Intrauterine Insemination

Kalyani Shrimali, Ritu Hinduja

INTRODUCTION

Intrauterine insemination (IUI) is one of the first lines of infertility treatments and assisted reproductive technologies (ART). It is the safest, least invasive, and cost-effective forms of assisted reproduction.[1]

Ovarian stimulation aims at development of one or more of the ovarian follicles to reach the stage of maturity culminating in release of one or more mature oocytes ready for fertilization. Ovarian stimulation has been shown to significantly improve the outcome in IUI cycles. With the help of ovulation-inducing drugs there is an increase in number of eggs for fertilization and also helping the patients with anovulatory cycles to overcome the subtle defect in the ovulatory function. When IUI is performed in unexplained subfertile couples, ovulation induction (OI) doubles the pregnancy rates, compared with IUI without OI.[2]

There are two mechanisms of ovarian stimulation, the first involves applying pharmacological agents that mimic endogenous gonadotropins (injectable gonadotropins) that directly stimulate ovarian follicular development through gonadotropin receptors. The second involves pharmacological agents that manipulate and moderate endogenous gonadotropin production. These are the oral ovulation through moderating estrogen action, a major regulator of endogenous gonadotropin production.[3]

ORAL AGENTS FOR OVARIAN STIMULATION

Oral agents modulate estrogen action, hence endogenous gonadotropin production through direct effect on estrogen receptors, i.e., selective estrogen receptor modulators [SERMs (clomiphene citrate or tamoxifen)], or through modulation of estrogen production (inhibition), i.e., aromatase inhibitors (AI; letrozole), or inhibition of the estrogen synthesis enzyme (the aromatase enzyme).

Clomiphene Citrate

Clomiphene citrate (CC) has been used as a first-line ovulation-inducing agent for over 40 years. CC is a nonsteroidal triphenylethylene derivative that exhibits both estrogen agonist and antagonist properties, i.e., SERM. CC mainly acts as antiestrogen.[4]

Mechanism of Action: The principal mechanism of action is a reduction in the negative feedback of endogenous estrogens due to prolonged depletion of hypothalamic and pituitary estrogen receptors. This action leads to the release of gonadotropin-releasing hormone (GnRH) from hypothalamus into hypothalamic-pituitary portal circulation, engendering an increase in the release of pituitary gonadotropins.

It is a SERM that stimulates endogenous follicle-stimulating hormone (FSH) production and secretion by interrupting estrogen feedback to the hypothalamus and pituitary. Increased FSH release drives folliculogenesis at the level of ovary.[4]

Regimens of Clomiphene Citrate for Ovarian Stimulation

The regimen usually starts from the early follicular phase that is second to the fifth day of the cycle for 5 days. There is no difference in pregnancy rate whether clomiphene is commenced on day 2, 3, 4, or 5 of the cycle; although, there is perhaps a tendency to multiple follicular development the closer the agent is commenced to menses.

The dose required for achieving ovulation is dependent on the body weight. Although the effective dose of CC ranges from 50 mg/day to 250 mg/day. Most women respond to treatment with 50 mg (52%) or 100 mg (22%). Although higher doses are sometimes required, the success rates are usually very low (150 mg, 12%; 200 mg, 7%; 250 mg, 5%). Most women who fail to respond to 150 mg of CC will ultimately require alternative or combination treatments.[5,6] The usual recommended dose is 100 mg per day.

Pregnancy rates are highest in the early cycles of CC treatment (usually first three cycles) with a significant decline in the chance of achieving pregnancy beyond the third treatment cycle down to a very low chance beyond the sixth treatment cycle.[5]

Outcome[5]

- Pregnancy: 30%
- Failure (No pregnancy despite ovulation): 40%
- Resistance (No ovulation): 25%
- Antiestrogenic effect: 5%

Generally speaking, failure to conceive after six ovulatory cycles of CC treatment should be regarded as a clear indication to expand the diagnostic evaluation to exclude other infertility factors or to change the treatment strategy when evaluation is already complete.[7]

Adverse Effects

Clomiphene citrate is in general a safe medication and usually well tolerated, with most of the side effects being relatively mild; multiple gestations, mild ovarian hyperstimulation being the most common. Other serious long-term adverse effects have been suggested, including increased risk of ovarian cancer.

- *Multiple gestation pregnancy:* The incidence reported for multiple pregnancy is approximately 8% with CC treatment. However, majority of multiple gestations are twins. Triplet and higher order pregnancies are rare.[8]
- Side effects such as vasomotor hot flashes10% also noted. Unusual visual symptoms (visual blurring or persistent after-images) are also noted in 1–2% of patients taking CC, which are likely due to antiestrogenic effects of CC on the visual cortex. These symptoms are rare, universally disappear upon cessation of CC.
- *Severe ovarian hyperstimulation syndrome (OHSS):* The incidence of severe OHSS is difficult to predict in CC treated group; though mild OHSS is relatively common, but does not require active management most of the time.[7]
- *Ovarian cancer:* There is an uncertain association of ovarian cancer that has been suggested in the past. The recent subsequent studies have been reassuring but the question of whether the treatment with ovulation-inducing drugs increases risk of ovarian tumors or cancer still remains unsettled and cannot be summarily dismissed.[9-11] It is best to limit a patients' lifetime exposure to CC to 12 treatment cycles, as additional cycles may place the patient at increased risk of borderline ovarian tumors.[12]

Failure of Clomiphene Citrate Treatment

In anovulatory infertility, the failure is divided into two groups:

1. *Clomiphene resistance:* Patient who fails to ovulate with CC ovarian stimulation, i.e., failure to achieve ovulation. This could be due to one of the two main reasons; insulin resistance [women with polycystic ovarian syndrome (PCOS)] and inappropriate indication for CC treatment, e.g., use in women with ovulatory dysfunction due to medical disorders or in women with WHO Type I or III anovulation.
2. *Clomiphene pregnancy failure:* The patients who ovulate in response to CC treatment but do not achieve pregnancy. These may be related to a variety of other underlying infertility causes such as male factor, endometriosis or tubal factor, or endometrial receptivity factors.

Clomiphene citrate exerts undesirable antiestrogenic effects in the periphery (endocervix, endometrium, ovary, ovum, and embryo) that cannot be avoided due to long half-life of CC isomers. This could explain the discrepancy between ovulation and conception rates observed in CC-treated patients, i.e., explain the clomiphene treatment failure (ovulation but no pregnancy).

Aromatase Inhibitors

Aromatase inhibitors have been used for the last decade as adjunctive treatments in breast cancer. They block the conversion of testosterone and androstenedione to estradiol and estrone, respectively, and hence inhibit the estrogen-negative feedback on the hypothalamic–pituitary axis. This leads to increased gonadotropin secretion, which in turn leads to ovarian follicular growth and development.[13]

Letrozole is the commonly used AI drug for ovulation induction. This is an off-label drug. According to the existing laws, the use of letrozole for ovulation induction alone is not allowed. Thus, it should be used only if the local Food and Drug Administration (FDA) approves it.

Ovulation and pregnancy rates with AI such as letrozole and anastrozole appear to be promising, and these agents appear to have less antiestrogen effect on the endometrium, but the evidence on endometrial effects is conflicting, and most studies show equivalence with CC.[13-16]

The addition of letrozole to gonadotropin stimulation protocols decreases the gonadotropin requirement and increases the number of preovulatory follicles.[17,18]

Dosage

Letrozole is administered in doses of 2.5–5 mg/day for 5 days, starting from day 3 of the cycle.

Extended Letrozole Therapy

In a recent study conducted by Badawy et al. extended letrozole therapy (2.5 mg daily from day 1 of menses for 10 days) was used in CC-resistant PCOS women. They observed that the long letrozole protocol (10 days) can produce more mature follicles and subsequently, more pregnancies than the short letrozole therapy (5 days).[19]

Letrozole Step-up Protocol

Recently, a new protocol known as the letrozole step-up protocol has been reported by Mitwally et al. In this protocol, letrozole was administered in the step-up doses consisting of one, two, three, and four tablets of letrozole (2.5 mg) daily on menstrual cycle days 2, 3, 4, and 5, respectively. When compared with the standard CC protocol (CC 100 mg for 5 days, starting on day 3), the step-up letrozole protocol was associated with multifollicular development and a higher clinical pregnancy rates per treatment cycle (27.3% vs. 11.8%, respectively).[20]

Adverse Effects

Reported side effects are bone pain (20%), hot flashes (18%), back pain (17%), nausea (17%), and dyspnea (14%). These side effects are typically observed after long-term administration.

One major concern is the possible teratogenicity as observed in animal models. There was one concerning report (publishes as an abstract only) of an increase in cardiac and nasal malformations. Following this, in 2005, Health Canada and the manufacturing company of letrozole issued a "Physician Warning Letter" on the off-label use of letrozole for fertility and the possibility of embryotoxicity, fetotoxicity, and teratogenicity found in rats.[21] US FDA banned letrozole for OI use.

More recently, however, Tulandi et al.[22] retrospectively evaluated 911 newborns from letrozole and CC pregnancies. They found a 2.4% incidence of congenital malformations and chromosomal abnormalities in the letrozole group versus 4.8% in the CC group.[22]

The argument in favor of using letrozole is its half-life is only 40–50 hours, means it is effectively cleared from the body by the time embryo implantation.[23]

Anastrozole

Anastrozole is approved only for breast cancer but used as "off-label" drug for OI. Mechanism of action is similar to letrozole.

Tamoxifen Citrate

It is used as an alternative to CC or with CC or in CC-resistant patients. It is structurally related to SERM which has weak estrogenic effect on cervical mucus and the endometrium. This drug also is used as an "off-label" drug.

Dosage: 20–40 mg/day to be started from day 2 to day 5.

Adverse effects: Similar to CC but also noted slight increase in endometrial hyperplasia and endometrial carcinoma.[24]

Contraindication: Liver toxicity, pituitary failure, gonadal failure pregnancies, ovarian cyst, and abnormal uterine bleeding.

Role of Adjuvants

There is no firm evidence of the role of adjuvants in improving the pregnancy rates, many physicians tend to use.

Metformin

This is an oral biguanide insulin-sensitizing agent.

It is supposed to improve ovulation in women with insulin resistance and hyperandrogenism associated with PCOS and in CC-resistant cases. [25]

Mechanism of Action: It reduces the hepatic gluconeogenesis, decreases intestinal absorption of glucose, and increases peripheral utilization of glucose.

Despite conflicting results, combination of metformin and CC should try in CC-resistance cares before attempting either ovarian drilling or gonadotropin use.

Dose: Recommended is 1,000–1,500 g/day in a step-up dose over 2–3 weeks.

Side effects: Nausea, diarrhea, flatulence, vomiting, lactic acidosis, megaloblastic anemia, and metallic taste.

Desirable side-effects especially in obese PCOS would be weight loss.

Contraindication: Liver toxicity during alcohol consumption and during contrast X-ray diagnostic procedure.

Corticosteroids: Dexamethasone (0.25–0.5 mg tablet) and prednisone (5–10 mg tablet) are the most common used drugs along with other OI drugs. The use of these medicines should be restricted to PCOS patients who has high dehydroepiandrosterone (DHEA) levels (>180 mg/dL).

Cabergoline

The routine use in normoprolactinemic anovulation is not recommended.

GONADOTROPINS

Use of gonadotropins has revolutionized the management of infertility.

Use of intramuscular gonadotropins began in the 1960s. Gonadotropins may be urinary derived (human menopausal gonadotropin or hMG) or manufactured using recombinant DNA technology (recombinant FSH or rFSH). Over the last decade, recombinant human FSH has been the main preparation, and it can be self-administered subcutaneously.[25] The rFSH is more expensive per unit dose but has been reported to have greater purity and, therefore greater efficacy of action.

Human menopausal gonadotropin also contains a degree of LH activity and some researcher claim that additional LH effect leads to better follicular/oocyte development and as a result, higher pregnancy rates compared to rFSH. However, there is no published evidence for this, particularly in IUI cycles where there is "background" pituitary production of FSH and LH. This is in contrast to ovarian stimulation for in vitro fertilization (IVF) where there is often concomitant pituitary down regulation using GnRH analogs.

Gonadotropins are used to treat infertility caused by anovulation, usually after other less complicated and costly methods have failed. Two groups of anovulatory disorders may require gonadotropin therapy: (1) hypogonadotropic amenorrhea [HA, also known as hypogonadotropic hypogonadism, hypothalamic amenorrhea, or World Health Organization (WHO) type I amenorrhea]; and (2) PCOS, also known as hyperandrogenic amenorrhea or WHO type II amenorrhea.[26,27]

A recent Cochrane review (2007) on the available results of gonadotropins suggested that gonadotropins might be the most effective drugs when IUI is combined with ovarian hyperstimulation.[28]

Choice of Gonadotropins

The choice of gonadotropin to be used depends upon the day 2 plasma luteinizing hormone (LH)/FSH/estradiol (E2) levels. If serum LH is elevated, FSH containing gonadotropins are indicated, whereas if serum FSH is elevated (>10 mIU/mL), a combination of LH and FSH is used for ovarian stimulation. For ovarian stimulation in patients with hypogonadotrophic hypogonadism, a combination of LH and FSH is used.

Gonadotropin Regimens

Conventional Regimen

In this protocol, a daily dose of 75–150 IU of gonadotropins is started from day 2 or day 3. Serial ultrasonography (USG) for follicular monitoring and serum estradiol (E2) estimation is performed from day 8 onward. This protocol has yielded acceptable pregnancy rates of up to 30%.

Low-Dose Step-Up

The use of a low-dose, step-up regimen of ovulation induction similar to that described by Franks and others (Messinis, 2005).[29] Following induction of menses with either progestagens or the oral contraceptive pill, FSH or hMG is commenced 2–3 days later at a dose no higher than 50–75 IU per day. The dose is not altered until an estrogen (and often ultrasound assessment) around 7 days later. If there is any evidence of an estrogen rise above baseline (even if no follicular development is seen), the existing dose is maintained and further assessment with ultrasounds and hormones are undertaken every 2–3 days. A rising estrogen level indicates follicular development. When there are 1–2 follicles, 17 mm in diameter or larger and the estrogen level is about 1,200 pmol/L or 350 pg/mL, human chorionic gonadotropin (hCG) 5,000–10,000 IU is administered (Fig. 1).

If no rise of estrogen above baseline is seen after 7 days of FSH/hMG, the dose can be cautiously increased by 25–50 IU per day above the previous dose. The process of further assessment 5–7 days later can be repeated, with further increases in FSH/hMG only being necessary in the absence of an estrogen/follicular response.

Step-down Regimen

In a step-down protocol, hMG/FSH therapy at a daily dose of 150 IU is started on day 2 and continued till a dominant follicle of more than 10 mm is observed on transvaginal sonography (TVS). After this, the dose is decreased to 112.5 units intramuscular (IM) per day for 3 days, followed by 75 units IM per day for the next 3 days. This dose is then continued till the day of hCG injection. The rest of the regimen is the same as in the step-up regime.

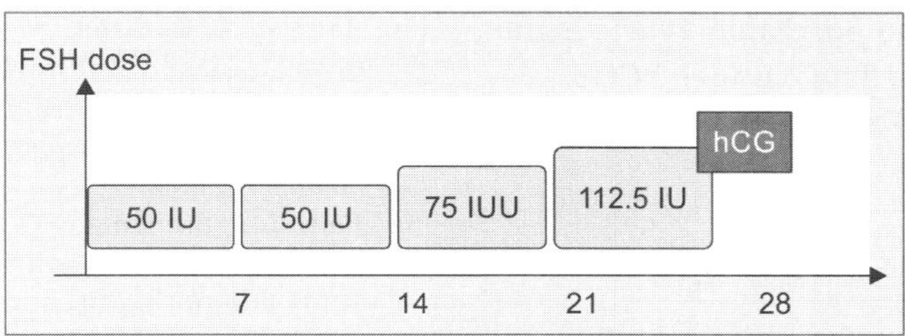

Fig. 1: Low-dose step-up regimen.[30]

In almost 15–20% of the cycles, which have been stimulated with gonadotropins or CC, the exaggerated estradiol level due to the multifollicular development often provokes higher LH levels during the follicular phase or an untimely LH hormone surge, which leads to cycle cancellation. Therefore, in order to avoid interference from endogenous gonadotropin secretion, a combination of gonadotropins and GnRH analogs have being used for ovulation induction. Although GnRH analogs are routinely used in IVF cycles, their routine use in IUI cycles is not recommended. A recent Cochrane review has concluded that GnRH analogs do not significantly improve pregnancy rates in IUI.

Gonadotropin-IUI is a successful treatment but the greatest risk lies with multiple pregnancy, as a result of multiple follicular development.

The aim of treatment is to develop one leading follicle but many times there are other smaller follicles. Additionally, most physicians would accept two codominant follicles as an appropriate result for triggering of ovulation. As a result, twin pregnancies are relatively common and represent about one-fifth of all ongoing pregnancies.

Unlike clomiphene, where pituitary FSH is initially stimulated and then gradually falls in serum level toward midcycle, gonadotropin injections maintain a constant level of serum FSH throughout the follicular phase. As a result the normal process of dominant follicle selection is overridden and even middle-sized follicles can contain an oocyte with the capacity to cause pregnancy. This leads to a higher risk of not only twins but also higher order multiple pregnancies

Gonadotropins Combined with Oral Ovulogens

Oral agents (CC, tamoxifem, letrozole) are given from day 2 to day 5 and hMG or FSH 75 IU or 150 IU is given daily or on alternated days till the desired follicular recruitment is achieved.

The rationale for using this regimen was that addition of gonadotropins on cycle days 7 to 9 would rescue the nondominant follicles.

There are no standardized protocols for the above regimen. The Gonadotropins can be added from cycle day 3 on alternate days or on daily basis from day 3 to 5 days.

The other regimen is to add the gonadotropin from day 7 to 9 or till the follicle reaches the adequate size for trigger.

Studies with CC + hMG or CC + FSH cycle have reported, PRs of 13–23% per cycle, "twin rates" of 7–18%.[31]

However, cancellation of cycles may still be required to prevent complications with excessive number of follcles.

Ovulation Trigger

The ovulation is triggered by the administration of hCG injection when the following conditions are met:

- Leading follicle is 18–20 mm.
- The number of follicles more than 16 mm is not more than four or follicles more than 12 mm are not more than eight in number.
- Serum E2 is not more than 1,500–2,000 pg/mL (serum estradiol level is estimated only if the total number of follicles exceed 12 and if there is a potential chance of OHSS).

CONCLUSION

Clomiphene citrate is an effective treatment for oligo-ovulation and anovulation. It helps to cause regular ovulation and increases pregnancy rates. It should be used only in properly selected patients and for the recommended amount of time. However, success rates with CC are low due to the antiestrogenic effects on the cervix (drying up the mucus) and endometrium.

Letrozole has been shown to be superior to clomiphene for patients with PCOS.

In women with infertility due to oligoanovulation where treatment with CC or metformin is unsuccessful, fair evidence shows that gonadotropin treatment is effective.

Fair evidence shows that the pregnancy rate is higher with hypothalamic amenorrhea than it is with PCOS.

Protocols should attempt to minimize risk of multiple pregnancy and OHSS.

REFERENCES

1. World Health Organization. Infecundity, infertility, and childlessness in developing countries. DHS Comparative Reports No 9. Calverton, Maryland, USA: ORC Macro and the World Health Organization; 2004.
2. Guzick DS, Carson SA, Coutifaris C, et al. Efficacy of superovulation and intrauterine insemination in the treatment of infertility. National Cooperative Reproductive Medicine Network. N Engl J Med. 1999;340:177-83.
3. Mitwally MF, Casper RF. Oral agents for ovarian stimulation: Mild forms of ovarian stimulation. In: Abolghar M, Rizk B (Eds). Ovarian Stimulation. Cambridge: Cambridge University Press; 2010. pp. 1-13.
4. Practice Committee of the American Society for Reproductive Medicine. Use of clomiphene citrate in women. Fertil Steril. 2004;82(Suppl 1):S90-S96
5. Garcia J, Jones GS, Wentz AC. The use of clomiphene citrate. Fertil Steril. 1977;28:707-17.
6. Athaullah N, Proctor M, Johnson NP. Oral versus injectable ovulation induction agents for unexplained subfertility. Cochrane Database Syst Rev. 2002;3.
7. Usadi RS, Fritz MA. Induction of ovulation with clomiphene citrate. In: Sciarra JJ (Ed). Gynaecology and Obstetrics. Philadelphia: Harper & Row;1986.
8. Schenker JG, Yarkoni S, Granat M. Multiple pregnancies following induction of ovulation. Fertil Steril. 1981;35:105-23.
9. Venn A, Watson L, Lumley J, et al. Breast and ovarian cancer incidence after infertility and in vitro fertilization. Lancet. 1995;346:995-1000.
10. Modan B, Ron E, Lerner-Geva L, et al. Cancer incidence in a cohort of infertile women. Am J Epidemiol. 1998;147: 1038-42.
11. Silva I dos S, Wark PA, McCormack VA, et al. Ovarian stimulation drugs and cancer risks: A long-term follow-up of British Cohort. Br J Cancer. 2009;100:1824-31.
12. Rossing MA, Daling JR, Weiss NS, et al. Ovarian tumors in a cohort of infertile women. N Engl J Med. 1994;331: 771-6.
13. Bayar U, Basaran M, Kiran S, et al. Use of an aromatase inhibitor in patients with polycystic ovary syndrome: A prospective randomized trial. Fertil Steril. 2006;86:1447-51.
14. Mitwally MFM, Casper RF. Use of aromatase inhibitor for induction of ovulation in patients with an inadequate response to clomiphene citrate. Fertil Steril. 2001;75:305-9.
15. Al-Fozen H, Al-Khadouri M, Tan SL, et al. A randomized trial of letrozole versus clomiphene citrate in women undergoing superovulation. Fertil Steril. 2004;82:1561-3.
16. Badawy A, Elnashar A, Totongy M. Clomiphene citrate or aromatase inhibitors for superovulation in women with unexplained infertility undergoing intrauterine insemination: A prospective randomized trial. Fertil Steril. 2009;92:1355-9.
17. Bancsi LF, Broekmans FJ, Eijkemans MJ, et al. Predictors of poor ovarian response in in vitro fertilization: A prospective study comparing basal markers of ovarian reserve. Fertil Steril. 2002;77:328-36.
18. Ng EH, Tang OS, Ho PC. The significance of the number of antral follicles prior to stimulation in predicting ovarian responses in an IVF programme. Hum Reprod. 2000;15:1937-42.
19. Badawy A, Mosbah A, Tharwat A, et al. Extended letrozole therapy for ovulation induction in clomiphene-resistant women with polycystic ovary syndrome: A novel protocol. Fertil Steril. 2009;92:236-9.
20. Mitwally MF, Said T, Galal A, et al. Letrozole step-up protocol: A successful superovulation protocol. Fertil Steril. 2008;89:S23-4.
21. Government of Canada. (2005). Health Canada Endorsed Important Safety Information on Femara (letrozole). [online] http://www.hc-sc.gc.ca/dhp-mps/medeff/advisories-avis/prof/_2005/ femara_hpc-cps-eng.php. [Accessed November 2018].
22. Tulandi T, Martin J, Al-Fadhli R, et al. Congenital malformations among 911 newborns conceived after infertility treatment with letrozole or clomiphene citrate. Fertil Steril. 2006;85:1761-5.
23. Casper RF. Letrozole versus clomiphene citrate: Which is better for ovulation induction? Fertil Steril. 2009;92(3):858-9.
24. Speroff L, Glass RH, Kase NG (Eds). Clinical Gynecologic Endocrinology and infertility. Baltimore: Williams and Wilkins; 1999. pp. 1-1200.
25. Guzick DS. Ovulation induction management of PCOS. Clin Obstet Gynecol. 2007;50:255-67.
26. Practice Committee of the American Society for Reproductive Medicine. Current evaluation of amenorrhea. Fertil Steril. 2006;86(Suppl 5):S148-55.
27. Reindollar RH, Novak M, Tho SP, et al. Adult-onset amenorrhea: A study of 262 patients. Am J Obstet Gynecol. 1986;155:531-43.
28. Cohlen BJ, Heineman MJ. Ovarian stimulation protocols (antiestrogens, gonadotropins with and without GnRH agonist/antagonist) for intrauterine insemination in women with subfertility. Cochrane Database Syst Rev. 2007;(2):CD005356.
29. Messinis IE. Ovulation induction: A mini review. Hum Reprod. 2005; 20:2688-97.
30. Bruyneel, Aude & Papas, Ralph & Delbaere, Anne. (2018). Ovulation Induction With Gonadotropins. 10.1016/B978-0-12-801238-3.65169-3.
31. Dickey RP. Strategies to reduce multiple pregnancies due to ovulation stimulation. Fertil Steril. 2009;91(1):1-17.

CHAPTER

22

Timing of Trigger and Insemination

PM Gopinath

INTRODUCTION

Intrauterine insemination (IUI) is the placing of especially prepared, concentrated "washed" sperm into the cavity of the uterus, bypassing the cervix. There are various reasons to consider IUI treatment.

Female Infertility

Unexplained Infertility

This is the most common indication for IUI. Whilst pregnancies can be achieved with natural "timed" intercourse in association with mild ovarian stimulation, better pregnancy rates occur with IUI.

Tubal Disease

There should be at least one normal tube and ovary.

Endometriosis

Intrauterine insemination is used for mild forms but not for severe endometriosis.

Age

This procedure has been shown to have good success in women under 40 years of age.

Male Infertility

Mild Sperm Abnormalities

Intrauterine insemination is an effective treatment where there are minor sperm abnormalities. Where the man has poor quality sperm (low numbers, reduced movement or abnormally shaped sperm), "natural cycle" IUI has very poor results but in that situation IUI can occasionally still be used in combination with ovarian stimulation of the female.

The rationale of IUI treatment is to increase the chances of pregnancy in the couple by increasing the chance that maximum number of healthy sperm reaches as close to the liberated ovum. Hence, it is very important to time the trigger and to effectively perform the IUI which can yield an optimum success rate.

TIMING OF TRIGGER

According to the World Health Organization analysis of natural cycles, ovulation takes place from 24 hours to 56 hours after the onset of the luteinizing hormone (LH) surge, with a mean time of 32 hours. Timing of ovulation in stimulated cycles also varies considerably and depends on the ovarian stimulation protocol used. Oocytes are fertilizable for only a period of 12–16 hours. It has been shown that the period when an oocyte can be successfully fertilized begins 6 hours after ovulation. This means that, even if spermatozoa meet the oocyte in the fallopian tube at the time of ovulation, there still are 6 hours to the fertilizable period of the oocyte to start. This suggests that IUI after observation of ovulation should be preferred to IUI prior to or even to the exact time of ovulation. Hence, IUI is done at either 24 hours or 36 hours after ovulation triggered by human chorionic gonadotropin (hCG) injection.

This is performed in an unstimulated cycle or stimulated with clomiphene citrate (CC) or stimulated cycle with gonadotropin or stimulated with gonadotropin and gonadotropin-releasing hormone (GnRH) analogs.

Unstimulated Cycle

It is illogical to plan an IUI cycle in an unstimulated cycle. However, there are some occasions where we will land up doing IUI in an unstimulated cycle. There is no need to use trigger in this situation. But it is important to predict the precise time of ovulation. Traditional methods for timing insemination were used; basal body temperature charts or cervical mucus assessment. In women who have regular periods and are undergoing unstimulated IUI treatment, IUI was done the day after detecting an LH surge in the urine or blood, which was tested 13–15 days before the next expected menstrual flow. Newer methods involve urine LH kits such as clearplan (Unipath, Bedford, UK), which provide a convenient and reasonably reliable method.[1-4]

Clomiphene-induced Cycle

Clomiphene citrate is the best treatment for majority of women whose infertility is associated with ovulatory dysfunction (anovulation, luteal phase deficiency). Combined with timed IUI, the intake of CC increases the fecundity of the couple. While using CC, it is useful to take the guidance of follicular monitoring with ultrasound. The mean follicular diameter and the trilaminar endometrial thickness are the key factors which guide one to time the trigger. The mean follicular diameter of 18–20 mm and the endometrial thickness of 8 mm will be the appropriate time to trigger.

Gonadotropins-induced Cycle

Induction of ovulation with gonadotropins and IUI are frequently used to treat infertility. Among infertile couple, treatment with induction of ovulation and IUI is three times as likely to result in pregnancy as is intracervical insemination and twice as likely to result in pregnancy as is treatment with either superovulation and intracervical insemination or IUI alone. Here again, the ultrasound follicular monitoring will be the key factor in timing the trigger. When the mean follicular diameter of 18–20 mm along with the endometrial thickness of more than 8 mm is achieved, the trigger can be administered.

Pregnancy rate per cycle of IUI with controlled ovarian hyperstimulation (COH; 9.8%) was significantly higher than that of IUI in natural cycles (3.3%) but approached significance when compared to IUI with CC cycles (5.4%). Also, unexplained infertility cases had a significantly higher pregnancy rate (58.7%) when compared to that of male factor cases (22.8%). IUI combined with COH, gives the best pregnancy rate although its benefit with natural or CC cycles remains obvious.[5]

Gonadotropin-releasing Hormone Analog Cycle

Given the aforementioned physiologic considerations, it follows reasonably that the women most likely to benefit from ovulation induction (OI) with pulsatile GnRH are those with an ovulatory defect resulting from deficient GnRH secretion. Thus, patients with hypogonadotropic hypogonadism will have the highest response rates. This group includes women with primary GnRH deficiency (e.g. Kallmann syndrome) as well as those with an intact hypothalamus but decreased GnRH release (e.g. hypothalamic amenorrhea). The success of GnRH stimulation in these patients led the Food and Drug Administration (FDA) to approve the use of intravenous (IV) pulsatile GnRH for OI in women with primary hypothalamic amenorrhea.

The midcycle LH surge in the reproductive cycle is an intriguing endocrinological phenomenon. The exact details of the mechanism in many species including human are still not known, while it is known that central signaling by hypothalamic GnRH is permissive.[4] Complete blockade of the GnRH receptor terminates the periovulatory LH surge, although alterations in the magnitude of GnRH secretion are not crucial for timing and size of the LH surge.[6]

A premature LH surge can be defined as a premature rise of LH (>10 IU/L) along with a concomitant rise in progesterone more than or equal to 1 ng/mL.[7] Premature LH surge in the natural cycle is very rare,[7] but may be more frequent in older women since their maximum follicle diameter at the time of ovulation is substantially smaller.[8,9]

Premature LH surges also occur in 25–30% of stimulated IUI cycles[7,10] and this may interfere with timing of the IUI or result in cancellation of the treatment and increased treatment failures. Administration of a GnRH antagonist almost completely prevents the premature luteinization but does not substantially improve the clinical pregnancy rate. The GnRH antagonists are used in IUI cycle to prevent the premature luteinization and to avoid untimely inseminations in the weekends. The monitoring and the timing of the trigger again depend on the follicular monitoring and endometrial thickness assessment. Probably premature luteinization is not the cause but one of the consequences of the poor quality of the growing follicle.[7] In seven randomized controlled trials (RCTs), the average ongoing pregnancy rate was only 5.3% greater with GnRH antagonist treatment [95% confidence interval (CI): 1.5, 9.2]. This means that it would take 20 cycles of GnRH antagonist administration to have one pregnancy more than without GnRH antagonist treatment.

CHOICE OF TRIGGER

The most commonly used agent for trigger in the IUI is injection hCG 5,000–10,000 IU. Nowadays, the choriogonadotropin alpha 250 µg in 0.5 mL (Ovitrelle-Merck Serono) or injection ganirelix 0.25 mg (Orgalutran-Schering-Plough), which is approximately equivalent to 6,500 IU of hCG being used in the place of hCG. When the stimulation is performed with gonadotropins and antagonist there is one more option of using GnRH agonist trigger of injection leuprolide acetate 1 mg or 2 mg (Lupride-Sun Pharma) instead of hCG.

Human Chorionic Gonadotropin versus Luteinizing Hormone

Human chorionic gonadotropin has been the universal trigger of final oocyte maturation for decades in assisted reproductive technologies (ARTs) due to structural and biological similarities with LH as both molecules bind to the same receptor, the LH or hCG receptor.[11] Importantly, however, the half-life of hCG is significantly longer than that of LH, more than 24 hours vs. 60 minutes,[12,13] facilitating ovarian hyperstimulation syndrome (OHSS) due to the sustained luteotropic activity and the production of vascular permeability mediators.[14,15] Moreover, even if bona fide OHSS is not diagnosed, luteal ovarian overstimulation is a significant source of physical discomfort during the luteal phase, increasing the treatment burden of the patient.[16] Interestingly, it has previously been reported that patients experience physical discomfort throughout the in vitro fertilization (IVF) treatment; however, even more discomfort is reported during the luteal phase compared with the stimulation phase.[17] Finally, a "standard" bolus of hCG has been shown to induce a significant histological advancement of the endometrium, which could negatively affect the receptivity.[18] This finding is in line with a recent prospective randomized trial, demonstrating the superiority of a spontaneous LH surge vs. an hCG-induced surge in natural cycle frozen embryo transfer cycles. The authors hypothesized that the administration of hCG in the late follicular phase might negatively affect endometrial receptivity by inducing endometrial events which would occur several days later after an endogenous LH surge.[5] Taken together, the ovulatory bolus of hCG increases the physical discomfort of the patient during the luteal phase, increases the risk of OHSS, and might hamper implantation.

The consented doses of hCG administered vary between 5,000 IU and 10,000 IU when urinary hCG is used and 6,500 IU (250 µg) when recombinant hCG is used. Although hCG has been the drug of choice to trigger final oocyte maturation until now, we believe that the time has now come to question this practice. The most natural compound with which to trigger final oocyte maturation and with an expected low incidence of OHSS would have been LH. Thus when recombinant LH (rLH) was introduced, a clinical trial was performed to explore the efficacy of rLH to trigger ovulation in a long GnRH agonist downregulation protocol. Doses differing between 5,000 IU and 30,000 IU were explored. However, apart from the significant increase in cost of treatment, a low implantation rate was seen after only one bolus of rLH to trigger ovulation; moreover, a disappointingly high OHSS rate (12%) was reported.[19,20]

TIMING OF INSEMINATION

Insemination can be performed at various time points around ovulation and can be done once or repeated several times. In the majority of the published studies, the insemination is done 32–38 hours following injection hCG administration[21] and it is believed that IUI at 32–38 hours post-hCG would provide the best results.[22] The scientific basis for 32–38 hours timing is derived from ultrasonographic and hormonal studies that have shown the occurrence of follicle rupture after day 2 post-hCG in 68% of cases in spontaneous cycles[23] and in 81% in stimulated cycles (95% CI; 76–86%).[24]

It is assumed that the timing of insemination relative to ovulation is critical for an optimal success rate, so it is rather surprising that few studies were designed to find the optimal time for insemination.[20] A systematic review found no difference in the pregnancy rate per couple with two inseminations compared with one. As shown in this study (Table 1), the incidence of follicular rupture shown by transvaginal ultrasound scanning (TVS) at the time of IUI ranged between 68% and 76%, which agrees with the above studies and lends credence to choosing the timing of IUI at 36 ± 2 hours post-hCG. The effects of timing of IUI in relation to ovulation and the number of inseminations on cycle pregnancy rate in common infertility etiologies.

Several retrospective studies have provided conflicting results with regard to the impact of the number of inseminations on clinical pregnancy rate. However, meta-analysis of all cycles of single and double IUI in three randomized trials with the husband's sperm seemed to show an increased probability of pregnancy with double IUI.[25] On the other hand, two systematic reviews found no difference in the pregnancy rate per couple with two inseminations when compared with one.[25] Moreover, a more recent randomized trial of single vs. double IUI

Table 1: Cycle outcome related to occurrence of ovulation at IUI 36 ± 2 hours post-hCG.

Parameter	*All cycles*	*Male*	*Nonmale total*	*Anovulation*	*Unexplained*
Cycle outcome known	1,146	428	718	226	492
Ovulation status known	1,114	422	692	212	480
Ovulation present (n)[a]	816	322	494	146	348
Ovulation absent (n)[a]	298	100	198	66	132
Ovulation rate (%)	73.2	76.3	71.3	68.3	72.5
All cycles with clinical pregnancy (n)[a]	116	30	86	34	52
Overall CPR[b] (%)	10.1	7.1	12.4	16.1	10.8
Pregnancies in positive ovulation cycles (n)[a]	96	24	72	28	44
CPR[b] in cycles with positive ovulation (%)	11.7	7.4	14.6	19.1	12.6
Pregnancies in negative ovulation cycles (n)[a]	20	6	14	6	8
CPR[b] with negative ovulation (%)	6.7	6	7	9.9	6
OR (95% CI) of pregnancy in positive ovulation vs. negative ovulation cycles	1.85 (1.12–3.06)	1.26 (0.52–2.95)	2.2 (1.23–4.08)	2.1 (0.91–4.85)	2.08 (1.01–4.31)
P	0.015[c]	0.82[c]	0.007[c]	0.071[c]	0.047[c]

(a: number; b: cycle pregnancy rate; c: X^2 test; CI: confidence interval; CPR: clinical pregnancy rate; hCG: human chorionic gonadotropin; OR: odds ratio; IUI: intrauterine insemination)

in multifollicular ovarian hyperstimulation cycles in unexplained and mild male infertility[26] found no difference.

Studies show that pregnancy rates and live birth rates are statistically and clinically significantly higher for 36 hours IUI than 24 hours after hCG administration. The live birth rate declines with age but OI–IUI still seems beneficial up to age 44. In conclusion, pregnancy and live birth rates are higher when IUI is performed 36 hours after hCG than at 24 hours.

Guzick[27] and Abdelkader and Yeh[28] reviewed the available evidence for single and double IUI and both agreed that double IUI adds more to cost and inconvenience to CPR and recommended a well-timed single IUI. However, we should remember that there are limitations to the use of meta-analysis in the context of IUI studies because of heterogeneity of the published trials.

REFERENCES

1. Vermesh M, Kletzky OA, Davajan V, et al. Monitoring techniques to predict and detect ovulation. Fertil Steril. 1987;47(2):259-64.
2. Robinson JN, Lockwood GM, Dalton JD, et al. A randomized prospective study to assess the effect of the use of home urinary LH detection on the efficiency of donor insemination. Hum Reprod. 1992;7(1):63-5.
3. Lashen H, Afnan M, Kennefik A. Early resort to ovarian stimulation improves the cost-effectiveness of a donor insemination programme. Hum Reprod. 1999;14(8):1983-8.
4. Khattab AF, Mustafa FA, Taylor PJ. Hum Reprod. 2005;20(9):2542-5.
5. Hannoun A, Abu-Musa A, Kaspar H, et al. Intrauterine insemination IUI: the effect of ovarian stimulation and infertility diagnosis on pregnancy outcome. Clin Exp Obstet Gynecol. 1998;25(4):144-6.
6. Dubourdieu S, Charbonnel B, D'Acremont MF, et al. Effect of administration of a gonadotropin-releasing hormone (GnRH) antagonist (Nal-Glu) during the periovulatory period: the luteinizing hormone surge requires secretion of GnRH. J Clin Endocrinol Metab. 1994;78(2):343-7.
7. Lambalk CB, Leader A, Olivennes F, et al. Treatment with the GnRH antagonist ganirelix prevents premature LH rises and luteinization in stimulated intra-uterine insemination: results of a double-blind, placebo-controlled, multicentre trial. Hum Reprod. 2006;21(3):632-9.
8. de Koning CH. McDonnell J, Themmen AP, et al. The endocrine and follicular growth dynamics throughout the menstrual cycle in women with consistently or variably elevated early follicular phase FSH compared with controls. Hum Reprod. 2008;23(6):1416-23.
9. Klein NA, Harper AJ, Houmard BS, et al. Is the short follicular phase in older women secondary to advanced or accelerated dominant follicular development? J Clin Endocrinol Metab. 2002;87(12):5746-50.
10. Cantineau AE, Heineman MJ, Cohlen BJ. Single versus double intrauterine insemination (IUI) in stimulated cycles for subfertile couples. Cochrane Database Syst Rev. 2003;(1):CD003854.
11. Kessler MJ, Reddy MS, Shah RH, et al. Structures of N-glycosidic carbohydrate units of human chorionic gonadotropin. J Biol Chem. 1979;254(16):7901-8.
12. Yen SS, Llerena O, Little B, et al. Disappearance rates of endogenous luteinizing hormone and chorionic gonadotropin in man. J Clin Endocrinol Metab. 1968;28(12):1763-7.

13. Damewood MD, Shen W, Zacur HA, et al. Disappearance of exogenously administered human chorionic gonadotropin. Fertil Steril. 1989;52(3):398-400.
14. Papanikolaou EG, Pozzobon C, Kolibianakis EM, et al. Incidence and prediction of ovarian hyperstimulation syndrome in women undergoing gonadotropin-releasing hormone antagonist in vitro fertilization cycles. Fertil Steril. 2006;85(1):112-20.
15. Delvigne A, Rozenberg S. Epidemiology and prevention of ovarian hyperstimulation syndrome (OHSS): a review. Hum Reprod Update. 2002;8(6):559-77.
16. Cerrillo M, Rodriguez S, Mayoral M, et al. Differential regulation of VEGF after final oocyte maturation with GnRH agonist versus hCG: a rationale for OHSS reduction. Fertil Steril. 2009;91(4 Suppl):1526-8.
17. Boivin J, Takefman JE. Impact of the in-vitro fertilization process on emotional, physical and relational variables. Hum Reprod. 1996;11(4):903-7.
18. Fanchin R, Peltier E, Frydman R, et al. Human chorionic gonadotropin: does it affect human endometrial morphology in vivo? Semin Reprod Med. 2001;19(1):31-5.
19. European Recombinant LH Study Group. Human recombinant luteinizing hormone is as effective as, but safer than, urinary human chorionic gonadotropin in inducing final follicular maturation and ovulation in in vitro fertilization procedures: results of a multicenter double-blind study. J Clin Endocrinol Metab. 2001;86(6):2607-18.
20. Aboulghar M, Al-Inany H. Triggering ovulation for IVF. Reprod Biomed Online. 2005;10(1):142.
21. The ESHRE Capri Workshop Group. Intrauterine insemination. Hum Reprod Update. 2009;15(3):265-77.
22. Ragni G, Somigliana E, Vegetti W. Timing of intrauterine insemination: where are we are? Fertil Steril. 2004;82(1):25-6.
23. Luciano AA, Peluso J, Koch EI, et al. Temporal relationship and reliability of the clinical, hormonal, and ultrasonographic indices of ovulation in infertile women. Obstet Gynecol. 1990;75(3 Pt 1):412-6.
24. Pearlstone AC, Surrey ES. The temporal relation between the urine LH surge and sonographic evidence of ovulation: determinants and clinical significance. Obstet Gynecol. 1994;83(2):184-8.
25. Duran HE, Morhedi M, Kruger T, et al. Intrauterine insemination: a systemic review on determinants of success. Hum Reprod Update. 2002;8(4):373-84.
26. Bagis T, Haydardedeoglu B, Kilicdag EB, et al. Single versus double intrauterine insemination in multi-follicular ovarian hyperstimulation cycles: a randomized trial. Hum Reprod. 2010;25(7):1684-90.
27. Guzick DS. For now, one well-timed intrauterine insemination is the way to go. Fertil Steril. 2004;82(1):30-1.
28. Abdelkader AM, Yeh J. The potential use of intrauterine insemination as a basic option for infertility: a review for technology-limited medical settings. Obstet Gynecol Int. 2009;2009:584837.

CHAPTER

23

Monitoring an IUI Cycle: Ultrasonography and Hormonal Parameters

Carlos Iglesias Sánchez, Juan A García-Velasco

INTRODUCTION

The intrauterine insemination (IUI) procedure consists of washing an ejaculated semen specimen to remove prostaglandins, concentrating the sperm in a small volume of culture media and injecting the sperm suspension directly into the upper uterine cavity using a small catheter that is inserted through the cervix.

Depending on the source of the semen sample, IUI can be performed with semen from a male partner or from a donor.

CLINICAL USE OF INTRAUTERINE INSEMINATION

Clinical use of IUI is based on the hypothesis that placing a large number of sperm in the reproductive tract enhances the likelihood of conception. The idea is that IUI improves three main factors that determine success rates:

1. We stimulate the ovaries so that we can obtain more than one oocyte in a single cycle. Notably, in a natural cycle only one follicle grows.
2. We avoid circumvent dysfunctions of the cervical mucus, since a catheter is passed into the endometrial cavity where the semen sample is deposited.
3. We employ techniques for sperm processing such as the "swim-up" method or density gradient centrifugation to select sperm with good motility and morphology that are then placed close to the fallopian tubes.

The pregnancy rate after IUI depends on male factors and technical factors, all of which are discussed in this chapter.

REQUIREMENTS FOR INTRAUTERINE INSEMINATION

To perform an IUI procedure, the following conditions must be met: the patient's ovaries must have adequate function so that an ovulation can be induced, at least one fallopian tube must be open, there must be an adequate number of motile sperm according to the World Health Organization (WHO) reference values and there must not be any documented or suspected active cervical, intrauterine, or pelvic infections.

- Even if the ovaries show adequate function, the woman's age must be considered, as multiple treatment cycles are not beneficial in older women.

Dovey et al. reported that on a per patient treated basis, cumulative pregnancy rates by age were 24.2% for women under age 35 years, 18.5% for women aged 35–37 years, 15.1% for women aged 38–40 years, 7.4% for women aged 41–42 years and 1.8% for women older than 42 years (one pregnancy in 55 patients). In that study, there were no pregnancies after the fourth cycle in women aged 41 years and older.[1]

As of 2012, in Instituto Valenciano de Infertilidad, the pregnancy rate after IUI using semen from the couple was 18.7% per cycle and the rate using semen from a donor was 23.2% per cycle. However, as women ages, these rates decrease to 10% for women older than 35 years and to less than 5% for women older than 40 years.

- Many techniques have been proposed to determine whether the woman's fallopian tubes are open.

We recommend using a hysterosalpingography, a technique that introduces a radiopaque medium through the cervix. X-rays are used to visualize whether the fluid can pass through the tubes.

Swart et al. determined that although hysterosalpingography is of limited use for detecting tubal patency because of its low sensitivity, its high specificity makes it a useful test for ruling in tubal obstruction.[2]

However, others like Malek-Mellouli et al. report better results using hysterosonography; this technique is less painful, patients tolerate it better and no ionizing radiation is used.[3]

Determination of the presence of anti-*Chlamydia trachomatis* antibodies have been proposed for excluding tubes obstruction. Raoofi et al. report a negative predictive value of 100% when using anti-*C. trachomatis* immunoglobulin G (IgG) antibody detection to predict at least one normal tube in infertile women without a history of abdominal or pelvic surgery, pelvic inflammatory disease or endometriosis.[4]

Notably, the use of laparoscopy should be limited to cases suspected of having etiologies other than intratubal occlusion, such as endometriosis or peritubal adhesions.

- The reference values of the WHO, 2010 should be used to determine whether a semen sample is adequate:[5]
  - *Sperm concentration:* There should be more than 15 million sperm/mL or more than 39 million in the semen sample
  - *Sperm motility rate:* At least 32% of the sperm should be motile
- *Morphology:* At least 4% of sperm should have normal morphology

Before starting IUI, two main issues should be considered, i.e. the number of previous IUIs and how long the couple has been infertile.

1. Depending on the number of IUI cycles that have been performed, in IVI, we recommend 3–4 IUI cycles using semen from the couple or 4–6 cycles using semen from a donor. The cumulative pregnancy rates do not increase if more IUI cycles are performed. If pregnancy is not achieved, we recommend starting with an in vitro fertilization (IVF) cycle.

   To determine the number of IUIs that should be performed, we should also consider the etiology of the infertility, since the prognosis is worse if anovulatory disorders, mild male factors or unexplained infertility are present.
2. The appropriate time to begin IUI depends on how long the couple has been infertile and on the age of the women.

In women younger than 35 years of age, we recommend starting with IUI once the couple has been infertile for a year despite regular sexual intercourse. However, in women older than 35 years of age, we recommend starting after 6 months of infertility despite regular sexual intercourse.

Currently, experts differ concerning the number of cycles of IUI that should be performed or how to proceed after IUI fails before trying an IVF cycle.

In 2006, the European guidelines (Denmark, England, Wales, France, the Netherlands) suggested 3–6 IUIs be performed, depending on the cause of infertility.[6]

The National Institute for Health and Care Excellence (NICE) guidelines of 2013 recommend that couples who have not conceived after six cycles of donor or partner insemination, despite evidence of normal ovulation, tubal patency and semen analysis, should consider trying a further six cycles of unstimulated IUI before IVF is considered.

The NICE guidelines also recommend that couples who are having regular unprotected sexual intercourse and who are diagnosed with unexplained infertility, mild endometriosis, or mild male factor infertility, should not routinely be offered IUI, either with or without ovarian stimulation.

The guidelines further suggest that couples try to conceive for a total of 2 years (including the year before they begin to investigate fertility options) before considering IVF.[7]

INDICATIONS FOR INTRAUTERINE INSEMINATION

Intrauterine insemination is indicated in the following situations:

- Couples who are having regular unprotected sexual intercourse but who are diagnosed with unexplained infertility
- *Women with anovulatory disorders*: Intrauterine insemination is indicated for patients diagnosed with polycystic ovarian syndrome or with hypothalamic or pituitary disorders that lead to anovulation.
- *Men with mild male factor infertility*: Intrauterine insemination is indicated when there is male infertility because of diminished semen (according to WHO semen sample value references: more than 15 million sperm/mL, at least 32% of the sperm should be motile, at least 4% of sperm should have normal morphology). IUI is indicated, when after processing the semen sample, the sample has at least 3 million motile sperm.

In IVI we perform IUI, irrespective of the teratozoospermia rate, if after processing the sample has more than 3 million of motile sperm/mL.

- *Women diagnosed with mild endometriosis*: Intrauterine insemination is indicated for women undergoing ovulation induction, including those with minimal or mild endometriosis, pregnancy rates are higher with IUI compared to timed natural intercourse (NIC). In such couples, surgery has historically been performed, both to improve pain and treat infertility in women with endometriosis.

However, IUI is often used as an intermediate level, cost-effective intervention prior to proceeding to superovulation and IVF, both of which have proven to be effective in assisting women with endometriosis, to conceive.[8]

- *Mild cervical factor infertility*: Intrauterine insemination is indicated when cervical factors are affecting fertility. IUI allows sperm to bypass potentially hostile cervical factors and increase the number of sperm that gain access to the uterine cavity and the oocyte.

On the basis of a meta-analysis of 980 IUI cycles in randomized and prospective studies, Zeyneloglu concluded that a patient's chances of becoming pregnant are greater with IUI with her husband's sperm than with timed intercourse in superovulated cycles with gonadotropins.[9]

In 2005, Helmerhorst conducted a Cochrane review of randomized and controlled trials, and found that IUI was no more effective than timed intercourse for treatment of subfertility attributed to abnormal cervical mucus.[10]

However, as we noted previously, pregnancy rates also depend on the age of the woman and how long infertility has persisted. Women younger than 35 years of age have better pregnancy rates than older women.

- *Couples who are unable to or who find it very difficult to have vaginal intercourse*: Intrauterine insemination is indicated when there is a clinically diagnosed physical disability or psychosexual problem, such as severe vaginismus, ejaculatory dysfunction, hypospadias, or neurologic impotency.
- Couples in same-sex relationships
- Couples with conditions that require special consideration in terms to the method of conception, such as when one partner has a sexually transmitted disease, like human immunodeficiency virus (HIV) or hepatitis C.

Intrauterine insemination is indicated for couples in which the male is infected in order to prevent the transmission of infection to his female partner and to the fetus.

The first option is to start IUI using prepared (washed) sperm from the infected male. However, after the wash, if the semen sample has mediocre or poor quality sperm according to the WHO parameters, we recommend proceeding with IVF-intracytoplasmic sperm injection (IVF-ICSI) treatment.

Many reports from our group shows that sperm wash with nested polymerase chain reaction (PCR) and ICSI is a cost-effective, safe, and effective procedure that can prevent HIV and hepatitis C virus (HCV) transmission, while offering reasonable pregnancy rates.[11-13]

If the woman is HIV infected and man is uninfected, the goal is to prevent transmission of the virus to the man. Pregnancy rates are similar to those in HIV-uninfected couples undergoing artificial reproductive techniques.

SPERM COLLECTION AND PROCESSING

Intrauterine insemination is usually performed using fresh sperm from the woman's partner.

Semen Collection

We ask men to provide a semen sample 2 hours before IUI following 2 days or 3 days of sexual abstinence. Notably, prolonged abstinence decreases pregnancy rates, independent of other sperm parameters, perhaps as a result of sperm senescence and functional damage that is not readily identified by standard semen analysis.[14]

However, there is controversy about the quality of the semen sample that is needed, and the minimum and maximum period of sexual abstinence prior to semen sample provision. Marshburn et al. established that an ejaculatory abstinence period of less than or equal to 2 days before IUI produced the highest pregnancy rates per cycle compared with longer intervals of ejaculatory abstinence.[15]

The semen specimen is produced by masturbation in a private room designated for this purpose. The entire ejaculate is collected in a sterile cup to minimize the risk of uterine infection from contaminants. We advise the avoidance of lubricants, as most are toxic to sperm.

Sperm Processing

It is critical to separate sperm in the ejaculate from the prostaglandin-rich prostatic secretions and seminal fluid, which can cause uterine cramping, and very often anaphylaxis, when placed directly into the uterine cavity.

In addition, sperm preparation maximizes the number of motile sperm for insemination, removes cellular debris and concentrates the specimen.

Two techniques for sperm processing that are commonly employed are the "swim-up" method and "density gradient centrifugation". Boomsma et al. published a systematic review of randomized trials that compared these two techniques and found no statistically significant differences in pregnancy rates.[16] However, the percentage of motile sperm recovered after processing is generally higher with density gradient centrifugation than with the swim-up technique.[17] Therefore, we prefer to use this method for men with oligo- or asthenospermia.

An aliquot of the processed sample is evaluated prior to insemination to ensure that an adequate number of moving sperm has been recovered.

The minimum post-wash total motile sperm count for IUI is controversial. In IVI, we established that a count total (washed) motile sperm greater than 3 million/mL is associated with higher pregnancy rates. A lower count warrants further evaluation. IVF-ICSI is the appropriate course of treatment for overcoming severe male factor infertility.

TIMING THE INSEMINATION

The luteinizing hormone (LH) surge can be detected in serum 36 hours before ovulation and in urine, 24 hours before ovulation. The oocyte can be fertilized up to 24 hours after ovulation and sperms are most capable of fertilization up to 48 hours after entering the female genital tract. Timing of the IUI is based on these relationships.

Evaluation of the effectiveness of different synchronization methods in natural and stimulated cycles for IUI in subfertile couples concluded that the choice of IUI timing should be based on hospital facilities, patient convenience, medical staff, costs and drop-out levels. No method was clearly superior to the other.

Zreik and García-Velasco reported that timing the IUI while monitoring folliculogenesis by ultrasound (US) and using human chorionic gonadotropin (hCG) induction of ovulation does not appear to produce an increased pregnancy rate over urinary LH monitoring of ovulation.[18,19]

However, the optimum time for IUI is controversial within the 24–36 hours after hCG triggering. Rahman et al. report that altering the timing of IUI after controlled ovarian stimulation does not enhance pregnancy rates. They found that IUI performed 36 hours after hCG has marginally better pregnancy rates than after 24 hours.[20] Recently, Dehghani-Firouzabai et al. have compared the fertility rates in women who had an hCG injection before and after IUI. They concluded that hCG administration after IUI did not improve the pregnancy rate. Therefore, hCG can be administered either before or after IUI.[21]

Performing one versus two IUIs is also controversial. Rahman et al. conducted a prospective randomized trial that compared the efficacy of two versus one IUI in a population of 160 couples with unexplained infertility in which the woman underwent a controlled ovarian hyper stimulation and IUI.

The pregnancy rates were similar and statistically there were no difference between the groups. This suggested that using two IUI has no added advantage over use of a single IUI.[22] In our research group, Matorras conducted a meta-analysis and found that no significant differences when two inseminations per cycle were performed, compared with one insemination.[23] For these reasons, we now perform a single IUI 36 hours after hCG injection.

HOW CAN FOLLICLE SIZE BE MONITORED?

The use of a transvaginal US is recommended because it allows better determination of the size of the follicles than an abdominal US approach.

Many authors recommend using US to obtain the highest quality images of the ovaries, fallopian tubes and uterus, and to avoid invasive diagnostic methods.[24] US can provide accurate diagnoses, is cost-effective, and is reliable and minimally invasive. Ekerhovd described an US-based approach for assessing infertilty.[25] A vaginal US scan is also useful for determining the status of the endometrial cavity and for detecting polyps or fibromas that could decrease pregnancy rates. Pérez-Medina determined that once a polyp is diagnosed by vaginal US, hysteroscopic polypectomy before IUI is an effective measure. In their study group, women were more likely to become pregnant after polypectomy, with a relative risk (RR) of 2.1 [95% confidence interval (CI), 1.5–2.9].[26]

Over time, new US techniques have been introduced to assess reproductive status, such as three-dimensional (3D) US, and Doppler and power Doppler US. Kupesic found that 3D US has increased accuracy compared to a conventional two-dimensional transvaginal scan and allows precise reconstruction of the uterine cavity.[27]

Wu reported that the detection of subendometrial blood flow by 3D power Doppler US might be a useful US parameter for predicting the IVF pregnancy rate.[28]

Schild studied the relationship between blood flow and fertility outcomes in IVF but concluded that neither Doppler US of the spiral or uterine arteries nor measurement of the endometrial thickness or volume reliably predicted subsequent IVF outcome.[29]

Bhal et al. used power Doppler to assess whether there was a relationship between perifollicular vascularity and outcome in vivo following hCG administration. A group of 182 unselected consecutive patients undergoing stimulated IUI cycles was recruited for a study in which the perifollicular vascularity of follicles greater than equal to 16 mm was examined using a subjective grading system and transvaginal power Doppler ultrasonography, 36 hours after hCG administration. Their findings suggested that perifollicular vascularity plays an important role in the outcome of IUI cycles, and that power Doppler has the potential to refine the management of assisted reproduction treatment cycles.[30]

Chang proposed using US to count the antral follicles in order to predict the response to stimulation.[31] Later, US was used to assess, more exactly, the ovarian response after stimulation by measuring the ovarian volume rather than the follicle-stimulating hormone (FSH) levels;[32-34] even to predict the ovarian response to ovulation induction.

However, these measures vary depending on the person who performs the US. To compare the interobserver reliability of antral follicle counts, Jayaprakasan et al. compared real-time two-dimensional US with offline counts performed on stored 3D images. Two observers conducted trans- vaginal US examinations in 45 subfertile women in the early follicular phase of their menstrual cycles. Antral follicles were counted using real-time two-dimensional US and the time it took to perform the count was recorded. A 3D volume was then acquired from each ovary and stored for subsequent offline analysis using the multiplanar view. They published that there was a significantly higher interobserver reliability for counts made using 3D (mean: 0.992; 95% CI, 0.986–0.996) compared with real-time two-dimensional (mean: 0.961; 95% CI, 0.940–0.977) ($P < 0.01$).[35]

Mercè et al. confirmed that the intraobserver and interobserver reproducibility of the ovarian volume, follicle counts and 3D power Doppler angiography indices is excellent. They employed a first observer who acquired two volumes for each ovary, plus a second observer who performed a second analysis of the volumes acquired by the first one. They analyzed ovarian volume, follicle number in the basal group, vascularization index, flow index and vascularization-flow index. The volumes were processed by the virtual organ computer-aided analysis imaging program using plane A and 15 degrees rotational steps.[36] Raine-Fenning also conclude that rotational measurement of ovarian volume from 3D US data is significantly more reliable between observers than volume estimation from two-dimensional parameters.[37]

Another paper from this group examined the intraobserver and interobserver reliability of the semiquantitative determination of ovarian, endometrial and subendometrial blood flow using 3D power Doppler angiography plus virtual organ computer-aided analysis (VOCAL). When ultrasounds were performed on two different subjects, the intraobserver reliability for two observers was extremely high. There were no differences in reliability between the observers for the measurements of volume and vascularity within the ovary or endometrium.[38] Two years later, this group supports the use of the inversion mode of US for the identification and classification of pathological processes that are associated with hypoechogenic fluid filled areas, such as hydrosalpinges and ovarian cysts.[39] Use of 3D US to study polycystic ovaries revealed that they have increased stromal volume and vascularity. This vascularity is significantly higher in women with polycystic ovary syndrome who are hirsute and of normal weight.[40]

Opinions differ about what constitutes adequate size for the leading follicle in terms of the size of the follicle on the day of the hCG injection. A retrospective cohort study conducted by Ghosh et al. concluded that the group of women who received hCG when the follicular diameters were 20 mm or bigger were less likely to become pregnant, compared to women with follicular diameters between 15–19.99 mm (RR 0.58; 95% CI, 0.35–0.97).[41]

In a retrospective analysis of 122 cycles of controlled ovarian stimulation, Silverberg et al. predicted the number of expected ovulations in any given cycle of controlled ovarian hyperstimulation. They reported that the percentages of follicles measuring less than or equal to 14 mm, 15–16 mm, 17–18 mm, 19–20 mm, and greater than 20 mm on the day of hCG administration that subsequently ovulated which were 0.5%, 37.4%, 72.5%, 81.2% and 95.5%, respectively. Thus, the closer the size of the follicle to 20 mm, the greater the possibility of ovulation.[42] Recently, Palatnik et al. investigated the optimal size of the leading follicle in ovulation induction with clomiphene citrate and letrozole and reported higher pregnancy rates when the leading follicles were in the 23–28 mm range.[43]

Merviel et al. analyzed 1,038 cycles of IUI to determine the predictive factors for successful IUI. They concluded that depending on the follicle size, the ideal stimulation cycle enables the recruitment of two follicles measuring greater than 16 mm with an estradiol concentration greater than 500 pg/mL on the day of hCG administration.[44]

In IVI, we trigger ovulation with hCG, once there is a leading follicle at least 17 mm of diameter.

INTRAUTERINE INSEMINATION IN UNSTIMULATED CYCLES

Natural cycle procedures are most appropriate for patients with ejaculatory dysfunction, vaginismus, stenosis of the cervix after surgery and for single women or couples who do not want a twin pregnancy. Ovulation should be documented prior to proceeding with an unstimulated cycle of IUI.

Kyrou et al. conducted a randomized trial that included 300 patients and reported that ovulation monitoring and spontaneous triggering of ovulation is associated with significantly higher ongoing pregnancy rates compared with administration of hCG in patients undergoing IUI in natural cycles (34/150 versus 16/150, P = 0.008; difference of 12%; 95% CI, 3.6–20.4).[45]

However, in IVI once we check we confirm by transvaginal US that there is a leading follicle that is 17 mm in diameter, we inject hCG and proceed with the IUI 36 hours later.

INTRAUTERINE INSEMINATION IN STIMULATED CYCLES

The aim of controlled ovarian hyperstimulation is to enhance follicular development in order to stimulate ovulation. Controlled ovarian hyperstimulation is commonly used with IUI for treating couples with unexplained infertility. The objective is to hyperstimulate the ovaries in order to increase the size of one, two or three follicles to improve the chances of pregnancy. If more than three follicles grow, we can offer the patients lower the doses to try to reduce the number of leading follicles that develop. Another possibility is to cancel the cycle by stopping the medication and using barrier methods to avoid the risk of a multiple pregnancy. A third option is to continue the medication and go ahead with an IVF cycle, so we do not lose the cycle, and multiple pregnancies can be avoided by transferring only one embryo and vitrifying the others.

WHAT ARE THE ADVANTAGES OF INTRAUTERINE INSEMINATION COMPARED WITH PROGRAMMED COITUS?

In a 2012 Cochrane review that included six trials where IUI was compared with timed intercourse, both using stimulated cycles, there was evidence of an increased chance of pregnancy after IUI [six randomized controlled trials (RCTs), 517 women, odds ratio (OR) 1.68; 95% CI, 1.13–2.50].

There was also a significant increase in the live birth rate for women who underwent IUI with ovarian stimulation compared with IUI in a natural cycle (four RCTs, 396 women, OR 2.07; 95% CI, 1.22–3.50).[46]

WHICH DRUGS SHOULD BE USED TO STIMULATE OVULATION?

Clomiphene Citrate

Clomiphene citrate is the standard first-line therapy; if it is unsuccessful, injectable gonadotropins are usually the next step. Clomiphene citrate is affordable and very well tolerated. However, pregnancy rates are lower than with the use of stimulating gonadotropins because of the anti-estrogen effect of clomiphene citrate on the endometrium (it damages the growth of the endometrial lining).

Berker et al. compared the efficacy of clomiphene citrate versus recombinant FSH (rFSH) protocols in ovarian stimulation in IUI cycles for couples with unexplained infertility or male subfertility. They concluded that FSH is superior to clomiphene citrate for enabling multifollicular development and that the pregnancy rate per cycle was 9.6% and 15.6% for the clomiphene citrate and the rFSH groups, respectively (P = 0.31).[47]

For most patients, the first-line approach is clomiphene citrate (50–150 mg) for five consecutive days, beginning on cycle day 5 to day 9 and starting with vaginal US to measure the size of the follicle on days 10–12, depending on the patient's usual menstrual cycle length.

In a prospective longitudinal study, Imani et al. developed a nomogram to predict the individual's chances of live birth after clomiphene citrate administration. The nomogram included the free androgen index (testosterone/sex hormone-binding globulin ratio), body mass index (BMI), cycle history (oligomenorrhea vs amenorrhea), and the woman's age.[48]

Despite the possibilities of ovulation using clomiphene citrate, in IVI, we begin the stimulation using gonadotropins as the pregnancy rates per cycle are higher.

Aromatase Inhibitors

Aromatase inhibitors continue to be investigated as a therapeutic option for women who fail to conceive with clomiphene-based approaches. Requena et al. conducted a meta-analysis of four RCTs that compared the overall effect of letrozole with clomiphene citrate in patients with polycystic ovary syndrome. They concluded that letrozole is as effective as other methods of ovulation induction but randomized-controlled studies are warranted to define more clearly the efficacy and safety of letrozole in human reproduction.[49] Tulandi et al. compared congenital malformations and chromosomal abnormalities between a group in which clomiphene citrate was used to induce ovulation and a group in which letrozole was used. They reported that 14 of 514 newborns in the letrozole group (2.4%) and that 19 of 397 newborns in the clomiphene citrate group (4.8%) showed abnormalities. They concluded that there was no difference in the overall rates of major and minor congenital malformations in newborns from mothers who conceived after letrozole versus clomiphene citrate treatments. Thus, the idea that letrozole has teratogenic effects, when used for ovulation induction, is unfounded based on their data.[50]

Although letrozole use is controversial, this drug is not Food and Drug Administration (FDA) approved for use in infertility treatment. We do not use in IVI to induce ovulation based on its potential teratogenic effect on embryo development.

Gonadotropins

For older and younger women with diminished ovarian reserve, we induce ovulation with injectable gonadotropins or we directly IVF.

We prefer to use rFSH because it is more effective than urinary FSH for inducing ovulation. In addition, it is highly pure without differences between lots, and it is easy to adjust the exact dose and administer without damaging women health. Matorras et al. concluded that rFSH is associated with a higher per cycle pregnancy rate than urinary FSH, when used at the same dose; whereas the pregnancy rate is similar when the dose of rFSH is 50% lower.[51]

A large clinical trial sponsored by the National Institute of Health (NIH) randomly assigned 932 infertile couples with unexplained infertility or early stage endometriosis to one of four treatment groups: NIC, IUI, FSH injections plus intracervical insemination (ICI), or FSH injections plus IUI. The pregnancy rate in the control ICI group was 2% per cycle, while in the FSH plus ICI and the FSH plus IUI groups the pregnancy rates per cycle were 4% and 9%, respectively. Thus, FSH plus ICI and FSH plus IUI are clearly effective for the treatment of unexplained infertility.[52]

In a trial of gonadotropin injections with or without IUI, 62 couples with unexplained infertility were randomly assigned to receive IUI alone, gonadotropin injections alone, or gonadotropin injections plus IUI. The per cycle pregnancy rate was 2.2% for IUI alone, 6.1% for gonadotropin injections alone and 26% for gonadotropin injections plus IUI.[53]

Injectable gonadotropins are introduced on cycle day 2 or day 3 once US confirms that there are no remaining cysts bigger than 10 mm. If there is a cyst, we can prescribe an oral contraceptive pill for 21 days, or we can wait until the next menstruation happens and then check whether the cyst has disappeared.

It is the standard of care to follow serum estradiol levels and ovarian follicle size using transvaginal ultrasounds. Once the follicle has grown to 17 mm of size, it may correspond with 150-200 pg/mL of serum estradiol level.

How Should the Gonadotropin Dose be Determined?

The usual dose of gonadotropins varies from 50–100 IU, depending on the age of the woman, her ovarian reserve markers, her BMI and the etiology of infertility.

In polycystic ovarian women, we start by giving 50 IU dose and continue with a step-down stimulation protocol that depends on the ovarian response. Clinicians must proceed very carefully because of the possibility of a hyperstimulation response. After 5 days of stimulation, the patient should have a vaginal US to check if there is an ovarian response and to determine the number of follicles that have been recruited, the endometrial thickness, and how the patient is tolerating the medication.

The patient should then have a vaginal US every 2–3 days to monitor the speed of the follicle growth and the number of follicle that are getting bigger. If there are more than three follicles that are at least 14 mm in diameter, we recommend the medication and cancel the cycle to avoid a high multiple pregnancy, or even an ovarian hyperstimulation syndrome. If this excessive response happens twice again, we recommend starting with an IVF cycle in which the number of embryos to be transferred can be controlled. This also prevents the development of ovarian hyperstimulation syndrome.

IS A MULTIFOLLICULAR RESPONSE DESIRABLE?

By increasing the number of follicles, we increase the possibility of pregnancy. However, we should avoid multiple pregnancies and the development of ovarian hyperstimulation syndrome.

Pregnancy rates are better with ovarian controlled stimulation than natural cycles (21.5% vs 12%). The 2009 European workshop of European Society of Human Reproduction and Embryology (ESHRE), recommended proceeding with stimulated cycles to obtain better results.

In cases of IUI, that uses a donor semen sample, we recommend follicular stimulation in which the gonadotropin dose is adjusted according to the woman's BMI, age and ovarian reserve markers. Patients younger than 35 years receive 50–75 IU, while those who are older than 35 years receive 75–100 IU during the first 5 days of stimulation. After the first vaginal US scan, we adjust the doses of medication if the ovarian response is not adequate.

The objective is to develop 1 or 2 follicles to be triggered with hCG when they reach 17 mm in diameter and proceed with the IUI 36 hours later. If the woman does not get pregnant, we can start a new cycle of stimulation on the second or third day of menstruation. In this new stimulation protocol, we can increase the doses by 25–50 IU in order to develop three follicles and thereby increase the chances of pregnancy.

HOW DO WE MONITOR FOLLICLE DEVELOPMENT?

After 5 days of stimulation, we perform the first determination of estradiol serum levels and a vaginal US scan to measure the size of each follicle. The mean of the two maximum diameters of the follicle are used.

The timing of the next vaginal US depends on how fast the follicles are growing. Generally speaking, patients receive an US scan to measure the follicles sizes every 2 days until they reach 17 mm in diameter.

TRIGGERING OVULATION AND INSEMINATION

When at least one follicle reaches a mean diameter of 17–19 mm, the patient self-administers 5,000–6,500 IU of hCG using a subcutaneous or intramuscular injection to trigger ovulation.

To better monitor the cycle we determine serum estradiol levels. Preovulatory levels should be around 150–200 pg/mL for each mature follicle. One IUI is performed 36 hours after hCG injection.

IS A DOUBLE INSEMINATION RECOMMENDED?

The question remains: Is two IUIs per cycle better than a single IUI? Some clinicians perform a single IUI the day after detection of a urinary LH surge (or 36 hours following hCG injection). Others prefer two IUIs: one on the day of the LH surge and next, the day after (12–18 hours and 36 hours after hCG injection). The idea is that double insemination (24 hours and 48 hours after hCG injection) provides intrauterine motile sperm in case of premature ovulation.

As we noted previously, several meta-analyses have concluded that there is no improvement in the pregnancy rate when a second IUI is performed.[22,23] Indeed, our pregnancy rates are similar for single versus double IUI. Thus, we recommend performing only one IUI 36 hours after hCG injection. It is more comfortable for the couple to have one visit at which a semen sample is provided, and it also means less work for the laboratory and lower consumption of materials and staff resources, and less time for the couple and the clinic.

Two weeks after, the IUI the patient undergoes a urine or blood test to determine if she is pregnant.

IS IT NECESSARY TO USE ULTRASOUND-GUIDED INTRAUTERINE INSEMINATION?

A randomized trial that we conducted did not find higher pregnancy rates when abdominal ultrasound-guided IUI was performed.

The study included 73 consecutive couples that underwent IUI and a total of 231 IUI cycles were performed. The patients were randomized into two groups: an US-guided IUI group (n = 33) and a clinical IUI group (n = 40). The pregnancy rate was 16% per cycle in the US-guided IUI group and 16.8% in the control group; there were no statistically significant differences between the groups. We concluded that eco-guided IUI does not produce better results than blind insemination, as the pregnancy rate per cycle is similar.[54] However, it may be useful when it is difficult to access the uterine cavity.

LUTEAL PHASE SUPPORT

After the IUI we suggest starting with vaginal tablets of 200 mg of natural micronized progesterone every 12 hours. However, progesterone supplementation in the luteal phase is still controversial.

Kyrou et al. studied the effect of luteal phase supplementation on pregnancy rates in hCG-induced natural frozen-thawed embryo transfer (FET) cycles. The study group consisted of 452 cycles: 243 cycles that were supplemented with progesterone administration (600 mg of natural micronized progesterone in three separate doses) and 209 cycles without progesterone. No statistically significant differences were observed in the pregnancy rates between the two groups (22% vs 21%, P = 0.8; difference = +1%; 95% CI, -6.5 to +8.7). Devreoy et al. concluded that there is no convincing evidence to support the use of luteal phase supplementation in hCG-induced natural FET cycles, since there is no luteal phase defect.[55]

Apart from progesterone, we do not administer any other medications, such as salicylic acid, heparin, or estradiol.

ARE GONADOTROPIN-RELEASING HORMONE ANTAGONISTS USEFUL?

The addition of a GnRH antagonist (GnRHa) to rFSH or menotropin during controlled ovarian stimulation may improve pregnancy rates by reducing the incidence of premature luteinization in women with some types of ovulatory dysfunction. These factors can be added to the controlled ovarian stimulation cycle when the lead follicle is 14 mm in size. This delays luteinization and allows the development of additional follicles, which is particularly useful if only one follicle has developed.

Martinez-Salazar et al. evaluated 662 patients who were undergoing IUI. The overall incidence of premature luteinization was 11.5%. In patients with and without premature luteinization, the pregnancy rates were 22.4% (17/76) and 17.7% (104/586), respectively. Patients with premature luteinization were divided into two groups: those with increased serum progesterone [the pregnancy rate was 10.7% (3/28) in this group]; and patients with elevated serum LH but normal progesterone concentrations [the pregnancy rate was 29.2% (14/48) in this group]. Patients in the first group who did not become pregnant (n = 22) were administered GnRHa in a second IUI cycle and the pregnancy rate was 18.1%; however, some patients (n = 6; 27.3%) in this group still had high serum progesterone concentrations. In the second group, patients (n = 26) with elevated serum LH in the previous cycle were administered GnRHa in another IUI and the pregnancy rate was 23.1%. Martinez-Salazar et al. concluded that the use of a GnRHa in patients with premature luteinization who had a previous unsuccessful IUI could be considered in future cycles.[56]

The use of a GnRHa may also be beneficial in preventing luteinization when IUI is delayed over a weekend or holiday in practices with staffing restrictions. To look at this, Matorras et al. compared the results of IUI plus the use of GnRHa to avoid IUI on the weekend versus the results of IUI obtained with the standard IUI protocol. The per cycle pregnancy rate were very similar in both groups, i.e. 15.7% in the IU free weekend group versus 16.5% in the standard IUI group. Thus, in IUI cycles with ovarian superstimulation with gonadotropins, the use of a GnRHa allows the manipulation of follicular development in such a way that it is possible to avoid inseminations on the weekends, apparently without reducing the pregnancy rate.[57]

Checa et al. confirmed this finding. Their study involved patients with an IUI US scan on a Friday that showed greater than one and less than three follicles greater than or equal to 17 mm, indicating that the IUI should be performed during the weekend. The patients received half of the dose of rFSH that had been receiving for two more days in addition to cetrorelix [0.25 mg subcutaneously (SC)] until the day of hCG administration. The researchers concluded that this is a useful alternative for medical centers in which an on call gynecologist is not available.[58]

NUMBER OF INTRAUTERINE INSEMINATION CYCLES

Pregnancy rates are significantly lower after the third IUI cycle, irrespective of the ovulation induction method. Smith et al. investigated how many IUIs are needed to achieve pregnancy before starting IVF stimulation. They determined the pregnancy rates of couples after one [Hazar Ratio (HR) 2.9 (1.4–5.8)], two [HR 2.0 (0.9–4.5)] and three IUI cycles [HR 4.5 (1.8–10.9)]. No additional benefit was seen for couples undergoing four or more IUI cycles [HR 1.0 (0.4–2.6)].[59]

As we explained earlier, after three IUIs without achieving a pregnancy, we generally move on to IVF treatment.

CONCLUSIONS

- Intrauterine insemination is a useful technique for achieving pregnancy in couples diagnosed with infertility due to unknown causes. It can also be useful when there is severe sexual dysfunction and for patients with cervical factor infertility, as long as at least one fallopian tube is open
- Whether IUI is performed during a natural cycle or a stimulated cycle, we suggest use of an hCG injection 36 hours prior to the IUI
- For patients with mild male factor infertility, early stage endometriosis or unexplained infertility, we suggest controlled ovarian hyperstimulation with IUI rather than natural cycle IUI
- Clomiphene may be used for ovarian stimulation. However, pregnancy rates are significantly better when gonadotropins are used for ovarian stimulation
- The best way to monitor follicular growth is to perform transvaginal USthe first day of stimulation. Subsequently, it should be performed every 2 days until the follicles reach a mean diameter of 17 mm. In this moment serum estradiol levels are 150–200 pg/mL for each mature follicle
- We recommend 3–4 cylces of IUI plus a unique insemination 36 hours after hCG injection.

REFERENCES

1. Dovey S, Sneeringer RM, Penzias AS. Clomiphene citrate and intrauterine insemination: analysis of more than 4100 cycles. Fertil Steril. 2008;90:2281-6.
2. Swart P, Mol BW, van der Veen F, et al. The accuracy of hysterosalpingography in the diagnosis of tubal pathology: a meta-analysis. Fertil Steril. 1995;64: 486-91.
3. Malek-Mellouli M, Gharbi H, Reziga H. The value of sonohysterography in the diagnosis of tubal patency among infertile patients. Tunis Med. 2013;91:387-90.

4. Raoofi Z, Barchinegad M, Haghighi L. The value of negative Chlamydia trachomatis antibody in prediction of normal tubes in infertile women. Clin Exp Obstet Gynecol. 2013;40:95-7.
5. Sarabia L, Munuce MJ. Updated reference values for sperm counts (WHO 2010). Rev Med Chile. 2011;139:548-9.
6. Haagen EC, Hermens RP, Nelen WL, et al. Subfertility guidelines in Europe: the quantity and quality of intrauterine insemination guidelines. Hum Reprod. 2006;21:2103-9.
7. National Institute for Health and Care Excellence (2013). Assessment and treatment for people with fertility problems. Available from http://www.nice.org.uk/ CG011. [Accessed January, 2014].
8. Bernardi LA, Pavone ME. Endometriosis: an update on management. Womens Health (Lond Engl). 2013;9:233-50.
9. Zeyneloglu HB, Arici A, Olive DL, et al. Comparison of intrauterine insemination with timed intercourse in superovulated cycles with gonadotropins: a meta-analysis. Fertil Steril. 1998;69:486-91.
10. Helmerhorst FM, Van Vliet HA, Gornas T, et al. Intra-uterine insemination versus timed intercourse for cervical hostility in subfertile couples. Cochrane Database Syst Rev. 2005;CD002809.
11. Garrido N, Meseguer M, Remohí J, et al. Semen characteristics in human immunodeficiency virus (HIV)-and hepatitis C (HCV)-seropositive males: predictors of the success of viral removal after sperm washing. Hum Reprod. 2005;20:1028-34.
12. Garrido N, Meseguer M, Bellver J, et al. Report of the results of a 2 year programme of sperm wash and ICSI treatment for human immunodeficiency virus and hepatitis C virus serodiscordant couples. Hum Reprod. 2004;19: 2581-6.
13. Meseguer M, Garrido N, Gimeno C, et al. Comparison of polymerase chain reaction-dependent methods for determining the presence of human immunodeficiency virus and hepatitis C virus in washed sperm. Fertil Steril. 2002;78:1199-202.
14. Jurema MW, Vieira AD, Bankowski B, et al. Effect of ejaculatory abstinence period on the pregnancy rate after intrauterine insemination. Fertil Steril. 2005;84:678-81.
15. Marshburn PB, Alanis M, Matthews ML, et al. A short period of ejaculatory abstinence before intrauterine insemination is associated with higher pregnancy rates. Fertil Steril. 2010;93:286-8.
16. Boomsma CM, Heineman MJ, Cohlen BJ, et al. Semen preparation techniques for intrauterine insemination. Cochrane Database Syst Rev. 2007;CD004507.
17. Morshedi M, Duran HE, Taylor S, et al. Efficacy and pregnancy outcome of two methods of semen preparation for intrauterine insemination: a prospective randomized study. Fertil Steril. 2003;79:1625-32.
18. Zreik TG, García-Velasco JA, Habboosh MS, et al. Prospective, randomized, crossover study to evaluate the benefit of human chorionic gonadotropin-timed versus urinary luteinizing hormone-timed intrauterine inseminations in clomiphene citrate-stimulated treatment cycles. Fertil Steril. 1999;71:1070-4.
19. Garcia-Velasco JA, Arici A, Zreik TG. Endogenous LH surge detection versus administration of hCG to correctly time intrauterine insemination: which provides a better pregnancy rate? Hum Reprod. 2000;15:975-6.
20. Rahman SM, Karmakar D, Malhotra N, et al. Timing of intrauterine insemination: an attempt to unravel the enigma. Arch Gynecol Obstet. 2011;284:1023-7.
21. Dehghani-Firouzabai R, Aflatoonian A, Davar R, et al. A comparison of pregnancy rate before and after the administration of hCG in intrauterine insemination. Arch Gynecol Obstet. 2014;289:429-32.
22. Rahman SM, Malhotra N, Kumar S, et al. A randomized controlled trial comparing the effectiveness of single versus double intrauterine insemination in unexplained infertility. Fertil Steril. 2010;94:2913-5.
23. Osuna C, Matorras R, Pijoan JI, Rodríguez-Escudero FJ. One versus two inseminations per cycle in intrauterine insemination with sperm from patients' husbands: a systematic review of the literature. Fertil Steril. 2004;82:17-24.
24. Nargund G. Time for an ultrasound revolution in reproductive medicine. Ultrasound Obstet Gynecol. 2002;20:107-11.
25. Ekerhovd E, Fried G, Granberg S. An ultrasound-based approach to the assessment of infertility, including the evaluation of tubal patency. Best Pract Res Clin Obstet Gynaecol. 2004;18:13-28.
26. Pérez-Medina T, Bajo-Arenas J, Salazar F, et al. Endometrial polyps and their implication in the pregnancy rates of patients undergoing intrauterine insemination: a prospective, randomized study. Hum Reprod. 2005;20:1632-5.
27. Kupesic S, Kurjak A. Diagnosis and treatment outcome of the septate uterus. Croat Med J. 1998;39:185-90.
28. Wu HM, Chiang CH, Huang HY, et al. Detection of the subendometrial vascularization flow index by three-dimensional ultrasound may be useful for predicting the pregnancy rate for patients undergoing in vitro fertilization-embryo transfer. Fertil Steril. 2003;79:507-11.
29. Schild RL, Knobloch C, Dorn C, et al. Endometrial receptivity in an in vitro fertilization program as assessed by spiral artery blood flow, endometrial thickness, endometrial volume, and artery blood flow. Uterine Fertil Steril. 2001;75:361-6.
30. Bhal PS, Pugh ND, Gregory L, et al. Perifollicular vascularity as a potential variable affecting outcome in stimulated intrauterine insemination treatment cycles: a study using transvaginal power Doppler. Hum Reprod. 2001;16: 1682-9.
31. Chang MY, Chiang CH, Hsieh TT, et al. Use of the antral follicle count to predict the outcome of assisted reproductive technologies. Fertil Steril. 1998;69: 505-10.
32. Syrop CH, Dawson JD, Husman KJ, et al. Ovarian volume may predict assisted reproductive outcomes better than follicle stimulating hormone concentration on day 3. Hum Reprod. 1999;14:1752-6.
33. Tomas C, Nuojua-Huttunen S, Martikainen H. Pretreatment transvaginal ultrasound examination predicts ovarian responsiveness to gonadotrophins in in-vitro fertilization. Hum Reprod. 1997;12:220-3.
34. Frattarelli JL, Lauria-Costab DF, Miller BT, et al. Basal antral follicle number and mean ovarian diameter predict cycle cancellation and ovarian responsiveness in assisted reproductive technology cycles. Fertil Steril. 2000;74:512-7.
35. Jayaprakasan K, Campbell BK, Clewes JS, et al. Three-dimensional ultrasound improves the interobserver reliability of antral follicle counts and facilitates increased clinical work flow. Ultrasound Obstet Gynecol. 2008;31:439-44.

36. Mercé LT, Gómez B, Engels V, et al. Intraobserver and interobserver reproducibility of ovarian volume, antral follicle count, and vascularity indices obtained with transvaginal 3-dimensional ultrasonography, power Doppler angiography, and the virtual organ computer-aided analysis imaging program. J Ultrasound Med. 2005;24:1279-87.
37. Raine-Fenning NJ, Campbell BK, Clewes JS, et al. The interobserver reliability of ovarian volume measurement is improved with three-dimensional ultrasound, but dependent upon technique. Ultrasound Med Biol. 2003;29:1685-90.
38. Raine-Fenning NJ, Campbell BK, Clewes JS, et al. The reliability of virtual organ computer-aided analysis (VOCAL) for the semiquantification of ovarian, endometrial and subendometrial perfusion. Ultrasound Obstet Gynecol. 2003; 22:633-9.
39. Raine-Fenning NJ, Lam PM. Assessment of ovarian reserve using the inversion mode. Ultrasound Obstet Gynecol. 2006;27:104-6.
40. Lam PM, Johnson IR, Raine-Fenning NJ. Three-dimensional ultrasound features of the polycystic ovary and the effect of different phenotypic expressions on these parameters. Hum Reprod. 2007;22:3116-23.
41. Ghosh C, Buck G, Priore R, et al. Follicular response and pregnancy among infertile women undergoing ovulation induction and intrauterine insemination. Fertil Steril. 2003;80:328-35.
42. Silverberg KM, Olive DL, Burns WN, et al. Follicular size at the time of human chorionic gonadotropin administration predicts ovulation outcome in human menopausal gonadotropin-stimulated cycles. Fertil Steril. 1991;56:296-300.
43. Palatnik A, Strawn E, Szabo A, et al. What is the optimal follicular size before triggering ovulation in intrauterine insemination cycles with clomiphene citrate or letrozole? An analysis of 988 cycles. Fertil Steril. 2012;97:1089-94.e1-3.
44. Merviel P, Heraud MH, Grenier N, et al. Predictive factors for pregnancy after intrauterine insemination (IUI): an analysis of 1038 cycles and a review of the literature. Fertil Steril. 2010;93:79-88.
45. Kyrou D, Kolibianakis EM, Fatemi HM, et al. Spontaneous triggering of ovulation versus hCG administration in patients undergoing IUI: a prospective randomized study. Reprod Biomed Online. 2012;25:278-83.
46. Veltman-Verhulst SM, Cohlen BJ, Hughes E, et al. Intra-uterine insemination for unexplained subfertility. Cochrane Database Syst Rev. 2012;9:CD001838.
47. Berker B, Kahraman K, Taskin S, et al. Recombinant FSH versus clomiphene citrate for ovarian stimulation in couples with unexplained infertility and male subfertility undergoing intrauterine insemination: a randomized trial. Arch Gynecol Obstet. 2011;284:1561-6.
48. Imani B, Eijkemans MJ, te Velde ER, et al. A nomogram to predict the probability of live birth after clomiphene citrate induction of ovulation in normogonadotropic oligoamenorrheic infertility. Fertil Steril. 2002;77:91-7.
49. Requena A, Herrero J, Landeras J, et al. Use of letrozole in assisted reproduction: a systematic review and meta-analysis. Hum Reprod Update. 2008;14:571-82.
50. Tulandi T, Martin J, Al-Fadhli R, et al. Congenital malformations among 911 newborns conceived after infertility treatment with letrozole or clomiphene citrate. Fertil Steril. 2006;85:1761-5.
51. Matorras R, Osuna C, Exposito A, et al. Recombinant FSH versus highly purified FSH in intrauterine insemination: systematic review and metaanalysis. Fertil Steril. 2011;95:1937-42.
52. Guzick DS, Carson SA, Coutifaris C, et al. Efficacy of superovulation and intrauterine insemination in the treatment of infertility. National Cooperative Reproductive Medicine Network. N Engl J Med. 1999;340:177-83.
53. Serhal PF, Katz M, Little V, et al. Unexplained infertility—the value of Pergonal superovulation combined with intrauterine insemination. Fertil Steril. 1988; 49:602-6.
54. Ramón O, Matorras R, Corcóstegui B, et al. Ultrasound-guided artificial insemination: a randomized controlled trial. Hum Reprod. 2009;24:1080-4.
55. Kyrou D, Fatemi HM, Popovic-Todorovic B, et al. Vaginal progesterone supplementation has no effect on ongoing pregnancy rate in hCG-induced natural frozen-thawed embryo transfer cycles. Eur J Obstet Gynecol Reprod Biol. 2010;150:175-9.
56. Martinez-Salazar J, Cerrillo M, Quea G, et al. GnRH antagonist ganirelix prevents premature luteinization in IUI cycles: rationale for its use. Reprod Biomed Online. 2009;19:156-61.
57. Matorras R, Ramón O, Expósito A, et al. GnRH antagonists in intrauterine insemination: the weekend-free protocol. J Assist Reprod Genet. 2006;23: 51-4.
58. Checa MA, Prat M, Robles A, et al. Use of gonadotropin-releasing hormone antagonists to overcome the drawbacks of intrauterine insemination on weekends. Fertil Steril. 2006;85:573-7.
59. Smith JF, Eisenberg ML, Millstein SG, et al. Fertility treatments and outcomes among couples seeking fertility care: data from a prospective fertility cohort in the United States. Fertil Steril. 2011;95:79-84.

CHAPTER

24

Sperm Preparation for Intrauterine Insemination

Naval Navin Shah

INTRODUCTION

Advancement in techniques of artificial reproductive technology (ART) has revolutionized the treatment of infertility. Over the years, with a shift of assisted reproduction from mere gynecological indications to more of andrological indications, there has been an urge by researchers to develop more sophisticated techniques to separate functional spermatozoa from those that are immotile, have poor morphology or are incapable of fertilizing oocytes.[1] The fact that fertilization can be achieved with very few spermatozoa by intracytoplasmic sperm injection (ICSI) should not prevent the need for greatest care while retrieving as many normal sperms as necessary for intrauterine insemination (IUI).[2] IUI is an inexpensive, noninvasive, and effective method of assisted reproduction for selected patients with idiopathic infertility or cervical factor with mild to moderate male factor and infertility with ejaculatory disorders. The procedure works by increasing the number of healthy motile sperm available for fertilization. With ART, semen samples must first be processed before they can be used for insemination.[3]

PURPOSE OF SEMEN PREPARATION

Normally in the female genital tract, motile spermatozoa separate themselves from seminal plasma, immotile spermatozoa, leukocytes, debris and pathogens by actively migrating through the cervical mucus. This active migration selects progressively motile spermatozoa and allows them to undergo capacitation. The same conditions can be achieved in vitro by means of sperm preparation techniques. It has the following advantages:

- It removes seminal fluid which may become an obstacle to the fertilization when the in vitro fertilization or the IUI are performed.[4] Sperm may also lose functional capacity during prolonged exposure to seminal plasma as it inhibits capacitation and acrosome reaction.
- It helps to eliminate dead sperms, leukocytes, other cellular debris, etc. which may release reactive oxygen species (ROS) which also affect integrated sperms.
- It is critical that the spermatozoa are separated from the seminal plasma within 1 hour of ejaculation, to limit any damage from products of nonsperm cells.[5] It also helps to remove microbes and prostaglandins from the semen sample.

Hence, spermatozoa need to be separated from seminal plasma for insemination.

SPERM PREPARATION TECHNIQUES

As we keep understanding the physiology of sperm and realize the importance of the integrity of male gamete in both fertilization and development of the embryo more do we realize the need for improving sperm separation techniques. An ideal sperm processing technique should be gentle and one that recovers a highly functional sperm population.[1] Serial centrifugation of the semen is known to induce sperm dysfunction mediated through production of ROS by spermatozoa and leukocytes.[6-8] Therefore, using proper sperm washing technique which will lend the least stress on sperms is very much essential. Over the years various methods have been developed for sperm selection with different advantages and disadvantages.

This chapter will discuss the various sperm preparation and selection techniques used to process sperm for use with

ART from commonly used ones as a simple wash, swim-up, and density gradient centrifugation to new technologies like magnetic-activated cell sorting (MACS). It will also explain the procedures used to prepare samples procured using assisted ejaculation and retrograde ejaculation.

Conventional Techniques

Swim-up

The swim-up technique is based on active self-migration of motile spermatozoa into the wash medium. This technique can be used only for the sample with a high proportion of progressively motile sperms. Originally described by Mahadeven and Baker,[9] this is a method of choice in the case where no male factor is present to mild male factor infertility, i.e. when semen sample is largely considered to be normal.

Protocol:

- Mix the liquefied semen sample in 14 mL rounded bottom tube, duly identified with the details of the patient. Add sperm washing (buffered) media in approximately 1:1 proportion and homogenize.
- Centrifuge for 10 minutes at 2,000 rpm (600 g).
- Discard the supernatant leaving only the formed pellet.
- According to the quality of the sample, slide through the wall of the tube 0.5 mL to 1 mL of sperm washing media (the media volume will be directly proportional to the concentration of the sample) without disturbing the pellet.
- Leave the tube with the cap tightened inside the carbon dioxide (CO_2) incubator for 20–45 minutes, with an angle of approximately 45° to facilitate the migration of the sperms.
- Pipet up approximately 0.5 mL from the top of the supernatant containing the motile sperm, and shift them in a 6 mL rounded bottom tube.
- Analyze the concentration and motility of the capacitated sample.
- Keep the tube with a tightened cap at 37 °C until its utilization (Fig. 1).

The swim-up method has been modified for the oligozoospermic sample[10] and is known as direct swim-up. In this method, you have to underlay the semen with buffer media and sperms swim-up from semen rather than cell pellet as in regular swim-up. Direct swim-up is the simplest and fastest method for separating sperm by migration. Round-bottom tubes work well for direct swim-up as it maximizes the surface area when tilted and kept in an incubator between the semen and medium.

The swim-up method is simple and relatively inexpensive.[1] It is also easy to perform and does not take highly specialized skills.

But it also has disadvantages and they are as follows:

- Centrifugation, which is performed to create a cell pellet before conventional swim-up is in close contact with cellular debris, leukocytes and dead or defective sperms, hence ROS generation is also high.[6]
- The number of motile spermatozoa retrieved is relatively low.
- Only limited number of the sperm cells which are at the upper surface of the pellet is subjected to swim-up are retrieved.
- When a concentrated cell pellet is used, some motile spermatozoa may be trapped in the middle of the pellet and thus may not travel as far as the sperm cells at the edges of the pellet.

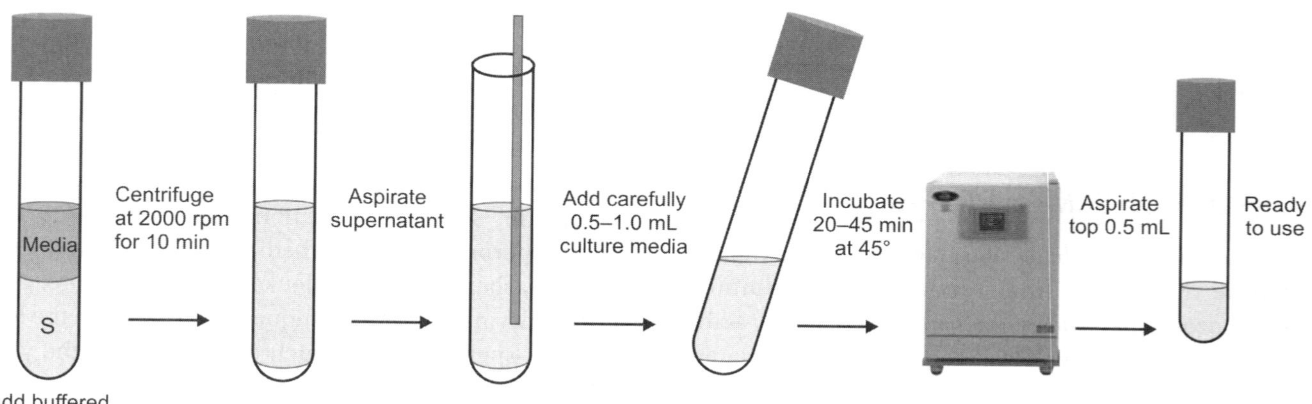

Fig. 1: The swim-up technique. Equal aliquots of semen and media are mixed together and after centrifugation pellet is incubated with media for approximately 45 minutes. Top approximately 0.5 mL of this is later used as a final aliquot.

Density Gradient

Density gradient centrifugation separates sperm cells based on their density. Thus, at the end of centrifugation, each spermatozoon is located at the gradient level that matches its density.[11] Morphologically normal and abnormal spermatozoa have different densities. A mature morphologically normal spermatozoon has a density of at least 1.10 g/mL whereas an immature and morphologically abnormal spermatozoon has a density between 1.06 g/mL and 1.09 g/mL.[12] As a result, the resulting interphases between seminal plasma and 45%, 45% and 90%, containing the leukocytes, cell debris and morphologically abnormal sperm with poor motility, are discarded. The highly motile, morphologically normal, and viable spermatozoa form a pellet at the bottom of the tube.

Protocol (Table 1 and Fig. 2):

- Prepare the gradients layers in conical tubes. Slide first between 0.5 mL and 1.5 mL (depending on the concentration and motility of the sample: use more medium as better the sample is) of the 90% gradient and thereupon the 45% gradient. After checking that both phases are properly formed, slide the semen sample. The volume of each phase has to be in the same proportion (1:1:1). In cases of poor samples (debris, a high number of immotile sperms, etc.) or high-volume samples, it is advisable to split the sample into more gradients (with a maximum of 1.5 mL of semen sample per tube of the gradient).
- Centrifuge for 10–15 minutes at 1,600 rpm (300 g; the time will be inversely proportional to the quality of the sample).
- Discard the supernatant and shift the pellet to a clean conical tube containing 2–3 mL of buffered media and mix it well.
- Centrifuge for 5–10 minutes at 2,000 rpm (600 g).
- Discard the supernatant and add a volume of 0.5 mL of buffered media to the pellet and resuspend.

Table 1: Advantages and disadvantages of density gradient.

Advantages	*Disadvantages*
We obtain a better fraction of morphologically normal sperms because of interphases through which sperms have to migrate	Production of good interphases between layers requires skill
Results in a higher recovery rate of motile sperm	Poor total motile sperm recovery may be seen in semen samples that are highly viscous, show sperm agglutination and have very poor sperm concentration and motility
As most of dead sperms and leukocytes are eliminated ROS production is significantly reduced	Some scientists have claimed that density gradient centrifugation negatively affects sperm DNA integrity. For instance, Zini et al.[13] found that spermatozoa recovered after density gradient centrifugation possess lower DNA integrity than spermatozoa recovered after swim-up
Spermatozoa from oligozoospermic semen can be effectively separated with density gradient centrifugation[1]	

(DNA: deoxyribonucleic acid; ROS: reactive oxygen species)

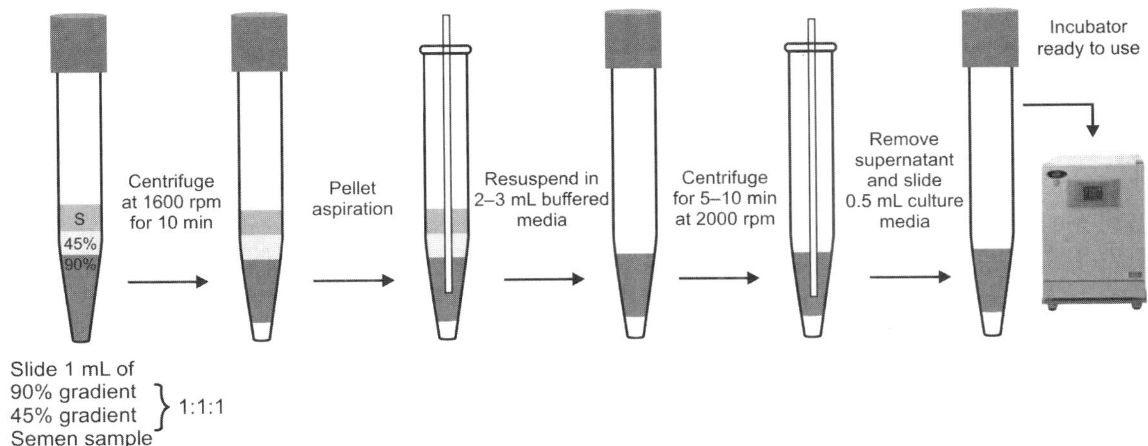

Fig. 2: The density gradient technique. Equal volume of density gradients along with semen sample is centrifuged. Pellet is resuspended in media for a second wash. Pellet obtained after the second wash is resuspended in approximately 0.5 mL of media and is ready for intrauterine insemination.

- Analyze the concentration and motility of the capacitated sample.
- Keep the tube with a tightened cap at 37 °C until its utilization.

Simple Wash

Though this method can also be implemented, for the best quality sperm samples, with respect to number and motility of sperms,[13,14] it is recommended to use this technique for the samples in which the aforementioned techniques cannot be performed due to a very low count or motility of sperm (cryptozoospermia or severe asthenozoospermia). The aim of this technique is to concentrate the sample in order to make easier the finding of motile sperm but without any kind of sperm selection.

Protocol:

- Mix the liquefied semen sample in 14 mL rounded bottom tube duly identified with the details of the patient and add buffered media in approximately 1:1 proportion and homogenize.
- Centrifuge for 10 minutes at 1,500 rpm (300 g).
- Discard the supernatant and add another 1 mL of buffered media. Resuspend the pellet and wash for 5 minutes at 1,500 rpm (300 g).
- Discard the supernatant and add a volume of 0.3–0.5 mL of buffered media to the pellet (the media volume will be directly proportional to the concentration of the sample) and resuspend it.
- Analyze the concentration and motility of the processed sample.
- Keep the tube with a tightened cap inside the incubator until its utilization (Fig. 3).

In spite of the simplicity of this procedure, the method involves repeated centrifugation without separation of good sperms from nonviable spermatozoa, leukocytes, and cellular debris. This along with centrifugation may result in the production of increased amount ROS and can damage sperm function of viable sperms too.[6] Additionally, the presence of large numbers of nonviable spermatozoa in the prepared sample can inhibit capacitation—a physiological process that confers spermatozoa with the ability to fertilize an oocyte.[15]

New Technique: MACS

All the techniques which have been discussed above, which are in routine practice, either increase the sperm concentration in final aliquot or increase the motile sperm count in the final aliquot. But none of the technique can actually assist in filtering sperm with the intact genetic material—deoxyribonucleic acid (DNA). Though we may be able to isolate physiologically normal sperm or morphologically normal sperm using different sperm preparation techniques, those may also have sperms with fragmented DNA. For the management of patients with unexplained infertility, failure of IUI necessitates further evaluation of biological properties of spermatozoa, such as apoptotic markers and DNA fragmentation.[16] Ejaculated human spermatozoa have been shown to display characteristics that are typical of apoptosis such as caspase activation, decreased mitochondrial membrane potential (MMP), and plasma membrane translocation of phosphatidylserine (PS).[17] MACS is a technique that with use of a magnetic field and special magnetic microparticles (microbeads), allows trapping of spermatozoa with damaged-fragmented DNA or spermatozoa that are already in their early stages of apoptosis.

Principle

The principle is that in the early steps of sperm apoptosis PS externalization occurs and the PS has a high affinity for the

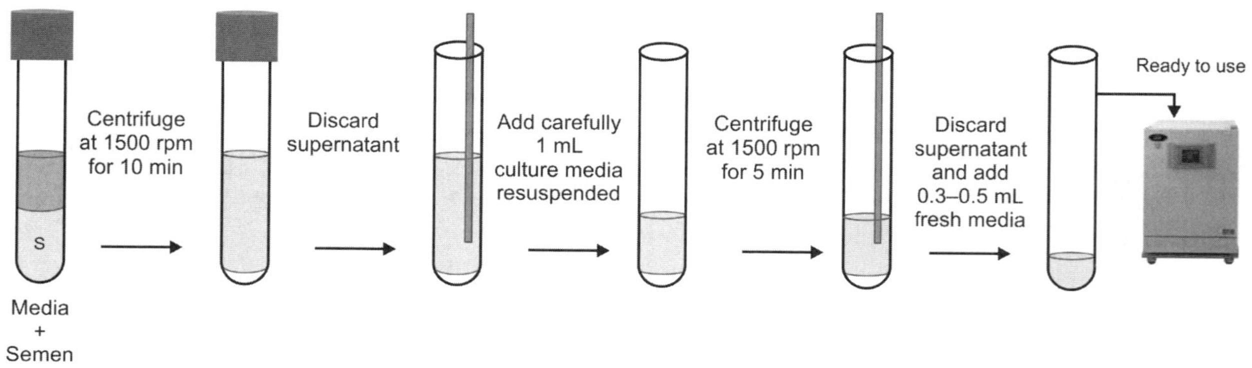

Fig. 3: Simple wash technique. Equal volume of sample and media are mixed and centrifuged. Pellet obtained is resuspended in media for a second wash. Pellet obtained after the second wash is resuspended in approximately 0.5 mL of media and is ready to use.

annexin V. This protein, conjugated with the microbeads, can be linked with the membranes of the compromised sperm, so the apoptotic sperms will be retained in the magnetic column as the annexin V positive fraction. The annexin V negative fraction (the healthy sperms) will be eluted through the column and can be then used for all fertilization techniques in assisted reproduction.

Protocol (Fig. 4)

- Dilute the annexin V binding buffer with distilled water (5%).
- To approximately 200 μL of capacitated sample add 300 μL of binding buffer solution.
- Add 100 μL of annexin beads to the mixture and wrap the tube with aluminum foil.
- Allow the mixture to incubate on a shaker at room temperature for 20–30 minutes.
- Rinse the mini MACS separator (MS) column with binding buffer 5 minutes before the incubation completes by letting the binding buffer pass through the column without any pressure.
- Pass the incubated mixture through MS column and let it elute on its own.
- All the unlabeled (annexin V negative) fraction, nonapoptotic sperms pass through the column and apoptotic (annexin V positive) fraction is retained in the column.
- Centrifuge the elution for 5 minutes at 1,500 rpm (300 g) and discard the supernatant.
- Add 0.3–0.5 mL of culture media to the pellet and incubate for at least 15 minutes before final use.

Note: For successful MACS separation always use the capacitated sample (either density gradient or swim-up). Minimum of 5 million/mL sample is required to guarantee the retrieval of sperms after elution. As much as possible pass minimum of 5 million/mL to a maximum of 10 million/mL sperms via MACS column. More count can be diluted and less count can be concentrated to get it adjusted within this limits before the final procedure (Fig. 5).

Annexin V-negative spermatozoa have a higher motility, lower caspase activation, lower membrane mitochondrial potential disruption, lower amounts of DNA damage, and higher oocyte penetration capacity than annexin V-positive spermatozoa.[18] The annexin-negative (nonapoptotic) spermatozoa separated by MACS following one-step wash had lower quality than those prepared by density gradient combined with MACS in all the assessed parameters and even compared with those prepared by density gradient only in terms of motility and PS externalization.[18] Therefore, it appears that one-step wash is not an optimal option for sperm preparation, regardless of the MACS integration.[18] The spermatozoa prepared by density gradient and MACS showed a reduced level of apoptotic markers. Improvement in the induced acrosome reaction test suggests a high fertilization potential of the processed spermatozoa. The identification of apoptotic markers and use of MACS may be helpful in directing the management plan for patients with unexplained infertility and multiple IUI failures (Table 2).[19]

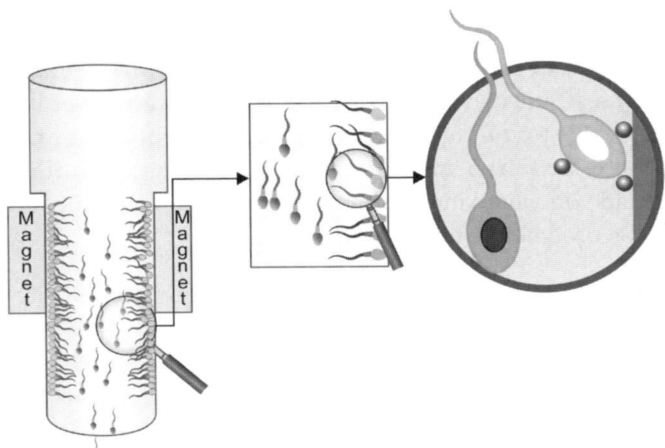

Fig. 4: Principle of MACS. Apoptic sperms get labeled with annexin V microbeads (magnetic) and will be retained in the strong magnetic field provided by separating columns as annexin V-positive fraction and healthy sperms will be eluted through the column as annexin V-negative fraction. (MACS: magnetic-activated cell sorting)

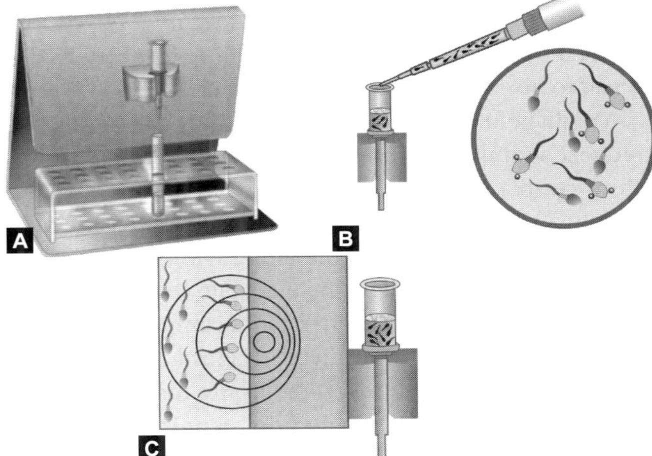

Figs. 5A to C: Assembly of MACS. (A) Magnetic collection device along with separating columns; (B) A mixed solution of sperms along with binding buffer and annexin V beads is passed through separating columns; and (C) Apoptotic sperms with annexin V beads (magnetic) are retained in columns whereas nonapoptotic sperms get eleuted out. (MACS: magnetic-activated cell sorting)

Table 2: Advantages and disadvantages of MACS.

Advantages of MACS	*Disadvantages of MACS*
MACS works at the molecular level in selecting viable sperm other than rest of sperm washing techniques.	To improvise outcome viable spermatozoa has to be separated from all other substance in ejaculate like leukocytes, cellular debris, etc.
MACS can be an ideal choice for frozen semen samples to improvise outcomes.	It has to be clubbed with sperm capacitation techniques like density gradient or swim-up.
MACS is convenient and noninvasive.	More expensive than other regular techniques.
Sperms retrieved after MACS has a higher percentage of motile and viable sperms with less amount of DNA fragmentation.	

(DNA: deoxyribonucleic acid; MACS: magnetic-activated cell sorting)

Occasionally Faced Conditions

Retrograde Ejaculations

In some men, semen passes directly into the urinary bladder at the moment of ejaculation resulting in absence of ejaculate or aspermia. The condition can occur as a result of congenital abnormality, spinal trauma, retroperitoneal lymph node dissection, diabetes mellitus, and bladder neck surgery or can be idiopathic.[20] For such patients, the postejaculatory urine sample has to be examined to assess the presence of sperms. But urine is very damaging to semen as it has acidic pH and can also have an effect on sperm with respect to osmotic change and toxicity. Hence it is recommended to alkalinize the urine pH in order to decrease the effects of urine on sperms. This can be achieved by prescribing sodium bicarbonate tablets as it is proved to be effective urine alkalinization.[21]

A night before sample collection patient can be advised to ingest sodium bicarbonate tablet and another 1 hour before sample collection. At the time of sample collection patient will be advised to urinate before sample collection to reduce the amount of urine along with sperms. Then he can be asked to produce the ejaculate (if possible) and then urinate again into another set of sample containers. As soon as containers are received in laboratory, centrifuge immediately, by distributing it equally in a number of tubes required after taking note of volume of sample. Centrifuge at 1,800 rpm (500 g). Discard the supernatant and resuspend the pellet in 0.5 mL of buffer media. Mix the resuspended pellet in one or maximum two tubes and centrifuge again at 1,800 rpm (500 g). Discard the supernatant and resuspend all the pellet in one tube in a maximum volume of 1 mL. Analyze the semen sample and according to the parameters analyzed, decide the sperm preparation technique to be used.

Note: It is advisable to do a trial analysis and wash before the day of the actual case and if possible to freeze the processed sample as a backup sample.

Electroejaculation

Ejaculatory dysfunction is an uncommon cause of male infertility in the general population.[22] However, ejaculatory dysfunction is the major cause of infertility in certain clinical situations such as in men with spinal cord injury (SCI), multiple sclerosis, diabetic neuropathy, idiopathic anejaculation or iatrogenic neurological lesions.[23] Indirect rectal stimulation is used to retrieve semen from men who have disturbed ejaculation or who cannot ejaculate due to such health issues.[5] Electroejaculation (EEJ) has been successfully used to induce ejaculation in men with such ejaculatory dysfunction. Any other conditions which affect the ejaculatory mechanism of the central and/or peripheral nervous system including surgical nerve injury may be treated successfully with EEJ.[23] Specimen obtained by EEJ can be processed by density gradients technique. Regardless of the method used for preparing these types of ejaculates will often contain a high percentage of immotile sperms.[5]

Donor Sperm

Donor semen sample procured from donor bank is generally cryopreserved after density gradient wash. Hence post-thaw simple wash technique can be used (with single wash) to just remove the cryoprotectants and sample can be prepared for IUI. Removing cryoprotectants by sequential dilution in small-volume steps avoids undue osmatic stresses[24] and may improve pregnancy results. However, it is advisable to communicate to respective sperm banks from where the frozen sperm samples are obtained to further decide on what kind of sperm preparation technique has to be used before final insemination.

Frozen-Thaw Sperm Preparation

Cryopreservation of spermatozoa has become one the most important part of many laboratories especially infertility clinics.[5] Male patients suffering from cancer and requiring chemotherapy for treatment, for example, can store their sperm for future fertility application by using sperm cryopreservation prior to chemotherapy.[25] It can also be utilized by patients who have severe oligoasthenoteratozoospermia (OAT), retrograde or EEJ problem or by a patient who cannot procure sample on the day of procedure as a backup sample.[5] A variety of cryopreservation protocol is now used with different cryoprotectants and freezing protocols.[5] The goal of sperm cryopreservation is to preserve a high number of post-thawing surviving normal sperms.[26] For sperm cryopreservation, several factors, such as the prefrozen sperm quality baseline, freezing and thawing method, and cryopreservative medium, and volume of cryopreserved specimen, have been previously demonstrated to be the crucial factors relating to post-thawing sperm outcome.[26] It can be advised to freeze the semen sample postcapacitation[26] and when required to be thawed and used with just simple wash technique (refer the washing techniques in the above mentioned text).

CHOICE OF TECHNIQUE

The aim of wash should be to enrich the final aliquot with a maximum number of motile sperms with intact chromatin to increase the chances of viable pregnancy. The choice of sperm preparation technique is dictated by the nature of the semen sample.[5] Swim-up technique is often used when the semen samples are considered to largely normal, whereas in cases of severe oligozoospermia, asthenozoospermia, or teratozoospermia, density gradients are usually preferred because of greater total number of motile spermatozoa recovered.[5] Each technique can be changed or improved with simple changes, in order to optimize the recovery of the sperms.[27]

A meta-analysis of five parallel randomized control trials (RCTs) comparing the effectiveness of gradient technique, swim-up, and sperm wash on clinical outcomes after IUI concluded that there are insufficient data to recommend any of these three techniques over each other.[14] Further research and RCTs are required to improve the efficiency and the safety of the sperm preparation methods.

CONCLUSION

The cut-off level of semen parameters in predicting the likelihood of successful IUI is still unequivocal.[28] Many new studies say that the post-wash total motile sperm count (TMSC) has been proposed as a test to help distinguish the couples who would benefit from IUI.[28] TMSC is obtained by multiplying the volume of the ejaculate in milliliters by the sperm concentration and the proportion of A (fast forward progressive) and B (slow progressive) motile sperms divided by 100%.[29] Mithad Hajder et al.[30] concluded that TMSC more than 5 million/mL are indicated for treatment for IUI whereas Elvan Koyun et al.[31] suggested that TMSC of 10 million/mL may be used as the threshold value. But though success is less, pregnancies are also reported with counts lesser than those and hence we can conclude that definitely, sperm processing improves the chances of viable pregnancy but success is dependent on many other factors. More studies are needed to confirm the effectiveness of different sperm preparation methods and to determine cut-off levels of semen parameters for a successful IUI.

REFERENCES

1. Henkel RR, Schill WB. Sperm preparation for ART. Reprod Biol Endocrinol. 2003;1:108.
2. Morris GJ, Acton E, Avery S. A novel approach to sperm cryopreservation. Hum Reprod. 1999;14(4):1013-21
3. Beydola T, Sharma R, Agarwal A. Sperm preparation and selection technique. In: Rizk B, Aziz N, Agarwal A, Sabanegh E Jr (Eds). Medical and Surgical Management of Male Infertility; 2014. pp. 244-51.
4. Björndhal L, Mohammadieh M, Pourian M, et al. Contamination of seminal plasma factors during sperm selection. J Androl. 2005;26(2):170-3.
5. World Health Organization. (2010). WHO manual laboratory manual for the examination and processing of human semen, 5th edition.
6. Aitken RJ, Clarkson JS. Significance of reactive oxygen species and antioxidants in defining the efficiency of sperm preparation techniques. J Androl. 1988;9(6):367-76.
7. Ivasaki A, Gagnon C. Formation of reactive oxygen species in spermatozoa of infertile patients. Fertil Steril. 1992;57(2):409-16.
8. Zalata A, Hafez T, Comhaire F. Evaluation of the role of reactive oxygen species in male infertility. Hum Reprod. 1995;10(6):1444-51.
9. Mahadevan M, Baker G. Assessment and preparation of semen for in vitro fertilization. In: Wood C, Trounsan A (Eds). Clinical In Vitro Fertilization. Berlin: Springer; 1984. pp. 83-97.
10. Jameel T. Sperm swim-up: a simple and effective technique of semen processing for intrauterine insemination. J Pak Med Assoc. 2008;58(2):71-4.
11. Malvezzi H, Sharma R, Agarwal A, et al. Sperm quality after density gradient centrifugation with three commercially available media: a controlled trial. Reprod Biol Endocrinol. 2014;12:121
12. Oshio S, Kaneko S, Iizuka R, et al. Effects of gradient centrifugation on human sperm. Arch Androl. 1987;19(1):85-93.
13. Zini A, Nam RK, Mak V, et al. Influence of initial semen quality on the integrity of human sperm DNA following semen processing. Fertil Steril. 2000;74(4):824-7.
14. Boomsma CM, Heineman MJ, Cohlen BJ, et al. Semen preparation techniques for intrauterine insemination. Cochrane Database Syst Rev. 2007;(4):CD004507.
15. Makker K, Agarwal A, Sharma R. Oxidative stress and male infertility. Indian J Med Res. 2009;129(4):357-67.
16. Aziz N, Agarwal A. Evaluation of sperm damage: beyond the World Health Organization criteria. Fertil Steril. 2008;90(3):484-5.

17. Said TM, Grunewald S, Paasch U, et al. Advantage of combining magnetic cell separation with sperm preparation techniques. Reprod Biomed Online. 2005;10(6):740-6.
18. Said T, Agarwal A, Grunewald S, et al. Selection of nonapoptotic spermatozoa as a new tool for enhancing assisted reproduction. Biol Reprod. 2006;74(3):530-7.
19. Lee TH, Liu CH, Shih YT, et al. Magnetic activated cell sorting for sperm preparation reduce spermatozoa with apoptotic markers and improves the acrosome reaction in couples with unexplained infertility. Hum Reprod. 2010;25(4):839-46.
20. Jefferys A, Siassakos D, Wardle P. The management of retrograde ejaculation: a systematic review and update. Fertil Steril. 2012;97(2):306-12.
21. Cohen B, Laish I, Brosh-Nissimov T, et al. Efficacy of urine alkalinization by oral administration of sodium bicarbonate: a prospective open-label trial. Am J Emerg Med. 2013;31(12):1703-6.
22. Dubin L, Amelar R. Etiologic factors in 1294 consecutive cases of male infertility. Fertil Steril. 1971;22(8):469-74.
23. Sonksen J, Ohl D. Penile vibratory stimulation and electroejaculation in the treatment of ejaculatory dysfunction. Int J Androl. 2002;25(6):324-32.
24. Gao Dy, Liu J, Liu C, et al. Prevention of Osmatic injury to human spermatozoa during addition and removal of glycerol. Hum Reprod. 1995;10(5):1109-22.
25. Nangia AK, Krieg SA, Kim SS. Clinical guidelines for semen cryopreservation in cancer patients. Fertil Steril. 2013;100(5):1203-9.
26. Petyim S, Neungton C, Thanaboonyawat I, et al. Sperm preparation before freezing improves sperm motility and reduces apoptosis in post-freezing-thawing sperm compared with post-thawing sperm preparation. J Assist Reprod Genet. 2014;31(12):1673-80.
27. Natali I. Sperm preparation techniques for artificial insemination—comparison of sperm washing, swim up, and density gradient centrifugation methods. In: Milad Minafi (Ed). Artificial Insemination in Farm Animals. 2011. pp. 115-22.
28. Nikbakht R, Saharkhiz N. The influence of sperm morphology, total motile sperm count of semen and the number of motile sperm inseminated in sperm samples on the success of Intrauterine insemination. Int J Fertil Steril. 2011;5(3): 168-73.
29. Hamilton J, Cissen M, Brandes M, et al. Total motile sperm count: a better indicator for severity of male factor infertility than the WHO sperm classification system. Hum Reprod. 2015;30(5):1110-21.
30. Hajder M, Hajdar E, Husic A. The effect of total motile sperm count on spontaneous pregnancy rate and pregnancy after IUI treatment in couples with male factor and unexplained infertility. Med Arch. 2016;70(1):39-43.
31. Ok EK, Dogan O, Okyay R, et al. The effect of post was total progressive motile sperm count and semen volume on pregnancy outcomes in intrauterine insemination cycles: a retrospective study. J Turk Ger Gynecol Assoc. 2013;14(3):142-5.

CHAPTER

25

Insemination: Tips and Tricks

Rohit Gutgutia, Arindam Rath

INTRODUCTION

Intrauterine insemination (IUI) remains a popular fertility treatment worldwide, especially in low resource settings.[1,2] However, there is great heterogeneity regarding patient selection, ovarian stimulation protocols and methods of sperm preparation leading to unpredictable outcomes. Here, in this chapter, we seek to discuss the procedural aspects of IUI and evaluate their impact on success rates.

TECHNIQUE OF INTRAUTERINE INSEMINATION

Essentially, IUI is injection of processed sperms into the woman's uterus around the time of ovulation.

The process involves:

Preprocedure Preparation

- Insemination room: It should be dedicated for the purposes of IUI. It should be located close to the andrology laboratory. The procedure table should accommodate lithotomy or modified lithotomy positions. Adequate light source should be made available. In absence of a dedicated insemination room, we can make do with the operation theater
- The instrument trolley should have the following sterilized instruments:
  - Cusco's bivalve vaginal speculum: They are laid out in three sizes and used as per clinician's discretion
  - Allis tissue forceps (long) or single tooth tenaculum
  - Sponge holding forceps (long)—two
  - Sterile gauze/cotton balls
  - Sterile gloves (preferably powder free)
  - Normal saline in a pot for cleaning
  - IUI catheter of choice.
- Identification: The identity of the sample as recorded in laboratory notes and on the tube is confirmed with both partners
- Post wash count and motility of the prepared semen sample is checked and recorded by the semenologist using standard operating protocols, ideally by the same person
- The sample is transferred to the insemination room in a test tube warmer/heating block keeping the temperature at 37°C. Alternatively, it can be held in the fist to keep it warm[3]
- The woman, if she so wishes, can have her partner join her in the room. She is made to lie down in the lithotomy position.

Procedure

- The clinician should scrub his hands and forearms with antiseptic solution or soap and put on cap and mask and the gloves. He should personally reconfirm the identity of the woman and match it with the semen sample.
- The vulva is cleaned with normal saline and sterile drapes put in place.
- Optimum sized speculum is introduced and the cervix exposed. The external os is gently cleaned with saline soaked cotton balls. Sometimes, the cervix needs to be held with Allis forceps/tenaculum to straighten the cervical canal.
- Loading of the IUI catheter is done by the semenologist who attaches the IUI catheter with 1 mL syringe and then draws up the washed semen. About 0.5–1 mL aspirate

is used. Most clinics use the Gynetics® catheter, which does not require preflushing with media. Consumables used in the laboratory including IUI catheters are made of material which is biologically safe.
- The catheter is then introduced through the cervix till the tip has crossed the internal os and lies in the uterine cavity. Care should be taken to avoid hitting the fundus but to deposit the semen below the fundus. It is a prudent habit to measure the uterocervical length when doing folliculometry scans and also to note the cervical angle. Then the blue marker on the IUI catheter can be placed accordingly so that catheter does not cross further into the cavity. This way, one can be better prepared when doing the insemination.
- The washed semen is slowly injected into the uterine cavity over 60–80 seconds by maintaining a gentle but continuous pressure on the piston of the syringe.[3] Eye should be kept on the woman to detect any uneasiness or discomfort that she may feel during this time.
- Once the entire volume is injected, the catheter is slowly withdrawn along with the speculum and Allis forceps. The woman is made comfortable and kept lying down in supine position for 5–10 minutes.

Postprocedure Instructions

- She is then free to get up and resume her normal life. Rest is not recommended.
- Luteal support is advised.
- She is asked to do a pregnancy test after 14 days and if pregnant, scheduled for an ultrasonography (USG) to confirm the viability.

DISCUSSION

Here we shall discuss a few practical issues concerning the process of IUI. Some of these do have a bearing on the results as well.

Choice of Catheters

The IUI catheter is a device that delivers washed semen in a concentrated form into the uterine cavity beyond the cervical barrier near the site of fertilization.[1] It should have the following attributes:
- Should be made of biologically safe material which does not affect sperm motility and is not reprotoxic[4]
- Should be easy to use
- Should be firm enough to negotiate the cervical canal yet soft enough to avoid trauma by injuring the endometrial lining[1]
- Should have a small intrauterine tip to avoid reflux of the inseminate back into the catheter after insemination[1]

Various types of IUI catheters are commercially available that satisfy the above criteria. They have been classified as soft and firm.

Soft Catheters

- Cook soft-pass artificial insemination catheter (Cook Women's Health, Spencer, In, USA)
- Gynetics® artificial insemination catheter (Gynetics® Medical Products, Hamont-Achel, Belgium)
- Labotect artificial insemination catheter (Labotect, Labor-Technik Göttingen, Germany)
- Wallace artificial insemination catheter (Smiths Medical International, London, UK)
- Various embryo transfer catheters.

Firm Catheters

- Makler IUI cannula and insemination device (Sefi Medical Instruments Ltd., Haifa, Israel)
- Tomcat™ artificial insemination catheter (Kendall Sovereign, Mansfield, USA)
- Metallic cannulas (local make).

Cases where entry into cervical canal is expected to be easy are best served by the soft catheters whereas in other cases firm catheters may be needed. Firm catheters are associated with more patient discomfort. However, there is no significant difference in clinical pregnancy rates and live birth rates with either catheter.[1,5,6]

Loading of the Catheter

The catheter has an inherent dead space within itself. When the catheter is attached to the loaded syringe containing the washed semen (usually 0.6 mL) even after fully pressing the piston, none of the washed semen is delivered into the uterus as the entire inseminate in held up in the catheter itself. Therefore, it is essential to load the catheter after attaching the syringe to it. This way, the entire aspirate is contained within the catheter and the dead space air is drawn into the syringe. Then if the pressure is put on the piston, the semen gets delivered first into the uterus and the dead space air stays in the catheter. Best way to ensure this is to load the catheter till a drop of washed semen is clearly seen sitting on the tip of the catheter.

Loading of the catheter should be followed immediately by insemination. Delay in depositing the washed semen affects the fertilizing capacity of sperms as energy sources in the media are used up prematurely by the activated sperms.[7]

Volume of Inseminate

There is some controversy as to what comprises ideal inseminate volume. Whereas most clinics use volumes between 0.6 mL and 1 mL, there are reports varying from 0.2 mL to 1 mL. The contention is that the exact volume needed for the sperms to be effectively present at the site of fertilization, in the ampulla of the fallopian tubes, is not known. Accordingly, studies have been designed with different volumes of inseminate. It has been found that a minimum volume of 0.4 mL is needed to reach the uterus and tubes. The impact on pregnancy rates, however, is not very clear. It has been seen that insemination with 1 mL volume gives similar results to insemination with 0.5 mL volume.[8]

Timing of Insemination

Timing the insemination close to ovulation would increase the probability of conception as because both ova and sperms have a limited survival span.[9] Most clinics perform IUI 24–36 hours post-luteinizing hormone surge, either spontaneous or induced with human chorionic gonadotropin (hCG) injection. But no significant differences in pregnancy rates have been seen with IUI done at 24 hours or at 36 hours. Cochrane review of the trials comparing different timing methods is also rather inconclusive. Basically, it is more an issue of patient and clinician's conveniences, availability of the staff and costs.[9] Some flexibility can be maintained to strike a balance between results and conveniences. However, for those so inclined, it seems that performing IUI after follicle rupture may give better results.[10]

Number of Inseminations in a Cycle

Single versus double insemination in cycle has always been a source of much discussion and debate. We are aware that bolus injection of sperms leads to nonphysiological concentration of sperms followed by rapid decay. Given that with ovarian stimulation, there are multiple follicles which do not ovulate all together, it makes eminent sense to consider double insemination in stimulated cycles. However, it does not translate in a big advantage in practice. Numerous studies exist on the subject but they are all handicapped by differences in ovulation induction protocols, semen preparation methods, patient selection bias,[11] etc. One study claims better results with double pre-ovulation insemination compared to single insemination in subfertile couples with male factor which can be possibly explained by the fact that in male factor subfertility, sperm survival for longer time may be a bigger issue.[12] Cochrane review shows no significant benefit for double insemination over single IUI in treatment of subfertile couples with husband's semen. A large well-controlled trial keeping all variables in mind is awaited. Till then, we can safely look at single well- timed insemination for most cases and double insemination in male factor cases.

Difficult Entry of the Catheter

At times, negotiating the cervical canal to enter the cavity becomes a vexing problem. There could be cervical stenosis, pinhole cervix or a false passage. Sometimes, the uterus may be acutely anteflexed or retroflexed as well.

We can look at tackling this problem in different ways. Pulling on the Allis forceps or the tenaculum applied to the anterior lip of cervix can straighten the canal and allow the catheter to go in.[13,14] The insemination can be attempted under USG guidance. If an acutely anteverted uterus is suspected, the woman is asked to hold the urine and IUI is done on full bladder. Even gentle pressure on the lower abdomen with one hand can sometimes help, both to relax the woman and to negotiate the catheter. We also resort to using the firmer embryo transfer catheters with a tough outer sheath to tackle difficult cervix. Even metallic catheters have been rarely used.

Most cases can be managed by using tricks as described above. If still unsuccessful, sometime, a simple change of hands works. Very rarely, however, especially in cases of apareunia, insemination needs to be done under general anesthesia.

Regurgitation of the Inseminate

Sometimes, the inseminate is seen to come out immediately after injecting. This happens when the internal os is open or when the tip of the catheter is coiled up inside the cervical canal. At times, it could also be because of a blocked catheter tip.

The trick to handle this is to rotate the catheter once we are inside the cavity. If the tip is coiled up, on rotation it shall come out and start showing. Another thing we can do is to go in and slowly inject the semen and stop midway to assess if there is reflux. If seen then, reposition the catheter, ask her to lift her pelvis, bring the table to the Trendelenburg position and then inject the rest. It is good practice to loosen the blades of the speculum so that they rest on the lips of the cervix thereby exerting a clamping effect. Sometimes, leaving the catheter behind for sometime also creates a stopper effect and retains the semen inside. Rarely, we can also clamp the cervix with Allis forceps to retain semen in cases of large patulous cervix.

Blood in the Catheter

Traumatic entry to the cavity may sometimes initiate bleeding from the cervix. In such cases, aspirating the blood with a syringe followed by insemination helps. Also, it is wise in these cases to put in the catheter first and then load with the semen. Here, after pushing we detach the syringe, take some air, push it further to disgorge the full contents of the catheter into the uterine cavity.

Poor Semen Parameters on the Day of Insemination

Sometimes, the partner fails to give an optimum sample on the day on insemination, even though previously the parameters may have been good. In these cases, giving a gap of hour or two followed by another attempt at collection is usually rewarded with a decent sample.[15] The volume may be low, but the count and motility is usually good.

Similarly, failure to ejaculate on day of insemination can be managed with freezing a sample prior to the procedure.

At times, cryopooling of samples in men with low volume ejaculate and then insemination is also rewarded with pregnancies.

CONCLUSION

Intrauterine insemination represents the first-line therapy in the fertility management algorithm. After trying honestly, if still there is no pregnancy; there is no shame in referring the couple for higher treatment modalities which offer a much higher likelihood of conception.

REFERENCES

1. Abou-Setta AM, Mansour RT, Al-Inany HG, et al. Intrauterine insemination catheters for assisted reproduction: a systematic review and meta-analysis. Hum Reprod. 2006;21(8):1961-7.
2. Hughes EG. The effectiveness of ovulation induction and intrauterine insemination in the treatment of persistent infertility: a meta-analysis. Hum Reprod. 1997;12(9):1865-72.
3. Allahbadia GN, Kadam K, Kaur K. Intrauterine insemination techniques. In: Allahbadia GN (Ed). Intrauterine Insemination. New Delhi: Jaypee Brothers Medical Publishers (P) Ltd; 2005. pp. 218-39.
4. Nijs M, Franssen K, Cox A, et al. Reprotoxicity of intrauterine insemination and in vitro fertilization-embryo transfer disposables and products: a 4-year survey. Fertil Steril. 2009;92(2):527-35.
5. Miller PB, Acres ML, Proctor JG, et al. Flexible versus rigid intrauterine insemination catheters: a prospective, randomized, controlled study. Fertil Steril. 2005;83(5):1544-6.
6. Fancsovits P, Toth L, Murber A, et al. Catheter type does not affect the outcome of intrauterine insemination treatment: a prospective randomized study. Fertil Steril. 2005;83(3):699-704.
7. Yavas Y, Selub MR. Intrauterine insemination (IUI) pregnancy outcome is enhanced by shorter intervals from semen collection to sperm wash, from sperm wash to IUI time, and from semen collection to IUI time. Fertil Steril. 2004;82(6):1638-47.
8. Tsai MY, Tsai YC, Chang JC, et al. Effect of postprepared sperm parameters and insemination specimen volume on the outcome of intrauterine insemination. Changgeng Yi Xue Za Zhi. 1998;21(3):265-70.
9. Cantineau AE, Janssen MJ, Cohlen BJ. Synchronised approach for intra-uterine insemination in subfertile couples. Cochrane Database Syst Rev. 2010;14(4):CD006942.
10. Kucuk T. Intrauterine insemination: is the timing correct? J Assist Reprod Genet. 2008;25(8):427-30.
11. Rahman SM, Malhotra N, Kumar S, et al. A randomized controlled trial comparing the effectiveness of single versus double intrauterine insemination in unexplained infertility. Fertil Steril. 2010;94(7):2913-5.
12. Ghanem ME, Bakre NI, Emam MA, et al. The effects of timing of intrauterine insemination in relation to ovulation and the number of inseminations on cycle pregnancy rate in common infertility etiologies. Hum Reprod. 2011;26(3):576-83.
13. Balci O, Acar A, Colakoglu MC. Does tenaculum application to the cervix during intrauterine insemination affect pregnancy rates? Acta Obstet Gynecol Scand. 2009;88(9):1053-6.
14. Park KE, Ku SY, Kim H, et al. The use of tenaculum during intrauterine insemination may not affect the pregnancy outcome. Yonsei Med J. 2010;51(6): 949-53.
15. Panpalia M, Parikh FR. IUI techniques and difficulties faced during insemination. In: Mukherjee GG, Chakravarty BN (Eds). Intrauterine Insemination. New Delhi: Jaypee Brothers Medical Publishers (P) Ltd; 2012. pp. 272-87.

CHAPTER

26

Donor Sperm Insemination: Do's and Don'ts

Richa Jagtap, Manjushri Kothekar

ABOUT DONOR INSEMINATION

Donor insemination refers to the placement of a donor sperm sample inside the female genital tract in an attempt to conception. Theoretically, it could be intracervical insemination or intrauterine insemination. It has been found that intracervical insemination has far lower success rate than intrauterine insemination.[1] The modern practice routinely followed is that of intrauterine insemination, i.e. placement of the donor sperm sample inside the uterine cavity. So we will restrict ourselves to donor insemination pertaining to intrauterine insemination.

HISTORY

Artificial insemination (AI) was the first great biotechnology applied to improve reproduction and genetics of farm animals. It is being widely used in dairy animals since many years. However, the application in humans has seen an interesting evolution, verging on scandalous to say in the least!

Unofficial history claims that crude attempts to artificially inseminate Juana, the wife of King Henry IV of Castile in the 1400s, was an early endeavor to artificially impregnate an infertile couple.[2]

Although we assume that artificial insemination is a modern technology, it has a documented history dating back to 1779, when Spallanzani's experiment established for the first time that there must be actual physical contact between the egg and the sperm for an embryo to develop. In human beings, John Hunter, British physiologist and surgeon, was the first to record a pregnancy and delivery of a child conceived by artificial insemination with a husband's semen in 1790.[2]

According to a letter in the American journal "Medical World" a doctor claimed that the first human donor insemination had been performed at the Jefferson Medical College in Philadelphia in 1884 without the couple's knowledge and it led to successful pregnancy. As can be expected, the can of worms was opened and it led to the disrepute which shrouds the procedure over the years.

In mid-1940s AI was allegedly widely practiced in Nazi Germany and the doctors were forced to perform AI experiments on Jews, gypsies, and concentration camp internees, in a bid to improve race. In 1953, the first successful pregnancy from AI of frozen sperm was reported.

Prior to the late 1980s, donor insemination was done using fresh semen samples. However, the need to prevent transmission of sexually transmitted diseases (including HIV) by donor insemination has led to the mandatory quarantine of donor sperm for 6 months by cryopreservation prior to its use.

As evident by the history, donor insemination is fraught with medical as well as social and legal issues that need proper evaluation before such a treatment is attempted. Further the advice of statutory bodies like Indian Council of Medical Research (ICMR) regarding the practice of donor insemination has to be followed. So there are certain Do's and Don'ts to be followed.

DO'S

Selection of the Patient

Donor insemination, being such a sensitive issue, should be offered to right kind of patient. It is indicated in:

- Patients with azoospermia
- Patients with severe male factor infertility not affording the intracytoplasmic sperm injection (ICSI)

- For certain infectious diseases in males e.g., HIV (if the viral load is very high)
- Cases with high risk of transmitting a genetic disease
- Single women
- Rh isoimmunization.

In case of azoospermia, the diagnosis should be confirmed by repeating the count at least two times 6 weeks apart. The semen should also be analyzed after centrifugation where in some cases a pellet will show a few sperms that can be used in ICSI.

Once azoospermia is confirmed, the cause needs to be pinpointed by investigating the male partner. It could either be obstructive azoospermia or nonobstructive azoospermia. Obstructive azoospermia can be primary, due to congenital bilateral absence of the vas deferens (CBAVD) or secondary due to infection, injury or previous surgeries like hernia/hydrocele. In secondary obstructive case the option of correction (if possible) should be explored. All these patients also have an option of ICSI after percutaneous testicular sperm extraction (PESA).

In case of nonobstructive azoospermia, i.e. spermatogenesis failure, it is worthwhile to examine the following:

- Testicular volume
- Follicle-stimulating hormone/luteinizing hormone (FSH/LH) levels
- Total testosterone.

If a case of hypogonadotropic hypogonadism is diagnosed (i.e. high FSH and low testosterone), it can benefit by gonadotropin therapy [FSH, human chorionic gonadotropin (hCG)]. It may not restore the sperm counts to normal levels for a natural conception but can definitely be sufficient for ICSI.

Option of donor insemination can be considered in couples where there is a high risk of transmitting infectious disease to the offspring or woman from the man.[3] This option can also be suggested if there is a history of severe Rh isoimmunization in the past.[3, 4]

Some single women may opt to conceive through donor insemination. According to ICMR, there would be no bar to the use of assisted reproductive technique (ART) by single women who wish to have a child and no ART clinic may refuse to offer its services to the above, provided other criteria are satisfied. The child thus born will have all the legal rights on the woman.[4]

It is equally important to ascertain the tubal patency of the female partner either by hysterosalpingography or laparoscopic chromopertubation. Atleast one tube should be patent to offer the insemination to the woman.

Rule out other possible contributory causes of female infertility. Things like age of the female partner, ovarian reserve, euthyroid status, and uterine pathology should be taken into consideration before offering treatment as all things are going to affect the success rate. It is a good practice to ensure that the female partner has immunity to Rubella by checking Rubella IgG. Also ensure absence of anemia and euglycemic status in female in view of the anticipated pregnancy.

Counseling and Legal Issues

For most couples it might be very difficult to accept donor sperm as an option. All possible modalities of treatment and the possible costs should be put forth them. The success rates of all these modalities should also be discussed. According to ICMR guidelines, success rates for a particular treatment for the last 6 months should be displayed in the clinic.[4] The couple should decide themselves, what treatment they want to opt for.

Then the couple should be offered counseling regarding all the physical and psychological implications of treatment for themselves and potential children.[3] They can be given an option of matching physical characteristics of the donor with the husband as far as possible. The sample will be from an anonymous donor and the anonymity will be maintained lifelong.

Legally the child born of donor insemination will be of the commissioning husband. However, the child will have a right to seek information about its genetic parent, and if so it can be given excepting information on name and address. It is not obligatory for the couple to disclose to the child that it is born out of donor insemination.[4]

The couple may also have certain issues about the safety of the procedure. They should be properly counseled that the sample is obtained from an accredited sperm bank and that all donors are tested negative for important viral infections, and the samples released after a window period of 6 months of first screening.

The couple may also have certain fears about passage of genetic disorder from the sperm donor. The sample will be checked for identifiable genetic disorder like thalassemia. In addition to this, if karyotype is checked it will rule out large deletions, translocations, and aneuploidies. But it is very difficult to check for small defects and uncommon single genetic disorder and diseases with multifactorial origin. Counseling should include this information.

Ovarian Stimulation and Monitoring the Cycle

After selecting the right kind of patient, doing the procedure itself the right kind of way is equally important.

The procedure can be done either in a natural cycle or a stimulated one. The success rate for a natural cycle donor insemination is less than the rate if it is coupled with clomiphene citrate or with gonadotropin stimulation.[5,6] But whether to go for a natural cycle or a stimulated cycle donor insemination is an individual decision.

Ideally a young ovulatory woman should be offered some nonstimulated cycles to decrease the chances of hyperstimulation and multiple pregnancies.[3] For anovulatory women, or those who have failed 2–3 natural cycles, stimulated intrauterine insemination (IUI) or SO-IUI (superovulation IUI) can be offered.

Clomiphene citrate is given in a dose of 50 mcg per day starting from third day of the cycle. One can increase the dose to 100 mcg a day in successive cycles if there is poor or no response. A day 2 follicular scan ideally should be done to rule out any cyst before starting stimulation.

Gonadotropins in the form of human menopausal gonadotropin (hMG) or recombinant FSH can be added in a clomiphene cycle or started from day 3 of menstrual cycle. They are added in lowest possible dose of 50–75 IU. The type of gonadotropins to be used constitutes another chapter all together; however, recombinant FSH is preferred for polycystic ovary (PCO) and young patients.

Donor insemination is planned in periovulatory phase. It is important to monitor the cycle to ascertain the time of ovulation. Monitoring can be done with LH kits, basal body temperature (BBT) method, or follicular monitoring. If LH kits are used, ask the female to start using the kit from 10th/11th day of cycle daily till she notices the LH surge in urine. Donor insemination is planned 24–36 hours after detection of LH in urine.

If follicular size is monitored on ultrasonography (USG) then an hCG trigger is given when dominant follicle reaches 18–20 mm in size and insemination is planned 36–40 hours after the trigger.

Consents

Taking an informed consent is an essential step in all procedures; however, the importance of the consent cannot be overstressed in a donor IUI. A written, valid, and timed consent is taken from both the partners in the format given by ICMR. Ideally the consent should be taken in local language. This should be countersigned by the doctor attending. If this procedure is done without the consent of husband it might be a ground for divorce in the court of law.[4] The consent for superovulation using gonadotropins should be taken if gonadotropin stimulation is planned.

Sourcing the Semen Sample

The couple can be given an option of matching husband's characteristics in terms of blood group, height, weight, color of the skin, and eyes with that of the donor. A sample from an accredited sperm bank should be used always. ICMR does not allow use of sperm from a known donor. ICMR has also prescribed a code of conduct for the sperm banks as well. They are as follows:[4]

- The individual must be free of HIV and hepatitis B and C infections, hypertension, diabetes, sexually transmitted diseases and identifiable and common genetic disorders such as thalassemia.
- The age of the donor must not be below 21 or above 45 years.
- An analysis must be carried out on the semen of the individual, preferably using a semen analyzer, and the semen must be found to be normal according to the World Health Organization (WHO) method manual for semen analysis, if intended to be used for ART.
- The blood group and the Rh status of the individual must be determined and placed on record.
- Other relevant information in respect of the donor, such as height, weight, age, educational qualifications, profession, color of the skin and the eyes, record of major diseases including any psychiatric disorder, and the family background in respect of history of any familial disorder, must be recorded in an appropriate proforma.
- According to ICMR, donors are not allowed to "father" more than 10 pregnancies. This means that the chance of consanguinity (the risk of a boy and girl from different families both fathered by the same donor meeting, marrying and having children) are extraordinarily remote—probably rather less than winning the lottery! But it is the responsibility of the clinic to inform about pregnancy from a donor to the sperm bank.

Ideally the screening should also include karyotype. In addition to all these, in some western countries, sperm donors need to be screened for autosomal recessive conditions (such as cystic fibrosis, beta-thalassemia, sickle-cell disease and Tay-Sachs disease) and rhesus antigens.[3] But as all these disorders are not so common in our country, ICMR stresses on testing for common disorders, viz. thalassemia.

Procedure

Donor insemination is an OPD procedure done without any kind of anesthesia. The patient is asked to report at the due time with partially full bladder, as a full bladder straightens the uterine axis and makes it easy to negotiate the uterine canal. The sample should be adequately thawed.

The patient is placed in lithotomy position and the perineal, vaginal area is gently cleaned with normal saline. Visualizing the cervix with the help of a Cusco's or Sim's speculum, clean it with normal saline. Load the thawed, washed semen sample inside an IUI catheter attached to a tuberculin syringe. Use a sterile catheter from a reliable source. Introduce the catheter in the cervix and gently push it forward inside the uterine cavity. Slowly inject the semen sample inside the uterine cavity and then slowly remove the catheter. The patient can then pass urine and go back to the normal routine lifestyle.

The patient should be given a copy of the certificate issued by the ART bank about donor specifications. It is preferable to confirm the ovulation on USG either on same day or next day; however, double inseminations have not been found to improve pregnancy rates. In any case, the second insemination if planned should *always* be of the same donor.[4]

Luteal Phase Support

It is debatable whether to give luteal phase support after the procedure. Especially in nondownregulated ovaries, the endogenous hormones are adequate. Patients with luteal phase insufficiency, PCO status, and those downregulated need the progesterone support essentially.

Preferably vaginal micronized progesterone can be prescribed in the luteal phase. Beyond this only requirement is for folic acid. The patient can confirm pregnancy by a serum beta hCG [if not urine pregnancy test (UPT)] 14 days after the procedure.

DON'TS

- Do not take any decision in haste and do not rush the couple for using this modality of treatment.
- Do not jump the "counseling part". Proceed with informed consents by the couple only.
- Do not use a sample from a known donor or a fresh, nonquarantined donor.
- While doing the procedure try not to use any antiseptic solution for cleaning as it might be toxic to the spermatozoa as well.
- It has been found that latex can affect the quality of spermatozoa. Use either plastic gloves or nonlatex gloves.
- Preferably do not catch the cervix with any instrument. Only if the insemination is very difficult, catch the cervix using Allis forceps and pull it gently to straighten the uterocervical canal. Preferably, do not lock the Allis forceps as it might initiate uterine contractions.
- There are chances of regurgitation or loss of the sperms into pelvis, if the semen is injected very fast. So try not to inject the semen sample very fast.
- Do not use a sample which is not thawed properly. Injecting a cold sample might cause pain and uterine contractions.

Optimizing Success Rate

Following things are important in deciding the success rate:

- *Age of the female partner*: The chances of success are less with older patients. Crude and expected cumulative delivery rate for women older than 40 years after six IUI cycles and three primary ICSI cycles (no previous IUI) were similar in both groups (24% versus 26% and 29% versus 35%, respectively).[5,6] There is no definitive cut-off but with patients who are older than 40 years, it is worthwhile to suggest an option of ICSI with donor semen because time to pregnancy is an important factor for that group.[7,8] For patients who are in late thirties this decision is a little complex, many factors are to be considered, e.g. ovarian reserve of the female [anti-Müllerian hormone (AMH)].
- *Donors*: History of a pregnancy from the donor is an important prognostic factor.[9] But, usually only those males with an excellent count are selected as donors.
- *Single or double insemination*: Evidence says that there is no statistically significant difference if insemination is done once or twice.[10] Further ICMR says that no woman should be treated in one cycle with gametes derived from more than one source.[4]
- *Timing of insemination*: Insemination should be planned periovulatory. It does not make any difference by which method you are monitoring the cycle for ovulation. Results do not change much if ovulation is monitored by urinary LH or USG.[11]
- *Stimulation protocols*: The success when gonadotropins are used for stimulation is almost 14–15% per cycle as compared to 6% when clomiphene is used.[6] In one study, it was found that no other thing but use of gonadotropins increases the success rate.[12]
- At the same time it should be noted that gonadotropins increase the chance of multiple pregnancy as well.
- *Type of catheter*: There was no significant difference observed in the success rates after using soft or firm catheters.[13,14]
- *Easy or difficult procedure:* When the procedure is difficult or when one has to catch the cervix during

procedure success rate drops. The success rate is also observed to be low if there is slight bleeding during the procedure.

- *Volume of inseminate*: The donor sample is centrifuged and the concentrated bolus postwash is introduced inside the uterine cavity. Live birth rate after a donor IUI is found to be not much different when the volume of sperm inseminate was 0.5 mL or 0.2 mL.[15]

Complications

Complications of the procedure per se are not there. But the complications can arise due to ovarian stimulation.

- *Ovarian hyperstimulation syndrome (OHSS):* One should exert caution while using gonadotropins for the stimulation. Minimum possible dose should be used. In case the situation seems to go out of hand, one can convert it into an IVF cycle after proper counseling. Use of antagonists and drugs like cabergoline should be considered also whenever hyperstimulation is anticipated.
- *Multiple pregnancies:* This situation also is more common when gonadotropins are used for ovarian stimulation (20%) than when clomiphene is used (12.5%).[6]

WHAT NEXT AFTER FAILED CYCLE

It is a difficult yet important question to answer. After three unsuccessful cycles definitely there is a need to review the situation. The best possible results with any donor insemination are within the first 3–6 cycles. But of course these three cycles should have a proper ovulation and insemination should have occurred at prescribed time. The couple can be offered an option of IVF using donor sperm in case of suspected fertilization defects and poor embryo quality. The final option, which should be brought up and discussed is of adoption. The decision has to be based on many factors including the couple's financial condition and other contributing factors for infertility.

REFERENCES

1. Wainer R, Merlet F, Ducot B, et al. Prospective randomised comparison of intrauterine and intracervical insemination with donor spermatozoa. Hum Reprod. 1995;10(11):2919-22.
2. Ombelet W, Van Robays J. Artificial insemination history: hurdles and milestones. Facts Views Vis Obgyn. 2015;7(2): 137-43.
3. National Institute for Health and Care Excellence. (2013). Fertility problems: assessment and treatment. (NICE Clinical Guideline No. 156). Retrieved from https://www.nice.org.uk/guidance/cg156.
4. Indian Council of Medical Research. The Assisted Reproductive Technologies [regulation] Bill 2010.
5. Lashen H, Afnan M, Kennefik A. Early resort to ovarian stimulation improves cost effectiveness of donor insemination. Hum Reprod. 1999;14(8):1983-8.
6. Matorras R, Diaz T, Corcostegui B, et al. Ovarian stimulation in intrauterine insemination with donor sperm: a randomised study comparing clomiphene citrate in fixed protocols with highly purified urinary FSH. Hum Reprod. 2002;17(8): 2107-11.
7. De Brucker M, Camus M, Haentjens P, et al. Assisted reproduction using donor spermatozoa in women aged 40 and above: The high road or the low road? Reprod Biomed Online. 2013;26(6):577-85.
8. Harris ID, Missmer SA, Hornstein MD. Poor success of gonadotropin-induced controlled ovarian hyper stimulation and intrauterine insemination for older women. Fertil Steril. 2010;94(1):144-8.
9. Boulard V, Charbit B, Brasseur F, et al. Prognostic factors of pregnancy in intra-uterine insemination with sperm of donor: A review of 535 cycles over 7 years. J Gynecol Obstet Biol Reprod (Paris). 2013;42(1):40-8.
10. Khalifa Y, Redgment CJ, Tsirigotis M, et al. The value of single vs. repeated inseminations in intrauterine donor insemination cycles. Hum Reprod. 1995;10(1):153-4.
11. Zreik TG, García-Velasco JA, Habboosh MS, et al. Prospective, randomized, crossover study to evaluate the benefit of human chorionic gonadotropin-timed versus urinary luteinizing hormone-timed intrauterine inseminations in clomiphene citrate-stimulated treatment cycles. Fertil Steril. 1999;71(6):1070-4.
12. Depypere HT, Gordts S, Campo R, et al. Methods to increase the success rate of artificial insemination with donor semen. Hum Reprod. 1994;9(4):661-3.
13. Van der Poel N, Farquhar C, Abou-Setta AM, et al. Soft versus firm catheters for intrauterine insemination. Cohrane Database Syst Rev. 2010;(11):CD006225.
14. Abou-Setta AM, Mansour RT, Al-Inany HG, et al. Intrauterine insemination catheter for assisted reproduction- a systematic review and meta-analysis. Hum Reprod. 2006;21(8):1961-7.
15. Rodriguez-Purata J, Latre L, Ballester M, et al. Clinical success of IUI cycles with donor sperm is not affected by total inseminated volume: A RCT. Hum Reprod Open. 2018;(2):2018.

CHAPTER

27

Complications of Ovarian Stimulation and Intrauterine Insemination

Antonia Tocino Díaz, Manuel Fernández

INTRODUCTION

The first paper entitled intrauterine insemination (IUI) was published by Cohen in 1962.[1] IUI is a noninvasive first-line therapy for selected patients with functionally normal tubes, and, infertility due to cervical factor, anovulation, moderate male factor, unexplained factors, immunological factor, or ejaculatory disorders with clinical pregnancy rates per cycle ranging from 10% to 20%.

Although IUI is less invasive and cheaper than in vitro fertilization (IVF), the safety and efficacy of IUI in combination with ovarian hyperstimulation (OH) is still debated. In fact, The National Institute for Health and Care Excellence (NICE) (2013) recommends unstimulated intrauterine insemination as a treatment option in some groups as an alternative to vaginal sexual intercourse and offer IVF treatment to women with unexplained infertility who have not conceived after 2 years (this can include up to 1 year before their fertility investigations) of regular unprotect sexual intercourse.[2]

COMPLICATIONS OF OVARIAN STIMULATION

Risk of Multiple Pregnancy

The high multiple pregnancy (MP) rate is still a major problem when performing IUI in stimulation cycles with standard gonadotropins dosage. A pregnancy case with 15 live fetuses after ovulation induction and intrauterine insemination should not occur again.[3]

In this century, physicians need to focus on another ART (assisted reproductive technology) goal, which is the healthy take-home baby rate.

European data of 2014 on intrauterine insemination using husband/partner's sperm (IUI-H) and donor (IUI-D) sperm have been reported from 26 and 21 countries, respectively (Table 1).[4]

Instituto Valenciano de Infertilidad (IVI) has a long experience in IUI. Multiple pregnancy rates were higher along the first years.

We have learned more about complications and presumptive risk factors for multiple pregnancy. Based on these practices, we have reduced the number of multiple pregnancies during the last few years of multiple pregnancies (IUI-H and IUI-D) from 2008 to 2017.

The prevention of multiple pregnancy is the best treatment. It is essential to know the risk factors in order to prevent them. Tur et al.[5] studied the risk factors for high-order multiple implantation in 1,878 consecutive pregnancies obtained in stimulation treatments with gonadotropins. They found that this risk correlates significantly with the total number of follicles. Moreover, the risk was significantly increased in women with a serum estradiol more than 862 pg/mL and women aged less than or equal to 32 years.

Dickey et al.[6] published an updated analysis in 2009, including references from 130 articles, and obtained several

Table 1: European data of 2014 on intrauterine insemination using husband/partner's sperm (IUI-H) and donor (IUI-D) sperm.

European	*IUI-H*	*IUI-D*
Cycles	120.789	49.163
Deliveries%	8.5	11.6
Twins%	9.5	7.7
Triplet%	0.3	0.3

conclusions. Risk factors for high-order multiple pregnancy included more than or equal to seven preovulatory follicles (≥10–12 mm), estradiol (E2) level more than 1,000 pg/mL, early cycles of treatment, age less than 32 years, low BMI, and the use of donor sperm.

However, Gleicher et al. noticed and published that the peak serum estradiol level and/or the number of preovulatory follicles were not useful to predict multiple pregnancy.[5,7]

The risk of MP may be minimized by carefully monitoring and adjusting the gonadotropin dosage or cancelling treatment when too many mature follicles develop. IVI group in a retrospective study (n = 6552) highlighted the importance of accounting for the presence of follicles that are 12 mm or more at the time of ovulation trigger, as they significantly increase the risk of multiple pregnancy as you can see in Table 2.[8]

Difficulties in the Selection of Ovulatory Follicle

Patients included in anovulation groups I or II according to the WHO (hypogonadotropic hypoestrogenic and normogonadotropic normoestrogenic) require more days of stimulation in order to select the ovulatory follicle. One frequent mistake is to raise the dose of gonadotropins at stimulation days 4–6 when we cannot detect a growing follicle.

In these patients, we recommend to start stimulation with a low-dose of gonadotropins (25–50 UI) and raise the dose when you cannot observe a dominant follicle. This is a way to avoid hyperstimulation syndrome and multiple pregnancy.[9-11]

Ovarian Hyperstimulation Syndrome

Ovarian hyperstimulation syndrome (OHSS) is infrequent in IUI cases when we use low doses of gonadotropins. OHSS involves an over response to the ovarian stimulation treatment. It can be classified in three degrees: mild, moderate, and severe:

1. Mild OHSS:
   i. *Grade 1:* Abdominal distension and discomfort.
   ii. *Grade 2:* Features of grade 1 plus nausea/vomiting and/or diarrhea. Ovaries enlarged to 5–12 cm.
2. Moderate OHHS:
   i. *Grade 3:* Features of mild OHSS plus ultrasonic evidence of ascites.
3. Severe OHSS:
   i. *Grade 4:* Features of moderate OHSS plus clinical evidence of ascites and/or hydrothorax (or breathing difficulties). Paracentesis due to OHHS symptoms.
   ii. *Grade 5:* All of above plus change in blood volume, increased blood viscosity due to hemoconcentration, coagulation abnormalities, diminished renal perfusion and function, and hospitalization due to OHSS symptoms. The polycystic ovary syndrome (PCOS) patients are at higher risk for OHSS. The risk relates to estradiol level and number of follicles at day of ovulation trigger with human chorionic gonadotropin (hCG). There are options to prevent OHSS in this case:
      a. Conversion of high-response (>4 follicles with a diameter larger than 14 mm or the level of E2 higher than 1,500 pg/mL)[12,13] to "rescue" IVF using a gonadotropin releasing hormone (GnRH) antagonist. This is a cost-effective strategy that produces better results than regular IVF with relatively minimal morbidity, and shorter duration to achieve pregnancy.[12,14]
      b. Use of a GnRH agonist to trigger the final follicular maturation in stimulated cycles of high responders. However, the rate of multiple pregnancies was found to be elevated, so it is not recommended.[15]

Table 2: Twin and high-order multiple pregnancies according to follicular size range in addition to one follicle measuring 16 mm or wider on the day of ovulation triggering per type of treatment.

Twin Pregnancies					
	Follicle ≤10 mm	*Follicle ≤12 mm*	*Follicle ≤14 mm*	*Follicle <16 mm*	*P-value*
IUI-H (n = 56)	1.8% (n = 1)	1.8% (n = 1)	10.7% (n = 6)	30.4% (n = 17)	<0.001
IUI-D (n = 71)	2.8% (n = 2)	2.8% (n = 2)	15.5% (n = 11)	40.8% (n = 29)	<0.001
High-order Multiple Pregnancies					
	Follicle ≤10 mm	*Follicle ≤12 mm*	*Follicle ≤14 mm*	*Follicle <16 mm*	*P-value*
IUI-H (n = 9)	0% (n = 0)	0% (n = 0)	44.4% (n = 4)	77.8% (n = 7)	<0.001
IUI-D (n = 10)	1% (n = 1)	1% (n = 1)	30% (n = 3)	50% (n = 5)	<0.001

(IUI-H: intrauterine insemination with husband's sperm; IUI-D: intrauterine insemination with donor's sperm.)

c. Aspiration of follicles before hCG administration.[16]
d. *Multiple pregnancy reduction:*[17] This should be avoided if possible, because of the psychological consequences. Fetal reduction is not good clinical practice. Also, a physician with a large clinical experience in fetal reduction and appropriate counseling for the couple need to be available.
e. Cancellation of the cycle and avoiding intercourse. This is the best option to avoid OHSS and multiple pregnancy.

Premature Luteinization

The LH surge is an absolute requirement for luteinization, final maturation of the oocyte, and follicle rupture. Premature luteinization (PL) can be defined as a premature rise of LH (>10 IU/L) accompanied by a concomitant rise in progesterone (>1 ng/mL or 3.2 nM/L).[18] Premature LH surges in natural cycles are rare, being more frequent in older women since their maximum follicle diameter at the time of ovulation is substantially smaller.[19]

The premature feedback of estradiol comes from progressive pituitary sensitization to GnRH in combination with a progressive and time-dependent increase in estradiol levels.

Premature LH surges occur in 25–30% of stimulated IUI cycles and theoretically may interfere with timing of the IUI or result in cancellation and more treatment failures.[18,20]

Premature luteinization could possibly be prevented with administration of a GnRH antagonist and low-dose gonadotropins but this does not substantially improve the pregnancy rate. It is likely that PL is not the cause but one of the consequences of the poor follicular maturation and quality.[18]

COMPLICATIONS OF INTRAUTERINE INSEMINATION TECHNIQUE

Problems with the Introduction of the Catheter

The inability to introduce the catheter through the cervix at the time of insemination may affect the results of IUI because it can cause bleeding and uterine contractions.

If the catheter cannot be placed into the endometrial cavity, the sperm can be deposited in cervical canal.[21] The possible causes of this problem are: the obstruction of the cervical opening secondary to adhesions from previous surgeries or infection; that the catheter is not soft and cannot pass through the endocervical canal; or that the cervical canal has an acute angle between the intracervical orifice and the endometrial cavity. Other anatomical causes of obstruction are endocervical polyps, endometrial polyps, submucous myomas, false channels secondary to prior surgery, or C-section or intrauterine adhesions.

How to avoid problems with the catheter and the insemination:

- Performing a mock transfer prior to starting treatment with IUI. If you have problems, you can try with a full or empty bladder. If it is still impossible to pass the catheter, a diagnostic hysteroscopy must be performed to correct any pathology and dilate the cervical canal.
- For IUI, the patient should be relaxed and comfortable, and be treated with a sterile technique and equipment.
- Patients with a full bladder can improve pregnancy rates because it is easier to pass the catheter when the uterus is in anteflexion. If patient has a retroflexed uterus, it is usually easier with an empty bladder.[22]
- Cleaning the ectocervical and endocervical canal to avoid infection and potentially reduce the introduction of harmful agents into the uterine cavity.
- Using a soft catheter which allows an easier intracervical canal passage into the uterine cavity without discomfort to the patient and without bleeding.
- Abdominal ultrasound imaging of the endocervical canal and uterus can assist physicians by showing where and how to introduce the insemination catheter and place the sperm.
- Gently pass the catheter through the cervical canal and then slowly place the sperm suspension into the uterine cavity.
- The recommended insemination volume is between 0.3 mL and 0.5 mL in order to prevent reflux of the sample. Amaral et al. found no differences when these two volumes were compared.[23]

Infection Post-insemination

Pelvic infection due to bacteria introduced with the sperm or by the insertion of the catheter through the cervix can occur. This is extremely rare.[24] The prevalence of pelvic infection has been reported to be 1.83 per 1,000 women undergoing IUI[25] from a review of 38 reported series. 2 cases, one of a ruptured pelvic abscess and the other an ovarian abscess following insemination, have been reported.[24,26]

- Possible sources of infection:
  - Media used for insemination
  - *Sperm sample:* The techniques used in sperm capacitation (swim-up or density gradient) eliminate most urethral and cutaneous microorganisms.[20,21]

Currently, antibiotics are added to the insemination media, such as penicillin, streptomycin or gentamicin. They are added in low concentrations to reduce the possibility of occurrence of anaphylactic reactions.
  - Microorganisms coming from the vagina, introduced with the catheter into the endometrial cavity.
- *Prophylactic antibiotics:* Yes or no?

The prevalence of infection is unaltered by the administration of prophylactic antibiotics or washing the semen sample with antibiotics. Therefore, IUI does not warrant routine antibiotic prophylaxis.[25]

- Advise to prevent infections:
  - Use a sterilized speculum
  - Sterile gloves
  - Cleaning the cervix
  - Sterile procedures in laboratory

Allergic Reaction

- *Seminal plasma:* It is removed through the sperm washing and capacitation.[27]
- Proteins in urine-derived gonadotropins could cause IgE-mediated hypersensitivity reactions in rare circumstances.[28]
- *Components of culture media:* Anaphylaxis after intrauterine insemination can be due to:
  - Antibiotics used in culture media.[29]
  - The bovine serum albumin (BSA). It is recommended to test the media prior to insemination if the patient has a history of allergies to animal epithelium.[27,30-33]

Antisperm Antibodies

Chymotrypsin can be used in the sperm pretreatment.[27]

Hemorrhage

- At the exocervix if patient has ectropion or a cervical polyp and we touch them with the inseminating catheter.
- When transfer is difficult and damage or trauma is inflicted to the intracervical canal.

PREGNANCY COMPLICATIONS AFTER INTRAUTERINE INSEMINATION

Ectopic Pregnancy

Risk of ectopic pregnancy is between 1.3% and 4–8% in small series.[34] The risk is greater with high estradiol levels and tuboperitoneal factor. IVI has an incidence of 0.37% in IUI-H and 0.29% in IUI-D.

Ovarian Torsion

There are only two published case reports of adnexal torsion.[35,36]

Risk of Transferring Infectious Diseases to Offspring

Significant reduction of the risk is possible in cases of Hepatitis C and HIV through sperm washing. This allows the use of the mobile fraction of sperm for IUI after eliminating components from the HIV and hepatitis C virus (HCV) from leukocytes in seminal plasma. Using polymerase chain reaction (PCR) prior to using the washed sample ensures the absence of virus.

Obstetric Problems

There is a higher incidence of pre-eclampsia in women conceiving by intrauterine insemination with washed donor sperm compared with intrauterine insemination with washed partner sperm.[37,38]

Twin pregnancy and multiple pregnancies have a higher incidence of premature delivery, low birth weight, and growth restriction.

Psychological Risks

Some couples experience anxiety symptoms and depression in one or both of the partners. In some cases, difficulties in the couple's relationship may arise. The waiting period between insemination and confirmation of the result as well as repeated failures with IUI create anxiety to the couple.

IVI group psychological support before, during, and after IUI treatment and patients appreciate of those efforts. A phone call while waiting to know the result of the procedure can help the couple feel more relaxed and comfortable.

CONCLUSION

- Successful pregnancy depends on careful control of the cycles with adjustment of the gonadotropin dosage. If there is risk of multiple pregnancy, the best option is cancellation of the cycle.
- Low-dose gonadotropin regimen combined with a GnRH antagonist may be an alternative treatment option for subjects with previous proven PL/ovulation.

- Mock transfer prior to the IUI cycle start and the use of sterile instruments and catheters to avoid technical problems and possible infection.
- The IUI procedure must be gentle and sterile.

REFERENCES

1. Cohen MR. Intrauterine insemination. Int J Fertil. 1962;7:235-40.
2. NICE Guidelines. (2013). Fertility problems: Assessment and treatment.
3. Abbas SM, Rouzi AA. Pregnancy with 15 live fetuses and severe ovarian hyperstimulation syndrome after ovulation induction and intrauterine insemination. Clin Exp Obstet Gynecol. 2013;40(2):297-9.
4. De Geyter Ch, Calhaz-Jorge C, Kupka MS, et al. Results generated from European registers by ESHRE. Hum Reprod. 2018;19:1-16.
5. Tur R, Barri PN, Coroleu B, Buxaderas R, Martinez F, Balasch J. Risk factors for high-order multiple implantation after ovarian stimulation with gonadotrophins: evidence from a large series of 1878 consecutive pregnancies in a single centre. Human Reproduction. 2001;16(10):2124-9.
6. Dickey RP, Taylor SN, Lu PY, et al. Risk factors for high-order multiple pregnancy and multiple birth after controlled ovarian hyperstimulation: Results of 4,062 intrauterine insemination cycles. Fertil Steril. 2005;83(3):671-83.
7. Gleicher N, Oleske DM, Tur-Kaspa I, et al. Reducing the risk of high-order multiple pregnancy after ovarian stimulation with gonadotropins. N Engl J Med. 2000;343(1):2-7.
8. Giles J, Cruz M, González-Ravina C, Caligara C, Prados N, Martínez JC, Vergara V, Requena A. Small-sized follicles could contribute to high-order multiple pregnancies: outcomes of 6552 intrauterine insemination. RBMO Volume 00 Issue 0 2018).
9. Lan VT, Norman RJ, Nhu GH, et al. Ovulation induction using low-dose step-up rFSH in Vietnamese women with polycystic ovary syndrome. Reprod Biomed Online. 2009;18(4): 516-21.
10. Homburg R, Levy T, Ben-Rafael Z. A comparative prospective study of conventional regimen with chronic low-dose administration of follicle-stimulating hormone for anovulation associated with polycystic ovary syndrome. Fertil Steril. 1995;63(4):729-33.
11. Orvieto R, Homburg R. Chronic ultra-low dose follicle-stimulating hormone regimen for patients with polycystic ovary syndrome: One click, one follicle, one pregnancy. Fertil Steril. 2009;91(4 Suppl):1533-5.
12. Zhong Y, Li J, Ying Y, et al. The efficacy of conversion from IUI to IVF-ET in infertility patients with hyper-response to ovulation induction: A retrospective study. Biomed Pap Med Fac Univ Palacky Olomouc Czech Repub. 2012;156(2):159-63.
13. Nisker J, Tummon I, Daniel S, et al. Conversion of cycles involving ovarian hyperstimulation with intra-uterine insemination to in-vitro fertilization. Hum Reprod. 1994;9(3):406-8.
14. Balayla J, Granger L, St-Michel P, et al. Rescue in vitro fertilization using a GnRH antagonist in hyperresponders from gonadotropin intrauterine insemination (IUI) cycles. J Assis Reprod Genet. 2013;30(6):773-8.
15. Awwad JT, Hannoun AB, Khalil A, et al. Induction of final follicle maturation with a gonadotropin-releasing hormone agonist in women at risk of ovarian hyperstimulation syndrome undergoing gonadotropin stimulation and intrauterine insemination: proof-of-concept study. Clin Exp Obstet Gynecol. 2012;39(4):436-9.
16. Albano C, Platteau P, Nogueira D, et al. Avoidance of multiple pregnancies after ovulation induction by supernumerary preovulatory follicular reduction. Fertil Steril. 2001;76(4):820-2.
17. Ombelet W, De Sutter P, Van der Elst J, et al. Multiple gestation and infertility treatment: registration, reflection and reaction—The Belgian project. Hum Reprod Update. 2005;11(1):3-14.
18. Lambalk CB, Leader A, Olivennes F, et al. Treatment with the GnRH antagonist ganirelix prevents premature LH rises and luteinization in stimulated intrauterine insemination: Results of a double-blind, placebo-controlled, multicentre trial. Hum Reprod. 2006;21(3):632-9.
19. de Koning CH, McDonnell J, Themmen AP, et al. The endocrine and follicular growth dynamics throughout the menstrual cycle in women with consistently or variably elevated early follicular phase FSH compared with controls. Hum Reprod. 2008;23(6):1416-23.
20. Cantineau AE, Cohlen BJ, Dutch IUISG. The prevalence and influence of luteinizing hormone surges in stimulated cycles combined with intrauterine insemination during a prospective cohort study. Fertil Steril. 2007;88(1):107-12.
21. Matorras R, Gorostiaga A, Diez J, et al. Intrauterine insemination with frozen sperm increases pregnancy rates in donor insemination cycles under gonadotropin stimulation. Fertil Steril. 1996;65(3):620-5.
22. Ayas S, Gurbuz A, Ayaz R, et al. Efficacy of passive uterine straightening during intrauterine insemination on pregnancy rates and ease of technique. J Obstet Gynaecol Res. 2012;38(1):291-6.
23. Do Amaral VF, Ferriani RA, Dos Reis RM, et al. Effect of inseminated volume on intrauterine insemination. J Assist Reprod Genet. 2001;18(8):413-6.
24. Sable DB, Yanushpolsky EH, Fox JH. Ruptured pelvic abscess after intrauterine insemination: A case report. Fertil Steril. 1993;59(3):679-80.
25. Sacks PC, Simon JA. Infectious complications of intrauterine insemination: A case report and literature review. Int J Fertil. 1991;36(6):331-9.
26. Kolb BA, Mercer L, Peters AJ, et al. Ovarian abscess following therapeutic insemination. Infect Dis Obstet Gynecol. 1994;1(5):249-51.
27. Iwahashi K, Miyazaki T, Kuji N, et al. Successful pregnancy in a woman with a human seminal plasma allergy. A case report. J Reprod Med. 1999;44(4):391-3.
28. Koh YI, Choi IS, Lee HC, et al. Desensitization to urine-derived gonadotropins in a woman with secondary infertility. Ann Allergy Asthma Immunol. 2001;87(5):434-8.
29. Al-Ramahi M, Leader A, Leveille MC. An allergic reaction following intrauterine insemination. Hum Reprod. 1998;13(12):3368-70.
30. Pagan JA, Postigo I, Rodriguez-Pacheco JR, et al. Bovine serum albumin contained in culture medium used in artificial insemination is an important anaphylaxis risk factor. Fertil Steril. 2008;90(5):2013.e17-9.

31. Sonenthal KR, McKnight T, Shaughnessy MA, et al. Anaphylaxis during intrauterine insemination secondary to bovine serum albumin. Fertil Steril. 1991;56(6): 1188-91.
32. Liccardi G, Asero R, D'Amato M, et al. Role of sensitization to mammalian serum albumin in allergic disease. Curr Allergy Asthma Rep. 2011;11(5):421-6.
33. Orta M, Ordoqui E, Aranzabal A, et al. Anaphylactic reaction after artificial insemination. Ann Allergy Asthma Immunol. 2003;90(4):446-51.
34. Zadehmodarres S, Oladi B, Saeedi S, et al. Intrauterine insemination with husband semen: an evaluation of pregnancy rate and factors affecting outcome. J Assist Reprod Genet. 2009;26(1):7-11.
35. Child TJ, Watson NR, Ledger WL. Sequential bilateral adnexal torsion after a single cycle of gonadotropin ovulation induction with intrauterine insemination. Fertil Steril. 1997;67(3):573-5.
36. Krishnan S, Kaur H, Bali J, et al. Ovarian torsion in infertility management—Missing the diagnosis means losing the ovary: A high price to pay. J Hum Reprod Sci. 2011;4(1):39-42.
37. Smith GN, Walker M, Tessier JL, et al. Increased incidence of preeclampsia in women conceiving by intrauterine insemination with donor versus partner sperm for treatment of primary infertility. Am J Obstet Gynecol. 1997;177(2):455-8.
38. Salha O, Sharma V, Dada T, et al. The influence of donated gametes on the incidence of hypertensive disorders of pregnancy. Hum Reprod. 1999;14(9):2268-73.

CHAPTER

28

Ethical and Psychosocial Aspects in Intrauterine Insemination

Mirudhubashini Govindarajan, Ramya Jayaram

INTRODUCTION

Infertile couples face several difficulties while undergoing infertility management.

Infertility and its management can be stressful from an emotional, physical, and financial point of view. It is the physician's responsibility to recognize and deal with these problems. In their keen interest and effort to deal with the clinical and medical problems, the other aspects may often be overlooked by the physicians.

Nearly 15% of all couples face the problem of infertility, and encounter feelings of depression, grief, chronic stress, and anxiety. Marital disharmony, mental, and sexual problems are often seen as issues among the infertile couples.

PSYCHOSOCIAL CONSEQUENCES OF INFERTILITY MANAGEMENT

- Isolation from social activities and friends
- Altered relationship with other family members who are fertile and have children
- Negative feeling toward medical establishment and abusive or critical of doctor's competence
- A feeling of intrusion into the sex life, affecting intimacy
- Feeling of loss of privacy leading to impotence and vaginismus
- Women become vulnerable and suffer from chronic depression with acute episodes of exacerbation
- Anger toward their husbands for having fertility problem
- Men may feel a loss of self-esteem and guilt about having to subject their wife to the pain and intrusion of insemination
- Either partner may develop a fear of losing their partner and/or instability in the marriage.

NEED FOR COUNSELING

Counseling becomes mandatory in the following situations:

- Persistent anxiety or depression
- Preoccupation with infertility
- Marital discord
- Sadness or guilt
- Loss of happiness
- Indecision regarding treatment options.

Objectives of Psychosocial Management/Counseling

- To impart knowledge about their specific problem, need for the procedure and the procedure itself
- To ensure that the patient understands the implications of their treatment choice
- To provide emotional support to deal with the outcome of the procedures
- Assuring privacy—a paramount concern
- To assure accessibility at any time—before, during, and after treatment.

Types of Counseling

Implication Counseling

- To enable couples to understand the implications of the treatment for themselves, their family and for any children born as a result
- Areas of concern such as anonymity, confidentiality, and risk of transmission from the donor of genetic and infectious diseases, etc. are dealt with
- Genetic counseling offered when there is an increased risk of passing on an inherited disease to the offspring

- Psychological counseling offered for partners suffering from psychosexual problems such as impotence and vaginismus.

Support Counseling

- To be aware of couple's individual needs and an effort to pursuit their peace of mind
- To give emotional support and information from the start of the treatment
- Alleviate feelings of isolation
- To help to deal with social and family pressure
- To enable couple to cope with stress by relaxation training and self-nurturing techniques
- To help infertile couples to process their feelings, to lead a normal life, and maintain marital harmony
- To understand and accept the limited success rates.

Therapeutic Counseling

- Help couples to understand their expectation, including the prospects of failure and adjusting to childlessness
- Focuses on sexual and menstrual problems.

SUMMARY

Psychological issues that need to be faced and sorted out are:

- Men
  - Loss of self-esteem
  - Fear of losing wife
- Women
  - Feeling of guilt
  - Feeling of anger
- Couple
  - Intimacy affected
  - Intrusion into sexual life.

ETHICAL GUIDELINES AS FORMULATED BY INDIAN COUNCIL OF MEDICAL RESEARCH

The following should be strictly adhered to for intrauterine insemination procedures:

- Complete and appropriate records should be maintained
- Appropriate consent forms should be signed by both partners
- Procedures should not be undertaken with unilateral consent alone
- No procedure shall be performed on a woman who is below 21 years of age
- The infrastructure of the facility, equipment, and procedure should conform to the norms as laid down by the guideline of Indian Council of Medical Research.

In case of donor IUI procedure, the following should be followed:

- The donor sample should be obtained only from the registered assisted reproductive technology (ART) banks
- A sample shall not be obtained from a friend, relative, or a known person
- Assisted reproductive technology center shall not mix semen samples of two individuals for insemination
- No woman shall be treated with gametes derived from more than one individual during any one treatment cycle
- One sample of semen supplied by an ART bank shall be used only once, on one recipient only.

LEGAL AND ETHICAL CONCERNS OF DONOR INSEMINATION

- Sperm donors and recipients should be informed about potential legal, medical, and emotional issues associated with donor insemination.
- Donors should be provided with the results of their medical evaluation. They should understand that they do not have control over the disposition of their sperm after it has been collected.
- Social fathers are legally recognized as the child's father. The donor has no legal rights or duties with respect to the children concerned. Moreover, donors and recipients have an obligation to authorize disclosure of nonidentifying medical information when appropriate.
- Disclosure of donor identity either to the recipient or to the offspring will remain a matter of controversy and varies from country to country.

CHAPTER

29

Medicolegal Aspects of Intrauterine Insemination

Arati Gupte Shah, Manish Banker, Pravin Patel

INTRODUCTION

Intrauterine insemination (IUI) involves the processing of semen in the laboratory so as to yield active sperm, devoid of seminal plasma, which are then directly placed into the uterus.

INDICATIONS FOR IUI-HUSBAND AND IUI-DONOR

- Cervical hostility
- Problems with intercourse or ejaculation
- Unexplained infertility
- Intrauterine insemination donor (IUI-D), if
  - Husband having nonobstructive azoospermia
  - Hereditary genetic defects in husband.

Although assisted reproductive technology (ART) in India has come of age, numerous gray areas still remain. In the last decade, the number of patients seeking treatment for infertility has gone up drastically mainly because of patient awareness and acceptance. IUI is now considered a routine practice and has generally gained acceptance among infertile patients.

Various countries have their own sets of rules and regulations to govern these procedures. This chapter deals with the medicolegal aspects of IUI in India.

To deal with issues regarding the clinical and ethical execution of these practices, and to make certain that they are resolved, the Indian Council for Medical Research (ICMR), under the Ministry of Health and Family Welfare, Government of India has come up with the draft of the ART Bill: Rules and Regulations in 2010. Parts of this bill were last updated in 2017. This has detailed laws in relation to all aspects of ART, including IUI covering medical, ethical, and moral issue. Although this bill is yet to become a law, it is being widely followed by Indian ART practitioners. This act has a code of practice related to every aspect of IUI.

CODE OF PRACTICE

This covers the following areas:

- Registration
- Facilities
- Confidentiality
- Information to patient
- Consent
- Counseling
- Use of gametes and embryos
- Storage and handling of gametes and embryos
- Research
- Complaints.

Registration

All clinics are to be registered under the National Registry of ART Clinics and Banks in India.

Facilities

This covers requirements of the location where insemination is done. The ICMR has divided the types of ART clinics according to their infrastructure and staffing.

Assisted reproductive technology clinics have been divided into three categories depending on the facilities they provide:

1. *Primary/level 1 clinics*: These clinics do not have facilities for IUI; only consultations, counseling,

and infertility treatment not involving collection or processing of gametes is carried out at these clinics. They do not require any registration

2. *Secondary/level 2 clinics*: These clinics have facilities for handling semen and performing IUI with self as well as donor sperm. They require facilities for hysteroscopy, laparoscopy, transvaginal ultrasound, and follicular monitoring, semen collection and processing, sperm function tests, and immunological tests. These clinics will require registration and accreditation. They are not, however, required to have facilities for oocyte handling, in vitro fertilization (IVF) or intracytoplasmic sperm injection (ICSI).
3. *Tertiary/level 3 clinics*: These clinics must have all facilities needed for handling oocytes, embryos, and sperms. They are to have provisions for genetic testing, cryopreservation, and surgical interventions. These clinics will also require registration and accreditation.

- Basic infrastructure requirements for level 2 clinic:
  - Waiting room
  - Examination room
  - Store room
  - Record room
  - Autoclave room
  - Steps for vermin proofing
  - Semen collection room
  - Semen processing laboratory
  - Clean room for IUI
  - Operation theater
  - *Laboratory facilities:* For hormonal assays, microbiology, and histopathology (which can be outsourced to an accredited laboratory)
  - Backup power supply
  - One room can double up for two purposes.
- Staffing:
  - Gynecologist
  - Andrologist/embryologist
  - Counselor
  - Program coordinator/director.

Confidentiality

Confidentiality of the patient undergoing treatment must be maintained at all costs, even from her family if required. In case of donor IUI, this confidentiality agreement works both ways. The donor is assured that his identity will not be revealed to the recipient. Similarly, sperm from a known donor is not permitted according to the Act. This is to avoid future disputes related to paternity and conflicts on property and ownership arising out of this.

Information

The patient or couple must be explained the technique of the procedure she is undergoing, the advantages or disadvantages, different methods available, the success rates, the time required, possible complications, postprocedure care, and costs. This helps the patient to make an informed decision about the treatment she is receiving.

There is some basic information that must be conveyed before starting treatment include the possibility of gametes losing their viability when in storage for too long, and the fact that over time, the type of treatments may change, depending primarily on the patient's age.

Informed Consent

The patient's consent is taken along with that of her spouse. In case of donor IUI, a separate consent form is required.

***Form-E:* Consent for Artificial Insemination or Intrauterine Insemination with Husband's Semen/Sperm**

We,_____and____, being husband and wife and both of legal age, authorize Dr.___ to inseminate the wife artificially or intrauterine with the semen or sperm of the husband for achieving conception.

We understand that even though the insemination may be repeated as often as recommended by the doctor, there is no guarantee or assurance that pregnancy or a live birth will result.

We have also been told that the outcome of pregnancy may not be the same as those of the general pregnant population, for example in respect of abortion, multiple pregnancies, anomalies or complications of pregnancy or delivery.

The procedure carried out does not ensure a positive result, nor does it guarantee a mentally and physically normal child. This consent holds good for all the cycles performed at the clinic.

Endorsement by the assisted reproductive technology clinic:

I/we have personally explained to____and____the details and implications of his/her/their signing this consent/approval form, and made sure to the extent humanly possible that he/she/they understand these details and implications.

Signed:_____(Husband)_____(Wife)

Name and signature of the doctor

Name, address and signature of the witness from the clinic Name and address of the ART clinic

Dated:

***Form-F:* Consent for Artificial Insemination or Intrauterine Insemination with Donor Semen**

We,_____and_____, being husband and wife and both of legal age, authorize Dr._____to inseminate the wife artificially or intrauterine with semen/sperm of a donor (ART bank's no. _____; obtained from_____ART bank with valid registration no. ______) for achieving conception.

We understand that even though the insemination may be repeated as often as recommended by the doctor, there is no guarantee or assurance that pregnancy or a live birth will result.

We have also been told that the outcome of pregnancy may not be the same as those of the general pregnant population, for example in respect of abortion, multiple pregnancies, anomalies or complications of pregnancy or delivery.

We declare that we shall not attempt to find out the identity of the donor. *I, the husband, also declare that should my wife bear any child or children as a result of such insemination(s), such child or children shall be as my own and shall be my legal heir(s).*

The procedure carried out does not ensure a positive result, nor does it guarantee a mentally and physically normal body. This consent holds good for all the cycles performed at the clinic.

Endorsement by the assisted reproductive technology clinic:

I/we have personally explained to_____and_____the details and implications of his/her/their signing this consent/approval form, and made sure to the extent humanly possible that he/she/they understand these details and implications.

Signed:_____(Husband)_____(Wife) Name and signature of the doctor

Name, address and signature of the witness from the clinic Name and address of the ART clinic

Dated:

Note: An appropriate modification of this form may be used for artificial insemination or IUI of a single woman with donor semen.

Counseling

The patient/couple should undergo a session with a professional counselor to relieve anxieties and answer questions. It is important to discuss with the patient, the emotional and psychological aspects of the treatment she is undergoing.

The counselor can discuss with the patient, side effects if any that this treatment can have, what effects it can have on her domestic life and routine. The patient can be taught stress relieving techniques and the importance of a positive mindset. Support from the patient's spouse is essential and should be explained to the couple.

When a report is negative, the counselor can empathize with their disappointment and help them look forward to start over.

The patient can be made aware of complications, and the possibility that at times, steps like fetal reduction or pregnancy termination might become essential.

In some cases, a patient can be counseled about where to draw the line and stop treatment.

In cases of donor IUI, the husbands especially might suffer from low self-esteem. They need to be counseled to make them understand that the children born from this treatment are still as much as their biological children would be. They also need to make them understand that the child has a right to want to know the identity of the donor once he/she reaches 18 years of age.

STORAGE AND HANDLING OF GAMETES AND EMBRYOS

Rules for storage and handling of sperm:

- Instructions for proper collection
- Meticulous labeling
- Liquid nitrogen containers for cryopreservation
- Duration for which semen can be stored (up to 10 years)
- Protocol for discarding frozen samples.

RIGHTS OF A CHILD BORN THROUGH INTRAUTERINE INSEMINATION

A child born through this process is considered to be the legitimate child of the parents. In case of donor IUI, the husband signs a consent stating that he accepts the child as his own. The child is granted the same legal rights and status as his own biological child. The birth certificate carries the names of both parents and makes no mention of the donor.

DONOR FOR INTRAUTERINE INSEMINATION

Rules for donor selection:

- The donor must be aged between 21 years and 45 years
- Donors must be rigorously screened for any chronic, transmissible or genetic diseases
- According to the draft ART Bill, a semen sample must be cryopreserved for a 6-month quarantine period, and then retested for HIV, before it is released for use
- The sperm of a single donor cannot be used more than 75 times

- One sample of semen must be used for one recipient only
- Mixing of semen of two separate individuals is prohibited under any circumstances. Special permission from the National Advisory Board is required if mixing is indicated for any reason.

Rights and Duties of Donors

A donor's identity cannot be revealed to the recipient or the offspring. The donor, on signing consent for sperm donation, legally relinquishes all parental rights over the child born through use of his sperm.

MANAGING COMPLICATIONS

Some of the complications that can occur are:

- *Multiple gestations*: If stimulation for IUI leads to development of more than three follicles, the patient should be explained the chances of multiple pregnancies, and the complications that can occur out of carrying more than one fetus. Ideally, such a cycle should either be cancelled or converted to an IVF cycle, where only up to three embryos can be transferred.
- *Abortions and ectopic pregnancies*: The patient must be explained about the risk of abortions and ectopic pregnancies. The patients should also be explained that the risk is the same as that for a normal conception.
- *Ovarian hyperstimulation syndrome*: Although this is rare in cases of IUI, it is possible especially in cases where gonadotropins are used for ovarian stimulation or in cases of polycystic ovary syndrome (PCOS).

The clinic where IUI is carried out should have the infrastructure and know-how to manage these complications.

OTHER ETHICAL ISSUES

Age Limit

The new version of the bill has introduced an age limit for couples seeking infertility treatment, and this applies to IUI as well.

Only men between the age of 21 years and 50 years and women between the age of 18 years and 45 years are legally entitled to avail treatment.

Consummation of Marriage

According to the draft Act, IUI does not amount to consummation of marriage and a woman can still seek divorce on grounds of impotency.

Adultery

Use of donor sperm for IUI does not amount to adultery. As long as the husband has consented to the procedure, it is considered legal. Donor IUI without the husband's consent can, however, be grounds for divorce.

Single Woman and Intrauterine Insemination Donor

The original bill of 2010 stated that an unmarried woman above the age of 21 years has the right to try for conception using an unknown donor sperm. Only the consent of the patient is sufficient. A child born through this process is considered a legitimate child of that parent with the same legal rights and privileges as a child born in wedlock.

Although the new modification in 2017 does not mention treatment for single women, many clinics have been known to refuse treatment on moral grounds.

Sex Selection and Intrauterine Insemination

Sex selection at any stage is prohibited under the Pre-Conception and Pre-Natal Diagnostic Techniques (PCPNDT) Act.

Intrauterine Insemination and Surrogacy

Traditional surrogacy, where a surrogate gives her eggs in addition to her womb is now considered illegal. Intrauterine insemination with surrogacy is thus prohibited by the draft ART Act.

POSTHUMOUS INTRAUTERINE INSEMINATION

Posthumous artificial insemination using the husband's semen sample stored in a semen bank is allowed and considered legitimate. Two types of posthumous insemination are defined:

1. The first where the sperms have been provided by the man before his death and with a written consent
2. The second, posthumous sperm retrieval, which is done after the death of a man without his prior consent.

According to the most recent International Federation of Fertility Societies (IFFS) surveillance, many countries legally recognize and allow both these types of posthumous artificial insemination by husband (AIH), but is rarely used in practice. India is one of these countries, as opposed to USA and UK, where posthumous AIH is practiced regularly.

The ART Bill of 2017 states that posthumous IUI is permitted legally only if prior consent from both partners is available.

RECENT ADVANCES

Use of stem cells to create male gametes has the potential to eliminate third party involvement thus opening up a whole new avenue of treatment.

There are currently no laws related to this technology since this is still under research.

SUGGESTED READING

1. National Ethical Guidelines for Biomedical and Health Research involving Human Participants. ICMR 2017. https://icmr.nic.in/sites/default/files/guidelines/ICMR_Ethical_Guidelines_2017.pdf
2. The Assisted Reproductive Technologies (Regulation) Bill 2010. www.icmr.nic.in/sites/default/files/guidelines/ART%20REGULATION%20Draft%20Bill1.pdf
3. The Assisted Reproductive Technologies Regulation (Rules) 2010. www.icmr.nic.in/sites/default/files/guidelines/ART%20REGULATION%20Draft%20Rules%201.pdf
4. The Assisted Reproductive Technology (Regulation) Bill 2017. https://dhr.gov.in/sites/default/files/Asssited%20Reproductive%20Technology%20%28Regulation%29%20Bill%2C2017.pdf
5. The Surrogacy (Regulation) Bill 2018. http://164.100.47.4/BillsTexts/LSBillTexts/PassedLoksabha/257-C%20_2016_Eng.pdf

CHAPTER

30

Design, Equipment and Personnel Management for Intrauterine Insemination Laboratory

Yolanda Minguez, Javier Herrero Zapata, Irene Rubio Palacios

INTRODUCTION

Designing an intrauterine insemination (IUI) laboratory involves the consideration of many aspects which can be encompassed into two groups. On one hand, recommendations and obligations applicable at the time of designing the laboratory and on the other, the setting of specific objectives for the services being offered. Laboratory set-up providing assisted reproductive technology (ART) services would have to be setup as per the guidelines of the reproductive medicine societies of the respective nations.[1] Regarding the latter, it should be taken into account that any unit focused on dealing with patients should be maintain the desired quality parameters. In medical field, the main attributes of quality are effectiveness, safety and robustness.[2] These attributes must be a part of the performances and processes at various levels, i.e. the quality of the process is ensured only if it is possible to prove the effectiveness and the safety of the process and if this process is robust or not. The latter means that the process works under various conditions and is not "defective".

Success of any IUI unit mainly depends on the infrastructure of the laboratory and the skill of the personnel working.[3] In this sense, a detailed layout and assessment of all laboratory furniture and equipment is essential prior to construction and can drastically improve the cost-benefit ratio. On his behalf, authorized technical staff shall demonstrate knowledge and competence in the concerned speciality.

The purpose of this chapter is to provide key aspects for the design of the IUI laboratory, the necessary equipment and personnel management in terms of requirements and safety, based on the specific procedures that an IUI laboratory can offer.

LABORATORY DESIGN

The laboratory should have adequate space to follow good laboratory practice as suggested by the "European Society of Human Reproduction and Embryology (ESHRE) guidelines for good practice in in vitro fertilization laboratories," as applicable for an IUI area.[4] There are different key points that should be taken into account. The first step is to determine the estimated number of cycles the laboratory is expected to perform in a given time period. Careful thought should go into the design and organization of the laboratory in order to minimize risks to gametes while maximizing embryologist/andrologist comfort, efficiency and use of space. To ensure an optimal handling of gametes during the treatment, the maintenance of cleanliness is an uncompromising issue. A water source is also required for hand washing, ideally it should be located in a corner and deep enough to avoid splashing. Air should be clean, free of dust, smoke, gases and microbes. For that purpose, the clinic and hence the laboratory should be located away from traffic, dust and fumes. The air supply in the laboratory should be equipped with filters, preferably high efficiency particulate absorbing filters to minimize the airborne contamination. All the individuals handling samples in the laboratory should change into clean clothes made up of cotton preferably, and wear slippers and non-powdered gloves while working in the laboratory.[5]

Another important point is the location of the semen collection room, if possible, adjacent to the laboratory, to facilitate the handling of the collected specimen. In fact, the ideal location of the IUI laboratory is between the semen collection room and the insemination room.

Regarding the laboratory building, the walls and ceiling should have absolute minimum number of penetrations.

The walls should reach the roof and be made of joint free stainless steel, covered with epoxy paint (no interior paint should contain materials like formaldehyde, acetaldehyde, benzene, etc.). Avoid false ceiling construction. Floor should be dust, crevices and crack free. It should be covered with large marble tiles, or granite tiles; alternately, with vitrified tiles. Bench surfaces should be resistant to acid, alkali, solvent and heat. Door will require seals and sweeps, and should be lockable. Another important issue is that electrical wiring should be concealed. Continuous power supply with power protection is essential. It is very important also to take into account that ducts and equipment must be laid out in such a way that routine and emergency maintenance and repair work can be performed outside the laboratory with minimum disruption.[3] Consideration should also be given to local health and safety requirements.

The location of storage areas and equipment such as incubators, centrifuges and cryo equipment should be logically planned for efficiency and safety within each working area. It should have enough space to store liquid nitrogen cylinders and tanks, disposables, media and other supplies. Thought should be given also to the most recent developments in equipment and facilities.

Separate office space should be provided for administrative work, such as record keeping and data entry.

Laboratory designer must keep in mind that laboratory personnel has to work for long hours, so it is essential to take into account aspects related to ergonomics such as bench height, adjustable chairs, microscope eyepiece height, efficient use of space and surfaces, sufficient air condition and the amount of daylight, all contribute to a working environment that minimizes distraction and fatigue. In this sense, humidity and temperature should be completely controlled according to climate and seasonal variation. As a reference, the temperature inside the laboratory should be around 20–24 °C and at less than 40% relative humidity.

EQUIPMENT

A detailed layout and assessment of all laboratory furniture is essential prior to construction in order to reach the best space achievement and create a distribution as more comfortable and functional as possible. Equipment should be suitably located in the laboratory so as to allow accessibility and sequential utilization thus minimizing the need for frequent movement of specimens or reagents.

A detailed list of equipment should be prepared out and checked against the planned location of each item, and should be of adequate capacity to meet workload requirement.

The essential items of equipment required for a laboratory are:

- A binocular phase contrast microscope with ×20, ×40 and ×100 objectives and ×10 eyepiece. Oil immersion lens should be available, and if possible also photography/video camera attached if training is desired (Fig. 1)
- A benchtop centrifuge for sperm processing with a rotor (calibrated in *g* or in revolutions per minute) and a timer, to control the speed and time (Figs 2 and 3)
- A refrigerator (around 4°C) and a freezer (–15 to –20°C) for the purpose of storing media, reagents and other materials that require refrigeration or be frozen (Figs 4 and 5)
- An incubator adjusted approximately to 35–37°C and 5% CO_2 to be used for the storage of bicarbonate based media and sperm capacitation, and a heater adjusted to 35–37°C for liquefaction of semen samples and warming of buffered media and mineral oil (Fig. 6)
- A laminar flow hood is recommended. The hood reduces contamination of semen samples as well as offering protection to laboratory personnel. A laminar flow hood can be either a vertical or a horizontal flow. Vertical flow is less harmful to the laboratory workers as the air flow is not directly aimed at their faces. On the other hand, a horizontal flow is more effective in reducing contamination (Fig. 7)
- Micropipettes 10–100 µL, 100–1,000 µL, automatic pipette (Figs. 8 and 9)
- Test tube racks to place the sample tubes (Fig. 10)
- Sperm counting chamber, such as Neubauer or Mackler (Fig. 11)
- Spirit burners (Fig. 12)
- Laboratory counter, to make easier the counting of the semen samples moreover in laboratories with a large volume of work (Fig. 13)
- Calculator (Fig. 14)
- Thermometers for both incubator/heater and fridge (Figs. 15A and B)
- Timer: It is used for control the time incubation of the sample, indicating the end of the processing (Fig. 16)
- Liquid nitrogen tank for storage of frozen samples and the related material as protective gloves and glasses (Figs. 17 and 18)
- Dustbins for the safe disposal of biological and laboratory materials; they can be made of paperboard, plastic sharped containers or waste plastic bags, always with the international "biohazard" symbol. If possible, glassware should be omitted in the laboratory, otherwise the Pasteur pipettes and broken glassware should be discarded in special containers (Fig. 19)

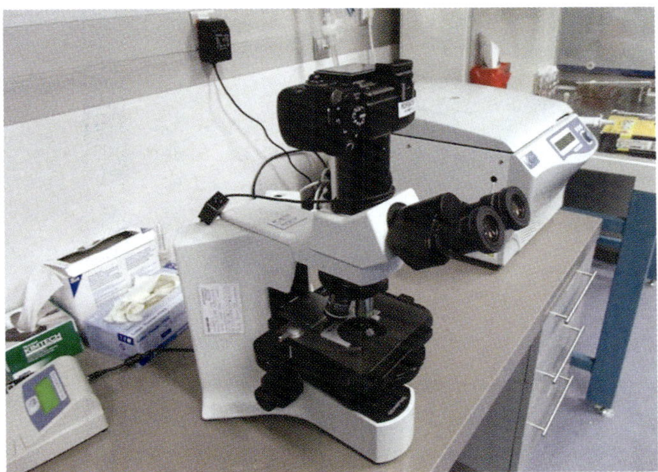

Fig. 1: Binocular phase contrast microscope

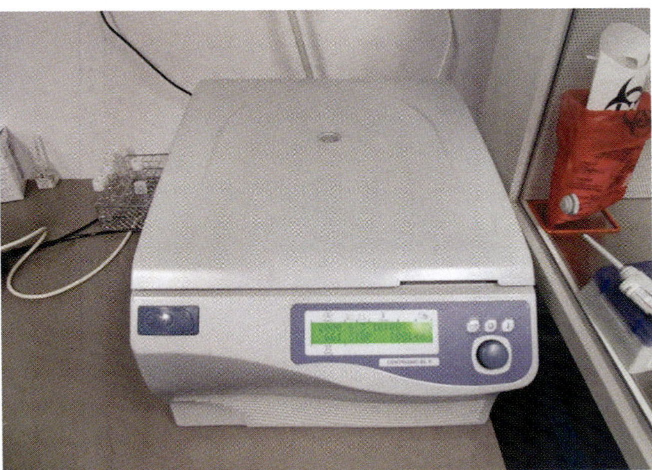

Fig. 2: A benchtop centrifuge for sperm processing

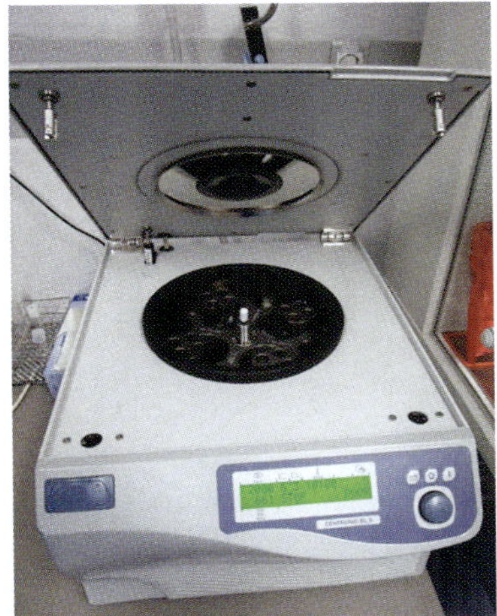

Fig. 3: Detail of the rotor (calibrated in g or in revolutions per minute) inside the centrifuge

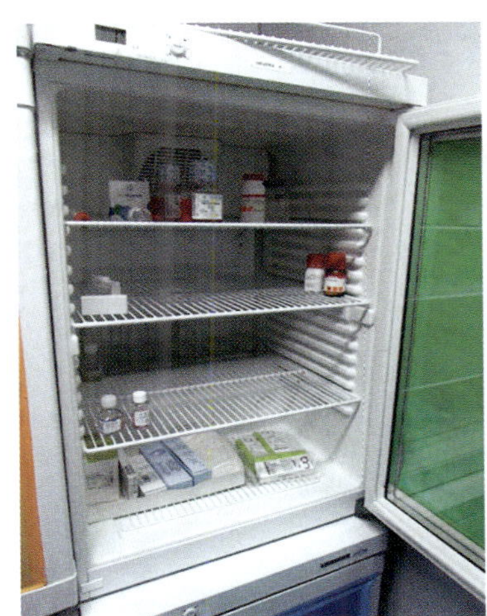

Fig. 4: A refrigerator (around 4°C) for storing media and reagents

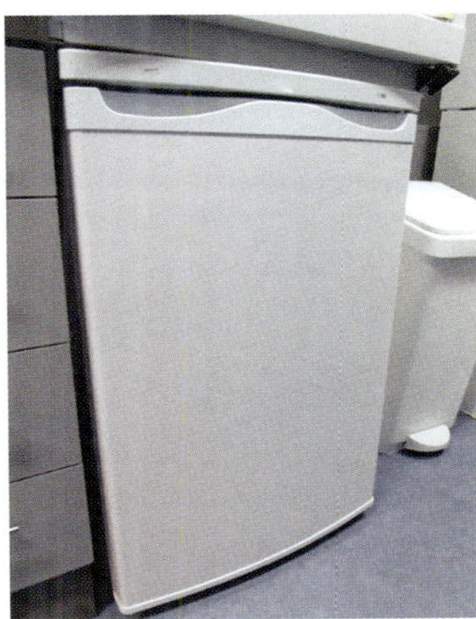

Fig. 5: A freezer (–15 to –20°C) to storage some media that requires lower temperatures

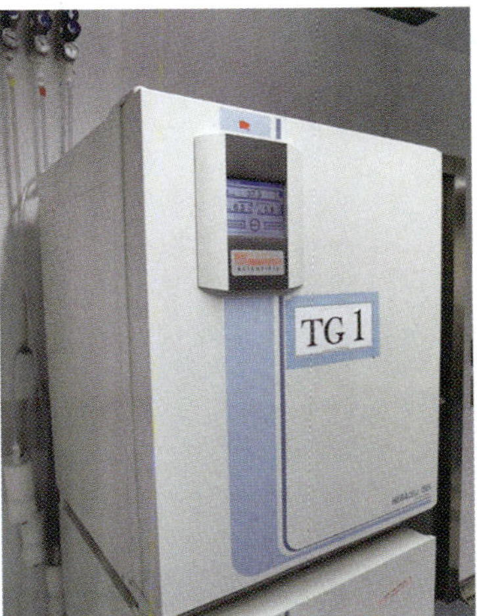

Fig. 6: Incubator for the equilibration of bicarbonate-based media and sperm capacitation

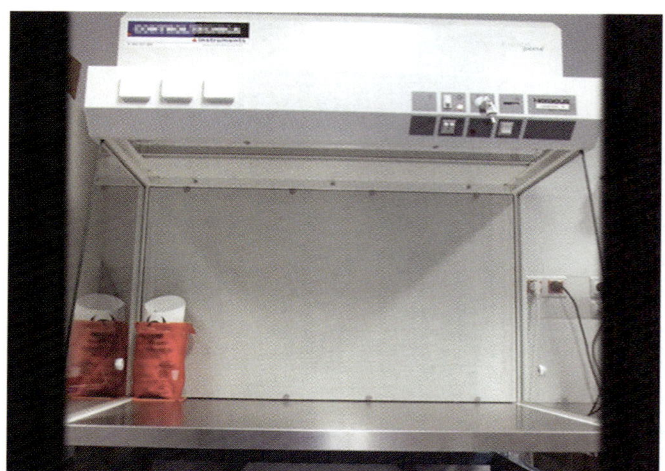

Fig. 7: A laminar flow hood (can be either a vertical or a horizontal flow) is recommended

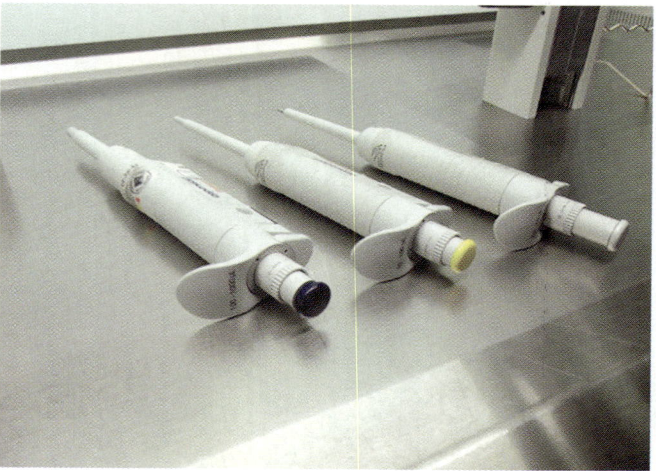

Fig. 8: Micropipettes of different volumes

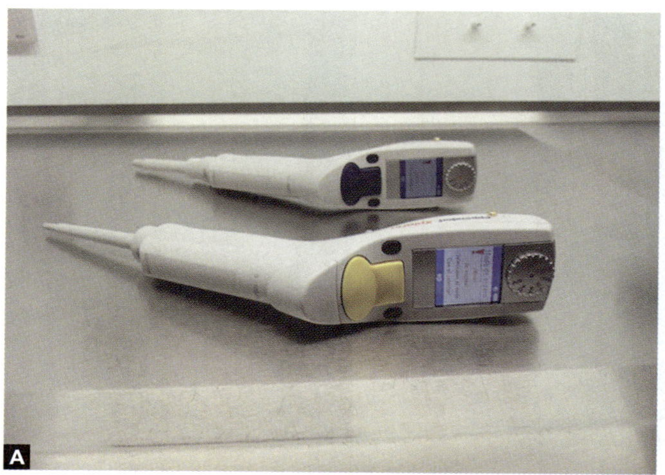

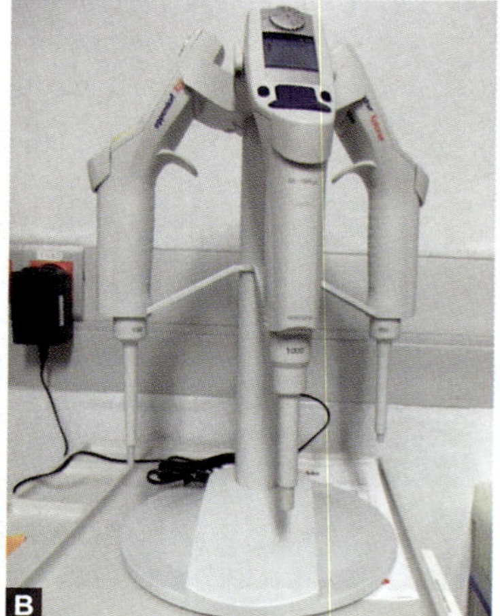

Figs. 9A and B: Automatic pipettes with different volumes

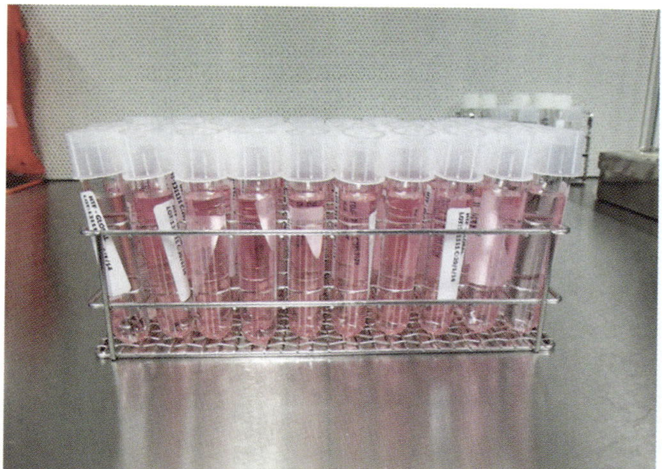

Fig. 10: Test tube racks to place the sample tubes. There are different models available for that purpose

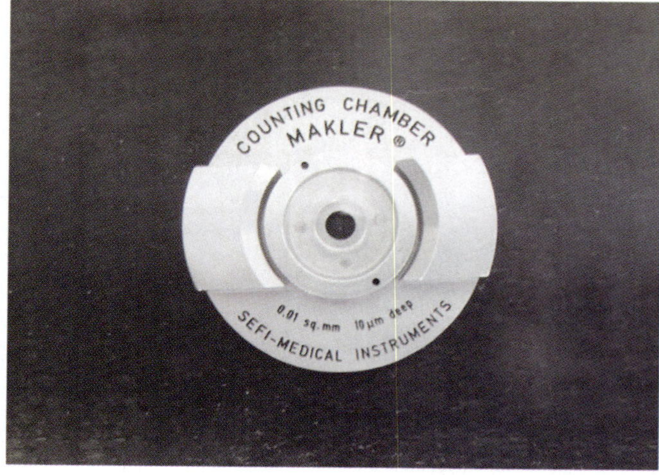

Fig. 11: Makler counting chamber for semen sample analysis

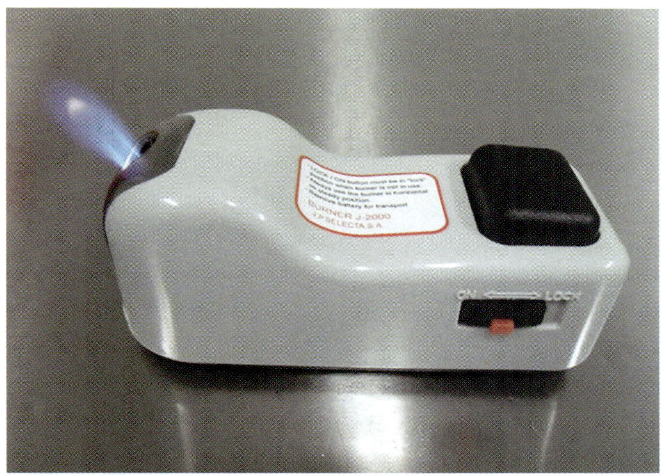

Fig. 12: Spirit burners

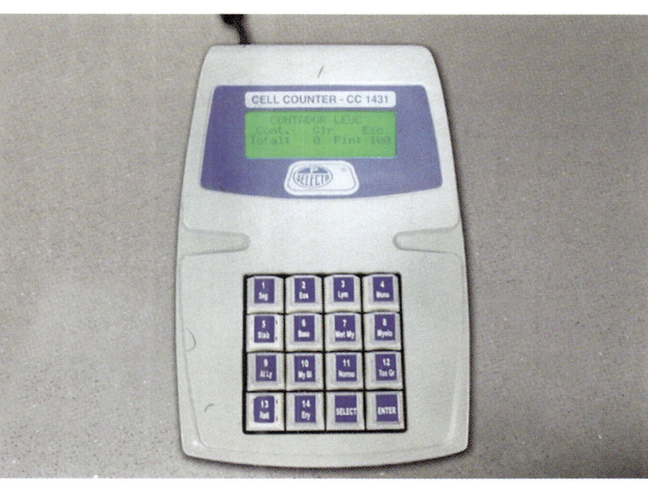

Fig. 13: A model of laboratory counter

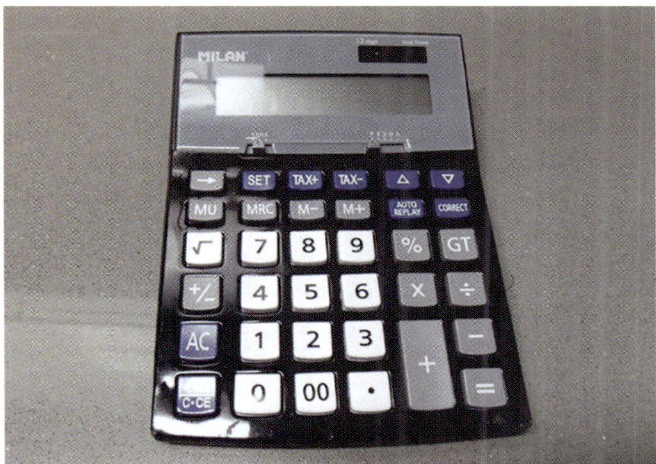

Fig. 14: Calculator

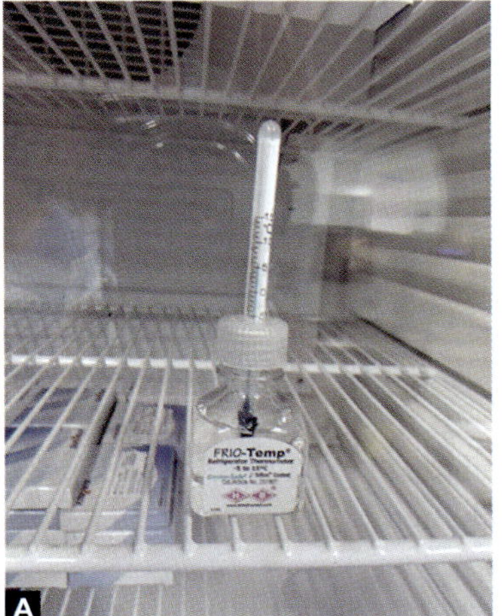

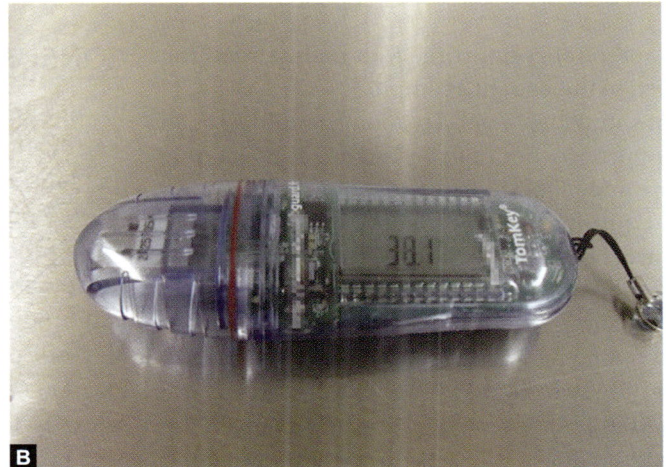

Figs. 15A and B: Thermometers for both incubator/heater and fridge

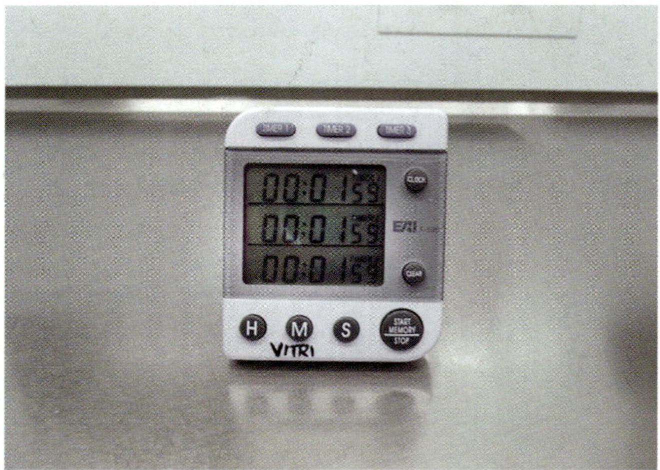

Fig. 16: Multitimer to control the duration of different procedures

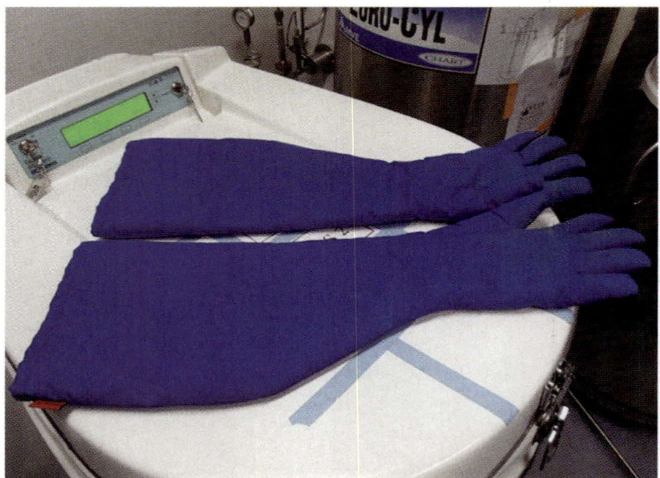

Fig. 18: Protective gloves to manipulate the material inside the nitrogen tank

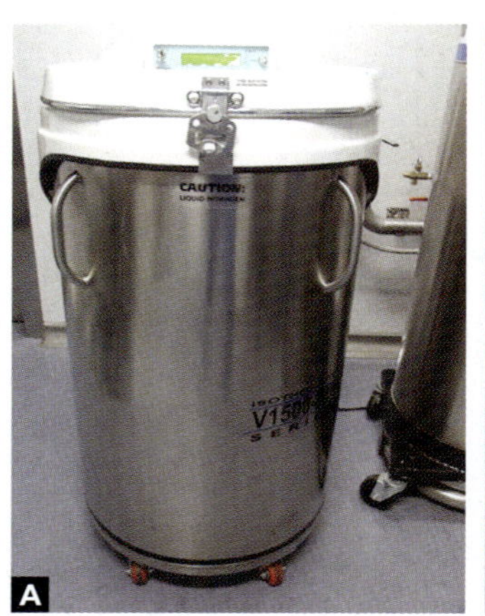

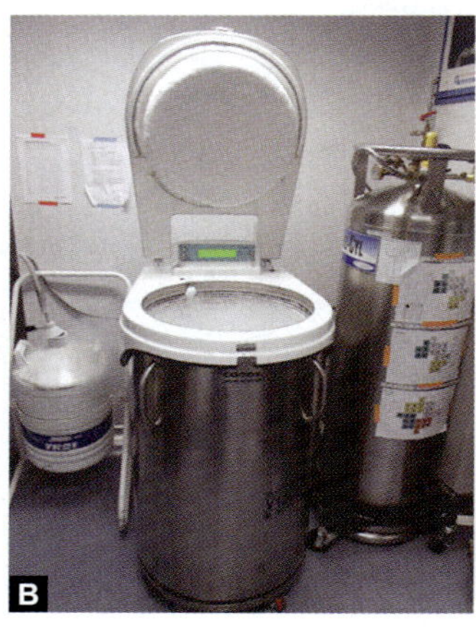

Figs. 17A and B: Liquid nitrogen tank, in this case it uses vapor nitrogen

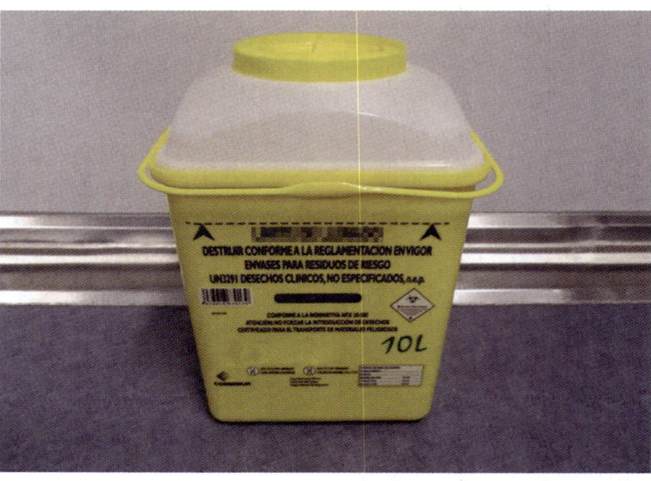

Fig. 19: Dustbins for the safe disposal of biological and laboratory materials

- Computer, preferably networked, to maintain all the date referred to the patient's sample.

Equipment should be in good working condition at all times; for this purpose, periodic inspection and cleaning should be done and at least once a year also a calibration check for all equipment using reference standards or reference material. The new equipment should be calibrated and validated before routine use.

Laboratories should have necessary instructions for operation and maintenance of equipment in the form of Standard Operating Procedures (SOPs) that should include also troubleshooting measures to be adopted for preventing equipment malfunction. In this sense, a copy of SOP should be readily available for the staff.[6]

CONSUMABLES AND MEDIA

In the laboratory, all supplies and materials must be sterilized and disposable, and must be tested also by the supplier as being nontoxic to sperm. This aspect is fundamental to prevent contamination and makes the whole process as safe as possible minimizing the risks. Most consumables and media have more than one manufacturer and model, but the specific branch to be used depends on costs, preference of laboratory and medical personnel, location of the manufacturer, and the availability of after-sales service.

The essential consumables include tips, pipettes, round bottom test tubes, conical bottom tubes, pH test

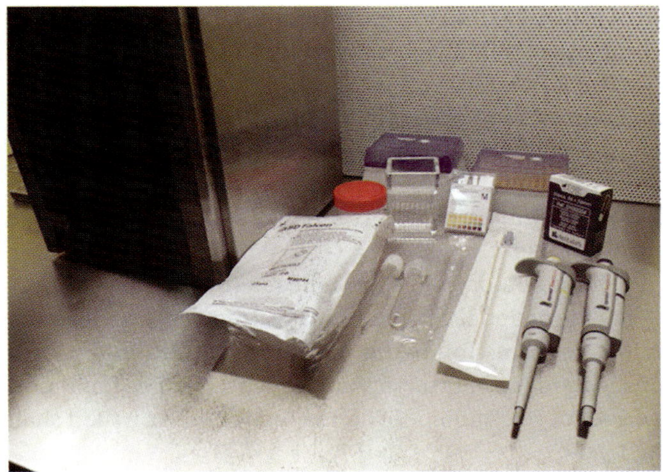

Fig. 20: Consumables and material most commonly used in the IUI laboratory

paper, slides and coverslips, IUI catheters, BD syringes and semen containers; also stains and jars to stain the slides for morphology assessment. Gloves to be used in the IUI unit should ideally be powder-free (Fig. 20).

Respect to media, the best option for IUI laboratories is to purchase buffer solutions and media that are sterile and already cell culture tested. Today it is uncommon that each laboratory prepares their own media, as the commercial ones offer all the necessary guarantees and are optimized to the maximum. These are easily available, nontoxic, tested for quality control (QC) and have consistent performance. The commonly used media are simple balanced salt solutions or complex solutions supplemented with proteins, vitamins, glucose and antibiotics, but can be supplemented with two different types of buffer: HEPES (4-(2-hydroxyethyl)-1-piperazineethanesulfonic acid) buffer (when exposed to atmosphere, it maintains the pH between 7.2 and 7.4 so these media do not require CO_2 incubation to maintain pH) or bicarbonate buffer (it requires a 5% CO_2 atmospheres to maintain the pH between 7.2 and 7.4).[5] Cryopreservation requires a ready supply of liquid nitrogen and its own special supplies and media.

PERSONNEL MANAGEMENT

Staff resources shall be adequate to carry out all the procedures and functions in the laboratory according to the level of facility and the workload. According to the Guidelines for good clinical laboratory practices from the Indian Council of Medical Research (ICMR), each laboratory should designate a Head of the laboratory who should be overall in-charge of the daily functioning of the laboratory including administration.[6] A quality manager should be designated for monitoring and maintaining of day-to-day quality management system. This laboratory manager shall have an organizational plan, personnel policies and job descriptions to define responsibility and authority of all personnel. A program for technical training and updating of skills on a regular basis should be in place. Laboratory management should be committed for providing continuing professional development and training opportunities to staff. Action plan for improvement in the laboratory should be determined and revised according to the feedback received from previous trainings and experiences, as reflected in the International Organization for Standardization (ISO) 15189:2007 and document 112 of National Accreditation Board for Testing and Calibration Laboratories (NABL).[7] Qualification level and experience required of the staff are also specified in the latter document.

The roles and responsibilities of the staff should be also clearly outlined, even more, policies defining the competency of each person to perform tasks such as using the computer system, access to patient data, enter and charge patient results or correct billing shall be established. However, confidentiality of info and data regarding patients shall be maintained by all personnel.

Laboratory should organize or conduct periodic staff evaluation, preferably once a year; frequency and method of evaluation should be decided by the laboratory.

LABORATORY SAFETY AND INFECTION CONTROL

As a general rule, procedures and policies on laboratory safety must be available to all laboratory personnel and should be reviewed annually by the laboratory director. The following guidelines are recommended:

- All patient worksheets should have clear patient identifying information as well as laboratory accession numbers that uniquely identify the patient during related procedures. All disposable material used during the preparation of the sample should be properly labeled or identified
- Protocols should be available for fire and electrical safety and internal and external disaster preparedness (including provisions for equipment back-up in the event of equipment failure)
- Semen samples should be handled using universal precautions (i.e. as if it were contaminated). All donor tissues and fluids should be subjected to appropriate infectious disease screens and quarantine periods where applicable
- All accredited laboratories are required to have an exposure control plan. A requirement of this plan is to offer and document hepatitis B vaccination to all

laboratory personnel. Testing for additional sexually transmitted infections (STIs) may be offered, but not required
- Extraordinary precautions should be taken to avoid accidental wounds from sharp instruments contaminated with body fluids. Accident/incident/injuries record of laboratory personnel should be maintained and reported to the designated authority. The report should include description of the event, factors contributing to the event and information on first aid or other health care provided. This information can be analyzed periodically toward effectively controlling and preventing future events
- Disposable, nontoxic (nonpowdered) gloves should be worn when handling fresh or frozen semen samples or any material that has come in contact with them. Gloves should be removed and discarded when leaving the laboratory or handling the telephone. Gloves should never be reused
- Hands should be washed after removing gowns and gloves and immediately if they become contaminated with body fluids. All hand washing should be done with disinfectant soap and hot water or alcohol-based solutions
- A laboratory coat or appropriate gown should be worn in the laboratory and removed upon leaving the laboratory
- Safety glasses or goggles are suggested where appropriated
- All the procedures and manipulation of semen sample should be performed to minimize the creation of aerosols. Complete facemask or the use of appropriate hoods is completely recommendable
- Disposable laboratory supplies must be used whenever possible
- All discarded body fluid samples and disposable laboratory supplies should be disposed of properly in a container marked "Biological hazard" and disposed of accordingly
- Contaminated laboratory equipment and/or work surfaces should be disinfected and sterilized after a spill
- Mechanical pipetting devices should be used for the manipulation of liquids in the laboratory. Mouth pipetting is never permitted
- Eating, drinking and smoking are not permitted in the laboratory.

RECORD MAINTENANCE

Records may include but not limited to request forms, report results, staff training, QC records, audit records, examination procedures, instruments printout, interlaboratory comparison or management reviews.

The laboratory will establish and implement policies and procedures for identification, indexing, access, storage and overall control of the registers. Records shall be legible and stored in a suitable environment to prevent damage, loss or unauthorized access but they should be retrievable in any moment.

The laboratory will decide the retention time of records as per the national, regional and local regulations. However, NABL requires following minimum retention time for ensuring the quality service and patient care. The minimum period for retention of IUI related test reports issued shall be 1 year.[7]

QUALITY CONTROL

Quality control is a process by which entities review the quality of all factors involved in lab functioning. An IUI laboratory QC should include aspects referred to equipment maintenance and calibration, validation and documentation of new protocols, vendor certification of media batch, safety laboratory procedures and record maintenance. Moreover, a written procedure manual must be readily available and followed by laboratory personnel. The laboratory director or designated supervisory personnel should review and update all procedures on at least annual basis. Any changes must be approved, signed and dated by the laboratory director or by designated proxy. The other hand refers to QC indicators that allows to identify problems or errors that exist in an attempt to improve the entire process. Indicators should be objective, relevant to the laboratory and measure a broad range of specific aspects that reflect quality of care. For each indicator incorporated, a threshold needs to be established for setting the critical level of quality laboratory performance. These markers may concern a wide variety of parameters such as technical aspects of the laboratory (e.g., temperature of working surfaces, percentage of CO_2 in incubators or pH in culture media) or clinical variables (e.g. concerning percentage of progressive mobile spermatozoa recovered per sample or gestational rates by group of analysis).[8]

REFERENCES

1. Pai RD. Pai´s Textbook of Intrauterine Insemination, 1st edition. New Delhi: Jaypee Brothers Medical Publishers (P) Ltd; 2011. pp. 39-54.
2. Keck C. Quality Management in Assisted Reproduction. Czech Republic: KAP CZ; 2003. pp. 11-8.
3. Mahmud N, Malhotra N, Malhotra J. Manual on IUI: What, When and Why. New Delhi: Jaypee Brothers Medical Publishers (P) Ltd; 2013. pp. 12-23.

4. Gianaroli L, Plachot M, van Kooij R. ESHRE guidelines for good practice in IVF laboratories. Committee of the Special Interest Group on Embryology of the European Society of Human Reproduction and Embryology. Hum Reprod. 2000;15(10):2241-6.
5. Mukherjee GG, Chakravarty BN. Intrauterine Insemination, 1st edition. Jaypee Brothers Medical Publishers (P) Ltd; 2012. pp. 62-75.
6. Indian Council of Medical Research. (2008). Guidelines for good clinical laboratory practices (GCLP). [online] Available from http://icmr.nic.in/ guidelines/GCLP.pdf [Accessed January, 2014].
7. National Accreditation Board for Testing and Calibration Laboratories (NABL). (2012). Specific criteria for accreditation of medical laboratories. [online] Available from http://www.nabl-india.org/nabl/file_download. php?filename=201210170522-NABL-112-doc.pdf [Accessed January, 2014].
8. Practice Committee of American Society for Reproductive Medicine, Practice Committee of Society for Assisted Reproductive Technology. Revised guidelines for human embryology and andrology laboratories. Fertil Steril. 2008;90(5 Suppl):S45-59.

Section 4

Endocrinology in Infertility

CHAPTER

31

Prevalence and Symptomatology of Polycystic Ovary Syndrome

Aviva Pinto Rodrigues

INTRODUCTION

Polycystic ovary syndrome (PCOS) is a heterogeneous ancient metabolic disorder of multifactorial causation. It is the most common endocrine dysfunction in reproductive age women. The first mention of PCOS comes from 5th century BC by Hippocrates who noted "Women whose menstruation is less than 3 days and are robust with healthy complexion and a masculine appearance; yet they are not concerned about bearing children nor do they conceive". Stein and Leventhal later in 1935 described the syndrome as one characterized by amenorrhea, sterility, bilateral polycystic ovaries and hirsutism.[1]

DEFINITION

Polycystic ovary syndrome is rightly a syndrome with the collection of signs and symptoms and the absence of a single definitive diagnostic test. PCOS continues to be an enigmatic disorder with a lot of controversy over its diagnosis and etiology. In the past, three societies have attempted to stipulate a definition suitable for clinical and research purposes. The first National Institutes of Health (NIH) sponsored meeting on PCOS was concluded at Bethesda in 1990 where a consensus was reached on the diagnostic criteria. These criteria (Table 1) were based on expert opinion rather than clinical evidence. Multiple trials subsequently piloted the need for a more inclusive definition.[2,3]

Nearly 15 years after the conference, the 2003 American Society for Reproductive Medicine/European Society of Human Reproduction and Embryology (ASRM/ESHRE) consensus met in Rotterdam and concluded "PCOS is a syndrome of ovarian dysfunction along with the cardinal features of hyperandrogenism and polycystic ovary (PCO) morphology" (Table 1) and that ovarian dysfunction could exist without hyperandrogenism. Insulin resistance and elevated serum luteinizing hormone (LH) levels were common features in PCOS, but however not necessary for diagnosis.

In 2006, androgen excess society appointed a task force to review all data on different phenotypes that constitute the PCOS. The task force recognized that PCOS is primarily a disorder of androgen excess after performing a meta-analysis of 527 studies.[4] A diagnosis of PCOS implies increased risk of infertility, diabetes, cardiovascular illness, dyslipidemia and cancer of the uterus, and as such it should never be assigned lightly. Metabolic dysfunction and insulin resistance are a unifying string amongst all PCOS phenotypes. The society recognized that although polycystic

Table 1: Definition.

NIH/NICHD 1992	*ASRM (Rotterdam) 2003*	*Androgen Excess Society 2006*
Exclusion of other androgen excess disorders with all of the below:	Exclusion of other androgen excess disorders with any two of three below:	Exclusion of other androgen excess disorders:
1. Clinical and/ or biochemical hyperandrogenism	1. Clinical and/ or biochemical hyperandrogenism	1. Clinical and/ or biochemical hyperandrogenism
2. Menstrual dysfunction	2. Oligo-anovulation	2. Oligo-anovulation and/or polycystic ovaries
	3. Polycystic ovaries	

(NIH: National Institute of Health; NICHD: National Institute of Child Health and Human Development; ASRM: American Society for Reproductive Medicine).

Table 2: Rotterdam's phenotypes (Prevalence in Indian adolescents).[12]

Phenotype I	*Phenotype II*	*Phenotype III*	*Phenotype IV*
Oligo-anovulation	Oligo-anovulation		Oligo-anovulation
Clinical and/or biochemical hyperandrogenism	Clinical and/or biochemical hyperandrogenism	Clinical and/ or biochemical hyperandrogenism	
Polycystic ovaries		Polycystic ovaries	Polycystic ovaries
27.4%	6.7%	13.3%	52.6%

ovaries were found in most women, PCOS and metabolic syndrome are less likely in the absence of androgen excess. It upheld the original 1990 consensus definition with minor variations (Table 1). All the three definitions agree that PCOS is also a diagnosis of exclusion of an androgen excess state secondary to androgen secreting tumors, congenital adrenal hyperplasia, Cushing's syndrome or acromegaly.

ADOLESCENT POLYCYSTIC OVARY SYNDROME

The last ASRM sponsored consensus meeting in Amsterdam in 2012 addressed knowledge gaps in women health issues. The investigators opined that all three features from the NIH definition must be present for at least 2 years to qualify for a diagnosis of PCOS. Ovarian volume greater than 10 cc and hyperandrogenemia, rather than hyperandrogenism should be used to label a girl PCOS.[5]

Prevalence

The reported prevalence of PCOS is 4–18% in women of reproductive age group.[5-8] The wide range in reporting of prevalence is due to the existence of different definitions and the gamut of expressions that the disorder can have at different ages and various races. It is now known to have repercussions in the postmenopausal period and is not necessarily limited to a syndrome of the reproductive age group.

Ethnicity and Polycystic Ovary Syndrome

Community based studies in Asian women (Rotterdam's definition) have reported a prevalence of 2–7.5% in China[9,10] and 6.3% in Sri Lanka.[11] In the Indian context, estimation of burden of illness can be gauged only from community based studies performed in adolescent girls in India. The prevalence of PCOS was 22.5% by Rotterdam and 10.7% by the Androgen Excess Society (AES) criteria in a community study performed by Indian Council of Medical Research (ICMR) in Mumbai.[12]

The Rotterdam criteria recognizes the existence of four different phenotypes (Table 2). The phenotype IV is less likely to be associated with insulin resistance, hence, the removal from the latest androgen excess task force definition. According to the ICMR study the maximum prevalence is of the phenotype IV (polycystic ovaries and oligo-anovulation) followed by phenotype III in India (Table 2).

HYPERANDROGENEMIA OR HYPERANDROGENISM

Androgen excess is an essential criterion of the syndrome. Androgens in the blood are elevated in 60–80% of PCOS women with free testosterone being the majority offender.[13-18] Additionally, 10% of women will have androstenedione levels elevated in the blood.

Hirsutism is a clinical sign of androgen excess as measured by the Ferriman-Gallwey scoring of 8 and above (Fig. 1). Hirsutism and its assessment is subjective and may

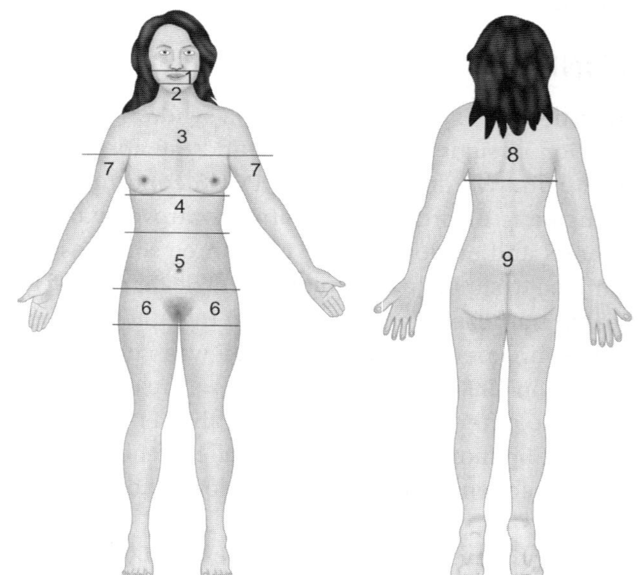

Fig. 1: Ferriman-Gallwey scoring: Each of the nine regions is graded for presence of male pattern terminal hair from 0 (minimum) to 4 (maximum). Mild hirsutism: < 8; Moderate hirsutism: 8–15; Severe hirsutism: > 15.

Table 3: Cut-off for defining androgen excess in blood.

Androgen	*Hyperandrogenemia*
Testosterone	> 60 ng/dL
Free testosterone	> 26 pmol/L
DHEA	> 350 µg/dL
Free androgen index	> 5%

(DHEA: Dehydroepiandrosterone).

be troublesome at the score of 3 as well. Hirsutism is present in 60% of women of black, white, Pacific and Southern Asian origin.[13,19-21] It is less predominant in women of East Asian descent and in adolescents with the same metabolic risk.[22] Acne is seen in 10–15% and androgenic alopecia in about 5–22% women.[3,7,23,24] However, unlike hirsutism isolated acne and alopecia are not as commonly associated with hyperandrogenemia and should not be regarded as a sign of androgen excess.[25] Evidence of androgen excess was seen in 47.6% of adolescent girls with PCOS (Rotterdam definition) in India.[12]

Acanthosis nigricans another dermatologic manifestation of PCOS is present in 5% of these[16,17] women and is characterized by velvety pigmentation at the nape, axilla and under the breasts.

The estimation of androgen levels (Table 3) in the blood is highly inaccurate at levels below the normal male range as in the case of PCOS women. The endocrine society issued a position statement in 2007 and recommended, to use methods involving mass spectrometry (MS) or organic extraction column chromatography radioimmunoassays (RIA) when values were expected to below.[25] The measurement of total testosterone has limited predictive value for distinguishing PCOS from normal women. Therefore, only free testosterone or free androgen index (total testosterone or sex hormone binding globulin (SHBG) × 100) should be used for diagnostic purposes.

POLYCYSTIC OVARY MORPHOLOGY

Polycystic ovaries were defined as presence of 12 or more follicles measuring 2 ± 9 mm in diameter in each ovary, and/or increased ovarian volume (> 10 mL).[26] These features if present in one ovary are sufficient for diagnosis. Stromal echogenicity and necklace appearance have been omitted from the definition. In the light of development of higher frequency probes the finding of PCO is becoming overtly common, and there is a need to revise these criterion and rightly so. It has been suggested in a few studies that a cut off of 20–25 small follicles should be more discriminating and realistic.[27] In adolescents and transabdominal sonography most researchers adhere to the old Rotterdam's definition of volume and follicle number. Additionally, many normal adolescent girls can have polycystic ovaries due to inefficient recruitment and anovulatory cycles. It is, therefore, suggested to use the ovarian volume as index for adolescent girls.[5] Youngster M, et al. however, did not find any significant prevalence of PCOS in normal adolescent girls.[28]

The polycystic morphology is present in up to 75% women[16,19,21,29] while 25–30% PCOS women will not have polycystic ovaries on ultrasound.[30] Indian studies have found a prevalence of 93% in the adolescent age group.[12]

Ovulatory and Menstrual Dysfunction

Women with PCOS have a 95% likelihood of having oligomenorrhea although up to 20% may have regular menstruation as well.[11] Ovulation can occur spontaneously in upto 32% of cycles in oligoamenorrheic women. Amenorrheic women are more hyperandrogenic and are likely to have complete metabolic derangements. Although ovulatory dysfunction in the absence of androgen excess has less severe metabolic phenotype, nonhyperandrogenic PCOS women also have increased cardiovascular and metabolic risk at a younger age.[31]

Infertility

Anovulation is the cause of infertility in 25% of women[32] and PCOS is the most common form of ovulatory dysfunction in them (90%). 50% of women with hyperandrogenic PCOS will have difficulty in conception as compared to 20% in normoandrogenic women with PCOS.[33]

Polycystic ovary syndrome is characterized by WHO type II anovulation or eugonadotropic eugonadism. Most women with PCOS will be able to conceive with clomiphene. 80% women ovulate on clomiphene, however, pregnancy rates are discrepantly lower at 50–60%.[34] Some women are resistant and require in vitro techniques (IVF/ICSI) for treatment. PCOS women have higher sensitivity to gonadotropins and, therefore, are also at risk of ovarian hyperstimulation syndrome and multiple pregnancies.

Insulin Resistance and Metabolic Syndrome

Metabolic syndrome has been defined by the International Diabetes Federation as increased central obesity with two of the four factors listed in Table 3. Polycystic ovary syndrome and metabolic syndrome are phenotypically overlapping but are not interchangeable. Both syndromes are heterogenous disorders of covert etiologies. 30–40% women with PCOS will have the metabolic syndrome.

In women with PCOS and normal glucose tolerance to start with, 16% converted to impaired glucose tolerance and 2% of them to type 2 diabetes per year.[35,36] Approximately, 30–40% of women with PCOS have impaired glucose tolerance and 7.5–10% have type 2 diabetes. In a study on 168 PCOS adolescent girls in India 36% had impaired glucose tolerance and 9% had diabetes.[37] The complex interplay between insulin resistance and PCOS is modulated by a third factor–"obesity". In one meta-analysis an increased risk of metabolic syndrome was found in PCOS women as compared to body mass index (BMI) matched controls, and this increased risk persisted in lean women.[38] Not all obese women develop PCOS and obesity has an additive rather than a causative role in PCOS.

Lipid and lipoprotein abnormalities are also common in 70% PCOS women.[39] PCOS women were observed to have raised low-density lipoprotein (LDL), triglyceride and decreased high-density lipoprotein cholesterol (HDL-C) in a meta-analysis by Wild RA, et al. In addition, highly atherogenic small dense LDL is found in women with PCOS.[29,40-43]

Women with PCOS have increased cardiovascular risk consistent with preponderance of dyslipidemia, insulin resistance and obesity. Very few studies estimate the risk these women are at due to the fact that most prevalence studies are among reproductive age group which is largely free of cardiovascular events. Nevertheless, women's ischemia evaluation study found more multivessel cardiovascular disease in women with history of menstrual irregularity and hyperandrogenemia.[44]

Familial Studies

There is familial clustering of PCOS in first degree relatives. In one study, 50% of sisters of PCOS women had elevated blood levels of testosterone.[17] Maternal heritability was stronger than paternal for fasting hyperglycemia in a parent of origin finding study.[45] This points out to the fact that although PCOS has a genetic basis it has complex polygenic inheritance with epigenetic and developmental influences.

Twin studies are relatively few but have found a higher preponderance of concordance among monozygotic than dizygotic twins, establishing a strong genetic component to the inheritance.[46]

Obesity

The relationship of obesity and PCOS is one of mutual symbiosis, obesity does not cause PCOS as is evident from the high prevalence of PCOS among lean women. Both entities are on the rise in the world population. In a study by Azziz, in an unselected population the prevalence of PCOS was similar across all BMI groups.[47] Obesity is not the sole cause of PCOS, clearly manifest from the fact that all obese women do not have PCOS. However, animal studies of knock out phenotypes lead to obesity as well as reproductive and menstrual irregularities in animal models. Moreover, body weight distribution is racially determined for example PCOS women in UK, and China tend to have lower BMIs.[41,48]

Clearly obesity modifies the phenotype and severity of PCOS by influencing insulin action and peripheral hormone metabolism. Obese women with PCOS are more likely to have impaired glucose tolerance, dyslipidemia and hyperandrogenism.

REFERENCES

1. Stein IF Sr. The Stein-Leventhal syndrome; a curable form of sterility. N Engl J Med. 1958;259:420-3.
2. Nestler JE, Jakubowicz DJ, Evans WS, et al. Effects of metformin on spontaneous and clomiphene-induced ovulation in the polycystic ovary syndrome. N Engl J Med. 1998;338:1876-80.
3. Azziz R, Ehrmann D, Legro RS, et al. Troglitazone improves ovulation and hirsutism in the polycystic ovary syndrome: a multicenter, double blind, placebo-controlled trial. J Clin Endocrinol Metab. 2001;86:1626-32.
4. Azziz R, Carmina E, Dewailly D, et al. Positions statement: criteria for defining polycystic ovary syndrome as a predominantly hyperandrogenic syndrome: an Androgen Excess Society guideline. J Clin Endocrinol Metab. 2006;91:4237-45.
5. Asunción M, Calvo RM, San Millán JL, et al. A prospective study of the prevalence of the polycystic ovary syndrome in unselected Caucasian women from Spain. J Clin Endocrinol Metab. 200085:2434-8.
6. Diamanti-Kandarakis E, Kouli CR, Bergiele AT, et al. A survey of the polycystic ovary syndrome in the Greek island of Lesbos: hormonal and metabolic profile. J Clin Endocrinol Metab. 1999;84: 4006-11.
7. Azziz R, Woods KS, Reyna R, et al. The prevalence and features of the polycystic ovary syndrome in an unselected population. J Clin Endocrinol Metab. 2004:89:2745-9.
8. March WA, Moore VM, Willson KJ, et al. The prevalence of polycystic ovary syndrome in a community sample assessed under contrasting diagnostic criteria. Hum Reprod. 2010:25:544-51.
9. Chen X, Yang D, Mo Y, et al. Prevalence of polycystic ovary syndrome in unselected women from southern China. Eur J Obstet Gynecol Reprod Biol. 2008;139:59-64.
10. Li R, Zhang Q, Yang D, et al. Prevalence of polycystic ovary syndrome in women in China: a large community-based study. Hum Reprod. 2013;28:2562-9.
11. Kumarapeli V, Seneviratne Rde A, Wijeyaratne CN, et al. A simple screening approach for assessing community

prevalence and phenotypes of polycystic ovary syndrome in a semi-urban population in Sri Lanka. Am J Epidemiol. 2008;168:321-8.

12. Chauhan S, Joshi B, Mukherjee S, et al. A cross-sectional study of polycystic ovarian syndrome among adolescent and young girls in Mumbai, India. Indian J Endocrinol Metab. 2014;18:317-24.
13. Orio F Jr, Matarese G, Di Biase S, et al. Exon 6 and 2 peroxisome proliferator-activated receptor-gamma polymorphisms in polycystic ovary syndrome. J Clin Endocrinol Metab. 2003;88:5887-92.
14. Chang WY, Knochenhauer ES, Bartolucci AA, et al. Phenotypic spectrum of polycystic ovary syndrome: clinical and biochemical characterization of the three major clinical subgroups. Fertil Steril. 2005;83:1717-23.
15. Hahn S, Tan S, Elsenbruch S, et al. Clinical and biochemical characterization of women with polycystic ovary syndrome in North Rhine-Westphalia. Horm Metab Res. 2005;37:438-44.
16. Conway GS, Honour JW, Jacobs HS. Heterogeneity of the polycystic ovary syndrome: clinical, endocrine and ultrasound features in 556 patients. Clin Endocrinol (Oxf). 1989;30:459-70.
17. Balen AH, Conway GS, Kaltsas G, et al. Polycystic ovary syndrome: the spectrum of the disorder in 1741 patients. Hum Reprod. 1995;10:2107-11.
18. Legro RS, Driscoll D, Strauss JF 3rd, et al. Evidence for a genetic basis for hyperandrogenemia in polycystic ovary syndrome. Proc Natl Acad Sci USA. 1998;95:14956-60.
19. Ferriman D, Purdie AW. The aetiology of oligomenorrhoea and/or hirsuties: a study of 467 patients. Postgrad Med J. 1983;59:17-20.
20. Falsetti L, Eleftheriou G. Hyperinsulinemia in the polycystic ovary syndrome: a clinical, endocrine and echographic study in 240 patients. Gynecol Endocrinol. 1996;10:319-26.
21. Khoury MY, Baracat EC, Pardini DP, et al. Polycystic ovary syndrome: clinical and laboratory evaluation. Sao Paulo Med J. 1996;114:1222-5.
22. Carmina E, Lobo RA. Polycystic ovaries in Hirsute women with normal menses. Am J Med. 2001;111:602-6.
23. Wijeyaratne CN, Balen AH, Barth JH, et al. Clinical manifestations and insulin resistance (IR) in polycystic ovary syndrome (PCOS) among South Asians and Caucasians: is there a difference? Clin Endocrinol (Oxf). 2002;57:343-50.
24. Quinn M, Shinkai K, Pasch L, et al. Prevalence of androgenic alopecia in patients with polycystic ovary syndrome and characterization of associated clinical and biochemical features. Fertil Steril. 2014; 101:1129-34.
25. Rosner W, Auchus RJ, Azziz R, et al. Position statement: Utility, limitations, and pitfalls in measuring testosterone: an Endocrine Society position statement. J Clin Endocrinol Metab. 2007;92:405-13.
26. Rotterdam ESHRE/ASRM-Sponsored PCOS consensus workshop group. Revised 2003 consensus on diagnostic criteria and long-term health risks related to polycystic ovary syndrome (PCOS). Hum Reprod. 2004;19:41-7.
27. Lujan ME, Jarrett BY, Brooks ED, et al. Updated ultrasound criteria for polycystic ovary syndrome: reliable thresholds for elevated follicle population and ovarian volume. Hum Reprod. 2013;28:1361-8.
28. Youngster M, Ward VL, Blood EA, et al. Utility of ultrasound in the diagnosis of polycystic ovary syndrome in adolescents. Fertil Steril. 2014;102:1432-8.
29. Legro RS, Myers ER, Barnhart HX, et al. The Pregnancy in Polycystic Ovary Syndrome (PPCOS) study: baseline characteristics of the randomized cohort including racial effects. Fertil Steril. 2006;86: 914-33.
30. Balen AH, Laven JS, Tan SL, et al. Ultrasound assessment of the polycystic ovary: international consensus definitions. Hum Reprod Update. 2003;9:505-14.
31. Daan NM, Louwers YV, Koster MP, et al. Cardiovascular and metabolic profiles amongst different polycystic ovary syndrome phenotypes: who is really at risk? Fertil Steril. 2014;102:1444-51.
32. ACOG Committee on Practice Bulletins-Gynecology. ACOG Practice Bulletin. Clinical management guidelines for obstetrician-gynecologists number 34, February 2002. Management of infertility caused by ovulatory dysfunction. Obstet Gynecol. 2002;99:347-58.
33. Medeiros SF, Gil-Junior AB, Barbosa JS, et al. New insights into steroidogenesis in normo- and hyperandrogenic polycystic ovary syndrome patients. Arq Bras Endocrinol Metabol. 2013;57:437-44.
34. Kousta E, White DM, Franks S. Modern use of clomiphene citrate in induction of ovulation. Hum Reprod Update. 1997;3:359-65.
35. Ehrmann DA, Liljenquist DR, Kasza K, et al. Prevalence and predictors of the metabolic syndrome in women with polycystic ovary syndrome. J Clin Endocrinol Metab. 2006;91:48-53.
36. Legro RS, Gnatuk CL, Kunselman AR, et al. Changes in glucose tolerance over time in women with polycystic ovary syndrome: a controlled study. J Clin Endocrinol Metab. 2005;90:3236-42.
37. Ganie MA, Khurana ML, Eunice M, et al. Prevalence of glucose intolerance among adolescent and young women with polycystic ovarian syndrome in India. Indian J Clin endocrinol metab. 2004;6:9-14.
38. Moran LJ, Misso ML, Wild RA, Norman RJ. Impaired glucose tolerance, type 2 diabetes and metabolic syndrome: a systematic review and meta-analysis. Hum Reprod Update. 2010;16(4):347-63.
39. Legro RS, Kunselman AR, Dunaif A. Prevalence and predictors of dyslipidemia in women with polycystic ovary syndrome. Am J Med. 2001;111:607-13.
40. Wild RA, Rizzo M, Clifton S, et al. Lipid levels in polycystic ovary syndrome: systematic review and meta-analysis. Fertil Steril. 2011;95:1073-9.
41. Legro RS, Blanche P, Krauss RM, et al. Alterations in low-density lipoprotein and high-density lipoprotein subclasses among Hispanic women with polycytic ovary syndrome: influence of insulin and genetic factors. Fertil Steril. 1999;72(6):990-5.
42. Dejager S, Pichard C, Giral P, et al. Smaller LDL particle size in women with polycystic ovary syndrome compared to controls. Clin Endocrinol (Oxf). 2001;54: 455-62.
43. Pirwany IR, Fleming R, Greer IA, et al. Lipids and lipoprotein subfractions in women with PCOS: relationship to metabolic and endocrine parameters. Clin Endocrinol (Oxf). 2001;54:447-53.

44. Shufelt CL, Johnson BD, Berga SL, et al. Timing of hormone therapy, type of menopause, and coronary disease in women: data from the National Heart, Lung, and Blood Institute-sponsored Women's Ischemia Syndrome Evaluation. Menopause. 2011;18(9):943-50.
45. Kobaly K, Vellanki P, Sisk RK, et al. Parent-of-origin effects on glucose homeostasis in polycystic ovary syndrome. J Clin Endocrinol Metab. 2014:99:2961-6.
46. Goodarzi MO, Dumesic DA, Chazenbalk G, et al. Polycystic ovary syndrome: etiology, pathogenesis and diagnosis. Nat Rev Endocrinol. 2011;7:219-31.
47. Yildiz BO, Knochenhauer ES, Azziz R. Impact of obesity on the risk for polycystic ovary syndrome. J Clin Endocrinol Metab. 2008;93:162-8.
48. Chen ZJ, Zhao H, He L, et al. Genome-wide association study identifies susceptibility loci for polycystic ovary syndrome on chromosome 2p16.3, 2p21 and 9q33.3. Nat Genet. 2011;43:55-9.

CHAPTER

32

Genetics and Pathophysiology

Paula Celada, Carmen Vidal, Juan Giles

INTRODUCTION

Polycystic ovary syndrome (PCOS) is a widespread reproductive disorder that encompasses many associated health conditions and has an impact on various metabolic processes. Hyperandrogenism, polycystic ovaries, and anovulation depict PCOS. It is often called the most common cause of anovulatory infertility in women.

The pathophysiology of this disease has not been well understood, but studies suggest a strong genetic component that is affected by gestational environment, lifestyle factors, or both. However, genetic research in PCOS is still new, and there are several inconsistencies among studies.

In this chapter, the current status of genetics and pathophysiology of PCOS will be discussed.

GENETICS

The more modest approach would target a gene of possible relevance to the pathology and compare either the full sequences or a known associated single nucleotide polymorphism (SNP), whereas the more robust approach involves what is called whole-genome analysis study or genome-wide association study (GWAS), which documents only a set of SNP. The GWAS approach provides the advantage of surveying large number of variants covering much of the genome at once, thus facilitating the discovery of novel genes, regardless of whether their function has previously been implicated in PCOS (Table 1).

Candidate Gene Association Studies

Genes Related to the General Metabolic Pathways

- *Fat and obesity associated gene (FTO):* There is an association of FTO genotype and PCOS status, which was attenuated by adjustment for body mass index (BMI).[1-3] This association was most evident in obese PCOS patients, but no relationship between FTO genotype and androgen concentration was seen. The predominant effect of FTO variants on PCOS susceptibility is probably mediated through adiposity, so possible effects of FTO in PCOS is limited to the metabolic phenotypes.[3,4]
- *Adiponectin gene (ADIPOQ):* Two SNP, C45G15G (T/G), and C276 (G/T), were significantly associated with PCOS, and C276 (G/T) appeared to affect fasting insulin concentration and insulin resistance in PCOS patients. Genotypes GG and GT had lower serum adiponectin, compared with TT.[5] In an additional study in Japanese women, in the resistin gene the 420GG homozygous variant genotype occurred significantly more frequently among the PCOS group than among the control group. Furthermore, women with 420GG had higher BMI compared with GC and CC.[6]
- *Peroxisome proliferator-activated receptors (PPAR):* PPARs have three isotypes operating as regulators of carbohydrate metabolism. A meta-analysis on a total

Table 1: Genes involved in polycystic ovary (PCO) pathogenesis.

Genes related to metabolism and steroid hormones	*Genes related to insulin*
CAPT 10	CAPT 10
ADIPO Q	ADIPO Q
RETN	RETN
FTO	INS
PPAR	INSR
FBN 3	IRS 1
LHCGR AND FSHR	AKT2 AND GDK3B
AR	MTNR1B
SHBG	THADA
YAP	
DENND1A	

of 17 case-control studies summarized that PPAR-c2 Pro12Ala polymorphism was capable of reducing PCOS risk in Europeans, but not in Asians.[7]

- *Fibrillin-3 gene (FBN3):* The susceptibility locus to chromosome 19p13.2 nears the dinucleotide repeat marker D19S884, D19S884 allele 8 (A8) within intron 55 of the fibrillin-3 (FBN3) gene, showed the strongest evidence for association with PCOS.[8] PCOS women carrying D19S884 allele 8 (A8) had significantly lower circulating total TGF-β1, and higher Inhibin B and aldosterone levels, compared to PCOS women without A8.[9] A recent study demonstrated expression of FBN3 in the stromal compartments of fetal ovaries during the first trimester of gestation when the follicles are forming, and declining significantly afterward, being undetectable in adult ovaries. This finding suggests that FBN3 may exert its effect during fetal development, and influence a person's predisposition to PCOS later in life, supporting previously proposed hypotheses on fetal origins for PCOS.[2]
- *Calpain-10 gene (CAPN-10):* Although the evidence for association with T2DM has weakened recently due to the fact that no significant association signal was observed in any GWAS, CAPN10 remained as one of the candidate genes most frequently investigated in PCOS research. Recent studies in diverse ethnic groups support a putative role for CAPN10 in PCOS.[10-12]

Insulin Signaling Genes

- *Insulin gene (INS):* INS is located at chromosome 11p5.5. A variable number tandem repeat (VNTR) polymorphism located in the 5′ regulatory element of the INS affects its transcriptional regulation, and is associated with hyperinsulinemia, fasting insulin levels, susceptibility to T2DM, birth weight, and childhood obesity and juvenile obesity. A significant association between class III VNTR alleles and PCOS was found in some studies; however, these findings have not been replicated consistently.[2,13]
- *Insulin receptor gene (INSR):* The tyrosine kinase domain of INSR is of particular interest, as mutations in this domain are associated with moderate hyperinsulinemia and insulin resistance.[14] A silent C-to-T substitution at His1058 position was previously shown to be associated with PCOS. However, a meta-analysis of the His1058 C/T polymorphism suggests that this variation is not a contributor to the etiology of PCOS.[15] Two studies showed an association of SNP and rs2252673, with PCOS.[16,17] This variant is located in intron 11 of the *INSR* gene, so it is unclear how this SNP might affect *INSR* expression or function to influence the PCOS phenotype.
- *Insulin receptor substrate 1 (IRS1):* A meta-analysis for association with IRS1 Gly972Arg polymorphism found that the Arg972 allele is a risk factor for PCOS, and suggested that PCOS susceptibility due to the Arg972 is mediated through increased levels of fasting insulin.[15]
- *AKT2 and GSK3b:* These two genes are pivotal in the insulin signal transduction pathway, since in response to insulin signaling, Akt2 phosphorylates and inhibits GSK3b, which facilitates glycogen synthesis. Carriers of the risk haplotypes for both AKT2 and GSK3b had further increased odds of PCOS.[18]
- *Resistin gene (RETN):* RETN 420GG is more frequent in PCOS. PCOS women with the RETN 420GG genotype also showed significantly higher BMI and greater insulin resistance.[6]
- *Melatonin receptor 1B gene (MTNR1B):* Intrafollicular melatonin concentrations are significantly lower in PCOS. Melatonin may reduce peripheral tissue tolerance to glucose and sensitivity to insulin. PCOS cases with the CG and GG genotypes in rs10830963 were associated with higher serum total testosterone concentration and glucose concentration at the oral glucose tolerance test.[19,20]

Steroidogenic and Steroid-regulated Genes

- *Androgen receptor gene (AR):* One study suggested that shorter CAG repeats increase the risk for precocious pubarche and subsequent ovarian hyperandrogenism.[18,21] The relationship between AR and PCOS has been studied by different groups, yet they have produced controversial results. Recently, a meta-analysis including 1,536 PCOS patients and 1,807 controls revealed that the lengths of CAG repeat contributed to hyperandrogenism in PCOS.[22]
- *Sex hormone-binding globulin (SHBG):* SHBG likely influences PCOS phenotype indirectly, perhaps by altering the bioavailable androgen levels in the target tissues; however, genetic variation in SHBG is not associated with PCOS per se.

In summary, although a large number of candidate gene studies have been conducted for PCOS, findings for these studies have been mostly inconclusive.

Genome-wide Association Studies

Since the first report on GWASs in 2005, more than 2,000 studies have been added to the catalogue of published

GWASs by 2013 (http://www.genome.gov/gwastudies/). GWASs have been successfully used to identify susceptibility loci for a number of common diseases. In recent years, GWASs have been used to examine female reproductive disorders such as PCOS, premature ovarian failure, and endometriosis.

The first GWAS in Han Chinese women was reported by Chen et al.[23] They discovered the first published set of three loci that were significantly associated with PCOS: 2p16.3 (rs13405728), 2p21 (rs13429458), and 9q33.3 (rs2479106).

- *Chromosome 2p16.3:* Several known genes are located nearby, among which are *GTF2A1L* and *LHCGR* genes, both in a small linkage-disequilibrium block, and FSHR, 211 kb downstream of rs13405728, but not in the block. Interestingly, markers mapping to FSHR were associated with FSH concentration in women with PCOS.
- *Chromosome 2p21:* Two independent associations, which can be represented by rs13429458 and rs12478601, were located in the *THADA* gene (thyroid adenoma-associated protein), known as a susceptibility gene for obesity and T2DM.[18]
- *Chromosome 9q33.3:* Two independent associations, represented by rs10818854 and rs2479106, both within DENND1A. It is conceivable that in PCOS patients the DENND1A risk variant might influence the pathogenesis of PCOS through misregulation of ERAP1.

There have been no published genome-wide associated variants for PCOS in European women. Indeed, these studies will be important because the susceptibility variants may differ in individual ethnic groups. Nevertheless, a number of groups using European cohorts have replicated a subset of the findings in Han Chinese women and found that loci corresponding to genes for DENND1A and THADA were strongly associated with PCOS.

In a second GWAS,[24] eight new PCOS association signals were identified: 9q22.32, 11q22.1, 12q13.2, 12q14.3, 16q12.1, 19p13.3, 20q13.2 and a second independent signal at 2p16.3 (the *FSHR* gene).

Two additional risk variants identified in the second GWAS of Han Chinese women have been replicated in European women.[25] The risk variant on chromosome 11 is located in an intron of *YAP1,* the studies suggest a role for YAP in the maintenance of the follicle complement and follicle growth. The variant at locus 12q13.2 is located between two genes; RAB5B is a member of the RAS oncogene family and SUOX, sulfite oxidase 12q13.2 has been reported as a susceptibility locus of T1D. It is not clear which gene, if either, might be affected by the associated variant.[26]

Two recently published GWAS in European cohorts have significantly increased the number of identified PCOS genes.

In the first report,[27] two novel loci were identified: 8p32.1 and 11p14.1. A causal transcript at the 8p32.1 locus is not clear; it has been shown to affect developmental pathways, including that of the gonads. The association interval extends across the regulatory elements of *FDFT1,* involved in the cholesterol synthesis pathway. The association signal at 11p14.1 extends across both *FSHB,* which encodes the beta subunit of FSH, and *ARL14EP,* which controls the export of major histocompatibility class II molecules via connection to the actin network.

The second study of white subjects, published by Day et al. in 2015, used a unique patient population.[28] Six loci were associated with PCOS at genome-wide significance: two previously reported loci in Chinese (*THADA* and *YAP1*); one previously reported locus in whites (*FSHB*), and three novel loci (*ERBB4, RAD50,* and *KRR1*).

The ultimate goal of GWASs is not to identify a variant associated with a disorder, but to find a causal variant that demonstrates a functional effect and a pathophysiology that explains how a variant predisposes a person to develop the disorder.[29]

In a large Chinese cohort, significant associations between rs13429458 from the *THADA* locus and increased LH, testosterone, and LH–FSH ratio were identified.[30] A second risk SNP from the *THADA* gene, rs12478601, was significantly associated with increased low-density lipoprotein levels. A single SNP in *DENND1A,* rs2479106, was associated with increased 2-hour insulin levels during oral glucose tolerance test.[30] The association between rs13429458 (*THADA*) and testosterone was not reported in the initial GWAS study. The two recent GWAS in white PCOS subjects reported associations between the lead PCOS risk SNP at the *FSHB* locus and LH level and, in a subset of subjects from the deCODE cohort, FSH level.[27,28]

Studies using theca cells isolated from normal cycling and PCOS women provided the first evidence to demonstrate a functional relationship between augmented DENND1A. V2 and *CYP17A1* expression and increased androgen biosynthesis in PCOS theca cells.[31] *DENND1A* SNPs have been reported to be associated with diverse phenotypes found in PCOS women, including elevated insulin levels and endometrioid carcinoma.[30,31] Additionally, quantitative trait analyses have linked the *DENND1A* locus with glucose and insulin levels and body weight in humans.[31] Thus, DENND1A.V2 could possibly contribute directly to or modify a number of PCOS phenotypes, which heretofore have not been tied to a single genetic locus.

Thus, it is conceivable that various GWAS candidates converge to regulate *CYP17A1* expression and androgen biosynthesis.

In the light of the relative disappointing scope of the insight afforded by GWAS and SNP association studies, one inevitably looks forward to the next generation techniques (proteomic and transcriptomic analysis and study of RNA interference studies). As compared with GWAS, next-generation sequencing (NGS) is not limited to gene chips and thereby enables genotyping of complete genes. Through this new technique, rare variants may be identified. These will contribute to the understanding of the pathogenesis of PCOS, and eventually lead to the development of risk prediction models and therapeutic strategies for patient care.

PATHOPHYSIOLOGY

Polycystic ovary syndrome is a multifactorial disorder that arises from interactions between genetic, environmental, and intrauterine factors.

Environmental factors associated with PCOS can be classified as prenatal (fetal developmental programming) or postnatal (diet, obesity, sedentary lifestyle, environmental toxins, and prescription drugs).[32]

Developmental Programming in the Pathogenesis of PCOS

The developmental programming of PCOS represents changes in gene expression that result from the presence of increased levels of steroid hormones in the fetal circulation at critical stages of fetal development and that result in permanent structural and functional modifications of the body organs.[33,34] This phenomenon might be caused either by the presence of excess glucocorticoids (resulting from fetal hypoxia and IUGR)[35,36] or by the elevation of maternal androgen levels during pregnancy.[37,38]

Glucocorticoid Excess

If fetal hypoxia develops because of dietary restrictions and/or maternal or placental disease, fetal blood flow is redirected to essential organs (heart, brain, and adrenal glands) in a phenomenon called centralization. Consequently, there is an increased production of glucocorticoids because of the hyperactivity of the hypothalamic-pituitary-adrenal (HPA) axis, which results in epigenetic modifications.

Fetuses with IUGR and born SGA show a predisposition to developing PCOS[39-41] and other pathologies in postnatal life after compensatory growth during the first 2 years of life: Type 2 DM,[42] systemic arterial hypertension (SAH),[43] dyslipidemia, obesity,[44] etc. (Flowchart 1).

Flowchart 1: Pathophysiology of PCOS: From intrauterine environment to reproductive age.

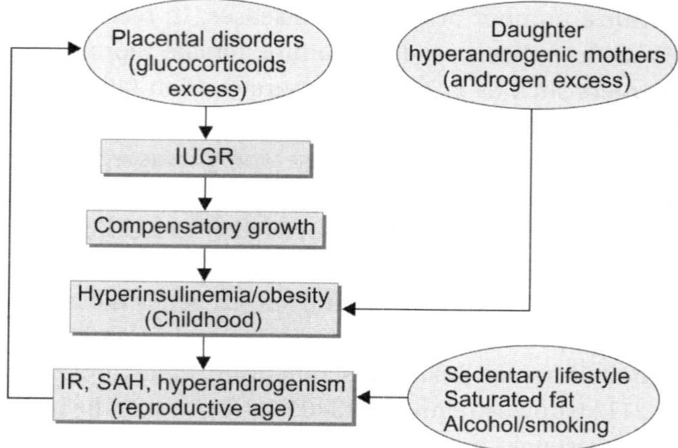

(IR: insulin resistance; IUGR: intrauterine growth restriction; PCOS: polycystic ovarian syndrome; SAH: systemic arterial hypertension)

Androgen Excess

Hyperandrogenism is a central feature of PCOS; however, only 80–85% of women with clinical hyperandrogenism have PCOS.[45] The androgens are secreted primarily by the ovaries and secondarily by the adrenals.[46]

As a consequence of dysregulation of androgen synthesis within the ovary, women with PCOS have ovarian hyper-responsiveness to gonadotropins: theca cells to LH explaining the excess androgens, and granulose cells to FSH leading to increased estrogens.[47]

The mechanism that determines excess numbers of follicles is unknown, but several lines of evidence implicate abnormal androgen signaling. Additionally, a polymorphism in the androgen receptor that affects the potency of its activity has been implicated in the disorder.[48]

In anovulatory women with PCOS, antral follicle growth stops when the follicle is less than 10 mm in diameter, which is the stage just before emergence of a dominant follicle. Follicular arrest is associated with excessive stimulation of follicular cells by insulin, LH, or both, in addition to a hyperandrogenic environment.[49]

However, PCOS can also occur in women who were born at appropriate weight for GA or in newborns of women without PCOS, which suggests that genetic variation and environmental factors play important roles in the development and maintenance of PCOS in a population.

Although the pathophysiology of PCOS is not clear, a variety of abnormalities have been described with this syndrome.

Hyperinsulinemia

Hyperinsulinemia, defined as impaired action of insulin on glucose transport and antilipolysis in adipocytes in the presence of normal insulin binding, causes or exacerbates hyperandrogenemia. Increased insulin levels at the ovarian level lead to increased androgen production from the ovarian thecal cells.

Hyperinsulinemia is noted in 50–70% of PCOS patients. The major defect is a decrease in insulin sensitivity secondary to a postbinding abnormality in insulin receptor-mediated signal transduction, with a decrease in insulin responsiveness.[50] It appears that decreased insulin sensitivity in PCOS is potentially an intrinsic defect in genetically susceptible women.

Although the insulin resistance might occur irrespective of BMI, the common association of PCOS and obesity has a synergistic deleterious impact on glucose homeostasis and can worsen both hyperandrogenism and anovulation.[47,51]

Insulin acts through multiple sites to increase endogenous androgen levels. Increased peripheral insulin resistance results in a higher serum insulin concentration. Excess insulin binds to the IGF-1 receptors and enhances the theca cells androgen production in response to LH stimulation.[52] Hyperinsulinemia also decreases the synthesis of SHBG by the liver. There is therefore an increase in the concentration of free testosterone (T) in the serum and consequent peripheral androgen action. In addition, hyperinsulinemia inhibits the hepatic secretion of IGF binding protein-1 (IGFBP-1), leading to increased bioavailability of IGF-1 and IGF-2,[53,54] the important regulators of ovarian follicular maturation and steroidogenesis.[55] Together with more IGF-2 secretion from the theca cells, IGF-1 and IGF-2 further augment ovarian androgen production by acting on IGF-1 receptors.[56,57]

Insulin might also increase endogenous androgen concentrations by increased cytochrome P450c17a enzyme activity, which is important for ovarian and adrenal steroid hormone biosynthesis.[58] Intraovarian androgen excess is responsible for anovulation by acting directly on the ovary, promoting the process of follicular atresia.[59]

Gonadotropin Abnormalities

Another key feature of PCOS is altered gonadotropin dynamic.

The increase in LH pulse frequency in patients with PCOS provides clear evidence for an increase in GnRH pulse frequency and therefore a hypothalamic defect.[60,61] Whether the hypothalamic defect is a primary cause of PCOS or secondary to other hormonal phenomenon remains to be determined.

However, high concentrations of androgens desensitize the hypothalamus,[60] suggesting that the abnormalities of gonadotropin release in PCOS are secondary to abnormal steroid release by the ovaries or adrenal glands.[61]

The influence of nonsteroidal factors on pituitary and hypothalamic function is still being elucidated. Further work is required to examine both the pathophysiology of hypersecretion of LH and its effects at the level of the oocyte.[47]

Although LH action at the ovarian level may be enhanced in PCOS, as the LH receptor is overexpressed in the thecal and granulose cells from PCOS.[62]

Environmental Postnatal Factors

The ethnic and geographic heterogeneity of PCOS demonstrates that this disorder is associated with environmental factors.[63] Dietary habits, exercise, and cultural, social and economic factors might modify environmental exposure.

The relevance of environmental factors to the development of PCOS is evidenced by the effect of lifestyle changes on obesity, which is a highly prevalent comorbidity among women with PCOS. Reduction in body weight is the first line of treatment in obese women with PCOS: restores the ovulatory cycle and improves clinical hyperandrogenism and metabolic disorders.[64]

Environmental endocrine disrupting chemicals also might disrupt ovarian and metabolic function, causing PCOS-like abnormalities. Bisphenol A (BPA) is one of them, owing to the decreased hepatic clearance that arises from androgen excess.[65]

CONCLUSION

Polycystic ovary syndrome is a heterogeneous condition. Pathogenesis remains unclear, with contributions from insulin resistance, adipose tissue dysfunction, abnormal steroidogenesis, and hypothalamic-pituitary-ovarian dysregulation, not all of which exist in any given patient. Genetic variants and developmental programming factors, probably contribute to the origin of this endocrinopathy (Flowchart 2).

Flowchart 2: Mechanism causing metabolic changes related with the pathophysiology of PCOS.

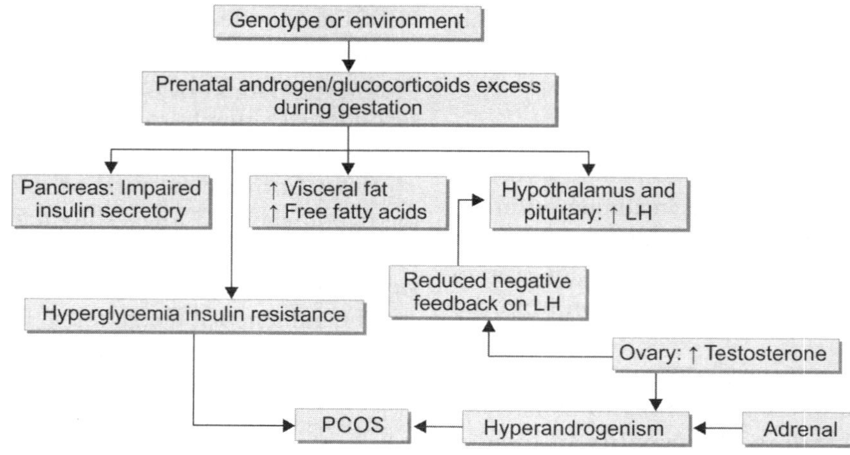

(LH: luteinizing hormone; PCOS: polycystic ovarian syndrome).

REFERENCES

1. Risch N, Merikangas K. The future of genetic studies of complex human diseases. Science. 1996;273:1516-7.
2. Kosova G, Urbanek M. Genetics of the polycystic ovary syndrome. Mol Cell Endocrinol. 2013;373(1-2):29-38.
3. Barber TM, Bennett AJ, Groves CJ, et al. Association of variants in the fat mass and obesity associated (FTO) gene with polycystic ovary syndrome. Diabetologia. 2008;51: 1153-8.
4. Tan S, Scherag A, Janssen OE, et al. Large effects on body mass index and insulin resistance of fat mass and obesity associated gene (FTO) variants in patients with polycystic ovary syndrome (PCOS). BMC Med Genet. 2010;11:12.
5. Zhang N, Shi YH, Hao CF, et al. Association of +45G15G(T/G) and +276(G/T) polymorphisms in the ADIPOQ gene with polycystic ovary syndrome among Han Chinese women. Eur J Endocrinol. 2008;158:255-60.
6. Baba T, Endo T, Sata F, et al. The contributions of resistin and adiponectin gene single nucleotide polymorphisms to the genetic risk for polycystic ovary syndrome in a Japanese population. Gynecol Endocrinol. 2009;25:498-503.
7. Zhang H, Bi Y, Hu C, et al. Association between the Pro12Ala polymorphism of PPAR-gamma gene and the polycystic ovary syndrome: A meta-analysis of case-control studies. Gene. 2012;503:12-7.
8. Urbanek, M, Sam S, Legro RS, et al. Identification of a polycystic ovary syndrome susceptibility variant in fibrillin-3 and association with a metabolic phenotype. J Clin Endocrinol Metab. 2007;92:4191-8.
9. Raja-Khan N, Kunselman AR, Demers LM, et al. A variant in the fibrillin-3 gene is associated with TGF-beta and inhibin B levels in women with polycystic ovary syndrome. Fertil Steril. 2010;94:2916-9.
10. Vollmert C, Hahn S, Lamina C, et al. Calpain-10 variants and haplotypes are associated with polycystic ovary syndrome in Caucasians. Am J Physiol Endocrinol Metab. 2007; 292:E836-44.
11. Marquez JL, Pacheco A, Valdes P, et al. Association between CAPN10 UCSNP-43 gene polymorphism and polycystic ovary syndrome in Chilean women. Clin Chim Acta. 2008;398:5-9.
12. Lee JY, Lee WJ, Hur SE, et al. 111/121 diplotype of Calpain-10 is associated with the risk of polycystic ovary syndrome in Korean women. Fertil Steril. 2009;92:830-3.
13. Fratantonio E, Vicari E, Pafumi C, et al. Genetics of polycystic ovarian syndrome. Reprod Biomed Online. 2005;10(6):713-20.
14. Taylor SI, Cama A, Accili D, et al. Mutations in the insulin receptor gene. Endocr Rev. 1992;13:566-95.
15. Ioannidis A, Ikonomi E, Dimou NL, et al. Polymorphisms of the insulin receptor and the insulin receptor substrates genes in polycystic ovary syndrome: A Mendelian randomization meta-analysis. Mol Genet Metab. 2010;99:174-83.
16. Lee EJ, Oh B, Lee JY, et al. A novel single nucleotide polymorphism of INSR gene for polycystic ovary syndrome. Fertil Steril. 2008;89:1213-20.
17. Goodarzi MO, Louwers YV, Taylor KD, et al. Replication of association of a novel insulin receptor gene polymorphism with polycystic ovary syndrome. Fertil Steril. 2011;95:1736-41.e11.
18. Ben-Shlomo I, Younis JS. Basic research in PCOS: Are we reaching new frontiers? Reprod Biomed Online. 2014;28(6):669-83.
19. Wang L, Wang Y, Zhang X, et al. Common genetic variation in MTNR1B is associated with serum testosterone, glucose tolerance, and insulin secretion in polycystic ovary syndrome patients. Fertil Steril. 2010b;94:2486-9.
20. Li C, Shi Y, You L, et al. Association of rs10830963 and rs10830962 SNP in the melatonin receptor (MTNR1B) gene among Han Chinese women with polycystic ovary syndrome. Mol Hum Reprod. 2011;17:193-8.
21. Ibanez L, Ong KK, Mongan N, et al. Androgen receptor gene CAG repeat polymorphism in the development of ovarian hyperandrogenism. J Clin Endocrinol Metab. 2003;88:3333-8.
22. Zhao H, Lv Y, Li L, et al. Genetic studies on polycystic ovary syndrome. Best Pract Res Clin Obstet Gynaecol. 2016;37: 56-65.
23. Chen ZJ, Zhao H, He L, et al. Genome-wide association study identifies susceptibility loci for polycystic ovary syndrome on chromosome 2p16.3, 2p21 and 9q33.3. Nat Genet. 2011;43:55-9.

24. Shi Y, Zhao H, Shi Y, et al. Genome-wide association study identifies eight new risk loci for polycystic ovary syndrome. Nat Genet. 2012;44:1020-5.
25. Goodarzi MO, Jones MR, Li X, et al. Replication of association of DENND1A and THADA variants with polycystic ovary syndrome in European cohorts. J Med Genet. 2012;49:90-5.
26. Welt CK, Duran JM. Genetics of polycystic ovary syndrome. Semin Reprod Med. 2014;32(3):177-82.
27. Hayes MG, Urbanek M, Ehrmann DA, et al. Genome-wide association of polycystic ovary syndrome implicates alterations in gonadotropin secretion in European ancestry populations. Nat Comm. 2015;6:7502.
28. Day FR, Hinds DA, Tung JY, et al. Causal mechanisms and balancing selection inferred from genetic associations with polycystic ovary syndrome. Nat Comm. 2015;6:8464.
29. Jones MR, Goodarzi MO. Genetic determinants of polycystic ovary syndrome: Progress and future directions. Fertil Steril. 2016;106(1):25-32.
30. Cui L, Zhao H, Zhang B, et al. Genotype-phenotype correlations of PCOS susceptibility SNPs identified by GWAS in a large cohort of Han Chinese women. Hum Reprod. 2013;28:538-44.
31. McAllister JM, Legro RS, Modi BP, et al. Functional genomics of PCOS: From GWAS to molecular mechanisms. Trends Endocrinol Metab. 2015;26(3):118-24.
32. Diamanti-Kandarakis E, Kandarakis H, Legro RS. The role of genes and environment in the etiology of PCOS. Endocrine. 2006;30:19-26.
33. de Melo AS, Dias SV, Cavalli Rde C, et al. Pathogenesis of polycystic ovary syndrome: Multifactorial assessment from the foetal stage to menopause. Reproduction. 2015;150(1):R11-24.
34. Goodarzi MO, Dumesic DA, Chazenbalk G, et al. Polycystic ovary syndrome: Etiology, pathogenesis, and diagnosis. Nat Rev Endocrinol. 2011;7(4):219-31.
35. Wells JC. The thrifty phenotype: An adaptation in growth or metabolism? Am J Hum Biol. 2011;23:65-75.
36. Longo S, Bollani L, Decembrino L, et al. Short-term and long-term sequelae in intrauterine growth retardation (IUGR). J Matern Fetal Neonatal Med. 2013;26:222-5.
37. Padmanabhan V, Veiga-Lopez A. Developmental origin of reproductive and metabolic dysfunctions: Androgenic versus estrogenic reprogramming. Semin Reprod Med. 2011;29:173-86.
38. Escobar-Morreale HF, Alvarez-Blasco F, Botella-Carretero JI, et al. The striking similarities in the metabolic associations of female androgen excess and male androgen deficiency. Hum Reprod. 2014;29:2083-91.
39. Pandolfi C, Zugaro A, Lattanzio F, et al. Low birth weight and later development of insulin resistance and biochemical/clinical features of polycystic ovary syndrome. Metabolism. 2008;57:999-1004.
40. Melo AS, Vieira CS, Barbieri MA, et al. High prevalence of polycystic ovary syndrome in women born small for gestational age. Hum Reprod. 2010;25:2124-31.
41. Hızlı D, Köşüş A, Köşüş N, et al. The impact of birth weight and maternal history on acne, hirsutism, and menstrual disorder symptoms in Turkish adolescent girls. Endocrine. 2012;41:473-8.
42. Willemsen RH, de Kort SW, van der Kaay DC, et al. Independent effects of prematurity on metabolic and cardiovascular risk factors in short small-for-gestational-age children. J Clin Endocrinol Metab. 2008;93:452-8.
43. Elting MW, Korsen TJ, Bezemer PD, et al. Prevalence of diabetes mellitus, hypertension and cardiac complaints in a follow-up study of a Dutch PCOS population. Hum Reprod. 2001;16:556-60.
44. Martinez-Aguayo A, Capurro T, Pena V, et al. Comparison of leptin levels, body composition and insulin sensitivity and secretion by OGTT in healthy, early pubertal girls born at either appropriate- or small-for-gestational age. Clin Endocrinol. 2007;67:526-33.
45. Azziz R, Carmina E, Dewailly D, et al. The androgen excess and PCOS society criteria for the polycystic ovary syndrome: The complete task force report. Fertil Steril. 2009;91:456-88.
46. Kumar A, Wood KS, Bartolucci AA, et al. Prevalence of adrenal androgen excess in patients with the polycystic ovary syndrome (PCOS). Clin Endocrinol (Oxf). 2005;62:644.
47. Balen A. The pathophysiology of polycystic ovary syndrome: Trying to understand PCOS and its endocrinology. Best Pract Res Clin Obstet Gynaecol. 2004;18(5):685-706.
48. Hickey T, Chandy A, Norman RJ. The androgen receptor CAG repeat polymorphism and X-chromosome inactivation in Australian Caucasian women with infertility related to polycystic ovary syndrome. J Clin Endocrinol Metab. 2002;87:161-5.
49. Franks S, Mason H, White D, et al. Etiology of anovulation in polycystic ovary syndrome. Steroids. 1998;63:306-07.
50. Dunaif A. Insulin resistance and the polycystic ovary syndrome: Mechanisms and implication for pathogenesis. Endocr Rev. 1997;18:774-800.
51. Matalliotakis I, Kourtis A, Koukoura O, et al. Polycystic ovary syndrome: Etiology and pathogenesis. Arch Gynecol Obstet. 2006;274(4):187-97.
52. Bergh C, Carlsson B, Olsson JH, et al. Regulation of androgen production in cultured human thecal cells by insulin-like growth factor I and insulin. Fertil Steril. 1993;59:323-31.
53. Leroith D, Werner H, Beitner-Johnson D, et al. Molecular and cellular aspects of the insulin-like growth factor I receptor. Endocrinol Rev. 1995;16:143-63.
54. De Leo V, la Marca A, Orvieto R, et al. Effect of metformin on insulin-like growth factor (IGF) I and IGF-binding protein I in polycystic ovary syndrome. J Clin Endocrinol Metab. 2000;85:1598-600.
55. Adashi E. Intraovarian regulation: The proposed role of insulin-like growth factors. Ann N Y Acad Sci. 1993;687:10-2.
56. Erickson GF, Magoffin D, Cragun J, et al. The effects of insulin and insulin-like growth factors-I and II on estradiol production by granulosa cells of polycystic ovaries. J Clin Endocrinol Metab. 1990;70:894-901.
57. Fauser B, Tarlatzis B, Chang J, et al. The Rotterdam ESHRE/ASRM-sponsored PCOS consensus workshop group. Revised 2003 consensus on diagnostic criteria and long-term health risks related to polycystic ovary syndrome (PCOS). Hum Reprod. 2004;19:41-7.
58. la Marca A, Egbe TO, Morgante G, et al. Metformin treatment reduces ovarían cytochrome P450c17 (response to human chorionic gonadotrophin in women with insulin resistance related polycystic ovary syndrome. Hum Reprod. 2000;15:21-3.

59. Uilenbroek JTJ, Wonlersen PJA, Van der Schoot P. Atresia in preovulatory follicles: Gonadotropin binding in steroidogenic activity. Biol Reprod. 1980;23:219-29.
60. Blank SK, McCartney CR, Marshall JC. The origins and sequelae of abnormal neuroendocrine function in polycystic ovary syndrome. Hum Reprod Update. 2006;12: 351-61.
61. McCartney CR, Eagleson CA, Marshall JC. Regulation of gonadotropin secretion: Implications for polycystic ovary syndrome. Semin Reprod Med. 2002;20:317-26.
62. Taylor AE, McCourt B, Martin KA, et al. Determinants of abnormal gonadotropin secretion in clinically defined women with polycystic ovary syndrome. J Clin Endocrinol Metab. 1997;82(7):2248-56.
63. Amsterdam ESHRE/ASRM-Sponsored 3rd PCOS Consensus Workshop Group. 2012 Consensus on women's health aspects of polycystic ovary syndrome (PCOS). Hum Reprod. 2012;27:14-24.
64. Thessaloniki ESHRE/ASRM-Sponsored PCOS Consensus Workshop Group. Consensus on infertility treatment related to polycystic ovary syndrome. Hum Reprod. 2008;23:462-77.
65. Takeuchi T, Tsutsumi O, Ikezuki Y, et al. Positive relationship between androgen and the endocrine disruptor, bisphenol A, in normal women and women with ovarian dysfunction. Endocr J. 2004;51:165-9.

CHAPTER

33

Adolescent Polycystic Ovarian Syndrome and Hyperandrogenism

Saroja Koppala

INTRODUCTION

Polycystic ovaries are common endocrinological problem that we encounter in our day-to-day life. In adult women, it affects 8–13% of women of reproductive age group.[1,2] Diagnosis of polycystic ovaries in adolescents can be difficult. The exact diagnosis of polycystic ovaries in adolescence is important because early diagnosis can prevent long-term complications.[3,4] And wrong diagnoses can cause lot of distress to the adolescent girl and her family. These girls present with myriad of symptoms and so they can to present to either the gynecologist, endocrinologist, dermatologist or general physicians. Hyperandrogenism is also one of the common presentations and they can present with hirsutism, menstrual disturbances, acne, alopecia, hoarseness of voice, and infertility.[1] Many conditions can present with hyperandrogenism and few of them could be life-threatening.

DEFINITION OF POLYCYSTIC OVARIAN SYNDROME

Polycystic ovaries have been described in the literature for many years. But it was Stein Leventhal who identified an entity consisting of oligomenorrhea, infertility, hirsutism, and bilateral enlarged polycystic ovaries.[5] National Institutes of Health (NIH) criteria for polycystic ovaries were oligoanovulation and biochemical or clinical hyperandrogenism.[6] In 2004, the Rotterdam consensus criteria for polycystic ovarian syndrome (PCOS) were (two out of three of oligoanovulation, clinical and/or biochemical hyperandrogenism or polycystic ovary appearance on ultrasound).[7] In 2009, the Androgen Excess Society (AES) new definition of PCOS is a disorder of clinical and/or biochemical androgen excess, plus either chronic oligoanovulation and/or polycystic ovaries.[8] Other endocrinological disorders should be excluded. In spite of these definitions, the diagnosis of polycystic ovaries in adolescents can be challenging.[9] In adolescents, strict criteria requiring both hyperandrogenism and irregular cycles, with ultrasound not indicated in adolescents, due to overlap with normal reproductive physiology (International evidence-based guideline for the assessment and management of polycystic ovary syndrome, 2018).

Physicians should be cautious of overdiagnosing of PCOS in adolescents. Adolescent girls who are obese, hirsute or having irregular menstrual cycles should be identified and followed.[10] Whenever the diagnosis is not clear they should be followed closely and diagnosis should be reconsidered[10] at or before full reproductive maturity, 8 years postmenarche. (International evidence-based guideline for the assessment and management of polycystic ovary syndrome 2018).[11]

DIAGNOSIS OF POLYCYSTIC OVARIAN SYNDROME IN ADOLESCENCE

Menstrual Disturbance

Menstrual irregularity is common in majority of the girls after menarche. Nearly 85% of the cycles are anovulatory in the first year after menarche.[12] In adolescent girls with menstrual irregularity only 40% of them have features of polycystic ovaries on ultrasound examination.[13] Adolescent girls who have oligomenorrhea 2 years after menarche have high probability of developing PCOS.[14,15] And also menarche in girls with PCOS can vary widely, from early menarche before the age of 9 years to primary amenorrhea.[16] Higher androgen levels are found in women with primary amenorrhea and were more likely to be overweight[17-19] or have a family history of overweight,[19] which exacerbates hyperandrogenemia. Persistence of anovulation was seen more in girls with increased body mass index (BMI).[10] Within 8 years of menarche, both hyperandrogenism[20] and ovulatory dysfunction are required, with ultrasound not recommended (International evidence-based guideline for the assessment and management of polycystic ovary syndrome 2018).

Ultrasound

In adolescent girls who are sexually not active transabdominal ultrasound is used which gives a less better picture compared to transvaginal scan. Also one of the criteria for the diagnosis of polycystic ovary is volume of the ovaries greater than 10 mL. In adolescents, normal girls also have larger volumes so it is difficult to diagnose PCOS based on volume alone.[21] So we need higher threshold values for ovarian volume for adolescents (Carmina et al., 2010) a task force report from the Androgen Excess and Polycystic Ovary Syndrome Society recommends that normal range should be available based on age, ethnicity, and body weight.[22] With the improvement in technology and with the better resolution of scan machines with transvaginal ultrasound and transducer frequency of more than or equal to 8 MHz, the threshold for diagnosis of PCOS should be more than 20 follicles per ovary and or an ovarian volume more than or equal to 10 mL after excluding cysts or dominant follicles. But higher frequency scans are not available in all centers. Ovarian volume and morphology that are used for diagnosis of PCOS in adults, may be of limited value in adolescence PCOS.[21] Features of PCOS are more common in overweight or obese girls.[12]

Hyperandrogenism

Hyperandrogenism is a common clinical presentation in women. They can present with hirsutism, menstrual disturbance or infertility.[1] It can be caused by many conditions like PCOS, congenital adrenal hyperplasia, androgen-secreting tumors, and Cushing' syndrome.[1,23] There is either more production of androgens or they are not converted into estrogens or they can be a combination of both in hyperandrogenism.[24] Modified Ferriman-Gallwey score (mFG) proposed by Hatch et al.[25] is commonly used for evaluation of hirsutism.[26] In adolescents, hyperandrogenemia may be a consistent marker for PCOS[27] and may represent an important symptom of PCOS.[12]

Acne

Acne can be a feature of hyperandrogenism but not all girls with acne have hyperandrogenism.[28] It can be a normal feature for adolescents. It can affect around 70% of girls and did not associate with other features of PCOS.[21]

Hirsutism

Hirsutism in women with PCOS can be caused by increased androgen production, increased circulating free T, or greater androgen activity within the pilosebaceous unit[10] and these should be addressed while treating. Hirsutism in adolescents takes longer to develop in the presence of increased androgens.[29] Acne and hirsutism can cause lot of distress to the young girls. Severity of hirsutism does not correlate well with the level of androgens.[30-33] Even mild hirsutism in women can be an indicator of an underlying androgen excess disorder.[34] Sometimes women with severe hyperandrogenemia may not have hirsutism.[8,35,36] Genetic counseling should be done in cases of nonclassical congenital adrenal hyperplasia where there is risk of heritable transmission.[37] The treatment of hirsutism can take longer, so women should be warned regarding this. Pharmacological treatment should aim to decrease androgen secretion and action. Physical exercise and diet are essential for the management of androgen excess and for the cardiovascular protection in women with PCOS.[8,36,38] Hirsutism is a chronic disorder in most cases, underlying disorder should be treated.[39] PCOS is cause of hirsutism in majority of cases but others like hyperthecosis, nonclassical adrenal hyperplasia, Cushing syndrome, thyroid dysfunction, and ovarian and adrenal androgen-secreting tumors have to be ruled out.[10]

Pathophysiology

Insulin resistance and hyperandrogenism play a key role in the pathophysiology of PCOS and insulin resistance affects 85% (75% of lean and 95% of overweight) of cases.[40] This increase in insulin leads to increases androgen production and reduces sex hormone-binding globulin (SHBG) leading to hyperandrogenism.[41]

Laboratory Evaluation

Can we diagnose PCOS confidently by laboratory tests? Exact criteria for diagnosis of hyperandrogenism were not specified by the consensus group.[42] Calculated free testosterone, free androgen index or calculated bioavailable testosterone should be used to assess biochemical hyperandrogenism in the diagnosis of PCOS.[43] High quality assays such as liquid chromatography–mass spectrometry (LCMS)/mass spectrometry and extraction/chromatography immunoassays, should be used for the most accurate assessment of total or free testosterone in PCOS (International evidence-based guideline for the assessment and management of polycystic ovary syndrome 2018).[44-46] There is no specific range for adolescent population. The value of the androgen levels should be interpreted based upon the method used for testing and also the reference value for the lab.

Anti-Müllerian hormone (AMH)—AMH concentrations are a questionable surrogate marker of polycystic ovarian morphology (PCOM) in adolescents.[47] AMH levels are not yet adequate for diagnosis (International evidence-based guideline for the assessment and management of polycystic ovary syndrome 2018).

Follow-up

Once the diagnosis is made, by early interventions long-term complications can be prevented.[3,4] Compared to women without PCOS, women with PCOS are at higher risk of depression[48] and at any age they are at higher risk of elevated cardiovascular disease (CVD) markers and they are magnified with obesity.[10]

Treatment

Main aim of treatment should be to treat the problem, maintain quality of life, and prevent long-term complications. Because of the varied presentation of PCOS to different specialties, all specialists should be aware of this, and management should start at the earliest. PCOS has a negative impact on the quality of life in adolescents.[49] Some adolescent girls with PCOS find hirsutism and acne more troublesome compared to the nonvisible effects of PCOS. Obesity, hirsutism, and irregular menses should be treated in adolescents.[10] Life style modification plays a very important role in the management of women with polycystic ovaries. Weight loss through modifications in diet, exercise can decrease severity of PCOS. Adolescent girls should be educated that with restriction in calorie intake and regular physical activity, improvement in hirsutism can be seen in 40–55% of women within 6 months of weight reduction. Life styles modifications should be considered as a primary line of management in these girls because they are effective and also some girls consider taking medications as a social stigma. Dieticians can be helpful in weight reduction. Medications like metformin, orlistat or bariatric surgery improves insulin resistance and reduces severity of PCOS.[50-52] Oral contraceptive pills play a very important role in the treatment of PCOS. Combined oral contraceptive pills with the lowest estrogen content and which is effective should be used. It improves acne, hirsutism, regularize the menstrual cycles and acts as a contraception in sexually active adolescent girls. Before prescribing the oral contraceptive pills, absolute contraindications should be considered. Metformin is useful in adolescent girls with glucose intolerance.[10] Metformin is very safe from a metabolic point of view especially in obese/overweight adolescents with impaired glucose metabolism, because it improves insulin sensitivity, serum triglycerides levels, and BMI. In these cases, its administration should be always associated to lifestyle modification programs.[53] For treatment of hirsutism, ovarian steroid production is reduced by the use of oral contraceptive pill play an important role in the treatment for PCOS.[10] Adolescent girls with PCO tend to have psychological issues like depression, anxiety, and eating disorders and they should be appropriately counseled.

CONCLUSION

Polycystic ovarian syndrome in adolescence should be defined, diagnosed, and followed up to improve the quality of life and to prevent short and long-term complications.

REFERENCES

1. Azziz R, Sanchez LA, Knochenhauer ES, et al. Androgen excess in women: Experience with over 1000 consecutive patients. J Clin Endocrinol Metab. 2004;89:453-62.
2. March WA, Moore VM, Willson KJ, et al. The prevalence of polycystic ovary syndrome in a community sample assessed under contrasting diagnostic criteria. Hum Reprod. 2010;25(2):544-51.
3. Palmert MR, Gordon CM, Kartashov AI, et al. Screening for abnormal glucose tolerance in adolescents with polycystic ovary syndrome. J Clin Endocrinol Metab. 2002;87:1017-23.
4. Ibanez L, Valls C, Marcos MV, et al. Insulin sensitization for girls with precocious pubarche and with risk for polycystic ovary syndrome: Effects of prepubertal initiation and postpubertal discontinuation of metformin treatment. J Clin Endocrinol Metab. 2004;89:4331-7.
5. Stein IF, Leventhal ML. Amenorrhea associated with bilateral polycystic ovaries. Am J Obstet Gynecol. 1935;29:181-91.
6. Zawadzki JK, Dunaif A. Diagnostic criteria for polycystic ovary syndrome: Towards a rational approach. In: Dunaif A (Ed). Polycystic Ovary Syndrome. Boston: Blackwell Scientific. 1995;377-84.
7. The Rotterdam ESHRE/ASRM-sponsored PCOS consensus workshop group. Revised 2003 consensus on diagnostic criteria and long-term health risks related to polycystic ovary syndrome (PCOS). Hum Reprod. 2004;19:41-7.

8. Azziz R, Carmina E, Dewailly D, et al. The Androgen Excess and PCOS Society criteria for the polycystic ovary syndrome: The complete task force report. Fertil Steril. 2009;91:456-88.
9. Khan U. Polycystic ovary syndrome in adolescents. J Pediatr Adolesc Gynecol. 2007;20:101-4.
10. Fauser BC, Tarlatzis BC, Rebar RW, et al. Consensus on women's health aspects of polycystic ovary syndrome (PCOS): The Amsterdam ESHRE/ASRM-Sponsored 3rd PCOS Consensus Workshop Group. Fertil Steril. 2012;97(1):28-38.
11. Cibula D, Hill M, Starka L. The best correlation of the new index of hyperandrogenism with the grade of increased hair. Eur J Endocrinol. 2000;143:405-8.
12. Blank SK, Helm KD, McCartney CR, et al. Polycystic ovary syndrome in adolescence. Ann N Y Acad Sci. 2008;1135:76-84.
13. Venturoli S, Porcu E, Fabbri R, et al. Longitudinal change of sonographic ovarian aspects and endocrine parameters in irregular cycles of adolescence. Pediatr Res. 1995;38:974-80.
14. Balen A, Creighton S, Martin-Hirsch P. Adolescent reproductive health. Editor's choice. BJOG. 2010;117(2).
15. Barth JH, Yasmin E, Balen AH. The diagnosis of polycystic ovary syndrome: The criteria are insufficiently robust for clinical research. Clin Endocrinol. 67:811-5.
16. Dahlgren E, Johansson S, Lindstedt G, et al. Women with polycystic ovary syndrome wedge resected in 1956 to 1965: A long-term follow-up focusing on natural history and circulating hormones. Fertil Steril. 1992;57:505-13.
17. Bekx MT, Connor EC, Allen DB. Characteristics of adolescents presenting to a multidisciplinary clinic for polycystic ovarian syndrome. J Pediatr Adolesc Gynecol. 2010;23:7-10.
18. Dramusic V, Goh VH, Rajan U, et al. Clinical, endocrinology, and ultrasonographic features of polycystic ovary syndrome in Singaporean adolescents. J Pediatr Adolesc Gynecol. 1997;10:125-32.
19. Rachmiel M, Kives S, Atenafu E, et al. Primary amenorrhea as a manifestation of polycystic ovarian syndrome in adolescents: A unique subgroup? Arch Pediatr Adolesc Med. 2008;162:521-5.
20. Barth JH, Field HP, Yasmin E, et al. Defining hyperandrogenism in polycystic ovary syndrome: Measurement of testosterone and androstenedione by liquid chromatography-tandem mass spectrometry and analysis by receiver operator characteristic plots. Eur J Endocrinol. 2010;162(3):611-5.
21. Hickey M, Doherty DA, Atkinson H, et al. Clinical, ultrasound and biochemical features of polycystic ovary syndrome in adolescents: Implications for diagnosis. Hum. Reprod. 2011;26(6):1469-77.
22. Dewailly D, Lujan M, Carmina E, et al. Definition and significance of polycystic ovarian morphology: A task force report from the Androgen Excess and Polycystic Ovary Syndrome Society. Hum Reprod Update. 2014;20(3):334-52.
23. Dennedy MC, Smith D, O' Shea D, et al. Investigation of patients with atypical or severe hyperandrogenaemia including androgen-secreting ovarian teratoma. Eur J Endocrinol. 2010;162:213-20.
24. Meek C, Bravis V, Don A, et al. Polycystic ovary syndrome and the differential diagnosis of hyperandrogenism. Obstet Gynaecol. 2013;15:171-6.
25. Hatch R, Rosenfield RL, Kim MH, et al. Hirsutism: Implications, etiology, and management. Am J Obstet Gynecol. 1981;140:815-30.
26. Yildiz BO, Bolour S, Woods K, et al. Visually scoring hirsutism. Hum Reprod Update. 2010;16:51-64.
27. Jeffrey CR, Coffler MS. Polycystic ovary syndrome: Early detection in the adolescent. Clin Obstet Gynecol. 2007;50:178-87.
28. Slayden SM, Moran C, Sams WJ, et al. Hyperandrogenemia in patients presenting with acne. Fertil Steril. 2001;75:889-92.
29. Lucky AW, Biro FM, Daniels SR, et al. The prevalence of upper lip hair in black and white girls during puberty: A new standard. J Pediatr Endocrinol Metab. 2001;138:134-6.
30. Carmina E, Lobo RA. The addition of dexamethasone to antiandrogen therapy for hirsutism prolongs the duration of remission. Fertil Steril. 1998;69:1075-9.
31. Legro RS, Schlaff WD, Diamond MP, et al. Total testosterone assays in women with polycystic ovary syndrome: Precision and correlation with hirsutism. J Clin Endocrinol Metab. 2010;95:5305-13.
32. Pfeifer M, Prezelj J, Kocijancic A. The correlation between clinical and hormonal parameters in androgenisation. Acta Eur Fertil. 1989;20:31-33.
33. Reingold SB, Rosenfield RL. The relationship of mild hirsutism or acne in women to androgens. Arch Dermatol. 1987;123:209-12.
34. Di Fede G, Mansueto P, Pepe I, et al. High prevalence of polycystic ovary syndrome in women with mild hirsutism and no other significant clinical symptoms. Fertil Steril. 2010;94:194-7.
35. Azziz R. Controversy in clinical endocrinology: Diagnosis of polycystic ovarian syndrome: The Rotterdam criteria are premature. J Clin Endocrinol Metab. 2006;91:781-5.
36. Wild RA, Carmina E, Diamanti-Kandarakis E, et al. Assessment of cardiovascular risk and prevention of cardiovascular disease in women with the polycystic ovary syndrome: A consensus statement by the Androgen Excess and Polycystic Ovary Syndrome (AE-PCOS) Society. J Clin Endocrinol Metab.2010;95:2038-49.
37. Speiser PW, Knochenhauer ES, Dewailly D, et al. A multicentre study of women with nonclassical congenital adrenal hyperplasia: Relationship between genotype and phenotype. Mol Genet Metab. 2000;71:527-34.
38. Villarroel C, Trejo L, Muñoz A, et al. Assessment of diagnostic competence of plasmatic androgens on polycystic ovary syndrome based on receiver operator characteristic curves. Gynecol Endocrinol. 2010;26:600-6.
39. Escobar-Morreale HF, Carmina E, Dewailly Gambineri DA, et al. Epidemiology, diagnosis and management of hirsutism: A consensus statement by the Androgen Excess and Polycystic Ovary Syndrome Society. Hum. Reprod. Update. 2012;18(2):146-70.
40. Stepto NK, Cassar S, Joham AE, et al. Women with polycystic ovary syndrome have intrinsic insulin resistance on euglycaemic-hyperinsulaemic clamp. Hum Reprod. 2013;28:777-84.
41. Teede HJ, Hutchison SK, Zoungas S. The management of insulin resistance in polycystic ovary syndrome. Trends Endocrinol Metab. 2007;18:273-9.
42. Bell A, Meek CL, Viljoen A. Evidence of biochemical hyperandrogenism in women: The limitations of serum testosterone quantitation. J Obstet Gynaecol. 2012;32:367-71.

43. Ho CK, Stoddart M, Walton M, et al. Calculated free testosterone in men: Comparison of four equations and with free androgen index. Ann Clin Biochem. 2006;43:389-97.
44. Kane J, Middle J, Cawood M. Measurement of serum testosterone on women; what should we do? Ann Clin Biochem. 2007;44:5-15.
45. Rosner W, Auchus RJ, Azziz R, et al. Position statement: Utility limitations and pitfalls in measuring testosterone: An Endocrine Society position statement. J Clin Endocrinol Metab. 2007;92:405-13.
46. Vermeulen A, Verdonck L, Kaufman JM. A critical evaluation of simple methods for the estimation of free testosterone in serum. J Clin Endocrinol Metab.1999;84:3666-72.
47. Hart R, Doherty DA, Norman RJ, et al. Serum antimullerian hormone (AMH) levels are elevated in adolescent girls with polycystic ovaries and the polycystic ovarian syndrome (PCOS). Fertil Steril. 2010;94:1118-21.
48. Bhattacharya SM, Jha A. Prevalence and risk of depressive disorders in women with polycystic ovary syndrome (PCOS). Fertil Steril. 2010;94:357-9.
49. Jones GL, Hall JM, Lashen HL, et al. Health-related quality of life among adolescents with polycystic ovary syndrome. J Obstet Gynecol Neonatal Nurs. 2011;40(5):577-88.
50. Jensterle M, Kocjan T, Kravos NA, et al. Short-term intervention with liraglutide improved eating behavior in obese women with polycystic ovary syndrome. Endocr Res. 2015;40:133-8.
51. Moran LJ, Hutchison SK, Norman RJ, et al. Lifestyle changes in women with polycystic ovary syndrome. Cochrane Database Syst Rev. 2011;CD007506.
52. Vosnakis C, Georgopoulos NA, Rousso D, et al. Diet, physical exercise and Orlistat administration increase serum anti-Mullerian hormone (AMH) levels in women with polycystic ovary syndrome (PCOS). Gynecol Endocrinol. 2013;29: 242-5.
53. Palomba S, Materazzo C, Falbo A, et al. Metformin, oral contraceptives or both to manage oligo-amenorrhea in adolescents with polycystic ovary syndrome? A clinical review. Gynecol Endocrinol. 2014;30(5):335-40.

CHAPTER

34

Lifestyle Management and Role of Insulin-sensitizing Drugs

Esther Santamaría López, Cinzia Caligara, Manuel Fernández-Sánchez

INTRODUCTION

Polycystic ovarian syndrome (PCOS) definition has been a controversial debate since its recognition, 70 years ago by Stein and Leventhal. Bilaterally and symmetrically enlarged ovaries were the first symptom recognized in the Stein-Leventhal syndrome.[1] Throughout the years, other signs and symptoms have been added to the PCOS definition. Nevertheless, the Rotterdam American Society for Reproductive Medicine or European Society of Human Reproduction and Embryology (ESHRE/ASRM)-sponsored PCOS consensus workshop group revised the criteria established in 2003 that PCOS is a syndrome with two main features: hyperandrogenism and polycystic ovary (PCO).[2]

Polycystic ovary syndrome affects up to 6–21% of women of reproductive age when the Rotterdam criteria are used.[3] This syndrome can be manifested by menstrual irregularities, androgen excess and obesity. On the one hand, PCOS is also associated to a higher incidence of insulin resistance with compensatory hyperinsulinemia, leading to increased testosterone levels directly by stimulating theca hyperplasia and indirectly via inhibition of hepatic sex hormone-binding globulin (SHBG) production. On the other hand, insulin resistance is closely related to the presence of metabolic syndrome, which is a cluster of several risk factors that confer an increased risk for cardiovascular disease (Fig. 1).[2]

Treatment of infertile women with PCOS has been surrounded by many controversies over the last years. On the basis of the currently available evidence, a group of experts reached a consensus in 2008 regarding the therapeutic challenges raised in these women. According to Thessaloniki consensus recommendation, before any intervention is initiated, preconceptional counseling should be provided emphasizing the importance of lifestyle, especially exercise and weight loss in overweight women, smoking and alcohol consumption.[4]

The recommended first-line treatment for ovulation induction remains the antiestrogen clomiphene citrate, which is an effective medication but is not free of adverse effects. Recommended second-line intervention would be represented by either exogenous gonadotropins or laparoscopic ovarian surgery and in vitro fertilization (IVF) should be reserved for women with PCOS who fail gonadotropin therapy or who have other indications for IVF treatment (Flowchart 1). However, other approaches should be developed for ovulation induction based on initial screening characteristics of women with PCOS, such as adjuvant therapies, leading to a deviation from the previous

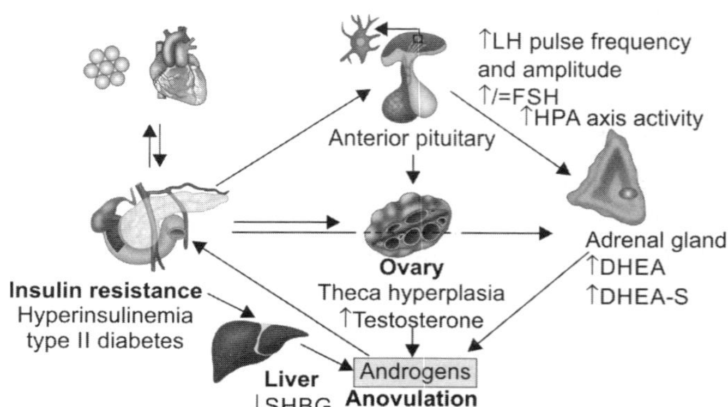

Fig. 1: Main associated disorders of PCOS women. (DHEA: dehydroepiandrosterone; DHEA-S: dehydroepiandrosterone sulfate; HPA: hypothalamic-pituitary-adrenal; FSH: follicle-stimulating hormone; LH: luteinizing hormone; SHBG: sex hormone-binding globulin).

Flowchart 1: Management of PCOS patients.

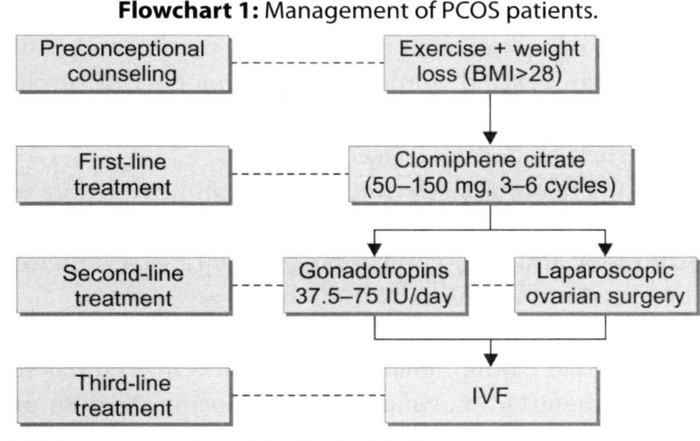

(BMI: body mass index; IVF: in vitro fertilization)

mentioned first-line, second-line or third-line strategies in well-defined subsets of patients.[4]

In this chapter, we will review the lifestyle management and the use of insulin-sensitizing drugs in PCOS patients.

LIFESTYLE

Diet and Exercise

Obesity adversely affects reproduction and is associated with anovulation, pregnancy loss, and late-pregnancy complications. The ideal amount of weight loss is unknown, but a 5% decrease of body weight might be clinically meaningful.[4,5]

For weight management, it has been proposed to add pharmacotherapy to lifestyle modifications "as a last resort" but more studies are necessary to confirm the effects.[3]

Exercise in PCOS women may improve ovulation, reduce insulin resistance and weight loss. Type of exercise, frequency and length of sessions are not significant. These studies are also limited and more well-designed studies are necessary.[6]

Antioxidants

Recently, a large number of medications have been shown to exert positive effects on different symptomatologies of PCOS. But unfortunately, nowadays, none of these treatments are fully able to combat the whole spectrum of the disorder.

However, clinical researches have been focused on the following treatments:

Simvastatin

Simvastatin belongs to the family of statins, competitive inhibitors of 3-hydroxy-3-methylglutaryl-coenzyme A reductase (HMG-CoA reductase), which is the enzyme limiting the rate of cholesterol synthesis. This blockade of the mevalonate pathway leads to a decreased availability of several downstream products, such as cholesterol and substrates of isoprenylation, interfering with several biological cell functions.

Simvastatin possess a broad range of biological properties, such as anti-inflammatory, antiproliferative and antioxidant agent in different tissues. However, little is known about the effect of simvastatin on ovary function.

First study showing effects on PCOS women resulted in a significant improvement of hormonal and lipid profiles, providing not only endocrine but also cardiovascular benefits. However, no significant changes were observed in glucose metabolism.[7]

These statin-induced beneficial effects of statins on PCOS women have also been demonstrated in the long run. A study comparing simvastatin with metformin treatments after 6 months showed for the first time that simvastatin improves menstrual regularity, reduces ovarian volume and induces progressive improvement of biochemical and clinical hyperandrogenism, being superior to metformin in the long run.[8]

However, effects of statins on PCOS should be viewed with caution since they may induce adverse effects (elevation of transaminases and myopathy) and may interact with other drugs (antibiotics and fibrates).

Moreover, statins are currently listed by the Food and Drug Administration (FDA) as pregnancy category X medications, being contraindicated in pregnancy. This is why sexually active women of reproductive age should use reliable contraception.

Finally, we have to take into account that the role of statins in glucose metabolism remains unknown and further studies are needed to clarify the effect of statins in the development of type 2 diabetes mellitus. One candidate for such adjuvant therapy is resveratrol.

Resveratrol

Resveratrol is a natural polyphenol synthesized by several medicinal plants and protects against ultraviolet and fungal infections. It is found in high concentration in grapes, berries, nuts, and red wine with potentially beneficial anticarcinogenic, cardioprotective, antioxidant, and anti-inflammatory properties. It has also been shown to be responsible for the French paradox, by which French people have a relatively low incidence of coronary heart disease (CHD), despite having a diet relatively rich in saturated fats, due to consumption of red wine, rich in resveratrol.[9]

Along with its antiaging properties, resveratrol also helps to prevent heart diseases, neurodegeneration and cancer.[10] Moreover, resveratrol treatment resulted in progressive time-dependent and concentration-dependent morphological changes consistent with apoptosis, such as nuclear shrinkage and cytoskeleton degradation.[11]

In addition, resveratrol also decreased androgen production, and this inhibitory effect correlated with a decrease in messenger RNA (mRNA) expression of genes regulating androgen production, especially CYP17A1 (cytochrome P450, family 17, subfamily A, polypeptide 1). Therefore, we can say that resveratrol decreases proliferation and steroidogenesis and exerts a proapoptotic effect on theca cell cultures.[12]

Moreover, resveratrol treatment resulted in a significant decrease of vascular endothelial growth factor (VEGF) expression, interesting finding bearing in mind that VEGF is a vasoactive molecule involved in the pathophysiology of ovarian hyperstimulation syndrome (OHSS), which is a clinical disorder with relatively high incidence in PCOS undergoing controlled ovarian hyperstimulation (COH). Therefore, we conclude that resveratrol exerts a cytostatic, but not cytotoxic, effect on granulosa cells and decreases VEGF expression.[13]

To summarize, resveratrol emerges as a potential therapeutic agent in conditions associated with highly vascularized theca-interstitial hyperplasia and abnormal angiogenesis, such as those seen in PCOS.

INSULIN-SENSITIZING DRUGS

These adjuvant therapies need to meet some requirements to be considered for clinical use:

- Long-term efficacy
- Tolerance pattern
- Simplicity
- Safety profile.

Current adjuvant therapies in PCOS are mainly represented by the group of insulin-sensitizing drugs, whereby metformin has classically played a prominent role.

Metformin

Metformin is recommended in addition or alone, primarily for management of metabolic features.[5] Many studies raised the question of whether metformin might be superior to clomiphene citrate for ovulation induction, and therefore, substitute clomiphene citrate as first-line treatment in PCOS. Trying to address this issue, several studies were published showing controversial results.[14]

Metformin use appears to have similar live birth rates when it is compared with placebo or no treatment, before or during an assisted reproductive technology (ART) cycle. Nevertheless, pregnancy rate is higher and OHSS risk is lower when metformin is used.[14]

Comparison of metformin with clomiphene citrate or combination of both therapies shows similar result in live birth rates, although clinical pregnancy rates are higher when metformin is used.[15]

These findings were widely accepted as definitive evidence that clomiphene citrate should remain the first-line treatment for anovulatory PCOS, closing the door on metformin.[14] Metformin use in PCOS should be restricted to women with glucose intolerance.[4] However, more studies are needed to confirm this fact.[15]

Regarding PCOS women treated with metformin during the first trimester of pregnancy, there is no evidence of an increased risk of problems at birth.[16]

These clinical findings were assimilated into the Thessaloniki consensus recommendation, stating:[4]

- Use of metformin in PCOS should be restricted to those patients with glucose intolerance. Decisions about continuing insulin sensitizers during pregnancy in women with glucose intolerance should be left to the obstetricians providing care and should be based on a careful evaluation of risks and benefits.
- Metformin alone is less effective than clomiphene citrate in inducing ovulation in women with PCOS.
- There seems to be no advantage to adding metformin to clomiphene citrate in women with PCOS.

D-Chiro-Inositol

Metformin has classically played a prominent role in adjuvant therapies in PCOS, mainly represented by the group of insulin-sensitizing drugs, however, there are also others.

Vitamin factors belonging to vitamin B complex that has emerged as a promising treatment for PCOS in the last years. Besides its beneficial effects on hormonal and metabolic profiles, inositol seems to play a role in oocyte quality.[17] For example, rodent studies have shown that the supplementation with myoinositol is positively related to meiotic progression of mouse germinal vesicle oocytes, enhancing intracellular Ca^{2+} oscillation.[18] Whereas in humans, higher concentrations of myoinositol in human follicular fluid have shown to provide a marker of good-quality oocytes.[19] This inositol-induced positive effect on oocyte quality has also been demonstrated in PCOS patients. Pretreatment with myoinositol and folic acid for 3 months has shown to reduce germinal vesicles and degenerated oocytes at ovum pick-up, without compromising the total number of retrieved oocytes.[20]

Polycystic ovary syndrome women undergoing IVF treatment present a mean number of oocyte retrieved similar to those women who use myoinositol, whereas in the group cotreated with myoinositol, the mean number of germinal vesicles (GV) and degenerated oocytes was significantly reduced. However, no significant changes were observed in either implantation or clinical pregnancy rates.[21]

Thus, we can conclude saying that myoinositol is a novel therapy that restores ovulation, improves glucose metabolism, and oocyte maturation but does not increase pregnancy rate in IVF cycles, being necessary further studies to evaluate its role in IVF treatment.[21]

Thiazolidinediones

Thiazolidinediones bind to peroxisome proliferator-activated receptor gamma (PPARγ) and activate it, increasing the expression of multiple genes encoding proteins and the insulin receptor substrate, accelerating the differentiation of adipose cells and increasing the response of surrounding tissues (especially in the insulin target tissue: skeletal muscle, liver, adipose) to insulin. Therefore, insulin resistance may be improved.[22]

"Resveratrol and simvastatin do not have the same risk of hepatotoxicity and are commonly used in clinical trials on women with PCOS."

However these two drugs are classified as pregnancy category C drugs according to the FDA due to the potential risk of causing fetal growth restriction in animal experiments.[22] However, due to the broad range of side effects associated with thiazolidinediones use, it is unlikely that these drugs would have a major role in treating PCOS women.[15]

CONCLUSION

Lifestyle modification and weight loss still remain being first-line intervention in overweight PCOS patients, while clomiphene citrate remains the treatment of first choice for induction of ovulation in most anovulatory women with PCOS.

Regarding antioxidants, simvastatin improves hormonal and metabolic profiles and decreases low-grade inflammation in PCOS patients and resveratrol might represent a novel therapeutic agent for conditions associated with excessive androgen production and highly vascularized theca-interstitial hyperplasia, such as PCOS.

At present, use of insulin-sensitizing drugs in PCOS, such as metformin should be restricted to those patients with glucose intolerance, because its improvement in other groups has not been demonstrated. Myoinositol restores ovulation, improves glucose metabolism and oocyte quality but does not increase pregnancy rate in IVF cycles. It is unlikely that thiazolidinediones would have a major role in treating PCOS women.

REFERENCES

1. Stein IF. Stein-Leventhal syndrome. Clin Obstet Gynecol. 1959;2(1):207-17.
2. Rotterdam ESHRE/ASRM-Sponsored PCOS Consensus Workshop Group. Revised 2003 consensus on diagnostic criteria and long-term health risks related to polycystic ovary syndrome. Fertil Steril. 2004;81(1):19-25.
3. Naderpoor N, Shorakae S, de Courten B, et al. Metformin and lifestyle modification in polycystic ovary syndrome: systematic review and meta-analysis. Hum Reprod Update. 2015;21(5):560-74.
4. Thessaloniki ESHRE/ASRM-Sponsored PCOS Consensus Workshop Group. Consensus on infertility treatment related to polycystic ovary syndrome. Hum Reprod. 2008;23(3): 462-77.
5. Teede HJ, Misso ML, Costello MF, et al. Recommendations from the international evidence-based guideline for the assessment and management of polycystic ovary syndrome. Fertil Steril. 2018;110(3):364-379.
6. Harrison CL, Lombard CB, Moran LJ, et al. Exercise therapy in polycystic ovary syndrome: a systematic review. Hum Reprod Update. 2011;17(2):171-83.
7. Duleba AJ, Banaszewska B, Spaczynski RZ, et al. Simvastatin improves biochemical parameters in women with polycystic ovary syndrome: results of a prospective, randomized trial. Fertil Steril. 2006;85(4):996-1001.
8. Banaszewska B, Pawelczyk L, Spaczynski RZ, et al. Effects of simvastatin and metformin on polycystic ovary syndrome after 6 months of treatment. J Clin Endocrinol Metab. 2011;96(11):3493-501.
9. Joe AK, Liu H, Suzui M, et al. Resveratrol induces growth inhibition, S-phase arrest, apoptosis, and changes in biomarker expression in several human cancer cell lines. Clin Cancer Res. 2002;8(3):893-903.
10. Brasnyó P, Molnár GA, Mohás M, et al. Resveratrol improves insulin sensitivity, reduces oxidative stress and activates the Akt pathway in type 2 diabetic patients. Br J Nutr. 2011;106(3):383-9.
11. Wong DH, Villanueva JA, Cress AB, et al. Effects of resveratrol on proliferation and apoptosis in rat ovarian theca-interstitial cells. Mol Hum Reprod. 2010;16(4):251-9.
12. Ortega I, Villanueva JA, Wong DH, et al. Resveratrol reduces steroidogenesis in rat ovarian theca-interstitial cells: the role of inhibition of Akt/PKB signaling pathway. Endocrinology. 2012;153(8):4019-29.
13. Ortega I, Wong DH, Villanueva JA, et al. Effects of resveratrol on growth and function of rat ovarian granulosa cells. Fertil Steril. 2012;98(6):1563-73.

14. Tso LO, Costello MF, Albuquerque LE, et al. Metformin treatment before and during IVF or ICSI in women with polycystic ovary syndrome. Cochrane Database Syst Rev. 2014;(11):CD006105.
15. Tang T, Lord JM, Norman RJ, et al. Insulin-sensitising drugs (metformin, rosiglitazone, pioglitazone, D-chiro-inositol) for women with polycystic ovary syndrome, oligo amenorrhoea and subfertility. Cochrane Database Syst Rev. 2012;(5):CD003053.
16. Cassina M, Donà M, Di Gianantonio E, et al. First-trimester exposure to metformin and risk of birth defects: a systematic review and meta-analysis. Hum Reprod Update. 2014;20(5):656-69.
17. Costantino D, Minozzi G, Minozzi E, et al. Metabolic and hormonal effects of myo-inositol in women with polycystic ovary syndrome: a double-blind trial. Eur Rev Med Pharmacol Sci. 2009;13(2):105-10.
18. Chiu TT, Rogers MS, Briton-Jones C, et al. Effects of myo-inositol on the in-vitro maturation and subsequent development of mouse oocytes. Hum Reprod. 2003;18(2):408-16.
19. Chiu TT, Rogers MS, Law EL, et al. Follicular fluid and serum concentrations of myo-inositol in patients undergoing IVF: relationship with oocyte quality. Hum Reprod. 2002;17(6):1591-6.
20. Ciotta L, Stracquadanio M, Pagano I, et al. Effects of myo-inositol supplementation on oocyte's quality in PCOS patients: a double blind trial. Eur Rev Med Pharmacol Sci. 2011;15(5):509-14.
21. Papaleo E, Unfer V, Baillargeon JP, et al. Myo-inositol may improve oocyte quality in intracytoplasmatic sperm injection cycles. A prospective, controlled, randomized trial. Fertil Steril. 2009;91(5):1750-4.
22. Du Q, Yang S, Wang YJ, et al. Effects of thiazolidinediones on polycystic ovary syndrome: a meta-analysis of randomized placebo-controlled trials. Adv Ther. 2012;29(9):763-74.

CHAPTER

35

Ovulation Induction in Polycystic Ovary Women

Nisha Thakre, Anil Gudi

INTRODUCTION

The polycystic ovary syndrome (PCOS) is the most common hyperandrogenic disorder in women and one of the most common causes of ovulatory infertility, with an estimated prevalence of 4–7%.[17] Of the women who fulfill criteria for PCOS, the majority are anovulatory. Almost 90% of ovulatory disorders are due to PCOS.[2] Obesity is present in over 50% of PCOS women which in turn increases the chances of anovulation.[1] Ovulation induction treatments are hence the first-line fertility treatment for women with PCOS.

PATHOPHYSIOLOGY OF PCOS

Polycystic ovary syndrome is a very heterogeneous syndrome as regards both clinical presentation and laboratory manifestations. While the basic dysfunction seems to lie within the ovary, the clinical expression and severity of the symptoms are dependent on extraovarian factors such as obesity, insulin resistance, and luteinizing hormone (LH) concentrations.[2.]

There are four main disturbances which may be involved in the pathophysiology of the syndrome:

1. *Abnormal ovarian morphology:* There are 6–8 times more preantral and small antral follicles are present in the polycystic ovary compared with the normal ovary. These are arrested in development at a small size of 2–9 mm but can be stimulated by gonadotrophins. In addition an enlarged stromal volume is present and a total ovarian volume more than 10 mL is common.
2. *Excessive ovarian androgen production:* Androgen excess is one of the premier presentations of this syndrome. The entire pathology is geared toward achieving increased androgen production. Insulin and LH individual and together worsen androgen production.
3. *Hyperinsulinemia* due to insulin resistance occurs in 80% of women with PCOS and central obesity, but also in 30–40% of lean women with PCOS.[2]
4. *Excessive serum concentrations of LH* are detected on single spot blood samples in 40–50% of women with PCOS. High LH concentrations are more commonly found in lean rather than obese women.

POLYCYSTIC OVARY SYNDROME AND ANOVULATION

Polycystic ovary syndrome involves a complex interaction between genetic and environmental factors that lead to various disturbances of this normal ovulatory cycle. Animal studies have provided some evidence that intrauterine exposure to increased androgen concentrations may be one of the predisposing factors to this condition.

Compared to the hormonal fluctuations that can be appreciated when considering the normal menstrual cycle, women with PCOS have relatively constant concentrations of several important reproductive hormones that are one explanation for anovulation. The average daily concentrations of both androgens and estrogens are increased in women with PCOS. LH secretion is generally greater than normal and follicle-stimulating hormone (FSH) levels are lower which may be caused by increased estrone and inhibin B concentrations. LH pulse frequency in PCOS women does not display the usually cyclical fluctuations but rather is constant at approximately one pulse per hour.

Table 1: WHO Classification of different types of endocrinological disorders.

WHO Classification	*Name*	*Hormonal profile*	*Incidence*
Group I	Hypogonadotropic hypogonadism, e.g. excessive exercise, anorexia nervosa, Kallmann syndrome, primary pituitary disorders	Decreased estrogen, decreased FSH	5–10%
Group II	Normoestrogenic, normogonadotropic, e.g. PCOS	Normal estrogen and FSH	80%
Group III	Hypergonadotropic hypogonadism, e.g. premature ovarian failure	Decreased estrogen, increased FSH	10%

(FSH: follicle-stimulating hormone; PCOS: polycystic ovary syndrome; WHO: World Health Organization)

Insulin resistance is seen in 50–75% of women with PCOS and is more prevalent in obese PCOS patients. These result in increased circulating levels of insulin which have been shown to stimulate androgen production. Hyperinsulinemia also inhibits sex hormone binding globulin (SHBG) production in the liver hence causing raised circulating androgen levels. This further increases the underlying insulin resistance.[3]

World Health Organization (WHO) type II anovulation is the most common cause of anovulation (Table 1). It is characterized by normal FSH and estradiol levels in an anovulatory woman. By far the most common case of WHO II anovulation is PCOS, accounting for approximately 75% of women with ovulatory disorders.

The clinical and laboratory findings of PCOS are variable, and the development of diagnostic criteria has helped to clarify the diagnosis. The Rotterdam criteria are given in Box 1.

Box 1: Rotterdam criteria for diagnosis of polycystic ovary syndrome.

Two of following three criteria must be met:

1. *Oligo or anovulation*:
   - *Oligo-ovulation*: The presence of ovulation not more than once every 35–180 days.
   - *Anovulation*: No ovulation for at least 6 consecutive months.
2. *Hyperandrogenism*: Clinical and/or biochemical:
   - *Clinical*: Hirsutism, acne, male pattern balding and/or frank virilization.
   - *Biochemical*: Raised androstenedione, free testosterone and/or free androgen index.
3. *Polycystic ovaries on ultrasound*: Greater than or equal to 12 follicles on one or both ovaries measuring 2–9 mm and/or ovarian volume ≥ 10 cm^3 on one or both ovaries.

OVULATION INDUCTION IN THE POLYCYSTIC OVARY SYNDROME PATIENT

Lifestyle Modifications

A discussion about treatments to restore ovulation in these women must begin with the role of weight loss and dietary modifications. Patients with PCOS have higher levels of insulin resistance than body mass index (BMI)-matched controls. Being overweight (BMI> 25) and obese (BMI > 30) worsens the fertility prognosis for women with PCOS and also increases the risk of other metabolic disturbances such as diabetes and hyperlipidemia. Weight loss of as little as 5–10% body weight has been shown to be effective at restoring ovulatory cycles.[4] Two small studies have compared a hypocaloric diet with high carbohydrate (55%), low protein (15%) versus high protein (30%), low carbohydrate (40%) content. No significant difference was found between these strategies.[5,6]

Several small studies have been performed to examine the effect of lifestyle modification on restoration of ovulation and natural conception. This was the subject of a Cochrane review which could not conclude upon the effect of lifestyle modification on reproductive outcomes but did find a reduction on the total testosterone levels and Ferriman-Gallwey (FG) scores as well as improvement in weight and adiposity distribution. This review also found that weight loss of 5–10% total body weight was clinically significant and led to reduction on impaired glucose tolerance and metabolic syndrome.[7]

Clomiphene Citrate

Clomiphene Citrate (CC) is a selective estrogen receptor modulator with both estrogenic and antiestrogenic properties. For many years, it was the first-line of treatment for ovulation induction. Clomiphene leads to a perceived deficit in estrogen concentrations in the bloodstream. Hence, FSH secretion is stimulated in order to restore estrogen concentrations, and in doing so, follicular development is also stimulated. It has both estrogen agonist and antagonist properties, which confer a unique range of benefits and drawbacks to its usage.

Clomiphene citrate is administered in doses from 50–150 mg/day for 5 days of the cycle beginning anytime from day 2 to day 5 of an induced or natural menstrual period, starting from the lowest dose and increasing, if an adequate response is not obtained. Success rates above 150 mg per day are less than 12% and alternative treatments should be advised. The first treatment cycle should be monitored by transvaginal ultrasound, starting from around day 10 of the cycle. Once a maximum of two follicles have reached 14 mm in mean diameter or more, the couple can be advised to have sexual intercourse. In order to document ovulation, the patient can self administer urinary LH kits and, once positive, can have a serum progesterone test 7 days thereafter. Where ovulation has not occurred despite the presence of an appropriately sized follicle, a human chorionic gonadotropin (HCG) trigger of 5,000 units can be used in a subsequent cycle, though this is not based on any randomized controlled trials.[2]

According to the National Institute of Clinical Excellence Guidelines in the United Kingdom, CC should be used for women with PCOS for up to 6 months.[8] CC induces ovulation in 60–85% of patients and approximately half of those that ovulate will conceive.

Women who are obese, insulin resistant and/or have raised basal LH levels are more likely to be clomiphene resistant.[2] Per cycle fecundability is approximately 15%.[3] Twin pregnancies occur in 7–9% of patients and tripletsin 0.3% of pregnancies. Side effects include hot flushes and in 1–2% of patients, visual disturbances.[4] As a manifestation of its estrogen antagonist properties, CC can cause impairment of endometrial growth and hence, in women whose peak preovulatory endometrial thickness does not exceed 5-6 mm, other options of treatment may be preferable.[3]

Several studies have reported on the incidence of birth defects in CC assisted pregnancies. One multicenter case control study involving data from 10 centers in the Unites States of America found an increased adjusted odds ratio (OR) of anencephaly (OR 2.3, 95% CI 1.1–4.7), Dandy-Walker malformation (OR 4.4, 95% CI 1.7–11.6), septal heart defects (OR 1.6, 95% CI 1.1–2.2) and several other anomalies. Despite the fact that this study included a group of 6,500 women, CC use was only described in 1.4%, hence the small number of women exposed to CC may make the results difficult to interpret.[9] Two larger studies have been started by the National Institute of Child Health and Human Development (NICHD) and will hopefully provide more clarity on this important issue.

Aromatase Inhibitors

Aromatase inhibition has the effect of reducing the conversion of androstenedione to estrogens by inhibiting the cytochrome P450 isozymes 2A6 and 2C19 of aromatase. This reduces the negative feedback effect of estrogen upon the hypothalamus and hence stimulates the production of FSH. Given that aromatase inhibitors do not have any effect on estrogen receptors, unfavorable effects on the endometrium is avoided and hence poses a potential benefit of this drug over clomiphene citrate. Another advantage of aromatase inhibitors is that it does not interfere with the negative feedback effect of estrogen; hence it is more likely to lead to monofollicular development. It also has a short half-life of around 48 hours, which further reduces the chances of antiestrogenic effects.

Letrozole is the most commonly used compound of this class for the purpose of ovulation induction. Its utility is the subject of a Cochrane systematic review, the findings of which shed a positive light upon the drug. As compared to clomiphene, clomiphene plus metformin and FSH injections, letrozole gave a higher live birth rate (OR 1.64, 95% CI 1.32–2.04) and higher clinical pregnancy rate (OR 1.40, 95% CI 1.18–1.65). There was no significant difference in the incidence of ovarian hyperstimulation syndrome (OHSS) or miscarriage. Aromatase inhibitors were associated with a lower incidence of multiple pregnancy than other ovulation induction agents (OR 0.38, 95% CI 0.87–0.84).

In the last decade Letrozole was not the first-line of treatment due to concern regarding its teratogenicity. In 2005, an abstract was presented at the American Society of Reproductive Medicine (ASRM) conference in which 150 babies conceived by letrozole ovulation induction were compared to 300 spontaneously conceived babies. It showed that the congenital anomaly rate in the letrozole group was 3–4%, which was not significantly different from that of the control l group.[11] It did, however, report an increased incidence of cardiac and locomotor defects. This abstract was not published owing to several methodological flaws in the study, most notable of which was the difference in baseline age and general health status between the two groups. In response to this evidence, despite its flaws, the pharmaceutical company, Novartis issued a warning that letrozole is not safe for use in premenopausal women. This strongly discouraged the use of the drug worldwide.[10]

Multiple systematic reviews and meta-analysis all failed to note an increased congenital anomaly rate with prevalence of anomalies with letrozole of clomiphene under 5% (the expected rate in this population is 5–8%).[18]

Letrozole is now as per the PCOS Evidence Based Guideline 2018 is the first-line of treatment for PCOS.

Gonadotropins

Gonadotropins can be used for women who are resistant to oral agents. To prevent overstimulation gonadotropins should always be started as the step up protocols and chronic low-dose protocols should be used. Pure FSH vs.

human menopausal gonadotropin (HMG) which offers LH activity along with FSH activity, has also not been shown to produce significantly different results in women with WHO II subfertility.[12,13]

It is generally advisable to start gonadotropin injections at a dose sufficient to induce follicular recruitment but as low as possible to reduce the risk of multifollicular development. In practice, a 50 IU–75 IU dose is usually started sometime within the first 5 days of a natural or progestin-induced menstrual period. A baseline ultrasound scan is advised to exclude ovarian cysts. While the presence of cysts is unlikely to affect the response to ovulation induction, it can cause difficulty in interpreting the response as follicles and cysts can be difficult to distinguish.

A scan to assess response can be performed 5–7 days after beginning the treatment. Once one follicle reaches 16–18 mm in size, the couple can be advised to have sexual intercourse and an ovulation trigger can be given. 5,000–10,000 IU of HCG is a common choice for this purpose. The dose is not changed for 14 days and 80% reach the criteria for trigger after 14 days.

Despite the advocacy for a low-dose regimen, the risk of multifetal gestation remains 5–10 fold higher with gonadotropin stimulated ovulation induction vs. spontaneously conceived pregnancy.[14] The risk of both OHSS and multiple pregnancy can be kept low by judicious dosing regimens, careful ultrasound surveillance and the willingness to abandon cycles with three or more dominant follicles.

Surgical Options

Surgical wedge resection was first described in 1939 as a technique of restoring ovulation in an ovulatory PCOS patients.[15] Surgical complications such as bleeding and adhesions led to a search for a less invasive surgical technique, leading to the development of laparoscopic ovarian drilling (LOD), which was first published in 1984.[16] Both laser and electrocautery have been used in various series to create multiple perforations in each ovary, typically form 4 to 10 each side. The purported mechanism of action is the destruction of androgen producing ovarian tissue which leads to a subsequent reduction in androgen and estrogen concentrations.

There have been several randomized controlled trials investigating the utility of LOD which have been the subject of a Cochrane systematic review. Most of the studies included patients who had CC-resistant PCOS. Most of the studies examined LOD with 4–6 but up to 10 punctures on each ovary with diathermy versus medical ovulation induction with either letrozole, clomiphene plus metformin or gonadotropins. One study compared LOD to conventional in vitro fertilization (IVF) and several studies compared unilateral to bilateral LOD.

There view showed that when LOD is compared to clomiphene plus metformin, the medical therapy appears more effective at producing live birth (OR 0.55, 95% CI 0.24–0.82). However, there is no significant difference when LOD is compared to aromatase inhibitors, gonadotropins or clomiphene plus tamoxifen. There was evidence, however, that LOD is less likely to be associated with multiple pregnancies than medical ovulation induction (OR 0.21, 95% CI 0.08–0.52). The majority of multiple pregnancies in the medical group were in cycles which used gonadotropin.

There were no significant differences in pregnancy rate per woman randomized or miscarriage rate. The review also found no significant difference in live birth, pregnancy or miscarriage rates in comparisons between unilateral versus bilateral LOD, LOD combined with second look laparoscopy and adhesiolysis or LOD followed by IVF versus IVF alone.

REFERENCES

1. Al-Azemi M, Omu FE, Omu AE. The effect of obesity on the outcome of infertility management in women with polycystic ovary syndrome. Arch Gynecol Obstet. 2004;270(4):205-10.
2. Homburg R. Ovulation Induction and Controlled Ovarian Stimulation: A Practical Guide, 2nd edition. USA: Springer International Publishing; 2014.
3. Fritz MA, Speroff L. Clinical Gynecologic Endocrinology and Infertility, 8th edition. Philadelphia: Lippincott Williams and Wilkins; 2011.
4. Vause TD, Cheung AP, Sierra S, et al. Ovulation induction in polycystic ovary syndrome. Int J Gynaecol Obstet. 2010;111(1):95-100.
5. Stamets K, Taylor DS, Kunselman A, et al. A randomized trial of the effects of two types of short-term hypocaloric diets on weight loss in women with polycystic ovary syndrome. Fertil Steril. 2004;81(3):630-7.
6. Moran LJ, Noakes M, Clifton PM, et al. Dietary composition in restoring reproductive and metabolic physiology in overweight women with polycystic ovary syndrome. J Clin Endocrinol Metab. 2003;88(2):812-9.
7. Moran LJ, Hutchison SK, Norman RJ, et al. Lifestyle changes in women with polycystic ovary syndrome. Cochrane Database Syst Rev. 2011.
8. National Collaborating Centre for Women's and Children's Health or National Institute for Health and Care Excellence. Fertility: assessment and treatment for people with fertility problems. London: RCOG Press; 2013.
9. Reefhuis J, Honein MA, Schieve LA, et al. Use of clomiphene citrate and birth defects, National Birth Defects Prevention Study, 1997-2005. Hum Reprod. 2011;26(2):451-7.

10. Kar S. Current evidence supporting "letrozole" for ovulation induction. J Hum Reprod Sci. 2013;6(2):93-8.
11. Tulandi T, Martin J, Al-Fadhli R, et al. Congenital malformations among 911 newborns conceived after infertility treatment with letrozole or clomiphene citrate. Fertil Steril. 2006;85(6):1761-5.
12. Yarali H, Bukulmez O, Gurgan T. Urinary follicle stimulating hormone (FSH) vs. recombinant FSH in clomiphene citrate-resistant, normogonadotropic, chronic anovulation: a prospective randomized study. Fertil Steril. 1999;72(2):276-81.
13. Weiss NS, Nahuis M, Bayram N, et al. Gonadotrophins for ovulation induction in women with polycystic ovarian syndrome. Cochrane Database Syst Rev. 2015:(9):CD010290.
14. Ratts VS, Pauls RN, Pinto AB, et al. Risk of multiple gestation after ovulation induction in polycystic ovary syndrome. J Reprod Med. 2007;52(10):896-900.
15. Stein IF, Cohen MR. Surgical treatment of bilateral polycystic ovaries. Am J Obstet Gynec. 1939;38:465-73.
16. Gjönnaess H. Polycystic ovarian syndrome treated by ovarian electrocautery through the laparoscope. Fertil Steril. 1984;41(1):20-5.
17. Asuncion M, Calvo RM, San Millan JL, et al. A prospective study of the prevalence of the polycystic ovary syndrome in unselected Caucasian women from Spain. J Clin Endocrinol Metab. 2000;85(7):2434-8.
18. Davies MJ, Moore VM, Willson KJ, et al. Reproductive technologies and risk of birth defects. N Engl J Med. 2012;366(19):1803-13.

CHAPTER
36

Surgical Management of Polycystic Ovarian Syndrome

Sujal Munshi, Jayesh Patel

INTRODUCTION

Anovulation is commonly associated with infertility, dysfunctional uterine bleeding (DUB), amenorrhea, hirsutism and increased risk of endometrial hyperplasia. Polycystic ovary syndrome (PCOS) is the most common cause of anovulatory infertility among the reproductive age group[1] with prevalence rate of 17–20% (Rotterdam diagnostic criteria).[2,3] It accounts for 19.92% of in vitro fertilization-intracytoplasmic sperm injection cycles (IVF-ICSI) in India [National Assisted Reproductive Technology (ART) Registry of India, Data for the year 2012]. PCOS presents with a heterogeneous range of clinical, biochemical and ultrasound features associated with: hyperandrogenism, chronic anovulation and insulin resistance.

- Though recognized about 50–60 years ago, scientific interest in PCOS continues. As a result, new concepts evolve with regard to changes in definition, pathophysiology, approach to diagnosis and investigations and much more in its management, be it surgical or medical. Polycystic ovaries and the clinical features of PCOS are due to follicular developmental dysfunction, resulting in chronic anovulation. In clinical practice, understanding the consequences of chronic anovulation and their effective management are far more important than just to assign a specific diagnosis of PCOS.
- Considering management of anovulatory infertility in PCOS, weight loss has a significant effect on the correction of endocrine milieu, ovulation and the chance of pregnancy.[4] Clomiphene citrate (CC), a selective estrogen modulator remains the first choice for ovulation induction (OI) and then gonadotropin therapy or laparoscopic ovarian surgery in clomiphene resistance cases. Metformin, an insulin sensitizer cotreatment has a controversial role. Ovulation induction with exogenous gonadotropins is effective, but requires monitoring to avoid risks of multiple pregnancy and ovarian hyperstimulation syndrome (OHSS), while laparoscopic ovarian drilling (LOD) with laser or diathermy is equally effective for restoring ovulatory function in PCOS,[5] but the risk of postoperative adnexal adhesions and decreased ovarian reserve should be considered.

SURGICAL MANAGEMENT

Aims of the surgical management of PCOS-associated infertility are: to induce ovulation, to correct hyperandrogenism and to avoid iatrogenic complications such as adhesions, multiple pregnancy and OHSS.

History

Polycystic ovarian syndrome is also known as Stein-Leventhal syndrome because in 1935, they have first reported this widely prevalent syndrome and proposed a possible therapy known as bilateral ovarian wedge resection.[6] From 1935 to the early 1960s, wedge resection of the ovary was the only treatment for PCOS.

Stein and Leventhal initially described wedge resection of the ovaries when polycystic ovaries were diagnosed during a laparotomy. It was found that ovarian biopsies taken to make the diagnosis led to subsequent ovulation. The rationale was to "normalize" ovarian size and hence the endocrinopathy by removing between 50% and 75% of each ovary with its hyperplastic capsule. A large review of 187 reports summarized data on 1,079 ovarian wedge resections, with overall rates of ovulation of 80% and pregnancy of 62.5% (range 13.5–89.5%).[7] Another 30 or so years later, Donesky and Adashi[8] have increased sample size to 1,766 treatments, with an average pregnancy rate of 58.8%. Because of the realization that significant postoperative adhesion formation occurred and that initial favorable effect on pregnancy rates were short-term, wedge resection became less popular in the 1970s, the same time medical therapies for OI appeared more successful.

Surgical approaches to OI have been developed from the traditional wedge resection [Stein and Leventhal (1935)] and ovarian biopsy and electrocautery[9,10] to modern day minimal access surgery [Huber J et al (1988)].[11] Multiple ovarian punctures performed either by diathermy (monopolar or bipolar) or by laser are known as LOD. There are various other surgical approaches available like transvaginal hydrolaparoscopy [bipolar or saline (fertiloscopic approach)], ultrasound guided transvaginal ovarian needle drilling (UTND), laparoscopic ovarian multi-needle intervention (LOMNI), no energy modality used, but LOD still remains the most commonly performed procedure in selected PCOS cases.

LAPAROSCOPIC OVARIAN DRILLING

The comparable success rate and the risks of medical treatment (like multiple pregnancy and OHSS) in women with PCOS, together with advances in minimal invasive surgery, made the concept of laparoscopic ovarian surgery highly acceptable. LOD with monopolar needle is a widely accepted approach among others.

Indications and Patient Selection

The main indication for LOD is CC-resistant PCOS, as a second-line therapy for anovulatory infertile PCOS cases, specifically, as an alternative to gonadotropins.

Royal College of Obstetricians and Gynecologists, American College of Obstetricians and Gynecologists, Society of Obstetricians and Gynecologists, Canada and the recent PCOS consensus working group, all recommend its use in highly selected cases, particularly in those with:

- Hypersecretion of luteinizing hormone (LH)
- Normal body mass index (BMI)
- Shorter duration of infertility
- Need for laparoscopic assessment of the pelvis
- When intensive monitoring during gonadotropin therapy is not possible.
- Polycystic ovarian syndrome women with pretreatment serum LH concentration of greater than or equal to 12 IU/L achieved significantly higher pregnancy rates postoperatively than those whose LH was less than 12 IU/L. After LOD, with restoration of ovarian activity, serum concentrations of LH and testosterone fall. This increases the chances of conception and reduces the risk of miscarriage.[12]

High BMI correlates with both increased rate of cycle disturbance and infertility.[13] Even moderate obesity (BMI greater than 27 kg/m^2) is associated with reduced chances of ovulation and pregnancy secondary to disturbances in insulin metabolism in PCOS.[14] It should be the policy to encourage obese women to lose weight by lifestyle modification even before undergoing LOD surgery. Loss of weight helps in a change in hormonal milieu as well as making surgery free of anesthesia risk. In a study of 200 patients who underwent LOD for anovulatory infertility due to PCOS, it was concluded that with increase in BMI (less than 29 kg/m^2, 29–34 kg/m^2, more than 34 kg/m^2), ovulation rate (81%, 84%, 44% respectively) and pregnancy rate (57%, 46%, 13% respectively) decreases.[15]

Munir et al. concluded that LOD is successful in PCOS patients who fail to ovulate on CC and is more effective in a subgroup of patients with age less than 25, duration of infertility less than 5 years and pretreatment serum LH concentration of greater than or equal to 12 IU/L.[16]

Laparoscopic ovarian drilling is not indicated for:

- Prevention of hyperresponsiveness to exogenous gonadotropin
- Nonfertility indications such as management of menstrual irregularities or hyperandrogenism (like acne or hirsutism).[17]

Morphological and Endocrinological Effects

The exact mechanism of action is yet to be elucidated, the plausible reasons are:

- Drilling causes destruction or removal of the ovarian theca and stroma, leading to:
  - Removal of the intraovarian block to follicular maturation, leading to recruitment of new cohort
  - Decrease in the crowding of the cortex, which allows progress of normal follicles to the surface resulting in resumption of normal ovulation
  - Destruction of stroma and release of androgen rich follicular fluid causing fall in local and circulatory levels of androgen[18]
  - Decrease in substrate for follicular aromatase and damage to the follicular wall itself, producing fall in the circulatory estradiol levels
  - A positive feedback leads to positive feedback on follicular stimulating hormone (FSH) at the pituitary

causing a secondary rise in FSH levels[19] and hence a decrease in LH/FSH ratio
 - Reduced concentration of LH and decreased LH bioavailability[20]
 - Temporary decrease in inhibin levels.
- Surgical trauma to the ovary leads to:
 - Production of insulin-like growth factor 1 (IGF-1) and other growth factors which increase ovarian sensitivity to circulating FSH[21]
 - Production of nonsteroidal factors which restores hypothalamic-pituitary-ovarian (HPO) axis function[22]

Vascular endothelial growth factor (VEGF) levels in women with PCOS are higher than in normal women, and ovarian drilling does not affect these levels. The procedure does not change insulin responses to oral glucose tolerance test.[23]

The beneficial effects of LOD appear to be sustained for up to 9 years in most patients.[24]

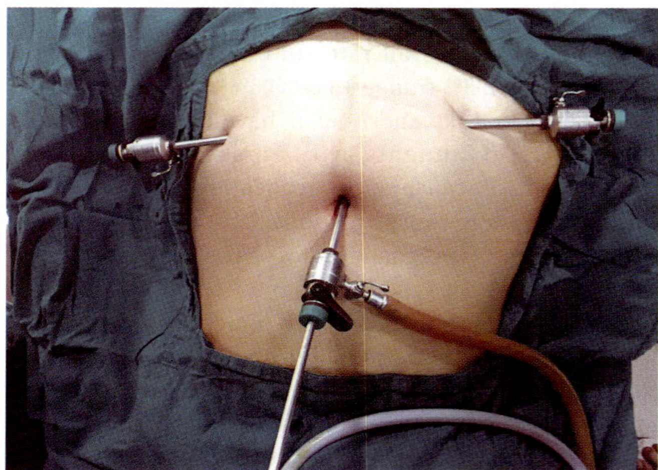

Fig. 1: Port placement for laparoscopic ovarian drilling. One 5 mm umbilical port for telescope and two 5 mm lateral ports for hand instruments.

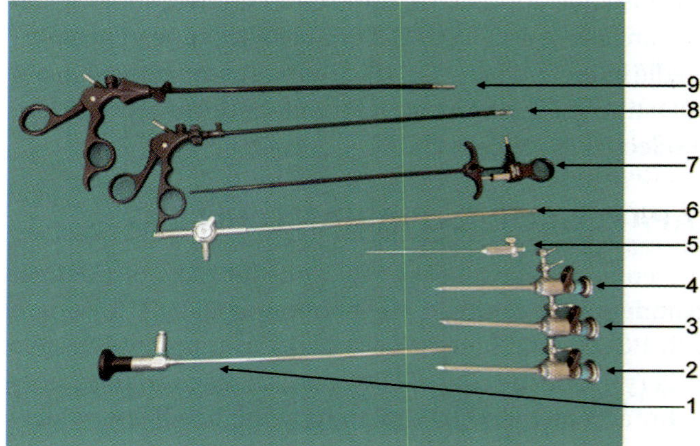

Fig. 2: Instruments for laparoscopic ovarian drilling. 1—Telescope (5 mm); 2,3,4—Trocar with cannula (5 mm); 5—Veress needle; 6—Suction irrigation cannula; 7—Monopolar PCO needle; 8—Maryland grasper; 9—Atraumatic grasper.

Techniques of Ovarian Drilling

The technique of wedge resection of the ovaries, previously performed by laparotomy, has now been abandoned due to high risk of postoperative ovarian adhesions and premature ovarian failure. Nowadays, polycystic ovaries have been drilled laparoscopically using electrocautery (monopolar or bipolar) or laser vaporization using carbon dioxide (CO_2), argon or neodymium-doped yttrium aluminum garnet (Nd:YAG; Nd:Y3Al5O12) crystal lasers. The idea was to reproduce the beneficial effects of ovarian wedge resection while avoiding its main adverse effect, pelvic adhesions. Reproductive outcomes are comparable with laser and diathermy.[25] Standardization of the surgical techniques is lacking in terms of use of energy source, wattage, number and depth of punctures and application time.

Electrocautery, using an insulated monopolar needle electrode with 1-2 cm distal noninsulated end, is the most commonly used method, although a few authors have reported similar ovulation and pregnancy rates with bipolar electrode.[26,27]

Laparoscopic Monopolar Needle Ovarian Drilling Technique

- Standard laparoscopic approach is utilized, with two ancillary lateral ports (Fig. 1).
- Instrumentation (Fig. 2): Veress needle, three 5 mm trocar with cannula, 5 mm telescope, atraumatic grasper, suction irrigation cannula, monopolar needle with cable
- Surgical steps:
 - Laparoscopic ovarian drilling is done under general anesthesia
 - Laparoscopy performed with one primary (5 mm) and two contralateral ancillary ports (5 mm)
 - Ovarian ligament is grasped using a grasper moving the ovary (towards anterior abdominal wall and in front of the uterus)
 - The double insulated retractable monopolar polycystic ovarian (PCO) drilling needle is introduced at a right angle with 40 watts cutting current, making 4-5 holes each lasting 4 seconds at a depth of 4 mm on both ovaries (Fig. 3)
 - Hilum being highly vascular should be avoided

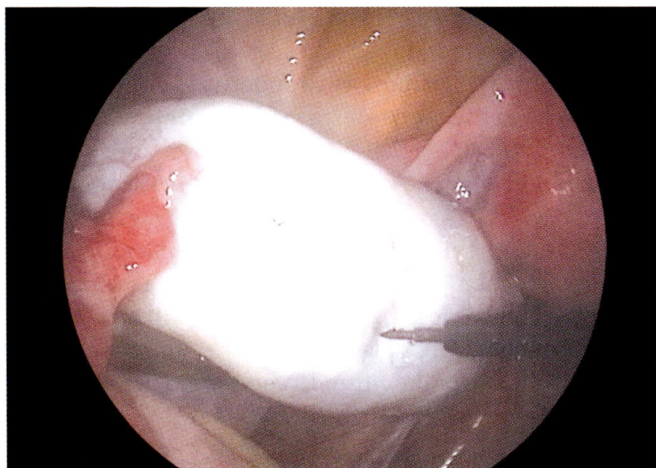

Fig. 3: Laparoscopic ovarian drilling (4–5 punctures with insulated monopolar needle).

- A thorough suction irrigation should be done to get a clean pelvis as the end result and minimize postoperative adhesions.

The relation between the extent of drilling (number, size and depth of punctures) and the success in inducing ovulation or length of maintenance of spontaneous ovulation has never been identified with any precision but our basic aim should be to damage ovarian tissue as minimal as possible to get optimum outcome.

Optimum Punctures and Dose

The techniques, instruments and settings used and accordingly the degree of ovarian thermal damage varies considerably and so its consequences. Gjönnaess[28] cauterized each ovary at 5–8 points for 5–6 seconds per point with 300–400 W. Using similar settings, Dabirashrafi et al.[29] reported mild to moderate adhesion formation in 20% of patients. Naether et al. cauterized 5–20 points per ovary with 400 W for nearly 1 second.[30] They found that the rate of adhesions was 19.3% and that this was reduced to 16.6% by saline peritoneal lavage.[31] They also reported that the postoperative fall in serum testosterone concentration was proportional to the degree of ovarian damage, with up to 40 cauterization sites being used in some patients.[32]

The greater the amount of damage to the surface of the ovary, the greater is the risk of periovarian adhesion formation. This led Armar to develop a strategy of minimizing the number of diathermy points.[33] This is a logical technique in which the ovary is simply cauterized at four points and the lowest effective dose is used. The high pregnancy rate (86% in those with no other pelvic abnormality) indicates that the small number of diathermy points used leads to a low rate of significant adhesion formation.[34] In a prospective cohort study on 63 CC resistance PCOS women, Malkawi et al.[35] have concluded that five, instead of greater than or equal to 10 punctures per ovary are sufficient to ameliorate the hyperandrogenic status and to improve their clinical and reproductive outcome.

The difficulty was to decide how to perform LOD, knowing about the dose response for a particular patient. Balen et al.[36] reported that LOD using 40 W for 4 seconds in four places on one ovary can lead to bilateral ovarian activity and ovulation (usually they perform bilateral drilling), their ovulation rate was 50% and conception rate 40% (some patients were sensitized to exogenous stimulation).

It has been proposed that the degree of ovarian destruction should be determined by the size of the ovary. Naether et al. in a series of 206 patients reported their method of laparoscopic electrocautery of the ovarian surface, which causes greater destruction of the ovary with application of 400 W at 5–20 sites on each ovary.[37] Despite such a large amount of ovarian destruction, 45.2% of women who conceived required additional ovarian stimulation (with an 8% multiple pregnancy rate) and 20% miscarriage rate. But in this series Naether has taken 24% women who had regular menstrual cycle and 15% were ovulating preoperatively.

Amer et al.[38] performed first retrospective assessment of the effect of the amount of energy used on the outcome of LOD and then proceeded to assess this prospectively.[39] They found in their analysis no difference between the uses of 3–10 punctures but suggested that two punctures were too few.[38] There are many variables in the potential for response, including the anthropometric characteristics of the patients and ovarian morphology.

In a prospective study using a standardized energy of 150 J/puncture, the rates of ovulation and pregnancy were, respectively, 67% and 67% with four punctures/ovary (n = 12), 44% and 56% with three punctures/ovary (n = 9), 33% and 17% with two punctures/ovary (n = 6), and 33% and 0% with one puncture/ovary (n = 12), indicating a clear dose response.[39]

Mahmoud et al. concluded that adjusted diathermy dose based on ovarian volume (60J/cm^3) for laparoscopic ovarian drilling of PCOS has a better reproductive outcome compared with fixed thermal dosage (600J/ovary).[40]

Laser versus Electrocautery

Aflatoonian et al.[41] reported comparable reproductive outcome following LOD using electrocautery and laser. Saleh et al.[42] also found that there was no statistically significant difference in the ovulation rate following LOD with diathermy and laser in anovulatory infertile women with PCOS (83% versus 77.5%); while there was a significantly higher cumulative pregnancy rate at 12 months after diathermy surgery (65% versus 54.5%). They concluded that LOD with diathermy is superior to laser drilling. Also, there are some points in favor of electrocautery like less cost, easy application and that it can be performed with basic endoscopy equipment which we should consider.

Different modifications of the classic needle electrode technique such as LOMNI, LOD using a monopolar hook electrode, LOD using the harmonic scalpel and office microlaparoscopic ovarian drilling are proposed. Various transvaginal methods such as transvaginal hydrolaparoscopy (fertiloscopy) and transvaginal sonography-guided ovarian interstitial laser treatment are also developed. However, larger prospective studies are needed to validate the use, safety, efficacy and long-term effects of these alternate techniques.

Complications

Surgery, of course, carries its own risks and should be performed only by properly trained laparoscopic surgeons. Considering ongoing concerns about the long-term effects of LOD on ovarian function, it should be performed judiciously in selected cases.

Intraoperative Complications

These mainly involve risks related to general anesthesia and being minimally invasive, risks related to laparoscopy like injury during trocar entry and very rarely bowel, bladder and major vessel injury. One isolated case report mentions external iliac vessel injury during ovarian drilling.[43] Apart from these risks, there is also a risk of an electrical accident, which can be avoided by moving the ovary away from adjacent organs when using monopolar current.

Postoperative Complications

These complications are related to the actual process of ovarian thermal drilling.

Periovarian adhesions: The risk of periovarian adhesion formation may be reduced by abdominal lavage and early second-look laparoscopy, with adhesiolysis if necessary.[44] Others have also used liberal peritoneal lavage to good effect.[33] Greenblatt and Casper[45] found no correlation between the degree of ovarian damage and subsequent adhesion formation, nor did they find benefit from the adhesion barrier Interceed® (Ethico, Inc.), as assessed by second-look laparoscopy. In another interesting study, 40 women undergoing laser photocoagulation of the ovaries using an Nd:YAG laser set at 50 W at 0–25 points per ovary were randomized to a second-look laparoscopy and adhesiolysis.[46] Of those who underwent a second-look laparoscopy, adhesions described as minimal or mild were found in 68%, yet adhesiolysis did not appear to be necessary because the cumulative conception rate after 6 months was 47% compared with 55% in the expectantly managed group; this difference was not significant.

Laser treatment seems to be as efficacious as diathermy and it has been suggested that it may result in less adhesion formation,[47,48] although the only study to compare the two techniques was nonrandomized, reported similar ovulation and pregnancy rates and did not examine adhesion formation.[48]

Various types of laser have been used, from the CO_2 laser to the Nd:YAG and potassium titanyl phosphate (KTP) lasers.

As in other spheres of laparoscopic surgery, whether laser or diathermy is employed, appears to depend upon the preference of the surgeon and the availability of the equipment.

- Varied incidence of postoperative adhesions 0–70%
- Flimsy adhesions on the ovarian surface of not much significance[48]
- Copious abdominal lavage and use of insulated needle electrocautery may help in reducing adhesions.

Decreased ovarian reserve or premature ovarian failure: Possibility of ovarian destruction leading to ovarian failure is an obvious disaster in women wishing to conceive, and is a matter of concern..

- Excessive use of energy in terms of high wattage settings, number of punctures or more application time per puncture may damage more ovarian tissue.
- An electrode introduced deep into the stroma may cause desiccation of hilar vessels and consequent ischemic damage.
- Large number of punctures leading to excessive destruction of ovarian follicular pool.
- Thermal damage produces anti-ovarian antibodies.[49]

Cases of ovarian failure have been reported after both open wedge resection and laparoscopic surgery. Even one isolated case of ovarian atrophy following high-energy drilling is reported.[50] Kandil et al.[51] showed a significant decrease in ovarian reserve (antral follicle counts and ovarian volume) after bilateral drilling but not after CC-induction of ovulation or unilateral drilling.

There is no concrete evidence of a decreased ovarian reserve (DOR) or premature ovarian failure (POF) associated with women undergoing proper LOD[52] as PCOS women had significantly greater ovarian reserve than age matched controls with normal ovulation.[53]

Results

In the first reported series, ovarian diathermy resulted in ovulation in 90% and conception in 70% of the 62 women treated.[28] The outcome of 62 pregnancies with the miscarriage rate of 15% was no different from the normal population.[54] Ovarian diathermy works by sensitizing the ovary to FSH and makes the clomiphene-resistant polycystic ovary sensitive to clomiphene.[55] After LOD, the reproductive performance improved and sustained for many years: 49% of women conceived within 1 year of treatment, this might be because 1 year period seems reasonable to wait for conception, beyond which patient might be advised to pursue alternative treatment such as gonadotropin ovarian stimulation or IVF.[56]

Despite its theoretical advantages, LOD is not superior to gonadotropins, neither as a first-line therapy for OI nor for CC-failure or prior to IVF. A recent Cochrane systematic review of 9 randomized controlled trials (RCTs) and 16 trials concluded that there was no evidence of a significant difference in rates of clinical pregnancy (39.7 versus 40.5%) or live birth (34 versus 38%) in women with clomiphene-resistant PCOS undergoing LOD compared to other medical treatments.[5] This implies that LOD is a valid, but not the sole option for CC-resistant PCOS.

There was no evidence of a significant difference in rates of live birth, pregnancy, ovulation or miscarriage when unilateral was compared with bilateral drilling.[5]

Based on the current evidence, LOD could be predicted to result in poor reproductive outcome in women with CC-resistant PCOS when they are obese (BMI more than 25 kg/m^2), long duration of infertility more than 3 years, low basal LH levels less than 10 IU/L, marked biochemical hyperandrogenism (testosterone levels greater than or equal to 4.5 nmol/L, free androgen index more than 15) and high basal antimullerian hormone (AMH) greater than or equal to 7.7 ng/mL. Setting eligibility criteria based on the existing evidence concerning predictors of success of LOD is critical not only for improving its outcome, but also to avoid unnecessary surgery.[57]

Laparoscopic Ovarian Drilling Compared with Exogenous Gonadotropins

Laparoscopic ovarian surgery is free of the risks of multiple pregnancy and ovarian hyperstimulation and does not require intensive ultrasound monitoring. Abdel Gadir et al.[58] suggested gonadotropin as a first-line treatment in cases of CC resistance and observed lower birth rate in the ovarian drilling group. But the recent Cochrane Database, 2012, recorded comparable live birth rates in both groups. These are some points in favor of LOD:

- Extensive monitoring is not required[59]
- No risk of multiple follicles and OHSS, therefore, decreased cycle cancellation rates
- The rate of multiple pregnancies was significantly lower in the LOD group compared with using gonadotropins (OR 0.13; 95% CI 0.03 to 0.52; P = 0.004).[5]
- Live birth rates in LOD and gonadotropin groups were similar[5]
- Lower treatment and delivery costs, Farquhar (2004),[60] reported that the costs of a live birth were one-third lower in the group that underwent LOD compared to those women who received gonadotropins
- Beneficial improvement in menstrual regularity, reproductive performance, endocrine effects after LOD continue for years.[61]

Long-term Efficacy of Laparoscopic Ovarian Drilling

The relevant parameters for long-term monitoring are the pregnancy rate and persistence of ovulation after drilling. Felemban et al.[62] reported a 100% follow-up rate of 112 patients at 36 months. Total pregnancy rate were 36% at 12 months, 54% at 18 months and 82% at 24 months of follow-up period. In a retrospective study, Amer et al.[61] have compared 116 women with PCOS who had undergone ovarian drilling and 34 women who had not undergone the procedure. The data showed that the relative risk of regular menstrual cycles after ovarian drilling was 1.6 at 1 year, 2.6 at 3 years and 2.2 at 9 years.

Gjönnaess (1998)[63] reported a very long-term follow-up of a group of 165 infertile PCOS patients who underwent ovarian drilling. Only 44 patients (26.6% of the initial cohort) were being followed after 6 months. Of the 31 patients monitored for more than 10 years, 74% were ovulating. Fifteen patients were monitored for 18–20 years and 67% continued to ovulate.

Although the data suggests that the effect of LOD may persist beyond the 1st year, these results must be confirmed by well controlled and larger studies.

CONCLUSION

Laparoscopic ovarian drilling is an option for management of anovulatory infertility in women with having with clomiphene resistant PCOS and not for nonfertility indications. The risks of surgery are minimal; however the major issue of concern is the long-term risk of diminished ovarian reserve due to destruction of normal ovarian tissue caused by the procedure, especially due to variations in the number of punctures to be made and the energy sources to be used. At the same time, the introduction of the gonadotropin-releasing hormone agonist (GnRH-a) trigger in high risk patients has made gonadotropins a much safer option today than what they used it used to be earlier. LOD should therefore be used very judiciously and in well selected cases and only after proper counseling.

REFERENCES

1. Overbeek A, Lambalk CB. Phenotypic and pharmacogenetic aspects of ovulation induction in WHO II anovulatory women. Gynecol Endocrinol. 2009;25(4): 222-34.
2. March WA, Moore VM, Willson KJ, Phillips DI, Norman RJ, Davies MJ. The prevalence of polycystic ovary syndrome in a community sample assessed under contrasting diagnostic criteria. Hum Reprod. 2010;25(2):544-51.
3. Yildiz BO, Bozdag G, Yapici Z, Esinler I, Yarali H. Prevalence, phenotype and cardiometabolic risk of polycystic ovary syndrome under different diagnostic criteria. Hum Reprod. 2012;27(10):3067-73.
4. Clark AM, Ledger W, Galletly C, Tomlinson L, Blaney F, Wang X, et al. Weight loss results in significant improvement in pregnancy and ovulation rates in anovulatory obese women. Hum Reprod. 1995;10(10):2705-12.
5. Farquhar C, Brown J, Marjoribanks J. Laparoscopic drilling by diathermy or laser for ovulation induction in anovulatory polycystic ovary syndrome. Cochrane Database Syst Rev. 2012;6:CD001122.
6. Stein IF, Leventhal ML. Amenorrhea associated with bilateral polycystic ovaries. Am J Obstet Gynecol. 1935;29:181-91.
7. Goldzieher JW, Axelrod LR. Clinical and biochemical features of polycystic ovarian disease. Fertil Steril. 1963;14:631-53.
8. Donesky BW, Adashi EY. Surgically induced ovulation in the polycystic ovary syndrome: wedge resection revisited in the age of laparoscopy. Fertil Steril. 1995;63(3):439-63.
9. Cohen J, Audebert A, De Brux J, Giorgi H. (1972a) Biopsie ovarienne d'une grossesse. Nouv. Presse Med. 1, 1294.
10. Cohen J, Audebert A, De Brux, J. and Giorgi H. (1972b) Les stérilités poar dysovulation: rôle pronotisque et thérapeutique de la biopsie ovairenne percoelioscopique. J Gynécol Obstet Biol Reprod. 657–71.
11. Huber J, Hosmann J, Spona J. Polycystic ovarian syndrome treated by laser through the laparoscope [letter]. Lancet. 1988;2:215.
12. Imani B, Eijkemans MJ, Fauser BC, te Velde ER, Habbema JD. Predictors of chances to conceive in ovulatory patients during clomiphene citrate induction of ovulation of induction in normogonadotrophic oligmenorrheic infertility. J Clin Endocrinol Metabol. 1999;84(5):1617-22.
13. Kiddy DS, Hamilton-Fairley, Bush A, Short F, Anyaoku V, Reed MJ, et al. Improvement in endocrine and ovarian function during dietary treatment of obese women with polycystic ovary syndrome. Clin Endocrinol. 1992;36(1): 105-11.
14. Conway GS. Insulin resistance and the polycystic ovary syndrome. Contemp Rev Obstet Gynaecol. 1990;2:34-9.
15. Amer SA, Li TC, Ledger WL. Ovulation induction using laparoscopic ovarian drilling in women with polycystic ovarian syndrome: predictors of success. Hum Reprod. 2004;19(8):1719-24.
16. Munir S, Amin D, Sultana M, Saeed T. Ovulation induction using laparoscopic ovarian drilling in women with polycystic ovarian syndrome : predictors of success Biomedica. 2010;26:130-34.
17. Johnson NP, Wang K. Is ovarian surgery effective for androgenic symptoms of polycystic ovarian syndrome? J Obstet Gynaecol. 2003;23(6):599-606.
18. Keckstein J, Borchers K, Wolf A. Is laparoscopic laser surgery an alternative treatment of polycystic ovarian disease? In: Donnez J, Nisolle M. (Eds). Laser Operative Laparoscopy and Hysteroscopy. New York:Nauwelaerts Printing; 1989. pp. 95-107.
19. Seow KM, Juan CC, Hwang JL, Ho LT. Laparoscopic surgery in polycystic ovary syndrome: reproductive and metabolic effects. Semin Reprod Med. 2008;26(1):101-10.
20. Liguori G, Tolino A, Moccia G, Scognamiglio G, Nappi C. Laparoscopic ovarian treatment in infertile patients with polycystic ovarian syndrome (PCOS): endocrine changes and clinical outcome. Gynecol Endocrinol. 1996;10(4):257-64.
21. Vizer M, Kiesel L, Szabó I, Arany A, Tamás P, Szilágyi A. Assessment of three-dimensional sonographic features of polycystic ovaries after laparoscopic ovarian electrocautery. Fertil Steril. 2007;88(4):894-9.
22. Rossmanith WG, Keckstein J, Spatzier K, Lauritzen C. The impact of ovarian laser surgery on gonadotrophin secretion in women with polycystic ovarian disease. Clin Endocrinol (Oxf). 1991;34(3):223-30.
23. Tulandi T, Saleh A, Morris D, Jacobs HS, Payne NN, Tan SL. Effects of laparoscopic ovarian drilling on serum vascular endothelial growth factor and on insulin responses to the oral glucose tolerance test in women with polycystic ovary syndrome. Fertil Steril. 2000;74(3):585-8.
24. Amer SA, Banu Z, Li TC, Cooke ID. Long term follow-up of patients with polycystic ovarian syndrome after laparoscopic ovarian drilling: endocrine and ultrasonographic outcomes. Hum Reprod. 2002;17(11):2051-7.
25. Farquhar C, Lilford RJ, Marjoribanks J, Vandekerckhove P. Laparoscopic 'drilling' by diathermy or laser for ovulation induction in anovulatory polycystic ovary syndrome. Cochrane Database Syst Rev. 2007;18(3):CD001122.
26. Fernandez H, Faivre E, Gervaise A, Deffieux X. Laparoscopic ovarian drilling using a 5-French bipolar energy probe. Fertil Steril. 2010;94(2):740-1.
27. Sharma M, Kriplani A, Agarwal N. Laparoscopic bipolar versus unipolar ovarian drilling in infertile women with resistant polycystic ovarian syndrome: A pilot study. J Gynaecol Surg. 2006;22:105-11.
28. Gjönnaess H. Polycystic ovarian syndrome treated by ovarian electrocautery through the laparoscope. Fertil Steril. 1984;41(1):20-5.
29. Dabirashrafi H, Mohamad K, Behjatnia Y, Moghadami-Tabrizi N. Adhesion formation after ovarian electrocauterization on patients with polycystic ovarian syndrome. Fertil Steril. 1991;55(6):1200-01.
30. Naether OG, Fischer R, Weise HC, Geiger-Kotzler L, Delfs T, Rudolf K, Delfs T. Laparoscopic electrocoagulation of the ovarian surface in infertile patients with polycystic ovarian disease. Fertil Steril. 1993;60(1):88-94.
31. Naether OG, Fischer R. Adhesion formation after laparoscopic electrocoagulation of the ovarian surface in polycystic ovary patients. Fertil Steril. 1993;60(1):95-9.
32. Naether O, Weise HC, Fischer R, Berger-Bispink S, Delfs T. Result of treatment with surface cauterization of polycystic

ovaries in sterility patients. Geburtshilfe Frauenheilkd. 1991;51(11):920-4.

33. Armar NA, McGarrigle HH, Honour J, Holownia P, Jacobs HS, Lachelin GC. Laparoscopic ovarian diathermy in the management of anovulatory infertility in women with polycystic ovaries: endocrine changes and clinical outcome. Fertil Steril. 1990;53:45-9.
34. Armar NA, Lachelin GC. Laparoscopic ovarian diathermy: an effective treatment for anti-oestrogen resistant anovulatory infertility in women with polycystic ovaries. Br J Obstet Gynaecol. 1993;100(2):161-4.
35. Malkawi HY, Qublan HS. Laparoscopic ovarian drilling in the treatment of polycystic ovary syndrome: how many punctures per ovary are needed to improve the reproductive outcome? J Obstet Gynaecol Res. 2005;31(2):115-9.
36. Balen AH, Jacobs HS. A prospective study comparing unilateral and bilateral laparoscopic ovarian diathermy in women with the polycystic ovary syndrome. Fertil Steril. 1994;62(5):921-5.
37. Naether OG, Baukloh V, Fischer R, Kowalczyk T. Long-term follow-up in 206 infertility patients with polycystic ovarian syndrome after laparoscopic electrocautery of the ovarian surface. Hum Reprod. 1994;9(12):2342-9.
38. Amer SAK, Li TC, Cooke ID. Laparoscopic ovarian diathermy in women with polycystic ovary syndrome: a retrospective study on the influence of the amount of energy used on the outcome. Hum Reprod. 2002;17:1046-51.
39. Amer SAK, Li TC, Cooke ID. A prospective dose-finding study of the amount of thermal energy required for laparoscopic ovarian. Hum Reprod. 2003;18(8): 1693-8.
40. Zakherah MS, Kamal MM, Hamed HO. Laparoscopic ovarian drilling in polycystic ovary syndrome: efficacy of adjusted thermal dose based on ovarian volume. Fertil Steril. 2011;95(3):1115-8.
41. Aflatoonian A, Maryam A, Naeimeh T. Comparison of laparoscopic drilling by diathermy and laser for ovulation induction in clomiphene citrate-resistant women with polycystic ovary syndrome. Middle East Fertility Society Journal. 2007;12(2):97-103.
42. Saleh AM, Khalil HS. Review of nonsurgical and surgical treatment and the role of insulin-sensitizing agents in the management of infertile women with polycystic ovary syndrome. Acta Obstet Gynecol Scand. 2004;83(7):614-21.
43. Ateş _S, Şevket O, Özsoy B, Zebitay AG, Kan A. External iliac artery injury during ovarian drilling procedure: A case report. Medical Bulletin of Haseki. 2014;52:120-2.
44. Naether OG. Significant reduction in of adnexal adhesions following laparoscopic electrocautery of the ovarian surface by lavage and artificial ascites. Gynaecol Endoscopy. 1995;4:17-9.
45. Greenblatt EM, Casper RF. Adhesion formation after laparoscopic ovarian cautery for polycystic ovarian syndrome: lack of correlation with pregnancy rate. Fertil Steril. 1993;60(5):766-70.
46. Gurgan T, Urman B, Aksu T, Yarali H, Develioglu O, Kisnisci HA. The effect of short internal laparoscopic lysis of adhesions in pregnancy rates following ND:YAG laser photocoagulation of polycystic ovaries. Obstet Gynecol. 1992;80(1):45-7.
47. Daniell JF, Miller W. Polycystic ovaries treated by laparoscopic laser vaporization. Fertil Steril. 1989;51(2):232-6.
48. Heylen SM, Puttemans PJ, Brosens IA. Polycystic ovarian disease treated by laparoscopic argon laser capsule drilling: comparison of vaporization versus perforation technique. Hum Reprod. 1994;9(6):1038-42.
49. Thessaloniki ESHRE/ASRM-Sponsored PCOS Consensus Workshop Group. Consensus on infertility treatment related to polycystic ovary syndrome. Fertil Steril. 2008;89(3):505-22.
50. Dabirashrafi H. Complications of laparoscopic ovarian cauterization. Fertil Steril. 1989;52(5):878-9.
51. Kandil M, Selim M. Hormonal and sonographic assessment of ovarian reserve before and after laparoscopic ovarian drilling in polycystic ovary syndrome. BJOG. 2005;112(10):1427-30.
52. Api M. Is ovarian reserve diminished after laparoscopic ovarian drilling? Gynecol Endocrinol. 2009;25(3):159-65.
53. Weerakiet S, Lertvikool S, Tingthanatikul Y, Wansumrith S, Leelaphiwat S, Jultanmas R. Ovarian reserve in women with polycystic ovary syndrome who underwent laparoscopic ovarian drilling. Gynecol Endocrinol. 2007;23(8): 455-60.
54. GjÖnnaess H. The course and outcome of pregnancy after ovarian electrocautery with polycystic ovarian syndrome: the influence of bodyweight. Br J Obstet Gynaecol. 1989;96(6):714-19.
55. Farhi J, Soule S, Jacobs HS. Effect of laparoscopic ovarian electrocautery on ovarian response and outcome of treatment with gonadotrophins in clomifene citrate-resistant patients with polycystic ovary syndrome. Fertil Steril. 1995;64(5):930-5.
56. Li TC, Saravelos H, Chow MS, Chisabingo R, Cooke ID. Factors affecting the outcome of laparoscopic ovarian drilling for polycystic ovarian syndrome in women with anovulatory infertility. Br J Obstet Gynaecol. 1998;105(3):338-44.
57. Abu Hashim H. Predictors of success of laparoscopic ovarian drilling in women with polycystic ovary syndrome: an evidence-based approach. Arch Gynecol Obstet. 2015;291(1):11-8.
58. Abdel Gadir A, Mowafi RS, Alnaser HM, Alrashid AH, Alonezi OM, Shaw RW. Ovarian electrocautery versus human menopausal gonadotropins and pure follicle stimulating hormone therapy in the treatment of patients with polycystic ovarian disease. Clin Endocrinol (Oxf). 1990;33(5):585-92.
59. Farquhar CM, Williamson K, Gudex G, Johnson NP, Garland J, Sadler L. A randomized controlled trial of laparoscopic ovarian diathermy versus gonadotrophin therapy for women with clomiphene-resistant polycystic ovarian syndrome. Fertil Steril. 2002;78(2):404-11.
60. Farquhar CM, Williamson K, Brown PM, Garland J. An economic evaluation of laparoscopic ovarian diathermy versus gonadotrophin therapy for women with clomiphene citrate resistant polycystic ovary syndrome. Hum Reprod. 2004;19:1110-5.
61. Amer SA, Gopalan V, Li TC, Ledger WL, Cooke ID. Long term follow-up of patients with polycystic ovarian syndrome after laparoscopic ovarian drilling: clinical outcome. Hum Reprod. 2002;17(8):2035-42.
62. Felemban A, Tan SL, Tulandi T. Laparoscopic treatment of polycystic ovaries with insulated needle cautery: a reappraisal. Fertil. Steril. 2000;73(2),266-9.
63. Gjönnaess H. Late endocrine effects of ovarian electrocautery in women with polycystic ovary syndrome. Fertil. Steril. 1998;69(4):697-701.

CHAPTER 37

Ovarian Hyperstimulation Syndrome: Identification and Management

Sulbha Arora, Ritu Hinduja

INTRODUCTION

Ovarian hyperstimulation syndrome (OHSS) is an iatrogenic, potentially life-threatening complication of ovarian stimulation, characterized by ovarian enlargement and fluid extravasation from the intravascular compartment to the third spaces (mainly to the thoracic and abdominal cavities). It is important to differentiate between a high ovarian response and clinically significant OHSS. While milder OHSS is relatively common and characterized by weight gain, abdominal discomfort and enlarged ovaries; severe OHSS is accompanied by severe ascites, pleural effusion, electrolyte imbalance, and hypovolemia with oliguria. Deep vein thrombosis and embolism are the most dreaded complications of severe OHSS.[1] Though less than 2% patients require hospitalization due to OHSS,[2] it can be life-threatening.

The aim of this chapter is to provide clinicians with information about the diagnosis and treatment of OHSS, based upon the best available evidence. This includes out-patient management, inpatient management and a brief glance at intensive care as well. The pathophysiology and prevention of OHSS lie outside the scope of this chapter and have not been discussed here.

DIAGNOSIS

Ovarian hyperstimulation syndrome is self-limiting and usually resolves spontaneously within several days, but may continue for longer duration, especially in conception cycles. The diagnosis is based on clinical criteria. The patient will give a history of ovarian stimulation followed by symptoms of abdominal distension, pain, rapid weight gain, nausea, vomiting and decreased urine output. The differential diagnoses in such situations must include complications of an ovarian cyst (torsion, hemorrhage), pelvic infection, intra-abdominal hemorrhage, ectopic pregnancy and appendicitis.

RISK FACTORS

Several factors increase the risk of developing severe OHSS:[3-8]

- Age less than 30 years
- Low body weight
- Polycystic ovaries or high basal antral follicle count
- Higher dose of gonadotropins
- Rapidly rising or high serum estradiol
- Previous history of OHSS
- Large number of growing follicles seen during ovarian stimulation
- Use of human chorionic gonadotropin (HCG) as opposed to progesterone for luteal phase support after in vitro fertilization (IVF)
- Large number of oocytes retrieved (more than 20)
- Early pregnancy.

CLINICAL PRESENTATION

Symptoms of OHSS may begin within 24 hours of HCG administration but exacerbate 7–10 days later with the rise of endogenous HCG from a growing pregnancy.[9] Mild manifestations of OHSS are relatively common and include transient lower abdominal discomfort, nausea, vomiting, diarrhea and abdominal distension (observed in up to a third of stimulation cycles).[10] Advancement of illness is recognized when symptoms persist, worsen or when pain is accompanied by one or more of the following:

- Rapid weight gain
- Ascites
- Oliguria
- Hemoconcentration
- Leukocytosis
- Intravascular hypovolemia
- Hemodynamic instability (orthostatic hypotension, tachycardia)
- Respiratory difficulty (tachypnea)
- Laboratory abnormalities including hyponatremia and hyperkalemia. Sequestration of protein-rich fluid and decreased vascular volume, oliguria or anuria due to reduced renal perfusion and/or tense ascites, and pulmonary compromise from an elevated diaphragm and/or hydrothorax can all lead to hypotension. Hemoconcentration, reduced peripheral blood flow and inactivity due to abdominal distension and pain increase the risk of thromboembolism. If the patient is not diagnosed early, ascites, pleural and pericardial effusions, severe respiratory failure and adult respiratory distress syndrome (ARDS), hypercoagulability with thromboembolism, hemorrhage from ovarian rupture and multiple organ system failure can occur, which could potentially be fatal.[11-13]

PATIENT ASSESSMENT

Careful assessment of the patient is needed to classify disease severity. This should include a review of her stimulation and a prediction of underlying risk based on age, onset of presentation, follicle number and size during stimulation, number of eggs retrieved, peak estradiol level and estradiol level at trigger. The history should include symptoms such as abdominal pain, bloating, shortness of breath, the ability to maintain oral hydration and include estimation of urine output and weight gain.

Physical examination should include measurement of vital signs, body weight, abdominal girth at the umbilicus, assessment for the presence of ascites, pleural effusion and signs of venous thromboembolic disease such as unilateral increase in calf diameter. Pelvic ultrasound should be included to measure ovarian size and check for ascites. Initial laboratory investigations should screen for hemoconcentration with hematocrit and/or hemoglobin measurement and urine specific gravity. Additional laboratory investigations that are helpful in assessing the severity are serum creatinine, electrolytes and liver function tests. Baseline values may help track the progress of the condition.

Review every 2–3 days is usually adequate. However, urgent clinical review is necessary if the woman develops increasing severity of pain, abdominal distension, shortness of breath and reduced urine output. If the woman conceives, prolonged monitoring may be necessary, whereas, in the absence of pregnancy, resolution would be anticipated by the time of the withdrawal bleed.

The first sign of impending severe OHSS is usually abdominal bloating due to a small amount of ascites that can generally be detected by physical examination with abdominal percussion for shifting dullness or through ultrasound. Early intraperitoneal fluid accumulation can only be visualized by vaginal ultrasound because enlarged superovulated ovaries make the pelvis difficult to assess on abdominal ultrasound. Once OHSS becomes severe, distension due to ascites is more readily apparent. Ultrasound will usually show ovaries 10–12 cm in diameter filled with multiple luteal cysts. On gross examination, ascitic fluid is clear and straw colored. Laboratory examination will show a high concentration of albumin and low leukocyte count. Red blood cells are often present, likely due to bleeding from the egg retrieval or the paracentesis itself. This extravascular albumin-rich exudate accumulates in the peritoneal cavity, occasionally in the pleura, and rarely in the pericardial space.[9] The loss of albumin from the intravascular compartment leads to decreased plasma oncotic pressure. An increase in urine specific gravity and hematocrit are useful in determining whether a patient is so dehydrated as to warrant hospital admission for intravenous hydration.

In general, leukocytosis is a harbinger of hemoconcentration and is thought to be due to monocyte tissue factor expression from the granulosa cells.[14] In severe OHSS, electrolyte imbalance is also often observed.[15] If pleural effusion develops, the woman will present with tachypnea or shortness of breath.

Once the diagnosis of OHSS is made, disease severity should be classified as mild, moderate, severe or critical.

CLASSIFICATION OF OVARIAN HYPERSTIMULATION SYNDROME

Golan et al. in 1989 classified OHSS into three categories (mild, moderate and severe) and five grades (Grade 1–5).[10] In 1992, the severe form was further categorized into two subgroups by Navot et al.[7] The practice committee of the American Society for Reproductive Medicine (ASRM) proposed a classification for OHSS of mild, worsening and serious.[4] However, as all women undergoing IVF have enlarged ovaries and varying levels of fluid in the cavity; it is clinically difficult to classify them into grades. Clinicians should be aware that OHSS is a dynamic condition and moderate OHSS may progress to severe OHSS within hours.[16,17]

A practical classification of OHSS severity was proposed by Navot et al.[7] and modified by Mathur et al.[18,19] as follows:

Mild Ovarian Hyperstimulation Syndrome

- Abdominal bloating
- Mild abdominal pain
- Ovarian size usually less than 8 cm.*

Moderate Ovarian Hyperstimulation Syndrome

- Moderate abdominal pain
- Nausea ± vomiting
- Ultrasound evidence of ascites
- Ovarian size usually 8–12 cm.*

Severe Ovarian Hyperstimulation Syndrome

- Clinical ascites (occasionally hydrothorax)
- Oliguria
- Hemoconcentration with hematocrit more than 45%
- Hypoproteinemia
- Ovarian size usually more than 12 cm.*

Critical Severe Ovarian Hyperstimulation Syndrome

- Tense ascites or large hydrothorax
- Hematocrit more than 55%
- White cell count more than 25,000/mL
- Oligo- or anuria
- Thromboembolism
- Acute respiratory distress syndrome.

MANAGEMENT

Management of OHSS depends on the severity of the condition. Every center that offers assisted reproductive techniques (ART) should develop agreed protocols for referral of women with suspected OHSS to hospital care, including written protocols for initial OHSS management. Specific complications, such as ARDS, renal failure and thromboembolism may require intensive care management. Anesthetic and medical colleagues should be involved at an early stage in all cases of critical OHSS.

Information and Communication

Every ART center should provide written information about OHSS including potential risks, signs and symptoms and actions to take in case of symptoms. Patients should be told how they can contact a physician with expertise in the diagnosis and management of OHSS.

Outpatient Management

Outpatient management is usually possible in women with mild and moderate OHSS.[7] A number of studies have shown that day care management in patients with severe OHSS with abdominal paracentesis and IV hydration is simple, safe and effective compared to traditional treatment with in-patient hospitalization and supportive measures.[20-23]

Recommendations by the ASRM Practice Committee[4] for the outpatient management of persistent and worsening OHSS include:

- Oral fluid intake should be maintained at no less than 1 L/day
- Strenuous physical activity should be avoided as risk of ovarian torsion increases when the ovaries are significantly enlarged. Light physical activity should be maintained to the extent possible. Strict bed rest is unwarranted and may increase risk of thromboembolism.
- Weight and urine output should be recorded daily. Weight gain greater than or equal to 2 pounds (roughly 1 kg) per day or decreasing urinary frequency should prompt repeated physical examination, ultrasound and laboratory evaluation to include hematocrit, electrolytes and serum creatinine.
- Pregnant patients with OHSS must be monitored very closely because risk of progressing to severe disease is particularly high for those further stimulated by rapidly rising serum concentrations of HCG.
- In ART cycles, it may be necessary to consider cryopreserving all embryos and deferring transfer to a remote cycle after symptoms have completely subsided. This approach reduces the risk of developing severe OHSS without a marked decrease in pregnancy rates.[24-26]

Pain Relief

Symptomatic relief of abdominal pain can be achieved with acetaminophen and if necessary oral or parenteral opiates. Nonsteroidal anti-inflammatory agents with antiplatelet properties should not be used because they may interfere with implantation and may also compromise renal

*Ovarian size may not correlate with severity of OHSS in cases of assisted reproduction because of the effect of follicular aspiration.

function in women with severe OHSS.[7] If opiates are used, particularly in women with reduced mobility, care should be taken to avoid constipation.

Paracentesis

Patients with tense ascites causing significant pain and/or respiratory compromise benefit from paracentesis. Intra-abdominal pressure may be measured via a urinary catheter with pressures greater than 20 mm Hg suggestive of the need for decompression.[27] Paracentesis will also improve oliguria that is secondary to reduced renal perfusion from ascites increasing intra-abdominal pressure and compromising blood flow to the kidneys.[13,28] Paracentesis should be performed under ultrasound guidance to avoid inadvertent puncture of vascular ovaries distended by large luteal cysts.

The optimal volume of fluid that should be removed on any one occasion and over what interval of time has not been well established. To avoid cardiovascular collapse from massive fluid shifts, the rate of ascitic fluid drainage should be controlled, IV colloid should be administered and pulse and blood pressure should be monitored. Serial paracentesis may be required to maintain adequate renal and pulmonary function. Drainage of ascites will also generally resolve a pleural effusion. Transabdominal aspiration is likely to be better tolerated than a vaginal approach.

Repeated paracentesis may be avoided by the use of pigtail or suprapubic catheters that can be left in place.[29] Pigtail catheters have been used for drainage in various clinical situations, and have been described for the percutaneous drainage of ascites caused by severe or critical OHSS in both outpatient and inpatient settings.[30]

Paracentesis causes relief of pressure on the inferior vena cava and improvement in venous return, cardiac output and renal perfusion.[31] It is also possible that removal of ascites decreases the amount of vascular endothelial growth factor (VEGF) and its effects on vascular permeability.

Treatment of worsening OHSS typically requires antiemetics and more potent analgesics. Most patients can still be effectively managed on an outpatient basis, but they require more careful and frequent evaluation. If symptoms do not resolve and severe OHSS develops, hospital admission should be considered.

Inpatient Management

Serious illness requiring hospitalization is relatively uncommon but by no means rare. Hospitalization may be required based on severity of symptoms, analgesic requirements and other social conditions. It is imperative to stress that an outpatient management protocol can only be used in patients who are motivated, reliable and have the necessary support at home to allow them to return to the clinic or go to the emergency room if the need arises. No one symptom or sign is an absolute indication but hospitalization should be considered when one or more of the following are present:[4]

- Severe abdominal pain or peritoneal signs
- Intractable nausea and vomiting that prevent ingestion of food and adequate fluids
- Severe oliguria or anuria
- Tense ascites
- Dyspnea and tachypnea
- Hypotension (relative to baseline), dizziness or syncope
- Severe electrolyte imbalance (hyponatremia, hyperkalemia)
- Hemoconcentration
- Abnormal liver function tests.

Laboratory findings in women with serious illness resulting from OHSS include:[7,11,28]

- Hemoconcentration (hemoglobin more than 14 g/dL; hematocrit more than 45%)
- Leukocytosis (white blood cell count more than 15,000)
- Electrolyte imbalances (sodium less than 135 mEq/L; potassium more than 5.0 mEq/L)
- Elevated liver enzymes
- Decreased creatinine clearance (serum creatinine more than 1.2; creatinine clearance less than 50 mL/min).

Monitoring

Admitted patients should be assessed by a physician at least once daily, with more frequent assessment in cases of critical OHSS. Physical examination should assess hydration, cardiorespiratory status, level of ascites and signs of thromboembolism.

Recommendations for the evaluation and monitoring of hospitalized patients with OHSS include:[4]

- Vital signs (every 2–3 hours according to the clinical status)
- Weight (recorded daily)
- Complete physical examination (daily, avoiding bimanual examination of the ovaries due to risk of ovarian rupture)
- Abdominal circumference (at the umbilicus, recorded daily)
- Monitoring of fluid intake and output (recorded daily or as often as needed)
- Ultrasound examinations (ascites, ovarian size), repeated as necessary to guide management or paracentesis

- Chest X-ray and echocardiogram (when pleural or pericardial effusion is suspected), repeated as necessary
- Pulse oximetry (for patients with symptoms of pulmonary compromise)
- Complete blood count (daily or as often as required to guide fluid management)
- Electrolytes (daily)
- Serum creatinine or creatinine clearance, urine specific gravity (repeated as necessary)
- Liver enzymes (repeated as necessary)
- Prothrombin time or activated partial thromboplastin time.

Urine output should be maintained at a minimum of 30 mL/hour. Output less than 1,000 mL/day or a persistent positive fluid balance is a cause for concern. Hemoconcentration is a measure of the severity of OHSS.[32] An increase in the white cell count may indicate an ongoing systemic stress response. Hyponatremia, observed in 56% cases of severe OHSS, may be dilutional as a result of antidiuretic hormone hypersecretion.[33] Although reduced renal perfusion may lead to oliguria in about one-third of women with severe OHSS, acute renal failure is rare. Abnormal liver function tests can be found in 25–40% of severe OHSS cases and usually normalize with resolution of the disease.[9]

Ultrasound of the pelvis assesses the extent of ovarian enlargement and the degree of abdominal fluid accumulation. Chest X-ray is indicated in women with respiratory symptoms and signs suggestive of hydrothorax, pulmonary infection or pulmonary embolism. An electrocardiogram (ECG) should be carried out if pulmonary embolism or pericardial effusion is suspected. A pericardial effusion may present with quieter heart sounds and reduced QRS voltages on ECG. A chest radiograph would demonstrate an increased size in the cardiac shadow, with the heart appearing globular or pear shaped.[34]

Careful and frequent re-evaluation of the hospitalized patient with severe OHSS is essential. Complaints of increasing abdominal pain and distension demand immediate attention, remaining mindful that pain and ascites can easily mask ovarian rupture and acute intra-abdominal hemorrhage. Serial clinical and laboratory evaluations provide the means to monitor progression of illness, to judge the response to treatment and to recognize evidence of resolution.

Fluids and Electrolytes

Allowing women to drink according to their thirst represents the most physiological approach to replacing volume,[35] avoiding the risk of hypervolemia and worsening ascites that may occur with vigorous IV therapy. Women may need antiemetics and analgesics to enable them to tolerate oral fluids. However, where oral intake cannot be maintained, IV crystalloids, such as normal saline, should be used. Most women will need a fluid intake of 2–3 liters in 24 hours, guided by a strict fluid balance chart. IV hydration with a crystalloid solution (100–150 mL/hour) should be instituted until diuresis occurs. Renal and pulmonary function must be carefully monitored. Women with hemoconcentration may need more intensive initial rehydration, such as 1 liter of physiological saline over 1 hour. Women with persistent hemoconcentration and/or urine output less than 0.5 mL/kg/hour may benefit from colloids. IV albumin (15–20 mL/hour of 25% albumin over 4 hours) should be initiated and repeated until hydration status improves.[36] Human albumin, 6% hydroxyethylstarch (Hespan), dextran, mannitol and Haemaccel® have been used for this purpose. Few comparative data exist to support the use of any one of these over the other in the specific situation of severe OHSS. If hemoconcentration and/or oliguria persist despite these measures, paracentesis should be considered. Further, fluid management may be guided by central venous pressure monitoring and an anesthetist should be involved.

Diuretics should not be used as they can further deplete intravascular volume, although they may have a role with careful hemodynamic monitoring in cases where oliguria persists despite adequate intravascular volume expansion and a normal intra-abdominal pressure.

Guidelines for fluid management for patients hospitalized with severe illness relating to OHSS include the following:[7,11,28]

- Strict monitoring of fluid intake and urine output is essential.
- Oral fluid intake should be carefully recorded and limited to those amounts necessary to maintain the patient's comfort.
- Rapid initial hydration may be accomplished with a bolus of IV fluid (500–1,000 mL). Thereafter, fluids should be administered judiciously, in the volumes necessary to maintain adequate urine output (more than 20–30 mL/hour) and reverse hemoconcentration. 5% dextrose in normal saline is preferable to lactated Ringer's solution, given the tendency to hyponatremia. Correction of hypovolemia, hypotension and oliguria has highest priority, accepting that fluid administration may contribute to the accumulation of ascites.
- Albumin (25%) in doses of 50–100 g, infused over 4 hours and repeated at 4–12 hour intervals as necessary, is an effective plasma expander when infusion of normal

saline fails to achieve or maintain hemodynamic stability and adequate urine output. In general, albumin is the preferred plasma expander,[37] although others (e.g., mannitol, fresh frozen plasma) may be used. Dextran has been associated with development of ARDS and is best avoided.[12]

- Treatment with diuretics (e.g., furosemide 20 mg IV) may be considered after an adequate intravascular volume has been restored (hematocritless than 38%). Premature or overzealous use of diuretics will aggravate hypovolemia and hemoconcentration, thereby increasing risk of thromboembolism.
- Intravenous fluid administration should be sharply curtailed and oral fluid intake increased, when there is evidence that the syndrome is resolving, generally heralded by improving symptoms and the onset of a brisk diuresis.
- Hyperkalemia is associated with risk of cardiac dysrhythmias. Acute management involves treatments that move potassium into the intracellular space (insulin and glucose, sodium bicarbonate, albuterol) or protect the heart from the effects of elevated potassium levels (calcium gluconate). ECG manifestations of hyperkalemia (prolonged PR and QRS intervals, ST segment depression and tall peaked T waves) indicate the need for immediate treatment with calcium gluconate. Kayexalate is a cation exchange resin that removes potassium from the body but works more slowly (onset of action 1–2 hours); it may be administered orally or rectally as a retention enema.

Intravenous Hespan

The use of Hespan instead of albumin has been shown by some investigators to be beneficial in reducing the incidence of severe OHSS.[38] By increasing the intravascular oncotic pressure, Hespan helps in decreasing the incidence of ascites and symptoms of severe OHSS. Hespan is also less expensive than albumin. However, Hespan is a category C drug with adverse effects in animals. Therefore, it is not suitable for patients who have late onset OHSS as a result of pregnancy, and its use should be discontinued once pregnancy is confirmed. Hespan should be used with caution in patients with late onset OHSS only when benefits outweigh risks.

Nausea and Vomiting

Antiemetic agents considered to be safe in early pregnancy should be used to alleviate nausea and/or vomiting.

Paracentesis and Thoracocentesis

Insertion of an indwelling pigtail catheter under ultrasound guidance circumvents the need for multiple attempts at drainage and limits potential infectious complications.[15] The drain output should be recorded daily. Clinical resolution is achieved when ascitic output starts to decrease and urine output increases. When drain output is less than 50 mL/day, the catheter can be removed. Severe ascites may be associated with hydrothorax, most commonly on the right resulting from transfer of abdominal fluid to the chest via the thoracic duct. Paracentesis will generally be effective in resolving hydrothorax and thoracocentesis may be reserved for those with bilateral or severe pleural effusions that persist.[13,39]

Prevention of Thromboembolic Complications

Thromboembolism is a life-threatening complication and prophylactic measures are warranted. Daily prophylactic doses of low-molecular weight heparin (e.g., dalteparin sodium 5,000 IU/day or enoxaparin sodium 40 mg/day) and use of thromboembolic deterrent stockings should be considered on admission and continued until discharge. The use of an intermittent pneumatic compression device is prudent when symptoms prevent ambulation and confine the patient to bed. Signs and symptoms suggesting thromboembolism demand prompt additional diagnostic measures (arterial blood gas measurements, ventilation or perfusion scans) and therapeutic anticoagulation when the diagnosis is confirmed or strongly suspected.[4] However, there are no randomized controlled trials demonstrating that prophylactic anticoagulation prevents venous thromboembolism in cases of severe OHSS. In addition, there have been several reports of thromboembolism in women with OHSS treated with thromboprophylaxis.[40-43]

Unusual neurological symptoms after ovarian stimulation should raise the possibility of a thrombotic episode in an uncommon location, prompting referral for appropriate expert opinion. The reported incidence of thrombosis with OHSS ranges between 0.7% and 10%, with an apparent preponderance of upper body sites and frequent involvement of the arterial system.[9]

In women who do not conceive, thromboprophylaxis may be discontinued with resolution of OHSS. The risk of thrombosis appears to persist into the first trimester of pregnancy and heparin prophylaxis may need to be continued until the end of the first trimester, or even longer, depending on the presence of risk factors and course of the OHSS.

Surgical Management

Pelvic surgery should be restricted to cases with adnexal torsion or coincident problems requiring surgery and only undertaken by an experienced surgeon after careful assessment. Patients with severe OHSS who may require surgery for a ruptured ovarian cyst with hemorrhage, torsion or an ectopic pregnancy present a unique challenge for the anesthetist who is unlikely to be familiar with the pathophysiology of the syndrome and must be quickly educated to minimize the additional risks involved.[44] OHSS, particularly if associated with pregnancy, may be a risk factor for ovarian torsion.[45,46] Torsion should be suspected in the presence of further ovarian enlargement, worsening pain especially unilateral, nausea, leukocytosis and anemia.[33] Color Doppler assessment of ovarian blood flow may help in diagnosis.[47] Untwisting of the twisted adnexa followed by observation of improved color at laparoscopy or laparotomy is associated with a favorable prognosis for ovarian function.[48]

MANAGEMENT OF COMPLICATIONS AND INTENSIVE CARE

Renal failure, thromboembolism, pericardial effusion and ARDS are potential life-threatening complications of OHSS. These conditions should be diagnosed early and managed by a multidisciplinary team according to the end-organ affected, possibly in an intensive care unit (ICU) setting, if they do not respond to supportive care and paracentesis. Renal failure will often respond to low-dose dopamine therapy (0.18 mg/kg/h) that will dilate renal vessels and increase renal blood flow.[49] Invasive monitoring of central venous pressure or pulmonary capillary wedge pressure and even short-term dialysis may be required. Pulmonary intensive care may involve oxygen supplementation, thoracocentesis and assisted ventilation when more conservative measures fail.

A few patients with critical late OHSS do not improve even after all these measures and the treating clinicians are left with very few difficult options namely, termination of pregnancy and less commonly, bilateral partial oophorectomy.[50]

COUNSELING

Women should be counseled and their partners should be made aware, that the management of OHSS is primarily supportive until the condition resolves spontaneously. They should be counseled regularly about the natural history of OHSS and are advised that their clinical course may be prolonged if they become pregnant and may require hospitalization for the same.[51] It is also important to provide reassurance that pregnancy would not be adversely affected by the OHSS, if complications of critical OHSS do not occur.[9]

CONCLUSION

The key pathophysiological feature of OHSS is a fluid shift with extravascular fluid accumulation combined with intravascular volume depletion and hemoconcentration. This state of effective dehydration (and its detection and management) is the main clinical problem in the care of women with OHSS. Knowledge of OHSS risk factors, clinical presentation and classification of severity are essential to the effective diagnosis and management of this disease. Mild manifestations of OHSS are common, occurring in up to one-third of women being stimulated for IVF. Patients with mild manifestations of OHSS can be managed on an outpatient basis. Treatment usually only requires oral analgesics and counseling regarding the signs and symptoms of progressing illness. Intercourse is best avoided as it may be painful and may increase the risk of ovarian rupture.

Treatment of worsening OHSS typically requires antiemetics and more potent analgesics. Most patients can still be effectively managed on an outpatient basis, but they require more careful evaluation. Serious illness resulting from OHSS is much less common but it can be life-threatening. Hospitalization may occasionally be necessary to prevent deterioration to clinical disease.

Continued research will further increase our understanding of the pathophysiology of OHSS and may advance our ability to altogether predict and prevent this potentially serious illness.

REFERENCES

1. Bulun SE, Adashi EY. The physiology and pathology of the female reproductive axis. In: Kronenberg HM, Melmed S, Polonsky KS, Larsen PR (Eds). Williams Textbook of Endocrinology, 11th edition. Philadelphia:Saunders; 2008. pp. 541-614.
2. Papanikolaou EG, Tournaye H, Verpoest W, et al. Early and late ovarian hyperstimulation syndrome: early pregnancy outcome and profile. Hum Reprod. 2005;20(3):636-41.
3. Navot D, Relou A, Birkenfield A, et al. Risk factors and prognostic variables in the ovarian hyperstimulation syndrome. Am J Obstet Gynecol. 1988;159(1):210-5.
4. The Practice Committee of the American Society for Reproductive Medicine. Ovarian hyperstimulation syndrome. Fertil Steril. 2008;90(5 Suppl):S188-93.
5. Brinsden PR, Wada I, Tan SL, et al. Diagnosis, prevention and management of ovarian hyperstimulation syndrome. Br J Obstet Gynaecol. 1995;102(10):767-72.

6. Enskog A, Henriksson M, Unander M, et al. Prospective study of the clinical and laboratory parameters of patients in whom ovarian hyperstimulation syndrome developed during controlled ovarian hyperstimulation for in vitro fertilization. Fertil Steril. 1999;71(5):808-14.
7. Navot D, Bergh PA, Laufer N. Ovarian hyperstimulation syndrome in novel reproductive technologies:prevention and treatment. Fertil Steril. 1992;58(2):249-61.
8. Asch RH, Li HP, Balmaceda JP, et al. Severe ovarian hyperstimulation syndrome in assisted reproductive technology: definition of high risk groups. Hum Reprod. 1991;6(10):1395-9.
9. Delvigne A, Rozenberg S. Review of clinical course and treatment of ovarian hyperstimulation syndrome (OHSS). Hum Reprod Update. 2003;9(1):77-96.
10. Golan A, Ron-el R, Herman A, et al. Ovarian hyperstimulation syndrome: an update review. Obstet Gynecol Surv. 1989;44(6):430-40.
11. Whelan JG, Vlahos NF. The ovarian hyperstimulation syndrome. Fertil Steril. 2000;73(5):883-96.
12. Zosmer A, Katz Z, Lancet M, et al. Adult respiratory distress syndrome complicating ovarian hyperstimulation syndrome. Fertil Steril. 1987;47(3):524-6.
13. Abramov Y, Elchalal U, Schenker JG. Pulmonary manifestations of severe ovarian hyperstimulation syndrome: a multicenter study. Fertil Steril. 1999;71(4):645-51.
14. Balasch J, Reverter JC, Fabregues F, et al. Increased induced monocyte tissue factor expression by plasma from patients with severe ovarian hyperstimulation syndrome. Fertil Steril. 1996;66(4):608-13.
15. Rahami M, Leader A, Claman P, et al. A novel approach to the treatment of ascites associated with ovarian hyperstimulation syndrome. Hum Reprod. 1997;12(12):2614-6.
16. Rizk B, Aboulghar M. Classification, pathophysiology and management of ovarian hyperstimulation syndrome. In: Brinsden P (Ed). A Textbook of In vitro Fertilization and Assisted Reproduction, 2nd edition. London:CRC Press;1999. pp. 131-55.
17. Rizk B. Symposium: Update on prediction and management of OHSS. Genetics of ovarian hyperstimulation syndrome. Reprod Biomed Online. 2009;19(1):14-27.
18. Mathur R, Kailasam C, Jenkins J. Review of the evidence base strategies to prevent ovarian hyperstimulation syndrome. Hum Fertil (Camb). 2007;10(2):75-85.
19. Mathur R, Evbuomwan I, Jenkins J. Prevention and management of ovarian hyperstimulation syndrome. Curr Obstet Gynecol. 2005;15:132-8.
20. Lincoln SR, Opsahl MS, Blauer KL, et al. Aggressive outpatient treatment of ovarian hyperstimulation syndrome with ascites using transvaginal culdocentesis and intravenous albumin minimizes hospitalization. J Assist Reprod Genet. 2002;19(4):159-63.
21. Shrivastav P, Nadkarni P, Craft I. Day care management of severe ovarian hyperstimulation syndrome avoids hospitalization and morbidity. Hum Reprod. 1994;9(5):812-14.
22. Csokmay JM, Yauger BJ, Henne MB, et al. Cost analysis model of outpatient management of ovarian hyperstimulation syndrome with paracentesis: "tap early and often" versus hospitalization. Fertil Steril. 2010;93(1):167-73.
23. Smith LP, Hacker MR, Alper MM. Patients with severe ovarian hyperstimulation syndrome can be managed safely with aggressive outpatient transvaginal paracentesis. Fertil Steril. 2009;92(6):1953-9.
24. Pattinson HA, Hignett M, Dunphy BC, et al. Outcome of thaw embryo transfer after cryopreservation of all embryos in patients at risk of ovarian hyperstimulation syndrome. Fertil Steril. 1994;62(6):1192-6.
25. Shaker AG, Zosmer A, Dean N, et al. Comparison of intravenous albumin and transfer of fresh embryos with cryopreservation of all embryos for subsequent transfer in prevention of ovarian hyperstimulation syndrome. Fertil Steril. 1996;65(5):992-6.
26. Ferraretti AP, Gianaroli L, Magli C, et al. Elective cryopreservation of all pronucleate embryos in women at risk of ovarian hyperstimulation syndrome: efficiency and safety. Hum Reprod. 1999;14(6):1457-60.
27. Meldrum DR, Moore FA, Moore EE, et al. Prospective characterization and selective management of the abdominal compartment syndrome. Am J Surg. 1997;174(6):667-72.
28. Borenstein R, Elhalah U, Lunenfeld B, et al. Severe ovarian hyperstimulation syndrome:a re-evaluated therapeutic approach. Fertil Steril. 1989;51(5):791-5.
29. Abuzeid MI, Nassar Z, Massaad Z, et al. Pigtail catheter for the treatment of ascites associated with ovarian hyperstimulation syndrome. Hum Reprod. 2003;18(2):370-3.
30. Abuzeid M, Warda H, Joseph S, et al. Outpatient management of severe hyperstimulation syndrome with placement of pigtail catheter. Facts Views Vis Obgyn. 2014;6(1):31-7.
31. Padilla SL, Zamaria S, Baramki TA, et al. Abdominal paracentesis for the ovarian hyperstimulation syndrome with severe pulmonary compromise. Fertil Steril. 1990;53(2):365-7.
32. Fábregues F, Balasch J, Manau D, et al. Haematocrit, leukocyte and platelet counts and the severity of the ovarian hyperstimulation syndrome. Hum Reprod. 1998;13(9):2406-10.
33. Fábregues F, Balasch J, Gines P, et al. Ascites and liver test abnormalities during severe ovarian hyperstimulation syndrome. Am J Gastroenterol 1999;94(4):994-9.
34. Haslett C, Chilvers ER, Hunter JAA, et al. Davidson's Principles and Practice of Medicine, 18th edition. London:Churchill Livingstone; 1999. pp. 300.
35. Evbuomwan IO, Davidson JM, Murdoch AP. Coexistent hemoconcentration and hypoosmolality during superovulation and in severe ovarian hyperstimulation syndrome: a volume homeostasis paradox. Fertil Steril. 2000;74(1):67-72.
36. Fluker MR, Copeland J, Yuzpe AA. An ounce of prevention: outpatient management of ovarian hyperstimulation syndrome. Fertil Steril. 2000;73(4):821-4.
37. Forman RG, Frydman R, Egan D, et al. Severe ovarian hyperstimulation syndrome using agonists of gonadotropin-releasing hormone for in vitro fertilization: a European series and a proposal for prevention. Fertil Steril. 1990;53(3): 502-9.
38. Youssef MA, Al-Inany HG, Evers JL, et al. Intra-venous fluids for the prevention severe ovarian hyperstimulation syndrome. Cochrane Database Syst Rev. 2011;16(2):CD001302.

39. Rinaldi ML, Spirtos NJ. Chest tube drainage of pleural effusion correcting abdominal ascites in a patient with severe ovarian hyperstimulation syndrome: a case report. Fertil Steril. 1995;63(5):1114-7.
40. Hignett M, Spence JE, Claman P. Internal jugular vein thrombosis: a late complication of ovarian hyperstimulation syndrome despite mini-dose heparin prophylaxis. Hum Reprod. 1995;10(12):3121-3.
41. Hortskamp B, Lubke M, Kentenich H, et al. Internal jugular vein thrombosis caused by resistance to protein C as a complication of ovarian hyperstimulation syndrome after in-vitro fertilization. Hum Reprod. 1994;11(2);280-2.
42. Todros T, Carmazzi CM, Bontempo S, et al. Spontaneous ovarian hyperstimulation syndrome and deep vein thrombosis in pregnancy: a case report. Hum Reprod. 1999; 14(9):2245-8.
43. Cil T, Tummon IS, House AA, et al. A tale of two syndromes: ovarian hyperstimulation and abdominal compartment. Hum Reprod. 2000;15(5):1058-60.
44. Reed AP, Tausk H, Reynolds H. Anesthetic considerations for severe ovarian hyperstimulation syndrome. Anesthesiology 1990;73(6):1275-7.
45. Mashiach S, Bider D, Moran O, et al. Adnexal torsion of hyperstimulated ovaries in pregnancies after gonadotropin therapy. Fertil Steril. 1990;53(1):76-80.
46. Gorkemli H, Camus M, Clasen K. Adnexal torsion after gonadotrophin ovulation induction for IVF or ICSI and its conservative treatment. Arch Gynecol Obstet. 2002;267(1): 4-6.
47. Gordon JD, Hopkins KL, Jeffrey RB, et al. Adnexal torsion: color Doppler diagnosis and laparoscopic treatment. Fertil Steril. 1994;61(2):383-5.
48. Oelsner G, Cohen SB, Soriano D, et al. Minimal surgery for the twisted ischaemic adnexa can preserve ovarian function. Hum Reprod. 2003;18(12):2599-602.
49. Ferraretti AP, Gianaroli L, Diotallevi L, et al. Dopamine treatment for severe ovarian hyperstimulation syndrome. Hum Reprod. 1992;7(2):180-3.
50. Rizk B. Ovarian hyperstimulation syndrome. In: Studd J (Ed). Progress in Obstetrics and Gynecology, 11th edition. Edinburgh:Churchill Livingstone; 1994. pp. 311-49.
51. Delvigne A, Demoulin A, Smitz J, et al. The ovarian hyperstimulation syndrome in in-vitro fertilization: a Belgian multicen- tric study.1. Clinical and biological features. Hum Reprod. 1993;8(9):1353-60.

CHAPTER

38

Polycystic Ovary Syndrome and Assisted Reproduction Techniques

Israel Ortega Sanchez, Juan A García-Velasco

INTRODUCTION

Polycystic ovary syndrome (PCOS) is one of the most common endocrine disorders, affecting 5–10% of women of reproductive age. Although the main hallmarks of the syndrome are the presence of hyperandrogenemia, enlarged ovaries, and oligo/anovulation; PCOS women frequently present additional features such as obesity, insulin resistance, and metabolic syndrome.[1]

Although significant progress has been made toward the development of universally accepted diagnostic criteria for the syndrome, the optimal treatment for infertile women with PCOS has not yet been defined. A broad range of interventions have been proposed, including lifestyle modifications, administration of ovulation-inducing agents such as clomiphene citrate, insulin-sensitizing drugs, gonadotropins and gonadotropin-releasing hormone (GnRH) analogs, laparoscopic drilling, and the application of assisted reproduction techniques (ART).

In vitro fertilization (IVF) is the most effective of existing fertility treatment strategies, although is also the most costly and invasive approach to infertility management. According to the European Society of Human Reproduction and Embryology/The American Society for Reproductive Medicine (ESHRE/ASRM) PCOS consensus, this strategy should be considered as third-line of treatment for those PCOS women who failed to achieve pregnancy following multiple attempts at ovulation induction after clomiphene citrate, gonadotropins and/or laparoscopic drilling. Moreover, IVF may be indicated in these patients in the presence of associated pathologies, such as in cases of tubal disease, severe male factor, severe endometriosis, and preimplantation genetic diagnosis.[2]

In the present review, we will discuss in detail the IVF protocols used in PCOS women, as well as the controversies surrounding their efficacy and safety. Furthermore, we will address the risks of ART in these patients, providing some guidelines for the management of infertility in PCOS undergoing IVF.

OVARIAN STIMULATION IN POLYCYSTIC OVARY SYNDROME

Gonadotropin-releasing Hormone Analogs

The concomitant use of a GnRH agonist with gonadotropin administration to improve pregnancy rates in patients undergoing ovulation induction has not yet been confirmed.[3] Moreover, recent studies have demonstrated that the use of GnRH antagonist in ovarian stimulation protocols is associated with a lower risk of ovarian hyperstimulation syndrome (OHSS). Lainas et al. carried out a randomized controlled trial including up to 220 PCOS patients allocated into two groups: long GnRH agonist downregulation protocol vs. flexible GnRH antagonist protocol. In this study, no differences between both study groups were observed in ongoing pregnancy rates. However, the incidence of OHSS was 20% significantly lower in the antagonist compared to the agonist group. In addition, duration of ovarian stimulation and the total amount of gonadotrophins required were also lower in the antagonist compared to the agonist protocol. Therefore, the use of GnRH antagonist protocol might represent the first choice treatment in PCOS patients undergoing IVF.[4]

In a similar study, the efficacy of the GnRH antagonist protocol (study group) in comparison with the GnRH agonist (control group) was evaluated in oral contraceptive pills (OCP) pretreated PCOS women undergoing their first ART cycle. Coasting or GnRH agonist trigger was used when estradiol levels were more than 3.000 pg/mL in the control and study group, respectively. Luteal phase support was based on daily administration of 800 mg of vaginal progesterone and 4 mg oral estradiol valerate. Although there were no significant differences in either fertilization or clinical pregnancy rates, the incidence of moderate OHSS in the control group was 22%, and severe 11.1% compared to lack of the syndrome in the study group. Additionally, the duration of the treatment and the total amount of gonadotropins used for ovarian stimulation were lower in the study group.[5]

In light of these findings, we may conclude that the use of GnRH antagonist protocol for ovarian stimulation in PCOS patients is more efficient and safe compared to the gold standard long GnRH agonist protocol, providing a shorter duration of treatment with fewer injections and with no negative effects on ART outcome. This leads to a significantly lower amount of gonadotropins required, which results in an improved patient compliance. Moreover, the use of GnRH agonist to trigger final oocyte maturation during a GnRH antagonist cycle has been shown to reduce and prevent the incidence of OHSS.[6]

Gonadotropins

Classically, it has been suggested that increased luteinizing hormone (LH) secretion in PCOS may exert a deleterious effect on fertility, due to the presence of premature oocyte maturation through inhibition of oocyte maturation inhibitor, negative LH effect on granulosa cell steroidogenesis and increased pregnancy loss.[7-9]

However, the findings of recent clinical studies are not consistent with this assumption. Platteau et al. published a prospective randomized study aimed to evaluate the noninferiority of highly purified urinary human menopausal gonadotropin (HP-hMG) compared to recombinant follicle stimulating hormone (rFSH) with respect to ovulation rate, in women with anovulatory infertility WHO group II. In this study, ovulation rates and singleton live birth rates were comparable between both groups. Moreover, significantly fewer intermediate-sized follicles together with a less frequency of OHSS and/or cancellation due to excessive response were observed after administration of HP-hMG. Therefore, this study demonstrates the noninferiority of HP-hMG compared to rFSH in the main clinical outcomes, suggesting a potential positive effect on the safety of ovulation induction protocols.[10]

This comparison between hMG and rFSH with respect to clinical outcomes and incidence of OHSS has also been evaluated in PCOS patients undergoing a long GnRH agonist protocol in an IVF cycle. In the hMG group, a significantly lower peak estradiol level, fewer intermediate-sized follicles, and lower number of retrieved oocytes were observed. However, both fertilization and pregnancy rates were comparable between both groups. Moreover, the incidence of OHSS was 11.9% in rFSH group patients, whereas no OHSS was observed in hMG group patients. Following this line of reasoning, a recent retrospective study demonstrated that high LH/FSH ratio has no adverse effect on pregnancy rates in PCOS women undergoing long agonist protocol, antagonist protocol or in vitro maturation. Therefore, both type of gonadotropins are associated with similar clinical outcomes in PCOS patients undergoing a long GnRH agonist protocol; however, hMG provides lower incidence of OHSS and decreased coasting requirements.[11]

With regard to the optimal type of FSH used in PCOS patients undergoing IVF, Aboulghar et al. carried out a prospective randomized study comparing urinary vs. recombinant FSH for IVF/intracytoplasmic injection in PCOS patients. In this study, there was no significant difference in total FSH used, duration of stimulation, number of retrieved oocytes, number of embryos transferred, and pregnancy rates.[12] Similarly, a recent review evaluated the safety and effectiveness of gonadotropins for ovulation induction in PCOS patients resistant to clomiphene citrate, and no differences were observed in terms of either live birth or OHSS rates between urinary-derived gonadotropins and rFSH or hMG/HP-hMG.[13]

RESULTS

Previously, PCOS women have been suggested to present impaired fertilization and pregnancy rates due to abnormal follicle development and poor oocyte quality.[9] However, these results have not been confirmed by subsequent studies. Heijnen et al. in a meta-analysis comparing the clinical outcomes of conventional IVF in PCOS patients and non-PCOS patients demonstrated that there were no significant differences in clinical pregnancy and live birth rates per cycle between both groups, whereas PCOS patients presented a higher number of retrieved oocytes, lower fertilization, and higher cancellation rates.[14] Similarly, a recent retrospective study demonstrated that PCOS patients presented reduced fertilization rates and higher incidence of OHSS with similar clinical pregnancy and miscarriage rates when compared to their counterparts with tubal factor infertility.[15]

Moreover, PCOS patients are also at high risk of pregnancy and neonatal complications. A meta-analysis that included a total of 15 studies involving 720 patients presenting PCOS and 4,505 controls demonstrated that PCOS patients present a significantly higher risk of developing gestational diabetes, pregnancy-induced hypertension, pre-eclampsia, and preterm birth. In addition, the newborns are at high risk of admission in neonatal intensive care unit and higher perinatal mortality, unrelated to multiple pregnancies.[16]

COMPLICATIONS

Ovarian hyperstimulation syndrome represents one of the most serious complications subsequent to controlled ovarian stimulation and can be life-threatening. After gonadotropin administration for IVF, the reported incidence for the mild forms of OHSS is 20–33%, while severe forms occur in 0.1–2% of IVF cycles.[17,18] The specific risk factors for OHSS include young age (<35 years), lean habitus, the presence of multiple small and intermediate follicles, excessively high levels of serum estradiol (E2 > 4000 pg/ml) on the day of human chorionic gonadotropin (hCG) administration, and signs of PCOS.[19]

The pathogenesis of OHSS is a complex process that may result from the interaction of endocrine and paracrine factors (cytokines).[20] Human chorionic gonadotropin exposure is thought to be one of the crucial mediators of the syndrome. The role of hCG can be further elucidated via the two distinct clinical patterns of OHSS: the "early" type that occurs 3–7 days after ovulation triggering by hCG, and the "late" type that occurs 12–17 days after hCG administration. Early onset of OHSS is an acute consequence of exogenous hCG administration and is due to an excessive ovarian response to ovarian stimulation, whereas late onset of OHSS is associated with an endogenous production of hCG from the trophoblast.[21] hCG is thought to play a key role in the pathophysiology of OHSS by mediating the release of vascular endothelial growth factor A (VEGF-A), which through its interactions with VEGF receptor-2 (VEGFR-2), promotes increased vascular permeability and endothelial migration at least partly through modulation of vascular endothelial cadherin function.[22] Other mediators such as angiotensin II, insulin-like growth factor 1, and interleukin-6 have also been implicated in the disease process.[23]

Severe OHSS is characterized by growth of multiple large follicles with massive extravascular protein rich fluid shift, leading to hypovolemia, hemoconcentration and oliguria, and electrolyte disturbance. In women who are identified as being at high risk of OHSS, the total amount of gonadotropins used throughout ovarian stimulation should be decreased to reduce the risk of excessive ovarian response. In addition, other prevention strategies should be taken into account:

- Coasting, that consists of the withdrawal when a certain estradiol concentration and/or a critical number of follicles is reached, postponing hCG administration until estradiol levels significantly reduce or plateau. It is generally employed for a period less than 3 days.
- Administration of low doses of hCG appears to prevent the development of OHSS without compromising the success rate.[24]
- Administration of GnRH agonist as the trigger for final follicular maturation will reduce the risk of OHSS by reducing the duration of luteal stimulation, lowering estrogen levels by inducing luteolysis and reducing the secretion of VEGF.[25]
- Oocyte or embryo vitrification and subsequent embryo transfer in a frozen-thawed cycle.
- Cycle cancellation and withholding of hCG.

There are alternative methods of prevention, including:

- Intensive luteal phase supported by administration of GnRH agonist after oocyte retrieval.[6]
- Continued administration of aromatase inhibitor to reduce the incidence of early-onset of OHSS after oocyte retrieval.[26]
- Administration of dopamine receptor agonists, which prevent excessive increase in VEGF-mediated vascular permeability through their antiangiogenic properties.[27]

Mild cases can usually be treated on an outpatient basis, as long as resolution is reported and review takes place every 2–3 days. The outpatient management is based on analgesia, avoidance of strenuous exercise, and hydration and should cover important aspects, including daily fluid balance, daily weight check and regular bloods and scans.

Women with symptoms of severe OHSS, such as intolerance of oral fluids, hypotension, vomiting or diarrhea, distended abdomen or peritonism, and thromboembolic event should be referred to and managed in a hospital. In these cases, the supportive management includes:

- Intravenous fluids such as normal saline with constant monitoring with the input/output balance.
- Prevention of thromboembolism based on prophylactic anticoagulant therapy with low molecular weight heparin.
- Pain relief.
- Plasma expanders such as hydroxyethyl starch.
- Albumin administration once hypoalbuminemia is proven, and especially during drainage of ascites.
- Paracentesis in those women with severe abdominal distension and renal impairment of dyspnea.

However, nowadays the combination of low doses of gonadotropins in a GnRH antagonist protocol and administration of GnRH agonist to trigger final oocyte maturation with subsequent oocyte/embryo vitrification has notably decreased the incidence of OHSS in PCOS patients.

ADJUVANT THERAPIES

Weight Loss

Obesity is present in 40% of PCOS population and correlates with increased rate of cycle disturbances and infertility.[28] Weight loss has been shown to be associated with improvements not only in metabolic profile, but also in spontaneous ovulation rates. Indeed, Kiddy et al. demonstrated that 40% of obese women with PCOS who lost 5% of the initial body weight with caloric restriction achieved spontaneous pregnancy.[29]

In addition to influencing the time to conception, which is often delayed in obese women, excess body mass is also related to suboptimal reproductive performance, such as increased duration of ovarian stimulation, higher requirements of gonadotropins, follicular asynchrony, and higher miscarriage and cancellation rates.[30] The relative ovarian resistance to gonadotropins in obese PCOS women might be due to several factors. First, the presence of altered pharmacokinetics of gonadotropins in obese women might impair reproductive outcomes, resulting in lower effective concentrations of exogenous FSH.[31] Another potential factor inducing gonadotropin resistance is the adipocyte-derived hormone, leptin, which inhibits the stimulatory effect of FSH on steroid synthesis in granulosa cells in vitro.[32]

Therefore, preconceptional counseling should be provided emphasizing the importance of lifestyle, especially weight reduction and exercise in overweight/obese PCOS women. Although the ideal amount of weight loss for a women prior to attempting infertility treatment remains unclear, strong consideration should be made for obese women to lose 5–10% of body weight before starting any medical therapy.

Metformin

Increased insulin resistance is observed in 20–30% of nonobese and 70–80% of obese women with PCOS, and is associated to hyperandrogenemia and resistance to ovulation-inducing agents.[33] Metformin is an Food and Drug Administration (FDA)-approved biguanide for the management of type 2 diabetes mellitus (T2DM), inhibiting hepatic production of glucose, reducing oxidation of fatty acids, and increasing peripheral tissue uptake of glucose.[34]

Classically, it has been suggested that the use of insulin-sensitizing drugs as adjuvant therapies in PCOS undergoing ART might improve the hormone and metabolic profiles and, thus, might induce a positive effect on reproductive outcomes. However, Legro et al. demonstrated that extended-release metformin, either alone or in combination with clomiphene citrate did not improve the rate of live birth in women with PCOS.[35] In addition, current evidence confirms that metformin does not carry a developmental risk for the fetus when used during the first trimester. These findings were inconsistent with data from other studies reporting benefits of metformin in stimulating ovulation in PCOS women, most of them coming from small, primarily single-center trials, focused on metabolic and hormonal measurements rather than live birth rates.[36,37]

To conclude, on the basis of the current available evidence, in an ESHRE Consensus on infertility treatment related to PCOS it was stated that the use of metformin should be restricted to those women diagnosed with glucose intolerance, and therefore, the routine use of this drug for ovulation induction is not recommended.[2]

Inositol

D-chiro-inositol (DCI), a compound belonging to vitamin B complex, has beneficial effects on ovulation and androgen production in women with PCOS due to its ability to increase insulin sensitivity. This drug has been associated with a reduction on insulin secretion and increased sex hormone-binding globulin (SHBG) levels, resulting in decreased serum testosterone and improved ovulatory function.[38]

In addition to inositol-induced positive effect on ovulation induction, treatment of PCOS women with this drug resulted in a significantly reduced number of immature oocytes and better oocyte quality.[39] These findings have been confirmed by Papaleo et al., who observed that myoinositol and folic acid decrease estradiol levels at hCG administration and reduce germinal vesicles and degenerated oocytes without compromising total number of retrieved oocytes.[40] However, a significant improvement in pregnancy rate has not yet been observed.

IN VITRO MATURATION OF OOCYTES

In vitro maturation (IVM) of human oocytes was first reported in 1965 and consists of the maturation of immature oocytes in culture after their recovery from small antral follicles at the stage prior to selection and dominance.[41] As IVM requires little or no FSH administration in vivo, this technique has been suggested to be an alternative to conventional IVF, since it reduces potential side effects due to controlled ovarian stimulation, including the life-threatening OHSS.

Immature oocyte recovery could be developed as a new method for the treatment of infertile PCOS patients, since their oocytes retain their maturational and developmental competence.[42] Nevertheless, clinical outcomes achieved with this technique are significantly worse when compared to conventional IVF. Indeed, Child et al. demonstrated that implantation, clinical pregnancy, and live birth rates were significantly lower in PCOS patients undergoing IVM patients compared to those patients following regular IVF.[43] However, clinical outcomes in these patients might be improved in mild stimulation protocols combining FSH and hCG priming.[44]

Previously, it has been suggested that the presence of chromosome abnormalities in embryos obtained through IVM might account for the low implantation rates observed in these patients. However, Requena et al. did not observe any significant difference in the incidence of miscarriage or congenital abnormalities in babies born after IVM compared to conventional IVF.[45] Therefore, although initial results of IVM are promising and suggest the potential for clinical application, IVM should only be performed as an experimental procedure in specialized centers for carefully selected patients evaluating both efficacy and safety.[46]

CONCLUSION

Management of infertility of PCOS still represents, nowadays, a challenge for physicians. Individualization of the treatment based on a detailed assessment and risk quantification should be done before any intervention is initiated. In infertile PCOS patients, IVF should be recommended as third-line treatment in case clomiphene citrate and gonadotropins fail to result in pregnancy. Although the optimal stimulation protocol is still under debate, growing evidence demonstrates that GnRH antagonist protocol is the first choice of treatment in PCOS patients, with fewer incidences of complications and similar clinical outcomes. However, recommendation regarding gonadotropin type is not yet clear, since both recombinant and human menopausal gonadotropins yield similar clinical outcomes. In those patients at high risk of OHSS, the combination of GnRH agonist triggering with oocyte/embryo vitrification seems to be the gold standard to avoid early- and late-onset OHSS. Although promising, IVM of oocytes should only be performed as an experimental procedure in specialized centers for carefully selected patients evaluating both efficacy and safety. The use of adjuvant therapies must be individualized and consideration for the long-term health of the patient and for the safety of the pregnancy should be the primary goal of all health-care providers.

REFERENCES

1. Fauser BC, Tarlatzis BC, Rebar RW, et al. Consensus on women's health aspects of polycystic ovary syndrome (PCOS): The Amsterdam ESHRE/ASRM-Sponsored 3rd PCOS Consensus Workshop Group. Fertil Steril. 2012;97:28-38.e25.
2. Thessaloniki ESHRE/ASRM-Sponsored PCOS Consensus Workshop Group. Consensus on infertility treatment related to polycystic ovary syndrome. Fertil Steril. 2008;89:505-22.
3. Dodson WC, Hughes CL, Whitesides DB, et al. The effect of leuprolide acetate on ovulation induction with human menopausal gonadotropins in polycystic ovary syndrome. J Clin Endocrinol Metab. 1987;65:95-100.
4. Lainas TG, Sfontouris IA, Zorzovilis IZ, et al. Flexible GnRH antagonist protocol versus GnRH agonist long protocol in patients with polycystic ovary syndrome treated for IVF: A prospective randomised controlled trial (RCT). Hum Reprod. 2010;25:683-9.
5. Tehraninejad ES, Nasiri R, Rashidi B, et al. Comparison of GnRH antagonist with long GnRH agonist protocol after OCP pretreatment in PCOs patients. Arch Gynecol Obstet. 2010;282:319-25.
6. Fusi FM, Arnoldi M, Bosisio C, et al. Ovulation induction and luteal support with GnRH agonist in patients at high risk for hyperstimulation syndrome. Gynecol Endocrinol. 2015;31:693-7.
7. Jacobs HS, Homburg RR. The endocrinology of conception. In: Frank S (Ed). Bailliere's Clinical Endocrinology and Metabolism. London: Bailliere's Tindall. 1990;195-205.
8. Willis DS, Watson H, Mason HD, et al. Premature response to luteinizing hormone of granulosa cells from anovulatory women with polycystic ovary syndrome: Relevance to mechanism of anovulation. J Clin Endocrinol Metab. 1998;83:3984-91.
9. Homburg R, Armar NA, Eshel A, et al. Influence of serum luteinising hormone concentrations on ovulation, conception, and early pregnancy loss in polycystic ovary syndrome. BMJ. 1988;297:1024-6.
10. Platteau P, Andersen AN, Balen A, et al. Similar ovulation rates, but different follicular development with highly purified menotrophin compared with recombinant FSH in WHO Group II anovulatory infertility: A randomized controlled study. Hum Reprod. 2006;21:1798-804.
11. Figen Turkcapar A, Seckin B, Onalan G, et al. Human menopausal gonadotropin versus recombinant FSH in polycystic ovary syndrome patients undergoing in vitro fertilization. Int J Fertil Steril. 2013;6:238-43.
12. Aboulghar M, Saber W, Amin Y, et al. Prospective, randomized study comparing highly purified urinary follicle-stimulating hormone (FSH) and recombinant FSH for in vitro fertilization/intracytoplasmic sperm injection in patients with polycystic ovary syndrome. Fertil Steril. 2010;94:2332-4.
13. Weiss NS, Nahuis M, Bayram N, et al. Gonadotrophins for ovulation induction in women with polycystic ovarian syndrome. Cochrane Database Syst Rev. 2015;9:CD010290.
14. Heijnen EM, Eijkemans MJ, Hughes EG, et al. A meta-analysis of outcomes of conventional IVF in women with polycystic ovary syndrome. Hum Reprod Update. 2006;12:13-21.
15. Okohue JE, Onuh SO, Ikimalo JI. Comparison of IVF/ICSI outcome in patients with polycystic ovarian syndrome or tubal factor infertility. Nigerian J Clin Pract. 2013;16:207-10.

16. Boomsma CM, Eijkemans MJ, Hughes EG,, et al. A meta-analysis of pregnancy outcomes in women with polycystic ovary syndrome. Hum Reprod Update. 2006;12:673-83.
17. Golan A, Ron-el R, Herman A, et al. Ovarian hyperstimulation syndrome: An update review. Obstet Gynecol Surv. 1989;44:430-40.
18. Morris RS, Miller C, Jacobs L, et al. Conservative management of ovarian hyperstimulation syndrome. J Reprod Med. 1995;40:711-4.
19. Navot D, Bergh PA, Laufer N. Ovarian hyperstimulation syndrome in novel reproductive technologies: Prevention and treatment. Fertil Steril. 1992;58:249-61.
20. Mathur R, Jenkins J. Ovarian hyperstimulation syndrome: An endocrinopathy? Curr Opin Obstet Gynecol. 2001;13:329-33.
21. Lyons CA, Wheeler CA, Frishman GN, et al. Early and late presentation of the ovarian hyperstimulation syndrome: Two distinct entities with different risk factors. Hum Reprod. 1994;9:792-9.
22. Villasante A, Pacheco A, Ruiz A, et al. Vascular endothelial cadherin regulates vascular permeability: Implications for ovarian hyperstimulation syndrome. J Clin Endocrinol Metab. 2007;92:314-21.
23. Pellicer A, Albert C, Mercader A, et al. The pathogenesis of ovarian hyperstimulation syndrome: In vivo studies investigating the role of interleukin-1beta, interleukin-6, and vascular endothelial growth factor. Fertil Steril. 1999;71:482-9.
24. Nargund G, Hutchison L, Scaramuzzi R, et al. Low-dose HCG is useful in preventing OHSS in high-risk women without adversely affecting the outcome of IVF cycles. Reprod Biomed Online. 2007;14:682-5.
25. Casper RF. Reducing the risk of OHSS by GnRH agonist triggering. J Clin Endocrinol Metab. 2015;100(12):4396-8.
26. He Q, Liang L, Zhang C, et al. Effects of different doses of letrozole on the incidence of early-onset ovarian hyperstimulation syndrome after oocyte retrieval. Syst Biol Reprod Med. 2014;60:355-60.
27. Ferrero H, García-Pascual CM, Pellicer N, et al. Dopamine agonist inhibits vascular endothelial growth factor protein production and secretion in granulosa cells. Reprod Biol Endocrinol. 2015;13:104.
28. Brewer CJ, Balen AH. The adverse effects of obesity on conception and implantation. Reproduction. 2010;140:347-64.
29. Kiddy DS, Hamilton-Fairley D, Bush A, et al. Improvement in endocrine and ovarian function during dietary treatment of obese women with polycystic ovary syndrome. Clin Endocrinol. 1992;36:105-11.
30. Maheshwari A, Stofberg L, Bhattacharya S. Effect of overweight and obesity on assisted reproductive technology—a systematic review. Hum Reprod Update. 2007;13:433-44.
31. Fridstrom M, Sjöblom P, Pousette A, et al. Serum FSH levels in women with polycystic ovary syndrome during ovulation induction using down-regulation and urofollitropin. Eur J Endocrinol. 1997;136:488-92.
32. Zachow RJ, Magoffin DA. Direct intraovarian effects of leptin: Impairment of the synergistic action of insulin-like growth factor-I on follicle-stimulating hormone-dependent estradiol-17 beta production by rat ovarian granulosa cells. Endocrinology. 1997;138:847-50.
33. Dunaif A, Segal KR, Futterweit W, et al. Profound peripheral insulin resistance, independent of obesity, in polycystic ovary syndrome. Diabetes. 1989;38:1165-74.
34. Diamanti-Kandarakis E, Zapanti E. Insulin sensitizers and antiandrogens in the treatment of polycystic ovary syndrome. Ann N Y Acad Sci. 2000;900:203-12.
35. Legro RS, Barnhart HX, Schlaff WD, et al. Clomiphene, metformin, or both for infertility in the polycystic ovary syndrome. N Engl J Med. 2007;356:551-66.
36. Legro RS, Myers E. Surrogate end-points or primary outcomes in clinical trials in women with polycystic ovary syndrome? Hum Reprod. 2004;19:1697-704.
37. Moll E, Bossuyt PM, Korevaar JC, et al. Effect of clomifene citrate plus metformin and clomifene citrate plus placebo on induction of ovulation in women with newly diagnosed polycystic ovary syndrome: Randomised double blind clinical trial. BMJ. 2006;332:1485.
38. Gerli S, Papaleo E, Ferrari A, et al. Randomized, double blind placebo-controlled trial: Effects of myo-inositol on ovarian function and metabolic factors in women with PCOS. Eur Rev Med Pharmacol Sci. 2007;11:347-54.
39. Ciotta L, Stracquadanio M, Pagano I, et al. Effects of myo-inositol supplementation on oocyte's quality in PCOS patients: A double blind trial. Eur Rev Med Pharmacol Sci. 2011;15:509-14.
40. Papaleo E, Unfer V, Baillargeon JP, et al. Myo-inositol may improve oocyte quality in intracytoplasmic sperm injection cycles. A prospective, controlled, randomized trial. Fertil Steril. 2009;91:1750-4.
41. Edwards RG. Maturation in vitro of mouse, sheep, cow, pig, rhesus monkey and human ovarian oocytes. Nature. 1965;208:349-51.
42. Trounson A, Wood C, Kausche A. In vitro maturation and the fertilization and developmental competence of oocytes recovered from untreated polycystic ovarian patients. Fertil Steril. 1994;62:353-62.
43. Child TJ, Phillips SJ, Abdul-Jalil AK, et al. A comparison of in vitro maturation and in vitro fertilization for women with polycystic ovaries. Obstet Gynecol. 2002;100:665-70.
44. Lin YH, Hwang JL, Huang LW, et al. Combination of FSH priming and hCG priming for in-vitro maturation of human oocytes. Hum Reprod. 2003;18:1632-6.
45. Requena A, Bronet F, Guillén A, et al. The impact of in-vitro maturation of oocytes on aneuploidy rate. Reprod Biomed Online. 2009;18:777-83.
46. Practice Committees of the American Society for Reproductive Medicine and the Society for Assisted Reproductive Technology. In vitro maturation: A committee opinion. Fertil Steril. 2013;99:663-6.

CHAPTER

39

Long-term Effects and Metabolic Syndrome in PCOS

Juan José Espinós

INTRODUCTION

Polycystic ovary syndrome (PCOS) is the most frequent endocrine disorder in women of childbearing age, affecting 6–20% of the female population.[1,2] PCOS is a heterogeneous entity of unknown origin characterized by an association of clinical and/or biochemical hyperandrogenism, chronic anovulation, infertility, and polycystic ovary.[3,4] The more frequently associated clinical symptoms are overweight or obesity (showing a specific accumulation of abdominal adipocytes) and hyperestrogenism secondary to peripheral aromatization of androgens. The reproductive alterations associated with PCOS tend to be present early on, just after menarche, manifesting to a greater or lesser extent during the second or third decade of the reproductive life and often go into spontaneous remission once subjects reach their 40s. It may be associated with, insulin resistance (IR), secondary hyperinsulinism (HI), and changes in the lipid profile.[5] As it is well-known, many of these disorders are risk factors for events that use to appear during the fifth or sixth decade of life, such as cardiovascular disease (CVD) or estrogen dependent reproductive neoplasms (Fig. 1). Not all patients are at equal risk, since every case has its own clinical profile and biochemical characteristics.[6] At the Rotterdam consensus meeting, four separate phenotypes of PCOS were identified, extended to 15 by the Androgen Excess Society (AES).[7,8] One of the most relevant common concepts emerging from these classifications is that the

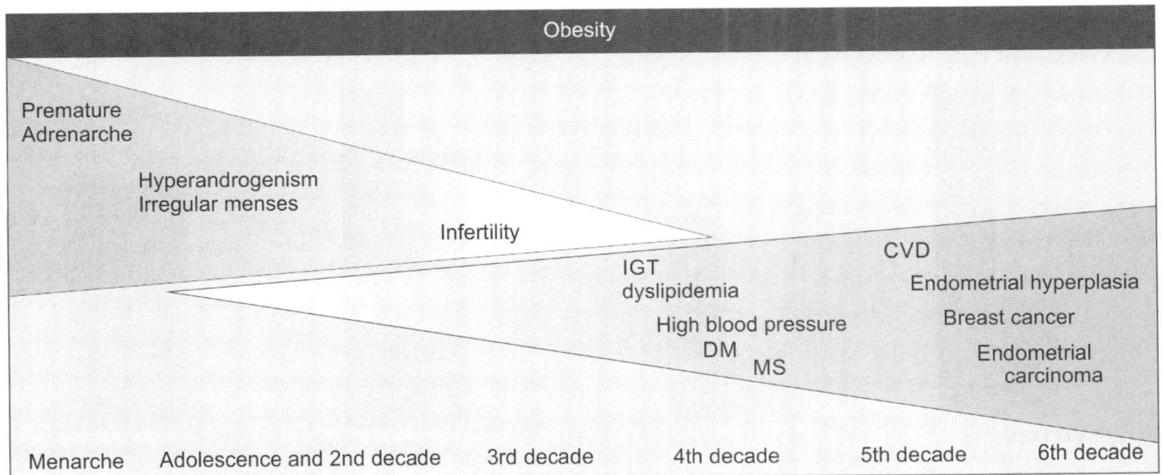

Fig. 1: Reproductive disorders and long-term effects associated with PCOS. (IGT: impaired glucose tolerance; DM: diabetes mellitus; MS: metabolic syndrome; CVD: cardiovascular disease)

classic phenotypes associated with hyperandrogenism and anovulation are those having the greatest number of long-term complications.[9]

INSULIN RESISTANCE, HYPERINSULINEMIA AND PCOS

The most relevant contribution to the understanding of the etiopathogeny of this syndrome is the identification of IR and the resulting HI as frequent accompanying endocrine changes to PCOS. Burghen et al. were the first to demonstrate the association between PCOS and HI, confirmed subsequently by others.[10,11] IR occurs in 50–80% of women with PCOS, and the differences between populations are attributable to different lifestyles and presence of genetic factors.[12-14] The prevalence also varies depending on the diagnostic criteria used, with 15–25% of the population affected when applying the Rotterdam criteria, whereas the figures rise to 20–45% if we choose the more classic classification of the National Institutes of Health (NIH).[15] There are also differences in terms of phenotype: 80% of women affected by the classical phenotype, 65% by the ovulatory, and 40% by the normoandrogenic.[16] Finally, there is a very tight connection with body mass index (BMI). The majority of insulin resistant women are overweight or obese, showing specifically an upper-body or central adiposity, although 10–15% of the PCOS women with normal weight may also be IR.[16]

In a study conducted in our center, including 299 consecutive PCOS patients evaluated between 2005 and 2010, the prevalence of IR was 48.8%, mainly in obese women (87%). This group of patients was somewhat older (27 years vs. 24.5 years), had a greater waist-hip ratio (WHR) (0.92 vs. 0.86) and a higher free androgen index (FAI) (12.3 vs. 8.1), consequence of a significant decrease in the levels of sex hormone binding globulin (SHBG; Fig. 2). In our population, the predictive factors for IR were a BMI above 25 kg/m^2 [sensitivity (S): 86.8%, specificity (Sp): 56.9%] and a SHBG below 31 nmol/L (S: 85.6%, Sp: 56.6%).

The potential mechanisms responsible for IR are a lower sensitivity of the insulin receptor and/or a postreceptor dysfunction. In many insulin resistant women, there is not a single identifiable factor, but rather, the origin of IR is multifactorial, with different degrees of genetic susceptibility associated to differing environmental and lifestyle factors. Intrinsic alterations in the processes of phosphorylation of the insulin receptors have been seen in women with PCOS. These changes are not linked to BMI or to the hormonal environment and lead to a lower insulin sensitivity and impaired glucose transport capacity.[11] The modern changes in lifestyle with a higher caloric intake not compensated by an increase in physical activity or impaired by sedentary influence negatively the situation.[17] Obesity, particularly of the upper body, also referred to as android or visceral, is the main cause of the increased frequency of IR that has been witnessed over recent decades. This relationship between central obesity and IR is mediated by an excess of free fatty acids (FFA). Abdominal adipocytes have a higher lipolytic activity as compared to those from other locations. The concentration and function of other factors, such as tumor necrosis factor α (TNFα), adiponectin, resistin or leptin in fat and at muscular tissue levels is also different in these cases.[18] The FFA, competes with glucose as a source of energy, inhibit glucose uptake via insulin, and promote the intracellular accumulation of lipids, ceramide, and diacylglycerol in muscle cells.[19,20]

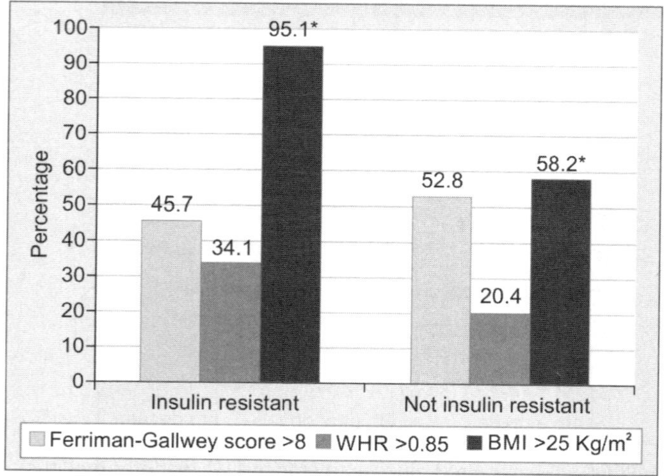

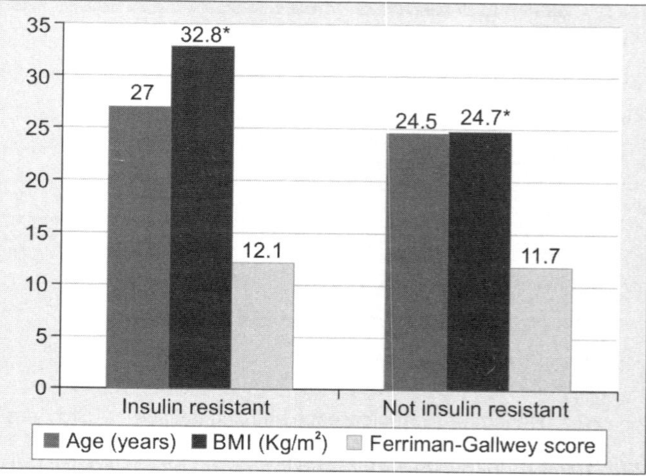

Fig. 2: General characteristics of PCOS patients in relation to the degree of insulin resistance (*P < 0.001).

The higher FFA disposal also increases the levels of hepatic triglycerides (TG), suppressing hepatic extraction of insulin and the inhibitory mechanisms on the hepatic production of glucose.[21,22] At long-term, the FFA activates apoptosis of the pancreatic β-cells leading to a reduction in their secretion capacity.[23] The high levels of TNFα found in obese women cause IR, by decreasing the autophosphorylation capacity of the insulin receptor and the insulin receptor substrate 1 (IRS 1). They also negatively regulate the genes responsible for the transport of glucose and the peroxisome proliferator-activated receptor γ (PPARγ), and induce lipolysis. Adiponectin, which is reduced in obese patients, increases the oxidation of fats and the phosphorylation of IRS in the muscle, reducing the expression of hepatic enzymes of gluconeogenesis, and inhibiting TNFα in the fatty tissue.[24,25]

OBESITY AND PCOS

Obesity is considered today one of the largest worldwide epidemics, affecting 60–75% of the adult population in developed countries, but also spreading in developing and undeveloped countries.[26,27] Its true prevalence in patients with PCOS is unknown, but it is estimated to be 2–3 times higher among these individuals than in the general population, and it is probably subjected to the same influences mentioned for IR.[28] It is more prevalent among the Caucasian population [RR (risk ratio) 10.79 (5.36–21.7)] than among other ethnicities, such as Asian women [RR 2.31 (1.33–4)]. The latter has also experienced an upward trend over recent decades, in some cases affecting up to 75% of the studied population. In our setting, a Western Mediterranean country, up to 64% of patients with PCOS are also found to be overweight or obese.[29]

Obese women suffering from PCOS have a higher incidence of menstrual disorders, hyperandrogenism, infertility, IR and HI, carbohydrate metabolism alterations and potentially greater cardiovascular risk than their normal weight counterparts. In the meta-analysis conducted by Lim et al., including 30 studies, it was demonstrated that these patients had lower levels of SHBG, higher levels of total testosterone (TT), FAI, insulin, the homeostasis model assessment (HOMA), glucose, total cholesterol (CT), low-density lipoprotein cholesterol (LCL-C) and TG and lower levels of high-density lipoprotein (HDL-C). This was more pronounced in cases of android obesity (upper body adiposity), probably due to the higher degree of IR. Obesity also contributes to the lower quality of life of these patients and the higher frequency of psychological disturbances including depression and anxiety.[29]

The influence of BMI on the severity of hirsutism or on the morphological characteristics of the ovary (ovarian volume and/or the presence of antral follicles) is not clear. In the case of hirsutism, it has been postulated that, in obese women, the peripheral conversion of androgens to estrogens is specially efficient and diminishes the amount of testosterone available to the androgenic receptor. Therefore, the relationship between obesity and phenotypic manifestations adopts a "J-shape".[30] It is also unclear if there are significant differences between overweight and obese women, in terms of the appearance and severity of the symptoms. Similarly happens in respect to establishing clear cut-off points allowing to consider the presence or absence of metabolic risk.

GLUCOSE INTOLERANCE AND DIABETES MELLITUS

Insulin resistance is recognized as an independent major risk factor for the development of impaired glucose tolerance (IGT) and type 2 diabetes mellitus (DM). Thus, PCOS is regarded as a risk factor for the development of abnormal glucose tolerance (AGT).

In the meta-analysis performed by Moran et al., the risk for IGT among PCOS women was 2.48 times higher than that found in the general population and more than four times higher [OR (odds ratio): 4.43 (4.06–4.82)] for DM.[31] These results were recently confirmed by a large Danish nationwide study [HR (heart rate) for DM of 4, 3.7–4.3, $p < 0.001$].[32] Among our population, AGT was present in 19% of the women: 11% had IGT and 8% had DM. These figures are clearly lower than those observed in Asian and American studies (ranging from 20% to 47%; Table 1).[33-41] The prevalence of AGT among patients with PCOS more than doubles that of non-PCOS women aged between 35 years and 44 years, with an incidence rate of 1.05% per women/year.[42,43] Glucose metabolism disturbances in PCOS patients tend to appear earlier and evolve more rapidly than in the general population.[44,45] Among women with PCOS, those with DM are older, more obese, have a higher waist/hip ratio and higher free testosterone levels than normal glucose tolerance (NGT) patients.[44,45]

As mentioned above, IR plays a leading role in the development of these disorders. Obesity, that is 3–4 times more prevalent in these cases, worsens the evolution to AGT. Thus a combination of genetic and environmental factors, such as dietary habits or sedentary lifestyle, seems to be determining in the development of AGT in PCOS patients.[46-50]

Table 1: Impaired glucose tolerance and diabetes mellitus in different PCOS population studies.[3]

Author	*Patients included (n)*	*Location*	*Age (years)*	*BMI (kg/m²)*	*IGT (%)*	*DM (%)*	*Normal (%)*
Legro RS et al.[33]	254	USA			31.1	7.5	61.4
Erhmann DA et al.[34]	122	USA	29	41	35	12	53
Weerakiet S et al.[35]	85	Thailand			20.3	17.7	62
Gambineri A et al.[36]	121	Italy	28.1	34.3	15.7	2.5	81.8
Chen X et al.[37]	102	China	25.4	23.07	20.5	1.9	77.6
Dabadghao P et al.[38]	372	Australia	30.3	35.1	15.6	4	80.4
Barcellos CR et al.[39]	85	Brasil	25.5	28.5	27	4.8	68.2
Espìnós JJ et al.[40]	103	Spain	26.7	30.2	10.7	7.7	81.6
Celik C et al.[41]	252	Turkey	24.8	26.1	14.3	2	83.7

(BMI: body mass index; DM: diabetes mellitus; IGT: impaired glucose tolerance)

METABOLIC SYNDROME

Gerard Reaven of the American Diabetes Association first described "Syndrome X" in 1988. Glucose intolerance was associated to hypertriglyceridemia, a decrease in HDL and arterial hypertension. Since then, this situation has been described with different names such as "resistance syndrome", "plurimetabolic syndrome", "the cardiovascular metabolic" or "the deadly quartet". Similarly, other components have been associated to the syndrome such as microalbuminuria, hyperferritinemia, hyperhomocysteinemia, hepatic steatosis, inflammatory markers or procoagulants such as C-reactive protein (CRP), plasminogen activator inhibitor-1 (PAI-1) or the fibrinogen or endothelial dysfunction markers.[51,52] Today, the most commonly used name is metabolic syndrome (MS), coined by the World Health Organization (WHO), which also proposed its first definition that has been subsequently updated.[53] There are up to five other ways of classifying this complex syndrome (Table 2), among them that of the National Cholesterol Education Program (NCEP) being the most frequently used in daily clinical practice.[53-58]

The prevalence of MS in the general population at a global level is virtually impossible to estimate. The percentage of affected women depends on the diagnostic criteria used (from 19% to 35%)[59] or on age (prevalence between 20 years and 29 years of 7%, increasing to 40% for 60–69 years olds).[17] There are also noteworthy geographical differences, with an average prevalence in the United States of 35%, slightly higher than in Europe (which is around 25%). The clinical importance of MS derives from its association with an increased risk (RR between 2 and 4) of coronary and/or cerebral disease, as well as a higher mortality rate due to cardiovascular events.[60-63]

The prevalence of MS in PCOS patients is higher than in the normal population, with an OR of 2.88 (2.4–3.45) and also in their relatives (parents and sisters).[64] The rates are varying depending on the country of origin (American studies had the highest percentages); age[65] or the PCOS diagnostic criteria used (the Rotterdam criteria leading to a lower prevalence) ranging from 0% to 46%.[66-71] In Spain, the overall prevalence of MS was 21.4% and the majority of the affected individuals were overweight or obese with 76.2% being insulin resistant.[72] Discrepancies exist on the extent to which obesity constitutes a determinant factor in the rising prevalence of MS in PCOS patients.[73] Of all the parameters defining MS, abdominal circumference or BMI are the most frequently altered (11–98%), followed by HDL-C (30–95%), arterial hypertension (7.7–70%), hypertriglyceridemia (5.5–56%) and hyperglycemia (0–43.5%). Thus, the most common association tends to be an abnormal abdominal circumference, high HDL-C and blood pressure (BP) or hypertriglyceridemia (Table 3).

PCOS AND CARDIOVASCULAR DISEASE

The evidences presented lead to assume that patients with PCOS have an increased risk of CDV appearing at an earlier age than among the nonpolycystic population. The most uniform and consistent observations are those relating PCOS to CDV risk factors or surrogate markers.[74] The association of PCOS with AGT and MS has already been mentioned. The results are less conclusive regarding hypertension or dyslipidemia.

PCOS patients have higher BP, TG and LDL-C and lower HDL-C than unaffected women[75-80] although the individual values tend to fall within the normal range. Holte et al. demonstrated that these patients had a higher prevalence of

Table 2: Definition of metabolic syndrome.

	WHO, 1999[53]	*EGIR, 1999*[54]	*NECP, 2001*[55]	*AAEC, 2003*[56]	*IDF, 2005*[57]	*AHA/NHLBI, 2005*[58]
Insulin resistance	Glucose captation < 25% after euglycemic clamp	Basal insulin > P75				
Basal glucose	≥ 6.1	≥ 6.1	≥ 6.1	≥ 6.1	≥ 5.6 or DM in treatment	≥ 5.6 or DM in treatment
2 hours glucose	≥ 7.8 or DM in treatment			≥ 7.8 Not in treatment of DM		
Abdominal circumference (cm) or WHR	> 0.85	≥ 80	≥ 88		≥ 80	> 88
BMI (kg/m^2)				≥ 25		
SBP/DBP (mm Hg)	≥ 140/90	≥ 140/90	≥ 130/85	≥ 130/85	≥ 130/85 or with treatment	≥ 130/85 or with treatment
TG (mmol/L)	≥ 1.7	≥ 2.0	≥ 1.7	≥ 1.7 or with treatment	≥ 1.7 or with treatment	≥ 1.7 or with treatment
HDL-C (mmol/L)	< 1	< 1	< 1.29	< 1	< 1.29 or with treatment	< 1.01 or with treatment
Diagnosis	IR, impaired fasting glucose or intolerance and two or more criteria including microalbuminuria	IR, and two or more criteria including glucose intolerance	Three or more criteria	Clinical	Central obesity and two or more criteria	Three or more criteria

(AACE: American Association of Clinical Endocrinologists; AHA: American Heart Association; BMI: body mass index; DBP: diastolic blood pressure; DM: diabetes mellitus; EGIR: European Group for the Study of Insulin Resistance; HDL-C: high-density cholesterol; IDF: International Diabetes Federation; NCEP: National Cholesterol Education Program; NHLBI: National Heart, Lung and Blood Institute; SBP: systolic blood pressure; TG: triglycerides; WHO: World Health Organization; WHR: waist-hip ratio)

Table 3: Performance measures for metabolic syndrome characteristics.[70]

	Patients (%)	*PPV*	*PNV*	*Specificity*	*Sensitivity*
WC > 88 cm	64.3	29	100	42.9	100
HDL-C < 1.30 mmol/L	43.9	40	98.1	65.8	94.7
TG ≥ 1.70 mmol/L	32.9	60	85.1	94.9	31.6
BP ≥ 130/85 mm Hg	9.2	43.8	92.3	72.7	77.8
Glucose ≥ 6.11 mmol/L	7.15	26	100	31.2	100

(BP: blood pressure; HDL-C: high-density cholesterol; PPV: predictive positive value; PNV: predictive negative value; WC: waist circumference)

labile BP with an increase in systolic pressure, mean blood pressure (MBP) and pulse, reflecting a prehypertensive state (Table 4).[81] Martins et al. found a two-fold higher prevalence of hypertension, as the consequence of an arterial muscle cells hypertrophy and a reduced vascular compliance related to the impairment of the endothelium dependent vasodilation.[82] Proinflammatory changes such as an increase in the levels of TNFα, interleukin-6 (IL-6), IL-17, IL-18 or CRP and a prothrombotic state due to an imbalance between the fibrinolytic and procoagulatory activities have also been described. The later are the result of modifications of factor VIIc, tissue plasminogen activator (tPA), fibrinogen, von Willebrand factor (vWF), PAI-1, thrombomodulin (TM), D-dimer or antithrombin III (AT-III).[83-87] Endothelial dysfunction with a lower nitrous oxide (N_2O)-dependent vasodilation capacity and an increase in reactivity, as shown by five-fold increase in the levels of endothelin-1[88-90] contribute to the vascular risk. A review by Sprung et al. reveals

Table 4: Differences in carbohydrate and lipid metabolisms and blood pressure among patients with PCOS in relation to the insulin sensitivity and a control group in our population (data not published).

	Insulin resistant PCOS (n = 42)	*Not insulin resistant PCOS (n = 56)*	*Control group (n = 51)*	*P-value*
Glucose (nmol/L)	5.8 ± 2[a]	4.8 ± 0.4[b]	4.8 ± 0.5[b]	[ab]p = 0.01
Insulin (pmol/L)	146 ± 61[a]	46.9 ± 20[b]	41.1 ± 17[b]	[ab]p < 0.001
SBP (mm Hg)	128.4 ± 18[a]	119.8 ± 13	118.4 ± 17[b]	[ab]p < 0.05
DBP (mm Hg)	80.7 ± 10.5[a]	75.1 ± 10.4	69.1 ± 12.2[b]	[ab]p = 0.01
TC (mmol/L)	4.9 ± 1	4.7 ± 0.9	4.6 ± 0.8	P = ns
Triglycerides (mmol/L)	1.43 ± 1.27[a]	0.92 ± 0.6	0.68 ± 0.22[b]	[ab]p < 0.05
HDL-C (mmol/L)	1.24 ± 0.3[a]	1.49 ± 0.4[b]	1.65 ± 0.3[b]	[ab]p < 0.001
LDL-C (mmol/L)	3.2 ± 1	3 ± 0.6	2.8 ± 0.7	p = ns
VLDL (mmol/L)	0.42 ± 0.2	0.66 ± 3	0.16 ± 0.1	p = ns
LDL size (nm)	25.9 ± 0.6[a]	26.2 ± 0.45	26.2 ± 0.5[b]	[ab]p < 0.05
Apo A (g/L)	1.36 ± 0.2[a]	1.46 ± 0.24	1.58 ± 0.2[b]	[ab]p = 0.001
Apo B (g/L)	0.91 ± 0.2[a]	0.82 ± 0.15	0.73 ± 0.2[b]	[ab]p = 0.002
Lp (a) (mg/L)	236 ± 267	372 ± 394	286 ± 250	p = ns
Homocysteine (mmol/L)	8.34 ± 2	8.9 ± 2.3	8.65 ± 2.1	p = ns
CRP (mg/L)	5.4 ± 5.5	4.6 ± 7.5	1.68 ± 1.9	p = ns

(Apo: Apo protein; CRP: C-reactive protein; DBP: diastolic blood pressure; HDL-C: high-density lipoprotein cholesterol; LDL-C: low-density lipoprotein cholesterol; Lp (a): Lipoprotein a; PCOS: polycystic ovary syndrome; SBP: systolic blood pressure; TC: total cholesterol; VLDL: very low-density lipoprotein)

a reduction of the brachial artery flow mediated dilatation which remains after controlling for age, BMI, and smoking. It may be related to hyperandrogenism and IR and worsens with increase in BMI.[91]

Different studies have been carried out with PCOS patients, assessing the degree of aortic and coronary calcification by angiography and tomography or evaluating the carotid intima-media thickness (CIMT) via ultrasound.[92,93] Guzick et al. found that in women over the age of 40, the CIMT was 0.68 mm, as compared to 0.63 mm in a control group.[94] However, a study by the same Pittsburg University group comparing 125 patients with 142 controls, found differences in CIMT only in the subgroup of women older than 45 years.[95] Meyer et al., reviewed 19 high quality studies and found, an increase of 0.072 (0.040–0.105), in the CIMT of patients with PCOS suggesting a higher risk of arteriosclerosis.[96] Wild et al., in 1990, were the first to discover that in women subjected to coronary catheterization, those having alterations, tended to have more frequently a history of hirsutism and acne.[97] Subsequently, Birdsall et al. reported that women with polycystic ovaries had more coronary segments with over 50% stenosis than women having normal follicle ovaries (1.7 as compared to 0.82).[98] Talbott et al. found, using tomographic techniques, that the prevalence and the extension of the coronary calcifications, were significantly higher in patients with PCOS. PCOS was predictive of coronary calcifications with an OR of 2.31.[99] Other related factors were obesity, smoking, HI or a low HDL-C.

The longitudinal prospective studies including patients from their early reproductive years until menopause and showing that PCOS patients have a greater prevalence of CVD are scarce. Retrospective studies do not lend uniform outcomes and lead to increased doubts. Dahlgren et al. in one of the first published studies, performed in a Swedish PCOS population with a mathematical model, found a RR of 7.4 for myocardial infarction (MI).[100] Talbott et al. identified women with hyperandrogenic anovulation and after a follow up of 10 years, found an OR for CVD events of 5.91.[101] Similar results were found by Shaw et al. (HR for fatal and nonfatal coronary heart disease (CHD) and stroke of 2.3 (1.4–3.8) or Solomon [RR 1.67 (1.35–2.06)].[102,103] Mani et al. found in a retrospective study with 2,300 women, that the prevalence of MI and angina was specifically increased in the group of women over the age of 65 years (27.3%).[104] The most recent data come from a Danish cohort of 18,112 PCOS patients and 52,769 controls between 1992 and 2012. The results show an HR of 1.4, confidence interval (CI) 95% 1.3–1.5, $p < 0.0001$ for CVD (excluding hypertension and dyslipidemia) with a number of total events of 6.4 in the study group vs. 4.5 in the control group. Age, BMI, BP, lipid profile and glycemic status were predictors of CVD.[105]

Four meta-analyses have been published until now with inconclusive results.[106-109] De Groot's study included five heterogeneous studies (two prospective and three retrospective) finding a RR for CHD or stroke of 2.02 (1.47–2.76), reduced to 1.55 (1.27–1.89) after adjusting by BMI. Anderson et al. included nine studies with no significant differences in regards to nonfatal CHD [OR of 1.63 (0.96–2.78)] or nonfatal stroke [OR of 1.6 (0.82–3.1)]. A subanalysis of the studies with only women over 45 years, showed an OR of 1.94 (1.19–3.17). Similar data were reported by Wild et al. showing a higher risk for stroke [OR 2.8 (1.1–7.1)].[105] Zhao et al. appreciated an increased risk of CVD after analyzing 10 studies that included 104,392 subjects (OR 1.3, 95% CI (1.13–1.84), however this was limited to CHD (OR = 1.44; 95% CI 1.13–1.84; p = 0.004) without significant association between PCOS and MI (OR = 1.01; 95% CI 0.68–1.51; p = 0.95). Finally, Zhou et al. found an increased risk of developing stroke (OR = 1.36; 95% CI 1.09–1.70; p = 0.007) but after pooling the five studies with risk estimates adjusted for BMI, the association between PCOS and stroke was attenuated, without reaching statistical significance (OR = 1.24; 95% CI 0.98–1.59). Neither was observed an increase of all-cause of death (OR = 1.21; 95% CI 0.88–1.66; p = 0.25). Wild et al. also showed a higher risk for stroke (OR = 2.8; 5% CI 1.1–7.1).[110]

Pierpoint et al., studying 800 women with pathological diagnosis of PCOS, did not find an increase in mortality due to coronary disease.[111] The same research group in a retrospective study with a 5 years follow-up period of a group with mean age of 56.7 years old failed to find differences in the prevalence of CHD (4.7% in women with PCOS as compared to 4% in the control group), in spite of a higher prevalence of risk factors in the study group.[110] Similar data were presented by Schmidt et al., in PCOS women ascertained by biopsy and older than 70 years, with a high prevalence of hypertension, hypercholesterolemia and hypertriglyceridemia, where the incidence of cardiovascular events and mortality rate was not different of that in a control population.[112]

These discrepancies could be the result of the lack of unification and consensus in the PCOS diagnostic criteria adopted by the different studies. It is interesting to note that the maximum incidence of CVD was found in women over the age of 60–65 years, with a temporary time gap with the reproductive disorders, questioning the causal link and also limiting the homogenization of the sample.[113,114] Furthermore, it should be noted that over time, the prevalence of risk factors such as obesity, hypertension, DM tend to be equivalent in all groups, regardless of the presence or not of PCOS.[115]

In summary, the lack of evidence does not necessarily imply its absence.[116] It might be argued that in lean not insulin resistant PCOS women, the negative impact of hyperandrogenism, particularly on the lipid profile, may lead to a significant increase in CVD risk that could be counterbalanced by the relative hyperestrogenism present in these patients. By contrast, obese women, particularly those having "central obesity" and sustained IR and HI, have clearly an increased risk.[117,118] Thus, PCOS, which in many cases is the consequence and not the cause of the metabolic alterations, should be considered to be a warning sign that appears early on and deserves specific cardio-healthy measures in order to prevent problems in older ages.

ONCOLOGIC RISK

Few studies have attempted to assess the risk of endometrial, ovarian, and breast cancer in patients suffering from PCOS, resulting in the publication of three meta-analyses.[119-121] The most consistent data refers to endometrial cancer, suggesting that PCOS patients have a risk that is 4–6 times greater than that of the general population, meaning an absolute risk of 13.1/100,000 women per year.[122] This has been attributed to the unopposed continuous estrogen stimulation. However, it has also been suggested that the increased risk may be caused by the coexistence of other risk factors such as obesity, common in this type of patients and independent risk factors for endometrial cancer. In the study by Fearnley et al., the RR of endometrial cancer was reduced from 4 (1.7–9.3) to 2.2 (0.9–5.7) after adjusting for BMI.[123] The concurrent presence of DM, MS, inflammation, infertility or the resulting nulliparity may also contribute to the increased risk. The majority of neoplasms detected in these cases use to be type I, which is that associated with an extended unopposed exposure to estrogens. These cases tend to appear at younger ages as compared to those of type II (associated with atrophy) and are well-differentiated and therefore have a good prognosis.

The results are less conclusive in respect to ovarian cancer. Infertility and nulliparity are known to favor an increased risk. However, many of these women do not ovulate and are contraceptive pills users for extended periods of time to regulate their menstrual cycles. These circumstances have been proven to be protective factors. In 1996, Schildkraut et al. reported a risk of 2.5, just the opposite to Pierpoint et al. who reported a lower mortality from ovarian cancer.[124,125] The meta-analysis of Barry et al., which included only three studies, found an OR of 1.41 (0.93–2.15). As with endometrial cancer, when women older than 54 years were excluded, the OR raised to 2.52

(1.08–5.89), suggesting that the risk was concentrated in the younger women. Recently, Gottschau et al. suggested a similar relationship, although the differences were not significant [OR 1.8 (0.8–3.2)].[126]

The data on breast cancer are limited suggesting a higher risk in PCOS patients almost two to three folds.[127,128] However Shobeiri and Jenabi in a review of eight studies including 45,470 participants and 243,064 person-year did not show any association between PCOS and the breast cancer risk in both, case-control studies (0.87; 95% CI 0.44–1.31) and cohort studies (1.18; 95% CI 0.93–1.43).[129]

There are in the literature some specific references to colon, kidney or brain cancers, but there are no biological bases to justify these associations.

RECOMMENDATIONS

The current evidence shows that some subsets of patients with PCOS could be at higher risk of CVD. These patients have been catalogued by the "Androgen Excess and Polycystic Ovary Syndrome Society" (AE-PCOS) as "at risk" when presenting with obesity, smoking, hypertension, dyslipidemia, subclinical vascular disease, IGT, family history of premature CVD (<55 years male and <65 years female) and "at high risk" if MS, DM, vascular or renal disease where accompanying disorders.

The main objective is to identify women eligible for prevention strategies. Therefore, the AE-PCOS recommends:[130]

1. Measure waist circumference, BMI and BP periodically.
2. Determine lipid profile including CT, LDL-C, HDL-C and TG every 2 years or earlier if there is a relevant weight increase.
3. Perform oral glucose tolerance test with 75 g in PCOS women if BMI more than 30 kg/m^2 or in normal weight females of 40 years and older, having family history of gestational diabetes or DM family members. Repeat every 2 years or earlier if additional risk factors are identified.
4. Periodic evaluation of the level of anxiety, depression and quality of life.

The Rotterdam group considered worth to screen all obese women (BMI ≥ 27 kg/m^2) with PCOS with an oral glucose tolerance test but a recent ESHRE/ASRM (European Society of Human Reproduction and Embryology/American Society for Reproductive Medicine) consensus meeting recommended to screen only in the following conditions: when hyperandrogenism coexist with anovulation, *Acanthosis Nigricans*, obesity (BMI > 30 kg/m^2, or > 25 kg/m^2 in Asian populations) and in women with a family history of DM.[131] There is a general agreement that fasting glucose or insulin measurements are not reliable to predict IGT or DM. Other options like the glucose:insulin ratio (G:I), quantitative insulin-sensitivity check index (QUICKI), homeostatic model assessment (HOMA) and hemoglobin A1c concentrations correlate well with glucose tolerance tests, but their predictive value is controversial (Table 5).

They have recently been published recommendations from a group led by the Australian National Health and Medical Research Council (NHMRC) Center for Research Excellence in Polycystic Ovary Syndrome in collaboration with ESHRE and ASRM and many other scientific societies and consumer groups. Based on all the evidences available to date, they recommend assessing for cardiovascular risk factors and global CVD risk all women with PCOS. The recommendations in relation to the prevention and detection of risk factors for CVD are given in the Table 6.[134]

The convenience to perform routine ultrasound evaluation or an endometrial biopsy in PCOS patients in order to rule out hyperplasia or endometrial cancer has not been conveniently evaluated. Its efficiency has not been proven in asymptomatic patients. Therefore, these studies should be reserved for cases with abnormal uterine bleeding.

Table 5: Cut-off points for the diagnosis of insulin resistance.

Study	*Population*	*Insulin (μU/mL)*	*G:I ratio*	*HOMA*	*QUICKI*
Kauffman et al.[47]	White women	>20	<7.2	>3.8	
Kauffman et al.[47]	Mexican American	>23	<4	>4.5	
Carmina and Lobo[132]	Italian	>12.1	<6.4	>47	<0.332
Legro et al.[133]	American		<4.5		
Espìnós et al.[40]	Spanish		<6.227	>2.643	<0.33

(HOMA: homeostasis model assessment; QUICKI: quantitative insulin-sensitivity check index)

Table 6: Summary of recommendations from the international evidence-based guideline group related to CVD risk.

- If screening reveals CVD risk factors (obesity, cigarette smoking, dyslipidemia, hypertension, impaired glucose tolerance, and lack of physical activity) women with PCOS should be considered at increased risk of CVD.
- Overweight and obese women with PCOS, regardless of age, should have a fasting lipid profile (cholesterol, LDL, HDL and triglyceride level at diagnosis). Thereafter, frequency of measurement should be based on the presence of hyperlipidemia and global CVD risk.
- All women with PCOS should have blood pressure measured annually, or more frequently based on global CVD risk.
- Glycemic status should be assessed at baseline in all women with PCOS. In high-risk women with PCOS (BMI > 25 kg/m^2 or in Asians > 23 kg/m^2, history of IFG, gestational diabetes, family history of DM, hypertension or high-risk ethnicity), an OGTT is recommended.
- Thereafter, assessment should be every 1–3 years, influenced by the presence of other diabetes risk factors.
- A 75 g OGTT should be offered in all women with PCOS preconception when planning pregnancy or seeking fertility treatment, given the high risk of hyperglycemia and the associated comorbidities in pregnancy. If not performed preconception, an OGTT should be offered at less than 20 weeks gestation, and all women with PCOS should be offered the test at 24–28 weeks gestation.

(BMI: body mass index; CVD: cardiovascular disease; DM: diabetes mellitus; IFG: impaired fasting glycemia; HDL: high-density lipoprotein; LDL: low-density lipoprotein; OGTT: oral glucose tolerance test; PCOS: polycystic ovary syndrome)

REFERENCES

1. Azziz R, Woods KS, Reyna R, et al. The prevalence and features of the polycystic ovary syndrome in an unselected population. J Clin Endocrinol Metab. 2004;89(6):2745-9.
2. Kauffman RP, Baker TE, Baker VM, et al. Endocrine and metabolic differences among phenotypic expressions of polycystic ovary syndrome according to the 2003 Rotterdam consensus criteria. Am J Obstet Gynecol. 2008;198(6):670.
3. Homburg R. What is polycystic ovarian syndrome? A proposal for consensus on the definition and diagnosis of polycystic ovarian syndrome. Hum Reprod. 2002;17(10):2495-9.
4. Azziz R. Androgen excess is the key element in polycystic ovarian syndrome. Fertil Steril. 2003;80(2):252-4.
5. Goodman NF, Cobin RH, Futterweit W, et al. American Association of Clinical Endocrinologists, American College of Endocrinology, and Androgen Excess and PCOS Society Disease State Clinical Review: guide to the best practices in the evaluation and treatment of polycystic ovary syndrome-part 1. Endocr Pract. 2015;21(11):1291-300.
6. Moran LJ, Norman RJ, Teede HJ. Metabolic risk in PCOS: phenotype and adiposity impact. Trends Endocrinol Metab. 2015;26(3):136-43.
7. Rotterdam ESHRE/ASRM-Sponsored PCOS Consensus Workshop Group. Revised 2003 consensus on diagnostic criteria and long-term health risks related to polycystic ovary syndrome. Fertil Steril. 2004;81(1):19-25.
8. Azziz R, Carmina E, Dewailly D, et al. Androgen Excess Society. Positions statement: criteria for defining polycystic ovary syndrome as a predominantly hyperandrogenic syndrome: an Androgen Excess Society guideline. J Clin Endocrinol Metab. 2006;91(11):4237-45.
9. Daan NM, Louwers YV, Koster MP, et al. Cardiovascular and metabolic profiles amongst different polycystic ovary syndrome phenotypes: who is really at risk? Fertil Steril. 2014;102(5):1444-51.
10. Burghen GA, Givens JR, Kitabchi AE. Correlation of hyperandrogenism with hyperinsulinism in polycystic ovarian disease. J Clin Endocrinol Metab. 1980;50(1):113-6.
11. Dunaif A. Insulin resistance and the polycystic ovary syndrome: mechanism and implications for pathogenesis. Endoc Rev. 1997;18(6):774-800.
12. Legro RS, Castracane VD, Kauffman RP. Detecting insulin resistance in polycystic ovary syndrome: purposes and pitfalls. Obstet Gynecol Surv. 2004;59(2):141-54.
13. Ciaraldi TP, el-Roeiy A, Madar Z, et al. Cellular mechanisms of insulin resistance in polycystic ovarian syndrome. J Clin Endocrinol Metab. 1992;75(2):577-83.
14. Nandi A, Chen Z, Patel R, et al. Polycystic ovary syndrome. Endocrinol Metab Clin North Am. 2014;43(1):123-47.
15. Diamanti-Kandarakis E, Dunaif A. Insulin resistance and the polycystic ovary syndrome revisited: an update on mechanisms and implications. Endocr Rev. 2012;33(6):981-1030.
16. Moghetti P, Tosi F, Bonin C, et al. Divergences in insulin resistance between the different phenotypes of the polycystic ovary syndrome. J Clin Endocrinol Metab. 2013;98(4):E628-37.
17. Ford ES, Giles WH, Dietz WH. Prevalence of the metabolic syndrome among US adults: findings from the third National Health and Nutrition Examination Survey. JAMA. 2002;287(3):356-9.
18. Lebovitz HE. Insulin resistance: definition and consequences. Exp Clin Endocrinol Diabetes. 2001;109 (Suppl 2):S135-48.
19. Adams JM II, Pratipanawatr T, Berria R, et al. Ceramide content is increased in skeletal muscle from obese insulin resistant humans. Diabetes. 2004;53(1):25-31.
20. Itani SI, Ruderman NB, Schmieder F, et al. Lipid induced insulin resistance in human muscle is associated with changes in diacylglycerol, protein kinase C, and IkappaB-alpha. Diabetes. 2002;51(7):2005-11.
21. Boden G, Cheung P, Stein TP, et al. FFA cause hepatic insulin resistance by inhibitin insulin suppression of glycogenolysis. Am J Physiol Endocrinol Metab. 2002;283(1):E12-9.
22. Wiesenthal SR, Sandhu H, McCall RH, et al. Free fatty acids impair hepatic insulin extraction in vivo. Diabetes. 1999;48(4):766-74.
23. Unger RH, Zhou YT. Lipotoxicity of beta-cells in obesity and in other causes of fatty acid spillover. Diabetes. 2001;50 (Suppl 1):S118-21.
24. Yamauchi T, Kamon J, Waki H, et al. The fat-derive hormone adiponectin reverses insulin resistance associated with both lipoatrophy and obesity. Nat Med. 2001;7(8):941-6.
25. Berg AH, Combs TP, Du X, et al. The adipocyte-secreted protein Acrp30 enhances hepatic insulin action. Nat Med. 2001;7(8):947-53.

26. Ruesten A, Steffen A, Floegel A, et al. Trend in obesity prevalence in European adult cohort populations during follow-up since 1996 and their predictions to 2015. PloS One. 2011;6(11):e27455.
27. Flegal KM, Carroll MD, Ogden CL, et al. Prevalence and trends in obesity among US adults, 1999-2008. JAMA. 2010;303(3):235-41.
28. Lim SS, Norman RJ, Davies MJ, et al. The effect of obesity on polycystic ovary syndrome: a systematic review and meta-analysis. Obes Rev. 2013;14(2):95-109.
29. Lim SS, Davies MJ, Norman RJ, et al. Overweight, obesity and central obesity in women with polycystic ovary syndrome: a systematic review and meta-analysis. Hum Reprod Update. 2012;18(6):618-37.
30. Marsden PJ, Murdoch AP, Taylor R. Tissue insulin sensitivity and body weight in polycystic ovary syndrome. Clin Endocrinol (Oxf). 2001;55(2):191-9.
31. Moran LJ, Misso ML, Wild RA, et al. Impaired glucose tolerance, type 2 diabetes and metabolic syndrome in polycystic ovary syndrome: a systematic review and meta-analysis. Hum Reprod Update. 2010;16(4):347-63.
32. Rubin KH, Glintborg D, Nybo M, et al. Development and risk factors of type 2 diabetes in a nationwide population of women with polycystic ovary syndrome. J Clin Endocrinol Metab. 2017;102(10):3848-57.
33. Legro RS, Kunselman AR, Dodson WC, et al. Prevalence and predictors of risk for type 2 diabetes mellitus and impaired glucose tolerance in polycystic ovary syndrome: a prospective, controlled study in 254 affected women. J Clin Endocrinol Metab. 1999;84(1):165-9.
34. Ehrmann DA, Barnes RB, Rosenfield RL, et al. Prevalence of impaired glucose tolerance and diabetes in women with polycystic ovary syndrome. Diabetes Care. 1999;22(1):141-6.
35. Weerakiet S, Srisombut C, Bunnag P, et al. Prevalence of type 2 diabetes mellitus and impaired glucose tolerance in Asia women with polycystic ovary syndrome. Internat J Gynecol Obst. 2001;75(2):177-84.
36. Gambineri A, Pelusi C, Manicardi E, et al. Glucose intolerance in a large cohort of Mediterranean women with polycystic ovary syndrome: phenotype and associated factors. Diabetes. 2004;53(9):2353-8.
37. Chen X, Yang D, Li L, et al. Abnormal glucose tolerance in Chinese women with polycystic ovary syndrome. Hum Reprod. 2006;21(8):2027-32.
38. Dabadghao P, Roberts BJ, Wang J, et al. Glucose tolerance abnormalities in Australian women with polycystic ovary syndrome. Med J Aust. 2007;187(6):328-31.
39. Barcellos CR, Rocha MP, Hayashida SA, et al. Prevalence of abnormalities of glucose metabolism in patients with polycystic ovary syndrome. Arq Bras Endocrinol Metabol. 2007;51(4):601-5.
40. Espinós-Gómez JJ, Corcoy R, Calaf J. Prevalence and predictors of abnormal glucose metabolism in Mediterranean women with polycystic ovary syndrome. Gynecol Endocrinol. 2009;25(3):199-204.
41. Celik C, Abali R, Bastu E, et al. Assessment of impaired glucose tolerance prevalence with hemoglobin A1c and oral glucose tolerance test in 252 Turkish women with polycystic ovary syndrome: a prospective, controlled study. Hum Reprod. 2013;28(4):1062-8.
42. Gambineri A, Patton L, Altieri P, et al. Polycystic ovary syndrome is a risk factor for type 2 diabetes: results from a long-term prospective study. Diabetes. 2012;61(9):2369-74.
43. Masia R, Sala J, Rohlfs I, et al. Prevalence of diabetes mellitus in the province of Girona, Spain: the REGICOR study. Rev Esp Cardiol. 2004;57(3):261-4.
44. Legro RS, Gnatuk CL, Kunselman AR, et al. Changes in glucose tolerance over time in women with polycystic ovary syndrome: a controlled study. J Clin Endocrinol Metab. 2005;90(6):3236-42.
45. Norman RJ, Masters L, Milner CR, et al. Relative risk of conversion from normoglycaemia to impaired glucose tolerance or non-insulin dependent diabetes mellitus in polycystic ovarian syndrome. Hum Reprod. 2001;16(9):1995-8.
46. Dunaif A, Sorbara L, Delson R, et al. Ethnicity and polycystic ovary syndrome are associated with independent and additive decreases in insulin action in Caribbean-Hispanic women. Diabetes. 1993;42(10):1462-8.
47. Kauffman R, Baker V, DiMarino P, et al. Polycystic ovarian syndrome and insulin resistance in white and Mexican American women: a comparison of two distinct populations. Am J Obstet Gynecol. 2002;187(5):1362-9
48. Wijeyaratne CN, Balen AH, Barth JH, et al. Clinical manifestations and insulin resistance (IR) in polycystic ovary syndrome (PCOS) among South Asians and Caucasians: is there a difference? Clin Endocrinol (Oxf). 2002;57(3):343-50.
49. DeUgarte CM, Bartolucci AA, Azziz R. Prevalence of insulin resistance in the polycystic ovary syndrome using the homeostasis model assessment. Fertil Steril. 2005;83(5):1454-60.
50. Carmina E, Koyama T, Chang L, et al. Does ethnicity influence the prevalence of adrenal hyperandrogenism and insulin resistance in polycystic ovary syndrome? Am J Obstet Gynecol. 1992;167(6):1807-12.
51. Reaven G. The metabolic syndrome or the insulin resistance syndrome? Different names, different concepts, and different goals. Endocrinol Metab Clin N Am. 2004;33(2):283-303.
52. Day C. Metabolic syndrome, or What you will: definitions and epidemiology. Diabetes Vasc Dis Res. 2007;4(1):32-8.
53. World Health Organisation Consultation. Definition, diagnosis and classification of diabetes mellitus and its complications. Part 1: diagnosis and classification of diabetes mellitus. Geneva: World Health Organisation; 1999. Report No. 9.2.
54. Balkau B, Charles MA. Comment on the provisional report from the WHO consultation. European Group for the Study of Insulin Resistance (EGIR). Diabet Med. 1999;16(5):442-3.
55. Executive summary of the third Report of the National Cholesterol Education Program (NCEP), Expert Panel on Detection, Evaluation, and Treatment of High Blood Cholesterol in Adults (Adult Treatment Panel). JAMA. 2001;285(19):2486-97.
56. Einhorn D, Reaven GM, Cobin RH, et al. American College of Endocrinology position statement on the insulin resistance syndrome. Endocr Pract. 2003;9(3):237-52.
57. 2006. The IDF consensus worldwide definition of the metabolic syndrome. [online] Available from http://www.idf.org/webdata/docs/MetS_def_update2006.pdf. [Accessed March, 2007].

58. Grundy SM, Cleeman JI, Daniels SR, et al. Diagnosis and management of the metabolic syndrome: an American Heart Association/National Heart, Lung and Blood Institute scientific statement. Circulation. 2005;112(17):2735-52.
59. The DECODE Study Group. Comparison of three different definitions for the metabolic syndrome in non-diabetic Europeans. Br J Diabetes Vasc Dis. 2005;5(3):161-8.
60. Hunt KJ, Resendez RG, Williams K, et al. National Cholesterol Education Program versus World Health Organization metabolic syndrome in relation to all-cause and cardiovascular mortality in the San Antonio Heart Study. Circulation. 2004;110(10):1251-7.
61. Ford ES. The metabolic syndrome and mortality from cardiovascular disease and all-causes: findings from the National Health and Nutrition Examination Survey II Mortality Study. Atherosclerosis. 2004;173(2):309-14.
62. McNeill AM, Rosamond WD, Girman CJ, et al. The metabolic syndrome and 11-year risk of incident cardiovascular disease in the atherosclerosis risk in communities study. Diabetes Care. 2005;28(2):385-90.
63. Rutter MK, Meigs JB, Sullivan LM, et al. C-reactive protein the metabolic syndrome prediction of cardiovascular events in the Framingham Offspring Study. Circulation. 2004;110(4):380-5.
64. Yilmaz B, Vellanki P, Ata B, et al. Metabolic syndrome, hypertension, and hyperlipidemia in mothers, fathers, sisters, and brothers of women with polycystic ovary syndrome: a systematic review and meta-analysis. Fertil Steril. 2018;109(2):356-64.
65. Apridonidze T, Essah PA, Iuorno NJ, et al. Prevalence and characteristics of the metabolic syndrome in women with polycystic ovary syndrome. J Clin Endocrinol Metab. 2005;90(4):1929-35.
66. Dokras A, Bochner M, Hollinrake E, et al. Screening women with polycystic ovary syndrome for metabolic syndrome. Obst Gynecol. 2005;106(1):131-7.
67. Ehrmann DA, Lijenquist DR, Kasza K, et al. Prevalence and predictors of the metabolic syndrome in women with polycystic ovary syndrome. J Clin Endocrinol Metab. 2006;91(1):48-53.
68. Vrbikova J, Vondra K, Cibula D, et al. Metabolic syndrome in young Czech women with polycystic ovary syndrome. Hum Reprod. 2005;20(12):3328-32.
69. Vural B, Caliskan E, Turkoz E, et al. Evaluation of metabolic syndrome frequency and premature carotid atherosclerosis in young women with polycystic ovary syndrome. Hum Reprod. 2005;20(9):2409-13.
70. Carmina E, Napoli N, Longo RA, et al. Metabolic syndrome in polycystic ovary syndrome (PCOS): lower prevalence in southern Italy than in the USA and the influence of criteria for the diagnosis of PCOS. Eur J Endocrinol. 2006;154(1):141-5.
71. Marcondes JA, Hayashida SA, Barcellos CR, et al. Metabolic syndrome in women with polycystic ovary syndrome: prevalence, characteristics and predictors. Arq Bras Endocrinol Metabol. 2007;51(6):972-9.
72. Espinós-Gómez JJ, Rodriguez-Espinosa J, Ordóñez-Llanos J, et al. Metabolic syndrome in Mediterranean women with polycystic ovary syndrome: when and how to predict its onset. Gynecol Endocrinol. 2012;28(4):264-8.
73. Panidis D, Macut D, Tziomalos K, et al. Prevalence of metabolic syndrome in women with polycystic ovary syndrome. Clin Endocrinol (Oxf). 2013;78(4):586-92.
74. Palomba S, Santagni S, Falbo A, et al. Complications and challenges associated with polycystic ovary syndrome: current perspectives. Int J Womens Health. 2015;7:745-63.
75. Legro RS, Blanche P, Krauss RM, et al. Alterations in low-density lipoprotein and high-density lipoprotein subclasses among Hispanic women with polycystic ovary syndrome: influence of insulin and genetic factors. Fertil Steril. 1999;72(6):990-5.
76. Legro RS, Kunselman AR, Dunaif A. Prevalence and predictors of dyslipidemia in women with polycystic ovary syndrome. Am J Med. 2001;111(8):607-13.
77. Elting MW, Korsen TJ, Bezemer PD, et al. Prevalence of diabetes mellitus, hypertension and cardiac complaints in a follow-up study of a Dutch PCOS population. Hum Reprod. 2001;16(3):556-60.
78. Lo JC, Feigenbaum SL, Yang J, et al. Epidemiology and adverse cardiovascular risk profile of diagnosed polycystic ovary syndrome. J Clin Endocrinol Metab. 2006;91(4):1357-63.
79. Pirwany IR, Fleming R, Greer IA, et al. Lipids and lipoprotein subfractions in women with PCOS: relationship to metabolic and endocrine parameters. Clin Endocrinol (Oxf). 2001;54(4):447-53.
80. Orbetzova MM, Shigarminova RG, Genchev GG, et al. Role of 24-hour monitoring in assessing blood pressure changes in polycystic ovary syndrome. Folia Med (Plovdiv). 2003;45(3):21-5.
81. Holte J, Gennarelli G, Berne C, et al. Elevated ambulatory day-time blood pressure in women with polycystic ovary syndrome: a sign of a pre-hypertensive state? Hum Reprod. 1996;11(1):23-8.
82. Martins Wde P, Soares GM, Vieira CS, et al. Cardiovascular risk markers in polycystic ovary syndrome in women with and without insulin resistance. Rev Bras Ginecol Obstet. 2009;31(3):111-6.
83. Wiltgen D, Spritzer PM. Variation in metabolic and cardiovascular risk in women with different polycystic ovary syndrome phenotypes. Fertil Steril. 2010;94(6):2493-6.
84. Samy N, Hashim M, Sayed M, et al. Clinical significance of inflammatory markers in polycystic ovary syndrome: their relationship to insulin resistance and body mass index. Dis Markers. 2009;26(4):163-70.
85. Yildiz BO, Haznedaroglu IC, Kirazli S, et al. Global fibrinolytic capacity is decreased in polycystic ovary syndrome, suggesting a prothrombotic state. J Clin Endocrinol Metab. 2002;87(8):3871-5.
86. Boulman N, Levy Y, Leiba R, et al. Increased C-reactive protein levels in the polycystic ovary syndrome: a marker of cardiovascular disease. J Clin Endocrinol Metab. 2004;89(5):2160-5.
87. Atiomo WU, Bates SA, Condon JE, et al. The plasminogen activator system in women with polycystic ovary syndrome. Fertil Steril. 1998;69(2):236-41.
88. Paradisi G, Steinberg HO, Hempfling A, et al. Polycystic ovary syndrome is associated with endothelial dysfunction. Circulation. 2001;103(10):1410-5.

89. Kelly CJ, Speirs A, Gould GW, et al. Altered vascular function in young women with polycystic ovary syndrome. J Clin Endocrinol Metab. 2002;87(2):742-6.
90. Diamanti-Kandarakis E, Spina G, Kouli C, et al. Increased endothelin-1 levels in women with polycystic ovary syndrome and the beneficial effect of metformin therapy. J Clin Endocrinol Metab. 2001;86(10):4666-73.
91. Sprung VS, Atkinson G, Cuthbertson DJ, et al. Endothelial function measured using flow-mediated dilation in polycystic ovary syndrome: a meta-analysis of the observational studies. Clin Endocrinol (oxf). 2013;78(3):438-46.
92. Luque-Ramirez M, Mendieta-Azcona C, Alvarez-Blasco F, et al. Androgen excess is associated with the increased carotid intima-media thickness observed in young women with polycystic ovary syndrome. Hum Reprod. 2007;22(12):3197-203.
93. Talbott EO, Zborowski JV, Rager JR, et al. Evidence for an association between metabolic cardiovascular syndrome and coronary and aortic calcification among women with polycystic ovary syndrome. J Clin Endocrinol Metab. 2004;89(11):5454-61.
94. Guzick DS, Talbott EO, Sutton-Tyrrell K, et al. Carotid atherosclerosis in women with polycystic ovary syndrome: initial results from a case-control study. Am J Obstet Gynecol. 1996;174(4):1224-9.
95. Talbott EO, Guzick DS, Sutton-Tyrrell K, et al. Evidence for association between polycystic ovary syndrome and premature carotid atherosclerosis in middle-aged women. Arterioscler Thromb Vasc Biol. 2000;20(11):2414-21.
96. Meyer ML, Malek AM, Wild RA, et al. Carotid artery intima-media thickness in polycystic ovary syndrome: a systematic review and meta-analysis. Hum Reprod Update. 2012;18(2):112-26.
97. Wild RA, Grubb B, Hartz A, et al. Clinical signs of androgen excess as risk factors for coronary artery disease. Fertil Steril. 1990;54(2):255-9.
98. Birdsall MA, Farquhar CM, White HD. Association between polycystic ovaries and extent of coronary artery disease in women having cardiac catheterization. Ann Intern Med. 1997;126(1):32-5.
99. Talbott EO, Guzick DS, Sutton-Tyrrell K, et al. Evidence for association between polycystic ovary syndrome and premature carotid atherosclerosis in middle-aged women. Arterioscler Thromb Vasc Biol. 2000;20(11):2414-21.
100. Dahlgren E, Janson PO, Johansson S, et al. Polycystic ovary syndrome and risk for myocardial infarction: evaluated from a risk factor model based on a prospective population study of women. Acta Obstet Gynecol Scand. 1992;71(8):599-604.
101. Talbott EO, Zborowski JV, Sutton-Tyrrell K, et al. Cardiovascular risk in women with polycystic ovary syndrome. Obstet Gynecol Clin North Am. 2001;28(1):111-33.
102. Shaw LJ, Bairey Merz CN, Azziz R, et al. Postmenopausal women with a history of irregular menses and elevated androgen measurements at high risk for worsening cardiovascular event-free survival: results from the National Institutes of Health-National Heart, Lung, and Blood Institute sponsored women's ischemia syndrome evaluation. J Clin Endocrinol Metab. 2008;93(4):1276-84.
103. Solomon CG, Hu FB, Dunaif A, et al. Menstrual cycle irregularity and risk for future cardiovascular disease. J Clin Endocrinol Metab. 2002;87(5):2013-7.
104. Mani H, Levy MJ, Davies MJ, et al. Diabetes and cardiovascular events in women with polycystic ovary syndrome: a 20-year retrospective cohort study. Clin Endocrinol (Oxf). 2013;78(6):926-34.
105. Glintborg D, Rubin KH, Nybo M, et al. Cardiovascular disease in a nationwide population of Danish women with polycystic ovary syndrome. Cardiovasc Diabetol. 2018;17(1):37.
106. De Groot PC, Dekkers OM, Romijn JA, et al. PCOS, coronary heart disease, stroke and the influence of obesity: a systematic review and meta-analysis. Hum Reprod Update. 2011;17(4):495-500.
107. Anderson SA, Barry JA, Hardiman PJ. Risk of coronary heart disease and risk of stroke in women with polycystic ovary syndrome: a systematic review and meta-analysis. Int J Cardiol. 2014;176(2):486-7.
108. Zhou Y, Wang X, Jiang Y, et al. Association between polycystic ovary syndrome and the risk of stroke and all-cause mortality: insights from a meta-analysis. Gynecol Endocrinol. 2017;33(12):904-10.
109. Zhao L, Zhu Z, Lou H, et al. Polycystic ovary syndrome (PCOS) and the risk of coronary heart disease (CHD): a meta-analysis. Oncotarget. 2016;7(23):33715-21.
110. Wild S, Pierpoint T, Jacobs H, et al. Long-term consequences of polycystic ovary syndrome: results of a 31 year follow-up study. Hum Fertil (Camb). 2000;3(2):101-5.
111. Pierpoint T, McKeigue PM, Isaacs AJ, et al. Mortality of women with polycystic ovary syndrome at long-term follow-up. J Clin Epidemiol. 1998;51(7):581-6.
112. Schmidt J, Landin-Wilhelmsen K, Brännström M, et al. Cardiovascular disease and risk factors in PCOS women of postmenopausal age: a 21-year controlled follow-up study. J Clin Endocrinol Metab. 2011;96(12):3794-803.
113. Legro RS. Polycystic ovary syndrome and cardiovascular disease: a premature association? Endocr Rev. 2003;24(3):302-12.
114. Cho LW, Randeva HS, Atkin SL. Cardiometabolic aspects of polycystic ovarian syndrome. Vasc Health risk Manag. 2007;3(1):55-63.
115. Welt CK, Carmina E. Clinical review: Lifecycle of polycystic ovary syndrome (PCOS): from in utero to menopause. J Clin Endocrinol Metab. 2013;98(12):4629-38.
116. Engin-Ustun Y, Ustun Y, Meydanli MM, et al. Are polycystic ovaries associated with cardiovascular disease risk as polycystic ovary syndrome? Gynecol Endocrinol. 2006;22(6):324-8.
117. Meyer C, McGrath BP, Teede HJ. Overweight women with polycystic ovary syndrome have evidence of subclinical cardiovascular disease. J Clin Endocrinol Metab. 2005;90(10):5711-6.
118. Haffner SM. Abdominal adiposity and cardiometabolic risk: do we have all the answers? Am J Med. 2007;120(9 Suppl 1):S10-6.
119. Chittenden BG, Fullerton G, Maheshwari A, et al. Polycystic ovary syndrome and the risk of gynaecological cancer: a systematic review. Reprod Biomed Online. 2009;19(3):398-405.

120. Haoula Z, Salman M, Atiomo W. Evaluating the association between endometrial cancer and polycystic ovary syndrome. Hum Reprod. 2012;27(5):1327-31.
121. Barry JA, Azizia MM, Hardiman PJ. Risk of endometrial, ovarian and breast cancer in women with polycystic ovary syndrome: a systematic review and meta-analysis. Hum Reprod Update. 2014;20(5):748-58.
122. Gottschau M, Kjaer SK, Jensen A, et al. Risk of cancer among women with polycystic ovary syndrome: A Danish cohort study. Gynecol Oncol. 2015;136(1):99-103.
123. Fearnley EJ, Marquart L, Spurdle AB, et al. Polycystic ovary syndrome increases the risk of endometrial cancer in women aged less than 50 years: an Australian case-control study. Cancer Causes Control. 2010;21(12):2303-8.
124. Schildkraut JM, Schwingl PJ, Bastos E, et al. Epithelial ovarian cancer risk among women with polycystic ovary syndrome. Obstet Gynecol. 1996;88(4 Pt 1):554-9.
125. Pierpoint T, McKeigue PM, Isaacs AJ, et al. Mortality of women with polycystic ovary syndrome at long-term follow-up. J Clin Epidemiol. 1998;51(7):581-6.
126. Gottschau M, Kjaer SK, Jensen A, et al. Risk of cancer among women with polycystic ovary syndrome: a Danish cohort study. Gynecol Oncol. 2015;136(1):99-103.
127. Shen CC, Yang AC, Hung JH, et al. A nationwide population-based retrospective cohort study of the risk of uterine, ovarian and breast cancer in women with polycystic ovary syndrome. Oncologist. 2015;20(1):45-9.
128. Kim J, Mersereau JE, Khankari N, et al. Polycystic ovarian syndrome (PCOS), related symptoms/sequelae, and breast cancer risk in a population-based case-control study. Cancer Causes Control. 2016;27(3):403-14.
129. Shobeiri F, Jenabi E. The association between polycystic ovary syndrome and breast cancer: a meta-analysis. Obstet Gynecol Sci. 2016;59(5):367-72.
130. Wild RA, Carmina E, Diamanti-Kandarakis E, et al. Assessment of cardiovascular risk and prevention of cardiovascular disease in women with the polycystic ovary syndrome: a consensus statement by the Androgen Excess and Polycystic Ovary Syndrome (AE-PCOS) Society. J Clin Endocrinol Metab. 2010;95(5):2038-49.
131. Fauser BC, Tarlatzis BC, Rebar RW, et al. Consensus on women's health aspects of polycystic ovary syndrome (PCOS): the Amsterdam ESHRE/ASRM-Sponsored 3rd PCOS Consensus Workshop Group. Fertil Steril. 2012;97(1):28-38.
132. Carmina E, Lobo RA. Use of fasting blood to assess the prevalence of insulin resistance in women with polycystic ovary syndrome. Fertil Steril. 2004;82(3):661-5.
133. Legro RS, Finegood D, Dunaif A. A fasting glucose to insulin ratio is a useful measure of insulin sensitivity in women with polycystic ovary syndrome. J Clin Endocrinol Metab. 1998;83(8):2694-8.
134. Teede HJ, Misso ML, Costello MF, et al. Recommendations from the international evidence-based guideline for the assessment and management of polycystic ovary syndrome. Fertil Steril. 2018;110(3):364-79.

CHAPTER

40

Thyroid Dysfunction and Infertility: An Intertwined Relationship

Shashank Joshi

THYROID DYSFUNCTION AND INFERTILITY: A SIGNIFICANT CORRELATION

Infertility is a worldwide issue that has been reported to affect approximately 8–10% of the couples.[1] As per the WHO estimates, the prevalence of primary infertility in India is reported to be around 3.5–16.8%.[2] Thyroid disease that is undiagnosed and untreated causes infertility as well as sub-fertility in women.[3] Thyroid disorders such as hyperthyroidism and hypothyroidism have profound effects on metabolism of androgen and estrogen, menstrual function, and fertility.[1] These affect fertility in various ways and result in luteal phase defect, high prolactin (PRL) levels, anovulatory cycles, imbalance of sex hormones, delayed onset of puberty, infertility, and miscarriages.[1,3] Therefore, normal functioning of the thyroid gland is essential for fertility during the earlier days of conception and sustaining a healthy pregnancy in women.[3]

Mechanism of ovulatory dysfunction in hypothyroidism is due to numerous interactions of thyroid hormones with the female reproductive system. Direct effect of thyroid hormones on the gonads occurs by modulation of T3 actions on follicle-stimulating hormone (FSH), luteinizing hormone (LH), and steroid biosynthesis. Thyroid hormones also synergize with the FSH-mediated LH/human chorionic gonadotropin (hCG) receptor to exert direct stimulatory effects on granulosa cell function and progesterone production. Figure 1 shows the different mechanisms for anovulation.

In hyperthyroidism, the serum thyroid-stimulating hormone (TSH) is suppressed and this was more frequent in all infertile women when thyroid peroxidase antibodies (Anti-TPO) were positive as compared to women who were not TPO-Abs positive (7 vs. 1%; P <0.05). It is also associated with reduced fertility and low progesterone levels.[4] Hormonal changes in thyrotoxicosis are given in the Figure 2.

Diagnosis and treatment of subclinical hypothyroidism is important in infertile women planning to conceive.[4,5]

Evaluation of thyroid function is essential in women wanting to conceive and having a family history of thyroid problem or irregular menstrual cycle or has had more than two miscarriages. Assessing the blood TSH levels can help in detecting hypothyroidism easily.

Priya et al. studied the prevalence of hypothyroidism in 95 infertile women and evaluated the response of treatment for hypothyroidism on infertility.[1]
Their study findings revealed that:

- Of all the infertile women, around 53.7% were found to be hypothyroid (TSH>4.6 μIU/mL; Fig. 3) which was high.

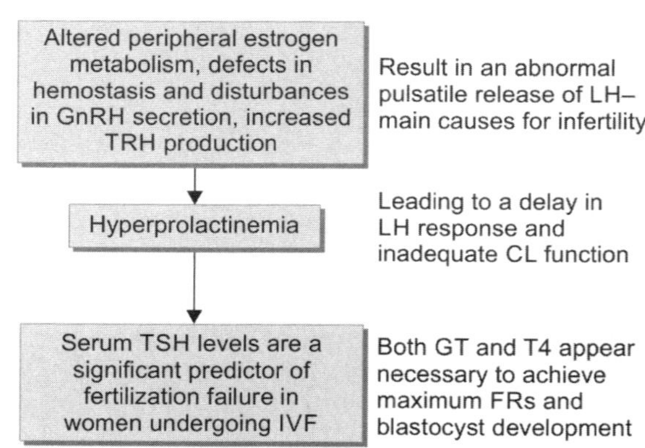

Fig. 1: Mechanism of thyroid dysfunction in hypothyroidism. (CL: corpus luteum; GT: gonadotropins; IVF: in vitro fertilization; LH: luteinizing hormone; TSH: thyroid-stimulating hormone; FRs: fertilization rates)

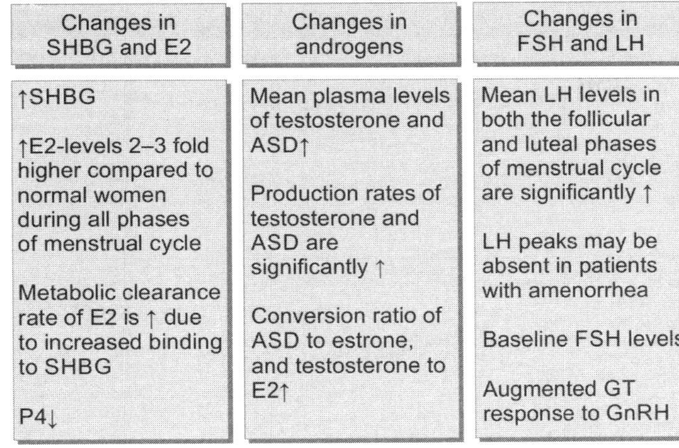

Fig. 2: Hormonal changes in hyperthyroidism. (ASD: androstenedione; E2: estradiol; FSH: follicle-stimulating hormone; GT: gonadotropins; GnRH: gonadotropin-releasing hormone; LH: luteinizing hormone; P4: progesterone; SHBG: sex hormone binding globulin)

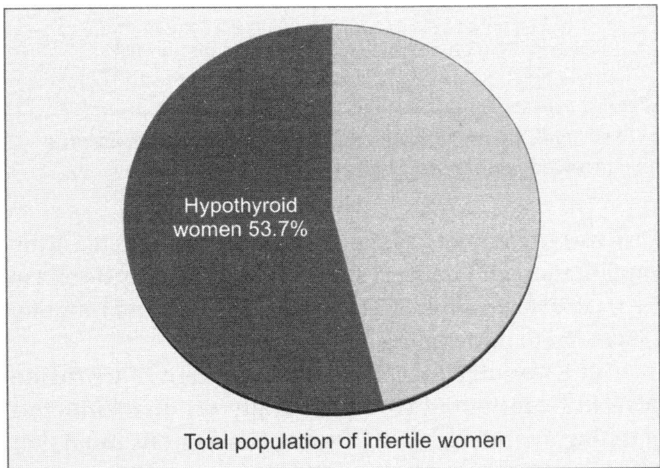

Fig. 3: Prevalence of hypothyroidism in infertile women.

- Of the hypothyroid women, around 50.5% had subclinical hypothyroidism and 3.2% had overt hypothyroidism.

INCREASED PREVALENCE OF HYPOTHYROIDISM IN WOMEN WITH INFERTILITY, PCOD, AND MENSTRUAL DISTURBANCES

Researchers determined thyroid disorders which were associated with reproductive disturbances in women.[6] Thyroid function profile including TSH, free T4 (FT4), and free T3 (FT3) were collected and analyzed. Findings were as follows:

- Of the 1192 patients, 63.8% were euthyroid, 27.5% were hypothyroid, 2.09% were hyperthyroid, and 6.54% of them had a mildly suppressed TSH. Of the hypothyroid patients, 6.7% of them were clinically hypothyroid and 20.8% subclinical hypothyroid.
- Around 34.9% of the patients were diagnosed for either primary or secondary infertility, 31.7% for polycystic ovarian disease (PCOD) and 33.3% for menstrual irregularities like oligomenorrhea, amenorrhea, polymenorrhagia, menorrhagia, and hypomenorrhea due to various causes.
- *The prevalence of hypothyroidism was observed to be on higher side among patients with infertility, PCOD, and menstrual disturbances compared with other thyroid dysfunctions (Table 1).*

BENEFITS OF THYROXINE TREATMENT IN INFERTILE WOMEN

Management of thyroid dysfunction can restore normal fertility in women. Hence, it is very important to regularly screen thyroid abnormalities among women with infertility.[7] The American Association of Clinical Endocrinologists and American Thyroid Association (AACE/ATA) clinical practice guidelines for hypothyroidism recommend thyroxine therapy in women of childbearing age and planning a pregnancy including assisted reproduction in the immediate future.[8]

Thyroxine Treatment Increases the Rates of Conception and Enhances Fertility

In the study by Priya et al., of the subclinical hypothyroid (50.5%) infertile women, 33.3% conceived after thyroxine treatment. Of these, 6.3% conceived within 6 months of therapy, 25% conceived after 6 months to 1-year of therapy and rest 68.7% conceived after 1–2 years of therapy. Around 50% of euthyroid women positive for antithyroid antibodies conceived.[1]

Yoshioka et al. determined the effects of thyroxine therapy on pregnancy rates and pregnancy outcomes in infertile patients with subclinical hypothyroidism (SCH). It was found that around 84.1% of women conceived successfully during the thyroxine treatment period (Group A) and the others remained infertile (Group B). Findings revealed:[9]

- A significant decrease was observed in the median TSH value in group A during thyroxine treatment (1.25 μIU/mL vs. 5.46 μIU/mL; $p<0.001$, Fig. 4A).
- A significantly shorter duration until pregnancy was observed after thyroxine treatment compared with estimated duration of infertility before treatment (0.9 ± 0.9 years vs. 2.8 ± 1.7 years; $p<0.001$, Fig. 4B).

Table 1: Distribution of thyroid disorders among reproductive problems.

	Euthyroid (%)	*Hypothyroid (%)*	*Hyperthyroid (%)*	*Mildly suppressed TSH (%)*
Infertility	58	32.3	3.1	6.4
Polycystic ovarian disease	68.5	24.8	1.0	5.8
Menstrual irregularities	65.4	24.9	1.2	7.3

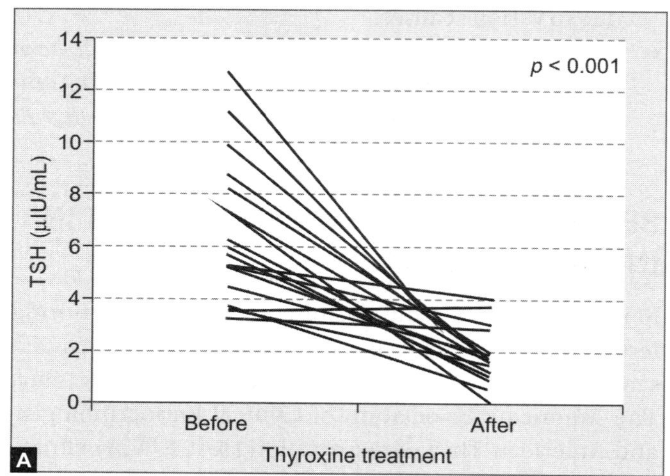

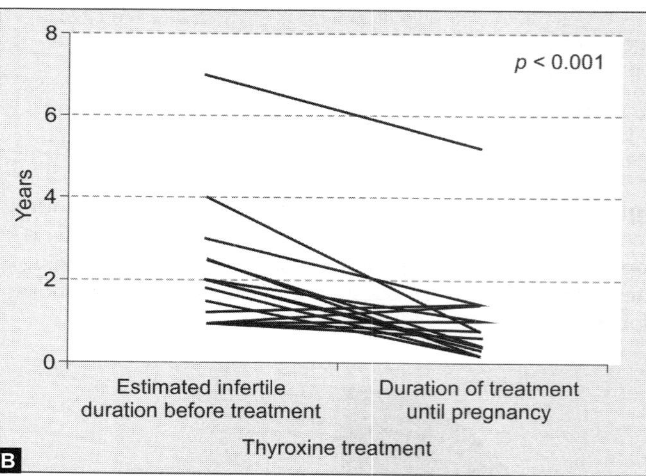

Figs. 4A and B: Comparison of serum thyroid-stimulating hormone (TSH) levels (A) and infertile duration (B) before and after the thyroxine treatment in patients who conceived spontaneously.[9]

- In group A, shortening of the infertile period was observed in patients treated with assisted reproductive technology (ART) as well as in those who conceived spontaneously after the thyroxine therapy.

Therefore, thyroxine therapy enhanced fertility in infertile patients with SCH as shown by high successful pregnancy rate and shorter duration of infertility until pregnancy.

GUIDELINE RECOMMENDATION FROM INTERNATIONAL SOCIETIES ON SCREENING AND TREATMENT OF THYROID DISORDERS IN INFERTILITY

The guideline recommendations are described in Table 2.

Interpreting Results

Results of thyroid evaluation are interpreted in Table 3.

When to Treat Subclinical Hypothyroidism in Infertile Patients?

Infertile women in whom thyroid function has been assessed by measuring TSH can be intervened. Most of the guidelines suggest thyroxine replacement in those with SCH. Thyroxine treatment has shown to significantly increase the implantation and delivery rate, and significantly decrease the miscarriage rate in SCH women, thyroid autoimmunity (TAI) or both undergoing ART.[8]

The ETA guidelines suggest adjustment of thyroxine dose in hypothyroid women already on thyroxine and planning to undergo ART.[8] A study has demonstrated that 84% of women on thyroxine replacement therapy required an increase of dosage during pregnancy achieved through IVF. This dosage adjustment was required very early, around 5–7 weeks of pregnancy.[11] Table 4 presents the recommendations of ASRM, ATA, Endocrine Society, and ETA on intervention policies in infertile women before conception or during pregnancy.[8]

Association of Prolactin Levels and Infertility

Hyperprolactinemia in woman is characterized as an abnormally high level of prolactin in the blood (normal level = 10–35 ng/mL). The prevalence of hyperprolactinemia among asymptomatic population with infertility is around 5%. Hyperprolactinemic patients usually have an inconstant ovulation, chronic anovulation, and defects in the luteal phase. Hyperprolactinemia impairs pulsatile secretion of gonadotropin-releasing hormone (GnRH) impairing the pituitary production of FSH and LH and hence interfering with ovulation.[11]

Table 2: Guidelines of international societies regarding investigation approaches in infertile women before or during pregnancy.[10]

Society	*Before ovarian stimulation*	*During ovarian stimulation*	*During (early) pregnancy*
ASRM	It is reasonable to test TSH in infertile women attempting pregnancy	No recommendation	No recommendation
ATA	Women with infertility should have screening with TSH, as part of their infertility work-up	There is insufficient evidence to recommend for or against screening for thyroid antibodies in women undergoing IVF	Serum TSH values should be obtained early in pregnancy in women at high risk for overt hypothyroidism (including those with infertility)
ES	Individuals at high risk for thyroid illness (including infertile women or those with known thyroid disease) should be identified before pregnancy and TSH should be measured Universal screening for anti-TPO antibodies before pregnancy is not recommended	No recommendation	No agreement regarding screening recommendations for all newly pregnant women Universal screening for anti-TPO antibodies during pregnancy is not recommended
ETA	No recommendation	No recommendation	Trimester-specific reference ranges for TSH and T4 (total or free) should be established in each antenatal hospital setting. If not available, the following reference range upper limits are recommended: *First trimester:* 2.5 mIU/mL, *Second trimester:* 3.0 mIU/mL, *Third trimester:* 3.5 mIU/mL In hypothyroid women, already treated with thyroxine before conception, TSH should be checked every 4 weeks during the first trimester and once during the second and third trimesters

(Anti-TPO: thyroid peroxidase antibodies; ASRM: American Society of Reproductive Medicine; ATA: American Thyroid Association; ES: Endocrine Society (US); ETA: European Thyroid Association; IVF: in-vitro fertilization; LT4: levothyroxine; SCH: subclinical hypothyroidism; T4: thyroxine; TSH: thyroid-stimulating hormone)

Table 3: Interpreting results of thyroid evaluation.

	High T4	*Normal T4*	*Low T4*
High TSH	Irregular use of thyroxine Amiodarone Pituitary hyperthyroidism (TSH-producing pituitary tumor-rare) Thyroid hormone resistance (rare)	Subclinical hypothyroidism T4 under replacement	Primary hypothyroidism
Normal TSH	As above Some drugs (steroids, β-blockers, NSAIDs) Non-thyroidal illness T4 replacement (sometimes stabilizes with normal TSH and ↑FT4)	Normal	Some drugs (anticonvulsants, anti-T3, anti-T4) Pituitary or hypothalamic hypothyroidism Severe nonthyroidal illness
Low TSH	Primary hyperthyroidism	Subclinical hyperthyroidism Subtle T4 over replacement Nonthyroidal illness	Pituitary or hypothalamic hypothyroidism Severe nonthyroidal illness

(TSH: thyroid-stimulating hormone; T4: thyroxine)

Correlation Between Hypothyroidism and Hyperprolactinemia

A close association is observed between hypothyroidism and hyperprolactinemia. In hypothyroidism, there is an increased production of thyrotropin-releasing hormone (TRH), which in turn stimulates pituitary to secrete TSH and prolactin, leading to hyperprolactinemia and infertility.[11] Clinical evidences suggesting the association of thyroid hormone imbalance and prolactin levels with infertility are given in Table 5.

Therefore, the measurement of thyroid hormones and serum prolactin has been considered an important component of infertility work-up in women.[12]

Table 4: Guidelines of international societies regarding intervention approaches in infertile women before or during pregnancy.[10]

Society	*Before ovarian stimulation*	*During ovarian stimulation*	*During (early) pregnancy*
ASRM	If TSH exceeds the nonpregnant laboratory reference range (typically >4mIU/mL) patients should be treated with thyroxine to maintain TSH <2.5 mIU/mL If TSH is between 2.5 mIU/mL and 4 mIU/mL, either monitor TSH and treat when TSH >4 mIU/mL, or treat to maintain TSH <2.5 mIU/mL If repeated TSH values are >2.5 mIU/mL or when other risk factors for thyroid disease are present, test for anti-TPO antibodies If anti-TPO antibodies are present, test TSH and treat if TSH is >2.5 mIU/mL	No recommendation	During the first trimester of pregnancy, it is advisable to treat when TSH is >2.5 mIU/mL
ATA	No recommendation	There is insufficient evidence to recommend for or against thyroxine therapy in euthyroid women with TAI undergoing ART	There is insufficient evidence to recommend for or against treating in the first trimester of pregnancy with thyroxine or IVIG, in women undergoing IVF
ES	If TSH is >2.5 mIU/mL, the test should be confirmed by repeat assay Low-dose thyroxine could be offered to bring TSH <2.5 mIU/mL, until the woman does not become pregnant or postpartum	No recommendation	All women on thyroxine should be verbally screened prenatally to assess their understanding of changing thyroxine requirements after conception An additional recommendation may be to increase their thyroxine dose by 30% which is often two additional tablets per week (nine tablets per week instead of seven tablets) until their serum TSH can be checked. Women with elevated anti-TPO antibodies are at increased risk for miscarriage, preterm delivery, progression of hypothyroidism, and PPT. If identified, such women should be screened for serum TSH abnormalities before pregnancy, as well as during the first and second trimesters of pregnancy. If serum TSH is >2.5 mIU/mL at the time of testing (or >3.0 mIU/mL in the second trimester) thyroxine therapy should be instituted. For overt hypothyroidism, if TSH concentration is 2.5–10 mIU/mL, starting thyroxine dose of 50 g/day or more is recommended.
ETA	SCH arising before conception should be treated with thyroxine	No recommendation	SCH arising during gestation should be treated with thyroxine. The thyroxine dose should be adjusted as necessary to reduce TSH to <2.5 mIU/mL or within the trimester-specific reference range. In hypothyroid women already treated with thyroxine before conception, the amount of increase in thyroxine may vary from 25% to 50% depending on the etiology of hypothyroidism and pre-pregnancy TSH level

(Anti-TPO: thyroid peroxidase antibodies; ART: assisted reproduction technologies; ASRM: American Society of Reproductive Medicine; ATA: American Thyroid Association; ES: Endocrine Society (US); ETA: European Thyroid Association; IVF: in vitro fertilization; IVIG: intravenous immunoglobulin; LT4: levothyroxine; PPT: postpartum thyroiditis; SCH: subclinical hypothyroidism; TAI: thyroid autoimmunity; TSH: thyroid-stimulating hormone)

Table 5: Clinical evidences suggesting the association of thyroid hormone imbalance and prolactin levels with infertility

Study	*Result and conclusion*
90 hyperprolactinemic infertile women, 90 normo-prolactinemic infertile women and 50 fertile women[13]	As compared to the fertile controls, a significantly higher mean serum prolactin and TSH were observed among the infertile groups (p<0.05) *In infertile women, hyperprolactinemia with thyroid dysfunction may be a major contributory hormonal factor*
30 women with primary infertility and 30 fertile women[14]	As compared to control group, the serum prolactin levels and serum TSH levels were significantly high in the infertile group (p<0.0001 for both) *In infertile women, there is a high incidence of hyperprolactinemia and thyroid disorders*

Fig. 5: Thyroid-stimulating hormone (TSH) levels in urinary incontinence and severe male factor group. Solid lines represent the median and first and third quartiles. Dotted line represents a TSH of 2.5 mIU/L.

Unexplained infertility is associated with high-normal TSH levels.

Thyroid-stimulating hormone and thyroid hormone are important factors during oocyte development and implantation. Increased risk of pregnancy loss is associated with TSH levels ≥2.5 mIU/L. But for nonpregnant women who are attempting to conceive, there are poor consensus regarding the normal range of TSH.

In a recent study, researchers evaluated the association between thyroid function, as estimated by TSH, with infertility in women with a completely normal fertility evaluation and no abnormal thyroid function.[12]

Researchers compared TSH and prolactin levels in women with urinary incontinence (UI) (n = 187, 31.5 ± 2.7 years) and women (n = 52, 30.1 ± 3.7 years) with a severe male factor infertility. Age of the patients and mean body mass index (BMI) was lower in the UI group as compared with the severe male factor group (p = 0.01 and p < 0.04, respectively).[12]

The results of the study revealed that:

- *TSH and prolactin levels:*
  - As compared to the severe male factor group, the TSH levels were significantly greater in the UI group [TSH 1.66 mIU/L, interquartile range: (1.25, 2.17) vs. TSH 1.95 mIU/L, interquartile range: (1.54, 2.61; p = 0.003, respectively] (Fig. 5). Even after controlling for BMI, age, and smoking status, the TSH levels remained significantly higher in the UI group.[12]
  - As compared with women in the severe male factor group, nearly twice as many women in the UI group had TSH values more than or equal to 2.5 mIU/L (13.5% vs. 26.9%, respectively; p < 0.05) (Fig. 6).[12]

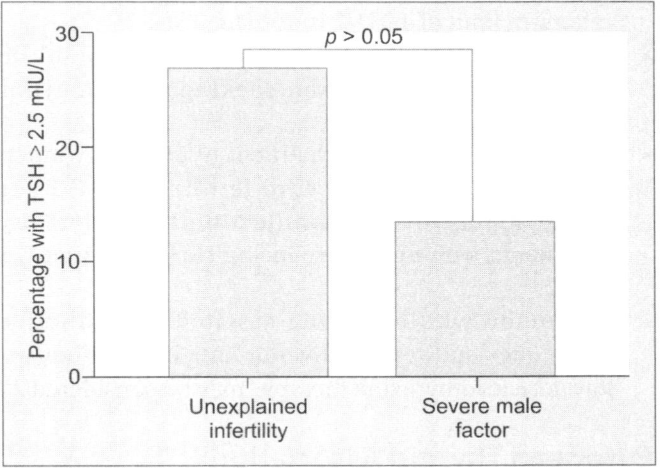

Fig. 6: Percentage of women in the urinary incontinence group and severe male factor group having a thyroid-stimulating hormone (TSH) level ≥2.5 mIU/L.

- *Thyroid peroxidase antibodies:*
  - After excluding the six subjects with positive TPO antibodies, the TSH level in the UI group (130) and the percentage of women with UI having a TSH more than or equal to 2.5 mIU/L were higher than the severe male factor group (n = 30) [UI TSH 1.94 mIU/L, interquartile range: (1.52, 2.54); severe male factor TSH 1.72 mIU/L, interquartile range: (1.32, 2.00); p = 0.01 and 25.4% vs. 6.7%, p < 0.03, respectively).[12]
- *Prolactin levels:* Between the groups, no difference in prolactin levels was observed.[12]

Therefore, this suggests that as compared to the control group, women with UI and without known thyroid dysfunction had higher TSH levels.

TSH levels should be maintained less than 2.5 mU/L: Thyroid-stimulating hormone more than 2.5 mU/L may be associated with reduced rates of fertilization during assisted conception, and reduced overall pregnancy rates. Clinical evidences suggest that, as compared with euthyroid controls, even following thyroid replacement therapy, egg numbers and fertilization rates, and implantation, pregnancy and live birth rates appear to be reduced. This indicates that in the subfertility setting, the serum TSH levels should be maintained less than 2.5 mU/L.

GUIDELINE RECOMMENDATIONS

American Thyroid Association

- The ATA 2017 guideline suggests that in the absence of specific population-based reference ranges, the upper reference limit of 4.0 U/L is used for TSH.[15]
- Thyroid-stimulating hormone testing should be performed for all women seeking treatment for infertility.[15]
- The ATA recommends treatment of SCH for women who are undergoing in vitro fertilization (IVF) or intracytoplasmic sperm injection (ICSI) fertility treatments, with a goal of reducing TSH to less than 2.5 mU/L.[15]
- In women who are using assisted reproductive techniques and test positive for anti-TPO antibodies, low dose levothyroxine therapy "may be considered".[15]

European Thyroid Association

- The ETA guideline suggests that in absence of specific reference range for TSH, in the first trimester of pregnancy, upper limit recommended is 2.5 mU/L.[16]
- Treatment with levothyroxine is suggested in SCH arising before conception.[16]

Practice Committee of the American Society for Reproductive Medicine[17]

TSH testing is reasonable in infertile women attempting pregnancy. If TSH concentrations are over the nonpregnant laboratory reference range (typically >4 mIU/L), patients should be treated with thyroxine to maintain levels below 2.5 mIU/L (Grade B).

If TSH levels before pregnancy are between 2.5 mIU/L and 4 mIU/L, it is essential to monitor and treat when TSH more than 4 mIU/L, or starting thyroxine treatment to maintain TSH less than 2.5 mIU/L (Grade C).

It is advisable to treat when the TSH is more than 2.5 mIU/L during the first trimester of pregnancy (Grade B).

Thyroid antibody testing is recommended for testing anti-TPO antibodies for repeated TSH values more than 2.5 mIU/L or when other risk factors for thyroid disease are present (Grade C).

Presence of anti-TPO antibodies indicates checking of TSH levels and considering treatment if the TSH level is over 2.5 mIU/L (Grade B).

Quality of evidence was evaluated as—Level I: Evidence obtained from at least one properly designed randomized controlled trial; Level II-1: Evidence obtained from well-designed controlled trials without randomization; Level II-2: Evidence obtained from well-designed cohort or case control analytic studies, preferably from more than one center or research group; Level II-3: Evidence obtained from multiple time series with or without the intervention. Dramatic results in uncontrolled trials might also be regarded as this type of evidence. Level III: Opinions of respected authorities based on clinical experience, descriptive studies, or reports of expert committees. Strength of evidence was evaluated as—Level A: Good evidence to support the recommendations, either for or against; Level B: Fair evidence to support recommendations, either for or against; Level C: Insufficient evidence to support recommendations, either for or against.

SUMMARY

- Thyroid hormones play an important part in normal reproductive function both through direct effects on the ovaries and indirectly by multiple interactions with other reproductive hormones.
- Undiagnosed and untreated thyroid disease is the cause of infertility as well as sub-fertility in women of reproductive age. Hyperthyroidism and hypothyroidism results in anovulatory cycles, imbalance of sex hormones, miscarriages, luteal phase defects, and high PRL levels.
- The prevalence of hypothyroidism is high, 53.7%, in infertile Indian women.
- Women with infertility, PCOD, and menstrual disturbances have high prevalence of hypothyroidism compared with other thyroid dysfunctions.
- Thyroxine therapy increases the rate of conception in hypothyroid women and those positive for antithyroid antibodies as well as shortens the duration until pregnancy for those conceiving spontaneously or with ART.
- Various guidelines have suggested screening for TSH levels before ovarian stimulation in infertile women attempting pregnancy. Those treated with levothyroxine daily had normalized mid-progesterone secretion and 20% became pregnant spontaneously. Thus, when thyroid dysfunction is detected, treatment is able to normalize prolactin and LH levels, restore normal fertility, and reduce the risk and requirement for ART.
- The ETA also suggests establishing trimester-specific reference ranges for TSH and T4 (total or free) during

early pregnancy. Intervention includes treatment with thyroxine to maintain TSH less than 2.5 mIU/mL before ovarian stimulation, and adjustment as necessary to reduce TSH to less than 2.5 mIU/mL or within the trimester-specific reference range during pregnancy. However, the amount of increase in thyroxine may vary from 25% to 50% depending on the etiology of hypothyroidism and prepregnancy TSH level in those treated before conception.

REFERENCES

1. Priya DM, Akhtar N, Ahmad J. Prevalence of hypothyroidism in infertile women and evaluation of response of treatment for hypothyroidism on infertility. Indian J Endocrinol Metab. 2015;19(4):504-6.
2. World Health Organization. (2004). Infecundity, Infertility and Childlessness in Developing Countries. DHS Comparative Reports No. 9. Calverton, Maryland, USA: ORC Marco and World Health Organization.
3. Verma I, Sood R, Juneja S, et al. Prevalence of hypothyroidism in infertile women and evaluation of response of treatment for hypothyroidism on infertility. Int J Appl Basic Med Res. 2012;2(1):17-9.
4. Poppe K, Velkeniers B, Glinoer D. The role of thyroid autoimmunity infertility and pregnancy. Nat Clin Pract Endocrinol Metab. 2008;4(7):394-405.
5. Trokoudes KM, Skordis N, Picolos MK. Infertility and thyroid disorders. Curr Opin Obstet Gynecol. 2006;18(4):446-51.
6. Priyatharshini M, Muraliswaran P, Kanagavalli P, et al. A retrospective study of thyroid disorders among women of reproductive age group in Puducherry. RJPBCS. 2014;5(6):748-53.
7. Rijal B, Shrestha R, Jha B. Association of thyroid dysfunction among infertile women visiting infertility center of Om Hospital, Kathmandu, Nepal. Nepal Med Coll J. 2011;13(4):247-9.
8. Garber JR, Cobin RH, Gharib H, et al. Clinical practice guidelines for hypothyroidism in adults: cosponsored by the American Association of Clinical Endocrinologists and the American Thyroid Association. Thyroid. 2012;22(12):1200-35.
9. Yoshioka W, Amino N, Ide A, et al. Thyroxine treatment may be useful for subclinical hypothyroidism in patients with female infertility. Endocr J. 2015;62(1):87-92.
10. Mintziori G, Goulis DG, Kolibianakis EM. Thyroid function and IVF outcome: when to investigate and when to intervene? Curr Opin Obstet Gynecol. 2016;28(3):191-7.
11. Crosignani PG, Management of hyperprolactinemic infertility. Middle East Fertility Society Journal. 2012;17:63-9.
12. Orouji Jokar T, Fourman LT, Lee H, et al. Higher TSH levels within the normal range are associated with unexplained fertility. J Clin Endocrinol Metab. 2018;103(2):632-9.
13. Bassey IE, Udoh AE, Essien OE, Isong IK, Gali RM, Archibong EE. Thyroid hormones and prolactin levels in infertile women in southern Nigeria. J Clin Diagn Res. 2015;9(3):OC13-5.
14. Turankar S, Sonone K, Turankar A, et al. Hyperprolactinaemia and its comparison with hypothyroidism in primary infertile women. J Clin Diagn Res. 2013;7(5):794-6.
15. Alexander EK, Pearce EN, Brent GA, et al. 2017 Guidelines of the American Thyroid Association for the diagnosis and management of thyroid disease during pregnancy and the postpartum. Thyroid. 2017;27(3):315-89.
16. Lazarus J, Brown RS, Daumerei C, et al. 2014 European thyroid association guidelines for the management of subclinical hypothyroidism in pregnancy and in children. Eur Thyroid J. 2014;3(2):76-94.
17. Practice Committee of the American Society for Reproductive Medicine. Subclinical hypothyroidism in the infertile female population: a guideline. Fertil Steril. 2015;104(3):545-53.

CHAPTER

41

Hyperprolactinemia and Infertility

Pooja Dhir Bhayana

If a women have milk, who is not with child, nor has brought forth, her menses are obstructed.

—Hippocrates: Aphorism 39, Section V

PHYSIOLOGY

Prolactin is a polypeptide hormone secreted by the lactotroph cells of the anterior pituitary gland.[1] The polypeptide chain consists of 198 amino acids with a molecular mass of 21,500 kDa.[2] Its secretion is under the control of a single gene located on chromosome 5. The hormone weakly resembles growth hormone and human placental lactogen.

Being secreted in a pulsatile manner from the pituitary gland, a marked diurnal variation in plasma concentrations was demonstrated, with highest values during sleep.[3] Its highest levels (up to 30 μg/L) are seen between 1.00 AM and 6.00 AM the morning.

The hormone is responsible for lactation in the females. During the last two trimesters of pregnancy and initial months of lactation, there occurs marked lactotroph cell hyperplasia under the influence of high levels of estrogen thereby leading to increased prolactin secretion.[4]

Prolactin levels are almost 10-fold higher during pregnancy and further decline after 2 weeks of child birth. Basal prolactin levels remain elevated if breastfeeding is initiated. There is a reflex increase in the prolactin levels during suckling, and these high levels may last for 30–45 minutes.

Prolactin control is an exception to the hypothalamic control of the hormones. While all other pituitary hormones are under positive control by the hypothalamus, prolactin is under inhibitory control via dopamine type 2 receptors. Dopamine, formed by neurons in the arcuate nucleus in the medial-basal hypothalamus and secreted into portal blood, is a major contributor to hypothalamic pituitary inhibitor factor activity.[5] That is why spontaneous prolactin hypersecretion occurs after pituitary stalk section.

Estrogen, thyrotropin-releasing hormone (TRH),[6] and vasoactive intestinal peptide act as stimulant for the secretion of prolactin while dopamine acts as an inhibitor.

Prolactin levels can be transiently elevated after meals, sexual activity, stressful situations (such as trauma and surgery),[7] or exercise.

Prolactin suppresses hypothalamic gonadotropin-releasing hormone (GnRH) and pituitary gonadotropin secretion. It aiso blocks folliculogenesis and inhibits granulosa cell aromatase activity causing hypoestrogenic state and anovulation. It also affects luteal phase leading to shortening of luteal phase.

HYPERPROLACTINEMIA

Hyperprolactinemia or prolactin hypersecretion is the most prevalent hypothalamic pituitary dysfunction. It is one of the most common causes of secondary amenorrhea in females. The condition could be present because of physiologic or pathologic causes. Various causes of hyperprolactinemia are discussed in Table 1.

Various physiologic causes that lead to hyperprolactinemia include pregnancy during which the levels gradually rise and reach peak at delivery.[8] Nipple stimulation, physical and psychological stress, and minor surgical procedures are other known physiologic causes of hyperprolactinemia.

Table 1: Causes of hyperprolactinemia.

Physiologic	*Drug induced*	*Pathologic*	*Others*
Pregnancy Postpartum Chest wall reflex (e.g. nipple stimulation) Wet nursing reflex (e.g. crying baby) Stress Sleep Physical activity	1. Dopamine receptor blockers Phenothiazines, e.g. chlorpromazine Metoclopramide Butyrophenones, e.g. haloperidol 2. Serotonin reuptake inhibitors, e.g. fluoxetine 3. H2 antagonists, e.g. cimetidine 4. Tricyclic antidepressants, e.g. amitriptyline 5. Dopamine synthesis inhibitors, e.g. methyldopa 6. Calcium channel blockers, e.g. verapamil 7. Hormones—estrogen	Pituitary disease Prolactinomas Acromegaly Hypothalamic pituitary disconnection/hypothalamic disease Tumors Nonfunctioning pituitary adenomas Meningioma Craniopharyngioma Empty sella syndrome Inflammatory, e.g. sarcoidosis, histiocytosis Stalk section Neurogenic Chest wall lesions Spinal cord lesions	Primary hypothyroidism Adrenal insufficiency Chronic renal failure Cirrhosis Pseudocyesis Epileptic seizures Paraneoplastic Idiopathic

Various drugs can also cause hyperprolactinemia. These include antipsychotics, e.g. phenothiazines, haloperidol, risperidone, selective serotonin reuptake inhibitors, and commonly used domperidone. Increase in serum prolactin concentrations can be seen within hours after their administration, but it returns to normal within 2–4 days after cessation of chronic therapy.[9]

Serum prolactin concentrations are in the range of 25–100 ng/mL in medication-induced hyperprolactinemia, exception being risperidone, which may raise the levels up to 200 ng/mL.[10,11]

Hypothalamic pituitary disorders are another cause for hyperprolactinemia, most common being prolactin secreting pituitary adenomas or prolactinomas. Prolactinomas are the most common pituitary tumors, with a prevalence of approximately 500 cases/million.[12] They comprise almost 25% of surgically removed pituitary adenomas. Depending upon their size, prolactinomas could be either microadenomas (<10 mm) or they could be macroadenomas (>10 mm). Almost 60% of prolactin secreting adenomas are microadenomas with a higher prevalence in females as compared to males. Microadenomas can have serum prolactin values ranging from 50 ng/mL to 300 ng/mL, whereas macroprolactinomas can have values between 200 ng/mL and 500 ng/mL.

Other hypothalamic pituitary disorders could be tumors, e.g. craniopharyngioma, infiltrative disorders, hypothalamic pituitary stalk section, etc.

Hypothyroidism can be associated with hyperprolactinemia. This is because of increased TRH and also increased pituitary sensitivity to TRH.[13]

In a large number of patients, who have serum prolactin in the range of 20–100 ng/mL, there is no detectable cause of hyperprolactinemia, thereby representing idiopathic hyperprolactinemia. Their prolactin levels remain almost the same over years of follow-up.

CLINICAL MANIFESTATIONS

Hyperprolactinemia in females can lead to oligomenorrhea or amenorrhea, galactorrhea, and infertility.

In a retrospective analysis of 104 patients with hyperprolactinemia by Bayrak et al., the reported symptoms from most to least common were infertility (48%), headaches (39%), oligomenorrhea (29%), galactorrhea (24%), and visual changes (13%).[14]

Hyperprolactinemia causes menstrual disturbances by causing inhibition of GnRH and thereby gonadotropin secretion. These could range from oligomenorrhea to amenorrhea. Hyperprolactinemia may be seen in about 20% of females with amenorrhea.[15]

Mild degrees of hyperprolactinemia can cause shortening of the luteal phase because of decreased progesterone secretion.[16]

Overtly high concentrations more than 100 ng/mL can cause hypogonadism and hypoestrogenism, thereby leading to hot flashes and vaginal dryness. The range of symptoms depending upon the prolactin levels have been summarized in Figure 1.

Hyperprolactinemic women may complain of loss of libido, dyspareunia, and psychological distress.[17] In long standing cases associated with hypogonadism, there may

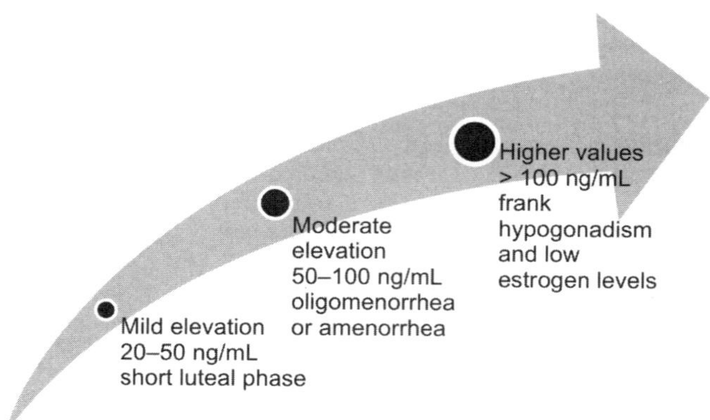

Fig. 1: Menstrual disturbances associated with varying serum prolactin levels.

Table 2: Symptoms of hyperprolactinemia.

Related to hyperprolactinemia	*Related to mass effect of the tumor*
Menstrual irregularities Oligomenorrhea/amenorrhea Infertility Sexual dysfunction Decreased libido, erectile dysfunction Osteoporosis Galactorrhea	Headache Visual disturbances–visual field defects Reduced visual acuity and ocular motility disturbances Rare manifestations—trigeminal neuralgia, hydrocephalus

be osteoporosis, relative risk of developing osteoporosis being 4.5%.[18]

Galactorrhea may be the presenting complaint, but it may not be present in all the women who present with hyperprolactinemia. The symptom can be seen in approximately 30% of patients with hyperprolactinemia.

Galactorrhea may be present in the absence of hyperprolactinemia. Kleinberg et al., in their series of patients with galactorrhea, reported that prolactin was normal in 46% of these patients.[19] Isolated galactorrhea in otherwise normal females does not require treatment if serum prolactin levels are within normal range. But in patients in whom the presence or the amount of secretion is physically or emotionally disturbing, then low-dose dopamine agonists are the treatment of choice.

Males with raised prolactin levels may have hypogonadotropic hypogonadism leading to infertility, loss of libido, erectile dysfunction, gynecomastia, and sometimes galactorrhea.[20,21]

Various clinical manifestations related to hyperprolactinemia are depicted in Table 2.

LABORATORY EVALUATION

Diagnosis of hyperprolactinemia is made by the measurement of serum prolactin levels. Most laboratories have a normal range of 5–20 ng/mL, normal values being higher in women than in men.

It can be measured at any time of the day. Mildly elevated values should be reconfirmed before putting the patient on treatment as levels may increase somewhat during any kind of physical or emotional stress, exercise, or breast stimulation.

Additional endocrine testing may be needed in cases of macroadenomas. This may include determining thyroid-stimulating hormone (TSH), total or free thyroxine, follicle-stimulating hormone, luteinizing hormone, insulin-like growth factor 1 (somatotroph adenomas), and 24-hour urinary free cortisol (corticotroph adenomas).

Artifacts that may lead to fallacies in diagnosis are the presence of macroprolactinemia and the hook effect.

Role of magnetic resonance imaging (MRI): MRI is the gold standard imaging modality for diagnosis and follow-up of adenomas. The present view is that it should be offered to all patients who show hyperprolactinemia, exception being drug-induced hyperprolactinemia. Most of the drugs cause hyperprolactinemia up to the range of 100 ng/mL so MRI should be done in pharmacologic hyperprolactinemia values above 100 ng/mL, exception being risperidone where it may be deferred till serum values of 300 ng/mL.

LABORATORY ARTIFACTS DURING PROLACTIN MEASUREMENT

Macroprolactinemia: There may be high serum prolactin levels in clinically normal patients. This may be due to heterogeneity in the size of prolactin molecule, with three forms in circulation that cannot be differentiated by routine immunoassay (23, 50, 150–170 kD).[22] Prolactin levels which are raised by the 150-170 kD prolactin, which is biologically less active, is labeled as macroprolactinemia. These patients typically will have high prolactin levels with minimal or no signs and symptoms related to hyperprolactinemia. Macroprolactinemia can be differentiated by asking the laboratory to pretreat the serum sample with polyethylene glycol.[23]

Hook effect: Sometimes patients having macroadenomas may have very low detectable prolactin levels. This could be because of the hook effect where large amounts of antigen (prolactin) saturate both the capture and signal antibodies used in immunoradiometric and chemiluminescent assays, preventing the binding of the two in a sandwich.[24,25] This can be avoided by repeating the assay using dilution method.

TREATMENT

A brief on the evaluation and management of hyperprolactinemia has been depicted in Flowchart 1.

Flowchart 1: Evaluation and treatment for hyperprolactinemia.

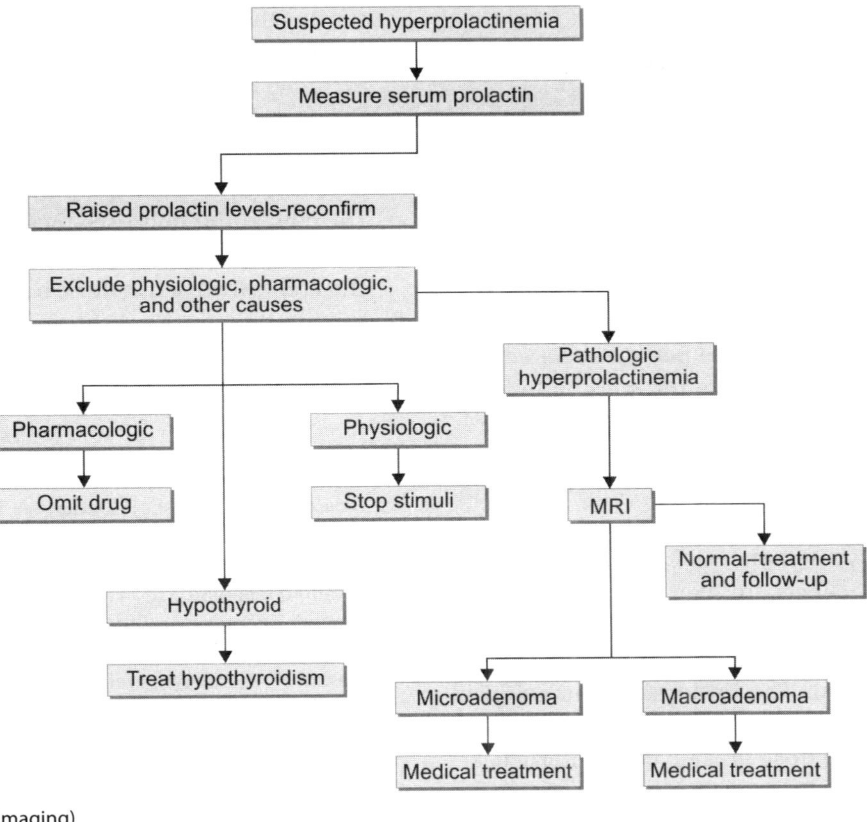

(MRI: Magnetic resonance imaging)

Before resorting to medical treatment, physiologic and pharmacologic causes should be excluded.

In patients with hypothyroidism, serum TSH values should be corrected. After exclusion of these, treatment should be planned for patients having mild degrees of hyperprolactinemia desiring to conceive, those presenting with hypogonadism or menstrual abnormalities or other signs of hyperprolactinemia, and if there are neurologic symptoms due to tumor mass effect.

Dopamine agonists are the treatment of choice for hyperprolactinemia including prolactinomas, because the drugs are effective in decreasing serum prolactin levels along with reduction in the size of the prolactinoma masses.[26] Cabergoline and bromocriptine are most commonly used drugs. Their administration leads to restoration of ovulatory function and restoration of menstrual cycles in most women with hyperprolactinemia. These drugs also lead to a decrease in breast secretion, but complete cessation may take a little longer time.

Cabergoline is the drug of first choice because of its better efficacy and lesser side effects.[27] It is better tolerated, with a lesser tendency to cause nausea as compared to bromocriptine,[28,29] and is more effective in inducing normoplactinemia.[30] Because of its longer duration of action, it needs to be administered once or twice a week. Cabergoline therapy leads to normalization of serum prolactin levels in almost 80% of the patients.[31,32] Starting dose should be 0.25 mg twice a week or 0.5 mg weekly.

Bromocriptine having a short half-life needs to be administered once or twice a day for better therapeutic efficacy. Being an ergot derivative, it can lead to gastrointestinal side effects including nausea, vomiting, and in some patients, postural hypotension. Other less common side effects are nasal congestion, headache, constipation, and psychotic events such as auditory hallucinations and mood changes.

To overcome the occurrence of side effects, treatment should be started with a low dose of 1.25 mg at bedtime after meal and then gradually increase the dose. Vaginal route is another effective treatment option for those who cannot tolerate oral dose as it is associated with fewer side effects.

Almost 25% of the patients show resistance to bromocriptine.[28,31] For those resistant to bromocriptine, cabergoline is the option, as resistance with cabergoline is seen in only 10% of the patients.[27]

Table 3: Drugs to treat hyperprolactinemia—dopamine agonists.

Drug	*Dose*	*Side effects*
Bromocriptine	2.5–10 mg/day 8–12 hourly	Nausea Headache Postural hypotension
Cabergoline	0.5–2 mg/week Once/twice weekly dose	Association with valvular heart disease with high doses
Quinagolide	0.075–0.6 mg/day Once/day	

One major side effect that has been associated with dopamine agonists (cabergoline and pergolide) is its association with hypertrophic valvular heart disease[33,34] when used in high doses (>3 mg/day) as in patients with Parkinson's disease. As a consequence pergolide which is another dopamine agonist had been voluntarily withdrawn from the United States in 2007. Although the major cardiovascular effects are seen when the drug has been used for high doses as in Parkinson's, it should be used in minimum effective dose to normalize serum prolactin concentration. The Endocrine Society in its recommendations advises for an echocardiogram in those who are on cabergoline dose greater than 2 mg/week.[27] Both the drugs appear to be safe in early pregnancy, so for those planning to conceive any of the two can be used.[35-37]

The drugs used in treatment for hyperprolactinemia are summarized in Table 3.

Surgical therapy: Surgical therapy is indicated in cases of adenomas if:

- Dopamine treatment has been unsuccessful in lowering serum prolactin concentration.
- When signs and symptoms persist or the size of the tumor does not decrease even after prolonged drug treatment.
- For those women who have large tumors more than 3 cm in size and wishing to conceive, as the size can substantially grow after cessation of drug therapy during pregnancy.

Postoperative radiation therapy: Radiation therapy is to be given postoperatively to prevent regrowth of residual tumors after surgery.

POINTS TO REMEMBER

- Hyperprolactinemia is one of the most common hypothalamic pituitary dysfunctions.
- Most common presenting complaints in females being oligomenorrhea, amenorrhea, galactorrhea, and infertility.
- Mildly elevated levels need to be reconfirmed before starting therapy.
- Physiologic and pharmacologic causes should be excluded before resorting to therapy.
- Magnetic resonance imaging is to be done to exclude microadenomas, macroadenomas, or other lesions in the brain leading to hyperprolactinemia.
- The most commonly used medications are cabergoline and bromocriptine. Cabergoline has a better tolerance and is effective even in those resistent to bromocriptine.
- Surgical therapy should be reserved for those who have large adenomas and/or those not responding to drug therapy.

REFERENCES

1. Pasteels JL, Ganesset P, Dangny A, et al. Morphology of the lactotropes and somatotropes of man and rhesus monkeys. J Clin Endocrinol Metab. 1972;34(6):959-67.
2. Niall HD, Hogan MC, Tregear GW, et al. The chemistry of growth hormone and the lactogenic hormone. Recent Prog Horm Res. 1973;29:387-416.
3. Sassin JF, Frantz AG, Weitzman ED, et al. Human prolactin: 24 hour pattern with increased release during sleep. Science. 1972;177(4055):1205-7.
4. Goluboff LG, Ezrin C. Effect of pregnancy on the somatotroph and the prolactin cell of the human adenohypophysis. J Clin Endocrinol Metab. 1969;29(12):1533-8.
5. Ben-Jonathan N, Oliver C, Weiner HJ, et al. Dopamine in hypophysial portal plasma of the rat during the estrous cycle and throughout pregnancy. Endocrinology. 1977;100(2):452-8.
6. Jacobs LS, Synder FJ, Utiger PD, et al. Prolactin response to thyrotropin-releasing hormone in normal subjects. J Clin Endocrinol Metab. 1973;36(6):1069-73.
7. Noel GL, Suh KK, Stone JG, et al. Human prolactin and growth hormone release during surgery and other conditions of stress. J Clin Endocrinol Metab. 1972;35(6):840-51.
8. Tyson JE, Hwang P, Guyda H, et al. Studies of prolactin secretion in human pregnancy. Am J Obstet Gynecol. 1972;113(1):14-20.
9. Rivera JL, Lal S, Ettigi P, et al. Effect of acute and chronic neuroleptic therapy on serum prolactin levels in men and women of different age groups. Clin Endocrinol (Oxf). 1976;5(3):273-82.
10. Ajmal A, Joffe H, Nachtigall LB. Psychotropic-induced hyperprolactinemia: a clinical review. Psychosomatics. 2014;55(1):29-36.
11. Kearns AE, Goff DC, Hayden DL, et al. Risperidone-associated hyperprolactinemia. Endocr Pract. 2000;6(6):425-9.
12. Miyai K, Ichihara K, Kondo K, et al. Asymptomatic hyperprolactinaemia and prolactinoma in the general population—mass screening by paired assays of serum prolactin. Clin Endocrinol. 1986;25(5):549-54.
13. Snyder PJ, Jacobs LS, Utiger RD, et al. Thyroid hormone inhibition of the prolactin response to thyrotropin-releasing hormone. J Clin Invest. 1973;52(9):2324-9.

14. Bayrak A, Saadat P, Mor E, et al. Pituitary imaging is indicated for the evaluation of hyperprolactinemia. Fertil Steril. 2005;84(1):181-5.
15. Franks S, Murray MA, Jequier AM, et al. Incidence and significance of hyperprolactinaemia in women with amenorrhea. Clin Endocrinol (Oxf). 1975;4(6):597-607.
16. Seppälä M, Ranta T, Hirvonen E. Hyperprolactinaemia and luteal insufficiency. Lancet. 1976;1(7953):229-30.
17. Kars M, van der Klaauw AA, Onstein CS, et al. Quality of life is decreased in female patients treated for microprolactinoma. Eur J Endocrinol. 2007;157(2):133-9.
18. Vartej P, Poiana C, Vartej I. Effects of hyperprolactinemia on osteoporotic fracture risk in premenopausal women. Gynecol Endocrinol. 2001;15(1):43-7.
19. Kleinberg DL, Noel GL, Frantz AG. Galactorrhea: a study of 235 cases, including 48 with pituitary tumors. N Engl J Med. 1977;296(11):589-600.
20. Carter JN, Tyson JE, Tolis G, et al. Prolactin-screening tumors and hypogonadism in 22 men. N Engl J Med. 1978;299(16):847-52.
21. Segal S, Yaffe H, Laufer N, et al. Male hyperprolactinemia: effects on fertility. Fertil Steril. 1979;32(5):556-61.
22. Sinha YN. Structural variants of prolactin: occurrence and physiological significance. Endocr Rev. 1995;16(3): 354-69.
23. Vieira JG, Tachibana TT, Obara LH, et al. Extensive experience and validation of polyethylene glycol precipitation as a screening method for macroprolactinemia. Clin Chem. 1998;44(8):1758-9.
24. St-Jean E, Blain F, Comtois R. High prolactin levels may be missed by immunoradiometric assay in patients with macroprolactinomas. Clin Endocrinol (Oxf). 1996;44(3): 305-9.
25. Petakov MS, Damjanović SS, Nikolić-Durović MM, et al. Pituitary adenomas secreting large amounts of prolactin may give false low values in immunoradiometric assays. The hook effect. J Endocrinol Invest. 1998;21(3):184-8.
26. Wang AT, Mullan RJ, Lane MA, et al. Treatment of hyperprolactinemia: a systematic review and meta-analysis. Syst Rev. 2012;1(1):33.
27. Melmed S, Casanueva FF, Hoffman AR, et al. Diagnosis and treatment of hyperprolactinemia: an Endocrine Society clinical practice guideline. J Clin Endocrinol Metab. 2011;96(2):273-88.
28. Webster J, Piscitelli G, Polli A, et al. A comparison of cabergoline and bromocriptine in the treatment of hyperprolactinemic amenorrhea. N Engl J Med. 1994;331(14):904-9.
29. Biller BM, Molitch ME, Vance ML, et al. Treatment of prolactin-secreting macroadenomas with the once-weekly dopamine agonist cabergoline. J Clin Endocrinol Metab. 1996;81(6):2338-43.
30. Vilar L, Freitas MC, Naves LA, et al. Diagnosis and management of hyperprolactinemia: results of a Brazilian multicenter study with 1234 patients. J Endocrinol Invest. 2008;31(5):436-44.
31. Verhelst J, Abs R, Maiter D, et al. Cabergoline in the treatment of hyperprolactinemia: a study in 455 patients. J Clin Endocrinol Metab. 1999;84(7):2518-22.
32. Ono M, Miki N, Kawamata T, et al. Prospective study of high-dose cabergoline treatment of prolactinomas in 150 patients. J Clin Endocrinol Metab. 2008;93(12):4721-7.
33. Schade R, Andersohn F, Suissa S, et al. Dopamine agonists and the risk of cardiac-valve regurgitation. N Engl J Med. 2007;356(1):29-38.
34. Zanettini R, Antonini A, Gatto G, et al. Valvular heart disease and the use of dopamine agonists for Parkinson's disease. N Engl J Med. 2007;356(1):39-46.
35. Robert E, Musatti L, Piscitelli G, et al. Pregnancy outcome after treatment with the ergot derivative, cabergoline. Reprod Toxicol. 1996;10:333.
36. Ricci E, Parazzini F, Motta T, et al. Pregnancy outcome after cabergoline treatment in early weeks of gestation. Reprod Toxicol. 2002;16(6):791-3.
37. Turkalj I, Braun P, Krupp P. Surveillance of bromocriptine in pregnancy. JAMA. 1982;247(11):1589-91.

Section 5

Ovarian Stimulation

CHAPTER

42

Oral Ovulogens

Mohan S Kamath, Korula George

INTRODUCTION

Ovulatory dysfunction is one of the common reasons for infertility and accounts for about 40% of female infertility.[1] According to World Health Organization (WHO) classification ovulatory dysfunctions are mainly categorized into: (1) Class I—consisting of hypothalamic pituitary failure, (2) Class II—being hypothalamic pituitary dysfunction, and (3) Class III—representing ovarian failure. The hypothalamic pituitary failure (5 - 10%) and ovarian failure (5%) are less common groups with majority of the ovulatory dysfunction belonging to the Class II category. Polycystic ovarian syndrome (PCOS), which belongs to WHO Class II, is the most common cause of ovulatory dysfunction.[1] Diagnosis of PCOS can be made using Rotterdam criteria or National Institute of Health (NIH) criteria. Out of the three criteria (oligo- and/or anovulation, clinical and/or biochemical signs of hyperandrogenism, and polycystic ovaries on ultrasound), presence of two are considered essential for diagnosis of PCOS under the Rotterdam criteria.[2] Additionally, other endocrine disorders such as congenital adrenal hyperplasia and androgen secreting tumors should be excluded.

Oral ovulogens are drugs, which are mainly used for inducing ovulation in women with anovulatory dysfunction. They are usually the first line of treatment for patients belonging to WHO Class II. They are also used to achieve super ovulation during intrauterine insemination (IUI) in couples with unexplained infertility.[3] During in vitro fertilization (IVF) treatment, they may also be combined with gonadotropins for controlled ovarian hyperstimulation (COH), commonly known as mild stimulation protocols.[4]

Most common oral ovulogens used in contemporary practice are clomiphene citrate (CC), aromatase inhibitors (e.g. anastrozole), and insulin sensitizers such as metformin.[1,5,6] Less commonly used drugs are tamoxifen, dexamethasone, and thiazolidinediones (e.g. rosiglitazone).[7,8]

ORAL DRUGS FOR OVULATION INDUCTION

Clomiphene Citrate

Clinical Case # 1

"A 23-year-old Mrs X and her husband Mr Y, aged 26 years, presented with complaints of inability to conceive from last 1 year. They have been married for 2 years. Menstrual cycles are irregular (40–45 days). No dysmenorrhea. No obvious clinical signs of excess androgen observed during examination. Body mass index 24 kg/m^2. On ultrasound, polycystic ovaries were seen. Thyroid-stimulating hormone (TSH) and serum prolactin levels were normal. Husband semen analysis reported as normozoospermia. Wife diagnosed as a case of PCOS. No previous treatment for infertility. The first pharmacological line of treatment for treatment naive PCOS woman is..."

Clomiphene citrate is the first-line drug used to induce ovulation in women with PCOS. It consists of two isomeric components: zuclomiphene and enclomiphene. Among the two, zuclomiphene is considered more potent for ovulation induction.[1] The estrogen receptors in hypothalamus are blocked by clomiphene citrate, which prevents a negative feedback of estrogen, causing a release of gonadotropin releasing hormone (GnRH). The release of GnRH results in increase in endogenous gonadotropins—follicle stimulating hormone (FSH) and luteinizing hormone (LH)—from the anterior pituitary, which promotes follicular development in the ovary. The negative impact of estrogen receptor blockade by CC at the endometrial and cervical level is considered to be the reason for lower pregnancy rates (30–40%) even though ovulation is achieved in almost 80% of the PCOS women.[1]

Though the starting dose is 50 mg daily for 5 days and can be initiated from anytime between day 2 to day 5 of menstrual cycle, many clinicians prefer 100 mg daily as the starting dose. The reason for this is higher ovulation rate (67%) with 100 mg compared to 46% following 50 mg dosage, without any apparent increase in multiple pregnancy rate.[9] The follicular development can be documented by an ultrasound by day 12–14 at least in the index cycle. Those with follicular development can be advised timed intercourse for at least 1 week after ultrasound. The routine administration of human chorionic gonadotropin (hCG) as a trigger for follicular rupture during ovulation induction with CC has not been found to be beneficial.[10]

Ultrasound monitoring helps in identifying those women who have responded to a particular dose of CC and the same dose can be adhered to for subsequent treatment cycles. In few cases, hyper-response can be noted and when more than three dominant follicles are noted, it is advisable to cancel the cycle and advise sexual abstinence for next 2 weeks.

In case no follicular development is noted, the daily dose of CC can be increased by 50 mg and a maximum of 150–200 mg per day is advised.

Women who do not respond to the maximum dose of CC are categorized under CC resistance, and those who respond but do not conceive after three to six treatment cycles are known as CC failure. It is advisable to restrict the number of CC cycles to a maximum of 12, due to potential threefold increase in risk of ovarian malignancy in future.[11]

For women with CC resistance which signifies a severe form of PCOS, next treatment options include aromatase inhibitors, gonadotropins, insulin sensitizers and in some cases, laparoscopic ovarian drilling.[1,12] In cases of CC failure, tubal evaluation is warranted to rule out tubal pathologies before moving to alternative options.

Clomiphene citrate may cause side effects such as nausea, hot flushes, and rarely visual disturbances.[1] In case any visual disturbance following CC is noted, it should be promptly discontinued and alternative ovulation induction agents should be offered.

Some of the less common CC regimens include stair step protocol and using CC for longer duration.

In stair step protocol, starting dose of CC (50 mg) is given for 5 days from day 2 of the menstrual cycle and ultrasound is done on day 11–14.[13] In case no follicle develops, the dose is increased by 50 mg (100 mg for 5 days) and started immediately while the ultrasound is planned 1 week after the first follicular ultrasound. If no response is noted again, then the daily dose is increased to 150 mg for 5 days and repeat ultrasound done 1 week later. In clinical practice, this protocol reduces time to ovulation (23–35 days) compared to standard cyclical protocol (55–88 days). PCOS women with anovulation are more suited for this protocol than oligo-ovulation.

Clomiphene citrate is sometimes used in couples with unexplained infertility. In the Cochrane review, no significant increase in clinical pregnancy rates following CC compared to expectant management after pooling results from two trials (OR 1.03, 95% CI 0.64–1.66).[11] In unexplained infertility, use of CC should be avoided since it has no proven benefit, and it increases risk of multiple pregnancies.

Aromatase Inhibitors

Clinical Case # 2

"A 27-year-old Mrs X and her husband Mr Y, age 36 years, presented with complaints of inability to conceive from last 6 years. They have been married for 7 years. Menstrual cycles are irregular (40–45 days). No dysmenorrhea. No obvious clinical signs of excess androgen observed during examination. Body mass index 26 kg/m^2. On ultrasound, polycystic ovaries were seen. TSH, serum prolactin, and testosterone levels were normal. Husband semen analysis reported as normozoospermia. Wife diagnosed as a case of PCOS. She gives history of ovulation induction with CC with no response at 200 mg daily dose (CC resistance). Hysterosalpingography demonstrated patent tubes. Sugar levels are normal. The next possible medical option for such women with CC resistance is..."

Aromatase inhibitors act at the ovarian level and prevent the conversion of androgen to estrogen. The reduced systemic levels of estrogen release the hypothalamo-pituitary axis from the negative feedback exerted by estrogen, thus resulting in increase in FSH levels. The higher androgen levels in the ovary also increases follicular sensitivity to FSH.[14] Unlike CC, aromatase inhibitors do not exert peripheral antiestrogenic action and are cleared from systemic circulation more rapidly due to shorter half-life (48 hours) compared to CC which has a prolonged half-life (2 weeks). Another advantage of aromatase inhibitor is reduced chances of multifollicular development due to intact estrogen negative feedback mechanism, which reduces FSH levels with rising estrogen.[14] With CC, this negative feedback mechanism is interrupted due to blockade of estrogen receptors by CC.

There were initial concerns about teratogenic effect of letrozole, an aromatase inhibitor. Subsequent studies have not shown increased congenital anomaly rate following the drug.[15]

Anastrozole, another aromatase inhibitor, is being used in clinical practice as an alternative oral ovulogen to CC. The recommended dose of anastrozole is 1 mg daily for 5 days from day 2 of menstrual cycle.[16] The ovulation rates following anastrozole are comparable to CC (67% vs. 68%).[5] It may have role in treating CC resistant PCOS women who constitute about 20–25%.[17,18]

Tamoxifen

Tamoxifen, a triphenylethylene derivative, is less commonly used drug for ovulation induction purpose. It is sometimes used in women who experience side effects following CC and rarely in CC resistant PCOS cases.[8,19] The dosage is between 20 mg and 40 mg daily from day 2 or day 3 of menstrual cycle for 5 days. Live birth rates following tamoxifen were not significantly different compared to CC.[8]

Dexamethasone

Clinical Case #3

"A 27-year-old Mrs X and her husband Mr Y, aged 36 years, presented with complaints of inability to conceive from last 6 years. They have been married for 7 years. Menstrual cycles are irregular (40–45 days). No dysmenorrhea. No obvious clinical signs of excess androgen observed during examination. Body mass index 26 kg/m^2. On ultrasound, polycystic ovaries were seen. TSH, serum prolactin, and testosterone levels were normal. Her dehydroepiandrosterone (DHEA) level is elevated. Husband semen analysis reported as normozoospermia. Wife diagnosed as a case of late onset congenital adrenal hyperplasia. She wants regularization of cycles and wishes to conceive. The recommended medical option for such women with late onset congenital adrenal hyperplasia (CAH) is..."

The role of dexamethasone as an ovulation induction agent is mainly confined to treating endocrinological conditions such as late onset congenital adrenal hyperplasia. However, it has been also offered in CC resistant PCOS case with normal levels of dehydroepiandrosterone sulfate (DHEAS). A randomized trial found significantly higher ovulation rates (75% vs. 15%; $p < 0.01$) with CC and dexamethasone compared to CC with placebo in women with CC resistance.[20] The low dosage of 0.5 mg per day from day 1 to day 14 of menstrual cycles is generally recommended. Earlier study has found better pregnancy rates with higher dose of 2 mg per day instead of low dose.[20]

Insulin Sensitizers

Clinical Case # 4

"A 28-year-old Mrs X and her husband Mr Y, aged 36 years, presented with complaints of inability to conceive from last 4 years. They have been married for 7 years. Menstrual cycles are irregular (40–45 days). No dysmenorrhea. No obvious clinical signs of excess androgen observed during examination. Body mass index 30 kg/m^2. On ultrasound, polycystic ovaries were seen. TSH, serum prolactin, and testosterone levels were normal. Husband semen analysis reported as normozoospermia. Wife diagnosed as a case of PCOS. She gives history of ovulation induction with CC with no response at 200 mg daily dose (CC resistance). Hysterosalpingography demonstrated patent tubes. She is diagnosed with impaired glucose tests. She has been advised weight reduction and given dietary advice. The next possible medical option for such women with CC resistance is.."

Most common insulin sensitizer used in PCOS women is metformin. Though its influence on weight reduction is not clearly established, it is commonly advised in PCOS women with impaired glucose.[2] It is also an option in women with CC resistant PCOS. In a randomized controlled trial (RCT) which included women with CC resistance, intervention arm consisted of metformin for 6 months followed by CC again. In the control arm, ovulation induction with gonadotropin was planned. No significant difference in clinical pregnancy rates was observed in the two groups and lower cost of metformin was an added advantage.[21] Recent update has reported improvement in menstrual cycle regularity and ovulation rate following metformin compared to placebo.[22] Metformin is associated with severe gastrointestinal side effects, which can lead to patient compliance issues. Usual recommended dose is 500–1,500 mg daily though it should be initiated with low dose and gradually titrated after assessing the tolerance.[22]

Since metformin is considered safe in pregnancy, clinicians continue its use during pregnancy once the woman conceives. This is done to help in improving metabolic profile and reduce the risk of gestational diabetes in PCOS women. A recent large trial however did not show any improvement in complication rate during pregnancy by continuing metformin throughout the gestation.[23]

There is paucity of trials evaluating other newer insulin sensitizers such as thiazolidinediones and d-chiro-inositol. Thiazolidinediones are mainly used for treating type 2 diabetes mellitus. Due to their beneficial action in improving insulin resistance, many clinicians have advocated its use in women with PCOS. A study found young PCOS women with pioglitazone had improvement in menstrual symptoms.[24]

However, there are ongoing concerns regarding side effects, weight gain, and safety during pregnancy with these drugs. Though many of these drugs showed initial promise, currently the evidence is insufficient to recommend their use for ovulation induction purpose.[22,25]

Oral Ovulogens for Ovarian Stimulation during Intrauterine Insemination

Commonly, ovarian stimulation is combined with intrauterine insemination (IUI) to achieve super ovulation (more than one follicle) in couples with unexplained infertility, mild male factor, or minimal endometriosis. Various agents are used for ovarian stimulation such as CC, aromatase inhibitors, gonadotropin or combination of oral ovulogens with gonadotropins.

Clomiphene or aromatase inhibitors are combined with gonadotropin to lower total dosage requirement of gonadotropin, which reduces the cost without compromising on IUI outcomes. Clomiphene citrate (100 mg) is started from day 2 of menstrual cycle and continued for 5 days. The gonadotropin (75 IU) is initiated from day 5 and given on alternate days and follicular monitoring is done from day 10. Satisfactory pregnancy rates are achieved using combination of CC and gonadotropin during IUI.[26] Similar combination protocol (CC and gonadotropin) also can be used for achieving ovulation induction instead of gonadotropin alone in CC resistant or CC failure cases as pregnancy rates are comparable.[12]

Use of Oral Ovulogens in Mild Stimulation Protocols

Clinical Case # 5

"A 37-year-old Mrs X and her husband Mr Y, aged 46 years, presented with complaints of inability to conceive from last 6 years. They have been married for 7 years. Menstrual cycles are regular. Body mass index 21 kg/m^2.

On ultrasound, normal ovaries and total antral follicle count of 5 was noted. TSH and serum prolactin levels were normal. Husband semen analysis reported as severe oligoasthenozoospermia. Couple underwent IVF with conventional stimulation of high gonadotropins. Three oocytes were retrieved and cycle was unsuccessful. The couple wishes to try another autologous IVF. The possible options for controlled ovarian hyperstimulation (COH) include..."

Oral ovulogens such as CC and aromatase inhibitors have been used for mild stimulation protocol during IVF. Use of CC in these protocols is quite common and some of the benefits include lower gonadotropin requirements and less cost during IVF.[27,28] They also are patient-friendly protocols and pregnancy rate for certain subset of patients is comparable to conventional IVF. The milder stimulation has added advantage of higher yield of euploid embryos compared to conventional high dose gonadotropins.[29]

The Cochrane review which included 12 trials and 2,536 participants found comparable live birth rates following CC and gonadotropin compared to gonadotropin alone during IVF (OR 0.93, 95% CI 0.69–1.24). The ovarian hyperstimulation syndrome (OHSS) rates were significantly lower in the CC and gonadotropin group (0.8–1.8%) compared to gonadotropin agonist protocol (3.5%).[4] The mild stimulation protocol has been advocated in women who had poor response or unsuccessful outcome in previous conventional IVF with high dose of gonadotropins. A recent systematic review which included four trials, evaluated CC with gonadotropin versus conventional gonadotropin alone in poor responders. They found no significant differences in live birth rates (OR: 0.71, 95% CI 0.22–2.2) and clinical pregnancy rates (OR: 1.11, 95% CI 0.80–1.55) following CC with gonadotropin compared to gonadotropin alone.[27]

Clomiphene citrate has also been used to prevent premature LH surge during IVF instead of GnRH analogs. In this protocol, CC is initiated from day 2 of the cycle and continued till the day hCG trigger is given. Continuous use of clomiphene citrate blocks estrogen receptors' sites at the hypothalamus and pituitary. Clomiphene used in this fashion mimics the action of a GnRH analog and prevents an LH surge due to rising estrogen levels, a result of follicular development. Low dose gonadotropins 75–150 IU are also added to enhance the response. Hence, conventional GnRH analogs are not required for prevention of premature LH surge.[30] This protocol is quite useful in low cost IVF program since the GnRH analogs are not used, and gonadotropin requirement is less.[28]

KEY SUMMARY POINTS

Lifestyle changes are the first line of therapy for ovulation induction in PCOS.

- Clomiphene citrate is the first choice for inducing ovulation medically in PCOS.
- For CC failure, alternatives are aromatase inhibitors or gonadotropins alone or in combination with CC or aromatase inhibitors.
- If resistant to CC, the next options are aromatase inhibitors, insulin sensitizers, gonadotropins, or surgical intervention for ovarian drilling.
- Metformin is recommended for women with PCOS who have impaired glucose tolerance and CC resistance. Currently other insulin sensitizers are not recommended

for routine ovulation induction due to insufficient evidence.

- Tamoxifen is another alternative antiestrogen which can be advised in CC failure.
- Dexamethasone can be offered as an adjuvant along with CC in women with CC resistance.
- Clomiphene citrate and aromatase inhibitors can be combined with gonadotropins in mild stimulation IVF protocols, especially in poor responders.

REFERENCES

1. Homburg R. Clomiphene citrate—end of an era? A mini-review. Hum Reprod. 2005;20(8):2043-51.
2. Thessaloniki ESHRE/ASRM-Sponsored PCOS Consensus Workshop Group. Consensus on infertility treatment related to polycystic ovary syndrome. Hum Reprod. 2008;23(3):462-77.
3. Kamath MS, Bhattacharya S. Demographics of infertility and management of unexplained infertility. Best Pract Res Clin Obstet Gynaecol. 2012;26(6): 729-38
4. Gibreel A, Maheshwari A, Bhattacharya S. Clomiphene citrate in combination with gonadotropins for controlled ovarian stimulation in women undergoing in vitro fertilization. Cochrane Database Syst Rev. 2012;11: CD008528.
5. Badawy A, Abdel Aal I, Abulatta M. Clomiphene citrate or anastrozole for ovulation induction in women with polycystic ovary syndrome? A prospective controlled trial. Fertil Steril. 2009;92(3):860-3.
6. Palomba S, Falbo A, Zullo F, et al. Evidence-based and potential benefits of metformin in the polycystic ovary syndrome: a comprehensive review. Endocr Rev. 2009;30(1):1-50.
7. Baillargeon JP, Jakubowicz DJ, Iuorno MJ, et al. Effects of metformin and rosiglitazone, alone and in combination, in nonobese women with polycystic ovary syndrome and normal indices of insulin sensitivity. Fertil Steril. 2004;82:893-902.
8. Brown J, Farquhar C. Clomiphene and other antioestrogens for ovulation induction in polycystic ovarian syndrome. Cochrane Database Syst Rev. 2016;12:CD002249.
9. Rostami-Hodjegan A, Lennard MS, Tucker GT, et al. Monitoring plasma concentrations to individualize treatment with clomiphene citrate. Fertil Steril. 2004;81(5):1187-93.
10. George K, Kamath MS, Nair R, et al. Ovulation triggers in anovulatory women undergoing ovulation induction. Cochrane Database Syst Rev. 2014;(1):CD006900.
11. Hughes E, Brown J, Collins JJ, et al. Clomiphene citrate for unexplained subfertility in women. Cochrane Database Syst Rev. 2010;(1): CD000057.
12. Abdelazim IA, Makhlouf HH. Sequential clomiphene citrate/hMG versus hMG for ovulation induction in clomiphene citrate-resistant women. Arch Gynecol Obstet. 2013;287(3):591-7.
13. Hurst BS, Hickman JM, Matthews ML, et al. Novel clomiphene "stair step" protocol reduces time to ovulation in women with polycystic ovarian syndrome. Am J Obstet Gynecol. 2009;200:510.e1-510.e4.
14. Mitwally M, Casper R. Aromatase inhibitors in ovulation induction. Semin Reprod Med. 2004;22:61-78.
15. Tulandi T, Martin J, Al- Fadhli R, et al. Congenital malformations among 911 newborns conceived after infertility treatment with Letrozole or Clomiphene citrate. Fertil Steril. 2006;85:1761-5.
16. Franik S, Kremer JA, Nelen WL, et al. Aromatase inhibitors for subfer- tile women with polycystic ovary syndrome. Cochrane Database Syst Rev. 2014;(2):CD010287.
17. Al-Omari WR, Sulaiman W, Al-Hadithi N. Comparison of two aromatase inhibitors in women with clomiphene-resistant polycystic ovary syndrome. Intern J Gynecol Obstet. 2004;85:289-91.
18. Badawy A, Mosbah A, Shady M. Anastrozole or letrozole for ovulation induction in clomiphene-resistant women with polycystic ovary syndrome? A prospective controlled trial. Fertil Steril. 2008; 89(5):1209-12.
19. Dhaliwal LK, Suri V, Gupta KR, et al. Tamoxifen: an alternative to clomiphene in women with polycystic ovary syndrome. J Hum Reprod Sci. 2011;4(2):76-9.
20. Elnashar A, Abdelmageed E, Fayed M, et al. Clomiphene citrate and dexamethazone in treatment of clomiphene citrate-resistant polycystic ovary syndrome: a prospective placebo-controlled study. Hum Reprod. 2006; 21(7):1805-8.
21. George SS, George K, Irwin C, et al. Sequential treatment of metformin and clomiphene citrate in clomiphene-resistant women with polycystic ovary syndrome: a randomized, controlled trial. Hum Reprod. 2003;18(2): 299-304.
22. Balen AH, Morley LC, Misso M, et al. The management of anovulatory infer- tility in women with polycystic ovary syndrome: an analysis of the evidence to support the development of global WHO guidance. Hum Reprod Update. 2016;22(6):687-708.
23. Vanky E, Stridsklev S, Heimstad R, et al. Metformin versus placebo from first trimester to delivery in polycystic ovary syndrome: a randomized, controlled multicenter study. J Clin Endocrinol Metab. 2010;95(12):E448-55.
24. Stabile G, Borrielli I, Artenisio AC, et al. Effects of the insulin sensitizer pioglitazone on menstrual irregularity, insulin resistance and hyperandrogenism in young women with polycystic ovary syndrome. J Pediatr Adolesc Gynecol. 2014;27(3):177-82.
25. Legro RS. Ovulation induction in polycystic ovary syndrome: current options. Best Pract Res Clin Obstet Gynaecol. 2016;37:152-9.
26. Brzechffa PR, Daneshmand S, Buyalos RP. Sequential clomiphene citrate and human menopausal gonadotrophin with intrauterine insemination: the effect of patient age on clinical outcome. Hum Reprod. 1998;13(8): 2110-4.
27. Song D, Shi Y, Zhong Y, et al. Efficiency of mild ovarian stimulation with clomiphene on poor ovarian responders during IVF\ICSI procedures: a meta-analysis. Eur J Obstet Gynecol Reprod Biol. 2016;204:36-43.
28. Aleyamma TK, Kamath MS, Muthukumar K, et al. Affordable ART: a different perspective. Hum Reprod. 2011;26(12):3312-8.
29. Baart EB, Martini E, Eijkemans MJ, et al. Milder ovarian stimulation for in-vitro fertilization reduces aneuploidy in the human preimplantation embryo: a randomized controlled trial. Hum Reprod. 2007;22(4):980-8.
30. Kato K, Takehara Y, Segawa T, et al. Minimal ovarian stimulation combined with elective single embryo transfer policy: age-specific results of a large, single- centre, Japanese cohort. Reprod Biol Endocrinol. 2012;10:35.

CHAPTER

43

Physiology and Pharmacology of Different Gonadotropins

Reena Gupta, Manish Banker

INTRODUCTION

Gonadotropins are hormones secreted by pituitary that have a stimulatory effect on gonads. This family includes follicle-stimulating hormone (FSH), luteinizing hormone (LH), and human chorionic gonadotropin (hCG). These hormones are central to the complex endocrine system that regulates normal growth, sexual development, and reproductive function. LH and FSH are secreted by the anterior pituitary gland, while hCG is secreted by the placenta in pregnant humans.

Gonadotropin therapy plays an integral role in ovarian stimulation for infertility treatments. It was introduced almost one century ago, and the last 25 years have yielded major advancements.

PHYSIOLOGY

The human ovarian follicular development depends on the synergistic and sequential effects of the two principal gonadotropins, FSH and LH. FSH stimulates the growth of a large preovulatory follicle that because of its FSH-dependent maturation is able to ovulate and to form a corpus luteum in response to the mid-cycle surge of LH.

At birth, ovaries contain 1–2 million follicles arrested at the primordial stage of development. But only about 400 follicles mature and ovulate during a woman's reproductive lifespan and rest of them undergo atresia.

Follicle development from the primordial to the preovulatory stage takes several months.[1] The initial growth of the primordial follicles to preantral follicles is independent of pituitary gonadotropins. However, antrum formation requires tonic stimulation by FSH. These early antral follicles are FSH responsive and constitute a pool of available follicles that can be stimulated to grow. During the luteal–follicular transition phase, a selective rise in FSH occurs that must reach a critical threshold for recruitment of follicles. Although several follicles begin to grow during this phase because of mitogenic action of FSH on granulosa cells, only one is selected and the rest are destined to undergo atresia.

At the mid-follicular phase, the dominant follicle reaches about 10 mm in diameter and is recognizable as the largest follicle in the ovary, which starts secreting estradiol at around 7th or 8th day of cycle. LH is capable of stimulating androgen-substrate production from theca cells, which is transformed to estrogen by FSH stimulated aromatase activity in granulosa cells (in accordance with two cell two gonadotropin therapy). This rise in estradiol (and inhibin) leads to fall in FSH levels through negative feedback on the pituitary. The mid-follicular fall in FSH concentration determines the atresia of less mature follicles that are unable to grow without adequate FSH concentrations. But, the mature selected follicle continues to grow which is likely to be due to its increased sensitivity to FSH itself. It has been demonstrated that FSH induces LH receptor formation on preovulatory follicle granulosa cells.[2] The action of LH on its receptors activates adenyl cyclase: the consequent production of cyclic adenosine monophosphate (cAMP) represents an additive response to FSH.[3] Therefore, the maturing follicle reduces its dependency on FSH by acquiring LH receptors and LH responsiveness.[4-8] On the other hand, lower concentrations of FSH bring less mature follicles to atresia. When mid cycle LH surge occurs, the LH–follicle interaction disrupts granulosa cells in cumulus oophorus and induces final oocyte maturation, causes follicular rupture, and finally luteinization of granulosa

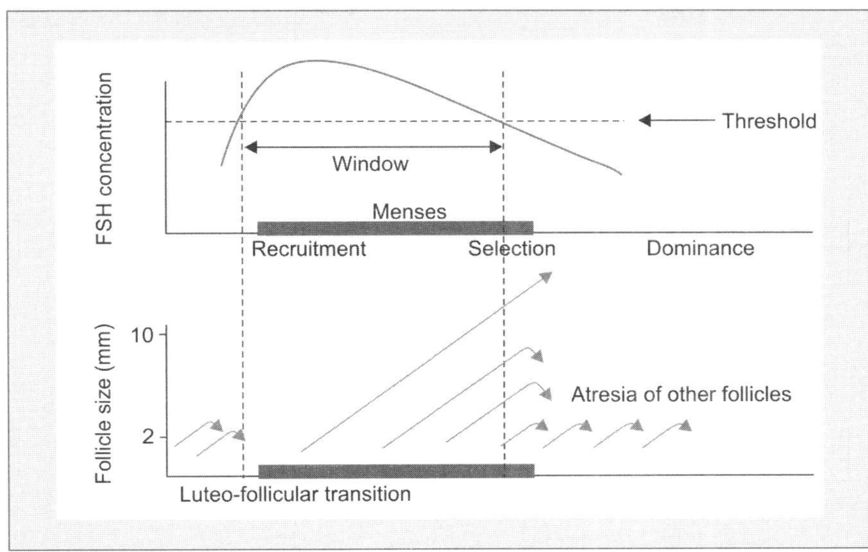

Fig. 1: Follicle-stimulating hormone (FSH) threshold and window concept in human follicle development.

cells. hCG has been used as surrogate to LH for final oocyte maturation and ovulation in artificially stimulated cycles (Fig. 1).

To summarize, FSH acts on the early antral follicles to stimulate cell growth, steroidogenesis, and the expression of LH receptors. Subsequently, LH, in conjunction with FSH, acts on the FSH-stimulated follicle to maintain growth, and is eventually responsible for the process of ovulation and luteinization.

HISTORY OF GONADOTROPINS

Pharmaceutical preparations containing biologically active gonadotropins for ovulation induction have been available in the market for 75 years. It was Aschheim and Zondek, in 1927, who first discovered a substance in the urine of pregnant women which had the same action as the gonadotropic factor in the anterior pituitary.[9] They called this substance gonadotropin or "prolan." Furthermore, they believed that there were two distinct hormones, prolan A and prolan B now called as FSH and LH. They subsequently used their findings to develop a pregnancy test. In 1930, Zondek reported that gonadotropins were also present in the urine of postmenopausal women and in the same year, Cole and Hart found gonadotropins in the serum of pregnant mares.[10] However, it was only in 1937 that Cartland and Nelson were able to produce a purified extract of this hormone. In 1948, Stewart, Sano, and Montgomery, discovered that gonadotropins in the urine of pregnant women were shown to originate from the chorionic villi of the placenta, rather than the pituitary, and subsequently designated it as "chorionic gonadotropin."[11] Within years, it became apparent that the use of gonadotropin extracts from nonprimate sources was of limited clinical value owing to the development of antibodies that neutralized their therapeutic effect. Then, efforts were made to produce these gonadotropins from urine of postmenopausal women. The first urine extract of gonadotropin contained LH and FSH and was named Pergonal, inspired by the Italian words "per gonadi" (for the gonads). In 1961, with the use of Pergonal treatment, first pregnancy was reported in a patient with secondary amenorrhea. Urinary FSH and highly purified FSH became available after 1980s with the development of new technologies using specific monoclonal antibodies that bind to FSH and LH molecules in the human menopausal gonadotropin (hMG) material in such a way that unknown urinary proteins can be removed. In 2000, a major evolution occurred in the field of infertility with the development of recombinant FSH which had many advantages over urinary preparations. With this evolution of gonadotropins from pituitary to urinary to highly purified and most recently recombinant products, the safety, purity, and specific activity have increased progressively (Fig. 2).

GONADOTROPIN STRUCTURE

The three gonadotropins, FSH, LH, and hCG are glycoproteins composed of two noncovalently-linked protein subunits, the alpha and beta subunits. The alpha subunit contains 92 amino acids (AA) and is identical in FSH, LH, and hCG. In contrast, the beta subunits are distinct and confer unique receptor specificity as well as differential biological properties. The subunits alone do not have any biological activity. It is the formation of

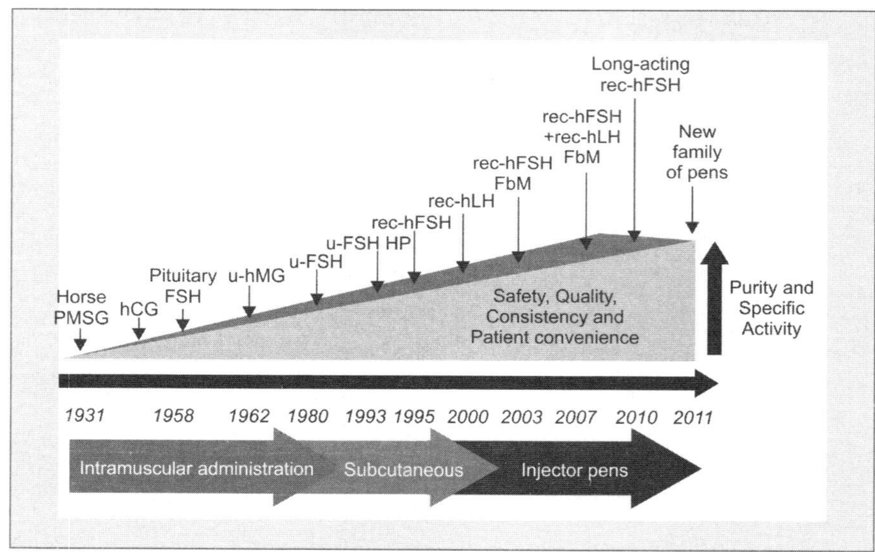

Fig. 2: Milestones in the development of gonadotropin preparations. (FSH: follicle-stimulating hormone; hCG: human chorionic gonadotropin; LH: luteinizing hormone; PMSG: pregnant mare's serum gonadotropin)
Source: Reproduced with permission from Leão R de BF, et al.[12]

Table 1: Characteristics of follicle-stimulating hormone (FSH) isoforms.

Isoform	*Estradiol (E2) levels*	*Sialic acid content*	*In vivo half-life*	*Receptor affinity*	*Predominance*
Acid	Low	High	Long	Low	Early/mid-follicular and luteal phase
Basic	High	Low	Short	High	Late follicular/preovulatory phase

heterodimers, by the attachment of carbohydrate moieties, which is responsible for biological activity. The extent and pattern of glycosylation conveys the spectrum of different charges, bioactivities, and half-lives for each glycoprotein. Glycoproteins have two basic types of glycosylation patterns: O-linked glycosylation, which is characterized by a carbohydrate N-acetylgalactosamine (GalNAc) attached to the hydroxyl group of the amino acid serine or threonine, and N-linked glycosylation, which is characterized by an N-acetyl glucosamine (GlcNAc) attached to the amide group of asparagine (Asn). The oligosaccharides often terminate with sialic acid and/or sulfonated b1-4-linked GalNAc (SO_3^{-4}GalNAc). Molecules with a large number of sulfonated Gal-NAcs disappear faster from the circulation than less-sulfonated isoforms due to their affinity for liver SO_3^{-4}GalNAc receptors. On the other hand, the more the sialylation, the more is the half-life.

Follicle-stimulating Hormone

The beta subunit of FSH is composed of 111 amino acids. There are four asparagine-linked glycosylation sites (two on the alpha subunit and two on the beta subunit). Each subunit is attached to two carbohydrate moieties with variable compositions that, in turn, create different isoforms. These multiple forms of FSH differ in their plasma half-lives (range: 3 hours) due to variations in their binding potentials. When FSH isoforms have more sialic residues, they have decreased receptor affinity and therefore remain in circulation longer. The distribution of isoform types is under endocrine control, and the amount of sialic acid present is influenced mainly by estradiol (E_2) levels—the higher the estradiol levels, the less glycosylated the FSH, the shorter the half-life, but the greater the receptor affinity (Table 1). Therefore, the isoform profile is more acidic during the early follicular to mid-follicular phase of the menstrual cycle, but shifts to become more basic shortly before ovulation. These dynamic changes in sialylation are not mimicked by current controlled ovarian gonadotropin stimulation regimens. It is unknown whether such modifications in follicular stimulation protocols would affect oocyte quality.

Luteinizing Hormone

Although the alpha subunit of LH is identical to FSH and hCG, it is the beta subunit composed of 121 amino acids, which confers specific biologic activity and facilitates its interaction with the LH receptor. LH beta-subunits contain a single site with N-linked glycosylation (Asn 30) and fewer sialic acid residues (only 1 or 2) because of which LH has a short half-life of only 20–30 minutes (Fig. 3).

Human Chorionic Gonadotropin

The beta subunit of LH and hCG has a similar amino acid sequence but, a notable difference is the presence of a long carboxy terminal segment with 24 amino acids containing four O-linked oligosaccharide sites in hCG (Fig. 1). In addition, hCG beta subunits contain two sites of N-linked glycosylation compared with one in LH. Due to the higher number of both glycosylation sites and sialic acid residues (approximately 20.) compared with LH, hCG has a markedly longer terminal half-life of 24 hours compared with approximately 30 minutes for LH. Due to the similarity in structure, hCG binds to the same receptor as LH.

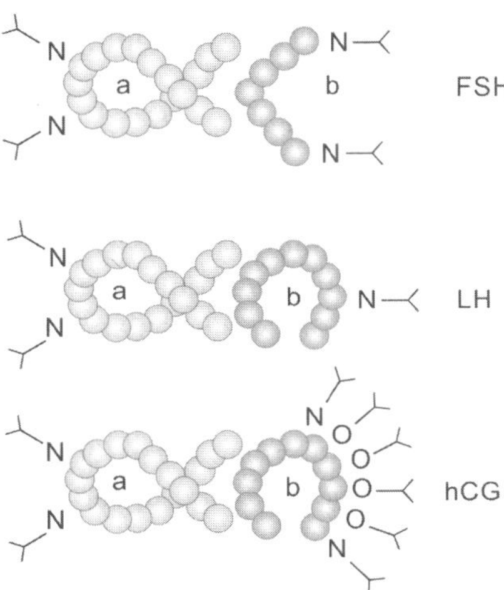

Fig. 3: Glycosylation patterns of FSH, LH and hCG. The alpha subunits of each hormone are identical in amino acid sequence and contain two sites of N-linked glycosylation. The beta subunit confers hormone specificity and contains variable amounts of N-linked glycosylation. LH beta subunit contains a single site of N-linked glycosylation, while FSH and hCG beta subunits contain two sites of N-linked glycosylation. In addition, hCG has an extended C-terminal that contains four sites of O-linked glycosylation. (FSH: follicle-stimulating hormone; hCG: human chorionic gonadotropin; LH: luteinizing hormone).
Source: Reproduced with permission from Esteves SC et al[13]

The structural characteristics of three glycoproteins are illustrated in Table 2.

DIFFERENT GONADOTROPIN PREPARATIONS

Human Menopausal Gonadotropin (Menotropin)

Human menopausal gonadotropin, or menotropin, was first extracted from the urine of postmenopausal women in 1949.[14] Urine was originally obtained from an Italian nunnery, and at that time preparations contained varying amounts of FSH, LH, and hCG with only 5% of pure forms, i.e. only 5% of protein content was gonadotropins.[15] The specific activity of these products usually does not exceed 150 IU/mg protein. Human menopausal gonadotropin preparations have both FSH and LH activity, in equal amounts, but the latter is primarily derived from the hCG component present in postmenopausal urine and concentrated during purification. Generally, hCG is added to achieve the desired amount of LH-like biological activity.

The different proteins found in various hMG preparations include tumor necrosis factor binding protein1, transferrin, urokinase, Tamm-Horsfall glycoprotein, epidermal growth factor, and immunoglobulin-related proteins. Urinary preparations are also found to have impurities such as prion proteins which are associated with transmissible spongiform encephalopathy (TSE) diseases, and if these Prion proteins are inactivated, it may also denature other proteins, including FSH. Local side effects, such as pain and allergic reactions are attributed to these nongonadotropin proteins. Later, improvements in the purification techniques led to standardization of FSH and LH activities to 75 IU for each type of gonadotropin in 1963, as measured by standard in vivo bioassays (Steelman–Pohley assay). According to this assay an ampoule of hMG, which has 75 IU of FSH, may actually contain 60 and 90 IU.

Table 2: Structural characteristics of FSH, LH and hCG molecules.

	Alpha subunit	*Beta subunit*	*N-linked glycosylation sites on alpha subunit*	*N-linked glycosylation site on beta subuit*	*O-linked glycosylation site on beta subunit*	*Carboxy terminal segment*	*Terminal half life*
FSH	92 AA	111 AA	2	2	0	Absent	3–4 hours
LH	92 AA	121 AA	2	1	0	Absent	20–30 minutes
hCG	92 AA	145 AA	2	2	4	Present	24 hours

(AA: amino acid; FSH: follicle-stimulating hormone; hCG: human chorionic gonadotropin; LH: luteinizing hormone)

In 1999, purified hMG gonadotropins were introduced, allowing its subcutaneous (SC) administration. Highly purified hMG (HP-hMG) contains more hCG and less LH than does traditional hMG. Both conventional and HP-hMG are now commercially available in a FSH:LH ratio of 1:1.

Urinary Follicle-stimulating Hormone (Urofollitropin)

In the 1980s, pure urinary FSH preparations were produced by removing LH with polyclonal antibodies but these preparations still contained high quantity of urinary proteins. Further technological advances made it possible to use highly specific monoclonal antibodies to extract FSH and produce HP-hFSH. The latter became commercially available in 1993. Such preparations contain less than 0.1 IU of LH and less than 5% of unidentified urinary proteins. FSH-specific activity is approximately 10,000 IU/mg protein compared to 100–150 IU/mg protein in the earlier urinary hMG preparations. In addition, the enhanced purity of HP-hFSH enabled subcutaneous administration. Subcutaneous administration had better acceptance and tolerability among patients.

Recombinant Follicle-stimulating Hormone

One of the major problems in the use of urinary-derived FSH preparation was limited supply of urinary products and because of their effective use in infertility the demand was constantly increasing. The other drawbacks were contamination due to presence of urinary proteins and the batch-to-batch variability in consistency which influences the real activity of the gonadotropins contained in the vials.

From 90s, recombinant technology overcame these disadvantages of urinary gonadotropins and fulfilled the need for a more reliable source of FSH. To manufacture recombinant products, first the genes coding for the human FSH alpha subunit and beta subunit were identified, which were then incorporated into the nuclear DNA of a host cell via a plasmid vector, using spliced DNA strings containing the FSH gene and segments of bacterial DNA. Initially *E. coli* was tried as a host but structural complexity of human gonadotropins which required post-translational modification of the molecule by protein folding and glycosylation, made functional protein production impossible in *E. coli*. The Chinese hamster ovary cell line was then chosen as the host to produce gonadotropins because it is genetically stable, fully characterized, and easily transfected with foreign DNA. Furthermore, it can be grown in cell cultures on a large scale and produce adequate levels of biologically active recombinant human follicle-stimulating hormone (rec-hFSH). In 1995, the first rec-hFSH (follitropin alpha) was licensed for clinical use in the European Union. One year later, a similar rec-hFSH (follitropin beta) was made available. In the manufacture of follitropin alpha, Serono (USA) used two separate vectors to construct an FSH-producing cell line, one vector for each subunit. Follitropin beta was manufactured by Organon Limited (Ireland), using a single vector containing the coding sequences of both subunit genes.

Initially a stable line of transformed cells was selected, which secreted high quantities of rec-hFSH. These cell lines were used to establish a master cell bank (MCB), which then serves as a source of working cell banks (WCB). The MCB consists of individual vials containing identical cells, which are cryopreserved until required. Thus a continuous supply of rec-hFSH with guaranteed consistency from MCB to WCB is now available. MCBs and WCBs are routinely tested for sterility, mycoplasma, and viral contamination.

Standardization of Gonadotropin Contents

Traditionally, quantification of gonadotropins was done by in vivo assays, most commonly used was Steelman–Pohley in vivo assay. FSH activity was quantified by rat ovarian weight gain and FSH vials or ampoules are subsequently filled according to the desired bioactivity, measured in IUs. However, this assay had many limitations: time consuming, cumbersome, uses large numbers of rats (ethical issues), and was limited in its precision—the European Pharmacopoeia defines an activity range (80–125% of the target value) within which an FSH batch is acceptable for clinical use.

Recent advances in the manufacturing process for rec-hFSH follitropin alpha enabled high batch to batch consistency in both isoform profile and glycan species distribution. The most significant advantage of this over other commercially available gonadotropins is that it permits FSH to be quantified by protein content (mass in mcg) rather than by biologic activity. A physicochemical assay (SE-HPLC) is used to assess the rhFSH content in the active drug substance and the drug product. The final drug formulation is based on the rhFSH protein content, thus ensuring a more precise content per vial [rhFSH filled by mass (FbM)].[16] The FbM rhFSH preparation showed a 1.6% batch-to-batch variability using the physicochemical assay versus 10% variability obtained with the bioassay.[16]

Some clinical studies assessed the clinical implications of this improvement in drug manufacturing. FbM rhFSH showed a better patient response consistency, improved control of follicular development, a reduced need for dose adjustment and fewer cancelled cycles, improved embryo quality and implantation rate with a trend to higher pregnancy rates, and fewer days of stimulation.[17,18] FbM rhFSH is probably the most consistent rhFSH in terms of protein content: this pharmaceutical FSH preparation is pure, low in degraded forms of FSH, and has a consistent isoform profile.

Gonadotropin Preparations with Luteinizing Hormone Activity

At present, we have three groups of commercially available gonadotropin preparations containing LH activity:

1. Urinary hMG in which LH activity is dependent on hCG rather than on pure LH glycoprotein
2. Pure LH glycoprotein produced by recombinant technology (lutropin alpha)
3. A combination of pure FSH and LH glycoproteins in a fixed ratio of 2:1 also manufactured by recombinant technology.

Recombinant LH (rec-hLH; lutropin alpha) came in the market in the year 2000 for use in women with gonadotropin insufficiency. The manufacturing process of rec-hLH is similar to rec-hFSH. It is administered subcutaneously in a dose of 75 IU. Rec-hLH is used not only to support follicular development during controlled ovarian stimulation (COS) in hypogonadotropic hypogonadic woman but also in other categories of female infertility, including poor responders, women over older than 35 years of age, and hyporesponders.

Recombinant LH has three major differences compared to urinary products containing LH activity:

- It has higher purity and specific activity because it is manufactured using recombinant technology
- It is associated with better dose precision due to filled-by-mass (FbM) technology that virtually eliminates batch-to-batch variation
- LH activity is derived directly from pure LH glycoprotein, unlike hMG, in which hCG is concentrated during purification or added to achieve the desired amount of LH-like biological activity.

In 2007, a new fixed combination of rec-hFSH and rec-hLH at 2:1 (150 IU + 75 IU) ratio was launched (follitropin alpha + lutropin alpha) as an alternative for those women who need LH supplementation. The 2:1 ratio of FSH and LH in a fixed dose combination was obtained by recombinant technology and vial filling using FbM. The bioequivalence of rec-hFSH and rec-hLH administrated alone or in combination has been found to be similar with the convenience of single injection.

Human Chorionic Gonadotropin

Human chorionic gonadotropin has been used traditionally to promote final follicular maturation in ovulation induction as a substitute for the mid-cycle LH surge. Due to structural and biological similarities, hCG and LH bind to and activate the same receptor. However, the luteotropic activity of hCG is markedly higher than that of LH due to its longer half-life and greater receptor affinity. Chorionic gonadotropins can be derived from urine of pregnant women or can be manufactured using recombinant technology. Currently, urinary hCG preparations are marketed in lyophilized vials with 5,000 or 10,000 IU for intramuscular use. Recombinant hCG (rec-hCG) is available in prefilled syringes containing 250 mcg of pure hCG, which is equivalent to approximately 6,500 IU of urinary hCG. Due to its higher purity, rec-hCG is better tolerated and used subcutaneously, thus allowing patient self-administration. Nevertheless, the clinical efficacy of both urinary and recombinant preparations does not seem to differ. In a Cochrane meta-analysis comparing rec-hCG vs. urinary hCG for triggering final oocyte maturation, no significant difference was detected in the live birth rate and incidence of ovarian hyperstimulation syndrome.[19]

Long-acting Follicle-stimulating Hormone (Corifollitropin Alpha)

Corifollitropin alfa is a synthetic recombinant follicle-stimulating hormone (rFSH) molecule containing a hybrid beta subunit, which provides a long plasma half-life of 65 hours while maintaining the pharmacodynamic properties of rFSH. It comprises an alpha subunit, which is identical to that of FSH and a beta subunit which is produced by the fusion of the C-terminal peptide from the beta-subunit of hCG (which provides a long half-life) to the beta subunit of FSH. The optimal dose is 100 µg for women less than 60 Kg and 150 µg for women with a body weight of more than 60 Kg. A single injection of corifollitropin alfa can replace first seven injections with standard daily gonadotropins and stimulation can then be continued with daily FSH injections if required. This makes corifollitropin alfa potentially more patient friendly as it reduces the number of injections, leading to more acceptance among patients. The disadvantage of corifollitropin alfa is that it is not suitable in situations where monofollicular development is the goal. Moreover, the dose of corifollitropin alfa cannot be reduced during one week interval treatment in case of hyperresponse. Hence, it may not be suitable for patients with expected hyperresponse such as PCOS or prior history of OHSS. According to recent Cochrane review in 2015, which included six randomized controlled trials (RCTs), a comparison of long-acting FSH versus daily FSH did not show evidence of difference in effect on overall live birth rate and OHSS.[20] There was no difference in the clinical pregnancy rate (any dose), ongoing pregnancy rate (any dose), multiple pregnancy rate (any dose), miscarriage rate (low or medium dose), ectopic pregnancy rate (any dose), congenital malformation rate; major or minor (low or medium dose). The authors concluded that the use of a medium dose (150–180 μg) of long-acting FSH is a safe treatment option and equally effective compared to daily FSH in women with unexplained subfertility. According to authors whether long-acting FSH is safe and effective for use in hyper- or poor responders still needs to be determined by further research.

Biosimilar Gonadotropins

As patents expire after 20 years from the launch of first recombinant FSH preparations (follitropin alpha), there is an increasing interest of other pharmaceutical companies in the resulting market opportunities through development of their own biosimilar products. Biosimilars are defined by FDA as biologic products (substances produced by living cells using biotechnology such as recombinant DNA technology) that are "highly similar to the reference product not withstanding minor differences in clinically inactive components and that there are no clinically meaningful differences between the biologic product and the reference product in terms of safety, purity, and potency of the product."[21] This means biosimilars contain similar active pharmaceutical ingredient, have to be used in same dose, same route of administration, and for similar indications in clinical practice.

The active substance of biologics is a collection of large complex protein isoforms and not a single small molecule and hence the active form of biosimilars are highly unlikely to be exactly the same as the originator product.[22] The cell lines used, the culture media, and the exact process of production are expected to vary between originator and different biosimilars resulting in differences in the final product. Biosimilar gonadotropins may differ in FSH isoform profile/glycosylation patterns as compared to originator product. These minor differences may result in major changes in terms of efficacy and safety of these products. As a result biosimilars, unlike a generic medicine, need to pass through the clinical trials and approval in as much the same way as is an originator product. Further, even after having shown similar safety and efficacy in trials, the distinct possibility of difference in safety and efficacy profiles of a biosimilar cannot be ruled out and this needs to be kept in mind while dealing with a biosimilar.

Biosimilar FSH has the potential to bring down the cost of infertility treatment by being cheaper than the originator product. However, the difference may not be as high as in case of generic products. Further, subtle differences in efficacy and safety can alter the overall cost-effectiveness of the treatment using biosimilar product and hence it is imperative to perform a formal cost-effective analysis for any biosimilar.

Urinary versus Recombinant Preparations

Many meta-analysis and randomized trials have been done till date comparing the efficacy of urinary vs. recombinant preparations, mostly concluding that both urinary and recombinant preparations have similar efficacy in terms of achieving a pregnancy or live birth per initiated cycle.[23-25] A recent Cochrane review in 2011 compared the effectiveness of recombinant gonadotropin (rFSH) with the three main types of urinary gonadotropins (i.e. hMG, FSH-P, and FSH-HP) for ovarian stimulation in women undergoing IVF or ICSI treatment cycles.[26] It included 42 trials with a total of 9,606 couples. The review did not find any statistically significant difference in live birth rate on comparing rFSH to any of the other gonadotropins irrespective of the protocol used [28 trials, 7,339 couples, odds ratio (OR) 0.97, 95% confidence interval (CI) 0.87–1.08], suggesting that for a group with a 25% live birth rate using urinary gonadotropins the rate would be between 22.5% and 26.5% using rFSH. There was also no evidence of a difference in the OHSS rate (32 trials, 7,740 couples, OR 1.18, 95% CI 0.86–1.61).[26]

Although the live birth rate per initiated cycle is the most important end result in IVF studies; however, in the present era of improved vitrification techniques and single embryo transfer, cumulative pregnancy rates could be better indicators of successful IVF, this in turn would depend upon the number of embryos formed and is directly proportional to the number of oocytes retrieved,[27] many studies recently have compared the efficacy of urinary gonadotropins with recombinant preparations in terms of oocyte yield. Revelli A et al. compared the efficacy of recombinant FSH (rFSH) plus recombinant LH (rLH) with urinary hMG.[28] They found that the pregnancy rate in both groups progressively improved according to the number of oocytes retrieved. When comparing patients within the same subgroup of oocyte yield, both groups showed a comparable outcome up to the reported highest yield (>8) of oocytes.[28] However, when more than eight oocytes were available, recombinant group had a significantly better pregnancy rate outcome.

Sykes et al. compared the cost-effectiveness of different gonadotropins, recombinant FSH (rFSH), highly purified urinary FSH (uFSH-HP), and human menopausal gonadotropins (hMG) in IVF stimulation.[29] They calculated the cost-effectiveness ratios for "the average cost per ongoing pregnancy" and "incremental cost per additional pregnancy" for women entering into IVF treatment for a maximum of three cycles. The predicted cumulative pregnancy rate after three cycles was 57.1% for rFSH and 44.4% for both uFSH-HP and hMG. The cost of IVF treatment was more for rFSH, as compared to uFSH-HP and hMG for index cycle but when assessed in association with ongoing pregnancy rate and cumulative pregnancy rate the average cost per ongoing pregnancy was more favorable with rFSH than with either uFSH-HP or hMG. The other studies comparing urinary vs. recombinant preparations have also concurred with these findings.[25,30-32]

Role of Luteinizing Hormone/Human Menopausal Gonadotropin

In view of the concepts of LH threshold and LH ceiling, there has been a lot of debate on who are the candidates to be benefitted by adding LH or hMG.[33] Optimal follicular development is supposed to occur when LH is above a threshold of 1.1 IU/L and below a ceiling of 5.1 IU/L.[34,35] Most women undergoing COS for IVF have adequate endogenous LH levels and thus do not require LH supplementation as only 1% of LH receptors must be occupied to drive an adequate ovarian steroidogenesis. However, LH supplementation is must in hypogonadotropic hypogonadism patients as they do not have any endogenous LH. The other group of patients who have been shown to be benefitted by adding LH are those with poor ovarian reserve, advanced maternal age (>35 years), and ones who show suboptimal response on day 6 of stimulation with recombinant FSH alone.[36-39] It has been hypothesized that these women would benefit from preparations containing LH, by an increase in androgen production for future aromatization into estrogens that could restore the follicular milieu and thus positively impact oocyte quality.

The MERIT (Menotrophin vs. Recombinant FSH In Vitro Fertilization Trial) group studied the effect of LH activity on IVF cycle outcomes and observed that, although the number of oocytes retrieved were more in rFSH group as compared to HP-hMG group (11.8 vs. 10), there were more top-quality embryos with HP-hMG (11.3%) than with rFSH (9.0%; $P = 0.044$).[40,41] They found lower estradiol (E2) ($P = 0.031$) and higher progesterone ($P < 0.001$) levels with rFSH at the end of stimulation even after adjusting for follicular response. The ongoing pregnancy rate per cycle was 27% with HP-hMG and 22% with rFSH which was not statistically significant. The live birth, ongoing pregnancy, and ongoing implantation rates for top-quality embryos were higher with HP-hMG than rFSH but did not reach statistical significance. The better implantation rates in the hMG group in this trial can be attributed to lower progesterone levels on the day of trigger, as the LH component in hMG converts the pregnenolone to androgens in theca cells which is later aromatized to estrogen. High serum progesterone on the day of trigger is found to be associated with reduced implantation rates due to detrimental effects on endometrium.[42,43] However, it has not been shown to have any adverse effect on embryo quality.[44] Contrary to the above findings, Thuesen et al. confirmed that hCG/LH activity even increases the progesterone production during the follicular phase rather than reducing it.[45] Some authors have proposed that the cause of premature progesterone elevation might be due to enhanced FSH stimulation in ART cycles and is not related to type of gonadotropin used.[8,46]

CONCLUSION

Gonadotropins are the sine qua non for IVF. Since last few decades, there have been continuous improvements in the manufacturing process of gonadotropins. Recombinant preparations are purer and safer than urinary-derived gonadotropins, and the introduction of FbM technology has virtually eliminated batch-to-batch variations, enabling accurate and consistent dosing.

As far as the outcome of treatment is concerned, no clear evidence of difference has been demonstrated between urinary and recombinant products, or between hMG/addition of LH and pure FSH alone. The final decision for choosing gonadotropins should be made by the treating clinician taking into consideration the patient profile, personal experiences, affordability, and availability of different preparations.

REFERENCES

1. Gougeon A. Regulation of ovarian follicular development in primates: Facts and hypotheses. Endocr Rev. 1996;17(2):121-55.
2. Zeleznik AJ, Hillier SG. The role of gonadotropins in the selection of the preovulatory follicle. Clin Obstet Gynecol. 1984;27(4):927-40.
3. Goff AK, Armstrong DT. Stimulatory action of gonadotropins and prostaglandins on adenosine-3',5'-monophosphate production by isolated rat granulosa cells. Endocrinology. 1977;101(5):1461-7.
4. Fauser BC, Van Heusden AM. Manipulation of human ovarian function: Physiological concepts and clinical consequences. Endocr Rev. 1997;18(1):71-106.
5. Willis DS, Watson H, Mason HD, et al. Premature response to luteinizing hormone of granulosa cells from anovulatory women with polycystic ovary syndrome: Relevance to mechanism of anovulation. J Clin Endocrinol Metab. 1998;83(11):3984-91.
6. Campbell BK, Dobson H, Baird DT, et al. Examination of the relative role of FSH and LH in the mechanism of ovulatory follicle selection in sheep. J Reprod Fertil. 1999;117(2):355-67.

7. Sullivan MW, Stewart-Akers A, Krasnow JS, et al. Ovarian responses in women to recombinant follicle-stimulating hormone and luteinizing hormone (LH): A role for LH in the final stages of follicular maturation. J Clin Endocrinol Metab. 1999;84(1):228-32.
8. Filicori M, Cognigni GE, Pocognoli P, et al. Modulation of folliculogenesis and steroidogenesis in women by graded menotrophin administration. Hum Reprod. 2002;17(8):2009-15.
9. Rohde W. The contributions of Aschheim and Zondek to endocrinology. Pediatr Endocrinol Rev. 2010;7(4):323-7.
10. Walker D. Laboratory methods of equine pregnancy diagnosis. Vet Rec. 1977;100(19):396-9.
11. Stewart HL, Sano ME, Montgomery TL. Hormone secretion by human placenta grown in tissue culture. J Clin Endocrinol Metab. 1948;8(2):175-88.
12. Leão R de BF, Esteves SC. Gonadotropin therapy in assisted reproduction: An evolutionary perspective from biologics to biotech. Clinics (Sao Paulo). 2014;69(4):279-93.
13. Esteves SC. Efficacy, efficiency and effectiveness of gonadotropin therapy for infertility treatment. Med Expr. 2015;2(3):1-11.
14. Lunenfeld B. Historical perspectives in gonadotrophin therapy. Hum Reprod Update. 2004;10(6):453-67.
15. Practice Committee of American Society for Reproductive Medicine, Birmingham, Alabama. Gonadotropin preparations: Past, present, and future perspectives. Fertil Steril. 2008;90(5 Suppl):S13-20.
16. Bassett RM, Driebergen R. Continued improvements in the quality and consistency of follitropin alfa, recombinant human FSH. Reprod Biomed Online. 2005;10(2):169-77.
17. Hugues J-N, Barlow DH, Rosenwaks Z, et al. Improvement in consistency of response to ovarian stimulation with recombinant human follicle stimulating hormone resulting from a new method for calibrating the therapeutic preparation. Reprod Biomed Online. 2003;6(2):185-90.
18. Balasch J, Fábregues F, Peñarrubia J, et al. Outcome from consecutive assisted reproduction cycles in patients treated with recombinant follitropin alfa filled-by-bioassay and those treated with recombinant follitropin alfa filled-by-mass. Reprod Biomed Online. 2004;8(4):408-13.
19. Youssef MA, Al-Inany HG, Aboulghar M, et al. Recombinant versus urinary human chorionic gonadotrophin for final oocyte maturation triggering in IVF and ICSI cycles. Cochrane Database Syst Rev. 2011;(4):CD003719.
20. Pouwer AW, Farquhar C, Kremer JAM. Long-acting FSH versus daily FSH for women undergoing assisted reproduction. Cochrane Database Syst Rev. 2015;(7):CD009577.
21. US Food and Drug Administration. (2012). Guidance for industry. Scientific considerations in demonstrating biosimilarity to a reference product. Available from http://www.fda.gov/downloads/Drugs/GuidanceComplianceRegulatoryInformation/Guidances/UCM291128.pdf [Accessed October 2018].
22. Sekhon BS, Saluja V. Biosimilars: An overview. Biosimilars. 2011;1:1-11.
23. Jee BC, Suh CS, Kim YB, et al. Clinical efficacy of highly purified hMG versus recombinant FSH in IVF/ICSI cycles: A meta-analysis. Gynecol Obstet Invest. 2010;70(2):132-7.
24. Al-Inany HG, Abou-Setta AM, Aboulghar MA, et al. Highly purified hMG achieves better pregnancy rates in IVF cycles but not ICSI cycles compared with recombinant FSH: A meta-analysis. Gynecol Endocrinol. 2009;25(6):372-8.
25. Devroey P, Pellicer A, Nyboe Andersen A, et al. A randomized assessor-blind trial comparing highly purified hMG and recombinant FSH in a GnRH antagonist cycle with compulsory single-blastocyst transfer. Fertil Steril. 2012;97(3):561-71.
26. van Wely M, Kwan I, Burt AL, et al. Recombinant versus urinary gonadotrophin for ovarian stimulation in assisted reproductive technology cycles. Cochrane Database Syst Rev. 2011;(2):CD005354.
27. Vaughan DA, Leung A, Resetkova N, et al. How many oocytes are optimal to achieve multiple live births with one stimulation cycle? The one and done approach. Fertil Steril. 2017;107(2):397-404.e3.
28. Revelli A, Pettinau G, Basso G, et al. Controlled ovarian stimulation with recombinant-FSH plus recombinant-LH vs. human menopausal gonadotropin based on the number of retrieved oocytes: Results from a routine clinical practice in a real-life population. Reprod Biol Endocrinol. 2015;13:77.
29. Sykes D, Out HJ, Palmer SJ, et al. The cost-effectiveness of IVF in the UK: A comparison of three gonadotrophin treatments. Hum Reprod. 2001;16(12):2557-62.
30. Lehert P, Schertz JC, Ezcurra D. Recombinant human follicle-stimulating hormone produces more oocytes with a lower total dose per cycle in assisted reproductive technologies compared with highly purified human menopausal gonadotrophin: A meta-analysis. Reprod Biol Endocrinol. 2010;8:112.
31. Wex J, Abou-Setta AM. Economic evaluation of highly purified human menopausal gonadotropin versus recombinant human follicle-stimulating hormone in fresh and frozen in vitro fertilization/intracytoplasmic sperm-injection cycles in Sweden. Clinicoecon Outcomes Res. 2013;5:381-97.
32. Levi Setti PE, Alviggi C, Colombo GL, et al. Human recombinant follicle stimulating hormone (rFSH) compared to urinary human menopausal gonadotropin (HMG) for ovarian stimulation in assisted reproduction: A literature review and cost evaluation. J Endocrinol Invest. 2015;38(5):497-503.
33. Shoham Z. The clinical therapeutic window for luteinizing hormone in controlled ovarian stimulation. Fertil Steril. 2002;77(6):1170-7.
34. Shoham Z, Smith H, Yeko T, et al. Recombinant LH (lutropin alfa) for the treatment of hypogonadotrophic women with profound LH deficiency: A randomized, double-blind, placebo-controlled, proof-of-efficacy study. Clin Endocrinol (Oxf). 2008;69(3):471-8.
35. The European Recombinant Human LH Study Group. Recombinant human luteinizing hormone (LH) to support recombinant human follicle-stimulating hormone (FSH)-induced follicular development in LH- and FSH-deficient anovulatory women: A dose-finding study. J Clin Endocrinol Metab. 1998;83(5):1507-14.
36. Laml T, Obruca A, Fischl F, et al. Recombinant luteinizing hormone in ovarian hyperstimulation after stimulation failure in normogonadotropic women. Gynecol Endocrinol. 1999;13(2):98-103.

37. De Placido G, Alviggi C, Perino A, et al. Recombinant human LH supplementation versus recombinant human FSH (rFSH) step-up protocol during controlled ovarian stimulation in normogonadotrophic women with initial inadequate ovarian response to rFSH. A multicentre, prospective, randomized controlled trial. Hum Reprod. 2005;20(2):390-6.
38. Lévy DP, Navarro JM, Schattman GL, et al. The role of LH in ovarian stimulation: exogenous LH: Let's design the future. Hum Reprod. 2000;15(11):2258-65.
39. Hill MJ, Levens ED, Levy G, et al. The use of recombinant luteinizing hormone in patients undergoing assisted reproductive techniques with advanced reproductive age: A systematic review and meta-analysis. Fertil Steril. 2012;97(5):1108-14.e1.
40. Andersen AN, Devroey P, Arce J-C. Clinical outcome following stimulation with highly purified hMG or recombinant FSH in patients undergoing IVF: A randomized assessor-blind controlled trial. Hum Reprod. 2006;21(12):3217-27.
41. Ziebe S, Lundin K, Janssens R, et al. Influence of ovarian stimulation with HP-hMG or recombinant FSH on embryo quality parameters in patients undergoing IVF. Hum Reprod. 2007;22(9):2404-13.
42. Van Vaerenbergh I, Fatemi HM, Blockeel C, et al. Progesterone rise on HCG day in GnRH antagonist/rFSH stimulated cycles affects endometrial gene expression. Reprod Biomed Online. 2011;22(3):263-71.
43. Elgindy EA. Progesterone level and progesterone/estradiol ratio on the day of hCG administration: Detrimental cutoff levels and new treatment strategy. Fertil Steril. 2011;95(5):1639-44.
44. Silverberg KM, Martin M, Olive DL, et al. Elevated serum progesterone levels on the day of human chorionic gonadotropin administration in in vitro fertilization cycles do not adversely affect embryo quality. Fertil Steril. 1994;61(3):508-13.
45. Thuesen LL, Smitz J, Loft A, et al. Endocrine effects of hCG supplementation to recombinant FSH throughout controlled ovarian stimulation for IVF: A dose-response study. Clin Endocrinol (Oxf). 2013;79(5):708-15.
46. Kyrou D, Al-Azemi M, Papanikolaou EG, et al. The relationship of premature progesterone rise with serum estradiol levels and number of follicles in GnRH antagonist/recombinant FSH-stimulated cycles. Eur J Obstet Gynecol Reprod Biol. 2012;162(2):165-8.

CHAPTER

44

Protocols for the Normoresponders

Sulbha Arora, Ashvini Deshmukh

INTRODUCTION

The first in vitro fertilization (IVF) baby was born from a natural or nonstimulated cycle.[1] However, it was soon realized that the success rates of natural cycle IVF were low, primarily due to the limited number of oocytes retrieved. To address this problem, stimulation of multiple follicular genesis by the ovaries was attempted by introducing urinary gonadotropin preparations. This resulted in a significant increase in both the number of oocytes retrieved as well as the success rates of IVF. Today, ovulation induction and controlled ovarian stimulation are integral parts of every assisted reproduction program.

As the popularity of ovarian stimulation grew, various problems started to surface. Premature luteinization and failure of synchronous follicular recruitment due to early dominant follicle selection were the two main problems limiting the success rates. Also, ovulation could occur at any time of the day, necessitating intensive monitoring and oocyte retrieval at inconvenient times of the day.[2] Gonadotropin-releasing hormone (GnRH) agonists were shown to result in pituitary down regulation and succeeded in overcoming these problems, becoming the next breakthrough in IVF treatment. Subsequently, GnRH antagonists, which have a similar function but require a shorter duration to achieve pituitary suppression (and prevent premature luteinizing hormone or LH surge) have been introduced and are now increasingly being used.

OBJECTIVES OF STIMULATION PROTOCOLS IN IN VITRO FERTILIZATION CYCLES

In stimulated cycles, our aim is to produce multiple follicles. In order to achieve this, we need to prevent dominant follicle selection. In natural cycles, estrogen secreted by the dominant follicle exerts a negative feedback on the pituitary that suppresses follicle-stimulating hormone (FSH) secretion below the threshold value, thereby causing atresia of the remaining follicles. In stimulated cycles, exogenous gonadotropins are used to achieve FSH levels above threshold during the phase of follicular recruitment to interfere with the selection of a single dominant follicle and encourage the growth of multiple follicles simultaneously.

Pituitary desensitization by using either GnRH agonists or GnRH antagonists, is an important part of IVF stimulation as it eliminates the possible interference by endogenous hormones, enabling synchronous follicular development. This prevents premature luteinization, and helps to reduce intensive and frequent monitoring allowing control over the timing of oocyte retrieval.

The LH surge is substituted by exogenous human chorionic gonadotropin (hCG), enabling clinics to time oocyte retrieval.

STIMULATION PROTOCOLS

- *Long protocol:* GnRH agonist + Gonadotropins FSH or human menopausal gonadotropin (hMG)
- *Short (flare-up protocol):* GnRH agonist + Gonadotropins
- *Antagonist protocol:* GnRH antagonist + Gonadotropins
  - Single dose
  - Multiple dose.

Various protocols have been used to achieve the goals of ovarian stimulation. The two agents used for downregulation include either the GnRH agonists or the GnRH antagonists. As the GnRH agonists cause an initial flare reaction, they need to be started earlier on, either in the mid-luteal phase of the previous cycle or at the start of the follicular phase. On the other hand, GnRH antagonists have an immediate suppressive effect, and therefore need to be started only toward the end of the follicular phase, that is just before the rise of the LH surge. They can be used either as a single dose or as multiple doses given daily.

Long Protocol

The long agonist protocol is the oldest stimulation protocol and has for many years also been the most common one to be used. It starts on day 21 of the previous cycle with a daily dose of GnRH agonist, which is then continued after the onset of menses and up to the day of trigger. Gonadotropin injections (hMG or FSH) are added with the onset of menses, that is, day 1 or 2 of the cycle. The gonadotropin doses are titrated by performing serial ultrasound measurements of the growing follicles. Follicular maturation is triggered by administering hCG, either urinary or recombinant, once at least three leading follicles have crossed 18 mm in diameter. Oocyte retrieval is scheduled 34.5 hours later (Fig. 1).

The advantage of this protocol is excellent cycle control, making it the desired protocol for first time patients as well as women with a previous normal response. However, the drawbacks include longer duration of injections, higher gonadotropin requirement and in turn added cost. Over repeated cycles, patients start getting fed up of the sheer number of injections required and compliance levels start to fall. Due to these reasons, this protocol has largely given way to the newer, more patient-friendly antagonist protocols.

Short Protocol

In the short protocol, GnRH agonists are started in a daily dose along with the gonadotropin injections on day 1 or 2 of the cycle, that is, in the early follicular phase. The timing and administration of the trigger injection and the subsequent scheduling of the oocyte retrieval is as for the long protocol (Fig. 2).

The benefit of this protocol is the initial flare up reaction of the GnRH agonist, which causes the stimulation of FSH secretion by the pituitary gland in the first few days. As the pituitary gland has not yet been suppressed, this protocol results in better follicular recruitment than the long protocol. However, a significant drawback of this protocol is the high progesterone level at the start of the cycle, which may be due to the rescue of the corpus luteum from the previous cycle. Studies have shown a lower pregnancy rate with this protocol than the long protocol.[3] Therefore, although this was a favored protocol for poor responders in the past, its popularity has reduced with the advent of antagonist protocols.

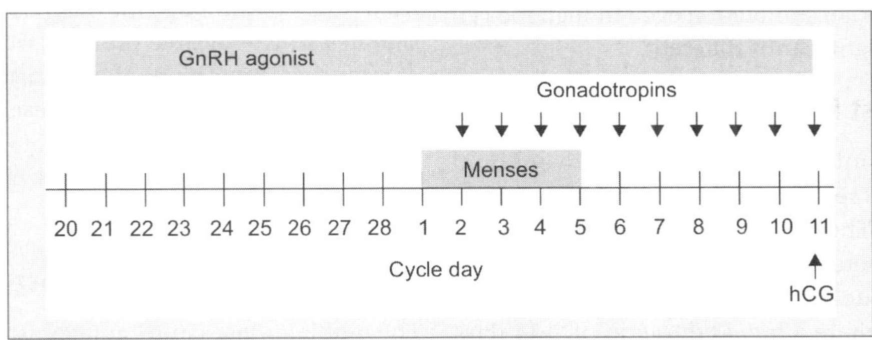

Fig. 1: Gonadotropin-releasing hormone (GnRH) agonist long protocol. (hCG: human chorionic gonadotropin).

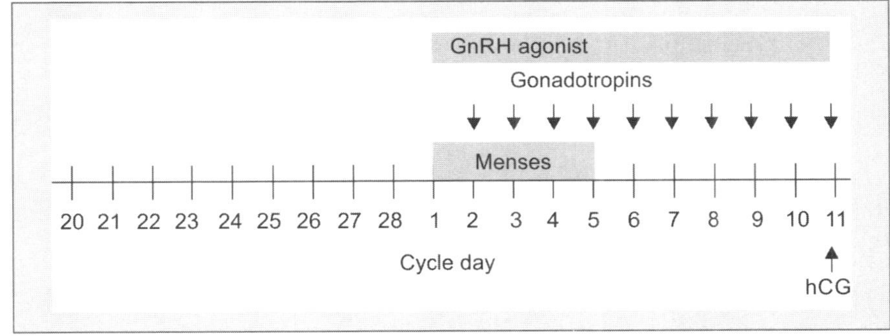

Fig. 2: Gonadotropin-releasing hormone (GnRH) agonist short protocol. (hCG: human chorionic gonadotropin).

GnRH Agonists used for Downregulation

Various different GnRH agonist preparations are available, and the choice of agent varies from one center to another based on the clinician's preference. They differ from each other mainly in potency and route of administration.

The most commonly used agents include buserelin, leuprorelin and triptorelin, which are administered in the form of a daily subcutaneous injection. Single dose subcutaneous depot preparations of the same are also available. Nafarelin and buserelin are available in the form of nasal sprays that need to be administered in multiple daily doses. Although patient compliance with the intranasal route is better, the drawback is fluctuating absorption of the agent resulting in an unpredictable response. However, it does appear to be sufficient to prevent a spontaneous LH surge.

Meta-analyses of trials comparing the different preparations have shown no difference in either the efficacy of pituitary suppression or IVF outcomes, measured in terms of the number of oocytes retrieved and the pregnancy rates respectively. However, women treated with nafarelin required lower doses of gonadotropins and shorter duration of ovarian stimulation, compared to leuprorelin, triptorelin and buserelin.[4] On the other hand, the use of depot preparations of GnRH agonists was associated with increased requirements for gonadotropins and a longer time required for ovarian stimulation even though the IVF outcomes were not significantly different.

GnRH Antagonist Protocols

Although GnRH agonists have been the conventional agents used for down regulation over the years, they have certain drawbacks. They have an initial flare reaction, which implies that there is an initial agonist action before the receptors get blocked and the antagonist reaction begins. Thus they require a longer duration of 7–14 days to achieve adequate down regulation. This also merits a larger number of injections, unless a depot preparation is used. Also, due to profound suppression of the pituitary, menopausal side effects are not uncommon and higher doses of gonadotropins are required for stimulation. In contrast, the GnRH antagonists have an immediate pituitary suppressive action by blocking of the receptors, causing an immediate fall in circulating Serum FSH and LH levels within 8 hours of administration. This action makes them beneficial over the GnRH agonists.

In the antagonist protocol, gonadotropins are started from Day 2 of the cycle. The GnRH antagonist may be added in one of two ways: (1) In the fixed protocol, the antagonist is started from day 6 of the cycle regardless of follicular size, (2) In the flexible protocol, the antagonist is started once the leading follicle crosses 14 mm in diameter. The antagonist is then continued till the day of the hCG trigger.

The two different agents used are cetrorelix and ganirelix, administered in a dose of 0.25 mg subcutaeonus daily, and both are equally effective. The follicular monitoring, timing of trigger injection and oocyte retrieval are the same as the agonist protocols.

Fixed versus Flexible

A meta-analysis of randomized studies comparing the fixed and the flexible protocols[5] concluded that a trend toward higher pregnancy rates was observed with the fixed protocol, although the difference was not statistically significant. The flexible protocol was beneficial in terms of requiring lesser number of antagonist doses and lower gonadotropin requirement. At present there is not enough evidence supporting either one protocol over the other, and the choice of protocol is a matter of personal preference (Fig. 3).

Single Versus Multiple Dose Protocols

The multiple-dose GnRH antagonist protocol involves the daily subcutaneous injections of 0.25 mg of antagonist from

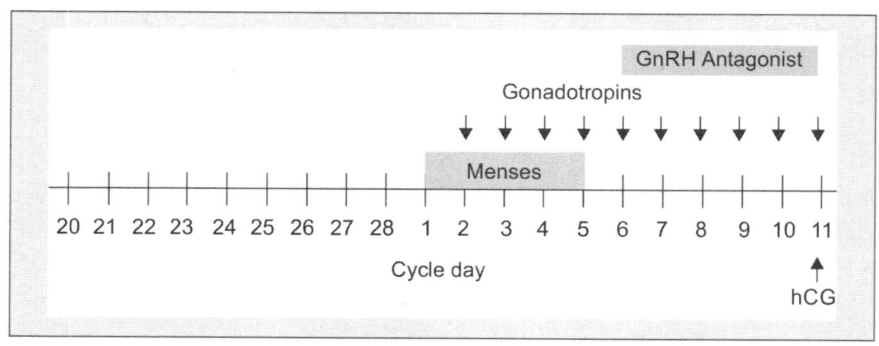

Fig. 3: Gonadotropin-releasing hormone (GnRH) antagonist fixed protocol. (hCG: human chorionic gonadotropin).

day 5 or 6 of stimulation (the fixed start) until administration of hCG. The single-dose protocol involves a single subcutaneous injection of 3 mg GnRH antagonist on day 7 or 8 of stimulation. This single dose provides 4 days of pituitary suppression. If the patient needs more days of stimulation, the daily 0.25 mg of antagonist injections are given until the hCG trigger. The monitoring, criteria for hCG administration and oocyte retrieval are similar to the agonist protocols.

GnRH Antagonists Versus GnRH Agonists

Gonadotropin-releasing hormone antagonist protocols have several advantages over the agonist protocols. The shorter duration of treatment, lesser number of injections required and lower incidence of menopausal side effects render the antagonists more patient-friendly, thereby increasing compliance and reducing dropout rates over repeated cycles. Cyst formation due to the initial flare-up reaction of the agonists is avoided when antagonists are used. Also, the gonadotropin requirement is higher when agonists are used as they can cause profound pituitary suppression. This allows the antagonist protocols to be less burdening financially as the gonadotropin requirement is correspondingly lower with their use. An important advantage, as shown in a 2007 Cochrane review,[6] is the significant reduction in the incidence of severe ovarian hyper stimulation syndrome (OHSS) in antagonist cycles as opposed to agonist cycles, as the former allow the use of a GnRH agonist trigger, eliminating the need of hCG which is known to aggravate the severity of OHSS.

On the other hand, the GnRH antagonist protocols are less programmable compared to the agonist protocols and this lack of flexibility may pose a problem at certain centers especially if planning batch IVF or if a couple has a tight traveling schedule. Although initially there was some skepticism about the possibility of lower success rates using antagonists, it is now well established that the success rates are not compromised by using the antagonist protocols. A large systematic review and meta-analysis that included results from 22 randomized controlled trials with 3,176 subjects found no significant difference in live birth rates between GnRH antagonists and agonists.[7]

OPTIMIZING OVARIAN STIMULATION

The response to stimulatory drugs during an IVF cycle depends on several factors: the number of recruitable follicles, their sensitivity to FSH as well as the bioavailability of FSH. While there are no strict criteria, "adequate response" to conventional ovarian stimulation usually means the retrieval of 8–10 oocytes. Failure to recruit an adequate number of follicles and retrieve 4–5 mature oocytes is termed "poor response," while recruitment of 20 or more follicles in high responders increases the risk of OHSS. Both are undesirable outcomes and hence an attempt is made to optimize ovarian stimulation to result in an adequate response.

The most important strategies to optimize ovarian stimulation include the following details.

Personalizing the Protocol

Different treatment protocols are suitable for different groups of women. The flare-up or antagonist protocols give better success rates in women with a poor ovarian reserve, e.g. patients with low antral follicle counts (AFCs) or low anti-Müllerian hormone (AMH) or women with a history of a poor response to the long protocol. The antagonist protocol has also been shown to reduce the risk of OHSS and may be the better choice in women at high risk of the same.

Optimal Starting Dose of Gonadotropin

In the first cycle, the important question is—what dose of gonadotropins will give an optimal response? Recent studies have demonstrated that predictive models can be useful in determining the optimal starting dose.[8]

A *standard patient* is one in whom we expect a normal response to ovarian stimulation and is usually defined as a patient aged less than 36 years, with a regular menstrual cycle, a normal basal FSH and a good AFC (>10 in both ovaries combined).

While the long protocol has so far been the oldest and the most popularly used protocol that gives good results in most "standard" patients, the GnRH antagonist protocol is more patient-friendly and is now increasingly being preferred by many centers for these "standard" patients.

Poor Responders

The long protocol gives poor results in patients with poor ovarian reserve, likely due to the profound pituitary suppression. While some studies have shown better results with the antagonist and microdose flare protocol in this group of patients, others have failed to demonstrate any benefit.

Many randomized trials have evaluated the use of various pituitary suppression regimens to improve outcome of poor responders undergoing IVF treatment. Sunkara et al.[9] conducted a systematic review of the trials of GnRH agonist long protocol, GnRH agonist short protocol and other pituitary suppression regimens in poor responders undergoing IVF/ICSI (intracytoplasmic sperm injection).

A total of 680 women considered as poor responders were included in 9 randomized controlled trials. Meta-analyses of the results of these studies did not show a consistent benefit of any one pituitary suppression regimen over the others in improving outcome measures. In a 2008 study conducted by Lainas et al.,[10] 270 patients with a previous poor response were randomized to receive either the GnRH agonist flare protocol or the GnRH antagonist flexible protocol. They found that the flexible GnRH antagonist protocol was associated with significantly higher ongoing pregnancy rates compared to the GnRH agonist flare protocol in poor responders. In 2011, a meta-analysis of the published data was performed by Pu et al.[11] to compare the efficacy of GnRH antagonist versus GnRH agonist protocols for ovarian stimulation in IVF poor response patients. Fourteen eligible studies were included in this meta-analysis. They concluded that a clear advantage was gained in duration of stimulation with GnRH antagonists in poor ovarian responders undergoing IVF, although there was no statistical difference in the number of oocytes retrieved, the number of mature oocytes retrieved, the cycle cancellation rate and clinical pregnancy rate between GnRH antagonist and GnRH agonist protocols.

Over-responders and Polycystic Ovarian Syndrome Patients

The GnRH antagonist protocol has the advantage of allowing GnRH agonist trigger to be used in place of hCG, thereby minimizing the incidence of OHSS in hyper-responders. Thus the antagonist protocol is preferred over the GnRH agonist long protocol in these patients. Women with polycystic ovarian syndrome (PCOS) are at risk of developing OHSS during ovarian stimulation. Current randomized controlled trials (RCTs) suggest that the flexible GnRH antagonist protocol is associated with a similar ongoing pregnancy rate, lower incidence of OHSS, lower gonadotropin requirement and shorter duration of stimulation, compared with GnRH agonist. The GnRH antagonist might be the treatment choice for patients with PCOS undergoing IVF.[12]

STARTING DOSE OF FSH/HMG

Safe and effective ovarian stimulation is a pivotal step in the success of assisted reproductive techniques (ART). It is important to categorize patients into normal, poor or high responders and accordingly select the starting dose so as to achieve an optimal yield of oocytes.[13] The appropriate starting dose usually depends on the clinician's experience rather than an objective calculated model.

The optimal yield of oocytes is also debatable. An appropriate response has been arbitrarily defined as retrieval of 8–10 oocytes as this should result in sufficient high quality embryos being available for transfer. In centers where cryopreservation is available the retrieval of 10–15 oocytes is considered a success as this allows multiple embryo transfer attempts per ovarian stimulation cycle and contributes to higher cumulative pregnancy rates.[14] While in centers where cryopreservation is not available or for patients who will not be able to afford it, choosing an appropriate dosage of gonadotropins that could yield a modest number of oocytes is considered crucial as it avoids oocyte and drug wastage.

At the same time, retrieval of less than 5 or more than 20 oocytes is regarded as an unfavorable response as the former would increase the incidence of cycle cancellation and the latter would increase the risk of OHSS.[15]

Many trials to develop a scoring system for calculating the appropriate gonadotropin dose have been attempted. Popovic-Todorovic in 2003 developed a model based on four predictors, the total number of antral follicles, total Doppler score, serum testosterone concentrations and smoking habit[8] but his scoring system was not widely adopted in clinical practice because of the inclusion of two predictive factors that are not measured routinely; Doppler score and testosterone concentrations. In addition smoking is not widespread in all communities to be included as a significant predictor of ovarian response.

In 2006, Howles and colleagues attempted another trial using a combination of 4 other variables that were identified as most important predictors of ovarian response. These included baseline serum FSH concentrations in the early follicular phase, body mass index (BMI), age and AFC.[16] These factors were modeled into a dosing algorithm to calculate the dose of recombinant FSH (rFSH) which was applied in a clinical trial in 2009.[17] Cancellation rate was high due to the application of a low starting dose of 75 IU for the stimulation of multiple follicular development in some cases which is an infrequent dose in routine clinical practice. In addition, the scoring system was very complicated. Olivennes and colleagues; the directors of the study advised modification of the algorithm and introduction of new variables that could yield a more practical model.

The main aspect of the "individualization" in IVF cycles is to offer every single patient the best therapy tailored on her own characteristics thus allowing a high chance of success and of course minimizing the risks deriving from ovarian stimulation. Choosing different doses of gonadotropins for different patients is the most important clinical decision in the personalization of therapy.[18] Usually clinicians choose the gonadotropin starting dose according to anamnesis and clinical criteria, the most important being the outcome of previous IVF cycles. If no previous cycles have been performed, the choice will be based on criteria as the women's age, BMI and markers of ovarian reserve.[19,20]

Currently used markers of ovarian reserve include FSH, AMH and AFC, with the last two markers having the best performance in predicting ovarian response to exogenous FSH.[21-23] AMH and AFC are nowadays considered two markers with similar diagnostic performance.[22-26] Indeed AMH and AFC actually measure the same thing: the pool of recruitable follicles. While AMH appears to have important advantages over AFC, as the lowest intra- and inter-menstrual cycle variability and the operator-independence, the great advantage of the AFC is the possibility of its measurement at the same moment in which clinicians examine the patient; hence, with great certainty we can assert that AFC will continue to be a widely used marker of ovarian reserve.

Rombauts performed a comprehensive search of the database in the Cochrane Library, MEDLINE, EMBASE, the NICE guidelines database and the reference lists of manuscripts.[27] A significant number of RCTs were identified that address the question of the FSH starting dose in expected normal responders. Using GnRH agonists for pituitary downregulation, five studies[28-32] compared a starting dose of 100 IU with 200 IU and three studies[33-35] compared a starting dose of 150 IU with 250 IU. Two studies were identified that used GnRH antagonists for pituitary suppression. One compared a starting dose of 150 IU with 200 IU,[36] whereas the other compared 150 IU with 225 IU.[37] All the studies were designed to detect differences in the number of oocytes collected and the total dose of FSH used and were of similar quality.

Taken together these RCTs suggest that higher starting doses do not lead to improved pregnancy rates, despite lower cancellation rates. One could argue that the higher oocyte numbers associated with higher starting doses will lead to more frozen embryos and therefore better cumulative pregnancy rates. However, 7 of the 10 RCTs found no significant difference. A higher number of frozen embryos was only found in 3 of the 5 studies comparing 100 versus 200 IU. Although it remains to be proven, it perhaps suggests that a starting dose of 100 IU may be associated with lower cumulative pregnancy rates per oocyte collection.

Even so, the improved egg yield was only apparent in younger patients, arguably those that need it the least. In a study by Out et al.[33] in the patient group of 30–33 years an average of four more eggs was collected (15 vs 11 eggs) if patients were given 250 IU instead of 150 IU. In the two other groups (34–36 years and 37–39 years) there was no difference. This observation was echoed by findings from the study from Yong et al.[34] They reported that approximately five more eggs were retrieved in women aged less than 33 years in the 225 IU compared with the 150 IU group, but in older women (≥33 years), the number of eggs retrieved in both groups was similar.

In view of the above, the higher rate of hormone-related side effects and extra cost associated with the higher dose protocol, it would be reasonable to conclude that most patients should start on a dose of 150 IU.

REGIMENS OF GONADOTROPIN USE

There are three regimens of gonadotropin use for ovarian stimulation:

1. In the *fixed dose regimen*, the gonadotropin dose is kept constant throughout the stimulation. If the optimal staring dose has been determined, this protocol is simple to follow and results in good outcomes.
2. In the "step-down" *regimen*, a high starting dose of gonadotropins (300–450 IU) is used for the first 2 days, followed by a dose reduction (150–225 IU/day). This enables supraphysiological levels of FSH required for maximal multifollicular recruitment during the critical period in the early follicular phase and seems to result in greater synchrony of follicles. The higher dose during the first few days theoretically increases the risk of over-response and OHSS, but the following dose reduction balances this risk.
3. In the "step-up" *regimen*, the starting dose of gonado-tropin is low and is then gradually increased on cycle day 5 or later, depending on the response. This protocol can result in high FSH serum levels in the late follicular phase leading to an asynchronous development of multiple follicles, an undesirable outcome.[38]

TYPE OF GONADOTROPIN USED

At present, several different gonadotropin preparations are used for ovarian stimulation. Follicle-stimulating hormone (FSH)-containing gonadotropin preparations are as follows:

- Human menopausal gonadotropins
- Urinary FSH (uFSH)
- Highly purified urinary FSH (HP-uFSH)
- Highly purified hMG (HP-hMG)
- Recombinant FSH

Human menopausal gonadotropin, containing approximately equal amounts of FSH and LH, was the first commercially available gonadotropin preparation, purified from postmenopausal urine. In the early period, after the introduction of rFSH, studies indicated that rFSH was superior to uFSH. The common assumption that if rFSH was superior to uFSH, it should be superior to hMG and was evident in a meta-analysis. However, a subsequent meta-analysis comparing rFSH and hMG pointed in the opposite direction.[39,40] Then, uFSH became largely unavailable and HP-hMG was introduced into the market. Simultaneously, several studies demonstrated the importance of LH in ovarian stimulation and studies comparing rFSH and HP-hMG found either no evidence of benefit of one product over the other or HP-hMG to be more effective than rFSH. The argument against hMG is that the use of urine as a source raises concerns about potential contamination with pathogenic microorganisms. With respect to pharmaceutical quality, the increased purity and batch-to-batch consistency of the recombinant proteins can be considered a breakthrough.[41] In the current era of "prion scare", this may be an important argument in favor of rFSH. However, it is important to note that urinary-derived gonadotropins have been available since the beginning of the 1960s and, so far, prion or other infectivity has never been ascribed to them.

The clinical choice of the gonadotropin preparation to be used for ovarian stimulation should depend on availability, convenience, and costs.

MONITORING IVF CYCLES

Cycle monitoring is an essential part of any IVF protocol as it can indicate over- or under-response, enabling dose adjustments to optimize response. When performing ovarian stimulation in IVF cycles there are obvious reasons why the cycle has to be monitored: to evaluate if the dose of gonadotropins is optimal; to avoid OHSS and to find the optimal time for hCG administration. Of all the methods described for monitoring IVF cycles, ultrasound imaging of the utero-ovarian response to gonadotropins has become the clinically most useful. With the use of GnRH analogs, there seems to be less need for extensive hormonal monitoring of IVF cycles.[42] Ultrasound alone or in certain cases combined with one or two serum estradiol (E_2) measurements seems to be sufficient in the majority of women entering an IVF cycle.[43]

The aims of monitoring are:

- To assess the ovarian response
- To enable optimal ovarian response by tailoring the dose during the course of the stimulation
- To time the ovulation trigger and hence, the time of the ovum pick-up (OPU)
- To monitor other factors, which may have a negative impact on the success rates of IVF.

SHORT PROTOCOL/ANTAGONIST PROTOCOL/MINIMAL STIMULATION PROTOCOL

In these protocols, the stimulation begins from the early follicular phase. Hence, the first monitoring begins on the first or second day of the cycle to ensure optimal conditions as follows:

- Endometrium less than 4 mm
- Absence of ovarian cysts or follicles more than 9 mm
- Serum progesterone less than 1 ng/mL
- Absence of factors known to have a negative impact, such as endometrial polyps, hydrosalpinx (that may have been missed previously), etc.

The AFC is assessed and the type of protocol and the dose of gonadotropins are decided at this time based on the need for ovarian stimulation and the necessity to prevent ovarian hyperstimulation. In case, the first progesterone level is more than 1 ng/mL, a GnRH agonist can be administered to the patient and continued till the progesterone levels drop to less than 1 ng/mL. Ovarian stimulation can then be commenced with gonadotropins in conjunction with the GnRH analog as in the short protocol.

Monitoring is individualized based on the clinic protocol and the ovarian response. The pelvic scan is repeated at the discretion of the clinician. Usually no changes in the gonadotropin dose are made for the first 5 days of stimulation, and therefore the first follow-up scan is done on day 6. Subsequent scans are done every 2–3 days or more frequently depending on the patient's response. The follicles are mapped on a graph. The trigger is given once the leading three follicles reach 18 mm (measured in two dimensions and the average dimension is calculated). On the day of trigger, serum E_2 and serum progesterone are measured.

A 2008 Cochrane review[44] concluded on the basis of the existent material that there is no significant difference in pregnancy rates and live birth in cycles monitored using ultrasound and serum E_2 or those monitored by ultrasound alone.

Long Protocol

Gonadotropin-releasing hormone analogs, such as leuprolide, buserelin and triptorelin, are commenced in the luteal phase of the preceding cycle. It is imperative to confirm downregulation prior to ovarian stimulation. This is usually done on the first or second day of the period following the commencement of analog. Alternatively, this scan can be done after 10 days of analog administration.

The conditions to be met prior to the ovarian stimulation are:

- Endometrial thickness of less than or equal to 4 mm
- Absence of ovarian follicles more than 9 mm
- Serum estradiol level less than or equal to 50 pg/mL
- Absence of factors, known to have a negative impact, such as endometrial polyps, hydrosalpinx (that may have been missed previously).

In case downregulation is not achieved, the patient is advised to continue the analog and follow-up after a week. In case downregulation is confirmed, the ovarian stimulation can start; otherwise, the patient may need to continue the analog. The patient can also be offered to restart the treatment afresh in the next cycle.

The monitoring of ovarian response once downregulation is confirmed is the same as that in the other protocols. It is also important to confirm the availability of the husband on the day of scheduled OPU as also of the clinic and laboratory staff. In case a delay is desired, the analog is continued till such time that the stimulation can start.

DOSE ADJUSTMENT

Recommendations during Stimulation

Most experts believe that the best results are obtained in cycles where the dose of the gonadotropin is maintained rather than increased. Hence, estimating the correct starting dose is extremely important for optimal results. The effectiveness of dose increases, though widely practiced, does not seem to be based on the evidence. Several studies have shown that in patients receiving a step-up dosing of gonadotropin following a low response after 5 days of stimulation, the number of oocytes retrieved as well as the pregnancy rates remain significantly lower than in patients treated with a fixed dose.

Increase in Dose of Gonadotropins

This is done in case of inadequate or slow response, based on the number and size of follicles in each of the ovaries. The increase in the dose is generally in increments of 75 IU.

Reduction in Dose of Gonadotropins

This is done in case of an exaggerated response, in terms of the number of follicles being stimulated in the ovaries. The number of all the follicles should be counted diligently along with the dimensions. The dose reduction is similarly in decrements of 75 IU. A sharp reduction in the dose is generally not recommended.

Freezing all Embryos

Freezing of all the embryos or oocytes retrieved may be recommended in a few scenarios:

- Serum estradiol more than 3,500 pg/mL on the day of trigger
- Serum progesterone more than 1 ng/mL on any day during the ovarian stimulation
- Any unexpected uterine bleeding
- Hitherto undiagnosed hydrosalpinx seen on ultrasound
- Significant endometrial polyps (>1 cm).

Cancellation/Conversion to an Intrauterine Insemination Cycle

Conversion to an intrauterine insemination (IUI) cycle may be offered in case of a poor ovarian response (<3 follicles of size ≥ 12 mm). Cycle cancellation may be required in case of no response or a poor response where IUI is not a possibility such as bilateral tubal block. This has to be after appropriate counseling regarding the pros and cons of IVF versus IUI.

Cycle Monitoring—OHSS

Ovarian hyperstimulation syndrome is a rare but serious complication of ovarian stimulation. Therefore, one of the main aims of cycle monitoring is to prevent its occurrence. If ovarian over-response is recognized during cycle monitoring, the dose of gonadotropin is reduced or stopped (coasting). Frequent (even daily) monitoring is performed to continually assess the response. If the risk of OHSS seems to be very high, an agonist trigger is used instead of an hCG trigger, and all embryos are cryopreserved for subsequent transfer in a thaw cycle.

A randomized trial with a sufficiently large sample size to test the effects of different monitoring protocols on a rare outcome like OHSS is difficult. Nevertheless, the 2008 Cochrane review[44] mentioned earlier suggested that cycle monitoring using transvaginal ultrasound plus serum estradiol be retained as a precautionary good practice point.

CONCLUSION

Safe and effective ovarian stimulation is a pivotal step in the success of ART. It is important to categorize patients into normal, poor or high responders and accordingly select the starting dose so as to achieve an optimal yield of oocytes. Recombinant gonadotropins represent a very obvious technical progress in comparison with the older urinary gonadotropins. This is evident in their relative ease of administration and lack of contamination. There is, however, no convincing evidence that rFSH improves the clinical outcome. The lower cost of urinary products represents a very significant factor in choosing a preferred gonadotropin. The clinical choice of the gonadotropin preparation to be used for ovarian stimulation should depend on availability, convenience and costs. A standard patient who is usually defined as a patient aged less than 36 years, with a regular menstrual cycle, a normal basal FSH and a good AFC (>10 in both ovaries combined) is usually treated with 150–225 IU/day as the starting dose. Patients with a poor response require a higher dose of 450 IU/day. Cycle monitoring is an essential part of any IVF protocol as it can indicate over- or under-response, enabling dose adjustments to optimize response. The best results are obtained in cycles where the dose of the gonadotropin is maintained rather than increased. Hence, estimating the correct starting dose is extremely important for optimal results.

REFERENCES

1. Steptoe PC, Edwards RG. Birth after the reimplantation of a human embryo. Lancet. 1978;2(8085):366.
2. Jones HW Jr, Jones GS, Andrews MC, et al. The program for in vitro fertilization at Norfolk. Fertil Steril. 1982;38(1):14-21.
3. Daya S. Gonadotropin releasing hormone agonist protocols for pituitary desensitization in in vitro fertilization and gamete intrafallopian transfer cycles. Cochrane Database Syst Rev. 2000;2:CD001299.
4. Wong JM, Forrest KA, Snabes SZ, et al. Efficacy of nafarelin in assisted reproductive technology: a meta-analysis. Hum Reprod Update. 2001;7(1):92-101.
5. Al-Inany H, Aboulghar MA, Mansour RT, et al. Optimizing GnRH antagonist administration: meta-analysis of fixed versus flexible protocol. Reprod Biomed Online. 2005;10(5):567-70.
6. Al-Inany HG, Abou-Setta AM, Aboulghar M. Gonadotrophin-releasing hormone antagonists for assisted conception: a Cochrane review. Reprod Biomed Online. 2007;14(5):640-9.
7. Kolibianakis EM, Collins J, Tarlatzis BC, et al. Among patients treated for IVF with gonadotrophins and GnRH analogues, is the probability of live birth dependent on the type of analogue used? A systematic review and meta-analysis. Hum Reprod Update. 2006;12(6):651-71.
8. Popovic-Todorovic B, Loft A, Bredkjaeer HE, et al. A prospective randomized clinical trial comparing an individual dose of recombinant FSH based on predictive factors versus a 'standard' dose of 150 IU/day in 'standard' patients undergoing IVF/ICSI treatment. Hum Reprod. 2003;18(11):2275-82.
9. Sunkara SK, Tuthill J, Khairy M, et al. Pituitary suppression regimens in poor responders undergoing IVF treatment: a systematic review and meta-analysis. RBM Online. 2007;15(5):539-46.
10. Lainas T, Sfontouris I, Papanikolaou E, et al. Flexible GnRH antagonist versus flare-up GnRH agonist protocol in poor responders treated by IVF: a randomized controlled trial. Hum Reprod. 2008;23(6):1355-8.
11. Pu D, Wu J, Liu J. Comparisons of GnR Hantagonist versus GnRH agonist protocol in poor ovarian responders undergoing IVF. Hum Reprod. 2011;26(10):2742-9.
12. Lainas TG, Sfontouris IA, Zorzovilis IZ, et al. Flexible GnRH antagonist protocol versus GnRH agonist long protocol in patients with polycystic ovary syndrome treated for IVF: a prospective randomized controlled trial (RCT). Hum Reprod. 2010;25(3):683-9.
13. Al-Azemi M, Killick S, Duffy S, et al. Multi-marker assessment of ovarian reserve predicts oocyte yield after ovulation induction. Hum Reprod. 2011;26(2):414-22.
14. Tiitinen A. Prevention of multiple pregnancies in infertility treatment. Best Pract Res Clin Obstet Gynaecol. 2012;26(6):829-40.
15. Inge G, Brindsen P, Elder K. Oocyte number per live birth in IVF: were Steptoe and Edwards less wasteful? Hum Reprod. 2004;20(3):588-92.
16. Howles C, Saunders H, Alam V, et al. Predictive factors and a corresponding treatment algorithm for controlled ovarian stimulation in patients treated with recombinant human follicle stimulating hormone (follitropin alfa) during assisted reproduction technology (ART) procedures. An analysis of 1378 patients. Curr Med Res Opin. 2006;22(5):907-18.
17. Olivennes F, Howles C, Borini A, et al. Individualizing FSH dose for assisted reproduction using a novel algorithm: the CONSORT study. RBM Online. 2009;18(2):195-204.
18. La Marca A, Grisendi V, Giulini S, et al. Individualization of the FSH starting dose in IVF/ICSI cycles using the antral follicle count. J Ovarian Res. 2013;6(1):11.
19. Fauser BC, Diedrich K, Devroey P, et al. Predictors of ovarian response: progress towards individualized treatment in ovulation induction and ovarian stimulation. Hum Reprod Update. 2008;14(1):1-14.
20. Alviggi C, Humaidan P, Ezcurra D. Hormonal, functional and genetic biomarkers in controlled ovarian stimulation: tools for matching patients and protocols. Reprod Biol Endocrinol. 2012;10:9.
21. Broekmans FJ, Kwee J, Hendriks DJ, et al. A systematic review of tests predicting ovarian reserve and IVF outcome. Hum Reprod Update. 2006;12(6): 685-718.
22. La Marca A, Sighinolfi G, Radi D, et al. Anti-Müllerian hormone (AMH) as a predictive marker in assisted reproductive technology (ART). Hum Reprod Update. 2010;16(2):113-30.
23. Nelson SM, Yates RW, Fleming R. Serum anti-Müllerian hormone and FSH: prediction of live birth and extremes of response in stimulated cycles—implications for individualization of therapy. Hum Reprod. 2007;22(9):2414-21.
24. Broekmans FJ, de Ziegler D, Howles CM, et al. The antral follicle count: practical recommendations for better standardization. Fertil Steril. 2010;94(3): 1044-51.
25. La Marca A, Spada E, Sighinolfi G, et al. Age-specific nomogram for the decline in antral follicle count throughout the reproductive period. Fertil Steril. 2011;95(2):684-8.
26. Broer SL, Dolleman M, Opmeer BC, et al. AMH and AFC as predictors of excessive response in controlled ovarian hyperstimulation: a meta-analysis. Hum Reprod Update. 2011;17(1):46-54.

27. Rombauts L. Is there a recommended maximum starting dose of FSH in IVF? J Assist Reprod Genet. 2007;24(8):343-9.
28. Tan SL, Child TJ, Cheung AP, et al. A randomized, double-blind, multicenter study comparing a starting dose of 100 IU or 200 IU of recombinant follicle stimulating hormone (Puregon®) in women undergoing controlled ovarian hyperstimulation for IVF treatment. J Assist Reprod Genet. 2005;22(2):81-8.
29. Out HJ, Lindenberg S, Mikkelsen AL, et al. A prospective, randomized, double-blind clinical trial to study the efficacy and efficiency of a fixed dose of recombinant follicle stimulating hormone (Puregon®) in women undergoing ovarian stimulation. Hum Reprod. 1999;14(3):622-7.
30. Out HJ, David I, Ron-El R, et al. A randomized, double-blind clinical trial using fixed daily doses of 100 or 200 IU of recombinant FSH in ICSI cycles. Hum Reprod. 2001;16(6):1104-49.
31. Pruksananonda K, Suwajanakorn S, Sereepapong W, et al. Comparison of two different fixed doses of follitropin-beta in controlled ovarian hyperstimulation: a prospective randomized, double blind clinical trial. J Med Assoc Thai. 2004;87(10):1151-5.
32. Asian Purgeon Study Group, Hoomans EH, Mulder BB. A group-comparative, randomized, double-blind comparison of the efficacy and efficiency of two fixed daily dose regimens (100- and 200-IU) of recombinant follicle stimulating hormone (rFSH, Puregon®) in Asian women undergoing ovarian stimulation for IVF/ICSI. J Assist Reprod Genet. 2002;19(10):470-6.
33. Out HJ, Braat DD, Lintsen BM, et al. Increasing the daily dose of recombinant follicle stimulating hormone (Puregon) does not compensate for the age-related decline in retrievable oocytes after ovarian stimulation. Hum Reprod. 2000;15(1):29-35.
34. Yong PY, Brett S, Baird DT, et al. A prospective randomized clinical trial comparing 150 IU and 225 IU of recombinant follicle-stimulating hormone (Gonal-F*) in a fixed-dose regimen for controlled ovarian stimulation in in vitro fertilization treatment. Fertil Steril. 2003;79(2):308-15.
35. Latin-American Puregon IVF Study Group. A double-blind clinical trial comparing a fixed daily dose of 150 and 250 IU of recombinant follicle-stimulating hormone in women undergoing in vitro fertilization. Fertil Steril. 2001;76(5):950-6.
36. Out HJ, Rutherford A, Fleming R, et al. A randomized, double-blind, multicentre clinical trial comparing starting doses of 150 and 200 IU of recombinant FSH in women treated with the GnRH antagonist ganirelix for assisted reproduction. Hum Reprod. 2004;19(1):90-95.
37. Wikland M, Bergh C, Borg K, et al. A prospective, randomized comparison of two starting doses of recombinant FSH in combination with cetrorelix in women undergoing ovarian stimulation for IVF/ICSI. Hum Reprod. 2001;16(8):1676-81.
38. Andoh K, Mizunuma H, Liu X, et al. A comparative study of fixed-dose, stepdown, and low-dose step-up regimens of human menopausal gonadotropin for patients with polycystic ovary syndrome. Fertil Steril. 1998;70(5):840-6.
39. Daya S, Gunby J, Hughes EG, et al. Follicle-stimulating hormone versus human menopausal gonadotropin for in vitro fertilization cycles: a meta-analysis. Fertil Steril. 1995;64(2):347-54.
40. Agrawal R, Holmes J, Jacobs HS. Follicle-stimulating hormone or human menopausal gonadotropin for ovarian stimulation in in vitro fertilization cycles: a meta-analysis. Fertil Steril. 2000;73(2):338-43.
41. Olijve W, de Boer W, Mulders JW, et al. Molecular biology and biochemistry of human recombinant follicle stimulating hormone (Puregon). Mol Hum Reprod. 1996;2(5):371-82.
42. Wikland M, Borg J, Hamberger L, et al. Simplification of IVF: minimal monitoring and the use of subcutaneous highly purified FSH administration for ovulation induction. Hum Reprod. 1994;9(8):1430-6.
43. Bergh C, Howles C, Borg K, et al. Recombinant human follicle stimulating hormone (r-hFSH; Gonal-F) versus highly purified urinary FSH (Metrodin HP): results of a randomized comparative study in women undergoing assisted reproductive techniques. Hum Reprod. 1997;12(10):2133-9.
44. Kwan I, Bhattacharya S, McNeil A, et al. Monitoring of stimulated cycles in assisted reproduction (IVF and ICSI). Cochrane Database Syst Rev. 2008;16(2):CD005289.

CHAPTER

45

Protocols for Management of Poor Responders

Ritu Hinduja, Nikita Banerjee, Kalyani Shrimali

INTRODUCTION

In the field of assisted reproductive technologies (ARTs), great steps forward have been made in recent years in terms of clinical knowledge and technological development. Over the past few decades poor ovarian response (POR) has emerged as a challenge. The incidence in a population undergoing assisted reproduction treatment is estimated to be 9–24%.

In patients defined "poor responders" the limited number of eggs obtained remains the main hurdle in optimizing the live birth rates. In fact, owing to the lower number of oocytes retrieved, there are fewer embryos to select and transfer, leading to lower pregnancy rates per transfer and lower cumulative pregnancy rates per cycle compared with normal responders. The Society of Human Reproduction and Embryology (ESHRE) working group on POR has finally given a common definition of "poor responder", where at least two of the following three features must be present:

1. Advanced maternal age or any other risk factor for POR
2. A previous POR
3. An abnormal ovarian reserve test.[1]

Two episodes of POR after maximal stimulation are sufficient to define a patient as poor responder in the absence of advanced maternal age or abnormal ovarian reserve testing. In such cases, the refined definition should be expected "poor responder".

POSEIDON group (**P**atient-**O**riented **S**trategies **E**ncompassing **I**ndividualize **D** **O**ocyte **N**umber) was recently established to focus specifically on the diagnosis and management of low prognosis patients.[2]

Four subgroups have been suggested based on quantitative and qualitative parameters, namely:

1. Age and the expected aneuploidy rate
2. Ovarian biomarkers [i.e. antral follicle count (AFC) and anti-Müllerian hormone (AMH)]
3. Ovarian response—provided a previous stimulation cycle was performed.

POSEIDON group 1: Young patients <35 years with adequate ovarian reserve parameters (AFC > 5; AMH >1.2 ng/mL) and with an unexpected poor or suboptimal ovarian response

Subgroup 1a: <4 oocytes

Subgroup 1b: 4–9 oocytes retrieved

After standard ovarian stimulation

POSEIDON group 2: Older patients > 35 years with adequate ovarian reserve parameters (AFC > 5; AMH > 1.2 ng/mL) and with an unexpected poor or suboptimal ovarian response.

POSEIDON group 3: Young patients, 35 years with poor ovarian reserve prestimulation parameters (AFC < 5; AMH < 1.2 ng/mL)

POSEIDON group 4: Older patients >35 years with poor ovarian reserve prestimulation parameters (AFC < 5; AMH < 1.2 ng/mL)

This is an important working and counseling tool for the ART specialist. Many protocols have been proposed for management of POR. Although high doses of gonadotropins have been used by vast majority of authors in the 1980s and early 1990s, results have been controversial and prospective randomized studies have shown little or no benefit.[3,4] In PORs, no superiority of recombinant follicle-stimulating hormone (rFSH) has been proved compared to urinary gonadotropins.[5,6] Flare-up gonadotropin-releasing hormone (GnRH) agonist protocol has been proposed to produce better results than standard long luteal protocols.[7,8] GnRH antagonist did not hold true to its initial promise.[9] Adjuvant therapy with growth hormone (GH) or GH-releasing factors resulted in no significant improvement.[9-12] Corifollitropin alfa followed by highly purified human menopausal gonadotropin (HP-hMG) stimulation has shown promising results in two pilot studies[13,14] when used in young poor responders fulfilling the Bologna criteria. Finally, natural cycle *in-vitro* fertilization (IVF) and mild or minimal stimulation IVF protocol have shown comparable result like those obtained in stimulated cycles in true poor responders.[15] However, well designed, large scale, randomized control trials are required to assess the efficacy of these different management strategies.

MAXIMAL GONADOTROPIN DOSAGE

The use of high doses of gonadotropins is the most extensively employed strategy to improve follicular response in "poor responders".[16-18] The obvious clinical approach when the standard dose of gonadotropins (225–300 IU) fails to induce a proper multifollicular growth approach is to increase the dose. In the literature, conflicting data are reported on the outcomes of this approach: some[19-21] but not all authors[22] did not report enhanced ovarian response and/or better pregnancy rates in prospective and retrospective studies when the starting dose of gonadotropins was increased up to 450 IU. It is today clear that these patients have a reduced ovarian reserve; the follicles that can be recruited are fewer and the gonadotropins, independently of the dosage administered, can only support the cohort of follicles receptive to stimulation without manufacturing follicles de novo. It is not effective to increase the starting dose of gonadotropin after an unexpected poor response in the first IVF cycle.[17] It may increase the oocyte retrieval rates and embryo transfer (ET) rates, but will not add any significant improvement in the number of oocytes retrieved and the number of transferable embryos. The only important benefit of increasing the dose is the low cancellation rate. Kovacs et al.[23] published a retrospective analysis of fresh ET cycles. Their analyses suggest detrimental influences of higher gonadotropin dose on the endometrium and confirmed the previously reported adverse association between higher dose and IVF outcome. Milder protocols may be of particular benefit in women less than and equal to 35 years of age. Low dose gonadotropin regimens have the benefit of reducing costs and risks of ovarian hyperstimulation without reducing the efficacy and in some cases, actually increasing the pregnancy rates.

GONADOTROPIN-RELEASING HORMONE ANALOGS

Combination of gonadotropins and GnRH agonists, started in the luteal phase of the previous cycle, has been considered the protocol of choice in normoresponders since the nineties. It lowers cancellation rate and raises the number of preovulatory follicles and the number of oocytes retrieved and good quality embryos for transfer, leading to better pregnancy rates.[24] However, in poor responders this protocol could have a detrimental effect as it may induce an excessive ovarian suppression that could lead to a reduced or absent follicular response.[25,26] In patients with POR the following options could be resorted to:

- Decrease the length of suppression by decreasing the duration of GnRH agonist use (short and ultrashort, mini- and microdose flare-up regimens).[27-29]
- Lower or stop (after pituitary suppression) the dose of GnRH agonists initiated during the luteal phase.[30,31]
- Use the GnRH antagonists in combination with gonadotropins to prevent premature luteinizing hormone (LH) rise during the mid-late follicular phase.[32,33]

The efficacy of the microdose flare-up and multiple-dose antagonist protocols for poor-responder patients in intracytoplasmic sperm injection-embryo transfer (ICSI-ET) cycles was compared by Demirol and Gurgan. The microdose flare-up protocol seemed to have a better, with a significantly higher mean number of mature oocytes retrieved and higher implantation rate.[34] Though short and ultrashort flare-up protocols are mostly used in poor responders for more than 20 years, prospective-nonrandomized trials, or retrospective studies[35,36] were unable to demonstrate any significant benefit on the clinical outcome in this group of patients. The rationale to lower the dose of GnRH agonists or to stop it completely in the follicular phase is to obtain a reduction of the inhibitory direct effect of the GnRH agonist on the gonads.[37,38]

BIRTH CONTROL PILL PRIMING

Kovacs et al.[39] conducted a retrospective analysis which revealed no improvement in IVF cycle outcomes in poor responders who received oral contraceptive pills (OCP) to achieve hypothalamic-pituitary suppression instead of GnRH analogs. Duvan et al.[40] on the other hand compared OCP pretreatment plus microdose GnRH agonists in flare-up protocol and non-OCP microdose GnRH agonists in flare-up protocol among poor responder ICSI patients which reflected no benefit of OCP pretreatment.

GONADOTROPIN-RELEASING HORMONE ANTAGONIST

Several authors suggest the use of GnRH antagonists along with gonadotropins as a suitable protocol for poor responders because they are not administered during follicular stage so the suppression of endogenous gonadotropins is not present at that time in contrast to GnRH agonists which is a possible advantage during ovarian stimulation in poor responders.[41] With GnRH antagonist the added benefit is that it is possible to assess the ovarian reserve by ultrasound on days two or third of the cycle in which ovarian stimulation is planned because there is absence of profound downregulation by GnRH agonist when resorting to a long protocol. This is beneficial in patients with a mean follicle count of less than five follicles as they are known to have significant cycle-to-cycle variability in AFC from –2 to +541 to –3 to +7.[42,43]

CORIFOLLITROPIN ALFA

Corifollitropin alfa, a new hybrid molecule with a prolonged half-life, supports the cohort of follicle receptive to stimulation for 7 days.[44] Corifollitropin can fully exploit the reduced ovarian reserve by rapidly increasing the serum follicle-stimulating hormone (FSH) concentration that consequently results in a significantly higher exposure of the small antral follicles to constant high levels of FSH during the early follicular phase. Polyzos et al.[45] conducted a retrospective study and compared laboratory and clinical results when corifollitropin alfa followed by rFSH in combination with GnRH antagonist with conventional stimulation protocols in poor responder patients according to the "Bologna criteria" and reported similar results in both groups. Finally, promising pregnancy rates were reported in a retrospective pilot study in young (less than 40 years) poor responder patients following a combination of corifollitropin alfa with HP-hMG in a GnRH antagonist protocol.[46]

GONADOTROPIN-RELEASING HORMONE ANTAGONIST OR LETROZOLE PROTOCOLS

Jovanovic et al.[47] evaluated the effect of adjunctive letrozole or clomiphene citrate (CC) in IVF stimulation protocols. Supplementation with CC in poor responders showed significant improvements in E2, number of dominant follicles, oocytes retrieved, and number of embryos transferred. It significantly improved biochemical pregnancy rates while reducing cycle cancellations. Letrozole supplementation showed similar effects. However, despite increasing oocyte yield and ET rates, the overall clinical and live birth rate in this population remained low and showed no measurable increase.

ALTERNATIVE APPROACHES

Several alternative approaches have been proposed as adjuvants with the aim of strengthening the effect of exogenous gonadotropins in women with POR.

ADDITION OF ESTRADIOL IN THE LUTEAL PHASE

A meta-analysis of eight selected studies reported a decreased risk of cycle cancellation and increased chances of clinical pregnancy in poor responder patients with the addition of estradiol in the luteal phase with or without the simultaneous use of GnRH antagonist.[48,49] The biological rationale might be that luteal estradiol priming could improve synchronization of the pool of follicles available to controlled ovarian stimulation. This meta-analysis has been strongly criticized because of important methodological pitfall randomized trials are needed before suggesting the addition of estradiol in the luteal phase.[50]

ADDITION OF RECOMBINANT LUTEINIZING HORMONE

Addition of recombinant LH during gonadotropin stimulation in poor responder patients has been suggested by some authors.[51] However, two meta-analyses[52,53] showed that the addition of recombinant LH does not increase the number of oocyte retrieved, the total dose of FSH, the cancellation rates, and the ongoing pregnancy rates in poor responder patients. A very recent meta-analysis of 40 randomized controlled studies,[54] on the other hand reported that significantly more oocytes were retrieved and significantly higher clinical pregnancy rates were observed with rFSH plus recombinant LH versus rFSH alone in poor responders.

ADDITION OF GROWTH HORMONE

It has been hypothesized that the use of GH might modulate the action of FSH on granulosa cells by upregulating the local synthesis of insulin-like growth factor-I (IGF-I).[55-57] The IGF-I amplifies the effect of FSH at the level of both granulosa and theca cells.[58,59] It has been suggested that addition of GH significantly increased the probability of live birth in poor responders by two recent meta-analyses of six randomized trials.[60] The frequency and dosage of GH varies from study to study. Up until now, there is not any robust data suggesting routine addition of GH in ovarian stimulation protocols for poor responders patients.[61,62] Because of the heterogeneity of the frequency and dosage of GH administered and the small number of patients enrolled in the studies, the recommendation of substituting ovarian stimulation with GH in poor responders is guarded.

ADDITION OF ANDROGENS

Theca cells produce androgens which play a critical role for an adequate follicular steroidogenesis and for a correct early follicular and granulosa cell development.[63] They are the substrate for the aromatase activity of the granulosa cells, which converts the androgens to estrogens. Androgens may increase FSH receptor expression in granulosa cells amplifying the effects of FSH and thus potentially enhance responsiveness of ovaries to FSH.[7,63,64] According to this hypothesis they may benefit poor responders when used as an adjuvant to gonadotropin for ovarian stimulation. Various modes of testosterone administration are known like dehydroepiandrosterone (DHEA), testosterone patches and testosterone gel or Androgel. Although DHEA has already found its way into the practice, use of Androgel seems to be the most promising due to acceptable safety profile and better convenience.

A recent meta-analysis of four randomized controlled trials of adjuvant androgens (DHEA and testosterone) in poor responder patients showed a significantly higher ongoing pregnancy rate in the androgen supplementation group.[65] There is an urgent need of robust data from randomized controlled studies that could justify the widespread use of DHEA before ovarian stimulation in poor responders. Androgel is to be used prior to ovarian stimulation. It has been used, in studies, for a variable time period of 4–6 weeks. The feasible and systematic way to use it would be from day 6 of previous cycle to day 2 of stimulated menstrual cycle.[66]

DEXAMETHASONE

Use of dexamethasone in patients aged over 35 years undergoing IVF/ICSI has shown to reduce the amount of HMG (*3-hydroxy-3-methylglutaryl*) needed to stimulate the ovaries in females at risk of POR. In a long agonist protocol, dexamethasone 1 mg/d is started from day 21 of previous cycle and continued till the day of oocyte retrieval. The outcome observed is reduction in cycle cancellation rate for poor response. Glucocorticoids are shown to sensitize ovary to gonadotropins. Dexamethasone is a substrate for the enzyme type 1, 11-hydroxysteroid dehydrogenase. This isoform is detected in luteinized granulosa cells and oocytes suggesting that dexamethasone can directly influence follicular development.[67,68]

ADDITION OF ASPIRIN

Increased intraovarian vascularity has been associated with improved delivery of gonadotropins and other growth factors required for folliculogenesis.[66,69] POR is associated with impaired ovarian blood flow.[70,61] Based on this rationale, by enhancing ovarian vascularization with vasoactive substances such as aspirin, the ovarian response could theoretically improve.[71,72] However, the evidence supporting the effect of a low dose of aspirin in women undergoing IVF is poor and controversial.[73]

OOCYTE VITRIFICATION, COFACCE

The major societies including European ESHRE, American Society for Reproductive Medicine (ASRM), and American Society of Clinical Oncologists (ASCO) acknowledged recently oocyte cryopreservation as a nonexperimental procedure which provides the required legal and moral support for widespread application. Different strategies are applicable for poor responder involving oocyte cryopreservation. Some authors have recently suggested obtaining a large cohort of oocytes in these patients by accumulating vitrified oocytes over several stimulation cycles creating a similar situation as in normal responder patients. According to the results presented in the study, it could be possible to obtain higher live birth rate per patient treated and potentially to reduce the dropout.

Co-transfer of fresh and collected cryopreserved embryos (COFACCE) can be performed for poor responders.[74] Oocytes retrieved in minimal stimulation or natural cycles were inseminated and 2 pronucleate zygotes were cryopreserved and collected. When fresh oocytes were retrieved and fertilized in the next cycle after two or three cryopreserved embryos were collected, cotransfer of a fresh and two or three cryopreserved-thawed embryos was performed 2-3 days after fresh oocyte retrieval.

NATURAL CYCLES IN VITRO FERTILIZATION

Some authors suggest that natural cycles IVF was a valid option for poor responder patients because it has the same chance in terms of pregnancy and implantation rates.[74]

Schimberni et al.[75] evaluated the IVF outcome in 500 patients and reported very encouraging results especially in young poor responders (less than 35 years). The pregnancy rate was 18% per started cycle, 29% per transfer, and 31% per patient in this group of women. In contrast, a recent paper studied the effect of natural cycles IVF in women defined as poor responders according to the "Bologna criteria": the data however showed that the cumulative live birth per patient does not exceed 8%. The contradictory data can be very likely associated to the diversity of patients selected before the application of "Bologna criteria".

CONCLUSION

In the last two decades, despite a large number of papers published suggesting the most efficient stimulation protocol for the management of patients with POR, it still remains the most challenging task in the field of assisted reproduction. The clear definition provided by expert committee ESHRE in Bologna in 2011 is highly appreciated. "Bologna criteria" can be considered an important step toward the identification of poor responder patients and consequently to find the most effective strategy in their management. Finally, we should consider the alternative strategies to be able to prevent the consequences of the POR. Oocyte cryopreservation for fertility preservation before the ovarian reserve decline is an important option that must be offered. Available evidence indicates no harmful consequence of oocyte vitrification,[77,78] hence it is not just a possibility but a moral duty to fully exploit its potentials especially in the prevention of poor ovarian response.[79]

REFERENCES

1. Ferraretti AP, La Marca A, Fauser BC, et al. ESHRE consensus on the definition of 'poor response' to ovarian stimulation for in vitro fertilization: the Bologna criteria. Hum Reprod. 2011;26(7):1616-24.
2. Humaidan P, Alviggi C, Esteves SC. The novel POSEIDON stratification of 'Low Prognosis Patients in Assisted Reproductive Technology' and its proposed marker of successful outcome. Version 1. F1000Res. 2016;5:2911.
3. Keay SD, Liversedge NH, Mathur RS, et al. Assisted conception following poor ovarian response to gonadotrophin stimulation. Br J Obstet Gynaecol. 1997;104(5):521-7.
4. Ben-Rafael Z1, Bider D, Dan U, et al. Combined gonadotropin-releasing hormone agonist/human menopausal gonadotropin therapy (GnRH-a/hMG) in normal, high, and poor responders to hMG. J In Vitro Fert Embryo Transf. 1991;8(1):33-6.
5. Jenkins JM, Davies DW, Devonport H, et al. Comparison of 'poor' responders with 'good' responders using a standard buserelin/human menopausal gonadotrophin regime for in-vitro fertilization. Hum Reprod. 1991;6(7):918-21.
6. Surrey ES, Schoolcraft WB. Evaluating strategies for improving ovarian response of the poor responder undergoing assisted reproductive techniques. Fertil Steril. 2000;73(4):667-76.
7. Kolibianakis EM, Venetis CA, Diedrich K, et al. Addition of growth hormone to gonadotrophins in ovarian stimulation of poor responders treated by in-vitro fertilization: a systematic review and meta-analysis. Hum Reprod Update. 2009;15(6):613-22.
8. Ferraretti AP, La Marca A, Fauser BC, et al. ESHRE consensus on the definition of "poor response" to ovarian stimulation for in vitro fertilization: the Bologna criteria. Hum Reprod. 2011;26(7):1616-24.
9. Benaglia L, Somigliana E, Tutuncu L, et al. Increasing the stimulation dose of rFHS in unexpected poor responders is not associated with better IVF outcome. Ginekol Pol. 2012;83(2):111-s5.
10. Streuli I, de Ziegler D, Gayet V, et al. In women with endometriosis anti-Müllerian hormone levels are decreased only in those with previous endometriomasurgery. Hum Reprod. 2012;27(11):3294-303.
11. Raffi F, Metwally M, Amer S. The impact of excision of ovarian endometrioma on ovarian reserve: a systematic review and meta-analysis. J Clin Endocrinol Metab. 2012;97(9):3146-54.
12. De Vos M, Devroey P, Fauser BC. Primary ovarian insufficiency. Lancet. 2010;376(9744):911-21.
13. Fritz MA, Speroff L. Clinical Gynecologic Endocrinology and Infertility. Philadelphia, PA: Wolters Kluwer Health/ Lippincott Williams & Wilkins; 2011.
14. Soto N, Iñiguez G, López P, et al. Anti-Müllerian hormone and inhibin B levels as markers of premature ovarian aging and transition to menopause in type 1 diabetes mellitus. Hum Reprod. 2009;24(11):2838-44.
15. Chang HH, Chen MJ, Lu MY, et al. Iron overload is associated with lowanti-müllerian hormone in women with transfusion-dependent β-thalassaemia. BJOG. 2011;118(7):825-31.
16. Check JH. Advantages of using a lower vs. higher dosage of gonadotropins forfollicular maturation including cycles of in vitro fertilization-embryo transfer. Clin Exp Obstet Gynecol. 2010;37(2):84-8.
17. Tutuncu L, Dundar O. Increasing the stimulation dose of rFHS in unexpected poor responders is not associated with better IVF outcome. Ginekol Pol. 2012;83(2):111-s5.
18. Kovacs P, Sajgo A, Kaali SG, et al. Detrimental effects of high-dose gonadotropin on outcome of IVF: making a case for gentle ovarian stimulation strategies. Reprod Sci. 2012;19(7):718-24.
19. Land JA, Yarmolinskaya MI, Dumoulin JC, et al. High-dose human menopausal gonadotropin stimulation in poor responders does not improve in vitro fertilization outcome. Fertil Steril. 1996;65(5):961-5.
20. Karande VC, Jones GS, Veeck LL, et al. High-dose follicle-stimulating hormone stimulation at the onset of the menstrual cycle does not improve the in vitro fertilization outcome in low-responder patients. Fertil Steril. 1990;53(3):486-9.
21. van Hooff MH, Alberda AT, Huisman GJ, et al. Doubling the human menopausal gonadotrophin dose in the course of an in-vitro fertilization treatment cycle in low responders: a randomized study. Hum Reprod. 1993;8(3):369-73.

22. Hofmann GE, Toner JP, Muasher SJ, et al. High-dose follicle-stimulating hormone (FSH) ovarian stimulation in low-responder patients for in vitro fertilization. J In Vitro Fert Embryo Transf. 1989;6(5):285-9.
23. Kovacs P, Sajgo A, Kaali SG, et al. Detrimental effects of high-dose gonadotropin on outcome of IVF: making a case for gentle ovarian stimulation strategies. Reprod Sci. 2012;19(7):718-24.
24. Hughes EG, Fedorkow DM, Daya S, et al. The routine use of gonadotropin-releasing hormone agonists prior to in vitro fertilization and gamete intrafallopian transfer: a meta-analysis of randomized controlled trials. Fertil Steril. 1992;58(5):888-96.
25. Yoshimura Y, Nakamura Y, Ando M, et al. Direct effect of gonadotropin-releasing hormone agonists on the rabbit ovarian follicle. Fertil Steril. 1992;57(5):1091-7.
26. Kowalik A, Barmat L, Damario M, et al. Ovarian estradiol production in vivo. Inhibitory effect of leuprolide acetate. J Reprod Med. 1998;43(5):413-7.
27. Surrey ES, Bower J, Hill DM, et al. Clinical and endocrine effects of a microdose GnRH agonist flare regimen administered to poor responders who are undergoing in vitro fertilization. Fertil Steril. 1998;69(3):419-24.
28. Schoolcraft W, Schlenker T, Gee M, et al. Improved controlled ovarian hyperstimulation in poor responder in vitro fertilization patients with a microdose follicle-stimulating hormone flare, growth hormone protocol. Fertil Steril. 1997;67(1):93-7.
29. Padilla SL, Dugan K, Maruschak V, et al. Use of the flare-up protocol with high dose human follicle-stimulating hormone and human menopausal gonadotropins for in vitro fertilization in poor responders. Fertil Steril. 1996;65(4):796-9.
30. Faber BM, Mayer J, Cox B, et al. Cessation of gonadotropin-releasing hormone agonist therapy combined with high-dose gonadotropin stimulation yields favorable pregnancy results in low responders. Fertil Steril. 1998;69(5):826-30.
31. Karande V, Gleicher N. A rational approach to the management of low responders in in-vitro fertilization. Hum Reprod. 1999;14(7):1744-8.
32. Craft I, Gorgy A, Hill J, et al. Will GnRH antagonists provide new hope for patients considered "difficult responders" to GnRH agonist protocols? Hum Reprod. 1999;14(12):2959-62.
33. Akman MA, Erden HF, Tosun SB, et al. Addition of GnRH antagonist in cycles of poor responders undergoing IVF. Hum Reprod. 2000;15(10):2145-7.
34. Demirol A, Gurgan T. Comparison of microdose flare-up and antagonist multiple-dose protocols for poor-responder patients: a randomized study. Fertil Steril. 2009;92(2):481-5.
35. Toth TL, Awwad JT, Veeck LL, et al. Suppression and flare regimens of gonadotropin-releasing hormone agonist: use in women with different basal gonadotropin values in an in vitro fertilization program. J Reprod Med. 1996;41(5):321-6.
36. Leondires MP, Escalpes M, Segars JH, et al. Microdose follicular phase gonadotropin-releasing hormone agonists (GnRH-a) compared with luteal phase GnRH-a for ovarian stimulation at in vitro fertilization. Fertil Steril. 1999;72(6):1018-23.
37. Yoshimura Y, Nakamura Y, Ando M, et al. Direct effect of gonadotropin-releasing hormone agonists on the rabbit ovarian follicle. Fertil Steril. 1992;57(5):1091-7.
38. Kowalik A, Barmat L, Damario M, et al. Ovarian estradiol production in vivo. Inhibitory effect of leuprolide acetate. J Reprod Med. 1998;43(5):413-7.
39. Kovacs P, Barg PE, Witt BR. Hypothalamic-pituitary suppression with oral contraceptive pills does not improve outcome in poor responder patients undergoing in vitro fertilization-embryo transfer cycles. J Assist Reprod Genet. 2001;18(7):391-4.
40. Duvan CI, Berker B, Turhan NO, et al. Oral contraceptive pretreatment does not improve outcome in microdose gonadotropin-releasing hormone agonist protocol among poor responder intracytoplasmic sperm injection patients. J Assist Reprod Genet. 2008;25(2-3):89-93.
41. Kenigsberg D, Littman BA, Hodgen GD. Medical hypophysectomy: I. Doseresponse using a gonadotropin-releasing hormone antagonist. Fertil Steril. 1984;42(1):112-5.
42. Scheffer GJ, Broekmans FJ, Dorland M, et al. Antral follicle counts by transvaginal ultrasonography are related to age in women with proven natural fertility. Fertil Steril. 1999;72(5):845-51.
43. Bancsi LF, Broekmans FJ, Looman CW, et al. Predicting poor ovarian response in IVF: use of repeat basal FSH measurement. J Reprod Med. 2004;49(3):187-94.
44. van Schanke A, van de Wetering-Krebbers SF, Bos E, et al. Absorption, distribution, metabolism and excretion of corifollitropin alfa, a recombinant hormone with a sustained follicle-stimulating activity. Pharmacology. 2010;85(2):77-87.
45. Polyzos NP, Devos M, Humaidan P, et al. Corifollitropin alfa followed by rFSH in a GnRH antagonist protocol for poor ovarian responder patients: an observational pilot study. Fertil Steril. 2013;99(2):422-6.
46. Polyzos NP, De Vos M, Corona R, et al. Addition of highly purified HMG after corifollitropin alfa in antagonist-treated poor ovarian responders: a pilot study. Hum Reprod. 2013;28(5):1254-60.
47. Jovanovic VP, Kort DH, Guarnaccia MM, et al. Does the addition of clomiphene citrate or letrozole to gonadotropin treatment enhance the oocyte yield in poor responders undergoing IVF? J Assist Reprod Genet. 2011;28(11):1067-72.
48. Reynolds KA, Omurtag KR, Jimenez PT, et al. Cycle cancellation and pregnancy after luteal estradiol priming in women defined as poor responders: a systematic review and meta-analysis. Hum Reprod. 2013;28(11):2981-9.
49. Fanchin R, Salomon L, Castelo-Branco A, et al. Luteal estradiol pre-treatment coordinates follicular growth during controlled ovarian hyperstimulation with GnRH antagonists. Hum Reprod. 2003;18(12):2698-703.
50. Polyzos NP, Tournaye H. Poor ovarian responders: to meta-analyse or not, that is the question. Hum Reprod. 2014;29(3):634-5.
51. Hill MJ, Levens ED, Levy G, et al. The use of recombinant luteinizing hormone in patients undergoing assisted reproductive techniques with advanced reproductive age: a systematic review and meta-analysis. Fertil Steril. 2012;97(5):1108-14.

52. Bosdou JK, Venetis CA, Kolibianakis EM, et al. The use of androgens or androgen-modulating agents in poor responders undergoing in vitro fertilization: a systematic review and meta-analysis. Hum Reprod Update. 2012;18(2):127-45.
53. Fan W, Li S, Chen Q, et al. Recombinant luteinizing hormone supplementation in poor responders undergoing IVF: a systematic review and meta-analysis. Gynecol Endocrinol. 2013;29(4):278-84.
54. Lehert P, Kolibianakis EM, Venetis CA, et al. Recombinant human follicle-stimulating hormone (r-hFSH) plus recombinant luteinizing hormone versus r-hFSH alone for ovarian stimulation during assisted reproductive technology: systematic review and meta-analysis. Reprod Biol Endocrinol. 2014;12:17.
55. Davoren JB, Kasson BG, Li CH, et al. Specific insulin-like growth factor (IGF) I- and II-binding sites on rat granulosa cells: relation to IGF action. Endocrinology. 1986;119(5):2155-62.
56. Hsu CJ, Hammond JM. Concomitant effects of growth hormone on secretion of insulin-like growth factor I and progesterone by cultured porcine granulosa cells. Endocrinology. 1987;121(4):1343-8.
57. Barreca A, Artini PG, Del Monte P, et al. In vivo and in vitro effect of growth hormone on estradiol secretion by human granulosa cells. J Clin Endocrinol Metab. 1993;77(1):61-7.
58. Adashi EY, Resnick CE, D'Ercole AJ, et al. Insulin-like growth factors as intraovarian regulators of granulosa cell growth and function. Endocr Rev. 1985;6(3):400-20.
59. Jia XC, Kalmijn J, Hsueh AJ. Growth hormone enhances follicle-stimulating hormone-induced differentiation of cultured rat granulosa cells. Endocrinology. 1986;118(4):1401-9.
60. Kyrou D, Kolibianakis EM, Venetis CA, et al. How to improve the probability of pregnancy in poor responders undergoing in vitro fertilization: a systematic review and meta-analysis. Fertil Steril. 2009;91(3):749-66.
61. Dor J, Seidman DS, Amudai E, et al. Adjuvant growth hormone therapy in poor responders to in-vitro fertilization: a prospective randomized placebo-controlled double-blind study. Hum Reprod. 1995;10(1):40-3.
62. Eftekhar M, Aflatoonian A, Mohammadian F, et al. Adjuvant growth hormone therapy in antagonist protocol in poor responders undergoing assisted reproductive technology. Arch Gynecol Obstet. 2013;287(5):1017-21.
63. Weil SJ, Vendola K, Zhou J, et al. Androgen receptor gene expression in the primate ovary: cellular localization, regulation, and functional correlations. J Clin Endocrinol Metab. 1998;83(7):2479-85.
64. Vendola KA, Zhou J, Adesanya OO, et al. Androgens stimulate early stages of follicular growth in the primate ovary. J Clin Invest. 1998;101(12):2622-9.
65. Sunkara SK, Coomarasamy A. Androgen pretreatment in poor responders undergoing controlled ovarian stimulation and in vitro fertilization treatment. Fertil Steril. 2011;95(8):e73-4.
66. Sunkara SK, Coomarasamy A, Arlt W, et al. Should androgen supplementation be used for poor ovarian response in IVF? Hum Reprod. 2012;27(3):637-40.
67. Weiner Z, Thaler I, Levron J, et al. Assessment of ovarian and uterine blood flow by transvaginal color Doppler in ovarian-stimulated women: correlation with the number of follicles and steroid hormone levels. Fertil Steril. 1993;59(4):743-9.
68. SD Keay, EA Lenton, ID Cooke, et al. Low dose Dexamethasone augments the ovarian response to exogenous gonadotrophins leading to a reduction in cycle cancellation rate in standard IVF programme. Hum Reprod. 2001;16(9):1861-65.
69. Bassil S, Wyns C, Toussaint-Demylle D, et al. The relationship between ovarian vascularity and the duration of stimulation in in-vitro fertilization. Hum Reprod. 1997;12(6):1240-5.
70. Pellicer A, Ballester MJ, Serrano MD, et al. Aetiological factors involved in the low response to gonadotrophins in infertile women with normal basal serum follicle stimulating hormone levels. Hum Reprod. 1994;9(5):806-11.
71. Battaglia C, Genazzani AD, Regnani G, et al. Perifollicular Doppler flow and follicular fluid vascular endothelial growth factor concentrations in poor responders. Fertil Steril. 2000;74(4):809-12.
72. Rubinstein M, Marazzi A, Polak de Fried E, et al. Low-dose aspirin treatment improves ovarian responsiveness, uterine and ovarian blood flow velocity, implantation, and pregnancy rates in patients undergoing in vitro fertilization: a prospective, randomized, double-blind placebo-controlled assay. Fertil Steril. 1999;71(5):825-9.
73. Nardo LG, Granne I, Stewart J, et al. Medical adjuncts in IVF: evidence for clinical practice. Hum Fertil (Camb). 2009;12(1):1-13.
74. Ubaldi FM, Rienzi L, Ferrero S, et al. Management of poor responders in IVF. Reprod Biomed Online. 2005;10(2):235-46.
75. Kim C-H, Jeon G-H, Lee H-A, et al. Co-transfer of fresh and collected cryopreserved embryos (COFACCE) obtained in minimal stimulation cycles for low responders. Fertil Steril. 2009;92:238.
76. Schimberni M, Morgia F, Colabianchi J, et al. Natural-cycle in vitro fertilization in poor responder patients: a survey of 500 consecutive cycles. Fertil Steril. 2009;92(4):1297-301.
77. Polyzos NP, Blockeel C, Verpoest W, et al. Live birth rates following natural cycle IVF in women with poor ovarian response according to the Bologna criteria. Hum Reprod. 2012;27(12):3481-6.
78. Noyes N, Porcu E, Borini A. Over 900 oocyte cryopreservation babies born with no apparent increase in congenital anomalies. Reprod Biomed Online. 2009;18(6):769-76.
79. Rienzi L, Cobo A, Paffoni A, et al. Consistent and predictable delivery rates after oocyte vitrification: an observational longitudinal cohort multicentric study. Hum Reprod. 2012;27(6):1606-12.

CHAPTER

46

The High Responder: Optimizing the Stimulation without Complications

Javier Martínez-Salazar Romero, Israel Ortega Sanchez, Juan Antonio García-Velasco

INTRODUCTION

Clinical practice has demonstrated that ovarian response to controlled ovarian stimulation with gonadotropins may present a broad range of biological actions in women. In this sense, clinical and biologically consensus exists to distinguish women with normal, low and high or multifollicular response, although there is no generally accepted definition for these different types of response.

One might think that a high ovarian response is desirable for in vitro fertilization (IVF), since it would provide multiple oocytes and embryos for subsequent embryo development, leading to a better selection of good-quality embryos for transfer and thus, improving reproductive outcomes. However, it has been shown that an excessive ovarian response to gonadotropins might exert a deleterious effect on endometrial receptivity and thus, on reproductive outcomes.[1] On the other hand, the problem of an excessive high response is mainly related to the administration of high doses of gonadotropins. However, this is partly true, since it has been shown that patient´s individual characteristics might account for a high ovarian response, regardless of the gonadotropin dose. This is especially relevant in patients with multifollicular ovaries or diagnosed with a polycystic ovary syndrome (PCOS).

The narrow threshold of the ovarian response to ovarian stimulation in PCOS patients is known, and the boundary between the minimum effective dose of gonadotropins and the ones inducing excessive follicular development is so narrow that small dose modifications might induce high ovarian response and clinical complications, being ovarian hyperstimulation syndrome (OHSS) the most relevant one.

In order to improve the prediction and management of these complications, better diagnostic criteria have been established to better identify these patients and predict their ovarian response. Moreover, the incorporation of new therapeutic strategies, such as the use of GnRH antagonist protocols and the clinical application of oocyte/embryo vitrification in current routine practice have dramatically decrease the incidence of OHSS, without compromising the reproductive outcomes.

DEFINITION AND IDENTIFICATION OF HIGH RESPONDERS

Since the beginning of assisted reproduction it has been known that the negative consequences and risks to which the high responder patients are exposed. Although, it has not been possible to reach a consensus on its definition. Over the past decade, several clinical criteria based on the number of follicles and serum estradiol levels obtained on the day of oocyte maturation have been proposed. Although a standard definition for high ovarian response is lacking, the clinical community has proposed that the following features must be present to define high ovarian response: more than 20 follicles in the final phase of stimulation, serum estradiol levels greater than 3,000 pg/mL and more than 15 oocytes obtained after oocyte retrieval.

Classically, the presence of risk factors such as age, body mass index, or the presence of polycystic ovaries have been used as good predictors of high ovarian response. According to the meta-analysis published by Broer et al.[2] these clinical markers together with the evaluation of the antral follicle count (AFC) by vaginal ultrasound, defined as the total number of follicles 2–10 mm in diameter at the beginning of the menstrual cycle, and determination of serum anti-Müllerian hormone (AMH) levels, are the best clinical markers to predict a high ovarian response in IVF with high sensitivity and specificity.

One of the most important advantages associated with the evaluation of AFC at the beginning of ovarian stimulation is that it presents limited intercycle variability, allowing a more accurate gonadotropin dose adjustment prior to the onset of ovarian stimulation. It has been proposed that an AFC more than 14 follicles per ovary might be a good predictor of high ovarian response, leading to a potential risk of developing OHSS.

Anti-Müllerian hormone is expressed in the granulosa cells of preantral and small antral follicles and is an excellent marker of ovarian reserve. Furthermore, it presents a low inter and intracycle variability, allowing its evaluation at any time of the menstrual cycle. Evaluation of serum AMH levels prior to the onset of ovarian stimulation is a good predictor of ovarian response, allowing physicians to customize the stimulation protocol according to patient's individual characteristics. However, there is a lack of consensus on the cut-off value of serum AMH level to define a high ovarian response. Based on our data, AMH levels less than 3 ng/mL (1 ng/mL = 7.14 pmol/L) might predict a high ovarian response, whereas levels greater than 7 ng/mL might predict a potential risk of developing OHSS.

Finally, the presence of more than 20 follicles greater than 14 mm at the end of the stimulation and/or serum estradiol levels greater than 3,000 pg/mL at the time of inducing oocyte maturation, are good predictors of high ovarian response, being useful to suspect a high risk of OHSS. However, the role of serum estradiol determination as a predictor of high ovarian response has recently been questioned.

CONSEQUENCES AND RISKS OF HIGH RESPONDERS

Ovarian Hyperstimulation Syndrome

The OHSS is the most important clinical complication in patients undergoing IVF, leading to potentially life-threatening situations, characterized by the presence of prolonged and persistent ovarian growth and accumulation of fluid in the serous cavities. It has been shown that the development of OHSS is directly related to the use of human chorionic gonadotropin (hCG) for triggering ovulation, which increases production of serum vascular endothelial growth factor and other mediators, such as ovarian renin-angiotensin system, interleukin-1 and interleukin-6, leading to increased vascular permeability.

Clinically, patients developing OHSS may present a broad range of clinical manifestations, including abdominal distension and pain, nausea and vomiting, oliguria and edema in the lower limbs. Regarding to laboratory abnormalities, the development of OHSS may be characterized by the presence of increased hematocrit (> 45%), leukocytosis (>15,000/mm^3), electrolyte disturbances (hyponatremia and hyperkalemia), increased liver enzymes, hypoalbuminemia and decreased creatinine clearance.

Although the evolution of OHSS is closely related to the levels of hCG, the underlying mechanisms of hCG clearance are still poorly characterized. Nowadays, OHSS can be classified into two forms:

1. *Early OHSS*: It appears between 3–7 days after hCG administration and is related with the exogenous hCG administration. It usually disappears within 10–14 days in the absence of pregnancy.
2. *Late OHSS*: It appears 10 days post-hCG administration and is related to the presence of gestation and endogenous production of trophoblastic hCG, which prolongs or aggravates the symptoms of the syndrome.

Oocyte and Embryo Quality

Currently, there is a controversy regarding oocyte and embryo quality in high responder patients, since a large number of immature oocytes and lower pregnancy rates together with higher miscarriage rates have been observed in these patients compared to normoresponders. Furthermore, patients diagnosed with PCOS should be differentiated from those non-PCOS high responder patients, since the presence of metabolic disturbances such as hyperandrogenism, low-grade inflammation, insulin resistance and obesity that might impair oocyte quality, leading to poorer reproductive outcomes.

There is growing evidence showing that hyperinsulinemia secondary to insulin resistance, might have a detrimental effect on oocyte quality, accounting for the lower implantation and pregnancy rates observed in these patients. This hyperinsulinemia-induced deleterious effect on oocyte quality has also been observed in PCOS fertile women donating their oocytes in an egg donation program.[3] Thus, the poorer reproductive outcomes observed in patients with hyperinsulinemia seem to be related with an impairment of oocyte quality, and not with the endometrial receptivity.

The presence of high rates of immature oocytes observed in most of high responder patients may be due to an alteration in the maturation of intermediate follicles, emerging as a potential cause of higher miscarriage rates in this case. Previously, it has been shown that there is an inverse relationship between the quality and the number of oocytes retrieved.[4] However, despite the presence of low oocyte quality and maturity that leads to lower fertilization rates, pregnancy rates are not necessarily impaired as embryo quality may not be affected.

Previously, it has been suggested that in high responder donors the aneuploidy rate for day 3 embryos rises up to 56.6%, after obtaining an average number of 25.9 oocytes.[5] However, it is not yet clear whether this increase in aneuploidy rate is due to the patient's characteristics or might be secondary to ovarian stimulation protocols. The abovementioned aneuploidy rate in high responder patients is in sharp contrast with the one observed in normoresponder patients (37.3%) and those undergoing moderate ovarian stimulations.[6] Taking these results into account, we may conclude that these patients present a high incidence of embryo aneuploidy due to high response to gonadotropin stimulation. Interestingly, Munne et al.[7] have demonstrated that normal donors present more than 50% of aneuploid embryos when tested by techniques of comparative genomic hybridization (CGH), and it has been suggested that the aneuploidy rate could be even greater in young donors.[8]

Currently, there is growing evidence demonstrating that embryo aneuploidy is closely related to the gonadotropin dose used in controlled ovarian stimulation. Our group conducted a crossover study[9] to evaluate the aneuploidy rate from embryos originated from donors with a previous cycle of high ovarian response. All donors underwent two cycles of ovarian stimulation with a GnRH-antagonist protocol, separated by at least 3 months. In the first cycle, ovarian stimulation was started with initial doses of recombinant follicle-stimulating hormone (rFSH) of 225 IU/day, being subsequently adjusted according to serum estradiol levels on day 5 of ovarian stimulation. However in the second cycle, a fixed rFSH dose of 150 IU/day was administered regardless of high estradiol levels on day 5 of stimulation. Out of the 32 donors initially included in the study, 10 had to be canceled during ovarian stimulation in the second cycle due to insufficient response. These results confirm a significant increase in fertilization rates and the number of chromosomally normal blastocysts in high responder donors receiving low doses of gonadotropins in the second cycle, although the live birth rates were similar in both stimulation protocols, since the higher number of oocytes and embryos counterbalanced the decline in egg quality.[6]

Endometrial Receptivity

Over the past decade, our group has demonstrated that high responder patients with elevated serum estradiol levels present impaired endometrial receptivity,[1] being eligible for embryo freezing to perform frozen-thawed embryo transfer in a subsequent cycle. Before the introduction of oocyte/ embryo vitrification in the routine clinical practice, the use of the slow freezing protocol in cases of high ovarian response avoided the incidence of OHSS. However, this cryopreservation technique was associated with low survival rates and poor reproductive outcomes.

Recently, several studies have shown that high responder patients exhibits increased serum progesterone levels during ovarian stimulation. Classically, this finding has been associated with the occurrence of premature luteinizing hormone (LH) surge during ovarian stimulation, but some studies indicate that this increase in progesterone levels is linked to excessive exposure to FSH during the follicular phase,[10] which induces paracrine changes leading to increased progesterone production in the late follicular phase. The presence of a high number of follicles and proliferation of granulosa cells leads to a higher progesterone concentrations in patients with high estrogen levels on the day of hCG,[11] suggesting that high response is frequently associated with elevated serum progesterone levels.

The consequences of such a progesterone increase during ovarian stimulation have been controversial. Several authors have suggested that elevated progesterone levels might exert a deleterious effect on IVF outcomes,[12] however such an association has not been confirmed by others.[13] The presence of high progesterone concentrations induces secretory changes in the endometrium and premature acceleration of endometrial maturation that might alter the window of implantation, impairing the clinical outcomes. In a recent study evaluating the cut-off of serum progesterone levels on the day of hCG in IVF patients, our group demonstrated that values greater than 1.5 ng/mL were associated with a significant decrease in pregnancy rates (31% vs. 19%).[14] Recently, a retrospective study published by our group evaluated the effect of serum progesterone levels on the day of hCG on clinical outcomes in 2,500 high responder patients, showing no differences in either implantation or pregnancy rates. However, there was a trend to lower implantation rates when progesterone levels were greater than 1.8 ng/mL. These findings might be due to the fact that high responder patients present fast developing embryos, that might be synchronized with an advanced endometrium, presenting optimal implantation and pregnancy rates. It should be noted that this study was finished in 2011, when embryo vitrification and the use of GnRH antagonist protocols were fully established in routine clinical practice.[15] A recent meta-analysis supports this hypothesis; however, it should be viewed with caution due to the presence of selection bias in the included studies.[11] Regardless of whether clinical outcomes are affected or not, these patients should be recommended to vitrify their oocytes/embryos and postpone embryo transfer, due to the high risk of developing OHSS.

STIMULATION PROTOCOL IN HIGH RESPONDERS

For several years, the use of GnRH agonist, either long or short protocol, has been the gold standard in ART to inhibit pituitary gonadotropin secretion, inhibiting the appearance of a premature LH surge. However, it requires the use of hCG for oocyte maturation induction, increasing the risk of high responder patients to develop OHSS. To overcome this, several strategies have been developed over the past decade:

- Use of low doses of gonadotropins, which is associated with a potential risk of cycle cancellation due to absence of ovarian response
- Use of half the dose of hCG to induce final oocyte maturation
- Coasting, which involves delaying hCG administration, while maintaining administration of GnRH analogs until estrogen levels drop to "safe" values
- Embryo freezing, postponing frozen-thawed embryo transfer to a subsequent cycle. In the past, the slow freezing protocol yielded poorer reproductive outcomes compared to vitrification technique
- Cycle cancellation, avoiding hCG administration. This strategy is associated with psychological burden and financial implications for the patient. The introduction of GnRH antagonists in stimulation protocols together with the incorporation of vitrification techniques in IVF laboratories represent one of the biggest breakthroughs in the management of these patients.

As previously discussed, both AMH levels and RFA allow us to predict high ovarian response in patients undergoing IVF using either GnRH agonists[2] or antagonist[16] protocols. It should be noted that GnRH antagonist protocol effectively suppresses endogenous LH secretion, while reducing the duration of ovarian stimulation and the dose of gonadotropins, leading to a reduction of complexity and cycle costs for the patient. Thus, the use of GnRH antagonist emerges as a safer approach to treat patients at risk of developing a high ovarian response compared to the GnRH agonist protocol, while maintaining similar ongoing and live birth rates.[17] Furthermore, the use of GnRH antagonist allows us to perform the induction of oocyte maturation with GnRH agonist, preventing the occurrence of early onset OHSS related to hCG administration. Taken together, the GnRH antagonist protocol represents nowadays the gold standard for those IVF patients at risk of developing a high ovarian response.

Taking into account the negative implications of high ovarian response, such as the high number of follicles, elevated serum estrogen and progesterone levels during ovarian stimulation, one might think that using half the dose of gonadotropins (150 IU of rFSH) with subsequent dose adjustment according to estradiol levels on day 3 of ovarian stimulation, might represent a valid strategy for these patients. Regarding the type of gonadotropin, several studies have demonstrated that there are not significant differences in clinical outcomes when comparing the use of both the urinary and recombinant gonadotropins.[18] However, the fact that most of these patients at risk of high ovarian response present PCOS with elevated basal LH levels, has led physicians to use rFSH, avoiding the effect of LH of urinary gonadotropins. However, further studies are necessary to establish the best gonadotropin protocol to be used in these patients.

In PCOS patients diagnosed with insulin resistance and hyperinsulinemia, the use of adjuvant therapies targeting glucose metabolism such as metformin, might improve oocyte hormonal environment and thus, improve oocyte quality.[19] Thus, according to current evidence, the use of metformin in association with gonadotropins is recommended in PCOS patients with impaired glucose tolerance.[20]

GNRH ANALOGS, OOCYTE MATURATION AND ITS CONSEQUENCES

It has been known for years that administration of a bolus of GnRH agonist at the end of ovarian stimulation induces trigger of oocyte maturation and reduces the incidence of OHSS.[21] However, this approach is not a valid strategy for those women undergoing a GnRH agonist long protocol. With the emergence of GnRH antagonists, the use of GnRH agonist as an agent to trigger ovulation has gained in importance,[22] being a dose of 0.2 mg of triptorelin acetate the optimal dose to yield a normal oocyte retrieval and produce good quality embryos. However, this approach was associated with some drawbacks, including high miscarriage rates and low ongoing pregnancy rates, secondary to a profound luteal phase insufficiency refractory to conventional luteal phase support protocols.

The underlying mechanism of such a profound luteal phase insufficiency after GnRH agonist administration is the inhibition of gonadotropin secretion, mainly LH, after initial flare-up. Humaidan et al.[22] confirmed that LH levels in the luteal phase when administering GnRH agonist to trigger ovulation were lower than in those patients who received hCG. However, hCG-induced luteotropic effect is enough to sustain the luteal phase, while low LH levels after GnRH agonist administration were not enough to maintain proper luteal phase.

Strategies in High Responders at Risk of OHSS

Given this background, there was an urgent need to establish new strategies in high responder patients at risk of OHSS after triggering oocyte maturation with GnRH agonist, aimed to avoid luteal phase insufficiency and unacceptable clinical outcomes.

To overcome this, over the past decade several alternatives have been suggested, including embryo freezing and subsequent embryo transfer at a later stage (also called "cycle segmentation"), or rescuing the insufficient luteal phase to allow fresh embryo transfer.

Freezing of all Oocytes/Embryos: Cycle Segmentation

This approach was already known at the time when hCG was administered to induce oocyte maturation in a GnRH antagonist protocol when the patients were at high risk of OHSS. By that time, the technique of oocyte freezing was not yet available and the slow freezing protocol offered limited results, but it was an alternative to avoid the risk of developing a severe OHSS.

Vitrification technique involves ultra-fast freezing, small volume and high concentration of cryoprotectants, and allows cryopreservation of both oocytes and embryos, yielding excellent survival rates of about 95%. Moreover, there are not significant differences in terms of clinical outcomes when comparing fresh embryo transfer with vitrified embryo transfer after thawing.[23] These optimal results together with its efficiency and safety have led the cryopreservation programs to become a crucial part in the routine practice in IVF laboratories.[24]

Embryo vitrification allows physicians to perform the frozen-thawed embryo transfer in a subsequent cycle with excellent clinical outcomes, either in a natural cycle or following hormonal replacement therapy.[25] Indeed, some studies have reported an improvement in obstetric and perinatal outcomes when using vitrified embryos compared to those obtained in the fresh cycle.[26]

The policy of cycle segmentation avoids the occurrence of severe late onset OHSS. In 2014, in IVI-Madrid there was only one case of early OHSS and 4 cases of late OHSS out of a total of 1,789 IVF cycles. Despite the use of vitrification, there is still a potential risk of developing an early OHSS, due to individual biological variability.[27]

It is still controversial whether high responder patients should freeze their oocytes or embryos. Oocyte vitrification has the advantage of limiting the number of surplus embryos, which might be beneficial not only for patients who have moral conflicts to generate supernumerary embryos, but also for embryologists, since the number of cryopreserved embryos decreases.

To clarify this issue, our group conducted a study[28] aimed to evaluate the pregnancy outcomes of 96 high responder patients after oocyte or embryo vitrification. All the patients followed a GnRH antagonist protocol with subsequent trigger with GnRH agonist, being randomized into two different groups: Group 1, oocyte vitrification was performed and ICSI was postponed in a subsequent cycle; Group 2, embryo vitrification was performed after ICSI, being thawed and transferred in a subsequent cycle. Baseline clinical characteristics were comparable between both groups.

Regarding the laboratory outcomes, there were no differences in either the number of retrieved oocytes or the maturation rate. Interestingly, a higher number of fertilized oocytes was observed in group 2 versus group 1 (14.8 vs. 10.7), as well as a higher number of transferable embryos in group 2 (6.4 ± 4.2) compared to group 1 (4.3 ± 2.7). However, no differences in either fertilization rate (68.3% vs. 73.3%) or in the transferable embryo rate (27.9% vs. 31.3%) were reported.

After the first embryo transfer, no significant differences in implantation, biochemical or clinical pregnancy rates (44% in group 1 vs. 50% in group 2) were observed. However, a significant increase in the miscarriage rate was observed in group 2 versus group 1 (30.4% vs. 4.5%). Interestingly, there were no cases of OHSS in both groups.

Embryo survival rates were similar in both groups (group 1, 87.5% and 89.4% in group 2). However, the oocyte survival rate in group 1 was 78.8%, slightly lower than the one published by our group,[23] possibly due to bad oocyte quality in these patients. This might be the cause of the difference in the number of transferable embryos in group 1, secondary to a lower number of mature oocytes for ICSI.

After three embryo transfers, clinical outcomes remained similar between groups, with live birth rates of 72% in group

1 compared to 69.6% in group 2. However, it should be noted that miscarriage rate remained higher in group 2 compared to group 1, 21.9% versus 9.7%, respectively. This finding is difficult to justify and, ruling out the potential deleterious effect of vitrification on cryopreserved embryos, the only plausible justification is that oocyte vitrification in group 1 might act as a filter of quality, while in group 2 the oocytes generate embryos with limited evolutionary potential, commonly associated with pregnancy loss.

In view of these considerations, oocyte freezing should be recommended to these patients since it offers similar clinical results compared to embryo freezing, avoiding legal and ethical concerns of generating surplus cryopreserved embryos. Moreover, oocyte vitrification also allows to better determine the number of oocytes to be fertilized, depending on patient's characteristics. Those couples interested in limiting the number of embryos, due to medical or ethical reasons, single women or presence of chronic diseases, would be eligible for oocyte vitrification, whereas those couples interested in having more children would be eligible for embryo freezing.

Luteal Phase Rescue

Given the luteal phase insufficiency after triggering oocyte maturation with GnRH agonist, some authors have suggested new strategies to perform fresh embryo transfer in the same cycle, avoiding the use of vitrification (Table 1). Among them, the most important approach to rescue the luteal phase in high responder patients is focused on administration of low doses of hCG, using 1,500 IU of hCG on the day of oocyte retrieval together with a conventional luteal phase support with progesterone and estradiol.[29] According to the current evidence, this protocol offers good pregnancy rates and low miscarriage rates, decreasing the number of cases of OHSS.[34] However, it has been shown that those patients with a high number of oocyte retrieval might develop an early OHSS due to hCG administration. Moreover, this strategy might be associated with a high risk of late OHSS in case a pregnancy occurs. Thus, this strategy should be viewed with caution when used in high responder patients, due to the potential risk of both and early and late OHSS.[35]

It has been proposed progesterone-free luteal phase support, using two subcutaneous bolus of 1,500 IU hCG separated by 4 days starting on the day of oocyte retrieval. However, this clinical approach seems to be more appropriate in cases of mild high ovarian response, since administration of hCG, even at low doses, might considerably increase the risk of these patients to develop OHSS.[30]

The administration of low doses of customized hCG (< 33 IU/kg) and GnRH agonist on the day of oocyte triggering (dual triggering), together with luteal phase support based on 6 mg orally administered estradiol and 800 mg vaginal progesterone, have been associated with optimal clinical results and low incidence of OHSS.[32] However, further studies are need to better evaluate the effectiveness of this approach before being integrated in the routine clinical practice.

It had been evaluated the potential beneficial effect of combined administration of high doses of progesterone in combination with transdermic estradiol as luteal phase support, achieving clinical pregnancy rates of up to 53% without the appearance of OHSS.[30,33,36,37]

Table 1: Strategies in high ovarian response. Final oocyte maturation with GnRHa.

GnRH agonist	*Day of oocyte retrieval*	*Oocyte/ embryo vitrification*	*Luteal phase support*	*Reference*
Yes	–	Yes	No	García-Velasco et al.[25]
Yes	1,500 IU hCG	No	6 mg oral estradiol + 600 mg of vaginal progesterone starting after ovarian retrieval	Humaidan et al.[29]
Yes	1,500 IU hCG	No	1500 IU hCG every 4 days starting on the day of oocyte retrieval	Kol et al.[30]
Yes	500 IU hCG	No	500 IU hCG every 3 days starting on the day of oocyte retrieval	Castillo et al.[31]
+hCG (<33 IU/kg) Dual triggering	–	No	6 mg oral estradiol + 800 mg vaginal progesterone	Shapiro et al.[32]
Yes	–	No	50 mg IM progesterone daily + 0.3 mg transdermic estradiol/day starting on the day oocyte retrieval	Engmann et al.[33]

CONCLUSION

Despite current knowledge about etiology and physiopathology of high ovarian response, the management of patients undergoing IVF at high risk of developing OHSS still represents a challenge for physicians. The use of GnRH antagonist protocol with low doses of rFSH (100–150 IU/day) represents the gold standard in the management of patients with high ovarian response. In cases of an excessive ovarian response (> 15 mature follicles on the day of oocyte maturation), administration of GnRH agonist to trigger final oocyte maturation together with oocyte vitrification avoids the development of both the early and late OHSS. Luteal phase rescue with hCG at low doses with or without steroids may represent an alternative for those women who want to undergo a fresh embryo transfer in the same cycle. In these cases, single embryo transfer should be recommended and the patient should be informed about the risk of developing late OHSS. However, it still remains unknown the best approach to rescue the luteal phase in those women receiving fresh embryo transfer after GnRH agonist trigger, as well as the patient profile that might benefit from this strategy.

REFERENCES

1. Simon C, Cano F, Valbuena D, et al. Clinical evidence for a detrimental effect on uterine receptivity of high serum oestradiol concentrations in high and normal responder patients. Hum Reprod. 1995;10(9):2432-7.
2. Broer SL, Dolleman M, Opmeer BC, et al. AMH and AFC as predictors of excessive response in controlled ovarian hyperstimulation: a meta-analysis. Hum Reprod Update. 2011;17(1):46-54.
3. Cano F, Garcia-Velasco JA, Millet A, et al. Oocyte quality in polycystic ovaries revisited: identification of a particular subgroup of women. J Assist Reprod Genet. 1997;14(5):254-61.
4. Giles J, Requena A, Garcia-Velasco JA, et al. GnRH analogue for the prevention of ovarian hyperstimulation syndrome: a pilot study. Fertil Steril. 2009;91(4 Suppl):1366-9.
5. Reis Soares S, Rubio C, Rodrigo L, et al. High frequency of chromosomal abnormalities in embryos obtained from oocyte donation cycles. Fertil Steril. 2003;80(3):656-7.
6. Labarta E, Bosch E, Alama P, et al. Moderate ovarian stimulation does not increase the incidence of human embryo chromosomal abnormalities in in vitro fertilization cycles. J Clin Endocrinol Metab. 2012;97(10):E1987-94.
7. Munne S, Ary J, Zouves C, et al. Wide range of chromosome abnormalities in the embryos of young egg donors. Reprod Biomed Online. 2006;12(3):340-6.
8. Keskintepe L, Sher G, Keskintepe M. Reproductive oocyte/embryo genetic analysis: comparison between fluorescence in-situ hybridization and comparative genomic hybridization. Reprod Biomed Online. 2007;15(3):303-9.
9. Rubio C, Mercader A, Alama P, et al. Prospective cohort study in high responder oocyte donors using two hormonal stimulation protocols: impact on embryo aneuploidy and development. Hum Reprod. 2010;25(9):2290-7.
10. Hofmann GE, Bentzien F, Bergh PA, et al. Premature luteinization in controlled ovarian hyperstimulation has no adverse effect on oocyte and embryo quality. Fertil Steril. 1993;60(4):675-9.
11. Griesinger G, Mannaerts B, Andersen CY, et al. Progesterone elevation does not compromise pregnancy rates in high responders: a pooled analysis of in vitro fertilization patients treated with recombinant follicle-stimulating hormone/gonadotropin-releasing hormone antagonist in six trials. Fertil Steril. 2013;100(6):1622-8. e1-3.
12. Bosch E, Valencia I, Escudero E, et al. Premature luteinization during gonadotropin-releasing hormone antagonist cycles and its relationship with in vitro fertilization outcome. Fertil Sterility. 2003;80(6):1444-9.
13. Yding Andersen C, Bungum L, Nyboe Andersen A, et al. Preovulatory progesterone concentration associates significantly to follicle number and LH concentration but not to pregnancy rate. Reprod Biomed Online. 2011;23(2):187-95.
14. Bosch E, Labarta E, Crespo J, et al. Circulating progesterone levels and ongoing pregnancy rates in controlled ovarian stimulation cycles for in vitro fertilization: analysis of over 4000 cycles. Hum Reprod. 2010;25(8):2092-100.
15. Requena A, Cruz M, Bosch E, et al. High progesterone levels in women with high ovarian response do not affect clinical outcomes: a retrospective cohort study. Reprod Biol Endocrinol. 2014;12:69.
16. Hamdine O, Eijkemans MJ, Lentjes EW, et al. Ovarian response prediction in GnRH antagonist treatment for IVF using anti-Müllerian hormone. Hum Reprod. 2015;30(1):170-8.
17. Al-Inany HG, Youssef MA, Aboulghar M, et al. Gonadotrophin-releasing hormone antagonists for assisted reproductive technology. Cochrane Database Syst Rev. 2011(5):CD001750.
18. Aboulghar M, Saber W, Amin Y, et al. Prospective, randomized study comparing highly purified urinary follicle-stimulating hormone (FSH) and recombinant FSH for in vitro fertilization/intracytoplasmic sperm injection in patients with polycystic ovary syndrome. Fertil Sterility. 2010;94(6):2332-4.
19. Legro RS. Metformin as adjuvant therapy to IVF in women with PCOS: when isintention-to-treat unintentional? Hum Reprod. 2011;26(8):2043-4.
20. Thessaloniki ESHRE/ASRM-Sponsored PCOS Consensus Workshop Group. Consensus on infertility treatment related to polycystic ovary syndrome. Hum Reprod. 2008;23(3):462-77.
21. Itskovitz-Eldor J, Kol S, Mannaerts B, et al. First established pregnancy after controlled ovarian hyperstimulation with recombinant follicle stimulating hormone and the gonadotrophin-releasing hormone antagonist ganirelix (Org 37462). Hum Reprod. 1998;13(2):294-5.
22. Humaidan P, Bredkjaer HE, Bungum L, et al. GnRH agonist (buserelin) or hCG for ovulation induction in GnRH antagonist IVF/ICSI cycles: a prospective randomized study. Hum Reprod. 2005;20(5):1213-20.
23. Cobo A, de los Santos MJ, Castello D, et al. Outcomes of vitrified early cleavage-stage and blastocyst-stage embryos in a cryopreservation program: evaluation of 3,150 warming cycles. Fertil Steril. 2012;98(5):1138-46 e1.

24. Mukaida T, Oka C. Vitrification of oocytes, embryos and blastocysts. Best Pract Res Clin Obstet Gynaecol. 2012;26(6):789-803.
25. Garcia-Velasco JA. Agonist trigger: what is the best approach? Agonist trigger with vitrification of oocytes or embryos. Fertil Steril. 2012;97(3):527-8.
26. Maheshwari A, Pandey S, Shetty A, et al. Obstetric and perinatal outcomes in singleton pregnancies resulting from the transfer of frozen thawed versus fresh embryos generated through in vitro fertilization treatment: a systematic review and meta-analysis. Fertil Steril. 2012;98(2):368-77. e1-9.
27. Fatemi HM, Popovic-Todorovic B, Humaidan P, et al. Severe ovarian hyperstimulation syndrome after gonadotropin-releasing hormone (GnRH) agonist trigger and "freeze-all" approach in GnRH antagonist protocol. Fertil Steril. 2014;101(4):1008-11.
28. Herrero L, Pareja S, Aragones M, et al. Oocyte versus embryo vitrification for delayed embryo transfer: an observational study. Reprod Biomed Online. 2014;29(5):567-72.
29. Humaidan P, Polyzos NP, Alsbjerg B, et al. GnRHa trigger and individualized luteal phase hCG support according to ovarian response to stimulation: two prospective randomized controlled multi-centre studies in IVF patients. Hum Reprod. 2013;28(9):2511-21.
30. Kol S, Humaidan P, Itskovitz-Eldor J. GnRH agonist ovulation trigger and hCG-based, progesterone-free luteal support: a proof of concept study. Hum Reprod. 2011;26(10):2874-7.
31. Castillo JC, Dolz M, Bienvenido E, et al. Cycles triggered with GnRH agonist: exploring low-dose HCG for luteal support. Reprod Biomed Online. 2010;20(2):175-81.
32. Shapiro BS, Daneshmand ST, Garner FC, et al. Comparison of "triggers" using leuprolide acetate alone or in combination with low-dose human chorionic gonadotropin. Fertil Steril. 2011;95(8):2715-7.
33. Engmann L, DiLuigi A, Schmidt D, et al. The effect of luteal phase vaginal estradiol supplementation on the success of in vitro fertilization treatment: a prospective randomized study. Fertil Steril. 2008;89(3):554-61.
34. Radesic B, Tremellen K. Oocyte maturation employing a GnRH agonist in combination with low-dose hCG luteal rescue minimizes the severity of ovarian hyperstimulation syndrome while maintaining excellent pregnancy rates. Hum Reprod. 2011;26(12):3437-42.
35. Seyhan A, Ata B, Polat M, et al. Severe early ovarian hyperstimulation syndrome following GnRH agonist trigger with the addition of 1500 IU hCG. Hum Reprod. 2013;28(9):2522-8.
36. Griffin D, Benadiva C, Kummer N, et al. Dual trigger of oocyte maturation with gonadotropin-releasing hormone agonist and low-dose human chorionic gonadotropin to optimize live birth rates in high responders. Fertil Steril. 2012;97(6):1316-20.
37. Orvieto R. Intensive luteal-phase support with oestradiol and progesterone after GnRH-agonist triggering: does it help? Reprod Biomed Online. 2012;24(6):680-1.

CHAPTER

47

Ovulation Trigger

Carlos Dosouto Capel, Haahr T, Peter Humaidan

INTRODUCTION

Ovulation trigger (OT) in assisted reproductive technology (ART) is a key factor for success, and OT agents aim at mimicking the final oocyte maturation of the natural cycle which is induced by the mid-cycle surge of gonadotropins [luteinizing hormone (LH) and follicle-stimulating hormone (FSH)]. However, stimulated in vitro fertilization (IVF) cycles are significantly different from the natural cycle due to the multifollicular development, supraphysiological follicular and luteal phase steroid level, and altered hypothalamic response due to either use of gonadotropin-releasing hormone (GnRH) analogs or to the supraphysiological steroid levels. A profound knowledge about pharmacokinetics and pharmacodynamics of all these agents enable fertility specialists to individualize OT to secure the correct timing of the oocyte retrieval as well as the most optimal luteal phase support (LPS).

The initial major OT agent used in ART as a surrogate of the natural mid-cycle LH surge was human chorionic gonadotropin (hCG) due to its molecular similarity with LH and, thus, its affinity for the luteinizing hormone/choriogonadotropin receptor (LHCG-R). The hCG is an excellent OT agent, seen from data on pregnancy outcomes in IVF cycles in which either fresh or frozen embryo transfer (ET) was performed. However, the major disadvantage of hCG relates to the pharmacological characteristics which in some patients—mainly high responder patients—induces a high risk of ovarian hyperstimulation syndrome (OHSS). OHSS remains a potential cause of death in women undergoing ART and the OHSS incidence ranges from 0.18% to 1.40%,[1] albeit it is well-established that OHSS is grossly underreported.[2] The condition is characterized by massive enlargement of the ovaries and the presence of ascites due to increased vascular permeability as a result of an hCG mediated up-regulation of vascular mediators.[3] OHSS occurs almost exclusively in the presence of prolonged LH activity which is seen after hCG trigger.[3,4] Furthermore, the severity of OHSS is proportional to the dose of hCG administered and the amount of follicles and corpora lutea (CL) obtained after ovarian stimulation, respectively.

During recent years, the gold standard hCG trigger for final oocyte maturation in IVF/ICSI (intracytoplasmic sperm injection) cycles has been challenged as first-line treatment with the introduction of the gonadotropin-releasing hormone agonist (GnRHa) trigger, which has been proven to almost eliminate the risk of OHSS.[5]

The most optimal strategy to prevent OHSS is the identification of high-risk patients before or during ovarian stimulation in order to modify the stimulation regimen accordingly, and subsequently plan the trigger agent, either hCG or GnRHa. Both trigger agents allow either a fresh transfer or a freeze-all policy (segmentation); however, only GnRHa trigger and segmentation will result in the virtually "OHSS free clinic".[6] Until now, the majority of fertility clinics plan segmentation for subgroups of patients, predominantly OHSS high-risk patients, and consequently the vast majority of IVF patients still undergo fresh ET after hCG trigger. However, patients with 15 or more preovulatory follicles less than or equal to 11 mm run a significantly higher risk of developing OHSS after hCG trigger than patient with fewer follicles;[7] thus, it is important to take the number of preovulatory follicles into account when the trigger agent (hCG or GnRHa) and the subsequent handling of the luteal phase is determined.

NATURAL OVULATORY CYCLE

At the end of every nonconception cycle an involution of the corpus luteum occurs, followed by a significant drop in the ovarian luteal steroid levels. The drop has a positive feedback effect at the level of the GnRH hypothalamic pulse generator which induces an early follicular raise in FSH levels. This phenomenon is the basis for the complex recruitment process of a new follicular cohort, which eventually ends up with monofollicular growth. The raise in estradiol (E) secreted by the leading follicle at a certain threshold induces a positive pituitary feedback, resulting in a mid-cycle surge of LH, and to a lesser degree FSH. This surge of gonadotropins triggers the resumption of meiosis, ovulation, and luteinization. Although the LH activity is crucial for final oocyte maturation, FSH also plays a role for oocyte maturation and, moreover, induces LH receptor formation in the luteinizing granulosa-theca cells which secures the function of the future corpus luteum.[3,8] Activation of the ovulatory cascade and luteinization of granulosa and theca cells do not occur as a result of the duration of the mid-cycle surge of gonadotropins, but rather the intensity of the signal (i.e. magnitude of increase in cAMP).[9] The secretion of both gonadotropins in a natural cycle is characterized by a three phased curve with a total duration of approximately 48 hours.[10] From the time of luteinization, the CL among other substances releases steroid hormones like progesterone (P) and E, and the function of the CL is entirely dependent on the pulsatile LH secretion from the pituitary.[8,11] However, LH also plays an important role during the luteal phase by upregulating cytokines and growth factors such as fibroblast growth factor 2 (FGF2), vascular endothelial growth factor A (VEGFA) and activating endometrial LH receptors—all factors which support implantation and early neovascularization.[3,8]

The functional life span of the CL in a nonconception cycle is usually 14 ± 2 days. During this time the CL produces 25–50 mg of P daily and its activity drops if no implantation has occurred.[12] However, in a conception cycle after implantation, which occurs approximately 7 days after ovulation, the trophoblast gradually begins to secrete hCG, which binds to and activates the same receptor as LH, the LHCG-R, securing an optimal CL function until approximately the 7th week of gestation at the so called luteo-placental shift.[12] The steroid production, of mainly P during the mid-luteal phase is mandatory to induce endometrial gland secretory transformation, prevent uterine contractions and enhance implantation. P deficiency at this point leads to early pregnancy loss (EPL).[5,8]

TRIGGERING AGENTS

Human Chorionic Gonadotropin

Human chorionic gonadotropin is a dimeric glycoprotein which shares the alpha subunit with FSH, LH and thyroid-stimulating hormone. The beta subunit is unique and confers specificity for the receptor. Moreover, the glycosylation degree of each hormone is variable and determines the receptor binding affinity and circulating half-life.[13] There is considerable structural homology between hCG and human LH and both hormones stimulate the same receptor—the LHCG-R.[13] For more than 30 years hCG extracted from the urine of pregnant women has proven to be useful for OT.[14] Urinary preparations, however, have some disadvantages, first and foremost uncontrolled source and low purity.[15] In recent years, recombinant human chorionic gonadotropin (rhCG), a genetically engineered hCG was developed with high purity and a more optimal consistency. Both urinary and rhCG are used in doses ranging from 5,000 to 10,000 IU for OT.[16]

Gonadotropin-releasing Hormone Agonist

Gonadotropin-releasing hormone agonist is a synthetic peptide modeled after the hypothalamic GnRH that interacts with the GnRH receptor to elicit its biological response, i.e. the release of LH and FSH. However, following the initial "flare" of gonadotropins, continued stimulation with GnRHa causes GnRH receptor downregulation and, thus, pituitary desensitization. GnRHa for OT is only possible in GnRH antagonist co-treated IVF/ICSI cycles or in cycles in which no GnRH analog is used during stimulation. GnRHa has an affinity coefficient 2–50 times higher than that of the endogenous GnRH for the GnRH receptor;[16] thus in a GnRH antagonist co-treated cycle a bolus of GnRHa will displace the GnRH antagonist from the receptor, inducing a flare of gonadotropins (LH and FSH) and subsequently, oocyte maturation and ovulation.[17] GnRHa most commonly used for OT are: leuprorelin, buserelin, nafarelin, and triptorelin.[18]

Kisspeptin

Kisspeptin (Kp), although until now not used in daily clinical practice, is an interesting peptide hormone which influences the human neuroendocrine regulation.[19] It is released in the hypothalamic infundibular nucleus and acts through the Kp receptor (KISS 1R) directly on GnRH neurons as a key regulator of GnRH-secretion, impacted by circulating E and P levels.[19,20] In humans, exogenously administered subcutaneous kisspeptin (1.6–12.8 nmol/kg)[21] induces a dose-dependent release of endogenous LH and to a lesser extent FSH.[19,22,23] In the first experimental trials the use of a kisspeptin trigger was associated with good results in terms of the oocyte maturity rate.[24] However, the luteal phase after kisspeptin trigger is even more impaired as compared to GnRHa trigger, as the LH surge elicited is significantly shorter and with lower amplitude than that induced by GnRHa trigger. This is contrasted by the long duration (6–10 days) of LH activity induced by an hCG trigger.[21] Thus, the future role of kisspeptin as an OT agent needs to be further determined.

OVULATION TRIGGER IN OVULATION INDUCTION CYCLES FOR INTRAUTERINE INSEMINATION OR PROGRAMMED INTERCOURSE

A combination of intrauterine insemination (IUI) or programmed intercourse (PI) after controlled ovarian stimulation (COS) or in spontaneous cycles remains an important first-line treatment option for indications like cervical factor, mild endometriosis, mild-to-moderate male factor, ovulatory dysfunction, and unexplained infertility.[25] In spontaneous cycles as well as in stimulated cycles hCG has been administered successfully as a substitute for the endogenous LH surge to induce final oocyte maturation.[26] Although pregnancy rates per cycle vary according to the indication, they are usually reported in a range from 8% to 22%.[27] GnRHa, although not commonly used, has also been proven useful for OT in IUI and ovulation induction (OI) cycles.[28] However, OT with GnRHa is followed by an inadequate production of P, which is not overcome with a standard LPS. Thus, the addition of luteal hCG was reported to be useful to overcome this deficiency.[29] Until now hCG still remains the most widely used OT in IUI or PI cycles.

OVULATION TRIGGER IN IVF/ICSI CYCLES

Stimulated IVF/ICSI Cycle Triggered with hCG

In controlled ovarian stimulation IVF cycles triggered with hCG, the early luteal supraphysiological steroid concentration (P and E) induces a negative feedback on the endogenous LH secretion by the pituitary. This results in a marked reduction in circulating LH levels and a subsequent disruption of the luteal phase, necessitating the use of LPS if ongoing pregnancies are to be obtained.[30] Thus, significant differences exist in the comparison between the luteal steroid levels of the natural cycle and the hCG triggered stimulated cycle due to the significantly longer half-life of hCG compared to LH.[26,31] As the endogenous LH level of the hCG triggered cycle is significantly reduced due to a negative feedback on the pituitary, the CL function relies completely on the exogenous administration of LH activity in the form of hCG.[5] However, at peri-implantation hCG levels and consequently P levels are decreasing, which makes exogenous P supplementation mandatory to overcome the peri-implantation gap that develops between the decrease of exogenous hCG activity and the increase in endogenous hCG production from an implanting embryo.[5]

Stimulated IVF/ICSI Cycles Triggered with GnRHa

Unlike the natural mid-cycle surge of gonadotropins which has three phases that last for a total of for 48 hours, the GnRHa-induced surge consists of two phases, only, with a duration of 24–36 hours. This results in a reduced total amount of circulating LH (and FSH) released after GnRHa trigger compared to the natural cycle.[4,5] Thus, the mean mid-luteal LH level of the natural cycle is approximately 6 IU/L whereas it is approximately 1.5 IU/L after GnRHa trigger.[5,10] This level is insufficient to support the function of the CL, leading to either implantation failure or early pregnancy loss in fresh ET cycles if a standard LPS is used.[5] After the initial introduction of the GnRHa trigger for IVF patients, several modified LPS policies have been suggested. One strategy is to administer exogenously administered steroid support (P + E). Another strategy is to boost the endogenous steroid support by adding LH activity either in the form of a small bolus of hCG after the initial trigger or by adding daily recombinant LH injections during the luteal phase.[11,32]

Although GnRHa trigger induces a luteal phase deficiency, the concomitant release of FSH may add further physiological benefits as FSH upregulates the LH receptors of the CL. Indeed, previous studies reported a higher maturity rate of oocytes and a lower incidence of empty follicle syndrome (EFS) when GnRHa trigger was compared to hCG trigger.[5,33-35] As for hCG triggered cycles, early luteal phase supraphysiological levels of P and E produced by multiple CL induce a negative feedback on the endogenous LH secretion, which after the initial flare-up will result in a CL demise and a short luteal phase. Moreover, a possible direct luteolytic action of GnRHa has previously been proposed, and data from in vitro studies suggested that GnRHa is capable of activating the apoptosis cascade in granulosa cells.[36-38] Taken together, due to significant differences in circulating LH activity during the early luteal phase induced by a GnRHa trigger compared to a hCG trigger and the natural mid-cycle surge of gonadotropins, an extended or modified LPS is mandatory to obtain optimal pregnancy rates after GnRHa trigger.[5,39]

Dual Trigger (GnRHa and hCG Trigger)

The use of GnRHa combined with low-dose hCG trigger, so called "dual trigger", was initially reported in a retrospective study including a total of 45 patients.[40] The hCG was administered concomitantly with a bolus of GnRHa in a dose ranging from 1,000 IU to 2,500 IU, depending on body weight of the patient and the individual risk of OHSS development. The authors reported an ongoing pregnancy rate of 53.3% and no OHSS cases. The dual trigger concept was subsequently investigated in a randomized controlled trial (RCT), in which a total of 200 patients who had failed at least one previous IVF-ET cycle using a long GnRHa downregulation protocol were included. The study group was triggered with both GnRHa (triptorelin 0.2 mg SC) and hCG (5,000 IU), whereas the control group was triggered with hCG (5,000 IU) only. The authors reported a significant increase in ongoing pregnancy rate per cycle in the dual trigger group.[41] Later a retrospective study was conducted in patients at risk of OHSS with peak serum estradiol (E2) levels less than 4,000 pg/mL. The use of dual trigger with GnRHa and a fixed dose of 1,000 IU hCG was compared to GnRHa trigger alone. In both groups an intensive LPS consisting of 50 mg intramuscular P daily and 0.3 mg transdermal E2 patches every other day starting from the day after the oocyte retrieval was used. Additional oral E and intramuscular P were given to maintain levels above 200 pg/mL and 20 ng/mL, respectively. The authors reported significantly higher live birth rates after dual trigger, and only one mild OHSS case occurred in the dual trigger group compared to none in the GnRHa trigger, only, group.[42] Similar results were reported in a retrospective study which included a total of 187 normal responder patients and compared dual trigger (GnRHa + hCG 6,500 IU) to hCG 6,500 IU alone.[43]

Interestingly the dual trigger concept has been proposed for the genuine EFS, and as previously mentioned the concept has also been shown to be an applicable OT strategy to improve the number of oocytes retrieved, especially in patients with a suboptimal follicle:oocyte ratio in a previous cycle (<50%) or a low proportion of mature oocytes (<66%).[44-46] Dual trigger combines the advantages of both agents (GnRHa and hCG): the direct intrafollicular LH activity mediated by hCG, the simultaneous induction of an endogenous FSH surge mediated by GnRHa and the support of the early luteal phase LH activity mediated by hCG.[47] Thus, dual trigger for a subgroup of patients might overcome existing impairments in granulosa cell function, oocyte maturation or cumulus expansion, resulting in the successful retrieval of mature oocytes.[48]

SAFETY AND EFFICACY OF TRIGGERING AGENTS (hCG AND GnRHa)

Ovulation Trigger, Optimal Oocyte Count and OHSS

The optimal OT should result in an optimal LH activity surge and a subsequent P rise.[49] A rule of thumb is that an optimal OT policy should result in more than 75% mature oocytes without increasing the risk of OHSS development.[19] GnRHa trigger effectively reduces OHSS rates due to the shorter half-life of the endogenous LH secretion compared to the long acting LH activity after an hCG trigger—approximately 33 hours versus 6–10 days respectively.[50,51] However, due to the short half-life, GnRHa trigger results in a defective CL formation and a decrease in the release of vasoactive peptides such as VEGF.[52] Although recent publications reported isolated cases of OHSS after GnRHa trigger in freeze-all cycles (segmentation),[53-55] OHSS after GnRHa trigger and segmentation is very rare and most probably related to unexpected mutations or polymorphisms of the GnRH, FSH or LH receptor.

In comparison with GnRHa triggered IVF cycles, the hCG triggered cycles have been reported to have equal or slightly lower number of mature oocytes retrieved.[5,56,57] The physiological background for this finding could be the result of a reduction in the release of EGF-like peptides after hCG trigger, which have been shown to be potent mediators of oocyte maturation.

Ovulation Trigger and Embryo Quality

Embryo quality can be measured by international score assessment, blastulation rate, aneuploidy rate, and above all the live birth rate. Good quality oocytes and embryos have been shown to be obtained after GnRHa as well as after hCG trigger as seen in the reproductive outcomes of oocyte donation frozen thawed cycles.[58-60] However, some earlier studies reported a negative impact on early embryonic development when a bolus of hCG was used for trigger.[61] The authors hypothesized that an exaggerated intrafollicular shift in steroids from androgens and estradiol to progesterone mediated by high concentrations of hCG in the theca cell might negatively affect the oocyte.[62,63] In general, there is a lack of solid evidence to show significant differences in embryo quality related to the trigger agent.

Ovulation Trigger and Endometrial Receptivity/Luteal Phase

The OT agents affect endometrial receptivity either through direct mechanisms or by affecting the physiology of the CL and its subsequent steroid production. Regarding the use of hCG for OT, some studies reported a potential negative impact of hCG on endometrial receptivity.[64-66] The average serum level of hCG in hCG triggered cycles is approximately 120 IU/L during the early luteal phase, slowly decreasing to 4–6 IU/L on day 6.[67] This supraphysiological LH activity level during the early luteal phase might hamper successful implantation due to interference with specific actions mediated by hyperglycosylated hCG (H-hCG) produced by the implanting embryo.[68] Moreover, after an hCG trigger, P levels peak significantly earlier than during natural cycle, in which P reaches its peak concentration during the mid-luteal phase. Hypothetically, this early P rise may lead to an endometrial advancement that might negatively impact endometrial receptivity at the time of implantation.[69] In contrast, after GnRHa trigger, the early to mid-luteal phase steroid level is closer to the physiological range.[5,30] Moreover, GnRH receptors are expressed in extra-pituitary tissue including the endometrium, and the use of GnRH antagonists results in inhibitory intracellular events on transforming growth factor-beta (TGF-β) pathway, interleukin-1β (IL-1β) and VEGF production.[70,71] In this aspect, earlier studies reported that the use of a mid-luteal bolus of GnRHa resulted in a significant improvement in implantation rates.[8,9] Thus, it was hypothesized that a mid-luteal bolus of GnRHa might displace the GnRHa attached to the endometrial GnRH receptor, activating the downregulated receptors and resulting in the upregulation of pro-implantation factors.[41]

Ovulation Trigger and Luteal Phase Symptoms

Human chorionic gonadotropin trigger results in a significant increase in luteal fluid retention and ovarian volume, which causes significantly more abdominal pain, bloating and discomfort. In contrast, GnRHa trigger is associated with less fluid retention,[72] reduced ovarian volume and reduced discomfort[52] and, thus, a higher patient convenience.[73]

LUTEAL PHASE AFTER OVULATION TRIGGER

In all fresh ET IVF cycles LPS is mandatory as previously described. LPS can be stratified into standard and modified.

Luteal Phase after hCG Triggered IVF/ICSI Cycles

In IVF/ICSI cycles triggered with hCG, there is a need for progesterone supplementation (either vaginal, intramuscular or subcutaneous) to avoid the peri-implantation gap in progesterone as mentioned earlier, however, there is no need for E supplementation.[74] The LPS used after hCG trigger is known as a standard LPS.

Luteal Phase after GnRHa Triggered IVF/ICSI Cycles

In IVF/ICSI cycles triggered with GnRHa, a standard LPS is not sufficient to counterbalance the luteal phase insufficiency induced by the trigger. In contrast, an intensive or modified LPS is mandatory. Thus, the early GnRHa trigger studies using a standard LPS found significantly lower implantation rates and significantly higher early pregnancy loss rates compared to hCG triggered cycles.[4,5,75,76] However, after the introduction of modifications of the standard LPS, subsequent trials showed good pregnancy and live birth rates.[77,78]

The use of hCG as a surrogate for LH activity to promote the endogenous steroid production by the remnant CL was recently referred to as "The European Approach".[78] Over the years, the main effort has been to find the minimum hCG dose needed to rescue the CL until the hCG produced by the implanting embryo covers the luteal LH activity deficiency without increasing the risk of OHSS.[56,77,78]

As it is physiologically plausible that a refractory period may occur after the initial GnRHa trigger, during which human granulosa cells do not respond to subsequent LH-like exogenous stimulation, a pilot RCT in which low dose hCG (1,500 IU) was administered at either 12 hours or 35 hours after GnRHa trigger was performed. The comparator was hCG trigger (10,000 IU).[77] Higher mid-luteal P levels and better pregnancy rates were reported in the 35 hours group compared with the 12 hours group. Importantly, no differences in pregnancy outcomes were seen between the GnRHa trigger 35 hours hCG group and hCG group. Thus, the ideal timing of the 1,500 IU hCG rescue bolus following GnRHa trigger seemed to be the day of the oocyte retrieval.

The CL rescue concept after GnRHa trigger was further explored in a small group of 12 OHSS high-risk patients, having 25 or more follicles more than or equal to 11 mm. Patients were administered a bolus of 1,500 IU hCG following GnRHa trigger, i.e. shortly after the oocyte retrieval, resulting in promising results in live birth rate (50%) and OHSS reduction.[79] In a subsequent RCT, a total of 302 normogonadotropic patients were triggered with either hCG or GnRHa followed by 1,500 IU hCG at 35 hours. Again, a nonsignificant difference in live birth rates between GnRHa and hCG trigger was seen: 24% versus 31%, respectively.[33] The OHSS rate (severe and moderate) was 2% in hCG group, whereas no OHSS cases occurred in the GnRHa group, despite the fact that more than one-third of the patients in each group were considered at risk of OHSS, above ≥ 14 follicles ≥ 11 mm.[7] Although not significant, a 7% difference in live birth rate in favor of hCG trigger encouraged the authors to further scrutinize their data, revealing an increase in early pregnancy losses in the subgroup of normal responders (< 14 follicles ≥ 11 mm) who were triggered with GnRHa. This finding prompted the authors to suggest an innovative concept of an individualized luteal phase support (iLPS) after GnRHa trigger, in which the luteal administration of hCG was correlated to the number of preovulatory follicles larger than 11 mm.[80]

Another LPS policy after GnRHa trigger was recently described as "The American Approach".[78] This approach is based on the luteal phase regimen used for oocyte recipients who are treated with intensive LPS using intramuscular P and transdermal or oral E after the transfer of donated oocytes. Thus, this concept disregards CL function and relies solely on exogenous LPS after GnRHa trigger. Over the years, pregnancy rates similar to those of hCG trigger have been reported, however, close luteal phase monitoring to maintain P levels above 20 ng/mL and E levels above 200 pg/mL is mandatory to obtain good reproductive outcomes.[42,52,81] Until now this protocol has mainly been reported for patients considered at high risk of OHSS development, and this particular subset of patients are known to have significantly increased LH levels during the luteal phase and a decreased sensitivity of the GnRH pulse generator to the inhibition by ovarian steroids,[82] which leaves the patient with higher endogenous serum LH levels in the luteal phase.

In conclusion, two main modified LPS strategies have been suggested for GnRHa triggered cycles:

1. A bolus of hCG administered either during the early luteal phase or at the time of trigger followed by a standard LPS. This strategy aims to rescue the CL with subsequent endogenous steroid production.[78]
2. Intensive daily exogenous E and P administration which disregards the CL function. To use this luteal phase concept close luteal phase monitoring of P and E2 levels is mandatory if good reproductive outcomes are to be obtained.[42,52,83]

SEGMENTATION (FREEZE-ALL POLICY)

Recently a "freeze-all" policy was proposed for all GnRHa triggered IVF cycles;[6,49,84] however, prior to implementing this concept, there are concerns that need to be addressed. Although laboratories worldwide develop fast, not all IVF units have an optimal cryopreservation program, which is clearly crucial for the success of a freeze-all policy. In addition, a higher early pregnancy loss rate related to frozen-thawed cycles has been reported,[85] as well as a higher risk of epigenetic changes.[86] Moreover, religious, ethical and financial reasons may preclude a freeze-all policy. Finally, the early embryonic stage is a vulnerable period in terms of epigenetic activity and, hypothetically, additional manipulations (freeze-thaw) might induce irreversible changes which only appear in adulthood.[87] Thus, a"freeze-all" policy should be adopted with caution, and results from large long-term follow-up trials in children conceived as a result of frozen-thaw ET are mandatory before a "freeze-all" policy can be advised as a first-line treatment. However, in OHSS risk patients the immediate benefits from segmentation already outweigh the known and unknown risks involved with this strategy.[88] This policy is also applicable in aging good ovarian reserve patients who due to biological aging have a high aneuploidy rate and for whom the retrieval of additional oocytes increases the chance of transferring one euploid embryo.

CONCLUSION

Success rates in ART improve day-by-day, due to the refinement of gonadotropins, OT concepts, LPS and laboratory techniques. Importantly, the stimulation protocol remains crucial to achieve the maximum number of mature oocytes to obtain a live birth with the minimum risk for the patient. In this aspect OT plays a crucial role, and individualization in OT strategy is important to minimize the risk of an IVF treatment without negatively affecting the reproductive outcome. Until now hCG and GnRHa have clinically proven their efficacy when used for OT whereas more trials are needed to reveal the possible future role of kisspeptin as a trigger agent in IVF.

REFERENCES

1. Kupka MS, Ferraretti AP, de Mouzon J, et al. Assisted reproductive technology in Europe, 2010: results generated from European registers by ESHRE†. Hum Reprod. 2014;29:2099-113.
2. Humaidan P, Nelson SM, Devroey P, et al. Ovarian hyperstimulation syndrome: review and new classification

criteria for reporting in clinical trials. Hum Reprod. 2016;31:1997-2004.

3. Humaidan P, Westergaard LG, Mikkelsen AL, et al. Levels of the epidermal growth factor-like peptide amphiregulin in follicular fluid reflect the mode of triggering ovulation: a comparison between gonadotrophin-releasing hormone agonist and urinary human chorionic gonadotrophin. Fertil Steril. 2011;95:2034-8.
4. Fauser BC, De Jong D, Olivennes F, et al. Endocrine profiles after triggering of final oocyte maturation with GnRH agonist after cotreatment with the GnRH antagonist ganirelix during ovarian hyperstimulation for in vitro fertilization. J Clin Endocrinol Metab. 2002;87:709-15.
5. Humaidan P, Bredkjaer HE, Bungum L, et al. GnRH agonist (buserelin) or hCG for ovulation induction in GnRH antagonist IVF/ICSI cycles: a prospective randomized study. Hum Reprod. 2005;20:1213-20.
6. Devroey P, Polyzos NP, Blockeel C. An OHSS-free clinic by segmentation of IVF treatment. Hum Reprod. 2011;26: 2593-7.
7. Papanikolaou EG, Pozzobon C, Kolibianakis EM, et al. Incidence and prediction of ovarian hyperstimulation syndrome in women undergoing gonadotropin-releasing hormone antagonist in vitro fertilization cycles. Fertil Steril. 2006;85:112-20.
8. Tesarik J, Hazout A, Mendoza-Tesarik R, et al. Beneficial effect of luteal-phase GnRH agonist administration on embryo implantation after ICSI in both GnRH agonistand antagonist-treated ovarian stimulation cycles. Hum Reprod. 2006;21:2572-9.
9. Pirard C, Donnez J, Loumaye E. GnRH agonist as luteal phase support in assisted reproduction technique cycles: results of a pilot study. Hum Reprod. 2006;21:1894-900.
10. Tavaniotou A, Albano C, Van Steirteghem A, et al. The impact of LH serum concentration on the clinical outcome of IVF cycles in patients receiving two regimens of clomiphene citrate/gonadotrophin/0.25 mg cetrorelix. Reprod Biomed Online. 2003;6:421-6.
11. Engmann L, Benadiva C, Humaidan P. GnRH agonist trigger for the induction of oocyte maturation in GnRH antagonist IVF cycles: a SWOT analysis. Reprod Biomed Online. 2016;32:274-85.
12. Duncan WC, McNeilly AS, Fraser HM, et al. Luteinizing hormone receptor in the human corpus luteum: lack of down-regulation during maternal recognition of pregnancy. Hum Reprod. 1996;11:2291-7.
13. Pierce JG, Parsons TF. Glycoprotein hormones: structure and function. Annu Rev Biochem. 1981;50:465-95.
14. Gemzell C. Induction of ovulation with human gonadotropins. Recent Prog Horm Res. 1965;21:179-204.
15. Penarrubia J, Balasch J, Fabregues F, et al. Recurrent empty follicle syndrome successfully treated with recombinant human chorionic gonadotrophin. Hum Reprod. 1999;14:1703-6.
16. Driscoll GL, Tyler JP, Hangan JT, et al. A prospective, randomized, controlled, double-blind, double-dummy comparison of recombinant and urinary HCG for inducing oocyte maturation and follicular luteinization in ovarian stimulation. Hum Reprod. 2000;15:1305-10.
17. Gonen Y, Balakier H, Powell W, et al. Use of gonadotropin-releasing hormone agonist to trigger follicular maturation for in vitro fertilization. J Clin Endocrinol Metab. 1990;71: 918-22.
18. van Loenen AC, Huirne JA, Schats R, et al. GnRH agonists, antagonists, and assisted conception. Semin Reprod Med. 2002;20:349-64.
19. Skorupskaite K, George JT, Anderson RA. The kisspeptin-GnRH pathway in human reproductive health and disease. Hum Reprod Update. 2014;20:485-500.
20. Millar RP, Newton CL. Current and future applications of GnRH, kisspeptin and neurokinin B analogues. Nat Rev Endocrinol. 2013;9:451-66.
21. Jayasena CN, Abbara A, Comninos AN, et al. Kisspeptin-54 triggers egg maturation in women undergoing in vitro fertilization. J Clin Invest. 2014;124:3667-77.
22. Jayasena CN, Comninos AN, Veldhuis JD, et al. A single injection of kisspeptin-54 temporarily increases luteinizing hormone pulsatility in healthy women. Clin Endocrinol (Oxf). 2013;79:558-63.
23. Jayasena CN, Abbara A, Veldhuis JD, et al. Increasing LH pulsatility in women with hypothalamic amenorrhoea using intravenous infusion of Kisspeptin-54. J Clin Endocrinol Metab. 2014;99:E953-61.
24. Jayasena CN, Comninos AN, Narayanaswamy S, et al. Acute and chronic effects of kisspeptin-54 administration on GH, prolactin and TSH secretion in healthy women. Clin Endocrinol (Oxf). 2014;81:891-8.
25. Duran HE, Morshedi M, Kruger T, et al. Intrauterine insemination: a systematic review on determinants of success. Hum Reprod Update. 2002;8:373-84.
26. Kessler MJ, Reddy MS, Shah RH, et al. Structures of N-glycosidic carbohydrate units of human chorionic gonadotropin. J Biol Chem. 1979;254:7901-8.
27. Guzick DS, Carson SA, Coutifaris C, et al. Efficacy of superovulation and intrauterine insemination in the treatment of infertility. National Cooperative Reproductive Medicine Network. N Engl J Med. 1999;340:177-83.
28. Balasch J, Fabregues F, Tur R, et al. Further characterization of the luteal phase inadequacy after gonadotropin-releasing hormone agonist-induced ovulation in gonadotrophin-stimulated cycles. Hum Reprod. 1995;10:1377-81.
29. Penarrubia J, Balasch J, Fabregues F, et al. Human chorionic gonadotrophin luteal support overcomes luteal phase inadequacy after gonadotrophinreleasing hormone agonist-induced ovulation in gonadotrophin-stimulated cycles. Hum Reprod. 1998;13:3315-8.
30. Humaidan P, Kol S, Papanikolaou EG. GnRH agonist for triggering of final oocyte maturation: time for a change of practice? Hum Reprod Update. 2011;17:510-24.
31. Mannaerts BM, Geurts TB, Odink J. A randomized three-way cross-over study in healthy pituitary-suppressed women to compare the bioavailability of human chorionic gonadotrophin (Pregnyl) after intramuscular and subcutaneous administration. Hum Reprod. 1998;13:1461-4.
32. Itskovitz J, Boldes R, Levron J, et al. Induction of preovulatory luteinizing hormone surge and prevention of ovarian hyperstimulation syndrome by gonadotropin-releasing hormone agonist. Fertil Steril. 1991;56:213-20.

33. Humaidan P, Ejdrup Bredkjaer H, Westergaard LG, et al. 1,500 IU human chorionic gonadotropin administered at oocyte retrieval rescues the luteal phase when gonadotropin-releasing hormone agonist is used for ovulation induction: a prospective, randomized, controlled study. Fertil Steril. 2010;93:847-54.
34. Lok F, Pritchard J, Lashen H. Successful treatment of empty follicle syndrome by triggering endogenous LH surge using GnRH agonist in an antagonist down-regulated IVF cycle. Hum Reprod. 2003;18:2079-81.
35. Oktay K, Türkçüoğlu I, Rodriguez-Wallberg KA. GnRH agonist trigger for women with breast cancer undergoing fertility preservation by aromatase inhibitor/FSH stimulation. Reprod Biomed Online. 2010;20:783-8.
36. Latouche J, Crumeyrolle-Arias M, Jordan D, et al. GnRH receptors in human granulosa cells: anatomical localization and characterization by autoradiographic study. Endocrinology. 1989;125:1739-41.
37. Minaretzis D, Jakubowski M, Mortola JF, et al. Gonadotropin-releasing hormone receptor gene expression in human ovary and granulosa-lutein cells. J Clin Endocrinol Metab. 1995;80:430-4.
38. Takekida S, Deguchi J, Samoto T, et al. Comparative analysis of the effects of gonadotropin-releasing hormone agonist on the proliferative activity, apoptosis, and steroidogenesis in cultured porcine granulosa cells at varying stages of follicular growth. Endocrine. 2000;12:61-7.
39. Humaidan P, Papanikolaou EG, Kyrou D, et al. The luteal phase after GnRH-agonist triggering of ovulation: present and future perspectives. Reprod Biomed Online. 2012;24: 134-41.
40. Shapiro BS, Daneshmand ST, Garner FC, et al. Gonadotropin-releasing hormone agonist combined with a reduced dose of human chorionic gonadotropin for final oocyte maturation in fresh autologous cycles of in vitro fertilization. Fertil Steril. 2008;90:231-3.
41. Schachter M, Friedler S, Ron-El R, et al. Can pregnancy rate be improved in gonadotropin-releasing hormone (GnRH) antagonist cycles by administering GnRH agonist before oocyte retrieval? A prospective, randomized study. Fertil Steril. 2008;90:1087-93.
42. Griffin D, Benadiva C, Kummer N, et al. Dual trigger of oocyte maturation with gonadotropin-releasing hormone agonist and low-dose human chorionic gonadotropin to optimize live birth rates in high responders. Fertil Steril. 2012;97:1316-20.
43. Lin MH, Shao-Ying Wu F, Kuo-Kuang Lee R, et al. Dual trigger with combination of gonadotropin-releasing hormone agonist and human chorionic gonadotropin significantly improves the live-birth rate for normal responders in GnRH-antagonist cycles. Fertil Steril. 2013;100:1296-302.
44. Kasum M, Kurdija K, Oreskovic S, et al. Combined ovulation triggering with GnRH agonist and hCG in IVF patients. Gynecol Endocrinol. 2016;32:861-65.
45. Haas J, Zilberberg E, Dar S, et al. Co-administration of GnRH-agonist and hCG for final oocyte maturation (double trigger) in patients with low number of oocytes retrieved per number of preovulatory follicles—a preliminary report. J Ovarian Res. 2014;7:77.
46. Zilberberg E, Haas J, Dar S, et al. Co-administration of GnRH-agonist and hCG, for final oocyte maturation (double trigger), in patients with low proportion of mature oocytes. Gynecol Endocrinol. 2015;31:145-7.
47. Beck-Fruchter R, Weiss A, Lavee M, et al. Empty follicle syndrome: successful treatment in a recurrent case and review of the literature. Hum Reprod. 2012;27:1357-67.
48. Haas J, Ophir L, Barzilay E, et al. Standard human chorionic gonadotropin versus double trigger for final oocyte maturation results in different granulosa cells gene expressions: a pilot study. Fertil Steril. 2016;106:653-9.e1.
49. Shapiro BS, Daneshmand ST, Garner FC, et al. Evidence of impaired endometrial receptivity after ovarian stimulation for in vitro fertilization: a prospective randomized trial comparing fresh and frozen-thawed embryo transfer in normal responders. Fertil Steril. 2011;96:344-8.
50. Damewood MD, Shen W, Zacur HA, et al. Disappearance of exogenously administered human chorionic gonadotropin. Fertil Steril. 1989;52:398-400.
51. Yen SS, Llerena O, Little B, et al. Disappearance rates of endogenous luteinizing hormone and chorionic gonadotropin in man. J Clin Endocrinol Metab. 1968;28:1763-7.
52. Engmann L, DiLuigi A, Schmidt D, et al. The use of gonadotropin-releasing hormone (GnRH) agonist to induce oocyte maturation after cotreatment with GnRH antagonist in high-risk patients undergoing in vitro fertilization prevents the risk of ovarian hyperstimulation syndrome: a prospective randomized controlled study. Fertil Steril. 2008;89:84-91.
53. Ling LP, Phoon JW, Lau MS, et al. GnRH agonist trigger and ovarian hyperstimulation syndrome: relook at "freeze-all strategy". Reprod Biomed Online. 2014;29:392-4.
54. Fatemi HM, Popovic-Todorovic B, Humaidan P, et al. Severe ovarian hyperstimulation syndrome after gonadotropin-releasing hormone (GnRH) agonist trigger and "freeze-all" approach in GnRH antagonist protocol. Fertil Steril. 2014;101:1008-11.
55. Gurbuz AS, Gode F, Ozcimen N, et al. Gonadotrophin-releasing hormone agonist trigger and freeze-all strategy does not prevent severe ovarian hyperstimulation syndrome: A report of three cases. Reprod Biomed Online. 2014;29: 541-4.
56. Humaidan P, Polyzos NP, Alsbjerg B, et al. GnRHa trigger and individualized luteal phase hCG support according to ovarian response to stimulation: two prospective randomized controlled multi-centre studies in IVF patients. Hum Reprod. 2013;28:2511-21.
57. Imoedemhe DA, Sigue AB, Pacpaco EL, et al. Stimulation of endogenous surge of luteinizing hormone with gonadotropin-releasing hormone analog after ovarian stimulation for in vitro fertilization. Fertil Steril. 1991;55:328-32.
58. Acevedo B, Gomez-Palomares JL, Ricciarelli E, et al. Triggering ovulation with gonadotropin-releasing hormone agonists does not compromise embryo implantation rates. Fertil Steril. 2006;86:1682-7.
59. Griesinger G, Kolibianakis EM, Papanikolaou EG, et al. Triggering of final oocyte maturation with gonadotropin-releasing hormone agonist or human chorionic gonadotropin. Live birth after frozen-thawed embryo replacement cycles. Fertil Steril. 2007;88:616-21.

60. Bodri D, Guillén JJ, Galindo A, et al. Triggering with human chorionic gonadotropin or a gonadotropin-releasing hormone agonist in gonadotropin-releasing hormone antagonist-treated oocyte donor cycles: findings of a large retrospective cohort study. Fertil Steril. 2009;91:365-71.
61. Hausdorff WP, Caron MG, Lefkowitz RJ. Turning off the signal: desensitization of beta-adrenergic receptor function. FASEB J. 1990;4:2881-9.
62. Dumesic DA. Reduced intrafollicular androstenedione and estradiol levels in early-treated prenatally androgenized female rhesus monkeys receiving follicle-stimulating hormone therapy for in vitro fertilization. Biol Reprod. 2003;69:1213-9.
63. Dumesic DA, Schramm RD, Peterson E, et al. Impaired developmental competence of oocytes in adult prenatally androgenized female rhesus monkeys undergoing gonadotropin stimulation for in vitro fertilization. J Clin Endocrinol Metab. 2002;87:1111-9.
64. Forman R, Fries N, Testart J, et al. Evidence for an adverse effect of elevated serum estradiol concentrations on embryo implantation. Fertil Steril. 1988;49: 118-22.
65. Fatemi HM, Kyrou D, Bourgain C, et al. Cryopreserved-thawed human embryo transfer: spontaneous natural cycle is superior to human chorionic gonadotropin-induced natural cycle. Fertil Steril. 2010;94:2054-8.
66. Fanchin R, Peltier E, Frydman R, et al. Human chorionic gonadotropin: does it affect human endometrial morphology in vivo? Semin Reprod Med. 2001;19:31-5.
67. Trinchard-Lugan I, Khan A, Porchet HC, et al. Pharmacokinetics and pharmacodynamics of recombinant human chorionic gonadotrophin in healthy male and female volunteers. Reprod Biomed Online. 2002;4:106-15.
68. Cole LA. Hyperglycosylated hCG and pregnancy failures. J Reprod Immunol. 2012;93:119-22.
69. Andersen CY, Elbaek HO, Alsbjerg B, et al. Daily low-dose hCG stimulation during the luteal phase combined with GnRHa triggered IVF cycles without exogenous progesterone: a proof of concept trial. Hum Reprod. 2015;30:2387-95.
70. Luo X, Xu J, Chegini N. Gonadotropin releasing hormone analogue (GnRHa) alters the expression and activation of Smad in human endometrial epithelial and stromal cells. Reprod Biol Endocrinol. 2003;1(1):125.
71. Meresman GF, Bilotas MA, Lombardi E, et al. Effect of GnRH analogues on apoptosis and release of interleukin-1β and vascular endothelial growth factor in endometrial cell cultures from patients with endometriosis. Hum Reprod. 2003;18:1767-71.
72. Garcia-Velasco JA, Motta L, Lopez A, et al. Low-dose human chorionic gonadotropin versus estradiol/progesterone luteal phase support in gonadotropin-releasing hormone agonist-triggered assisted reproductive technique cycles: understanding a new approach. Fertil Steril. 2010;94:2820-3.
73. Cerrillo M, Rodríguez S, Mayoral M, et al. Differential regulation of VEGF after final oocyte maturation with GnRH agonist versus hCG: a rationale for OHSS reduction. Fertil Steril. 2009;91:1526-8.
74. Fatemi HM. The luteal phase after 3 decades of IVF: what do we know? Reprod Biomed Online. 2009;19 Suppl 4:4331.
75. Beckers T, Bernd M, Kutscher B, et al. Structure-function studies of linear and cyclized peptide antagonists of the GnRH receptor. Biochem Biophys Res Commun. 2001;289:653-63.
76. Kolibianakis EM, Schultze-Mosgau A, Schroer A, et al. A lower ongoing pregnancy rate can be expected when GnRH agonist is used for triggering final oocyte maturation instead of HCG in patients undergoing IVF with GnRH antagonists. Hum Reprod. 2005;20:2887-92.
77. Humaidan P, Bungum L, Bungum M, et al. Rescue of corpus luteum function with peri-ovulatory HCG supplementation in IVF/ICSI GnRH antagonist cycles in which ovulation was triggered with a GnRH agonist: a pilot study. Reprod Biomed Online. 2006;13:173-8.
78. Humaidan P, Engmann L, Benadiva C. Luteal phase supplementation after gonadotropin-releasing hormone agonist trigger in fresh embryo transfer: the American versus European approaches. Fertil Steril. 2015;103:879-85.
79. Humaidan P. Luteal phase rescue in high-risk OHSS patients by GnRHa triggering in combination with low-dose HCG: a pilot study. Reprod Biomed Online. 2009;18:630-4.
80. Fatemi HM, Polyzos NP, van Vaerenbergh I, et al. Early luteal phase endocrine profile is affected by the mode of triggering final oocyte maturation and the luteal phase support used in recombinant follicle-stimulating hormone-gonadotropin-releasing hormone antagonist in vitro fertilization cycles. Fertil Steril. 2013;100:742-7.
81. Iliodromiti Z, Antonakopoulos N, Sifakis S, et al. Endocrine, paracrine, and autocrine placental mediators in labor. Hormones. 2012;11:397-409.
82. McCartney CR, Eagleson CA, Marshall JC. Regulation of gonadotropin secretion: implications for polycystic ovary syndrome. Semin Reprod Med. 2002;20:317-26.
83. Iliodromiti S, Lan VT, Tuong HM, et al. Impact of GnRH agonist triggering and intensive luteal steroid support on live-birth rates and ovarian hyperstimulation syndrome: a retrospective cohort study. J Ovarian Res. 2013;6:93.
84. Ozgur K, Humaidan P, Coetzee K. Segmented ART—The new era in ART? Reprod Biol. 2016;16:91-103.
85. Tomas C, Alsbjerg B, Martikainen H, et al. Pregnancy loss after frozen-embryo transfer—a comparison of three protocols. Fertil Steril. 2012;98:1165-9.
86. Henningsen AK, Romundstad LB, Gissler M, et al. Infant and maternal health monitoring using a combined Nordic database on ART and safety. Acta Obstet Gynecol Scand. 2011b;90:683-91.
87. Rimoldi SF, Sartori C, Rexhaj E, et al. Vascular dysfunction in children conceived by assisted reproductive technologies: underlying mechanisms and future implications. Swiss Med Wkly. 2014;144:w13973.
88. Krishna D, Dhoble S, Praneesh G, et al. Gonadotropin-releasing hormone agonist trigger is a better alternative than human chorionic gonadotropin in PCOS undergoing IVF cycles for an OHSS free clinic: a randomized control trial. J Hum Reprod Sci. 2016;9:164-72.

CHAPTER

48

Luteal Phase Support: ART and Non-ART Cycles

Barbara Lawrenz, Human M Fatemi

INTRODUCTION

The luteal phase of a menstrual cycle is the time between ovulation and, in case of conception, the establishment of a pregnancy or otherwise the onset of menses. In a natural cycle, under the influence of luteinizing hormone (LH) formation of the corpus luteum will occur after ovulation. The corpus luteum is characterized by the production of up to 40 mg progesterone per day and also estradiol. Progesterone induces the secretory transformation of the endometrium in the luteal phase, promotes local vasodilatation and relaxation of the uterine muscle.[1]

After conception the developing embryo will secrete human chorionic gonadotropin (hCG) which has structural similarities with LH and activates the same receptor. The role of hCG produced by the embryo is to maintain the corpus luteum and its secretions until the shift of progesterone production from the corpus luteum to the placenta around 9 weeks of pregnancy has taken place.[2]

For a pregnancy to occur, a receptive endometrium, a functional embryo at blastocyst developmental stage and synchrony between the embryo and the endometrium is required.[3] Failure to achieve receptivity and synchrony results in infertility and this is also a limiting factor for success in in-vitro fertilization (IVF) treatment.

Endometrial receptivity is driven by time of progesterone exposure after sufficient exposure to estrogen. The so called "window of implantation" (WOI), i.e. the time frame in which the endometrium is receptive and able to support trophoblast-endometrial interactions, is very limited in time. In a natural and idealized 28-day cycle, it is thought to occur during a time around day 22 to day 24.[4] It is assumed, that the WOI is constant in time in all women. However, displacement of the WOI might not bear are caused in infertility patients, especially in the patients with repeated implantation failure.[5]

STEROID PRODUCTION OF THE OVARY IN NATURAL AND STIMULATED CYCLES

Throughout the menstrual cycle, the ovary is producing the steroid hormones estradiol and progesterone. They are essential for human reproduction, which is demonstrated by the fact, that pregnancies with oocyte donation can be achieved after preparation of the endometrium with estradiol and progesterone,[6] even in women without ovaries.

In a natural cycle, estradiol synthesis increases progressively from the dominant follicle and initiates LH surge. Even before the LH surge, a small increase in progesterone levels is seen, which reflects the increasing LH pulse amplitude and frequency leading up to the surge. A LH surge of 24–36 hours is sufficient to initiate the resumption of oocyte meiosis, luteinization of granulosa cells, ovulation, and the initial phase of corpora lutea a development. Progesterone and 17α-hydroxyprogesterone (17α-OHP) plasma concentrations increase rapidly after the LH surge or administration of hCG,[7] indicating the beginning of granulosa and theca cell luteinization. As well as granulosa cells, the thecal cells produce significant amounts of progesterone. The corpus luteum is producing up to 40 mg of progesterone per day and additional a significant amount of androgens and estradiol. This is unique to the corpus luteum of many primates, including humans.[8]

Progesterone biosynthesis requires two enzymatic steps: firstly the conversion of cholesterol to pregnenolone (P5), catalyzed by the enzyme cytochrome P450scc and secondly its subsequent conversion to progesterone, which is catalyzed by 3β-hydroxysteroid dehydrogenase (3βHSD).[9] Progesterone is further metabolized to androgens by the action of CYP17 in the thecal cells under the influence of LH. This step takes only place in the thecal cell compartment. However, during early follicular phase, the enzymatic activity necessary to convert 17-OH-progesterone to androstenedione, is absent or very low. Therefore, this process leads to increasing concentrations of progesterone and estradiol, as the follicular diameter increases.[10]

Whereas in natural cycle with development of a single dominant follicle, mid-follicular follicle-stimulating hormone (FSH) levels are declining toward ovulation,[11] in ovarian stimulation for IVF, multifollicular development is achieved by administration of high daily gonadotropin concentrations. Stimulation dosage usually remains unchanged throughout the stimulation duration, unless the patient's individual response requires a change in the dosage. Therefore, ovarian stimulation will result in a large number of growing follicles and each follicle will contribute to the progesterone in the systemic circulation. Progesterone concentration often reflects the number of preovulatory follicles and patients with high estradiol concentrations have significantly more oocytes and significantly higher progesterone concentrations.[12]

In a natural cycle without conception, luteolysis occurs due to a lack of hCG support. The corpus luteum undergoes a process of regression with the loss of functional and structural integrity[13] leading to a decrease in progesterone production. In case of conception, the trophoblast produces hCG which prevents the regression of the corpus luteum and stimulates corpus luteum progesterone production which is necessary for maintenance of the pregnancy until placental progesterone production is adequate. Despite the fact, that serum hCG is detectable around the time of implantation approximately day 8 after ovulation, the hormonal characteristics of conception and nonconception cycles are different from the early luteal phase. Both LH and E2 levels are significantly higher in conception cycles on day 4 and 5 after the LH peak in urine compared to nonconception cycles.[14]

Influence of Progesterone on the Endometrium in Natural and Stimulated Cycles

The physiologic effects of P are primarily mediated by interaction with the progesterone receptor (PR). There are two classic PR isoforms, PR-A and PR-B and PR-A is required for normal ovarian and uterine function.[15] They are identical in structure except that the PR-B isoform contains a 164-amino acid N-terminal sequence, which is lacking in the PR-A isoform.[16] After binding to the nuclear receptors, steroid receptors activate their transcription genes.

The mitogenic effect of progesterone in the stroma is mediated by upregulating as well, PR-A as PR-B isoforms of the receptor.[17,18]

The different histological appearances of the endometrium, depending on the influence of estrogen or progesterone, have already been studied by Noyes et al. in 1950.[19] Whereas the proliferative phase under the influence of estradiol does not allow recognition of sub-phases other than early, middle or late proliferative phase, progressive changes occur in the endometrium of the secretory phase. In the period 36–48 hours directly after ovulation, no changes of the endometrium are visible. Further on under the influence of progesterone, the epithelial glands and vasculature continue to grow and become spiral, whereas the endometrial thickness is relatively unchanged, resulting in a denser endometrium. The morphological changes, observed on histology for each specific day after ovulation, established the classic endometrial dating paradigm that still serves as the gold standard for clinical evaluation of luteal function.[20] An endometrial biopsy that shows a difference of more than 2 days between the histologic dating and actual day after ovulation is considered to be "out of phase".[21]

Comparison of endometrial steroid receptors and proliferation index between natural cycles and gonadotropin-releasing hormone (GnRH)-agonist or human menopausal gonadotropin (hMG)-stimulated cycles for IVF have revealed distinct alterations in endometrial maturation. In stimulated cycles, a more advanced secretory endometrial maturation combined with reduced estrogen receptors (ERs) and PR and a low proliferation index in glands and stroma has been found on the day of oocyte retrieval, when compared to endometrial maturation in natural cycles on the day of ovulation.

Endometrial biopsies taken 2 days after oocyte pickup (OPU) in stimulated cycles showed a further reduction in steroid receptors and proliferation despite a similar histological maturation as compared to biopsies from natural cycles on day 2 after ovulation.[22] It can be assumed that supraphysiological hormonal levels during stimulation lead to a reduced number of ER and PR and a low proliferation index in glands and stroma. Those functional endometrial alterations might affect the proliferative potential of the endometrium.[22] However, solely from the serum progesterone concentrations and/or the absolute value of serum progesterone increase, the exact endometrial development on the day of OPU in stimulated cycles cannot be predicted.[23]

Besides the aforementioned advancement of endometrial maturation, in patients with a progesterone level above 1.5 ng/mL on the day of hCG-administration, differences in endometrial gene expression profile were found, when compared to the gene expression pattern be low this threshold.[24] These changes might explain the impairment of endometrial receptivity in the presence of elevated progesterone, reflected in the lower pregnancy rates reported in the literature.[25]

The influence of elevated progesterone levels on the endometrial gene expression pattern was also analyzed by Labarta et al.[26] In a study, comparing the endometrial dating as well as the endometrium gene expression pattern during the WOI in 12 healthy oocyte donors. Six patients had progesterone levels above and six patients below the progesterone threshold of 1.5 ng/mL. Out of 370 genes, 140 were dysregulated by more than two-fold in women with high serum progesterone levels. A large number of those genes represent biological processes like cell adhesion, immune system and organ development. Therefore, dysregulation of those genes could affect the endometrium and the implantation process.

Interestingly, at day 7 after trigger, no more endometrial advancement was found in the group with elevated progesterone levels on the day of final oocyte maturation. It was shown previously that no pregnancies are achieved in case of an endometrial advancement of more than 3 days, when the embryo transfer is performed on day 3.[23,27] However, the detrimental effect of elevated progesterone level on the day of final oocyte maturation subsidies when the transfer is delayed until the blastocyst stage.[28] This suggests that the endometrium could recover during the WOI period.

Endocrine Profile in IVF Cycles after Oocyte Retrieval, Depending on the Type of Trigger

Ovulation induction in ovarian stimulation for IVF with GnRH-agonist protocols has to be performed by the administration of hCG to mimic the LH surge, whereas within GnRH-antagonist-protocols the use of GnRH-agonist for final oocyte maturation is possible with the advantage of reducing the risk for ovarian hyperstimulation syndrome (OHSS). Due to the different ways of action of hCG and GnRH-agonist, different endocrine profiles are seen after oocyte retrieval procedure. Patients, who were triggered with only hCG or GnRH-agonist plus 1,500 IU hCG had lower LH levels compared to patients, triggered with GnRH-agonist only. Progesterone levels on day 5 after oocyte retrieval procedure were highest in patients triggered with either hCG alone or a combination of GnRH-agonist plus 1,500 IU hCG and lowest in patients after GnRH-agonist only without any luteal phase support. This difference is caused by the fact, that after hCG-application progesterone production of the theca cells is sustained to approximately at least 5 days due to the LH-activity and the half-life time of hCG of more than 24 hours.[29,30] After GnRH-agonist trigger severe luteal phase insufficiency occurred due to low levels of endogenous LH and therefore of progesterone.[31]

LUTEAL PHASE SUPPORT IN ASSISTED REPRODUCTIVE TECHNIQUES

As previously described, progesterone will be produced by the corpus luteum after LH surge in normal, unstimulated cycle. Correction of a dysfunctional corpus luteum with the symptoms shortened luteal phase and premenstrual spotting by administration of progesterone was first described in 1949[32] and a defective luteal phase was defined, if the serum mid-luteal progesterone levels are less than 10 ng/mL.[33] Prevalence of luteal phase defect (LPD) in natural cycles in normo-ovulatory patients with primary or secondary in fertility was demonstrated to be about 8.1%.[34] However in 2012, the American Society for Reproductive Medicine (ASRM) stated that there is no reproducible, physiologically relevant, and clinically practical standard to diagnose LPD or distinguish fertile from infertile women.[35] The minimum threshold of progesterone level that is essential for the maintenance of a pregnancy is unknown and successful pregnancies have been reported even when the concentration of progesterone was never above 15 nmol/L for the first 14 days.[36] After ovarian stimulation for IVF/intracytoplasmic sperm injection (ICSI) treatment it seems that patients having a progesterone levels at the day of implantation of more than 30 ng/mL and estradiol levels of more than 100 pg/mL, are more likely to have a viable and ongoing pregnancy compared to patients with hormone levels below those thresholds.[37]

In stimulated cycles for IVF, a defective luteal phase occurs in almost all patients[23,27,38] and different theories have been discussed.[39] However, the reason for the luteal phase insufficiency seen after controlled ovarian stimulation seems to be the multifollicular development achieved during the follicular phase, resulting in supraphysiological luteal levels of P and E2 which inhibit LH secretion by the pituitary via negative feedback actions at the level of the hypothalamic-pituitary axis.[40-44] Besides the defective luteal phase due to the supraphysiological levels of estradiol and progesterone the WOI might be shorter in IVF-cycles compared to a natural cycle.[45]

To counterbalance the luteal phase insufficiency after ovarian stimulation, different ways of luteal phase support can be applied. Either direct substitution of progesterone via different routes of administration or indirect substitution of progesterone via the stimulation of the remaining corpora lutea to sustain progesterone production.

WAYS OF PROGESTERONE ADMINISTRATION

Oral Progesterone

Natural progesterone is rapidly metabolized after oral intake and has been shown to be ineffective in inducing a sufficient secretory transformation. Synthetic progesterone derivates are associated with side-effects, especially regarding the impact on the lipids[46] and on the psyche[47] which will limit their use. Micronization of progesterone reduces the particle size and improves absorption and bioavailability.[48] After oral digestion of 200 mg micronized progesterone maximal progesterone concentrations within the range of luteal phase are reached within 2–4 hours and will remain elevated then for approximately 6–7 hours.[48] Even higher doses of micronized progesterone have failed to induce sufficient secretory transformation. It seems that progesterone metabolites produced by the first liver passage lead to cross-reactions and are therefore responsible for those high progesterone levels.

Progesterone Intramuscular

Progesterone is rapidly absorbed after intramuscular (IM) injection. High progesterone plasma concentrations are reached after approximately 2 hours and peak concentrations will be achieved after around 8 hours. To achieve serum progesterone concentrations, which are equivalent to those during luteal phase in natural cycle, injection of 25 mg progesterone is required. It has been suggested, that the IM site of the injection might serve as a depot with progesterone accumulation in the fat tissue, leading to more sustained serum concentrations of progesterone.[49] The disadvantage of IM application of progesterone is that injection is painful and daily injections are required to sustain sufficient progesterone concentrations. Also swelling, redness and even sterile abscess formation are not uncommon side-effects.

Vaginal Progesterone

Progesterone plasma concentrations reach maximal levels approximately 3–8 hours after vaginal application and then fall continuously over the next 8 hours. Compared to IM progesterone, vaginal progesterone is faster cleared out of the circulation. To achieve luteal phase plasma levels, higher dosages of vaginal progesterone are needed and in most cases, 300–600 mg of progesterone is administered daily divided into 2 or 3 dosages,[50] depending on the formula, e.g. tablets, creams, suppositories. Vaginal mucosa absorbs proteins and lipids, however absorption is influenced by the kind of formula preparation and absorption is enhanced after previous estrogenization.[51]

After vaginal administration of progesterone, the serum levels are lower compared to IM application and sometimes even lower than measured in a natural cycle. However, despite the low serum levels, adequate secretory endometrial transformation was achieved. This suggests that vaginally administered progesterone exerts a direct local effect on the endometrium before entering the systemic circulation, the so called "first uterine pass" effect. The mechanism behind the "first uterine pass" effect is not fully understood and different ways of action are discussed: absorption of progesterone into the rich venous or lymphatic vaginal system and/or possibly counter current transfer between uterovaginal lymph vessels or veins and arteries, direct drug diffusion through the tissues or even due to intraluminal transfer from the uterus to the vagina similar to sperm transport. As the vaginal route is effective in providing sufficient luteal phase support and additional almost without any side-effects, it is a valuable and nowadays the preferred route of progesterone administration.[52]

Human Chorionic Gonadotropin for Luteal Phase Support

With the application of hCG, no luteolysis occurs as the corpora lutea will be stimulated and will sustain progesterone production. For a long time, the hCG-administration was the standard luteal phase support, however the disadvantage of this approach is the possible development of OHSS, especially in the good responder patients.[53]

Timing of Luteal Phase Support with Progesterone

Timing of luteal phase support in assisted reproductive technology (ART) cycles is crucial, as it has to be initiated before endogenous progesterone levels are decreasing or low. On the other hand, preovulatory exposure of the endometrium to progesterone may have a negative impact on the endometrial receptivity as already described.

When luteal phase support was started before oocyte retrieval, a decreased likelihood of pregnancy was found, when compared to start on the day of oocyte retrieval. When P was initiated on the evening of oocyte retrieval versus start on day 1–3 after oocyte retrieval, no difference in clinical PR was found. However, when progesterone administration was started on day 6, a decreased likelihood of pregnancy was found. Therefore, initiation of progesterone supplementation between the evening of oocyte retrieval and day 3 after retrieval seems to be ideal.[54]

Duration of Luteal Phase Support

In early pregnancy, the embryo is producing a significant and rapidly increasing amount of hCG which will replace a possible lack of endogenous LH after ovarian stimulation. Later on in the pregnancy, between 7 and 9 weeks, progesterone production will shift from the corpora lutea toward the placenta. Studies evaluating the duration of progesterone administration after a positive pregnancy test did not find any influence on the miscarriage rate and the delivery rate when progesterone application was continued or discontinued for 3 weeks after positive pregnancy test.[55,56]

Luteal Support after GnRH Trigger

Meanwhile the use of GnRH-agonist for final oocyte maturation is common in high responder patients as development of OHSS can almost completely be avoided. Following the introduction of GnRH-agonist for final oocyte maturation in GnRH-antagonist protocols, the first large randomized controlled trials reported a very poor reproductive outcome with the use of GnRH-agonist trigger in combination with a standard luteal phase support,[57] whereas administration of high doses of steroids[58] can counterbalance luteolysis.

In most patients, final oocyte maturation by GnRH-agonist causes severe luteolysis as a result of reduced pulsatile LH secretion due to supraphysiologic hormonal levels.[59,60] However, lately it was shown that the severity of luteolysis after GnRH agonist trigger is patient-specific and will not follow the same pattern. Longer stimulation duration as well as a higher level of progesterone on the day of final oocyte maturation and more retrieved oocytes will result in higher levels of progesterone in the early luteal phase. These findings point toward a sustained secretory capability of the corpora lutea even after GnRHa trigger.[61]

There is an ongoing debate on the adequate luteal phase support in this scenario. Luteolysis occurs when LH support from the primate corpus luteum is withdrawn for more than or equal to 3 days,[62] hence corpus luteum function can be rescued, if LH activity is reinitiated within 3 days, suggesting that corpus luteum viability can be preserved without LH support for atleast 72 hours.[63] In order to sustain progesterone production from the corpora lutea and therefore rescue the luteal phase different treatment options have been described.

Following the concept that GnRH-agonist-induced luteolysis can be reverted with the administration of hCG, low-doses of hCG can be given during luteal phase. However it was found, that the rescue of the corpora lutea for up to 3 days of gonadotropin deprivation is hCG dose dependent, i.e. more than or equal to 1,500 IU.[64] The approach of administration of 1,500 IU of hCG 35 hours after GnRH-agonist trigger result in comparable pregnancy rates in respect to hCG-trigger, but unfortunately with this dosage, OHSS in the high-responder group occurred.[65,66] Other authors[67] applied low-dose hCG in different dosages in the luteal phase after GnRH-agonist triggering and could demonstrate that those dosages were effective in normalizing the reproductive outcome. Despite the low dosages of hCG, OHSS could not be completely avoided.

A proof-of-concept study evaluated a luteal phase support by application of daily low hCG-dosages (125 IU rhCG) from the day of OPU without the use of exogenous progesterone. Significant differences during the luteal phase were observed with progesterone levels being significantly higher in the groups receiving daily low-dose hCG supplementation.[68] Hence even with this low hCG dosage, OHSS occurred in 3% of the patients, hence no hospitalization was needed.

Lately, the concept of "luteal coasting" has been introduced to reduce the risk of the development of OHSS due to hCG administration as luteal phase support in high responder patients with GnRH-agonist trigger.[69,70] This concept individualizes the luteal phase support after GnRH-agonist administration for final oocyte maturation by monitoring the progesterone concentrations closely and administering a rescue dosage of hCG, when progesterone concentrations drop significantly. It seems that in cases with a less severe luteolysis, a hCG-dosage below 1,500 IU is sufficient to maintain adequate progesterone-levels in early and mid-luteal phase and to allow implantation.[71] From day 7 of fertilization, the embryo will start producing hCG by itself[72] and from that point of time, endogenous produced hCG will cover the LH-deficit.

Ovarian hyperstimulation syndrome can be almost completely avoided by the use of GnRH-agonist (200 mg of GnRH-agonist nasal spray twice daily; a total of 400 mg/day) for luteal phase support after GnRH-agonist trigger without exogenous progesterone and mid-luteal progesterone levels of around 190 nmol/L (approximately 59.7 ng/mL) can be achieved.[73]

Luteal Phase Support in Insemination Cycles

Intrauterine insemination (IUI) is a frequently applied techniques to increase the probability of conception in couples with subfertility or unexplained infertility, however the necessity of luteal support is addressed only in a few studies.

Intrauterine insemination can be performed in either natural cycles or stimulated cycles by using clomifene citrate or gonadotropins for stimulation.

In natural IUI-cycles, it can be assumed, that no luteal phase in sufficiency should be present and therefore there is no biological or empirical evidence that treatment with hCG or progesterone in the luteal phase is necessary or improves the pregnancy rate.[74] Nevertheless the addition of progesterone, hCG and/or other substances became established clinical practice even in the absence of any robust evidence of effectiveness.[75]

In patients, who undergo mild ovarian stimulation for IUI, it can be assumed that due to supraphysiological hormonal levels, endogenous LH will below, leading possibly to a luteal phase in sufficiency. However, it is crucial to differentiate between the kind of stimulation done, as after clomifene citrate administration, an increase in LH pulse frequency will result in a significant increase of serum E2 and progesterone levels, with a lengthening of the luteal phase. A study, evaluating a beneficial impact of progesterone application in normo-ovulatory patients stimulated with clomifene citrate for IUI, did not find higher ongoing pregnancy rates in patients receiving progesterone after IUI compared to those, who had no luteal phase support.[76] However, as after gonadotropin-stimulation, comparable to ovarian stimulation for IVF, supraphysiological hormonal levels will lead to suppression of endogenous LH, development of luteal phase in sufficiency can be expected. It was shown that after IUI in a gonadotropin-stimulated cycle, the chance of pregnancy and livebirth is higher, when progesterone application is done after IUI.[77]

Luteal Phase Support in Frozen Embryo Transfer Cycles

Due to the improvement of the cryoconservation-techniques in the IVF-laboratory with the introduction of vitrification, worldwide more and more frozen embryo transfer (FET) or warmth oocyte embryo transfer cycles are performed.[78] The advantage of this technique is to improve the chance of a pregnancy in patients with surplus oocytes or embryos without performing a new ovarian stimulation cycle.

To optimize the pregnancy rates, synchronization of the embryo development and the endometrium is crucial. A simple way of endometrium preparation is the use of the natural cycle with endogenous production of estradiol of the growing follicle. However, in a natural cycle the LH-surge has to be detected in order to plan the correct timing for the embryo thawing and embryo transfer. A study, designed to compare the pregnancy rates between natural cycles and modified natural cycles with application of hCG to end the follicular phase showed significantly higher pregnancy rates in the natural cycle. However, for the natural cycle, patients were monitored closely by blood tests to detect ovulation and plan the thawing and transfer of the embryo(s) accordingly. To define ovulation, LH surge was deemed to have begun when the concentration rose by 180% above the latest serum value available in that patient and continued to rise thereafter. Day 1 after the LH rise, a drop of E2 and concomitant rise of P more than 1.5 nmol/L confirmed the ovulation.[79] Unfortunately, detection of LH-surge with tests performed in the urine is too unreliable to be used for accurate planning of frozen embryo transfer.

In modified natural cycle for FET, hCG is administered to induce ovulation and luteinization. However, it seems that hCG-administration to end the follicular phase results in significant lower pregnancy rates compared to natural cycles with the detection of LH-surge. It is assumed, that hCG may have a negative effect on endometrium receptivity.[79,80]

A more common approach is the use of a hormonal-replacement cycle with the administration of exogenous estradiol and progesterone, as the advantages of this approach are that disturbances due to cycle-variation can be avoided and also planning of the embryo transfer is possible, which will smoothen the workflow for the IVF-laboratory. Hormonal replacement cycle can be performed with or without cotreatment with GnRH-agonists.

Until now, the best approach for FET is still under discussion and there is an urgent need for randomized controlled trials to compare the correctly conducted natural cycle with correct determination of LH-surge and the hormonal replacement cycle.

CONCLUSION

Estradiol and progesterone are essential for human production. Whereas in a natural cycle, progesterone is produced by the corpus luteum, luteal phase of ovarian stimulation cycles for IVF/ICSI are mostly characterized by severe luteal phase in sufficiency. Multifollicular follicle growth leads to unphysiological high hormonal levels, which inhibit LH secretion from the pituitary via negative feedback actions at the level of the hypothalamic-pituitary axis.

To counterbalance the luteal phase insufficiency after ovarian stimulation luteal phase support has to be applied, either by direct substitution of progesterone or indirect via the stimulation of the remaining corpora lutea to sustain progesterone production. Progesterone can be applied orally, as IM injection or vaginally. The latter one is nowadays the preferred route of progesterone administration. The hCG-administration has the disadvantage of a possible development of ovarian hyperstimulation syndrome, especially in a good responder patient. Luteal phase support should be initiated within 1–3 days after oocyte retrieval procedure and is not required any more after the progesterone production shifted to the placenta between 7 and 9 weeks of gestation. In case of final oocyte maturation with GnRH-agonist in a GnRH-antagonist protocol, the optimal luteal phase support is still under discussion.

REFERENCES

1. Bulletti C, de Ziegler D. Uterine contractility and embryo implantation. Curr Opin Obstet Gynecol. 2005;17:265-76.
2. Csapo AI, Pulkkinen MO, Ruttner B, et al. The significance of the human corpus luteum in pregnancy maintenance. I. Preliminary studies. Am J Obstet Gynecol. 1972;112:1061-7.
3. Simon C, Martın JC, Pellicer A. Paracrine regulators of implantation. Baillieres Best Pract Res Clin Obstet Gynaecol. 2000;14:815-26.
4. Bergh PA, Navot D. The impact of embryonic development and endometrial maturity on the timing of implantation. Fertil Steril. 1992;58:537-42.
5. Ruiz-Alonso M, Galindo N, Pellicer A, et al. What a difference two days make: "personalized" embryo transfer (pET) paradigm: a case report and pilot study. Hum Reprod. 2014;29:1244-7.
6. Devroey P, Pados G. Preparation of endometrium for egg donation. Hum Reprod Update.1998;4:856-61.
7. Christenson LK, Devoto L. Cholesterol transport and steroidogenesis by the corpusluteum. Reprod Biol Endocrinol. 2003;1:90.
8. Devoto L, Fuentes A, Kohen P, et al. The human corpus luteum: life cycle and function in natural cycles. Fertil Steril. 2009;92:1067-79.
9. Chaffin CL, Dissen GA, Stouffer RL. Hormonal regulation of steroidogenic enzyme expression in granulosa cells during the peri-ovulatory interval in monkeys. Mol Hum Reprod. 2000;6:11-8.
10. Yding Andersen C, Bungum L, Nyboe Andersen A, et al. Preovulatory progesterone concentration associates significantly to follicle number and LH concentration but not to pregnancy rate. Reprod Biomed Online. 2011;23:187-95.
11. Fleming R, Jenkins J. The source and implications of progesterone rise during the follicular phase of assisted reproduction cycles. Reprod Biomed Online. 2010;21:446-9.
12. Kyrou D, Al-Azemi M, Papanikolaou EG, et al. The relationship of premature progesterone rise with serum estradiol levels and number of follicles in GnRH antagonist/recombinant FSH-stimulated cycles. Eur J Obstet Gynecol Reprod Biol. 2012;162:165-8.
13. Stocco C, Tellerıa C, Gibori G. The molecular control of corpus luteum formation, function and regression. Endocr Rev. 2007;28:117-49.
14. Chen J, Oiu O, Lohstroh PN, et al. Hormonal characteristics in the early luteal phase of conceptive and nonconceptive menstrual cycles. J Soc Gynecol Investig. 2003;10:27-31.
15. Kastner P, Krust A, Turcotte B, et al. Two distinct estrogen-regulated promoters generate transcripts encoding the two functionally different human progesterone receptor forms A and B. EMBOJ. 1990;9:1603-14.
16. Wei LL, Gonzalez-Aller C, Wood WM, et al. 5'-Heterogeneity in human progesterone receptor transcripts predicts a new amino-terminal truncated. "C"-receptor and unique A-receptor messages. Molecular Endocrinol. 1990;4:1833-40.
17. Salmi A, Pakarinen P, Peltola AM, et al. The effect of intrauterine levonorgestrel use on the expression of c-JUN, oestrogen receptors, progesterone receptors and Ki-67 in human endometrium. Mol Hum Reprod. 1998;4:1110-5.
18. Tseng L, Zhu HH. Regulation of progesterone receptor messenger ribonucleic acid by progestin in human endometrial stromal cells. Biol Reprod. 1997;57:1360-6.
19. Noyes RW, Hertig AT, Rock J. Dating the endometrial biopsy. Fertil Steril. 1950;1:3-25.
20. Noyes RW, Hertig AT, Rock J. Dating the endometrial biopsy. Am J Obstet Gynecol. 1975;122:262-3.
21. Wentz AC. Endometrial biopsy in the evaluation of infertility. Fertil Steril. 1980;33:121-4.
22. Bourgain C, Ubaldi F, Tavaniotou A, et al. Endometrial hormone receptors and proliferation index in the periovulatory phase of stimulated embryo transfer cycles in comparison with natural cycles and relation to clinical pregnancy outcome. Fertil Steril. 2002;78:237-44.
23. Ubaldi F, Bourgain C, Tournaye H, et al. Endometrial evaluation by aspiration biopsy on the day of oocyte retrieval in the embryo transfer cycles in patients with serum progesterone rise during the follicular phase. Fertil Steril. 1997;67:521-6.
24. Van Vaerenbergh I, Fatemi HM, Blockeel C, et al. Progesterone rise on hCG day in GnRH antagonist/rFSH stimulated cycles affects endometrial gene expression. Reprod Biomed Online. 2011;22:263-71.
25. Bosch E, Valencia I, Escudero E, et al. Premature luteinization during gonad-otropin-releasing hormone antagonist cycles and its relationship with in vitro fertilization outcome. Fertil Steril. 2003;80:1444-9.
26. Labarta E, Martínez-Conejero JA, Alamá P, et al. Endometrial receptivity is affected in women with high circulating progesterone levels at the end of the follicular phase: a functional genomics analysis. Hum Reprod. 2011;26:1813-25.
27. Kolibianakis EM, Devroey P. The luteal phase after ovarian stimulation. Reprod Biomed Online. 2002a;5:26-35.

28. Papanikolaou EG, Kolibianakis EM, Pozzobon C, et al. Progesterone rise on the day of human chorionic gonadotropin administration impairs pregnancy outcome in day 3 single-embryo transfer, while has no effect on day 5 single blastocyst transfer. Fertil Steril. 2009;91:949-52.
29. Damewood MD, Shen W, Zacur HA, et al. Disappearance of exogenously administered human chorionic gonadotropin. Fertil Steril.1989;52:398-400.
30. Yen SS, Llerena O, Little B, et al. Disappearance rates of endogenous luteinizing hormone and chorionic gonadotropin in man. J Clin Endocrinol Metab. 1968;28:1763-7.
31. Fatemi HM, Polyzos NP, van Vaerenbergh I, et al. Early luteal phase endo-crine profile is affected by the mode of triggering final oocyte maturation and the luteal phase support used in recombinant follicle-stimulating hormone–gonadotropin-releasing hormone antagonist in vitro fertilization cycles. Fertil Steril. 2013;100:742-7.
32. Jones GES. Some new aspects of management of infertility. JAMA. 1979;141:1123.
33. Jordan J, Craig K, Clifton DK, et al. Luteal phase defect: the sensitivity and specificity of diagnostic methods in common clinical use. Fertil Steril. 1994;62:54-62.
34. Rosenberg SM, Luciano AA, Riddick DH. The luteal phase defect: the relative frequency of, and encouraging response to, treatment with vaginal proges- terone. Fertil Steril. 1980;34:17-20.
35. Practice Committee of the American Society for Reproductive Medicine. Current clinical irrelevance of luteal phase deficiency: a committee opinion. Fertil Steril. 2015;103:e27-32.
36. Csapo AI, Pulkkinen M. Indispensability of the human corpus luteum in the maintenance of early pregnancy. Luteectomy evidence. Obstet Gynecol Surv. 1978;33:69-81.
37. Liu HC, Pyrgiotis E, Davis O, et al. Active corpus luteum function at pre-, peri- and postimplantation is essential for a viable pregnancy. Early Pregnancy. 1995;1:281-7.
38. Macklon NS, Fauser BC. Impact of ovarian hyperstimulation on the luteal phase. J Reprod Fertil. 2000;55:101-8.
39. Fatemi HM, Popovic-Todorovic B, Papanikolaou E, et al. An update of luteal phase support instimulated IVF cycles. Hum Reprod Update. 2007;13:581-90.
40. Beckers NG, Macklon NS, Eijkemans MJ, et al. Nonsupplemented luteal phase characteristics after the administration of recombinant human chorionic gonadotropin, recombinant luteinizing hormone, orgonadotropin-releasing hormone (GnRH) agonist to induce final oocyte maturation in in vitro fertilization patients after ovarian stimulation with recombinant follicle-stimulating hormone and GnRH antagonist cotreatment. J Clin Endocrinol Metab. 2003;88:4186-92.
41. Fatemi HM. The luteal phase after 3 decades of IVF: what do we know? Reprod Biomed Online. 2009;19:4331.
42. Fauser BC, Devroey P. Reproductive biology and IVF: ovarian stimulation and luteal phase consequences. Trend sEndocrinol Metab. 2003;14:236-42.
43. Tavaniotou A, Devroey P. Effect of human chorionic gonadotropin on luteal luteinizing hormone concentrations in natural cycles. Fertil Steril. 2003;80:654-5.
44. Tavaniotou A, Albano C, Smitz J, et al. Comparison of LH concentrations in the early and mid-luteal phase in IVF cycles after treatment with HMG alone or in association with the GnRH antagonist Cetrorelix. Hum Reprod. 2001;16:663-7.
45. Bourgain C, Devroey P. The endometrium in stimulated cycles for IVF. Hum Reprod Update. 2003;9:515-22.
46. Hirvonen E, Mälkönen M, Manninen V. Effects of different progestogens on lipoproteins during postmenopausal replacement therapy. N Engl J Med. 1981;304:560-3.
47. Dennerstein L, Burrows GD, Hyman GJ, et al. Hormone therapy and affect. Maturitas. 1979;1:247-59.
48. Norman TR, Morse CA, Dennerstein L. Comparative bioavailability of orally and vaginally administered progesterone. Fertil Steril. 1991;56:1034-9.
49. Nillius SJ, Johansson, ED. Plasma levels of progesterone after vaginal, rectal, orintra-muscular administration of progesterone. Am J Obstet Gynecol. 1971;110:470-7.
50. Devroey P, Palermo G, Bourgain C, et al. Progesterone administration in patients with absent ovaries. Int J Fertil. 1989;34:188-93.
51. Villanueva B, Casper RF, Yen SS. Intravaginal administration of progesterone: enhanced absorption after estrogen treatment. Fertil Steril. 1981;35:433-7.
52. Tavaniotou A, Smitz J, Bourgain C, et al. Comparison between different routes of progesterone administration as luteal phase support in infertility treatments. Hum Reprod Update. 2000;6:139-48.
53. Ludwig M, Diedrich K. Evaluation of an optimal luteal phase support protocol in IVF. Acta Obstet Gynecol Scand. 2001;80:452-66.
54. Connell MT, Szatkowski JM, Terry N, et al. Timing luteal support in assisted reproductive technology: a systematic review. Fertil Steril. 2015;103:939-46.
55. Nyboe AA, Popovic-Todorovic B, Schmidt KT, et al. Progesterone supplementation during early gestations after IVF or ICSI has no effect on the delivery rates: arandomized controlled trial. Hum Reprod. 2002;17:357-61.
56. Schmidt KL, Ziebe S, Popovic B, et al. Progesterone supplementation during early gestation after in vitro fertilization has no effect on the delivery rate. Fertil Steril. 2001;75:337-41.
57. Humaidan P, Bredkjaer HE, Bungum L, et al. GnRH agonist (buserelin) or hCG for ovulation induction in GnRH antagonist IVF/ICSI cycles: a prospective randomized study. Hum Reprod. 2005;20:1213-20.
58. Engmann L, Benadiva C. Agonist trigger: what is the best approach? Agonist trigger with aggressive luteal support. Fertil Steril. 2012;97:531-3.
59. Fatemi HM, Polyzos NP, van Vaerenbergh I, et al. Early luteal phase endocrine profile is affected by the mode of triggering final oocyte maturation and the luteal phase support used in recombinant follicle-stimulating hormone–gonadotropin-releasing hormone antagonist in vitro fertilization cycles. Fertil Steril. 2013;100:742–747.
60. Tannus S, Burke Y, McCartney CR, et al. GnRH-agonist triggering for final oocyte maturation in GnRH-antagonist IVF cycles induces decreased LH pulse rate and amplitude in early luteal phase: a possible luteolysis mechanism. Gynecol Endocrinol. 2017;33(9):741-745.
61. Lawrenz B, Garrido N, Samir S, et al. Individual luteolysis pattern after GnRH-agonist trigger for final oocyte maturation. PLoS One. 2017;12(5):e0176600.

62. Hutchison JS, Zeleznik AJ. The rhesus monkey corpus luteum is dependent on pituitary gonadotropin secretion throughout the luteal phase of the menstrual cycle. Endocrinology. 1984;115;1780-6.
63. Hutchison JS, Zeleznik AJ. The corpus luteum of the primate menstrual cycle is capable of recovering from a transient withdrawal of pituitary gonadotropin support. Endocrinology.1985;117:1043-9.
64. Dubourdieu S, Charbonne lB, Massai MR, et al. Suppression of corpus luteum function by the gonadotropin-releasing hormone antagonist Nal-Glu: effect of the dose and timing of human chorionic gonadotropin administration. Fertil Steril. 1991;56:440-512.
65. Humaidan P. Luteal phase rescue in high-risk OHSS patients by GnRHa trig- gering in combination with low-dose HCG: a pilot study. Reprod Biomed Online. 2009;18:630-4.
66. Seyhan A, Ata B, Polat M, et al. Severe early ovarian hyperstimulation syndrome following GnRH-agonist trigger with the addition of 1500 IU hCG. Hum Reprod. 2013;28:2522-8.
67. Castillo JC, Dolz M, Bienvenido E, et al. Cycles triggered with GnRH-agonist: exploring low-dose HCG for luteal support. Reprod Biomed Online. 2010;20:175-81.
68. Andersen CY, Elbaek HO, Alsbjerg B, et al. Daily low-dose hCG stimulation during the luteal phase combined with GnRH a triggered IVF cycles without exogenous progesterone: a proof of concept trial. Hum Reprod. 2015;30:2387-95.
69. Lawrenz B, Humaidan P, Fatemi HM. GnRHa trigger and luteal coasting - A new approach for the OHSS high-risk patient? Repro Biomed Online. 2018;36(1):75-7.
70. Kol S, Breyzman T, Segal L, et al. Luteal coasting after GnRH-agonist trigger - individualized, HCG-based, progesterone-free luteal support in high responders': a case series. Reprod Biomed. Online. 2015;31(6),747-51.
71. Lawrenz B, Samir S, Fatemi HM, et al. Luteal coasting and individualization of human chorionic gonadotropin dose after gonadotropin-releasing hormone agonist triggering for final oocyte maturation-a retrospective proof-of-concept study. Front Endocrinol (Lausanne). 2018;15;9:33
72. Fishel SB, Edwards RG, Evans CJ. Human chorionic gonadotropin secreted by preimplantation embryos cultured in vitro. Science. 1984;11:816-8.
73. Bar-Hava I, Mizrachi Y, Karfunkel-Doron D, et al. Intranasal gonadotropin-releasing hormone agonist (GnRHa) for luteal-phase support following GnRHa triggering, an ovel approach to avoid ovarian hyperstimulation syndrome in high responders. Fertil Steril. 2016;106:330-3.
74. Ragni G, Vegetti W, Baroni E, et al. Comparison ofluteal phase profile in gonadotrophin stimulated cycles with or without a gonadotrophin-releasing hormone antagonist. Hum Reprod. 2001;16:2258-62.
75. ESHRE Capri Workshop Group. Intrauterine Insemination. Hum Reprod Update. 2009;15:265-77.
76. Kyrou D, Fatemi HM, Tournaye H, et al. Luteal phase support in normo-ovulatory women stimulated with clomiphene citrate for intrauterine insemination: need or habit? Hum Reprod. 2010;25:2501-6.
77. Oktem M, Altinkaya SO, Yilmaz SA, et al. Effect of luteal phase support after ovulation induction and intrauterine insemination. Gynecol Endocrinol. 2014;30:909-12.
78. LeLannou D, Griveau JF, Laurent MC, et al. Contribution of embryocryo preservation to elective single embryotransfer in IVF-ICSI. Reprod Biomed Online. 2006;13:368-75.
79. Fatemi HM, Kyrou D, Bourgain C, et al. Cryopreserved-thawed human embryotransfer: spontaneous natural cycle is superior to human chorionic gonadotropin-induced natural cycle. Fertil Steril. 2010;94:2054-8.
80. Montagut M, Santos-Ribeiro S, De Vos M, et al. Frozen-thawed embryo transfers in natural cycles with spontaneous or induced ovulation: the search for the best protocol continues. Hum Reprod. 2016;31:2803-10.

CHAPTER

49

Role of Luteinizing Hormone in Controlled Ovarian Stimulation

Carlo Alviggi, Alessandro Conforti, Giuseppe De Placido, Sandro C Esteves

INTRODUCTION

Physiologically, a fine interplay between follicle-stimulating hormone (FSH) and luteinizing hormone (LH) promotes follicle growth and maturation. According to the "two cells, two gonadotropin theory" FSH and LH regulate two distinct compartments. While FSH modulates proliferation of granulosa cells, LH exerts its activity in theca cells stimulating the androgen synthesis pathway. Nonetheless, evidence indicates that granulosa cells express LH receptors in late follicular phase, thus suggesting that LH has a role in the final steps of follicle maturation.[1] Despite its pivotal role in follicular growth on natural cycles, the effect of LH in stimulated cycle is more equivocal. It has been demonstrated that LH supplementation is not necessary during controlled ovarian stimulation (COS) for all in vitro fertilization (IVF) women.[2,3] For example, the addition of LH to COS does not seem to offer any benefit to young normogonadotropic women with an adequate ovarian response, irrespective of the type of gonadotropin-releasing hormone (GnRH) analog used. On the other hand, emerging data indicates that selected patients might benefit from exogenous LH supplementation.[4]

The purposes of this chapter are: (1) to illustrate the molecular and biologic action of LH, (2) to describe the gonadotropin preparations containing LH activity, and (3) to present the clinical evidence with regards the use of LH supplementation to selected patients undergoing COS.

STRUCTURE AND FUNCTION OF LUTEINIZING HORMONE

Luteinizing hormone is a pituitary glycoprotein hormone which together with FSH regulates gonadal function. LH is synthesized and secreted by gonadotrophs cells localized in the lateral portion of pituitary gland under stimulation of GnRH.[5] Through a calcium-dependent mechanism, GnRH stimulates LH and FSH synthesis using inositol 1,4,5 triphosphate and 1,2 diacylglycerol as second messengers. The LH molecule comprises two noncovalently linked protein subunits, alpha and beta maintained by internal disulfide bonds with molecular weights of approximately 30,000 Da.[6] The alpha subunit contains 92 amino acids (AA) and is identical in all glycoprotein hormones [LH, FSH, human chorionic gonadotropin (hCG), and thyroid-stimulating hormone (TSH)]. The alpha subunit is encoded by a single gene located on chromosome 6 (6q12-q21).[7] The beta subunit confers a unique receptor specificity as well as differential biological and immunological properties (Figs. 1A and B).[8] The LH beta subunit gene is located on chromosome 19 (19q13.32). Glycosylation, which is achieved by the attachment of carbohydrate moieties forming heterodimers, is fundamental for the differential spectrum of charges, bioactivities and half-lives of LH.[8,9] Moreover, the biological activity of LH is influenced by the addition of a sialic acid (sialylation) or sulfonic group (sulfonation) to the carbohydrate moieties.[8,10] The LH beta subunit has a single site of glycosylation (Asn 30) and few sialic acid residues (only 1 or 2) (Fig. 2). Native LH has a short half-life of only 20–30 minutes.[9,11] Pulsatile secretion of LH during the menstrual cycle varies: frequency is higher whereas amplitude is lower during follicular phase than the luteal phase. Moreover, LH bioactivity markedly differs: alkaline LH products with higher in vitro biological or immunological ratios are predominant in young women whereas long-lived acidic isoforms are found during menopause.[12,13]

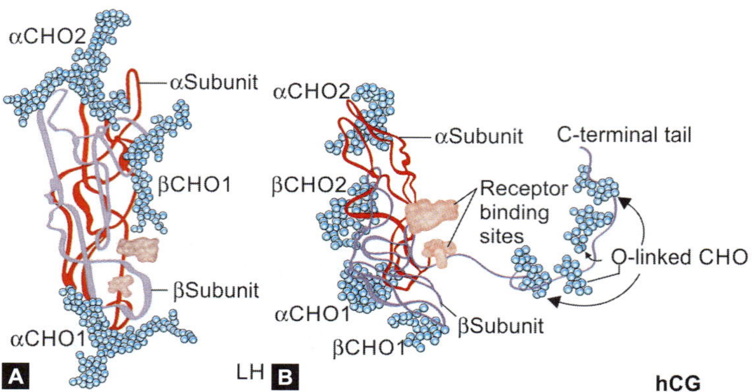

Figs. 1A and B: Luteinizing hormone and human chorionic gonadotropin molecules. (A) LH is a glycoprotein with two subunits, the alpha subunit (red), similar to that of FSH and hCG with two carbohydrate attachment sites, and the beta subunit (blue), with only one carbohydrate attachment site. The light purple balls represent the carbohydrate chains. (B) hCG is similar in its structural attributes to LH. A notable exception is the presence of a long carboxy-terminal segment that is O-glycosylated (O-linked CHO), conferring longer half-life to hCG. The alpha and beta subunits are represented in red and blue strands, respectively, whereas the light purple balls represent the carbohydrate chains. (FSH: Follicle-stimulating hormone; hCG: Human chorionic gonadotropin; LH: Luteinizing hormone)
Source: Leao Rde B, Esteves SC. Gonadotropin therapy in assisted reproduction: an evolutionary perspective from biologics to biotech. Clinics (Sao Paulo). 2014;69:279-93.

This phenomenon is due to physiologic fluctuations in isoform profile during the menstrual cycle. Indeed, the degree of sialylation and sulfation affects LH half-life and determines in vivo and in vitro biopotency. More basic LH isoforms are observed at midcycle due to decreased sulfonation and increased sialylation. These changes increase LH half-life, thus explaining the increased levels of serum LH at this period. This shift in isoform profile seems to be physiologically important for ovulation triggering.[14]

Luteinizing hormone binds to specific G protein-coupled receptors (GPCRs) characterized by seven transmembrane domains and a large N-terminal extracellular region (Fig. 3).[15] As a distinctive feature of this glycoprotein hormone receptor, receptor activation requires that the hormone binds to the extracellular domain at the N-terminal region. Like FSH and TSH receptors, the LH receptor belongs to a large group of GPCRs. Whereas a single ligand activates FSH and TSH receptors, the LH receptor has both LH and hCG as its ligands.

The LH signaling pathway involves stimulation of adenylyl cyclase via G-protein receptor coupling, resulting in elevation of intracellular cAMP levels.[15] Furthermore, other second messengers are involved such as inositol triphosphate, calcium and mitogen-activated protein kinases.[16] LH receptors are expressed in both granulosa and theca cells. In the former, they reach their maximum concentration in preovulatory follicles. Antral follicles express these receptors at approximately 10% of the maximum.[17] Interestingly, recent data indicate that in granulosa cells, LH and FSH receptors can constitute functional heterodimer. This heterodimer could have specific functional characteristics, which differ from those of each homodimer.[15]

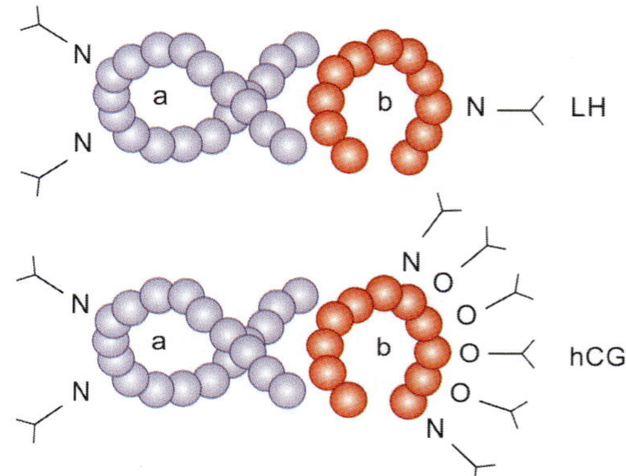

Fig. 2: Glycosylation patterns of LH and hCG. The alpha subunits of each hormone are identical in amino acid sequence and contain two sites of N-linked glycosylation. The beta subunit confers hormone specificity and contains variable amounts of N-linked glycosylation. LH beta subunit contains a single site of N-linked glycosylation, while hCG beta subunit contains two sites of N-linked glycosylation. Also, hCG has an extended C-terminal that includes four sites of O-linked glycosylation. (LH: Luteinizing hormone; hCG: Human chorionic gonadotropin)
Source: Leao Rde B, Esteves SC. Gonadotropin therapy in assisted reproduction: an evolutionary perspective from biologics to biotech. Clinics (Sao Paulo). 2014;69:279-93.

Metabolic and Physiological Function of Luteinizing Hormone

Luteinizing hormone is the central regulator of steroidogenesis in theca cells. The starting point of steroid

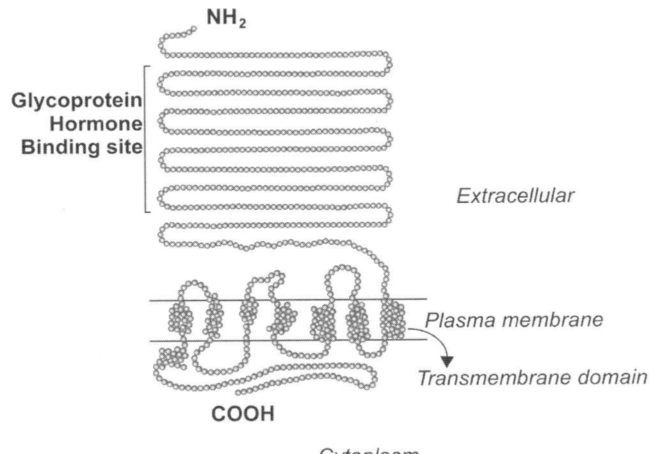

Fig. 3: The LH/hCG receptor. LH receptors are included in the subgroup of G-protein coupled receptors. Such receptors are characterized by having seven-transmembrane domains and a large N-terminal extracellular region, which is the predominant site of hormone binding.

biosynthesis is cholesterol, a carbon 27 (C27) steroid. Cholesterol is converted to pregnenolone (C21) by P450scc (CYP11A—cytochrome P450, family 11, subfamily A, polypeptide 1), whose regulation is mediated by steroidogenic acute regulatory protein (StAR).[10,18,19]

Pregnenolone metabolism is characterized by two routes. In the primary route (delta-5 pathway), pregnenolone is hydroxylated at the C17a and subsequently deacetalized to the androgen precursor dehydroepiandrosterone (DHEA). This action is mediated by CYP17 which has both hydroxylase and lyase activity. Lastly, DHEA is converted to androstenedione by 3 beta-hydroxysteroid dehydrogenase (3β-HSD).[19,20] In the secondary route of metabolism (delta-4 pathway), pregnenolone is converted to progesterone by the action of 3β-HSD. Progesterone is then converted to 17-hydroxyprogesterone by CYP17.[20] CYP17 is located exclusively in thecal and interstitial cells, whereas CYP19 (aromatase), which converts androgens to estrogens, is expressed only in granulosa cells.[20,21] Thus, aromatization of androgens to estrogens is carried out only granulosa cells induced by FSH receptor activation of the P450 aromatase *(P450arom)* gene. Androgens produced in the theca layer must diffuse into the granulosa layer to be converted to estrogens.

Theca and granulosa cells also secrete peptides that act as both autocrine and paracrine factors. Among these, insulin-like growth factor (IGF-I) and IGF-II, which are expressed in both granulosa and theca cells throughout folliculogenesis, are important in promoting follicular maturation.[22,23] IGFs enhance LH-mediated androgen production within the thecal compartment and FSH-mediated aromatization in granulosa cells.[24] Inhibin and activin are also two important modulators of steroidogenesis and follicle development. While inhibin stimulates androgen synthesis, activin has an opposite effect and sustains FSH action by increasing the expression of FSH receptors.[24]

Luteinizing hormone also acts in granulosa cells to stimulate progesterone production. Indeed, approximately 95% of progesterone is produced by the granulosa cells via the action of 3β-HSD that catalyzes the conversion of pregnenolone (delta-4 pathway); this pathway is under the influence of LH stimulation.[19,21,25] Peripheral concentrations of progesterone is limited by active liver metabolism. Progesterone can be further converted to 17-hydroxyprogesterone by CYP17 (delta-4 pathway). However, 17-hydroxyprogesterone is essentially the final product of delta-4 pathway in humans. The preovulatory rise in progesterone induces the positive feedback action of estrogen which in turn is the key factor to promote the midcycle LH peak in the natural cycle. Finally, progesterone also fosters a midcycle FSH surge, critical for supporting LH receptors expression in the granulosa layer.[26,27]

Role of Luteinizing Hormone during Folliculogenesis and Luteal Phase Support

During folliculogenesis LH plays two essential functions. The first, as explained in the previous session, consists in androgen production in the theca compartment. The second starts in the intermediate to late follicular phase[28,29] in which FSH induces LH receptor expression in the granulosa cells of developing follicles.[30] Progressively, the maturing follicle reduces its dependency on FSH by acquiring LH receptors and LH responsiveness.[31,32] FSH and LH cooperate in inducing the local production of various molecules necessary for follicular growth, including IGF-I, important for promoting follicular maturation,[23] and fibroblast growth factors which maintain calcium homeostasis and granulosa cell viability.[33] Additional growth modulators include endothelial-like growth factors (EGFs) that are also involved in granulosa cells proliferation, differentiation, and corpus luteum survival.[34,35] Finally, LH contributes to deselection of nondominant follicles. In fact, the developing follicles have specific LH requirements beyond which the maturation process is ceased.[1] In other words, each follicle has an established LH ceiling to continue the maturation process. LH ceiling may be higher in larger follicles and lower in those destined to atresia. Consequently, the increasing LH concentrations during folliculogenesis sustain progression of the leading follicles and favor degeneration of secondary follicles.[4] Notwithstanding, some investigators advocate that

Table 1: Differences in luteinizing hormone (LH) activity among gonadotropin

	Purity (LH content)	*FSH activity (IU/vial)*	*LH activity (IU/vial)*	*hCG content (IU/vial)*	*Specific activity (LH/mg protein)*
Lutropin alfa	> 99%	0	75	–	22,000
Follitropin alfa + lutropin alfa 2:1 ratio	> 99%	150	75	–	22,000
HP-hMG	Unknown*	75	75*	~8	–

(FSH: Follicle-stimulating hormone; hCG: Human chorionic gonadotropin; HP-hMG: Highly purified human menopausal gonadotropin).
1 µg of lutropin alfa = 22 IU
*Derives primarily from the hCG component, which preferentially is concentrated during the purification process and sometimes was added to achieve the desired amount of LH-like biological activity.

LH receptor expression governs the selection of dominant follicles; in other words, because small follicles do not express LH receptors, LH may indirectly promote their degeneration.[29,36]

During the luteal phase, LH sustains steroidogenic activity and corpus luteum.[37] LH induces the upregulation of growth factors, like vascular EGF-A,[37,38] which are implicated in luteal angiogenesis, and epidermal growth factor-like ligands (amphiregulin and epiregulin), which modulate apoptosis in luteinized human granulosa cells and sustains corpus luteum survival.[35] Furthermore, LH stimulates expression of cytokines involved in implantation[39] and seems to affect endometrial receptivity independently of ovarian functions.[40]

In conclusion, LH has a pivotal role in follicular development and maturation and is critical for maintaining corpus luteum function during the luteal phase.

GONADOTROPIN PREPARATIONS CONTAINING LUTEINIZING HORMONE ACTIVITY

Currently, there are three commercially available gonadotropin preparations containing LH activity: (1) conventional and highly purified human menopausal gonadotropin (hMG), in which LH activity is dependent on hCG rather than LH, (2) pure recombinant LH glycoprotein (lutropin alfa) and (3) a combination of recombinant FSH and LH in a fixed ratio of 2:1 also manufactured by recombinant technology (Table 1).

Menotropin

Human menopausal gonadotropin is obtained from the urine of postmenopausal women.[41,42] In the beginning, the preparations contained varying amounts of FSH, LH, and hCG, and only 5% of pure forms.[41,42] Improvements in the purification techniques standardized FSH and LH activities to 75 IU for each type of gonadotropin.

Luteinizing hormone activity in this preparation is primarily derived from hCG.[41,43] Sometimes hCG is added to achieve the desired amount of LH-like biological activity.[41]

At present, both conventional hMG and highly purified hMG (HP-hMG) are commercially available in vials containing FSH and LH at 1:1 ratio.[10] The enhanced purity of HP-hMG enabled subcutaneous delivery.[10]

Lutropin Alfa

Recombinant LH glycoprotein (lutropin alfa) was introduced in 2000. The manufacturing process of lutropin alfa involves recombinant technology in which the genes coding for human LH alpha and beta subunits are incorporated into the nuclear DNA of hamster ovary cells via a plasmid vector.[10]

Lutropin alfa is highly pure and has high biological activity (Table 1). It is presented in vials of 82.5 IU lyophilized pure glycoprotein powder to be reconstituted with a diluent before administration using a conventional syringe and needle (75 IU of lutropin alfa is delivered per vial). Lutropin alfa is intended for daily subcutaneous self-injections with good tolerability regarding pain at injection site. Due to the relatively short half-life (about one day), daily doses of lutropin alfa are needed during the stimulation period.[10,44]

Follitropin Alfa in Combination with Lutropin Alfa

A preparation containing both recombinant human follicle-stimulating hormone (r-hFSH) (follitropin alfa) and recombinant human luteinizing hormone (r-hLH) (lutropin alfa) at 2:1 ratio was introduced about 10 years ago.[45] The 2:1 ratio of FSH and LH in a fixed dose combination was obtained by recombinant technology and vial filling using protein mass (FbM). It is intended for daily subcutaneous injections and is presented in vials of lyophilized pure glycoprotein powder to be reconstituted with a diluent before administration using a conventional syringe and needle (150 IU of follitropin alfa and 75 IU of lutropin alfa is delivered per vial). This fixed 2:1 combination was demonstrated to be bioequivalent to r-hFSH and r-hLH administered separately, thus allowing the administration of both recombinant gonadotropins in a single injection.[46]

LUTEINIZING HORMONE SUPPLEMENTATION IN CLINICAL PRACTICE

On the one hand, fair evidence indicates that most normogonadotropic women do not need LH supplementation.[3,47] Indeed, residual circulating levels of endogenous LH after pituitary suppression are usually adequate to support multiple follicular growth in stimulated cycles.[48,49] It has been estimated that a minimum amount of LH is necessary to guarantee optimal follicle development during COS as only 1% of LH receptors need to be occupied to drive adequate ovarian steroidogenesis. According to some authors, the "LH window" for optimal androgen production of follicle maturation resides between 1.1 and 5.1 IU/L.[50,51]

On the other hand, there are distinct subgroups of women in which endogenous levels of LH are suboptimal during COS. For instance, patients with hypogonadotropic hypogonadism are not able to sustain adequate steroidogenesis by stimulation with FSH alone but resume sufficient estradiol production when LH is added.[50]

Moreover, response to FSH only-containing gonadotropins has shown to be suboptimal in normogonadotropic women with the following characteristics: (i) advanced reproductive age (≥ 35 years old),[52] (ii) poor ovarian reserve,[2,53] and (iii) highly suppressed levels of endogenous LH during COS.[54,55] Furthermore, normogonadotropic patients who require a high amount of FSH or show a steady response during COS, so-called "hypo-responders", seemed to benefit from LH supplementation.[56,57]

The possible clinical role of LH supplementation in the subgroups mentioned above could be explained by several factors, including reduced paracrine ovarian activity,[58] genetically-determined reduced LH bioactivity,[59] reduced androgen secretory capacity,[60] and decreased number of functional LH receptors.[61]

Furthermore, LH has also a direct effect on follicle growth and maturation, as already discussed, via different signaling pathways that positively impact oocyte quality.[62] Finally, recent data seemed to support the addition of LH for the prevention of ovarian hyperstimulation syndrome (OHSS),[63] as will be discussed later.

Hypogonadotropic Hypogonadism

The European Recombinant Human LH Study Group investigated the efficacy of recombinant LH in hypogonadotropic hypogonadal (WHO group I anovulation—LH levels of <1.2 IU/L; WHO group I anovulation).[50] Thirty-eight patients were randomized to receive 0, 25, 75, or 225 IU/day of r-hLH in addition to a fixed dose of r-hFSH (150 IU/day). In this study, r-hLH was able to promote a dose-related increase in estradiol and androstenedione. Furthermore, an increased ovarian sensitivity to FSH was observed in women who receive r-hLH. In detail, the proportion of women who developed follicles substantially increased according to the varying doses of r-hLH (42.8% in 25 IU, 77.8% and 80% in 75 IU and 225 IU, respectively).

A daily dose of 75 IU r-hLH was effective in the majority of women in promoting follicular development and endometrial growth.

The use of recombinant LH instead of HP-hMG seems to be the preferable option. In a recent randomized control trial, the efficacy of r-hFSH plus r-hLH in a 2:1 ratio was compared with HP-hMG urinary extract, in women with hypogonadotropic hypogonadism. In this study, pregnancy rates were significantly higher in r-hFSH + r-hLH group (55.6%) than in HP-hMG group in (23.3%) ($p = 0.01$).[64]

In conclusion, exogenous LH activity, preferably in the form of recombinant formulations, is mandatory in stimulation protocols applied to women with hypogonadotropic hypogonadism.

Advanced Age Women (More than 35 Years Old)

The impact of LH administration on the ovarian response of advanced age women was studied using both the agonist and antagonist protocols.[52,65-70]

The addition of r-hLH to advanced age women undergoing COS has shown to offer advantages. Specifically, exogenous LH can increase androgen production, which levels are decreased in such patients.[71] As previously demonstrated, r-hFSH monotherapy cannot restore androgen synthesis in advanced age women.[72] LH supplementation may also counteract the increased apoptosis rate observed in granulosa cells,[62] which increases with aging. In detail, LH up-regulates several growth factors located in theca and granulosa,[73] thus exerting anti-apoptotic effects.[35] Lastly, recent studies demonstrated that endometrial LH receptors might modulate the embryoendometrium crosstalk during implantation.[74]

This phenomenon could partially explain the higher implantation rate observed in women of an advanced age supplemented with exogenous LH.[65]

The larger randomized controlled trial published to date comparing the effect of r-hLH during COS in GnRH antagonist cycles was carried out Bosch and colleagues. Their study involved 720 women undergoing their first or second IVF cycle.[65] The authors compared cycle outcome according to the use of r-hFSH or r-hFSH + r-hLH in an age-adjusted analysis. In the young population (up to 35-year-old), implantation rates and ongoing pregnancy rate per started cycle were similar. On the other hand, in older women (between 36 years to 39 years), the implantation rate was significantly higher in the r-hFSH + r-LH group than in r-hFSH alone [odds ratio (OR) 1.56; 95% confidence interval (CI): 1.04–2.33, $p < 0.05$], albeit ongoing pregnancy rates per started cycle were not statistically different (33.5% vs. 25.3%, $p > 0.05$).

Contrary results were reported by Konig et al. in a randomized controlled trial (RCT) involving 253 couples undergoing IVF/ICSI (intracytoplasmic sperm injection), and Vuong et al. in a RCT involving 240 women.[75] In the former, women of 35 years of age or greater received ovarian stimulation in a GnRH antagonist protocol with either r-hFSH or r-hFSH + r-hLH 150 IU/day starting on stimulation day 6. The intention-to-treat analysis revealed that implantation rates (18.8% vs. 20.7%; mean difference 1.9%, 95% CI: –8.0 to 11.7) and clinical pregnancy rates (28.0% vs. 29.7%; mean difference 1.5%, 95% CI: –9.4 to 12.7) did not differ between groups.

In the latter, Vuong et al. (2015)[70] conducted a RCT involving 240 women older than 34 years old (BMI < 28 kg/m^2 and ≤ 3 IVF attempts) who received ovarian stimulation with r-hFSH starting from cycle day 2 or day 3 in a GnRH antagonist protocol. On day 6, patients were randomized to either continue r-hFSH stimulation alone or r-hLH supplementation in a 2:1 r-hFSH/r-hLH ratio (150/75 IU/day). Live birth rates were not different between the groups (16.7% vs. 17.5%, respectively), nor were the differences in the number of oocytes retrieved, implantation rate, miscarriage rate and clinical pregnancy rate.

The discrepancies in the results between the study of Bosch et al. and the other two studies may be related to the different r-hLH timing adopted (day 1 in Bosch study versus day 6 in Konig and Vuong studies). Moreover, the latter enrolled women with various age ranges whereas Bosch et al. only included women up to 39 years old.

Likewise, several trials have investigated the effect of r-hLH in advanced age women using the GnRH agonist long protocol.[66-69,76,77]

A positive effect regarding implantation rate, clinical pregnancy rate, and live birth rate was observed by Marrs et al., Humaidan et al., and Matorras et al. trials.[68,69,76] On the other hand, no significant differences between r-hFSH alone regimen and r-FSH + r-hLH were detected by Fabregues et al. and Nyboe Andersen et al.[66,67,77] Moreover, Fabregues et al. reported significantly fewer oocytes retrieved and fewer MII oocytes in r-LH supplemented group than in the non-supplemented group. Notably, a positive effect of r-hLH was observed in those studies including only women between 35-year and 40-year-old.

The most recent systematic review and meta-analysis of the studies examining the age-related effect of LH supplementation in COS was conducted by Hill and colleagues in 2012.[52] The authors demonstrated that LH supplementation in women aged more than 34-year-old undergoing COS was beneficial. This meta-analysis included 7 RCTs (902 women) and compared COS using r-hFSH alone or in combination with r-hLH in both GnRH-agonist (five trials) downregulation and GnRH-agonist microflare (two trials). The dose and day of starting r-hLH supplementation varied among trials. Implantation (OR = 1.36; 95% CI: 1.05–1.78, $p < 0.05$) and clinical pregnancy rates (OR = 1.37; 95% CI: 1.03–1.83, $p < 0.05$) were significantly higher for women who received r-hLH in addition to r-hFSH compared with those in whom r-hFSH was administered alone.

In conclusion, evidence suggests that r-hLH supplementation has a positive effect on cycle outcome of older women between 35 years and 39 years. In women above 40 years old, it seems that the impact of age on ovarian reserve and oocyte quality (aneuploidy rates) become too relevant to be compensated by the r-hLH administration.

In antagonist regimen is preferable to adopt LH supplementation from the start of COS instead of the late follicular phase. Nevertheless, given the heterogeneity of the published data additional large RCTs are needed to drawn conclusive recommendations.

Poor Responders

The definition of poor responder women has been debated for several years. Up to 2010, 41 different definitions have been used in published RCTs. No more than three trials used the same definition, whereas even trials from the same research groups used different definitions. Only in 2011, an attempt to identify a specific definition of poor response was carried out. Nonetheless, even the new Bologna criteria were criticized for including heterogeneous populations with different characteristics and clinical prognosis.[78-80] Very recently, in 2016, another classification has been proposed by a panel of experts. This new classification introduced by the Poseidon group (Patient-Oriented Strategies Encompassing Individualized Oocyte Number) advocates patient subgrouping according to low prognosis categories rather than poor ovarian response (POR).[79] Nonetheless, the utility of these new criteria in clinical practice is still under investigation.

As for poor responders, several RCTs and meta-analysis investigated the effect of r-hLH.[2,53,81-84] A meta-analysis by Mochtar et al. showed higher ongoing pregnancy rates (OR = 1.85; 95% CI: 1.1–3.11) in patients treated with r-hFSH plus r-hLH than r-hFSH alone. These authors pooled three RCTs including 310 participants. Another meta-analysis by Bosdou et al. which included 7 RCTs and 603 patients classified as poor responders, failed to detect differences in clinical pregnancy between patients receiving LH supplementation or not.[84] However, the definition criteria for poor responders was not uniform in the studies mentioned above. Moreover, even patients with adequate ovarian reserve but slow/hypo-response to gonadotropin stimulation were included as "poor responders". Lastly, the protocols of stimulation, LH dosage, and starting day of r-hLH differed or were not described, thus limiting the validity of the findings.

Recently, a large meta-analysis assessed the outcomes of r-hFSH plus r-hLH versus r-hFSH alone in poor responders undergoing ovarian stimulation in association with GnRH analogs for ART.[53] Although the studies included in meta-analysis were published prior to Bologna consensus, in 10 of the 14 studies, the definition of POR was aligned with Bologna criteria definition. In this meta-analysis, significantly more oocytes were retrieved (12 studies, n = 1077; weighted mean difference +0.75 oocytes; 95% CI: 0.14–1.36) and higher clinical pregnancy rates [14 studies, n = 1179; relative risk (RR): 1.30; 95% CI: 1.01–1.67; intention to treat population] were obtained with r-hFSH plus r-hLH versus r-hFSH.

Collectively, the literature is mixed regarding the clinical effect of r-hLH supplementation in poor responder women. Although it seems that the number of oocytes retrieved and clinical pregnancy rates are higher in the poor responder population undergoing r-hFSH plus r-hLH stimulation, caution should be given to interpreting results for the extensive heterogeneity in the criteria with which the poor responder population is classified.

In addition, preliminary results from Efficacy and Safety of Pergoveris in Assisted Reproductive Technology (ESPART) study failed to find any differences in terms of oocytes retrieved between poor ovarian responders receiving fixed-ratio combination r-hFSH plus r-hLH and those receiving r-hFSH alone in women classified as poor responders according to Bologna criteria.[85]

Hyporesponders

The concept of "hypo-response" to COS has been proposed to identify normogonadotropic young women with normal ovarian reserve and at first hand with good prognosis for COS who turn out to (i) require high amounts of r-hFSH (e.g. > 2,500 IU total dose) to obtain an adequate number (i.e. >4) of oocytes retrieved or (ii) who show a steady response during COS in terms of number of follicles and/ or estradiol levels.[56,57] These women differ from classical poor responders because they are usually young (< 39 years) and ovarian biomarkers [anti-Müllerian hormone (AMH)/ antral follicle count (AFC)] are within normal ranges. The pathogenesis of hypo-response to FSH monotherapy is not entirely understood, but it has been hypothesized that hypo-response could be a genetically determined condition.[86,87] Some evidence indicates that this condition is associated with the presence of specific genetic polymorphism involving beta chain of LH (v-beta LH), and FSH receptor (FSH-R).[88,89]

In detail, a recent systematic review and meta-analysis confirmed that FSH-R Ser 680 polymorphism (rs 6166) reflects an ovarian resistance to exogenous gonadotropin with lower number of oocytes retrieved during COS.[90]

The role of LH supplementation in hypo-responders was evaluated by Ferraretti and colleagues, who conducted a RCT involving 184 patients (age < 38 years).[91] The mean number of oocytes retrieved was significantly lower in hypo-responders treated with r-hFSH step-up versus the group in which recombinant LH was added during ovarian stimulation. Pregnancy rates were also substantially higher in the group treated with r-hLH plus r-hFSH dose compared with both the patients receiving r-hFSH alone and hMG. Finally, live birth rates in r-hLH (40.7%) group were two-fold higher than the r-hFSH alone group (22%); however, this difference did not reach statistical significance.

These results were confirmed later by De Placido and colleagues, in a multicenter RCT involving a total of 117 IVF/ICSI cycles.[56] In detail, the number of oocytes retrieved was significantly higher in the patients who received r-hLH supplementation (9.0 ± 4.3) compared with those in whom an increased dose of r-hFSH was administered (6.1 ± 2.6; $p < 0.01$). Furthermore, implantation and ongoing pregnancy rates were similar in "hypo-responders" treated with r-hLH and "normal responders" women.

Ruvolo et al. performed an RCT to verify whether r-hLH could improve oocyte quality in women with a hypo-response profile.[62] In this study, only women with a history of previous stimulation with high r-hFSH doses (> 3,000 IU) was included. The apoptosis rate in cumulus cells was significantly lower in women who received r-hLH than those in the r-hFSH-alone group. Also, pregnancy and implantation rates were significantly higher in the r-hLH-supplemented group than in the nonsupplemented group.

Recently, a single center prospective study confirmed the results mentioned above.[92] The authors explored the effect of r-hLH supplementation in hypo-responders, according to the classification of De Placido et al.[56,57] Implantation rates were significantly higher in the r-hLH supplementation (36.1%) group than in the increased-dose r-hFSH group (15%, $p < 0.02$). The pregnancy rates were also higher in the former group than in the latter group.

In conclusion, these studies reinforced the idea that hypo-responders may benefit from LH supplementation. In this scenario, r-hLH can be started at the mid-follicular phase in the attempt to rescue the ongoing cycle or at stimulation day one in a subsequent cycle. The role of recombinant LH supplementation in hypo-responder women undergoing COS in association with the GnRH antagonist protocol remains to be established.

Deeply Suppressed Luteinizing Hormone Levels

Profound suppression of LH levels after GnRH agonist downregulation is found in 7–48% of normogonadotrophic women undergoing COS.[93-96] This variation might be related to the type of molecules and dosage adopted. For instance, intranasal administration of buserelin resulted in significantly less depressed levels of mid-follicular LH than subcutaneous administration. Also, suppressed steroidogenesis and follicular development seem to be more evident with buserelin than leuprolide acetate.[93,96]

Preliminary studies suggested that ovarian response and IVF cycle outcome could be impaired when mid-follicular serum LH levels are between 0.5 UI/L and 0.7 UI/L after downregulation with GnRH agonist.[97,98]

Westergaard and colleagues[94] observed that 49% women stimulated with r-hFSH after pituitary suppression with buserelin acetate (0.5 mg SC daily) achieved very low concentrations of LH for 14 days in the mid-follicular phase (< 0.5 IU/L). Compared with the normal LH group, these women had significantly lower serum estradiol concentrations on stimulation day 8 (1349 ± 101 vs. 2908 ± 225 pmol/L; $p < 0.001$). Furthermore, a five-fold higher risk of early pregnancy loss was observed in the low LH group (45% vs. 9%; $p < 0.005$).

On the other hand, Fleming and colleagues[95] found that 26% of women treated with highly purified or recombinant FSH and GnRH agonist (type and dose not reported) had LH levels less than 0.7 IU/L on stimulation day 7. Nonetheless, no effect on pregnancy outcome was observed irrespective of the level of LH suppression.

Humaidan and colleagues also evaluated the effect of LH levels on stimulation day 8 on ovarian response and pregnancy outcome.[61] In this study, only 12% of the patients showed LH concentration below 0.5 IU/L. Notably, the frequency of fertilized oocytes was significantly lower in the group with profound LH suppression than the group with normal LH levels ($p < 0.05$). Likewise in the study of Fleming and colleagues, pregnancy and implantation rates were not significantly affected by profound mid-follicular LH suppression. Altogether, these data indicate that deeply-suppressed LH levels in GnRH agonist treated women could play a role on the ovarian response of stimulated cycles.

Nonetheless, the utility of LH supplementation in those women during COS is still a matter of debate. The only study specifically investigating this issue suggested that women with LH levels below 0.5 IU/L might benefit from r-hLH supplementation as regards the clinical pregnancy rates.[55] However, the higher number of embryos transferred in r-hLH (2.72 ± 0.22 vs. 1.97 ± 0.91, $p < 0.001$) could have influenced the results of the study mentioned above. Interestingly, even studies carried out by the same group have shown conflicting results. For instance, in their first study Lisi et al. observed an increased implantation rate in women with levels of LH below 1.0 mIU/mL;[54] this effect, however, was not confirmed in their subsequent study.[99]

In conclusion, the evidence is not sufficiently high to suggest r-hLH supplementation in women with suppressed endogenous LH after GnRH agonist suppression.

Luteinizing Hormone in the Prevention of Ovarian Hyperstimulation Syndrome

Many strategies have been proposed to prevent or limit the occurrence of OHSS.[100] Recently, the clinical utility of adding r-hLH to good prognosis normogonadotropic women undergoing ART has been investigated in a large RCT.[63] A possible explanation for the beneficial effect observed may relate to the fact that these selected patients achieved a "ceiling effect" after the addition of r-hLH, which resulted in a reduction of the number of selected follicles.[4] In this study, the authors investigated 999 infertile women aged less than or equal to 40 years old with basal FSH levels less than or equal to 12 mIU/m. The study population was randomized to receive r-hFSH alone (n = 501) or r-hFSH + r-hLH (n = 498). r-hLH supplementation was given at a dose of 75 IU/day from stimulation day 7 onward. The proportion of canceled cycles due to OHSS risk (8.3% vs.

2.4%, $p < 0.001$) and clinical OHSS was significantly higher in the r-hFSH alone group than in the r-hFSH + r-hLH group (1.6% vs. 0.2%, $p < 0.05$).

While these preliminary results are encouraging, more trials are necessary before a firm conclusion can be drawn.

CONCLUSION

Although FSH is the key gonadotropin to promote follicular recruitment and growth during COS, the importance of LH has been revisited. At present, the consensus is that most women have sufficient levels of endogenous LH to support ovarian stimulation with FSH alone. However, 15–40% of the patients undergoing ART have less sensitive ovaries, and fair evidence suggests that LH supplementation to FSH regimen can be advantageous during COS. Currently, three gonadotropin formulations deliver LH activity: (1) hMG (with LH activity originated from hCG), (2) r-hLH and (3) a fixed combination of r-hFSH and r-hLH at 2:1 ratio. The patients most likely to benefit from LH supplementation include (i) older patients (between 35 years and 39 years), (ii) hypo-responders.[101] The utility of recombinant LH supplementation in the prevention of OHSS syndrome need to be confirmed by further trials; however, the preliminary evidence is encouraging. Nevertheless, the specific requirements regarding LH dosages for optimal follicular development during the follicular phase of stimulated cycles have not been defined yet. Future clinical research should consider these aspects to aid in the development of better therapeutic strategies.

REFERENCES

1. Hillier SG, Whitelaw PF, Smyth CD. Follicular oestrogen synthesis: the 'two-cell, two-gonadotrophin' model revisited. Mol Cell Endocrinol. 1994;100:51-4.
2. Mochtar MH, Van der Veen, Ziech M, et al. Recombinant Luteinizing Hormone (rLH) for controlled ovarian hyperstimulation in assisted reproductive cycles. Cochrane Database Syst Rev. 2007;2:CD005070.
3. Kolibianakis EM, Kalogeropoulou L, Griesinger G, et al. Among patients treated with FSH and GnRH analogues for in vitro fertilization, is the addition of recombinant LH associated with the probability of live birth: a systematic review and meta-analysis. Hum Reprod Update. 2007;13:445-52.
4. Alviggi C, Clarizia R, Mollo A, et al. Who needs LH in ovarian stimulation? Reprod Biomed Online. 2011;22:S33-41.
5. Speroff L, Fritz M. Neuroendocrinology. In: Wilkins LW. (Ed). Clinical gynecologic Endocrinology and Infertility. 2005. pp. 157-99.
6. Palermo R. Differential actions of FSH and LH during folliculogenesis. Reprod Biomed Online. 2007;15:326-37.
7. Fiddes JC, Goodman HM. Isolation, cloning and sequence analysis of the cDNA for the alpha-subunit of human chorionic gonadotropin. Nature. 1979;281:351-6.
8. Ulloa-Aguirre A, Espinoza R, Damian-Matsumura P, et al. Immunological and biological potencies of the different molecular species of gonadotrophins. Hum Reprod (Oxford, England). 1988;3:491-501.
9. Wide L, Naessen T, Sundstrom-Poromaa I, et al. Sulfonation and sialylation of gonadotropins in women during the menstrual cycle, after menopause, and with polycystic ovarian syndrome and in men. J Clin Endocrinol Metabol. 2007;92:4410-7.
10. Leao Rde B, Esteves SC. Gonadotropin therapy in assisted reproduction: an evolutionary perspective from biologics to biotech. Clinics (Sao Paulo, Brazil). 2014;69:279-93.
11. Campbell RK. Molecular pharmacology of gonadotropins. Endocrine. 2005;26:291-6.
12. Fauser BC, Pache TD, Hop WC, et al. The significance of a single serum LH measurement in women with cycle disturbances: discrepancies between immunoreactive and bioactive hormone estimates. Clin Endocrinol. 1992;37:445-52.
13. Imse V, Holzapfel G, Hinney B, et al. Comparison of luteinizing hormone pulsatility in the serum of women suffering from polycystic ovarian disease using a bioassay and five different immunoassays. J Clin Endocrinol Metabol. 1992;74:1053-61.
14. Combarnous Y. Molecular basis of the specificity of binding of glycoprotein hormones to their receptors. Endocr Rev. 1992;13:670-91.
15. Costagliola S, Urizar E, Mendive F, et al. Specificity and promiscuity of gonadotropin receptors. Reproduction. 2005;130:275-81.
16. Themmen APN, Huhtaniemi IT. Mutations of gonadotropins and gonadotropin receptors: elucidating the physiology and pathophysiology of pituitary-gonadal function. Endocr Rev. 2000;21:551-83.
17. Jeppesen JV, Kristensen SG, Nielsen ME, et al. LH-receptor gene expression in human granulosa and cumulus cells from antral and preovulatory follicles. J Clin Endocrinol Metabol. 2012;97:E1524-31.
18. Alviggi C, Mollo A, Clarizia R, et al. Exploiting LH in ovarian stimulation. Reprod Biomed Online. 2006;12:221-33.
19. Wickenheisser JK, Nelson-DeGrave VL, McAllister JM. Human ovarian theca cells in culture. Trends Endocrinol Metab. 2006;17:65-71.
20. Smyth CD, Miro F, Whitelaw PF, et al. Ovarian thecal/interstitial androgen synthesis is enhanced by a follicle-stimulating hormone-stimulated paracrine mechanism. Endocrinology. 1993;133:1532-8.
21. Whitelaw PF, Smyth CD, Howles CM, et al. Cell-specific expression of aromatase and LH receptor mRNAs in rat ovary. J Mol Endocrinol. 1992;9:309-12.
22. Zhou J, Bondy C. Anatomy of the human ovarian insulin-like growth factor system. Biol Reprod. 1993;48:467-82.
23. Huang ZH, Clayton PE, Brady G, et al. Insulin-like growth factor-I gene expression in human granulosa-lutein cells. J Mol Endocrinology. 1994;12:283-91.
24. Speroff L, Fritz MA. Hormone biosynthesis, metabolism, and mechanisms of action. Steroidogenesis. In: Wilkins LW (Ed). Clinical Gynecologic Endocrinology and Infertility. Philadelphia: Lippincott Williams & Wilkins; 2005. pp. 109-16.
25. Miller WL. Steroidogenic enzymes. Endocr Dev. 2008;13:1-18.

26. Filicori M, Cognigni GE, Taraborrelli S, et al. Luteinizing hormone activity supplementation enhances follicle-stimulating hormone efficacy and improves ovulation induction outcome. J Clin Endocrinol Metab. 1999;84:2659-63.
27. Couzinet B, Brailly S, Bouchard P, et al. Progesterone stimulates luteinizing hormone secretion by acting directly on the pituitary. J Clin Endocrinol Metab. 1992;74:374-8.
28. Willis DS, Watson H, Mason HD, et al. Premature response to luteinizing hormone of granulosa cells from anovulatory women with polycystic ovary syndrome: relevance to mechanism of anovulation. J Clin Endocrinol Metab. 1998;83:3984-91.
29. Filicori M, Cognigni GE, Pocognoli P, et al. Current concepts and novel applications of LH activity in ovarian stimulation. Trends Endocrinol Metab. 2003;14:267-73.
30. Zeleznik AJ, Hillier SG. The role of gonadotropins in the selection of the preovulatory follicle. Clin Obstet Gynecol. 1984;27:927-40.
31. Sullivan MW, Stewart-Akers A, Krasnow JS, et al. Ovarian responses in women to recombinant follicle-stimulating hormone and luteinizing hormone (LH): a role for LH in the final stages of follicular maturation. J Clin Endocrinol Metabol. 1999;84:228-32.
32. Campbell BK, Dobson H, Baird DT, et al. Examination of the relative role of FSH and LH in the mechanism of ovulatory follicle selection in sheep. J Reprod Fertil. 1999;117:355-67.
33. Peluso JJ, Pappalardo A, Fernandez G. Basic fibroblast growth factor maintains calcium homeostasis and granulosa cell viability by stimulating calcium efflux via a PKC delta-dependent pathway. Endocrinol. 2001;142:4203-11.
34. Park JY, Su YQ, Ariga M, et al. EGF-like growth factors as mediators of LH action in the ovulatory follicle. Science. 2004;303:682-4.
35. Ben-Ami I, Armon L, Freimann S, et al. EGF-like growth factors as LH mediators in the human corpus luteum. Hum Reprod. 2009;24:176-84.
36. Filicori M, Cognigni GE, Ciampaglia W. What clinical evidence for an LH ceiling? Hum Reprod. 2003;18:1556-7.
37. Wang TH, Horng SG, Chang CL, et al. Human chorionic gonadotropin-induced ovarian hyperstimulation syndrome is associated with up-regulation of vascular endothelial growth factor. J Clin Endocrinol Metabol. 2002;87:3300-8.
38. Sugino N, Kashida S, Takiguchi S, et al. Expression of vascular endothelial growth factor and its receptors in the human corpus luteum during the menstrual cycle and in early pregnancy. J Clin Endocrinol Metabol. 2000;85:3919-24.
39. Licht P, Russu V, Wildt L. On the role of human chorionic gonadotropin (hCG) in the embryo-endometrial microenvironment: implications for differentiation and implantation. Semin Reprod Med. 2001;19:37-47.
40. Tesarik J, Hazout A, Mendoza C. Luteinizing hormone affects uterine receptivity independently of ovarian function. Reprod Biomed Online. 2003;7:59-64.
41. Lunenfeld B. Historical perspectives in gonadotrophin therapy. Hum Reprod Update. 2004;10:453-67.
42. Beall SA, DeCherney A. History and challenges surrounding ovarian stimulation in the treatment of infertility. Fertil Steril. 2012;97:795-801.
43. Cole LA, Khanlian SA, Muller CY. Normal production of human chorionic gonadotropin in perimenopausal and menopausal women and after oophorectomy. Int J Gynecol Cancer. 2009;19:1556-9.
44. Practice Committee of American Society for Reproductive Medicine. Gonadotropin preparations: past, present, and future perspectives. Fertil Steril. 2008;90:S13-20.
45. Bosch E. Recombinant human follicular stimulating hormone and recombinant human luteinizing hormone in a 2:1 ratio combination. Pharmacological characteristics and clinical applications. Expert Opin Biol Ther. 2010;10:1001-9.
46. Picard M, Rossier C, Papasouliotis O, et al. Bioequivalence of recombinant human FSH and recombinant human LH in a fixed 2:1 combination: two phase I, randomised, crossover studies. Curr Med Res Opin. 2008;24:1199-208.
47. Esteves SC, Schertz JC, Verza S Jr, et al. A comparison of menotropin, highly-purified menotropin and follitropin alfa in cycles of intracytoplasmic sperm injection. Reprod Biol Endocrinol. 2009;7:111.
48. Loumaye E, Engrand P, Howles CM, et al. Assessment of the role of serum luteinizing hormone and estradiol response to follicle-stimulating hormone on in vitro fertilization treatment outcome. Fertil Steril. 1997;67:889-99.
49. Sills ES, Levy DP, Moomjy M, et al. A prospective, randomized comparison of ovulation induction using highly purified follicle-stimulating hormone alone and with recombinant human luteinizing hormone in in-vitro fertilization. Hum Reprod. 1999;14:2230-5.
50. Recombinant human luteinizing hormone (LH) to support recombinant human follicle-stimulating hormone (FSH)-induced follicular development in LH- and FSH-deficient anovulatory women: a dose-finding study. The European Recombinant Human LH Study Group. J Clinical Endocrinol Metab. 1998;83:1507-14.
51. Shoham Z, Smith H, Yeko T, et al. Recombinant LH (lutropin alfa) for the treatment of hypogonadotrophic women with profound LH deficiency: a randomized, double-blind, placebo-controlled, proof-of-efficacy study. Clin Endocrinol (Oxf). 2008;69:471-8.
52. Hill MJ, Levens ED, Levy G, et al. The use of recombinant luteinizing hormone in patients undergoing assisted reproductive techniques with advanced reproductive age: a systematic review and meta-analysis. Fertil Steril. 2012;97:1108-14.e1.
53. Lehert P, Kolibianakis EM, Venetis CA, et al. Recombinant human follicle-stimulating hormone (r-hFSH) plus recombinant luteinizing hormone versus r-hFSH alone for ovarian stimulation during assisted reproductive technology: systematic review and meta-analysis. Reprod Biol Endocrinol. 2014;12:17.
54. Lisi F, Rinaldi L, Fishel S, et al. Use of recombinant LH in a group of unselected IVF patients. Reprod Biomed Online. 2002;5:104-8.
55. Pezzuto A, Ferrari B, Coppola F, et al. LH supplementation in down-regulated women undergoing assisted reproduction with baseline low serum LH levels. Gynecol Endocrinol. 2010;26:118-24.
56. De Placido G, Alviggi C, Perino A, et al. Recombinant human LH supplementation versus recombinant human FSH (rFSH) step-up protocol during controlled ovarian stimulation in normogonadotrophic women with initial inadequate ovarian

response to rFSH. A multicentre, prospective, randomized controlled trial. Hum Reprod. 2005;20:390-6.

57. De Placido G, Alviggi C, Mollo A, et al. Effects of recombinant LH (rLH) supplementation during controlled ovarian hyperstimulation (COH) in normogonadotrophic women with an initial inadequate response to recombinant FSH (rFSH) after pituitary downregulation. Clin Endocrinol. 2004;60:637-43.
58. Hurwitz JM, Santoro N. Inhibins, activins, and follistatin in the aging female and male. Semin Reprod Med. 2004;22:209-17.
59. Alviggi C, Clarizia R, Pettersson K, et al. Suboptimal response to GnRHa long protocol is associated with a common LH polymorphism. Reprod Biomed Online. 2009;18:9-14.
60. Piltonen T, Koivunen R, Ruokonen A, et al. Ovarian age-related responsiveness to human chorionic gonadotropin. J Clinical Endocrinol Metabol. 2003;88:3327-32.
61. Vihko KK, Kujansuu E, Morsky P, et al. Gonadotropins and gonadotropin receptors during the perimenopause. Eur J Endocrinol. 1996;134:357-61.
62. Ruvolo G, Bosco L, Pane A, et al. Lower apoptosis rate in human cumulus cells after administration of recombinant luteinizing hormone to women undergoing ovarian stimulation for in vitro fertilization procedures. Fertil Steril. 2007;87:542-6.
63. Caserta D, Lisi F, Marci R, et al. Does supplementation with recombinant luteinizing hormone prevent ovarian hyperstimulation syndrome in down regulated patients undergoing recombinant follicle stimulating hormone multiple follicular stimulation for IVF/ET and reduces cancellation rate for high risk of hyperstimulation? Gynecol Endocrinol. 2011;27:862-6.
64. Carone D, Caropreso C, Vitti A, et al. Efficacy of different gonadotropin combinations to support ovulation induction in WHO type I anovulation infertility: clinical evidences of human recombinant FSH/human recombinant LH in a 2:1 ratio and highly purified human menopausal gonadotropin stimulation protocols. J Endocrinol Invest. 2012;35:996-1002.
65. Bosch E, Labarta E, Crespo J, et al. Impact of luteinizing hormone administration on gonadotropin-releasing hormone antagonist cycles: an age-adjusted analysis. Fertil Sterility. 2011;95:1031-6.
66. Fabregues F, Creus M, Penarrubia J, et al. Effects of recombinant human luteinizing hormone supplementation on ovarian stimulation and the implantation rate in down-regulated women of advanced reproductive age. Fertil Steril. 2006;85:925-31.
67. Fabregues F, Iraola A, Casals G, et al. Evaluation of two doses of recombinant human luteinizing hormone supplementation in down-regulated women of advanced reproductive age undergoing follicular stimulation for IVF: a randomized clinical study. Eur J Obstet Gynecol Reprod Biol. 2011;158:56-61.
68. Marrs R, Meldrum D, Muasher S, et al. Randomized trial to compare the effect of recombinant human FSH (follitropin alfa) with or without recombinant human LH in women undergoing assisted reproduction treatment. Reprod Biomed Online. 2004;8:175-82.
69. Matorras R, Prieto B, Exposito A, et al. Mid-follicular LH supplementation in women aged 35-39 years undergoing ICSI cycles: a randomized controlled study. Reprod Biomed Online. 2009;19:879-87.
70. Vuong TN, Phung HT, Ho MT. Recombinant follicle-stimulating hormone and recombinant luteinizing hormone versus recombinant follicle-stimulating hormone alone during GnRH antagonist ovarian stimulation in patients aged >/= 35 years: a randomized controlled trial. Hum Reprod. 2015;30:1188-95.
71. Davison SL, Bell R, Donath S, et al. Androgen levels in adult females: changes with age, menopause, and oophorectomy. J Clin Endocrinol Metabol. 2005;90:3847-53.
72. Welt CK, Jimenez Y, Sluss PM, et al. Control of estradiol secretion in reproductive ageing. Hum Reprod. 2006;21: 2189-93.
73. Rimon E, Sasson R, Dantes A, et al. Gonadotropin-induced gene regulation in human granulosa cells obtained from IVF patients: modulation of genes coding for growth factors and their receptors and genes involved in cancer and other diseases. Int J Oncol. 2004;24:1325-38.
74. Gridelet V, Tsampalas M, Berndt S, et al. Evidence for cross-talk between the LH receptor and LH during implantation in mice. Reproduction, fertility, and development. 2013;25: 511-22.
75. Konig TE, van der Houwen LE, Overbeek A, et al. Recombinant LH supplementation to a standard GnRH antagonist protocol in women of 35 years or older undergoing IVF/ICSI: a randomized controlled multicentre study. Hum Reprod. 2013;28:2804-12.
76. Humaidan P, Bungum M, Bungum L, et al. Effects of recombinant LH supplementation in women undergoing assisted reproduction with GnRH agonist down-regulation and stimulation with recombinant FSH: An opening study. Reprod Biomed Online. 2004;8:635-43.
77. Nyboe Andersen A, Humaidan P, Fried G, et al. Recombinant LH supplementation to recombinant FSH during the final days of controlled ovarian stimulation for in vitro fertilization. A multicentre, prospective, randomized, controlled trial. Hum Reprod. 2008;23:427-34.
78. Venetis CA. The Bologna criteria for poor ovarian response: the good, the bad and the way forward. Hum Reprod. 2014;29:1839-41.
79. Alviggi C, Andersen CY, Buehler K, et al. A new more detailed stratification of low responders to ovarian stimulation: from a poor ovarian response to a low prognosis concept. Fertil Steril. 2016;105:1452-3.
80. Papathanasiou A. Implementing the ESHRE 'poor responder' criteria in research studies: methodological implications. Hum Reprod. 2014;29:1835-8.
81. Barrenetxea G, Agirregoikoa JA, Jimenez MR, et al. Ovarian response and pregnancy outcome in poor-responder women: a randomized controlled trial on the effect of luteinizing hormone supplementation on in vitro fertilization cycles. Fertil Steril. 2008;89:546-53.
82. Berkkanoglu M, Isikoglu M, Aydin D, et al. Clinical effects of ovulation induction with recombinant follicle-stimulating hormone supplemented with recombinant luteinizing hormone or low-dose recombinant human chorionic gonadotropin in the midfollicular phase in microdose cycles in poor responders. Fertil Steril. 2007;88:665-9.

83. Ferraretti AP, Gianaroli L, Motrenko T, et al. LH pretreatment as a novel strategy for poor responders. Biomed Res Int. 2014;2014:926172.
84. Bosdou JK, Venetis CA, Kolibianakis EM, et al. The use of androgens or androgen-modulating agents in poor responders undergoing in vitro fertilization: a systematic review and meta-analysis. Hum Reprod Update. 2012;18:127-45.
85. Humaidan P, Chin W, Rogoff D. Abstracts of the 32nd Annual Meeting of the European Society of Human Reproduction and Embryology. Human Reproduction. 2016;31:i1-i513.
86. Alviggi C, Conforti A, Esteves SC. Impact of mutations and polymorphisms of gonadotrophins and their receptors on the outcome of controlled ovarian stimulation. In: Ghumman S (Ed). Principles and Practice of Controlled Ovarian Stimulation in ART. India, New Delhi: Springer; 2015. pp. 147-56.
87. Alviggi C, Conforti A, Fabozzi F, et al. Ovarian stimulation for IVF/ICSI cycles: A pharmacogenomic approach. Medecine Therapeutique Medecine de la Reproduction, Gynecologie et Endocrinologie. 2009;11:271-7.
88. Alviggi C, Conforti A, Caprio F, et al. In Estimated Good Prognosis Patients could Unexpected "Hyporesponse" to Controlled Ovarian Stimulation be Related to Genetic Polymorphisms of FSH Receptor? Reprod Sci. 2016;23:1103-8.
89. Alviggi C, Pettersson K, Longobardi S, et al. A common polymorphic allele of the LH beta-subunit gene is associated with higher exogenous FSH consumption during controlled ovarian stimulation for assisted reproductive technology. Reprod Biol Endocrinol. 2013;11:51.
90. Alviggi C, Conforti A, Santi D, et al. Clinical relevance of genetic variants of gonadotrophins and their receptors in controlled ovarian stimulation: a systematic review and meta-analysis. Hum Reprod Update. 2018 [Epub ahead of print].
91. Ferraretti AP, Gianaroli L, Magli MC, et al. Exogenous luteinizing hormone in controlled ovarian hyperstimulation for assisted reproduction techniques. Fertil Steril. 2004;82:1521-6.
92. Yazici Yilmaz F, Gorkemli H, Colakoglu MC, et al. The evaluation of recombinant LH supplementation in patients with suboptimal response to recombinant FSH undergoing IVF treatment with GnRH agonist down-regulation. Gynecol Endocrinol. Official journal of the International Society of Gynecological Endocrinology. 2015;31:141-4.
93. Humaidan P, Bungum L, Bungum M, et al. Ovarian response and pregnancy outcome related to mid-follicular LH levels in women undergoing assisted reproduction with GnRH agonist down-regulation and recombinant FSH stimulation. Hum Reprod. 2002;17:2016-21.
94. Westergaard LG, Laursen SB, Andersen CY. Increased risk of early pregnancy loss by profound suppression of luteinizing hormone during ovarian stimulation in normogonadotrophic women undergoing assisted reproduction. Hum Reprod. 2000;15:1003-8.
95. Fleming R, Rehka P, Deshpande N, et al. Suppression of LH during ovarian stimulation: effects differ in cycles stimulated with purified urinary FSH and recombinant FSH. Hum Reprod. 2000;15:1440-5.
96. Balasch J, Vidal E, Penarrubia J, et al. Suppression of LH during ovarian stimulation: analysing threshold values and effects on ovarian response and the outcome of assisted reproduction in down-regulated women stimulated with recombinant FSH. Hum Reprod. 2001;16:1636-43.
97. Esposito MA, Barnhart KT, Coutifaris C, et al. Role of periovulatory luteinizing hormone concentrations during assisted reproductive technology cycles stimulated exclusively with recombinant follicle-stimulating hormone. Fertil Steril. 2001;75:519-24.
98. Nakagawa K, Ohgi S, Nakashima A, et al. The ratio of late-follicular to mid-follicular phase LH concentrations efficiently predicts ART outcomes in women undergoing ART treatment with GnRH-agonist long protocol and stimulation with recombinant FSH. Journal of Assisted Reproduction and Genetics. 2008;25:359-64.
99. Lisi F, Rinaldi L, Fishel S, et al. Evaluation of two doses of recombinant luteinizing hormone supplementation in an unselected group of women undergoing follicular stimulation for in vitro fertilization. Fertil Steril. 2005;83:309-15.
100. Humaidan P, Quartarolo J, Papanikolaou EG. Preventing ovarian hyperstimulation syndrome: guidance for the clinician. Fertil Steril. 2010;94:389-400.
101. Alviggi C, Conforti A, Esteves SC, and International Collaborative Group for the Study of r-hLH (iCOS-LH). Recombinant luteinizing hormone supplementation in assisted reproductive technology: a systematic review. Fertil Steril. 2018;109:644-64.

CHAPTER

50

Adjuvant Treatments in Low Ovarian Response

Alfredo Guillén, Guillermo Martínez Canillas

INTRODUCTION

The management of patients with low ovarian reserve is one of the most important challenges in everyday practice in the infertility clinic. The percentage of this subgroup of patients is variable among centers and the prevalence in the literature ranges between 9% and 24%.[1] There is a clear tendency to delay the age of the first pregnancy and patients are referred or decide to go to fertility units at more advanced ages. Those are the main reasons why the percentage of patients with a low response to ovarian stimulation is increasing.

Due to the fact that conventional stimulation protocols provide low pregnancy rates, and similar results with no superiority of one over the others, some alternatives have been described.

It is also well known by clinicians that sometimes patients start an active and intense search for different alternatives. Needless to say, that new treatments or procedures have to be performed according to the good clinical practice (GCP) guidelines in controlled clinical trials in order to provide patients objective data about adjuvant treatments to improve their prognosis based in scientific conclusions.

One of the unsolved problems in this matter was the lack of a unique definition for low ovarian response. More than 40 different definitions have been included in the available literature. Fortunately, a consensus definition has been available since 2011. The Bologna Criteria[2] definition can be used in the studies, although it has many critics.

The different treatment options throughout the chapter are summarized in Table 1.

Table 1: Alternatives in low response.

- Androgenization
- Aromatase inhibitor—letrczole
- Dehydroepiandrosterone
- Transdermal testosterone
- Growth hormone

FOLLICULAR ANDROGENIZATION

Physiological Basis

The creation of a reversible pseudopolicystic endocrine state with the use of androgens would be the fundamental element of this therapeutic approach. Women with polycystic ovaries often show high responses to ovarian stimulation that lead to the development of multiple growing follicles. These follicles have been exposed to high androgen levels for a long time, which makes them develop a high sensitivity to FSH that can lead to a high response.

According to the two cell-two hormones theory, androgens play a critical role in the steroidogenesis process. They act as a substrate for the aromatase in granulosa cells, where they are transformed into estrogens.

First data on mice models confirmed that elevated androgen levels induced atresia in developing follicles,[3] nevertheless primate studies have shown an opposite effect.

Androgen receptors are present in granulosa and theca cells in human and primate ovaries. These androgen receptors are highly expressed in granulosa cells in preantral and antral follicles. Primate studies have shown that androgens can enhance the ovarian response to gonadotropins.[4]

Other papers have also suggested that androgens have a positive regulatory role in follicular development, since the treatment with testosterone or dehydroepiandrosterone (DHEA) increases FSH receptor expression in granulosa cells.[5,6] It has also been demonstrated that androgens promote the beginning of the development of the primordial follicle, and cause an increase in the number of developing preantral and antral follicles.[7]

Another evidence in humans is available. In male-to-female trans-sexuals, a high exposure to exogenous testosterone is used, and it is associated with polycystic ovary related morphological changes, with a significant increase in the number of antral follicles.

Apart from this evidence in patients with polycystic ovaries, a high production of androgens is sometimes present, and there is a positive correlation between the number of follicles and the androgen levels.

In patients with congenital adrenal hyperplasia or with androgen producing tumors (non-ovarian hyperandrogenism causes) some similar polycystic ovaries related changes have been described.

All these observations and data suggest that androgens promote follicular development by an indirect amplification of the ovarian response to FSH.

Aromatase Inhibitors

Aromatase inhibitor, letrozole has been used in patients with low ovarian response. For more than a decade letrozole has taken part in different protocols for ovulation induction, insemination, and IVF. A Canadian group was the first to publish their experience with letrozole in ovulation induction in 2000. This work was awarded with the prize of the Society for Reproductive Endocrinology and Infertility.[8]

This molecule inhibits the androgen aromatization to estrogens and releases the hypothalamus-pituitary axis from the estrogenic feedback on gonadotropin secretion. The increased gonadotropin concentration would enhance follicular development. There is also a second hypothesis in which a peripheral action would involve an amplified follicular sensitivity to FSH. The temporary accumulation of ovarian androgens would increase the follicular expression of FSH and IGF I receptors.[9]

From the first papers published by Mitwally and Casper[10] many studies with letrozole[11-16] in patients with low response were published. They are summarized in Table 2.

Significant differences in clinical outcomes can be found in two publications. Implantation rate is higher in the group that was treated with letrozole in Garcia-Velasco paper[12] and the ongoing pregnancy rate is also better in Schoolcraft[15] work.

Unfortunately, differences in letrozole dose and the variety of stimulation protocols make the comparison and conclusions more difficult. Dose ranged between 2.5 mg/day and 5 mg/day orally during the first five days of the gonadotropin administration.

In the case of poor responders letrozole was used in combination with recombinant follicle-stimulating hormone (rFSH) and highly purified human menotropin (HP-hMG) in antagonist protocol.

Safety issues with letrozole have been a matter of discussion since 2005. Bijlan[17] showed his data with a 4.7% malformation rate in 150 babies born after a treatment with letrozole versus a 1.8% malformation rate in a database of 36,050 babies born after spontaneous conception in low risk community hospital. The incidence of cardiac and muscular malformations was significantly higher in the letrozole

Table 2: Letrozole in low response.

Study	*Protocol*	*Ovarian stimulation*	*Case/ Control*	*Dose*	*Pregnancy rate (%)*	*Implantation rate (%)*	*Ongoing pregnancy rate (%)*
Goswami 2004	Agonist	rFSH + letrozol/rFSH	13/25	2.5 mg/day 5 days	23/24	Unknown	Unknown
Garcia-Velasco 2005	Antagonist	rFSH + hMG + letrozol/ rFSH + hMG	71/76	2.5 mg/day 5 days	22.4/15.2	25/9.4	Unknown
Ozmen 2009	Antagonist	rFSH + Letrozol/rFSH	35/35	5 mg/day 5 days	32.3/24	Unknown	Unknown
Schoolcraft 2008	Antagonist/ agonist microdose flare	rFSH + hMG + letrozol/ rFSH + hMG	179/355	2.5 mg/day 5 days	Unknown	15/21	37/52
Davar 2010	Antagonist/ Agonist	rFSH-hMG + letrozol/rFSH or hMG	45/49	5 mg/day 5 days	5.3/14.3	3.8/7.7	Unknown
Lee 2011	Antagonist	hMG + letrozol/hMG	26/27	2.5 mg/day 5 days	Unknown	21.7/13.9	19.2/7.4

(rFSH: recombinant follicle-stimulating hormone; hMG: human menopausal gonadotropin).

group. As a result of this data Novartis Pharmaceutical issued a statement to physicians in Canada and a worldwide advising that letrozole in premenopausal women was contraindicated. More recently, Tulandi[18] published another study of five centers in Canada with 911 newborns comparing letrozole and clomiphene citrate. Congenital malformations and chromosomal abnormalities were found in 2.4% of babies born after a treatment with letrozole and 4.8% in the clomiphene group. The rate of congenital cardiac malformations was also significantly higher (1.8%) in the clomiphene group compared to the letrozole group (0.2%). During that time letrozole was also used by our group in ovulation induction, insemination and IVF. Our data were presented in ESHRE meeting in 2006[19] and no significant number of malformations were found in 64 newborns.

Concerns about a teratogenic effect of letrozole are unfunded with the available data.[20] Its short half-life (approximately 45 hours) and its exposition (5 days at the beginning of the stimulation) limit its presence during the time of conception, implantation or organogenesis.

Dehydroepiandrosterone

Dehydroepiandrosterone (DHEA) is an endogenous steroid that is mainly produced in the reticular zone of the adrenal cortex, and in small amounts by the theca cells in the ovary. It is essential in follicular steroidogenesis and increases insulin-like growth factor I (IGF-I), which facilitates gonadotropic effect.[21]

A first publication of the benefit of DHEA in low response was done in five patients undergoing intrauterine insemination.[22]

Barad and Gleicher have extensively used this molecule later as an adjuvant treatment in low response. Their first case was a 42 years old patient.[23]

A few controlled or randomized trials are available on DHEA. The first meta-analysis on the effect of DHEA in patients with low ovarian reserve was published in 2013.[24] The clinical pregnancy rate was chosen as the main outcome and two studies were included.[25,26] No significant difference was found on the clinical pregnancy rate between patients treated with DHEA or not, however the result was marginally superior in the group treated with DHEA with a relative risk of 1.87 (95% CI 0.96–3.64; p = 0.07). This tendency can be explained due to the low number (198) of patients included in both studies. With respect to the number of retrieved oocytes three studies were included,[25-27] and a lower number of oocytes was obtained in the group treated with DHEA.

In 2016, a systematic review was published[28] including 21 studies. DHEA pretreatment increased the clinical pregnancy rate (RR 1.53, 95% CI 1.25–1.86), live birth rate (RR 1.87, 95% CI 1.22–2.88), implantation rate (RR 1.56, 95 % CI 1.20–2.01). They concluded that based on the limited available evidence, DHEA supplementation seems to improve ovarian reserves and IVF/ICSI outcome in patients with low ovarian response.

Also a meta-analysis[29] was published in 2017 with a total of nine studies, four were randomized controlled trials (RCTs), four retrospective studies, one prospective study, including 540 cases and 668 controls. The pooled analysis showed that the clinical pregnancy rates were increased significantly in patients with low ovarian response who were pre-treated with DHEA (OR = 1.47, 95% CI: 1.09–1.99). However, it is worth noting that when data were restricted to RCTs, there was a nonsignificant difference in the clinical pregnancy rate (OR = 1.08, 95% CI: 0.67–1.73).

The lack of homogeneity in the study populations, the dose and time of DHEA administration are the main limiting factors to obtain solid conclusions on the role of this molecule in low response. In most of the studies, DHEA is used at a dose of 25 mg three times a day during 5 to 16 weeks. There is no sufficient evidence to know the optimal duration for the treatment with DHEA, serum or follicular fluid DHEAS or testosterone levels with different regimens.

The another important factor that could make the use of DHEA attractive is a possible improvement in the oocyte quality with a decrease in the miscarriage rate[30] and lower proportion of aneuploid embryos.[27] The small sample size in these papers makes the results inconclusive.

Another paper[31] in an animal model evaluates the effect of DHEA in vivo in the early follicular development. A higher proportion of follicle population in the ovary after DHEA treatment has been found. These data support the general hypothesis that DHEA can be a useful adjuvant treatment in the case of a low ovarian reserve.

Further research is required to clarify the effect of DHEA exposure in assisted reproduction technology, although no serious adverse events have been reported on patients or babies.

Transdermal Testosterone

Transdermal testosterone administration in patches or gel has also been used as an adjuvant treatment in patients with low ovarian response with the objective to increase the ovarian androgen concentration.

The application of testosterone gel was first described in two papers.[32,33] The main characteristics of the testosterone gel treatment are summarized in Table 3.

In these two studies, a total number of 163 patients were included and when data are pooled, an increase in 15% in the clinical pregnancy rate and in 11% in the live birth rate is shown in the group of patients treated with testosterone gel.[34] Also transdermal testosterone pretreatment resulted in an increase of 1.5 cumulus-oocyte complexes (COCs) as compared with no pretreatment. However, this effect was based on the analysis of only two RCTs including a small sample size.

In 2016, the same research group published a RCT.[35] They evaluated if pretreatment with transdermal testosterone increase the number of COCs retrieved by more than 1.5 in poor responders undergoing intracytoplasmic sperm injection (ICSI) and they concluded that the pretreatment failed to increase the number of COCs. In this study due to sample size restrictions, no conclusions can be drawn regarding the probability of live birth.

One of the most cited papers on the use of testosterone patches in the treatment of low response is by Fábregues.[36] In this prospective randomized trial, 62 patients with a previous cancellation of a stimulated cycle due to low response were included. Testosterone patches of 2.5 mg were used daily for 5 days during the GnRH agonist down-regulation in a long protocol. In group 1 (with testosterone patches) the ovarian stimulation was done with 400 and 350 IU of recombinant FSH during the first two days followed by 150 IU on stimulation days 3 and 4, and with an individualized dose from day 5 onwards. Group 2 (control) was also stimulated with a long agonist protocol with 300 IU of recombinant FSH with 300 IU of highly purified HP-hMG on days 1–2, followed by 300 IU of HP-hMG on days 3–4, and with an individualized dose from day 5 onwards. It was shown that in the group that was treated with testosterone, the proportion of cycles with a low response was lower when compared with the control group (32% vs. 71%). A higher number of patients with oocyte retrieval tended to be higher in the group with the testosterone patches (60.6% vs. 58.1%), reaching statistical significance in the group of patients with normal basal FSH levels (81.2% vs. 41.1%).

A long agonist protocol was used in Fábregues paper, but this is not the most usual protocol in our daily practice. That is the reason why we decided to perform a prospective randomized trial with testosterone patches in an antagonist protocol.[37] Patients from 18 years to 39 years with a low response (<5 oocytes and/or a cancellation due to less than 5 follicles of more than 14 mm) in 1–2 previous IVF cycles were included. They were pretreated with an oral contraceptive pill with 30 μg of ethinylestradiol and levonorgestrel for 15–19 days and were randomized before starting the stimulation. Patients on group 1 used a testosterone patch (2.4 mg) 12 hours/day during 5 days from the last pill until the first day of stimulation. Patients on group 2 had no treatment during the 5 days after the pill. The ovarian stimulation was done with a fixed dose of 225 IU of recombinant FSH and 75 IU of hp-hMG. Sixteen patients were included in the group with testosterone and 17 in the control group. No significant difference between both groups was shown in the duration, total gonadotropin dose, number of follicles more than 14 mm, endometrial thickness or estradiol level the day of the hCG. There were no differences in the number of retrieved oocytes, number of mature oocytes, fertilization rate or good quality day 3 embryos. No significant difference in the pregnancy rate per embryo transfer (36.3% vs. 31.25%) or the implantation rate (29.4% vs. 17.8%) was demonstrated.

A meta-analysis[38] reviews the role of transdermal testosterone and includes the three papers with the best methodology (Massin, Kim and Fábregues). Pooled data of the studies show that in the groups of patients treated with transdermal testosterone, there was a significant increase in the live birth rate when compared with the control groups (RR 1.91, 95% CI 1.01 to 3.63, $I^2 = 0\%$) and a similar result was shown for the clinical pregnancy rate (RR 2.07, 95% CI 1.13 to 3.78, $I^2 = 0\%$).

Table 3: Testosterone in low response.

Study	*Type*	*Dose*	*Timing*	*Duration*	*Protocol*	*Stimulation doser*	*Type of study*	*Case/ control*
Massin et al. 2006	Testosterone gel 1%	10 mg/ day thigh	15–20 days before stimulation	15–20 days before stimulation	Mainly long agonist but also short agonist	rFSH/ 300–450 IU	RCT	26/27
Kim et al 2011	Testosterone gel 1%	12.5 mg/ day arm	6th day of a previous cycle with E2 + P	21 days	Antagonist	rFSH/ 300 IU	RCT	55/55

(rFSH: recombinant follicle-stimulating hormone; RCT: randomized controlled trial)

The heterogeneity in the ovarian stimulation protocols and the variation in the duration and exposition to the study drug are the most important limiting factors for the conclusions.

One of the remaining questions of the use of transdermal testosterone is if the duration of the treatment is enough to cause an action in the ovary that led to a clinical significant difference.

No serious side effects of transdermal testosterone have been reported. Although the duration of this alternative is shorter than the duration of the DHEA pre-treatment.

GROWTH HORMONE

The last adjuvant treatment used in the low response in this review is the growth hormone (GH). This hormone has a role in early and late follicular development stimulating granulosa cell proliferation and differentiation, and increasing estradiol production in animal and human models.[39,40]

Two meta-analysis concludes that the use of GH in combination with ovarian stimulation may be beneficial in patients with low response.[41,42]

The groups of patients treated with GH showed a significant increase of the live birth rate of +17%, and +16% respectively in the first[41] and second[42] meta-analysis.

The Cochrane review[43] showed a statistically significant difference in the live birth rate and pregnancy rate using GH as an adjuvant treatment in patients with low response.

Two parallel randomized, controlled, open-label trials were performed to evaluate the use of GH in an antagonist protocol[44] and a long down regulation protocol.[45] The conclusions in both studies are similar. GH adjuvant treatment increases the number of retrieved oocytes and number of mature oocytes. Also increase fertilization rate and numbers of embryo transferred or cryopreserved. However, there was no significant difference in the live birth rate whether fresh or cumulative.

The GH is used during the follicular phase with a dose that ranges between 4 IU/day and 24 IU/day. It is started at the beginning of the administration of gonadotropins until the day of the hCG.

Growth hormone as an adjuvant treatment in IVF/ICSI cycles for poor responders should be cautiously used because there is still no identified impact on pregnancy outcomes. The increase of the cost of the GH treatment associated with gonadotropins is an important factor that cannot be forgotten.

Data on security for patients and babies are reassuring although they are limited.

REFERENCES

1. Venetis CA, Kolibianakis EM, Tarlatzi TB, et al. Evidence-based management of poor ovarian response. Ann N Y Acad Sci. 2010;1205:199-206.
2. Ferraretti a P, Fauser BCJM, Tarlatzis B, et al. ESHRE consensus on the definition of "poor response" to ovarian stimulation for invitro fertilization: the Bologna criteria. Hum Reprod. 2011;26(7):1616-24.
3. Hillier SG, Ross GT. Effects of exogenous testosterone on ovarian weight, follicular morphology and intraovarian progesterone concentration in estrogen-primed hypophysectomized immature female rats. Biol Reprod. 1979;20:261-8.
4. Harlow CR, Hillier SG, Hodges JK. Androgen modulation of follicle-stimulating hormone induced granulosa cell steroidogenesis in the primate ovary. Endocrinology. 1986;119,1403-5.
5. Weil S, Vendola K, Zhou J, et al. Androgen and follicle stimulating hormone interactions in primate ovarian follicle development. J Clin Endocrinol Metab. 1999;84,2951-6.
6. Weil SJ, Vendola K, Zhou J, et al. Androgen receptor gene expression in the primate ovary: cellular localization, regulation, and functional correlations. J Clin Endocrinol Metab. 1998;83:2479-85.
7. Vendola KA, Zhou J, Adesanya OO, et al. Androgens stimulate early stages of follicular growth in the primate ovary. J Clin Invest. 1998;101:2622-9.
8. Mitwally MFM, Casper RF. The Aromatase Inhibitor, Letrozole: a Promising Alternative for Clomiphene Citrate for Induction of Ovulation. SREI Prize Paper. Fertil Steril. 2000;S35.
9. Casper RF, Mitwally MF. Aromatase inhibitors for ovulation induction. J Clin Endocrinol Metab. 2006;91:760-71.
10. Mitwally MF, Casper RF. Aromatase inhibition improves ovarian response to follicle-stimulating hormone in poor responders. Fertil Steril. 2002;4:776-80.
11. Goswami SK, Das T, Chattopadhyay R, et al. A randomized single-blind controlled trial of letrozole as a low-cost IVF protocol in women with poor ovarian response: a preliminary report. Hum Reprod. 2004;19:2031-5.
12. Garcia-Velasco JA, Moreno L, Pacheco A, et al. The aromatase inhibitor letrozole increases the concentration of intraovarian androgens and improves in vitro fertilization outcome in low responder patients: a pilot study. Fertil Steril. 2005;84:82-7.
13. Ozmen B, Sonmezer M, Atabekoglu CS, et al. Use of aromatase inhibitors in poor-responder patients receiving GnRH antagonist protocols. Reprod Biomed Online. 2009;19:478-85.
14. Davar R, Oskouian H, Ahmadi S, et al. GnRH antagonist/letrozole versus microdose GnRH agonist flare protocol in poor responders undergoing in vitro fertilization. Taiwan J Obstet Gynecol. 2010;49:297-301.
15. Schoolcraft WB, Surrey ES, Minjarez D a, et al. Management of poor responders: can outcomes be improved with a novel gonadotropin-releasing hormone antagonist/letrozole protocol. Fertil Steril. 2008;89(1):151-6.
16. Chi V, Lee Y, Chi C, et al. Sequential use of letrozole and gonadotrophin in women with poor ovarian reserve : a randomized controlled trial. Reprod Biomed Online. 2011;23:380-8.

17. Biljan MM, Hemmings R, Brassard N. The outcome of 150 babies following the treatment with letrozole or letrozole and gonadotropins. Fertil Steril. 2005;84:S64-S65.
18. Tulandi T, Martin J, Al-Fadhli R, et al. Congenital malformations among 911 newborns conceived after infertility treatment with letrozole or clomiphene citrate. Fertil Steril. 2006;85:1761-5.
19. Guillén A, Vidal C, Pellicer A, et al. Perinatal outcome in cycles with letrozole Abstracts of the 22nd Annual Meeting of the ESHRE, Prague, Czech Republic. Hum Reprod. 2006;21(Suppl 1):341.
20. Requena A, Herrero J, Landeras J, et al. Use of letrozole in assisted reproduction: a systematic review and meta-analysis. Hum Reprod Update. 2008;14(6):571-82.
21. Casson PR, Santoro N, Elkind-Hirsch K, et al. Postmenopausal dehydroepiandrosterone administration increases free insulin-like growth factor-I and decreases high-density lipoprotein: a six-month trial. Fertil Steril. 1998;70(1):107-10.
22. Casson PR, Lindsay MS, Pisarka MD, et al. Dehydroepiandrosterone supplementation augments ovarian stimulation in poor responders: a case series. Hum Reprod. 2000;15(10):2129-32.
23. Barad DH, Gleicher N. Increased oocyte production after treatment with dehydroepiandrosterone. Fertil Steril. 2005;84(3):756.
24. Narkwichean A, Maalouf W, Campbell BK, et al. Efficacy of dehydroepiandrosterone to improve ovarian response in women with diminished ovarian reserve: a meta-analysis. Reprod Biol Endocrinol. 2013;11:44.
25. Wiser A, Gonen O, Ghetler Y, et al. Addition of dehydroepiandrosterone (DHEA) for poor-responder patients before and during IVF treatment improves the pregnancy rate: a randomized prospective study. Human Reprod. 2010;25:2496-500.
26. Barad D, Brill H, Gleicher N. Update on the use of dehydroepiandrosterone supplementation among women with diminished ovarian function. J Assist Reproduction Genet. 2007;24(12):629-34.
27. Gleicher N, Weghofer A, Barad DH. Dehydroepiandrosterone (DHEA) reduces embryo aneuploidy: direct evidence from preimplantation genetic screening (PGS). Reprod Biol Endocrinol. 2010;8:140-4.
28. Zhang M, Niu W, Wang Y, et al. Dehydroepiandrosterone treatment in women with poor ovarian response undergoing IVF or ICSI: a systematic review and meta-analysis. J Assist Reprod Genet. 2016;33:981-91.
29. Qin JC, Fan L, Qin AP. The effect of dehydroepiandrosterone (DHEA) supplementation on women with diminished ovarian reserve (DOR) in IVF cycle: Evidence from a meta-analysis. J Gynecol Obstet Hum Reprod. 2017;46(1):1-7.
30. Gleicher N, Ryan E, Weghofer A, et al. Miscarriage rates after dehydroepiandrosterone (DHEA) supplementation in women with diminished ovarian reserve: a case control study. Reprod Biol Endocrinol. 2009;7:108.
31. Narkwichean A, Jayaprakasan K, Maalouf WE, et al. Effects of dehydroepiandrosterone on in vivo ovine follicular development. Human Reprod. 2014;29:146-54.
32. Massin N, Cedrin-Durnerin I, Coussieu C, et al. Effects of transdermal testosterone application on the ovarian response to FSH in poor responders undergoing assisted reproduction technique: a prospective, randomized, double-blind study. Human Reprod. 2006;5:1204-11.
33. Kim CH, Howles CM, Lee HA. The effect of transdermal testosterone gel pretreatment on controlled ovarian stimulation and IVF outcome in low responders. Fertil Steril. 2011;95(2):679-83.
34. Bosdou JK, Venetis CA, Kolibianakis EM, et al. The use of androgens or androgen-modulating agents in poor responders undergoing in vitro fertilization: a systematic review and meta-analysis. Hum Reprod Update. 2012;18:127-45.
35. Bosdou JK, Venetis CA, Dafopoulos K, et al. Transdermal testosterone pretreatment in poor responders undergoing ICSI: a randomized clinical trial. Human Reprod. 2016;31:977-85.
36. Fabregues F, Penarrubia J, Creus M, et al. Transdermal testosterone may improve ovarian response to gonadotrophins in low-responder IVF patients: a randomized, clinical trial. Human Reprod. 2009;24(2):349-59.
37. Guillen A, Ortega I, Bou C, et al. Testosterona transdermica con protocolo antagonista en baja respuesta ovárica. Comunicación Oral XXIX Congreso Nacional SEF, Granada 2012 Revista Iberoamericana de Fertilidad y Reproducción Humana. 2012;29:144.
38. Gonzalez-Comadran M, Duran M, Sola I, et al. Effects of transdermal testosterone in poor responders undergoing IVF: systematic review and meta-analysis. Reprod Biomed Online. 2012;25(5):450-9.
39. Langhout DJ, Spicer LJ, Geisert RD. Development of a culture system for bovine granulosa cells: effects of growth hormone, estradiol, and gonadotropins on cell proliferation, steroidogenesis, and protein synthesis. J Anim Sci. 1991;69(8):3321-34.
40. Lanzone A, Fortini A, Fulghesu AM, et al. Growth hormone enhances estradiol production follicle-stimulating hormone-induced in the early stage of the follicular maturation. Fertil Steril. 1996;66:948-53.
41. Kolibianakis EM, Venetis CA, Diedrich K, et al. Addition of growth hormone to gonadotrophins in ovarian stimulation of poor responders treated by in-vitro fertilization: a systematic review and meta-analysis. Hum Reprod Update. 2009;15: 613-22.
42. Kyrou D, Kolibianakis EM, Venetis CA, et al. How to improve the probability of pregnancy in poor responders undergoing in vitro fertilization: a systematic review and meta-analysis. Fertil Steril. 2009;91(3):749-66.
43. Duffy JM, Ahmad G, Nardo LG, et al. Growth hormone for in vitro fertilization. Rev Cochrane Database Syst. 2009;(4):CD000099.
44. Bassiouny YA, Dakhly DMR, Bayoumi YA, et al. Does the addition of growth hormone to the in vitro fertilization/ intracytoplasmic sperm injection antagonist protocol improve outcomes in poor responders? A randomized, controlled trial. Fertil Steril. 2016;105:697-702.
45. Dakhly DMR, Bassiouny YA, Bayoumi YA, et al. The addition of growth hormone adjuvant therapy to the long down regulation protocol in poor responders undergoing in vitro fertilization: randomized control trial. Eur J Obstet Gynecol Reprod Biol. 2018;228:161-5.

CHAPTER

51

Freeze-all in Assisted Reproductive Technology

Natalia Basile, Juan Antonio García-Velasco

INTRODUCTION

There is a new concept in assisted reproductive technology (ART) called "freeze-all". It appears as a consequence of great advancements in the vitrification protocols allowing us to "electively" defer an embryo transfer from a fresh to a frozen cycle. Beyond the most common indications: ovarian hyperstimulation syndrome (OHSS) prevention, high progesterone levels, genetic screening, etc. the freeze-all concept has shifted from a solution when there is an indication to a routine practice in many programs around the world. However, we should analyze when and for who is this freeze-all approach most appropriate. Based on the principle that controlled ovarian stimulation (COS) may cause a less physiological milieu for embryos to implant, the freeze-all concept represents an opportunity to provide a more natural environment for the embryo. However, we must balance this against the possible non-natural changes that we may be causing the embryo as a result from freezing. Physician's treatment choices are influenced by a number of factors, including guidelines, evidence-based medicine, past experience and, to a certain extent, habit.[1] This chapter will go over the different milestones that may have led to the establishment of the freeze-all concept, the critical review of published data, and the conclusion whether the shift should be reverted or not.

FACTORS IN ASSISTED REPRODUCTIVE TECHNOLOGY CONTRIBUTING TO THE FREEZE-ALL POLICY

Introduction of Vitrification: A Safe Technique

Cryopreservation is of crucial importance in reproductive medicine. Advancements in cryopreservation techniques have resulted in similar quality and implantation potential between fresh and frozen embryos.[2,3] Slow freezing was the method of choice for decades for cryopreservation of cleavage stage embryos and blastocysts. In term of oocytes, however, even though a number of pregnancies and births have been reported following the transfer of embryos derived from slow-freezed oocytes;[4-6] survival rates are only close to 50%[7-10] and fertilization rates of frozen-thawed oocytes are low compared to fresh ones (just over 50% overall).[11] Vitrification on the other hand has proven to be more effective than slow freezing in terms of survival rates and clinical outcomes for oocytes and embryos[12-14] representing with no doubt the method of choice in practically every IVF clinic today. Vitrification is a fast cryopreservation method that involves exposure of oocytes/embryos to high concentrations of cryoprotectants and ultra-rapid cooling rates causing an instant solidification (vitrous state) that avoids damages to the cell due to ice crystal formation. It is here where the major advantage with respect to slow freezing relies. Given the excellent results provided by this technique, vitrification can no longer be taken as a complement to IVF treatments but as a fundamental tool for the management of our patients. Low responders, for instance, can benefit from accumulation of oocytes through vitrification allowing them to achieve similar clinical outcomes as normoresponders.[15] Moreover, this strategy is also attractive for patients with advance maternal age (a more difficult group to treat) who, in addition to being low responders, require preimplantation genetic screening (PGS).[16] On the contrary, the vitrification of oocytes (and embryos) has also proven to work with patients at risk of developing OHSS representing a solution when an embryo transfer needs to be delayed.[17,18] Last but not least oocyte vitrification allows women to preserve their fertility today, the so called "social freezing", and clinics to establish egg donor banks with similar results than with fresh oocytes.[19]

In terms of live birth rates a population-based cohort study comparing cryopreservation by vitrification or slow freezing in a large data set (over 30,000 cases between the two groups) revealed that vitrified blastocyst transfer cycles resulted in a significantly higher live delivery rate [adjusted relative risk (ARR): 1.41, 95% confidence interval (CI): 1.34–1.49] compared with slow frozen blastocyst transfer cycles, although a limitation of this study is the lack of information available on clinic-specific cryopreservation protocols and processes for slow freezing-thaw and vitrification-warm of blastocysts and the potential impact on outcomes.[20]

Given all these facts it would be plausible to discuss the introduction of freeze-all policies involving the elective vitrification of all the viable embryos from a fresh cycle. The objective of a future transfer of vitrified-warmed embryos would be to place them in a more favorable intrauterine environment, without facing the possible adverse effects of supraphysiologic hormonal levels over the endometrial receptivity.[21]

Implementation of Ovarian Hyperstimulation Syndrome-free Clinics

Ovarian hyperstimulation syndrome represents one of the major complications encountered during COS in IVF. The syndrome has a broad spectrum of clinical manifestations, from mild illness needing only careful observation to severe disease requiring hospitalization and intensive care.[22] It occurs in approximately 1–14% of ART cycles and is related to increased vascular permeability (VP).[23,24] Human chorionic gonadotropin (hCG), either exogenous or endogenous, is the most probable triggering factor of this syndrome.[25] Following the administration of hCG, the expression of vascular endothelial growth factor (VEGF) and VEGF receptor 2 (VEGFR-2) mRNA increases significantly, rising to a maximum level that coincides with peaked VP. These findings suggest that the syndrome can be prevented by inducing ovulation with a gonadotropin-releasing hormone agonist (GnRH) instead of hCG, preventing VEGF overexpression.[26] This strategy would prevent the early, but not the late, onset of OHSS.

For many years GnRH agonists were considered the "gold standard" protocol especially in young normoresponders, but a major drawback of these protocols was the risk of OHSS. The introduction of GnRH antagonists on the other hand seemed to open up a new way toward a more "friendly IVF".[27] Unlike the indirect pituitary suppression induced by GnRH agonists, GnRH antagonists administration causes immediate and dose-related suppression of gonadotropins release by competitive occupancy of the GnRH receptors in the pituitary[28] resulting in a much shorter duration of stimulation and absence of the side-effects caused by profound hypoestrogenemia.[29,30] In addition, COS with antagonists protocols can be combined with complementary measures to avoid even further the risk of OHSS like triggering ovulation induction with GnRH agonist instead of hCG.[31-34] Still, this approach is not 100% safe considering that a few anecdotal cases of severe OHSS following GnRH agonist triggering without any luteal supplementation have been reported.[35-37] Moreover, GnRH agonists triggering has been associated with luteal phase defects presumably due to an excessive negative steroid feedback.[38-40] Two consecutive Cochrane reviews by the same author state that: "GnRH agonist triggering is associated with a lower ongoing pregnancy rate compared with conventional hCG".[34,41,42] This conclusion was qualified as premature and mistaken based on (1) that Cochrane reviews should not be conducted during the research phase when new concepts are being developed, and (2) the authors missed the fact that the variable that affects results is the luteal phase support itself and not the use of GnRH agonist trigger for final oocyte maturation.[40] Therefore, if triggering with GnRH agonist (which is the preferred strategy to reduce the risk of OHSS) is associated with luteal phase defects, then a fresh embryo transfer should not take place, the treatment needs to be segmented and the concept of freeze-all becomes attractive.

Rise in Genetic Screening

Preimplantation genetic screening is increasingly being used to improve implantation rates after IVF. The European Society of Human Reproduction and Embryology (ESHRE) preimplantation genetic diagnosis (PGD) consortium collects PGD data from a number of clinics worldwide and according to the last report 52% of the PGD cycles in 2010 were used as PGS. The most common indications for PGS in IVF include patients with advanced maternal age (AMA), repeated implantation failure (RIF), recurrent pregnancy loss (RPL) and, to a lesser extent, patients with partners with male factor infertility[43,44] and egg donors.[45] From a technical point of view genetic screening has evolved from the early fluorescence in situ hybridization (FISH) years to the use of array comparative genomic hybridization (CGH) and next generation sequencing (NGS). Moreover, the stage in which embryos are being biopsied has also changed from biopsies of the oocyte's first and second polar bodies[46,47] to biopsies on cleavage stage embryos and blastocysts. The first clinical studies with biopsies on cleavage-stage embryos showed higher implantation and ongoing pregnancy rates as well as lower abortion rates.[48,49] The initial thinking about day 3 biopsy was that it gave the laboratory plenty of time to do the actual testing and still be able to do a fresh embryo transfer on day 5; however, there were several drawbacks including mosaicism and embryo damage due to removal of a large percentage of the embryo's cells.[50] Fortunately, advancements in culture media formulations allowed embryologists to culture embryos to later stages of development and the first cases of trophectoderm biopsy took place in 2005.[51] Today, trophectoderm biopsy is the method of choice not only due to a decreased likelihood of mosaicism but also to an increase in the amount of DNA available for testing and less damage to the embryo. The use of comprehensive chromosome screening (CCS) in blastocyst stage with elective single embryo transfer (eSET) has been proposed as effective as double-embryo transfer of unscreened embryos with the advantage of dramatically reducing the risk of twins.[52] However, it is unclear if the screened embryo transfer results in better outcomes when performed in fresh or frozen embryo transfer (FET) cycles.

From a practical point of view we should consider that not all the programs are able to obtain a 24-hour turn around and perform a fresh embryo transfer following a trophectoderm biopsy. In addition, those embryos requiring a day 6 biopsy may not be eligible for fresh transfer due to an asynchrony between the embryo and the endometrium. It is within this context that the idea of freeze-all plays a role overcoming time restraints and allowing us to biopsy the embryos at later stages of development, vitrify them immediately after, send the cells to be tested, wait for the results to come back and schedule the transfer of a normal embryo in a subsequent cycle. Needless to say that a good vitrification program is mandatory and that the logistics of an IVF laboratory will change the more genetic screening we offer to our patients, not only due to the biopsy process but due to a significant increase in the percentage of patients being vitrified.

Concern on Perinatal and Obstetric Outcomes

There is a growing body of evidence highlighting concerns regarding perinatal and obstetric outcomes after ART, and in particular following fresh transfers.

Different studies have shown that children born ART have poorer outcomes in terms of preterm birth (PTB), low birthweight (LBW), small for gestational age (SGA) and perinatal mortality when compared with newborns of natural conceptions.[53-55] Within those undergoing IVF, results between fresh and FETs in terms of obstetric perinatal outcome are still unclear.[56-58] A systematic review and meta-analysis based on 11 observational studies concluded that singleton pregnancies after the transfer of frozen thawed embryos resulted in lower risk of antepartum hemorrhage [relative risk (RR) = 0.67, 95% CI 0.55–0.81], PTB (RR = 0.84, 95% CI 0.78–0.90), SGA (RR = 0.45, 95% CI 0.30–0.66), LBW (RR = 0.69, 95% CI 0.62–0.76), and perinatal mortality (RR = 0.68, 95% CI 0.48–0.96) than with fresh embryos.[59] A Scandinavian study including three different countries,[57] corroborated some of these findings but also observed that frozen-thawed embryos had a higher risk of post-term birth [adjusted odds ratio (aOR) 1.40, 95% CI 1.27–1.55], large for gestational age (LGA) (aOR 1.45, 95% CI 1.27–1.64), macrosomia (aOR 1.58, 95% CI 1.39–1.80) and perinatal mortality (aOR 1.49, 95% CI 1.07–2.07) which was in line with other large-population-based studies.[60,61] More recent evidence from another large observational study in Australia[62] confirmed that embryo transfers of vitrified-warmed blastocysts yield equivalent live birth rates than fresh blastocysts but significantly improved neonatal outcomes in terms of gestational age, being on average weeks longer, and for live birth weight with babies born on average 145 g heavier as compared with fresh transfers; however, we may ask ourselves what is the clinical relevance of this. Finally, this year a report from a group in Brussels analyzed 1,072 singletons and twins born after embryo vitrification on day 3 and day 5 concluding that neonatal health parameters, including the prevalence of congenital malformations were similar to or slightly better than after fresh embryo transfer.[63] It should be acknowledged that the majority of these studies are observational and that vitrified embryos are always second choice for transfer. We could assume that elective FET with first choice embryos could yield even better results but these studies are yet to be performed. Therefore, the published data suggest that it is still unclear if perinatal and obstetric outcomes are better with FETs compared to fresh ones (Table 1).

EVIDENCE IN FAVOR OF FREEZE-ALL

There is not much evidence backing up the freeze-all policy. A recent meta-analysis[64] concluded that: "the use of FET, compared with fresh embryo transfer, significantly improves clinical and ongoing pregnancy rates in patients submitted to ART". However, this conclusion is highly questionable due to different factors:

Table 1: Perinatal and obstetric outcomes of frozen embryo transfers.

Reduced risks in FET	*Increased risks with FET*	*Unclear*
LBW (<2,500 g)	Macrosomia (> 4,500 g)	Ectopic pregnancy
SGA (<10%)	Large for GA	Preeclampsia
Placental abruption	Placenta accreta	Congenital abnormalities
Placenta previa	C-section delivery	NICU
Antepartum hemorrhage		VLBW (<1,500 g)
Perinatal mortality		VPTB (<32 weeks)

(FET: frozen embryo transfer; LBW: low birth weight; SGA: small for gestational age; GA: gestational age; NICU: neonatal intensive care unit; VLBW: very low birth weight; VPTB: very preterm birth).

- *First,* the meta-analysis includes only three small studies. A proper meta-analysis should involve at least 3–4 RCTs with no less than 1,000 participants.[65] This was not met in this review considering that the total number of patients included wasonly 633. In addition, one of the studies,[66] in fact, the largest one was retracted at the request of the editor and the ASRM Publications Committee, due to serious methodological flaws, diminishing even more the total number to backup such conclusion.
- *Second,* the three studies are very heterogeneous in terms of the types of patients included (normo and high responders) as well as some technical aspects. Normo and high responders represent two different entities in terms of clinical approach, management and IVF outcomes, not to mention safety issues, which are very different from one group of patients to the other. In addition, the cryopreservation technique and the stage of development at which the embryos were cryopreserved were different. Both studies by Shapiro et al.[67,68] performed slow freezing of 2PNs whereas Aflatoonian et al. did vitrification on day 2 of development.
- *Third,* the study by Shapiro et al.[68] including normo-responders was underpowered (the required sample size was 411 patients and the study randomized only 67 patients for fresh transfer and 70 for FET), involved co-interventions such as dual trigger for final oocyte maturation and led to pregnancy rates in the FET group of 84% which were far higher than those reported from European or American registries.
- *Fourth,* none of these RCTs were able to provide data on live birth rates, cost-effectiveness and acceptability from the patient.

In our opinion, there is no doubt that patients at risk of OHSS are good candidates for this approach. For this type of patients, the combination of the right stimulation protocol plus the vitrification of oocytes/embryos has transformed what was a high-risk situation into an anecdotic one.[69,70] As described by Devroey et al.,[71] the strategy to obtain an OHSS-free clinic is closely related to the concept of segmentation. It consists of: Segment A, stimulation with GnRH antagonist and triggering with GnRH agonist; Segment B, optimum cryopreservation of oocytes or embryos through vitrification; and Segment C, embryo replacement into a receptive, non-stimulated endometrium in a natural cycle or with artificial endometrial preparation. With respect to Segment B a common question is whether if we should vitrify oocytes or embryos. According to a prospective comparison by Herrero et al., both approaches are safe since they result in similar ongoing pregnancy rates and live births after three transfers.[17] Therefore, the decision to do one or the other will most likely depend on the individual patient's preferences as well as ethical and cultural issues and not on clinical outcomes. A trial regarding the expectations and perceptions of frozen embryo holders revealed that many couples are concerned about frozen embryo disposition for ethical reasons.[72] Given these concerns, in the end, oocyte vitrification may be a more attractive and realistic alternative for certain groups of society.[73] With respect to segment C, there is little consensus on the most effective method of endometrium preparation prior to FET. A systematic review and meta-analysis published in 2013 compared clinical and ongoing pregnancy rates as well as live birth rates in (a) true natural cycle FET (NC-FET), (b) modified NC-FET with hCG, (c) artificial cycle FET (AC-FET), and (d) AC-FET supplemented with GnRH agonists. The study revealed no significant advantage of one specific approach to prepare the endometrium for FET in terms of clinical pregnancy rates or live birth rates.[74] Results were in line with the previous systematic review published in 2008.[75] Either way and independently of the particular characteristics of segment B and C, there is no doubt that the segmentation approach for patients with OHSS works[69,70,76,77] and the freeze-all policy is without controversy in this situation.

On the other side, controversy does exist when it comes to normoresponders. The benefits of the freeze-all policy on patients at risk of OHSS cannot be extrapolated to safe normoresponders. A recent study by our group[78] revealed no difference in terms of ongoing pregnancy and live birth rates between normoresponder patients that underwent fresh and deferred embryo transfers. This was a retrospective study including 882 patients aged 20–44 undergoing their first or second IVF/ICSI (intracytoplasmic sperm injection) cycle, in which a normal oocyte yield (4–20) was obtained. Patients were divided in two groups: 364 (41.3%) had a fresh embryo transfer and 518 (58.7%) were submitted to freeze-all according to the doctor's preference. No differences were observed between both patients groups in terms of demographic characteristics and ovarian stimulation parameters. The raw analysis showed that ongoing pregnancy (36.2% vs. 33.8%, p = 0.51) and live birth (33.2% vs. 32.9%, p = 0.94) rates for freeze-all versus fresh cycles respectively were similar. When adjustments were made for patient age and other variables likely to affect results, there was still no evidence of any impact of freezing. All the patients in the study were considered "normal responders" and were thus representative of a routine IVF patient population. Opposite to these results, a different study by Roque et al.[79] did find better ongoing pregnancy rates using freeze-all policy in patients with progesterone levels less than or equal to 1.5 ng/mL on the day of triggering. However, the sample size was lower than our study (total 530 patients: 351 in fresh group and 179 in FET group). In addition, the retrospective design of this study does not allow us to understand if poor responders were transferred and normo and high responders were frozen, which would have biased the results.

It should be acknowledged that a normal response per se is not exclusive of freeze-all. Normoresponders can face situations where this policy may apply like those undergoing genetic screening, presenting high progesterone levels, impaired endometrium, etc. But, out of an indication, the question whether freeze-all represents a benefit for the general IVF population still remains and further well-designed prospective studies will answer this question. This is the case of an ongoing randomized controlled trial taking place in UK (E-FREEZE trial). In this multicentric study, 1,086 women (543 in each arm) will be randomized in a period of 2 years to show (or not) an absolute difference in the primary outcome of at least 9% (with 90% power and a two-sided 5% level of statistical significance). The primary outcome has been defined as, "a live singleton baby born at term with an appropriate weight for gestation (AGA)". A composite primary outcome has been chosen to reflect safety (single, term and AGA) and effectiveness (live birth) as the goal of modern IVF is accepted to be a healthy baby and a healthy mother (with no OHSS), for details visit website at http://www.nets.nihr.ac.uk/ projects/ hta/1311582.

What About Costs?

Regardless of the evidence in favor or against the freeze-all policy, a not minor issue to take in consideration is the additional cost that this policy entails. Unfortunately there are no studies evaluating the cost-effectiveness of elective FET when compared to fresh embryo transfer. It is necessary to conduct these studies to determine whether a change in policy (performing elective FET instead of fresh embryo transfer) is cost-effective taking in consideration (a) the cryopreservation costs, (b) the costs associated with endometrial priming, and (c) the emotional cost associated to the distress arising in patients not undergoing a fresh ET.

CONCLUSION

Freeze-all, Freeze-none or Freeze-some?

A change in practice should be based on good evidence and sufficiently powered studies. As of today, the benefits of the freeze-all policy are based mainly on high responder patients and they cannot be extrapolated to the general IVF population. An interesting opinion paper published last year performed a SWOT (strengths, weaknesses, opportunities and threats) analysis of the freeze-all policy shedding light to the different aspects of this strategy. The authors concluded that although the major advantage or strength of a freeze-all strategy is the potential for eliminating OHSS, several other factors also support a move toward this approach including: enhanced cycle scheduling and improved organization of the IVF unit. However, potential threats were also presented including: costs and outcomes (LGA).[80]

We are entering the era of individualized treatments in IVF, not only from a clinical point of view but also from the laboratory technologies that we are offering our patients. Why would the freeze-all policy be exempt from this individualization, especially since there is not enough data to justify it?

Clear indications should be specified (Box 1). In our center, indications for freeze-all are not only restricted for patients at risk of OHSS but also for any type of patient with

Box 1: Indications for frozen embryo transfers.

- OHSS
- Elevated progesterone
- Genetic screening
- Low responders
- Inadequate uterine cavity
- Hypertension
- Zica virus (areas affected)

(OHSS: ovarian hyperstimulation syndrome).

a clear indication: patients seeking for genetic screening; patients with an altered endocrine and cardiovascular profile at the moment of transfer (elevated progesterone, hypertension, etc.); patients with inadequate uterine cavity for embryo transfer (i.e. fluid in cavity), and low-responders seeking for a strategy to accumulate oocytes or embryos. In addition, in some areas around the world, especially Latin America, the endemic situation of the Zica virus is causing patients to either postpone or interrupt their IVF treatments to avoid infection during pregnancy. However, postponing is not a choice for some of our patients since they are already fighting with their biological clock, therefore initiating the treatment and freezing all the embryos represents a solution.

The importance of a good laboratory should be emphasized. Implementation of the freeze-all policy will not work unless high survival rates for oocytes and embryos are guaranteed. This aspect is not minor and it is the essence for this policy to work. Any embryologist would agree that vitrification is a laborious process, requiring a lot of focus and it is inevitably affected by a long learning curve. In this context, perhaps the introduction of automatic systems may help in the standardization of results and the easier implementation of freeze-all policies. Finally, we should consider the following: would IVF patients accept this shift? Are we ready to handle their expectations? A study evaluating patients attitudes toward eSET clearly showed that even though informed patients are sufficiently concerned about the adverse outcomes of multiple pregnancies they become less risk concerned when faced with multiple IVF failures and economic burden.[72] Then the question is—"why would elective freezing be any different than eSET?"

Enough questions still need to be answered and more well-designed trials are still necessary to confirm the clinical benefits of this policy and to justify a shift in current ART practice. Therefore, we believe that the freeze-all policy should only be implemented when there is a real indication for it.

REFERENCES

1. Lode H, Torres A, Cockle A. What drives our choices? Evidence, guidelines or habit? Int J Antimicrob Agents. 2007;29:S17-22.
2. Cobo A, de los Santos MJ, Castello D, et al. Outcomes of vitrified early cleavage-stage and blastocyst-stage embryos in a cryopreservation program: evaluation of 3,150 warming cycles. Fertil Steril. 2012;98:1138,46.e1.
3. Herrero L, Martinez M, Garcia-Velasco JA. Current status of human oocyte and embryo cryopreservation. Curr Opin Obstet Gynecol. 2011;23:245-50.
4. Tucker MJ, Wright G, Morton PC, et al. Birth after cryopreservation of immature oocytes with subsequent in vitro maturation. Fertil Steril. 1998;70:578-9.
5. Borini A, Bonu MA, Coticchio G, et al. Pregnancies and births after oocyte cryopreservation. Fertil Steril. 2004;82:601-5.
6. De Santis L, Cino I, Rabellotti E, et al. Oocyte cryopreservation: clinical outcome of slow-cooling protocols differing in sucrose concentration. Reprod Biomed Online. 2007;14:57-63.
7. Porcu E, Fabbri R, Seracchioli R, et al. Birth of a healthy female after intracytoplasmic sperm injection of cryopreserved human oocytes. Fertil Steril. 1997;68:724-6.
8. Chia CM, Chan WB, Quah E, et al. Triploid pregnancy after ICSI of frozen testicular spermatozoa into cryopreserved human oocytes: case report. Hum Reprod. 2000;15:1962-4.
9. Miller KA, Elkind-Hirsch K, Levy B, et al. Pregnancy after cryopreservation of donor oocytes and preimplantation genetic diagnosis of embryos in a patient with ovarian failure. Fertil Steril. 2004;82:211-4.
10. Greco E, Iacobelli M, Rienzi L, et al. Birth of a healthy boy after fertilization of cryopreserved oocytes with cryopreserved testicular spermatozoa from a man with nonmosaic Klinefelter syndrome. Fertil Steril. 2008;89:991.e5, 991.e7.
11. Gook DA, Edgar DH. Human oocyte cryopreservation. Hum Reprod Update. 2007;13:591-605.
12. Rezazadeh Valojerdi M, Eftekhari-Yazdi P, Karimian L, et al. Vitrification versus slow freezing gives excellent survival, post warming embryo morphology and pregnancy outcomes for human cleaved embryos. J Assist Reprod Genet. 2009;26:347-54.
13. Stehlik E, Stehlik J, Katayama KP, et al. Vitrification demonstrates significant improvement versus slow freezing of human blastocysts. Reprod Biomed Online. 2005;11:53-7.
14. Cobo A, Perez S, De los Santos MJ, et al. Effect of different cryopreservation protocols on the metaphase II spindle in human oocytes. Reprod Biomed Online. 2008;17:350-9.
15. Cobo A, Garrido N, Crespo J, et al. Accumulation of oocytes: a new strategy for managing low-responder patients. Reprod Biomed Online. 2012;24:424-32.
16. Milan M, Cobo AC, Rodrigo L, et al. Redefining advanced maternal age as an indication for preimplantation genetic screening. Reprod Biomed Online. 2010;21:649-57.
17. Herrero L, Pareja S, Aragones M, et al. Oocyte versus embryo vitrification for delayed embryo transfer: an observational study. Reprod Biomed Online. 2014;29:567-72.
18. Herrero L, Pareja S, Losada C, et al. Avoiding the use of human chorionic gonadotropin combined with oocyte vitrification and GnRH agonist triggering versus coasting: a new strategy to avoid ovarian hyperstimulation syndrome. Fertil Steril. 2011;95:1137-40.
19. Cobo A, Kuwayama M, Perez S, et al. Comparison of concomitant outcome achieved with fresh and cryopreserved donor oocytes vitrified by the Cryotop method. Fertil Steril. 2008;89:1657-64.
20. Li Z, Wang YA, Ledger W, et al. Clinical outcomes following cryopreservation of blastocysts by vitrification or slow freezing: a population-based cohort study. Hum Reprod. 2014;29:2794-801.

21. Shapiro BS, Daneshmand ST, Garner FC, et al. High ongoing pregnancy rates after deferred transfer through bipronuclear oocyte cryopreservation and postthaw extended culture. Fertil Steril. 2009;92:1594-9.
22. Practice Committee of American Society for Reproductive Medicine. Ovarian hyperstimulation syndrome. Fertil Steril. 2008;90:S188-93.
23. Nastri CO, Ferriani RA, Rocha IA, et al. Ovarian hyperstimulation syndrome: pathophysiology and prevention. J Assist Reprod Genet. 2010;27:121-8.
24. Youssef MA, van Wely M, Hassan MA, et al. Can dopamine agonists reduce the incidence and severity of OHSS in IVF/ICSI treatment cycles? A systematic review and meta-analysis. Hum Reprod Update 2010;16:459-66.
25. Humaidan P, Quartarolo J, Papanikolaou EG. Preventing ovarian hyperstimulation syndrome: guidance for the clinician. Fertil Steril. 2010;94:389-400.
26. Gomez R, Soares SR, Busso C, et al. Physiology and pathology of ovarian hyperstimulation syndrome. Semin Reprod Med. 2010;28:448-57.
27. Olivennes F, Frydman R. Friendly IVF: the way of the future? Hum Reprod. 1998;13:1121-4.
28. Huirne JA, Homburg R, Lambalk CB. Are GnRH antagonists comparable to agonists for use in IVF? Hum Reprod. 2007;22:2805-13.
29. Borm G, Mannaerts B. Treatment with the gonadotrophin-releasing hormone antagonist ganirelix in women undergoing ovarian stimulation with recombinant follicle stimulating hormone is effective, safe and convenient: results of a controlled, randomized, multicentre trial. The European Orgalutran Study Group. Hum Reprod. 2000;15:1490-8.
30. Fluker M, Grifo J, Leader A, et al. Efficacy and safety of ganirelix acetate versus leuprolide acetate in women undergoing controlled ovarian hyperstimulation. Fertil Steril. 2001;75:38-45.
31. Kolibianakis EM, Schultze-Mosgau A, Schroer A, et al. A lower ongoing pregnancy rate can be expected when GnRH agonist is used for triggering final oocyte maturation instead of hCG in patients undergoing IVF with GnRH antagonists. Hum Reprod. 2005;20:2887-92.
32. Kolibianakis EM, Tarlatzis B, Devroey P. GnRH antagonists in IVF. Reprod Biomed Online. 2005;10:705-12.
33. Griesinger G, Diedrich K, Devroey P, et al. GnRH agonist for triggering final oocyte maturation in the GnRH antagonist ovarian hyperstimulation protocol: a systematic review and meta-analysis. Hum Reprod Update. 2006;12:159-68.
34. Youssef MA, Van der Veen F, Al-Inany HG, et al. Gonadotropin-releasing hormone agonist versus hCG for oocyte triggering in antagonist-assisted reproductive technology. Cochrane Database Syst Rev. 2014;10:CD008046.
35. Fatemi HM, Popovic-Todorovic B, Humaidan P, et al. Severe ovarian hyperstimulation syndrome after gonadotropin-releasing hormone (GnRH) agonist trigger and "freeze-all" approach in GnRH antagonist protocol. Fertil Steril. 2014;101:1008-11.
36. Gurbuz AS, Gode F, Ozcimen N, etal. Gonadotrophin-releasinghormoneagonist trigger and freeze-all strategy does not prevent severe ovarian hyperstimulation syndrome: a report of three cases. Reprod Biomed Online. 2014;29:541-4.
37. Santos-Ribeiro S, Polyzos NP, Stouffs K, et al. Ovarian hyperstimulation syndrome after gonadotropin-releasing hormone agonist triggering and "freeze-all": in-depth analysis of genetic predisposition. J Assist Reprod Genet. 2015;32:1063-8.
38. Segal S, Casper RF. Progesterone supplementation increases luteal phase endometrial thickness and oestradiol levels in in-vitro fertilization. Hum Reprod. 1992;7:1210-3.
39. Casper RF. Introduction: Gonadotropin-releasing hormone agonist triggering of final follicular maturation for in vitro fertilization. Fertil Steril. 2015;103:865-6.
40. Kol S, Humaidan P, Alsbjerg B, et al. The updated Cochrane review 2014 on GnRH agonist trigger: repeating the same errors. Reprod Biomed Online. 2015;30:563-5.
41. Hamamah S, Matha V, Berthenet C, et al. Comparative protein expression profiling in human cumulus cells in relation to oocyte fertilization and ovarian stimulation protocol. Reprod Biomed Online. 2006;13:807-14.
42. Huirne JA, Lambalk CB, van Loenen AC, et al. Contemporary pharmacological manipulation in assisted reproduction. Drugs. 2004;64:297-322.
43. Silber S, Escudero T, Lenahan K, et al. Chromosomal abnormalities in embryos derived from testicular sperm extraction. Fertil Steril. 2003;79:30-8.
44. Platteau P, Staessen C, Michiels A, et al. Comparison of the aneuploidy frequency in embryos derived from testicular sperm extraction in obstructive and non-obstructive azoospermic men. Hum Reprod. 2004;19:1570-4.
45. Munne S, Fischer J, Warner A, et al. Preimplantation genetic diagnosis significantly reduces pregnancy loss in infertile couples: a multicenter study. Fertil Steril. 2006;85:326-32.
46. Munne S, Dailey T, Sultan KM, et al. The use of first polar bodies for preimplantation diagnosis of aneuploidy. Hum Reprod. 1995;10:1014-20.
47. Verlinsky Y, Kuliev A. Preimplantation polar body diagnosis. Biochem Mol Med. 1996;58:13-7.
48. Munne S, Chen S, Fischer J, et al. Preimplantation genetic diagnosis reduces pregnancy loss in women aged 35 years and older with a history of recurrent miscarriages. Fertil Steril. 2005;84:331-5.
49. Gianaroli L, Magli MC, Ferraretti AP, et al. Preimplantation diagnosis for aneuploidies in patients undergoing in vitro fertilization with a poor prognosis: identification of the categories for which it should be proposed. Fertil Steril. 1999;72:837-44.
50. Cohen J, Wells D, Munne S. Removal of 2 cells from cleavage stage embryos is likely to reduce the efficacy of chromosomal tests that are used to enhance implantation rates. Fertil Steril. 2007;87:496-503.
51. McArthur SJ, Leigh D, Marshall JT, et al. Pregnancies and live births after trophectoderm biopsy and preimplantation genetic testing of human blastocysts. Fertil Steril. 2005;84:1628-36.
52. Forman EJ, Hong KH, Ferry KM, et al. In vitro fertilization with single euploid blastocyst transfer: a randomized controlled trial. Fertil Steril. 2013;100:100,7.e1.
53. Helmerhorst FM, Perquin DA, Donker D, et al. Perinatal outcome of singletons and twins after assisted conception: a systematic review of controlled studies. BMJ. 2004;328:261.

54. Henningsen AK, Pinborg A, Lidegaard O, et al. Perinatal outcome of singleton siblings born after assisted reproductive technology and spontaneous conception: Danish national sibling-cohort study. Fertil Steril. 2011;95:959-63.
55. Bloise E, Feuer SK, Rinaudo PF. Comparative intrauterine development and placental function of ART concepti: implications for human reproductive medicine and animal breeding. Hum Reprod Update. 2014;20:822-39.
56. Pelkonen S, Koivunen R, Gissler M, et al. Perinatal outcome of children born after frozen and fresh embryo transfer: the Finnish cohort study 1995-2006. Hum Reprod. 2010;25:914-23.
57. Wennerholm UB, Henningsen AK, Romundstad LB, et al. Perinatal outcomes of children born after frozen-thawed embryo transfer: a Nordic cohort study from the CoNARTaS group. Hum Reprod. 2013;28:2545-53.
58. Ishihara O, Araki R, Kuwahara A, et al. Impact of frozen-thawed single-blastocyst transfer on maternal and neonatal outcome: an analysis of 277,042 single-embryo transfer cycles from 2008 to 2010 in Japan. Fertil Steril. 2014;101:128-33.
59. Maheshwari A, Pandey S, Shetty A, et al. Obstetric and perinatal outcomes in singleton pregnancies resulting from the transfer of frozen thawed versus fresh embryos generated through in vitro fertilization treatment: a systematic review and meta-analysis. Fertil Steril. 2012;98:368-77. e1-9.
60. Pinborg A, Loft A, Aaris Henningsen AK, et al. Infant outcome of 957 singletons born after frozen embryo replacement: the Danish National Cohort Study 1995–2006. Fertil Steril. 2010;94:1320-7.
61. Sazonova A, Kallen K, Thurin-Kjellberg A, et al. Obstetric outcome in singletons after in vitro fertilization with cryopreserved/thawed embryos. Hum Reprod. 2012;27(5):1343-50.
62. Roy TK, Bradley CK, Bowman MC, et al. Single-embryo transfer of vitrifiedwarmed blastocysts yields equivalent live-birth rates and improved neonatal outcomes compared with fresh transfers. Fertil Steril. 2014;101:1294-301.
63. Belva F, Bonduelle M, Roelants M, et al. Neonatal health including congenital malformation risk of 1072 children born after vitrified embryo transfer. Hum Reprod. 2016;31:1610-20.
64. Roque M, Lattes K, Serra S, et al. Fresh embryo transfer versus frozen embryo transfer in in vitro fertilization cycles: a systematic review and meta-analysis. Fertil Steril. 2013;99:156-62.
65. Humaidan P, Polyzos NP. (Meta)analyze this: systematic reviews might lose credibility. Nat Med. 2012;18:1321.
66. Aflatoonian A, Oskouian H, Ahmadi S, et al. Can fresh embryo transfers be replaced by cryopreserved-thawed embryo transfers in assisted reproductive cycles? A randomized controlled trial. J Assist Reprod Genet. 2010;27:357-63.
67. Shapiro BS, Daneshmand ST, Garner FC, et al. Evidence of impaired endometrial receptivity after ovarian stimulation for in vitro fertilization: a prospective randomized trial comparing fresh and frozen-thawed embryo transfers in high responders. Fertil Steril. 2011;96:516-8.
68. Shapiro BS, Daneshmand ST, Garner FC, et al. Evidence of impaired endometrial receptivity after ovarian stimulation for in vitro fertilization: a prospective randomized trial comparing fresh and frozen-thawed embryo transfer in normal responders. Fertil Steril. 2011;96:344-8.
69. Griesinger G, Kolibianakis EM, Papanikolaou EG, et al. Triggering of final oocyte maturation with gonadotropin-releasing hormone agonist or human chorionic gonadotropin. Live birth after frozen-thawed embryo replacement cycles. Fertil Steril. 2007;88:616-21.
70. Griesinger G, Schultz L, Bauer T, et al. Ovarian hyperstimulation syndrome prevention by gonadotropin-releasing hormone agonist triggering of final oocyte maturation in a gonadotropin-releasing hormone antagonist protocol in combination with a "freeze-all" strategy: a prospective multicentric study. Fertil Steril. 2011;95:2029,33, 2033.e1.
71. Devroey P, Polyzos NP, Blockeel C. An OHSS-Free Clinic by segmentation of IVF treatment. Hum Reprod. 2011;26:2593-7.
72. Nachtigall RD, Mac Dougall K, Lee M, et al. What do patients want? Expectations and perceptions of IVF clinic information and support regarding frozen embryo disposition. Fertil Steril. 2010;94:2069-72.
73. Heng BC. Oocyte cryopreservation as alternative to embryo cryopreservation— some pertinent ethical concerns. Reprod Biomed Online. 2007;14:402-3.
74. Groenewoud ER, Cantineau AE, Kollen BJ, et al. What is the optimal means of preparing the endometrium in frozen-thawed embryo transfer cycles? A systematic review and meta-analysis. Hum Reprod Update. 2013;19:458-70.
75. Ghobara T, Vandekerckhove P. Cycle regimens for frozen-thawed embryo transfer. Cochrane Database Syst Rev. 2008;1:CD003414.
76. Atkinson P, Koch J, Ledger WL. GnRH agonist trigger and a freeze-all strategy to prevent ovarian hyperstimulation syndrome: a retrospective study of OHSS risk and pregnancy rates. Aust N Z J Obstet Gynaecol. 2014;54:581-5.
77. Borges E Jr, Braga DP, Setti AS, et al. Strategies for the management of OHSS: Results from freezing-all cycles. JBRA Assist Reprod. 2016;20:8-12.
78. Celada P, Bosch E, De los Santos MJ, et al. Elective frozen embryo transfer does not improve reproductive outcome in normo-responder patients. Hum Reprod. 2015;30:i112.
79. Roque M, Valle M, Guimaraes F, et al. Freeze-all policy: fresh vs. frozen-thawed embryo transfer. Fertil Steril. 2015;103:1190-3.
80. Blockeel C, Drakopoulos P, Santos-Ribeiro S, et al. A fresh look at the freeze-all protocol: a SWOT analysis. Hum Reprod. 2016;31:491-7.

CHAPTER

52

Ideal Protocol for Egg Donors

Pilar Alamá Faubel, Diana Collado Muñoz

INTRODUCTION

Selecting the best stimulation protocol is essential for adequate ovarian response. In egg donation program, the stimulation protocol besides being cost-effective should be short and safe. In egg donors, the best stimulation protocol is chosen based on: body mass index, age, antral follicle count (AFC) and response to previous stimulation cycles. The AFC is the most important parameter to decide the starting dose of gonadotropin for stimulation in egg donors.

At present, the optimal protocol for donors is a protocol with gonadotropin-releasing hormone (GnRH) antagonist. This protocol has been shown to offer an advantage over standard long agonist protocol in terms of decreasing incidence of ovarian hyperstimulation syndrome (OHSS), short duration of treatment, lower cost, lesser doses of gonadotropins required and being more patient friendly. There are no differences in terms of ovarian response and outcomes depending on the type of gonadotropins used. In GnRH antagonist, GnRH analogs are used for triggering in all cases, avoiding OHSS in these patients. Frequently contraceptives can be used to avoid weekend retrievals and to distribute the oocyte retrievals during the week.

The ovarian stimulation protocol is very important in order to obtain a good ovarian response. Although, the number of oocytes is important, it is equally important the quality of oocytes. The main goal of assisted reproductive technology (ART) is live birth.

In egg donor population, we take into account: ovarian reserve, age, BMI and response to stimulation in previous cycles. Egg donors are young people, most of them have their own fertility, who undergo voluntary stimulation treatment, to give all the oocytes obtained in the pickup to other couple.

For this reason in egg donation programs, we need to consider the efficiency of the protocol (good ovarian response and good ovarian quality), as well as short and safe protocols in order to achieve greater adherence of women to stimulation treatments.

OVARIAN STIMULATION DRUGS FOR EGG DONOR PROGRAM

Four different types of drugs are needed to perform an ovarian stimulation:

1. Pretreatment in luteal phase,
2. Pituitary desensitization,
3. Gonadotropins for ovarian stimulation, and finally
4. Drugs for ovarian triggering.

Pretreatment in Luteal Phase

Gonadotropin-releasing hormone agonists were introduced in assisted reproductive treatments in the1980s, to reversibly block pituitary function and prevent a luteinizing hormone surge.

The major benefits of the Gonadotropin-releasing hormone agonists include decreased cancellation rate through prevention of premature luteinizing hormone (LH) surge and luteinization, enhancement of follicular recruitment, allowing the recovery of a larger number of oocytes, and the improvement in routine patient treatment schedule. The long protocol, starting Gonadotropin-releasing hormone agonists (GnRH agonists) in the midluteal phase of the preceding cycle had been considered the gold standard protocol in young normogonadotropic women.

Gonadotropin-releasing hormone agonist long protocol induces profound suppression of endogenous release of gonadotropins during the early follicular phase, allowing the early antral follicles to grow coordinately in response to exogenous gonadotropins to accomplish simultaneous maturation. This leads to an extended widening of the follicle-stimulating hormone (FSH) window, an increased number of recruited mature follicles and a higher number of retrieved oocytes and pregnancy rates and take home baby rates.

The introduction of GnRH antagonists in ART to prevent LH surge, seemed to open up a new way toward a more "friendly in vitro fertilization (IVF)": The GnRH antagonist offers a viable alternative to the long agonists, providing a shorter duration of treatment with fewer injections and with less frequent occurrence of side effects (e.g. hot flushes, headache, bleeding, and cyst development) during the desensitization period.

In the GnRH antagonist protocol, the gonadotropins are started on day 2–3 of the cycle. This fact makes it difficult to schedule the clinic's activity to avoid weekend oocyte retrievals.

Some authors have proposed to advance or delay the triggering date according to classical criteria to pick-up and avoid weekend oocyte retrievals, but this strategy was not useful.[1]

There are different strategies for planning the start of the stimulation cycle. The most used are combined oral contraceptive (OC) and estradiol valerate pretreatment in luteal phase. Both are based on suppressing the rise of FSH that takes place during the transition of the luteal phase and the initial proliferative phase, to achieve a synchronization of the follicular cohort, and thus to obtain a more synchronized response.

In egg donor population, the best strategy to make easier the planning of the stimulation cycle is the use of OC. All of them are young women of childbearing age and in many cases already use OC as a contraceptive method.

According to a survey conducted in 2016 on contraceptive habits in Spain, 26.8% of women of childbearing age used hormonal contraceptives in any of their routes of administration. It is also estimated that about three millions women use OCs not only for contraceptive protection but also for their additional benefits to regulate the menstrual cycle.[2]

There are several published studies on the use of OCs before a stimulation cycle with GnRH antagonists. Early retrospective studies showed that pretreatment with OC had no effect on the results of the stimulation. In 2008, Griesinger et al.[3] published a meta-analysis showing that gonadotropin doses, days of stimulation, as well as cycle outcomes (pregnancy and implantation rate) were worse with pretreatment with OCs. This publication generated a great debate in the scientific population, due to the results it showed, but when studying the review in detail, there was a great heterogeneity in the included studies, so caution should be exercised when interpreting the results. The reason for which pregnancy rates were supposed to decrease with OCs pretreatment was related to deleterious effect on the endometrial implantation.

A subsequent study by Bermejo in egg donors found no difference in the expressive pattern of the genes involved in endometrial receptivity depending on whether or not they used OCs in the previous cycle.[4]

Another fact to emphasize is the days that pass between the last pill of OCs and the start of the stimulation. Starting the stimulation early or late after the stop of OCs may have an impact on the outcome of the stimulation. At the present time, the studies defend to start the stimulation at the 5th day after stopping the last pill of OCs,[5] since it is the period necessary for the normalization of the hormones previously inhibited by the use of COs.

A study in by the IVI group compared estradiol valerate pretreatment with OCs in cycles with GnRH antagonists in patients 18–38 years of age, finding no significant difference in cycle parameters and clinical outcomes. The only significant difference found was the duration of treatment in favor of estrogens.[6]

We can conclude that in egg donors, we can use the OCs to be able to assure a better planning of the cycle, without that, it has impact in the results of the cycle.[7]

Gonadotropin-releasing Hormone Analog for Pituitary Desensitization

Through the early 1980s, GnRH agonist was applied to prevent the LH surge during ovarian stimulation. By the end of the decade, the so-called long down regulation protocol with GnRH agonist was established IVF practice, significantly reducing the rate of cycle cancellation, improving outcomes and enabling some flexibility to schedule oocyte retrieval.[8] Two decades later, GnRH antagonists have been introduced into IVF and have emerged as an alternative in preventing premature LH surges. There are a number of advantages of GnRH antagonists versus GnRH agonists: (1) less FSH dosage required for ovarian stimulation;[9] (2) fewer secondary effects due to hypoestrogenism; (3) less stimulation days; (4) less consumption of gonadotropins with the subsequent relation with the cost of the cycle; (5) reduction in a 50% of the OHSS.

For all these reasons, it was evident a change in the stimulation protocols in favor of the usage of the GnRH antagonists. Nevertheless, a review published in 2006 by Al-Inany et al.[10] showed worst rates on live births on cycles with GnRH antagonists than those with agonists. Some authors consider that the initial results difference was due to the learning curve of the GnRH antagonist usage, and also due to the usage of GnRH antagonist with patients of advanced age, low response and worst diagnosis.

Nevertheless, on the last review published by Cochrane in 2011 about the use of GnRH agonists and antagonists conclude that significant differences are not there in the live birth rates between both protocols; and there is a relevant decrease in the incidence of the OHSS in cycles with GnRH antagonists.[11]

Although, the debate between GnRH agonist and GnRH antagonist still continues 12 years later, in the oocyte donor population, in addition to the advantages described above in this text, GnRH antagonists allow to trigger the ovulation with GnRH agonists, keeping in mind that the OHSS can almost be completely let aside.

As far as the introduction of the GnRH antagonists in a fixed or flexible protocol is concerned, different trials have shown that the introduction of a flexible protocol with 13–14 mm follicles could improve the performance of the stimulation cycles, since it helps to reduce the dosage of gonadotropins used, as well as the number of antagonist vials.[12]

New ovarian stimulation regimens are emerging thanks to freeze all strategies. Progesterone is actually used as part of the protocol. There are two ways of using progesterone, whether it be endogenous, as with luteal stimulation, or exogenous, as with the use of progesterone in the follicular phase [progestin primed ovarian stimulation (PPOS)]. Medroxyprogesterone acetate, micronized progesterone or others gestagens are added to gonadotropins in follicular phase stimulation. More research is needed with randomized controlled trials to confirm the absolute control of LH surge and to confirm the outcomes.[13]

Induction of the Multiple Follicle Development in Oocyte Donors

Taking the previous criteria into account, during the selection of the suitable stimulation protocol for donors, we will evaluate:

- Initial FSH dosage
- Controversy respect to recombinant and urinary gonadotropins.

Initial FSH Dosage

The initial FSH dosage is decided in a personalized way by the specialist dealing with the patient, depending on her age, body mass index, ovarian response in previous cycles and ovarian reserve previous to the stimulation— including, at least, the antral follicle count (AFC).[14] Although, the anti-Mullerian hormone (AMH) was correlated with the number of oocytes retrieved, it demonstrates a modest ability in discriminating women with low or excessive ovarian response.[15]

This initial evaluation has a vital importance when it is time to reach adequate results in the oocyte donation program in order to reduce the number of cancellations due to low response.

We should not forget that we are dealing with young patients, healthy, normoresponders and without fertility problems. One study published by Melo et al. in 2009 established the cut-off point in AFC to predict a bad response to the stimulation in 12 antral follicles in both ovaries. Under this AFC, the possibility of a cancellation of an ovarian stimulation cycle could reach up to a 40%, depending on the criteria of the cancellation of the cycle.[16] That is the reason why the initial dosage of gonadotropins usually ranges:

- When the AFC is more than 20 in both ovaries: 150 IU of FSH or 187/225 of highly purified human menopausal gonadotropin (HP-hMG).
- When the AFC is between 12 and 20 in both ovaries: Between 200 and 225 IU of FSH or 150 IU of FSH/75 IU of HP-hMG. In the case of using corifollitropin alfa, the selection dosage will vary depending on the weight of the patient: When more than 60 kg, 150 µg of corifollitropin alfa; when the weight is less than 60 kg: 100 µg of corifollitropin alfa.

In the case of using medication with urinary origin, in both FSH and HP-hMG, the starting dosages use has to be slightly higher.

Controversy Respect to Recombinant and Urinary Gonadotropins

In relation to the controversial question about the usage of recombinant or urinary gonadotropins, there are many reviews and all of them conclude that there are not differences in the gonadotropin to be used.

In 2011, the last Cochrane review was published, where Van Welyet al.[17] compared recombinant and urinary gonadotropins in normoresponder patients under 35, including 42 trials with 9,606 couples and clearly similar results as far as effectiveness and security are concerned. One exception arises when the hMG/HP-hMG group is compared with the recombinant FSH group, the results show a 3% higher number of live births with FSH than with hMG.

Another study performed by Melo et al.,[18] in our group compared three different protocols in long agonist cycles: recombinant FSH alone, HP-hMG alone and a combination of the two. Nevertheless, the protocols where HP-hMG was used were more cost efficient than the rest.

It is also relevant to mention a recent study performed by our group in the oocyte donor population where it was compared the use of corifollitropin alfa with rFSH daily dosage. Although there were no differences between the number of retrieved oocytes and the final results, it was found that 75% of women stimulated with corifollitropin alfa preferred the same protocol in a subsequent cycle, as opposed to just 25% of those stimulated with rFSH.[19]

Therefore, as a conclusion, choosing the best gonadotropin for ovarian stimulation protocol for oocyte donors must depend on the availability, convenience and cost of the treatment.

Ovulation Induction: Final Oocyte Maturation with GnRH Agonists

The introduction of GnRH antagonists in stimulation protocols was a key factor to open the option to use a single GnRH agonist bolus as the trigger to the oocyte maturation at the end of the stimulation.

The LH[20]surge that goes with the *flare* effect after the GnRH agonist administration promotes the periovulatory changes that lead to the oocyte maturation and the ovulation triggering.

ADVANTAGES IN THE USE OF GnRH AGONIST

- The amount of gonadotropins released during the surge promoted by the GnRH agonist is reduced drastically when it is compared to the ones released during the natural cycle.[21]
- Triggering with GnRH agonist, compared to the use of hCG, is responsible for FSH wave compared to the one of a spontaneous cycle. Some studies have remarked a greater number of mature oocytes retrieved when the final maturation is completed with GnRH agonist; and a possible explanation for that would be the change which produced, is more physiologic and natural since it includes the FSH wave along with the LH[20] surge.
- But no doubt about this, its main advantage is the great reductionof a potentially dangerous situation such as OHSS[22,23] and it will neither harm the ovarian quality nor the pregnancy rates in recipient patients.
- The luteal phase defect linked to this oocyte maturation option does not present an inconvenience, but it brings another advantage in the oocyte donors, since the menstruation will take place 4–6 days after the follicle pickup.
- There are no cut-off levels of LH or progesterone on the day of the pick-up to identify cases of empty follicle syndrome or cases with suboptimal response to GnRH agonist.[24]

CONCLUSION

In the daily practice in our clinics, all the patients included in the donation program are stimulated with a protocol with daily dosage antagonists with the different options of available gonadotropins in the market.

In most of the cases, donors will use contraceptive pills (OCs) in the previous month to the stimulation start which, in our case, will take place from Friday to Sunday since the goal is to redistribute pick-ups throughout the week.

The final oocyte maturation will happen when the follicles reach diameters around 17–22 mm, which is a range that allows—in most of the cases— to program the pickup in those days where the clinics have more activity, avoiding to have pick-ups during the weekend and additional workloads for the IVF laboratory—improving, therefore, its performance.

We carry out the oocyte maturation with triptorelin 0.2 mg in a single dosage under skin, programming the ovarian pick up 36 hours after its administration.

The use of luteal protocols or follicular protocols with progestins is being studied in the context of oocyte donation because progesterone levels are not important for cycle outcomes and above all, because these protocols are easier and with fewer injections.

REFERENCES

1. Tremellen K, Lane M. Avoidance of weekend oocyte retrievals during GnRH antagonist treatment by simple advancement or delay of hCG administration does not adversely affect IVF live births outcomes. Hum Reprod. 2010;25:1219-24.
2. De la Cuesta, Benjumea R, Franco Tejeda C, et al. Actualización en anticoncepción hormonal. del Sistema Nacional de Salud. 2011;35(3):75-87.
3. Griesinger G, Venetis CA, Marx T, et al. Oral contraceptive pill pretreatment in ovarian stimulation with GnRH antagonists for IVF: a systematic review and meta-analysis. Fertil Steril. 2008;90:1055-63.

4. Bermejo A, Iglesias C, Ruiz-Alonso M, et al. The impact of using the combined oral contraceptive pill for cycle scheduling on gene expression related to endometrial receptivity. Hum Reprod. 2014;29:1271-8.
5. Cedrin-Durnerin I, Bstandig B, Parneix I, et al. Effects of oral contraceptive, synthetic progestogen or natural estrogen pre-treatments on the hormonal profile and the antral follicle cohort before GnRH antagonist protocol. Hum Reprod. 2007;22:109-16.
6. Hauzman EE, Zapata A, Bermejo A, et al. Cycle scheduling for in vitro fertilization with oral contraceptive pills versus oral estradiol valerate: a randomized controlled trial. Reprod Biol Endocrinol. 2013;11:96.
7. Garcia-Velasco JA, FatemiH. To pill or not to pill in GnRH-antagonist cycles: still an open debate. Reprod Biomed Online. 2015;31(3):39-42.
8. Tarlatzis BC, Kolibianakis EM. GnRH agonists vs antagonists. Best Pract Res Clin Obstet Gynaecol. 2007;21:57-65.
9. Borm G, Mannaerts B. Treatment with the gonadotrophin-releasing hormone antagonist ganirelix in women undergoing ovarian stimulation with recombinant follicle stimulating hormone is effective, safe and convenient: results of a controlled, randomized, multicentre trial. The European Orgalutran Study Group. Hum Reprod. 2000;15:1490-8.
10. Al-Inany HG, Abou-Setta AM, Aboulghar M. Gonadotrophin-releasing hormone antagonists for assisted conception. Cochrane Database Syst Rev. 2006;3:CD001750.
11. Al-Inany HG, Youssef MA, Aboulghar M, et al. Gonadotrophin releasing hormone antagonists for assisted reproductive technology. Cochrane Database Syst Rev. 2011;5:CD001750.
12. Ludwig M, Katalinic A, Banz C, et al. Tailoring the GnRH antagonist cetrorelix acetate to individual patients' needs in ovarian stimulation for IVF: results of a prospective, randomized study. Hum Reprod. 2002;17:2842-5.
13. Massin N. New stimulation regimens: endogenous and exogenous progesterone use to block the LH surge during ovarian stimulation for IVF. Hum Reprod Update. 2017;23(2):211-20.
14. Broekmans FJ, de Ziegler D, Howles CM, et al. The antral follicle count: practical recommendations for better standardization. Fertil Steril. 2010;94:1044-51.
15. Nikolaos P Polyzos, Stoop D, et al. Anti-Müllerian hormone for the assessmentof ovarian response in GnRH-antagonist-treated oocyte donors. Reprod BioMedi Online. 2012;24:532-9.
16. Melo MA, Garrido N, Álvarez C, et al. Antral follicle count (AFC) can be used in the prediction of ovarian response but cannot predict the oocyte/embryo quality in the IVF outcome in egg donation programme. Fertil Steril. 2009;91:148-56.
17. van Wely M, Kwan I, Burt AL, et al. Recombinant versus urinary gonadotrophin for ovarian stimulation in assisted reproductive technology cycles. Cochrane Database Syst Rev. 2011;2:CD005354.
18. Melo M, Bellver J, Garrido N, et al. A prospective, randomized, controlled trial comparing three different gonadotropin regimens in oocyte donors: ovarian response, in vitro fertilization outcome, and analysis of cost minimization. 2010;94:958-64.
19. Requena A, Cruz M, Collado D, et al. Evaluation of the degree of satisfaction in oocyte donors using sustained-release FSH corifollitropina. Reprod Biomed Online. 2013;26(3):253-9.
20. Humaidan P, Bredkjaer HE, Bungum L, et al. GnRh agonist (buserelin) or hCG for ovulation induction in GnRH antagonist IVF/ICSI cycles: a prospective randomized study. Hum Reprod. 2005;20(5):1213-20.
21. Aboulghar MA, Mansour RT, Serour GI, et al. Oocyte quality in patients with severe ovarian hyperstimulation syndrome. Fertil Steril. 1997;68(6):1017-21.
22. Bodri D, Guillen JJ, Trullenque M, et al. Early ovarian hyperstimulation syndrome is completely prevented by gonadotropin releasing-hormone agonist triggering in high-risk oocyte donor cycles: a prospective, luteal-phase follow-up study. Fertil Steril. 2010;93:2418-20.
23. Melo M, Busso CE, Bellver J, et al. GnRH agonist versus recombinant hCG in an oocyte donation programme: a randomized, prospective, controlled, assessor-blind study. Reprod Biomed Online. 2009;19:486-92.
24. Blazquez A, Guillén JJ1, Colomé C, . Empty follicle syndrome prevalence and management in oocyte donors. Hum Reprod. 2014;29(10):2221-7.

CHAPTER

53

Protocols for Thaw Embryo Transfer

Krithika Devi J

INTRODUCTION

Cryopreservation heralded a new era in assisted reproductive technology. Trounson and Mohr in 1983 reported the first live birth following frozen embryo transfer (FET). Despite the growing importance of FET in the treatment of subfertility, there is little consensus on the best method for endometrial preparation.[1] Different in vitro fertilization (IVF) clinics have different protocols for giving these medications, and there is no definite consensus over an ideal protocol.

Key Points for a Successful Frozen Embryo Transfer

- Selecting proper embryos
- Accurate synchronization of endometrium and embryos
- Luteal support.

The various available options for endometrial preparation for a FET cycle are described in Table 1.

Table 1: Protocols for a thaw embryo transfer cycle.

S No.	*Protocols*	*Drugs*
1.	Natural cycle	No drugs
2.	Modified natural cycle	hCG trigger ± progesterone
3.	Stimulation cycle	Clomiphene citrate /hMG/FSH
4.	Hormone replacement cycle	Estrogens and progesterones/ GnRH analogs

(hCG: human chorionic gonadotropin; hMG: human menopausal gonadotropin; FSH: follicle-stimulating hormone; GnRH: gonadotropin-releasing hormone).

NATURAL CYCLE FROZEN EMBRYO TRANSFER

In patients with predictable menstrual cycles, we can carefully monitor the cycle to determine the precise timing of ovulation. Once the precise date of ovulation is set, then the uterine lining should be receptive to embryo transfer 3/5 days later depending on the day it was frozen. In this way, the embryos can be replaced at approximately the time when they would normally be arriving in the uterus. Pregnancy rates in natural cycle frozen embryo transfer (NC-FET) are closely dependent on the timely identification of ovulation and calculation of the likely subsequent period of optimal endometrial receptivity.[2,3]

Natural cycle frozen embryo transfer poses the risk of unobserved ovulation. If ovulation occurs without notice, accurate planning of embryo thawing and transfer is not possible, which results in cycle cancellation (7–12%).[4]

Natural cycle frozen embryo transfer involves frequent monitoring of urine and/or blood luteinizing hormone (LH) levels, early luteal serum progesterone levels, and ultrasound monitoring of the developing dominant follicle. For optimal FET results precise identification of the LH surge and adequate natural corpus luteum function are required which may be difficult for logistic reasons.

The advantages and disadvantages of the natural cycle thaw embryo transfer are shown in Figure 1.

Luteinizing Hormone Monitoring—Practical Challenges in a Natural Cycle

- Possible only in women with perfect ovulatory cycles
- Luteinizing hormone surges in urine lag up to 21 hours behind the appearance of the surge in blood, and this

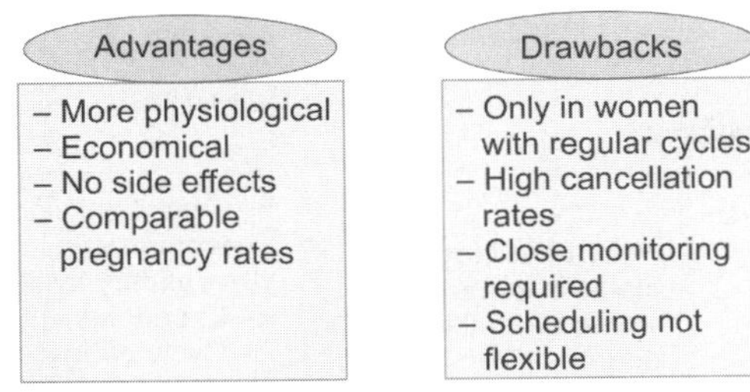

Fig. 1: Natural cycle—Thaw embryo transfer.

should be taken into consideration when interpreting urinary measurements[5-8]

- Variation in timing of LH surge occurrence between cycles and between patients[9]
- Luteinizing hormone levels needs to be assessed daily and preferably twice a day around ovulatory period. LH urine kits have a large variation in thresholds, which involve the risk of up to 30% of false-negative testing.[8,10,11]

Drawbacks of Natural Cycle Frozen Embryo Transfer

- Planning NC-FET carries the risk of unexpected ovulation and difficulty in ensuring timely thawing and transfer of the embryo
- It demands frequent monitoring around the time of ovulation
- The optimal time for implantation may fall at an unpredictable time during the laboratory work schedule, so some clinics choose not to offer NC-FET.

MODIFIED NATURAL CYCLE FROZEN EMBRYO TRANSFER

To overcome the disadvantages of LH monitoring, human chorionic gonadotropin (hCG) triggering of ovulation is often employed in NC-FET in what is termed "modified NC-FET". Modified natural cycles do not require LH monitoring, but regular ultrasound evaluation of the dominant follicle is required to ensure appropriate timing of hCG administration.

Ultrasound measurements of the endometrial stripe and monitoring of serum hormone levels is also done. As soon as the dominant follicle is of sufficient size (17–18 mm), hCG is administered as a surrogate to the endogenous LH surge to trigger final oocyte maturation and ovulation, which takes place approximately 36–38 hours later.[5]

This approach allows for precise definition of the ovulation trigger for scheduling FET, and also provides luteal support in the form of hCG in case of possible luteal dysfunction.

True Natural Cycle versus Modified Natural Cycle Using hCG

It is important to make a distinction between natural and modified natural FET protocols because of the inherent additional luteal phase support provided by hCG injection in the modified NC protocols. In both true and modified NC, thawing and transfer of the embryo should be performed 3–5 days after ovulation depending on the stage of the embryo when frozen.[12,13] The advantages of modified NC-FET are its simplicity with no injections (besides the hCG trigger shot) and minimal additional medications with an overall cost savings compared with a medicated FET.

Five studies, representing 1,965 cycles, were identified comparing true NC-FET with modified NC-FET.[4,14-16] The pooled result of all studies analysed showed no significant difference with regard to clinical pregnancy [odds ratio (OR) 0.91, 95% confidence interval (CI) 0.74–1.1], ongoing pregnancy (OR 1.0, 95% CI 0.66–1.6) and live birth (OR 1.0, 95% CI 0.63–1.6).

Role of Luteal Phase Progesterones in Natural Cycles

In fertility proven women, endogenous production of progesterone from the corpus luteum is sufficient to support the embryo implantation in a natural ovulatory cycle. However, the women undergoing FET are often subfertile or infertile, and their corpus luteal progesterone production may be insufficient during their natural cycles in some women. Inadequate progesterone production during the luteal phase or early pregnancy period can result in implantation failure or spontaneous abortion.

In the prospective randomized controlled trial (RCT) by Bjuresten et al.[17] and in other studies,[18,19] progesterone supplementation showed higher live birth rates and reduced miscarriage rates in patients undergoing NC-FET with luteal support. However, there are few studies published regarding luteal phase support in NC-FET including Kyrou et al.,[20] and Eftekhar et al.[21] who showed in their analysis no benefit of luteal phase support in patients undergoing modified NC-FET.

Based on the conflicting results of the studies it can be concluded that currently there is too little evidence supporting a positive effect of luteal phase support in patients undergoing NC-FET.

STIMULATED CYCLE FROZEN EMBRYO TRANSFER

Stimulated cycle is where fertility drugs such as gonadotropin injections are usually recommended for women who did not ovulate regularly and did not respond to hormone replacement treatment (HRT) in a previous cycle.

Stimulated FET cycles consist of the administration of human menopausal gonadotropins (hMG) or follicle-stimulating hormone (FSH) in low doses 50 or 75 IU/day from cycle day 2 or day 3. Sizes of follicles are monitored with ultrasound, and ovulation is induced with exogenous hCG administration when the dominant follicle reaches more than 17–18 mm in diameter and estradiol levels exceed 300 pg/mL. Embryo transfer is undertaken when these criteria are met. Progesterone is provided for luteal support (Fig. 2).[22]

Cochrane review on treatment regimes in FET concluded that current evidence does not demonstrate a significant difference in pregnancy rates between these methods of endometrial preparation.[23]

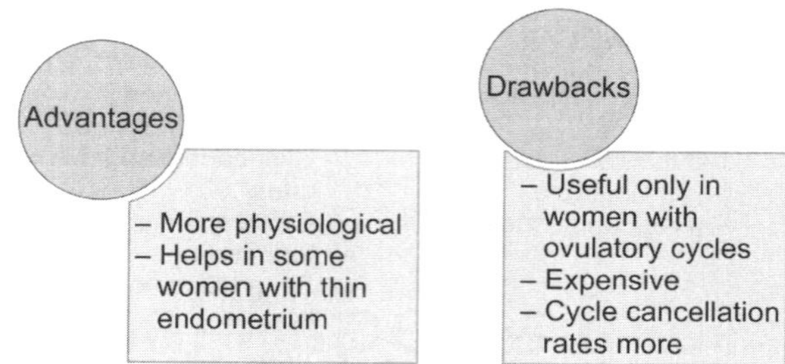

Fig. 2: Stimulation cycle for thaw embryo transfer.

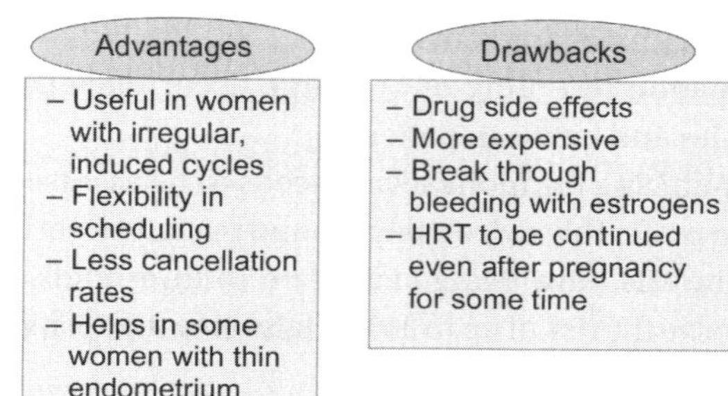

Fig. 3: HRT cycle for thaw embryo transfer. (HRT: hormone replacement treatment).

HORMONE REPLACEMENT FROZEN EMBRYO TRANSFER CYCLE

Hormone replacement cycle (HRT) allows the couple to avoid some of the pitfalls associated with a NC-FET. Medicated FETs do allow for advance scheduling, which both patients and physicians find attractive. The patient and medical team can focus on preparing the uterine lining and will thaw the embryos when the patient's lining is most likely to allow for implantation.

HRT carries some advantages over natural cycles. By using HRT, fewer times of visits were needed during the cycles—which considerably benefits the patients. The day of embryo thawing and transfer can be scheduled in advance. Treatment cancellation rates are limited in HRT, due to the programmed exogenous hormone replacement and suppression of ovulation. HRT constitutes a more suitable option for some specific patients, such as women who are more than 40 years old, women with premature ovarian failure, and oligomenorrhea (Fig. 3).

In programmed FET, estrogen and progesterone are administered in a sequential regimen, which aims to mimic the endocrine exposure of the endometrium in the normal cycle. Initially, estradiol is given in order to cause proliferation of the endometrium, while suppressing the development of the dominant follicle. This is continued until the endometrium is observed to be 7–9 mm thick on ultrasound, at which time progesterone assay is done and after ascertaining it is low (preferred cut off—less than 0.5 ng/mL), progesterone is added to initiate secretory changes.[24] The physiological mid-cycle shift from estrogen to progesterone is thus emulated.[25,26] The day progesterone is started is considered ovulation/OPU day and the time of thaw/transfer is planned accordingly.

When to Start and Stop Estrogen

The moment of commencing estrogen (E2) supplementation can differ, but all studies are suggesting to start before the 4th day of the cycle. Timely starting of E2 reduces the chance of unwanted follicular development and thus ovulation. In artificial endometrial preparation cycles without GnRH agonist use, it is better to start estrogens early at day 1–2 of menstrual cycle, after this time the inhibition of spontaneous ovulation is questionable.

If the pregnancy test is positive estrogen supplementation is maintained until 10–12 weeks of pregnancy. The dose can be reduced, tapered and stopped around that time.

Estrogen Administration

In patients who are unable to tolerate oral route, vaginal and transdermal route seemed to be an equally effective alternative (Table 2).

Table 2: Estrogen administration.

S No.	*Route*	*Dose*	*Benefits*	*Drawbacks*
1.	Oral	2–8 mg/day	Easy intake	Multiple doses
2.	Vaginal	2–8 mg/day	Higher endometrial concentrations	Inconve-nient
3.	Transdermal	100–400 μg/24 hours	Simple/ 24 hours administration	Expensive

Zhihong Niu et al.[27] suggested step-up protocol estradiol instead of fixed high dose estrogen because the former protocol is more similar to physiologic pattern and it is more suitable for endometrial maturation and then embryo implantation. Navot et al.[28] reported that shorter (5–10 days) and lower dosage protocols of estradiol priming of the endometrium could result in higher abortion rates. Borini et al.[29] also found a proliferative phase of less than 10 days is related to a higher abortion rate. This indicates an optimal endometrial proliferation, which is necessary to enable optimal development of progesterone receptors and subsequent transformation into an endometrium receptive to the transferred embryo. Devroey and Pados[30] presumed that an adequate period of estrogen administration is necessary in order to achieve a subsequent normal secretory endometrium.

HORMONE REPLACEMENT CYCLE WITH GnRH AGONIST

In some women GnRH agonists may be given in addition to hormone replacement to suppress any hormone production by the ovaries, which may interfere with the treatment.

The administration of estrogen and progesterone does not guarantee complete pituitary suppression, and a dominant follicle may therefore occur. If the follicle undergoes spontaneous lutenization, it may cause premature exposture of the endometrium to progesterone and affect the synchrony between the endometrium and the embryo implantation. For this reason, GnRH agonist co-treatment may be used to downregulate the pituitary and prevent follicular growth. However, it remains unclear whether any one of these approaches is superior to another with regard to ongoing pregnancy rate and patients preference.

The aim of pretreatment with GnRH agonist is to avoid spontaneous ovulation, but it is costly and there is a risk of hypoestrogenic side effect that would lengthen the preparation. Many published studies compared the two artificial protocols and showed similar clinical outcome.[24,31,32] Van de Vijveret al.[33] in his study retrospectively analyzed 1,129 frozen transfer cycles and concluded that live birth rates after cryopreserved embryo transfer in artificial cycles did not increase when a GnRH agonist was administered.[34]

Givens et al.[35] observed no difference in pregnancy rates between NC-FET and HRT-FET. Pregnancy rates did not differ significantly between both groups.

HRT-FET with or without GnRH: Both require medication and are there-fore less "physiological", but the cycles are easier to plan making it popular among many patients and their doctors.

ROLE OF PROGESTERONE ASSAY IN HORMONE REPLACEMENT FROZEN EMBRYO TRANSFER CYCLES

Since programmed FET does not guarantee complete downregulation, luteinization may occur in 5% of the cases and can affect the pregnancy rates.[24] Doing a progesterone assay before the start of progesterone in the cycle helps in identifying premature luteinization and cycle cancellation is recommended if the value is more than 0.5 ng/mL.

In cases where progesterone hormone levels are too high, the delicate synchronization of the embryo and the endometrium are disturbed. Increased levels of progesterone can result in "advancement" of the endometrium, such that the uterus is no longer optimally receptive when the embryo is ready to implant. From a cost-efficiency perspective, this aspect is of great importance and should be taken into account.

Whether an ovulatory HRT cycle should be cancelled constitutes a dilemma in practice of FET treatment. The unsuppressed follicle development and ovulation may alter the hormone profile, and thus impair the endometrial receptivity and pregnancy. Studies have found decreased implantation rates and pregnancy rates in ovulatory patients. This finding has clinical implication that the HRT cycle with unsuppressed ovulation may need to be cancelled.

OPTIMAL ENDOMETRIAL THICKNESS/ ENDOMETRIAL PATTERN

Endometrial thickness and pattern still remain the most researched parameters for their predictive value in IVF. An endometrial thickness of less than 7 mm at the time of embryo implantation is considered suboptimal in ART.

Kumbak et al.[36] looked at the cycle characteristics and outcomes of 175 patients with an endometrial thickness of less than 7 mm on the day of oocyte retrieval. Patients were stratified according to three endometrial thickness groups ≥4 mm and <5 mm, ≥5 mm and <6 mm, and ≥6 mm and <7 mm. Pregnancy rate and implantation rate did not show a statistically significant difference among the three groups though an increasing trend in values was observed as endometrial thickness increased.

A contrary view was given by Kasius et al.,[37] based on a systematic review and meta-analysis of 1,170 studies. Their review suggests that endometrial thickness cannot be used as a parameter to decide on cycle cancellation, freezing of all embryos or discontinuing IVF treatment. One can conclude from this review that *endometrial thickness can give us probability but cannot be predictive of pregnancy.*

In all studies, the start of progesterone was determined based on the endometrial thickness (7–8 mm). This is in-line with the fact that not duration of estrogen supplementation, but the endometrial thickness should be the leading factor in determining the start of progesterone.[12,38]

Endometrial thickness was not significantly associated with clinical outcomes of euploid embryos. A type-3 endometrial pattern at trigger day suggests a prematurely closed window of implantation.[39]

EXTENDED ESTROGEN SUPPORT

Endometrial thickness can be improved by extending the estrogen administration for 14–60 days, in HRT-FET cycles. A receptive endometrium should reach a thickness of at least 7–8 mm. Above this threshold, the endometrium can maintain its receptivity for up to 40–60 days, as has been shown by oocyte donation programs.[40]

IS ASSESSMENT OF FUNCTIONALITY IMPORTANT?

As suggested by various case reports and studies—thin endometrium is not necessarily nonreceptive. The endometrial receptivity array (ERA) test is a molecular test that defines the window of endometrial receptivity. This test can be used to confirm the receptivity of a thin endometrium before planning FET. In case of a changed window of receptivity, a personalized embryo transfer can be performed. A study done on patients with thin endometrium less than or equal to 6 mm revealed that ERA was nonreceptive in 23% (3/13) and receptive in 77% (10/13). The proportion of receptive to nonreceptive endometrium was not different from patients with endometrial thickness more than 6 mm. The overall pregnancy rate in the thin endometrium group—who underwent embryo transfer after ERA was 33.3% (6/9).[41]

The burning question regarding treatment of thin refractory endometrium remains unanswered. A number of treatments have been tried. Intrauterine insertion of granulocyte-colony stimulating factor (G-CSF), sildenafil, tocopherol, aspirin, and L-arginine have been used to improve endometrial vascularity but none validated so far.

Thin endometrium may not necessarily be secondary to a disease process. It can result from individual uterine architecture or the intrinsic properties of endometrium that affect its growth.[42]

MONITORING THE FROZEN EMBRYO TRANSFER CYCLE

Involves a baseline ultrasound for all the patients irrespective of the protocol used. Baseline hormone profile to exclude cysts in selective cases after scan. In HRT cycles, estradiol valerate is started at a dose of 4 mg/day, and stepped-up to 6 mg/day. An ultrasound assessment of the endometrial lining is made between the 9th day and 11th day and estradiol dose can be increased up to 8–10 mg/day if required. A trilaminar pattern with a thickness of 7–9 mm or above is indicative of good proliferation. A blood test for serum progesterone is done, and vaginal progesterone is started. Embryo transfer is carried out 3/5 days later depending on the day it was frozen.

WHEN TO STOP PROGESTERONES?

The available data has been insufficient to determine the optimal duration of therapy, and prolonged progesterone protocols have been the rule, with most clinicians following the dictum, "better safe than sorry". A growing body of evidence, however, has challenged this concept and adds to the increasing concern that progesterone supplementation of early pregnancy after IVF/ ICSI might be unnecessary.

Frozen embryo transfer cycles with HRT and donor oocyte recipient cycles are different from stimulated IVF cycles in that there is no endogenous progesterone production, and therefore instead of luteal phase supplementation, there is a need for luteal phase "creation" or replacement.

Vaginal progesterone supplementation is equally effective and better tolerated by patients than intramuscular preparations. Sufficient evidence of efficacy and tolerability to make vaginal supplementation the main route of progesterone support in stimulated IVF cycles exists. Food and Drug Administration (FDA) has approved vaginal gel for supplementation at once daily dose and for replacement at twice daily dose.

Once daily vaginal gel, or twice or thrice daily micronized progesterone 200 mg thrice a day are optimal doses of vaginal progesterone for luteal phase support in IVF. Patients should have a choice about which preparation to use based on convenience and cost considerations.

CONCLUSION

A properly powered RCT is much needed to establish the best endometrial preparation protocol for FET cycles. Until then, based on the limited prospective data and conflicting retrospective results, it can be concluded that:

- Natural FET cycles are most appropriate for patients with regular ovulatory cycles who are able to comply with strict regimen of frequent urine and blood hormonal measurements. Luteal phase support with progesterone does not appear to increase pregnancy rates.
- Modified natural FET cycles require ultrasound monitoring and blood hormonal measurements for optimal timing of hCG trigger. Because of the luteotrophic effect of hCG, progesterone support after embryo transfer could be optional and should use the most convenient and cost-effective preparation.
- Programmed FET cycles are the most convenient with respect to limited monitoring requirements and ease and flexibility of scheduling. However, they have not been shown to be superior to properly timed natural or modified natural FET protocols.

Based on the current literature including the ANTARCTICA trial study with large numbers, it is not possible to identify one method of endometrial preparation in FET as being more effective than another.[43,44] Therefore, patients' individual patient factor and convenience, as well as costs should be considered when choosing the method of endometrial preparation.

REFERENCES

1. Ghobara T, Vandekerckhove P. Cycle regimens for frozen-thawed embryo transfer. Cochrane Database Syst Rev. 2008;1:CD003414.
2. Harper MJ. The implantation window. Baillieres Clin Obstet Gynaecol. 1992;6:351-71.
3. Tabibzadeh S, Shea W, Lessey BA, et al. From endometrial receptivity to infertility. J Semin Reprod Endocrinol. 1999;17:197-203.
4. Fatemi HM, Kyrou D, Bourgain C, et al. Cryopreserved-thawed human embryo transfer: spontaneous natural cycle is superior to human chorionic gonadotropin-induced natural cycle. Fertil Steril. 2010;94:2054-8.
5. Andersen AG, Als-Nielsen B, Hornnes PJ, et al. Time interval from human chorionic gonadotropin (hCG) injection to follicular rupture. Hum Reprod. 1995;10:3202-5.
6. Hoff JD, Quigley ME, Yen SS. Hormonal dynamics at midcycle: a reevaluation. J Clin Endocrinol Metab. 1983;57:792-6.
7. Frydman R, Testart J, Feinstein MC, et al. Interrelationshipof plasma and urinary luteinizing hormone preovulatory surge. J Steroid Biochem. 1984;20:617-9.
8. Miller PB, Soules MR. The usefulness of a urinary LH kit for ovulation prediction during menstrual cycles of normal women. Obstet Gynecol. 1996;87:13-7.
9. Park SJ, Goldsmith LT, Skurnick JH, et al. Characteristics of the urinary luteinizing hormone surge in young ovulatory women. Fertil Steril. 2007;88:684-90.
10. Guermandi E, Vegetti W, Bianchi MM, et al. Reliability of ovulation tests in infertile women. Obstet Gynecol. 2001;97:92-6.
11. O'Connor KA, Brindle E, Miller RC, et al. Ovulation detection methods for urinary hormones: precision, daily and intermittent sampling and a combined hierarchical method. Hum Reprod. 2006;21:1442-52.
12. Nawroth F, Ludwig M. What is the 'ideal' duration of progesterone supplementation before the transfer of cryopreserved-thawed embryos in estrogen/progesterone replacement protocols? Hum Reprod. 2005;20:1127-34.
13. Paulson RJ. Hormonal induction of endometrial receptivity. Fertil Steril. 2011;96:530-5.
14. Weissman A, Horowitz E, Ravhon A, et al. Spontaneous ovulation versus hCG triggering for timing natural-cycle frozenthawed embryo transfer: a randomized study. Reprod Biomed Online. 2011;23:484-9.
15. Chang EM, Han JE, Kim YS, et al. Use of the natural cycle and vitrification thawed blastocyst transfer results in better in-vitro fertilization outcomes: cycle regimens of vitrification thawed blastocyst transfer. J Assist Reprod Genet. 2011;28:369-74.
16. Tomax C, Alsbjerg B, Martikainen H, et al. Pregnancy loss after frozen-embryo transfer—a comparison of three protocols. Fertil Steril. 2012;98:1165-9.
17. Bjuresten K, Landgren BM, Hovatta O, et al. Lutealphase-progesteroneincreases live birth rate after frozen embryo transfer. Fertil Steril. 2011;95:534-7.
18. You-Jeong Lee, Kyung-Hee Lee, Su-Kyung Kwon, et al. The effect of luteal phase progesterone supplementation on natural frozen-thawed embryo transfer cycles. Obstet Gynecol Sci. 2014;57:291-6.
19. Bjuresten K, Landgren BM, Hovatta O, et al. Luteal phase progesterone increases live birth rate after frozen embryo transfer. Fertil Steril. 2011;95:534-7.
20. Kyrou D, Fatemi HM, Popovic-Todorovic B, et al. Vaginal progesterone supplementation has no effect on ongoing pregnancy rate in hCG-induced natural frozen-thawed embryo transfer cycles. Eur J Obstet Gynecol Reprod Biol. 2010;150:175-9.
21. Eftekhar M, Rahsepar M, Rahmani E. Effect of progesterone supplementation on natural frozen-thawed embryo transfer cycles: a randomized controlled trial. Int J Fertil Steril. 2013;7:13-20.
22. Karen P, Couck I, Debrock S, et al. Frozen-thawed embryo transfer in a natural or mildly hormonally stimulated cycle in women with regular ovulatory cycles: a RCT. Hum Reprod. 2015;30:2552-62.

23. Dal PL, Borini A. Best protocol for frozen-thawed embryo transfer-cost benefit analysis needed. Fertil Steril. 2006;86:1554-5.
24. El-Toukhy T, Taylor A, Khalaf Y, et al. Pituitary suppression in ultrasound-monitored frozen embryo replacement cycles. A randomized study. Hum Reprod. 2004;19:874-9.
25. Dor J, Rudak E, Davidson A, et al. Endocrine and biological factors influencing implantation of human embryos following cryopreservation. Gynecol Endocrinol. 1991;5:203-11.
26. Jaroudi KA, Hamilton CJ, Willemsen WN, et al. Artificial endometrial stimulation for frozen embryo replacement. Fertil Steril. 1991;55:835-7.
27. Niu Z, Feng Y, Sun Y, et al. Estrogen level monitoring in artificial frozen-thawed embryo transfer cycles using step-up regime without pituitary suppression: is it necessary? J Exp Clin Assist Reprod. 2008;5:4.
28. Navot D, Bergh PA, Williams M, et al. An insight into early reproductive processes through the in vivo model of ovum donation. J Clin Endocrinol Metab. 1991;72:408-14.
29. Borini A, Dal Prato L, Bianchi L, et al. Effect of duration of estradiol replacement on the outcome of oocyte donation. J Assist Reprod Genet. 2001;18:187-92.
30. Devroey P, Pados G. Preparation of endometrium for egg donation. Hum Reprod Update. 1998;4:856-61.
31. Hill MJ, Miller KA, Frattarelli JL. A GnRH agonist and exogenous hormone stimulation protocol has a higher live-birth rate than a natural endogenous hormone protocol for frozen-thawed blastocyst-stage embryo transfer cycles: an analysis of 1391 cycles. Fertil Steril. 2010;93:416-22.
32. Azimi Nekoo E, Chamani M, Shahrokh Tehrani E, et al. Artificial endometrial preparation for frozen-thawed embryo transfer with or without pretreatment with depot gonadotropin releasing hormone agonist in women with regular menses. J Family Reprod Health. 2015;9(1):1-4.
33. van de Vijver A, Polyzos NP, Van Landuyt L, et al. Cryopreserved embryo transfer in an artificial cycle: is GnRH agonist down-regulation necessary? Reprod BioMed Online. 2014;29:588-94.
34. Trounson A, Mohr L. Human pregnancy following cryopreservation, thawing and transfer of an eight-cell embryo. Nature. 1983;305:707-9.
35. Givens CR, Markun LC, Ryan IP, et al. Outcomes of natural cycles versus programmed cycles for 1677 frozen-thawed embryo transfers. Reprod Biomed Online. 2009;19:380-4.
36. Kumbak B, Erden HF, Tosun S, et al. Outcome of assisted reproduction treatment in patients with endometrial thickness less than 7 mm. Reprod Biomed Online. 2009;18:79-84.
37. Kasius A, Smit JG, Torrance HL, et al. Endometrial thickness and pregnancy rates after IVF: a systematic review and meta-analysis. Hum Reprod Update. 2014;20:530-41.
38. ElToukhy T, Coomarasamy A, Khairy M, et al. The relationship between endometrial thickness and outcome of medicated frozen embryo replacement cycles. Fertil Steril. 2008;89:832-9.
39. Gingold JA, Lee JA, Rodriguez-Purata J, et al. Endometrial pattern, but not endometrial thickness, affects implantation rates in euploid embryo transfers. Fertil Steril. 2015;104:620-8.e5.
40. Chen MJ, Yang JH, Peng FH, et al. Extended estrogen administration for women with thin endometrium in frozen-thawed in-vitro fertilization programs. J Assist Reprod Genet. 2006;23:337-42.
41. Mahajan N. Endometrial receptivity array: Clinical application. J Hum Reprod Sci. 2015;8:121-9.
42. Scioscia M, Lamanna G, Lorusso F, et al. Characterization of endometrial growth in proliferative and early luteal phase in IVF cycles. Reprod Biomed Online. 2009;18:73-8.
43. Groenewoud ER, Cohlen BJ, Al-Oraiby A, et al. A randomized controlled, non-inferiority trial of modified natural versus artificial cycle for cryo-thawed embryo transfer. Hum Reprod. 2016;31:1483-92.
44. Groenewoud ER, Macklon NS, Cohlen BJ, et al. Cryo-thawed embryo transfer: natural versus artificial cycle. A non-inferiority trial (ANTARCTICA trial). BMC Womens Health. 2012;12:27.

CHAPTER

54

Ovarian Stimulation Protocols in Fertility Preservation

Puneet R Arora

CANCER AND FERTILITY

Improvement in cancer therapies has led to improvement in cancer survival rates. This has not only led to increase in life expectancy but also highlighted issues affecting long-term survivors. The toxic effects of some of the chemotherapeutic agents like alkylating agents (e.g. cyclophosphamide, busulfan, and ifosfamide), which are common components of chemotherapy for breast cancer, lymphomas, leukemia, and sarcomas are well documented. Pelvic radiation therapy is also known to cause follicular destruction, and exposure to 5–10 Gy pelvic radiation appears to be toxic to oocytes, resulting in premature ovarian insufficiency in many women. These effects are dependent on age of the women at the time of treatment and the baseline ovarian reserve prior to starting the treatment for cancer. The potential adverse effect of the disease process itself remains unknown.

Oncofertility, a new sub-specialty bridging oncology care with reproductive medicine, addresses essential parts of comprehensive reproductive patient care prior to cancer therapy.

OPTIONS OF FERTILITY PRESERVATION IN CANCER PATIENTS

There is importance of reproduction for many cancer patients especially those who are young. In a survey conducted on young women affected by breast cancer,[1] more than half of respondents were concerned with infertility as side effect. As a part of cancer care and counseling, patient should be made aware of the possible long-term consequences of cancer therapy in the form of impairment of fertility. Available fertility preservation options should be discussed as a part of cancer counseling. The discussion with regard to fertility preservation at the time of diagnosis of cancer might not be taken that well and can pose a challenge. This should be done in a best possible way jointly with the treating oncologist. Embryo cryopreservation and oocyte cryopreservation are the standard options available at present. Embryo cryopreservation and oocyte cryopreservation both need ovarian stimulation prior to oocyte recovery. Other options such as cortical tissue cryopreservation, in vitro maturation of the immature oocytes and ovarian cryopreservation are very promising but at this stage are experimental and need further trials. Use of medical therapies like gonadotropin-releasing hormone (GnRH) agonist is controversial and needs further robust randomized controlled trials. The time interval available between the diagnosis and the initiation of the cancer therapy is an important aspect as to which available option to be utilized prior to starting cancer treatment.

EFFECT OF CANCER ON OVARIAN STIMULATION

Controlled ovarian hyperstimulation (COH) is essential for embryo and oocyte cryopreservation. This can be achieved with either conventional methods of ovarian stimulation or with random-start ovarian stimulation protocols (ROS). Recent studies[2,3] have demonstrated no significant change in ovarian reserve or response to gonadotropins in patients with different cancers who are undergoing in vitro fertilization (IVF) treatment. By contrast, others[4,5] have found a decline in ovarian response in cancer patients who are undergoing ovarian stimulation protocols to preserve their fertility prior to cancer therapy.

A recent meta-analysis[6] found a reduced number of oocytes in patients with malignancies undergoing COH for fertility preservation. One of the theories behind this varied response to ovarian stimulation is put down to the fact that cancer is typically a catabolic state increasing stress hormone levels and altering the hypothalamic pituitary axis thereby impairing reproductive capacity. Many patients also experience weight loss that could also affect hypothalamic pituitary axis. Stress can lead to increase in prolactin and endogenous opioids, which could also affect ovary and its responsiveness. Another study[7] to evaluate COH in women with cancer compared with healthy women found no significant differences in the number of oocytes retrieved, number of mature oocytes retrieved and the number of oocytes fertilized. However, the patients with cancer had longer duration of stimulation and higher total dose of gonadotropin, which could be explained by some element of hypothalamic dysfunction. There is also varied stimulation response seen in cancer patients positive for BRCA mutations. Mutations in BRCA genes are associated with an increased risk of breast and ovarian cancers. A low response to ovarian stimulation in BRCA mutation positive breast cancer patients was seen in another study.[8]

OVARIAN STIMULATION PROTOCOLS IN CANCER PATIENTS

Proper understanding of the reproductive endocrinology is essential when planning ovarian stimulation protocols for such group of women as they may present in any part of their menstrual cycle and patients are not advised to delay the start of preservation. At the same time, achieving optimal reproductive outcome is of paramount importance in such group of women as well as they may not get another chance of considering their reproductive potential. Protocols for ovarian stimulation can be broadly divided into:

1. Conventional protocols of ovarian stimulation (COS)
2. Random start ovarian stimulation protocols (ROS).

Conventional methods of ovarian stimulation are related with onset of menstrual cycle. It involves initiation of the gonadotropins for ovarian stimulation in the follicular phase of the menstrual cycle for approximately 10–14 days to achieve multi-follicular development. The suppression of luteinizing hormone (LH) surge for spontaneous ovulation has been successfully achieved either with GnRH agonist started in the preceding luteal phase or with GnRH antagonist started when the dominant follicle has attained diameter of 14 mm or on day 6 of ovarian stimulation. GnRH antagonist protocols may offer advantage in ovarian stimulation for cancer patients by shortening the time frame from patient presentation to embryo/oocyte cryopreservation, but this protocol still requires onset of menses before initiating ovarian stimulation. Waiting for onset of menstrual cycle prior to starting ovarian stimulation for fertility preservation prior to initiation of cancer treatment can increase the stress and anxiety of patient and treating oncologist with regards to outcome of cancer therapies and hence prevent patients from forgoing fertility preservation treatment. This has been overcome by ROS.

With better understanding of the reproductive physiology, endocrinology and ovarian folliculogenesis, ROS have been developed to minimize the time interval needed for initiation of ovarian stimulation and hence with a hope to increase the uptake of these fertility preserving strategies. It is no longer felt that there is a single wave of folliculogenesis initiating in the follicular phase but there are two to three waves in one interovulatory cycle. Studies on changes in ovarian follicular dynamics during the human menstrual cycle have now well documented that there are wave like changes in follicle number rather than a single cohort of antral follicles occurring only during the follicular phase of the menstrual cycle. This concept has been used in providing ovarian stimulation in any part of the menstrual cycle and has been extrapolated to providing ovarian stimulation prior to cancer therapies, as this subgroup of women can present in any part of the menstrual cycle. The rest of the pattern of stimulation with regards to dose and type of gonadotropins is very much similar as in conventional protocols.

Depending on the timing of presentation in relation to menstrual cycle, random start protocols can be divided into starting controlled ovarian stimulation in early follicular phase, late follicular phase, early luteal phase, and late luteal phase (Figs. 1A to E).[9] Early follicular phase is defined as presentation within first 7 days of onset of menstruation. Late follicular phase is primarily defined as presentation after 7 days of onset of menstrual cycle, or presence of dominant follicle of more than 12 mm diameter or progesterone level less than 2 ng/mL. Early luteal phase is defined as presentation within first 7 days after ovulation. Late luteal phase is presentation within last 7 days of the last menstrual cycle. Late follicular phase and early luteal phase are the most challenging time for random start ovarian stimulation protocol.

Presentation in early follicular phase can very similarly be treated like conventional stimulation regimens with GnRH antagonist protocol provided there is no dominant follicle more than 12 mm. If there is already dominant follicle more than 12 mm, it can then be treated as being in late follicular phase, which will be discussed subsequently.

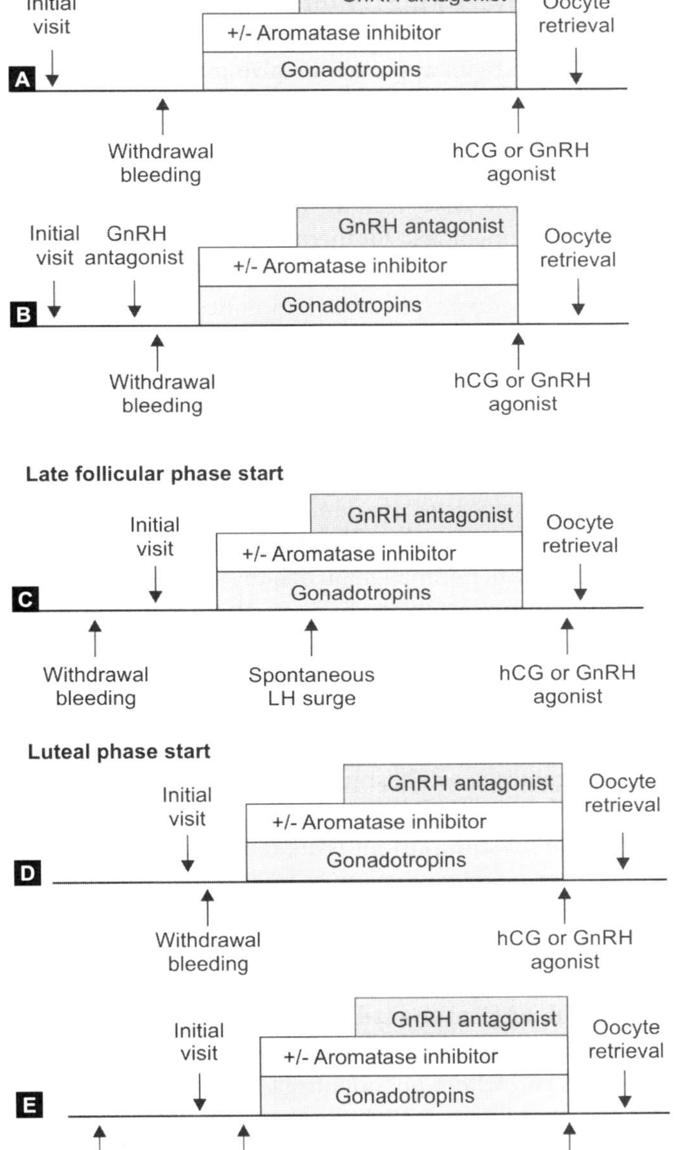

Figs. 1A to E: Conventional and random-start antagonist in vitro fertilization (IVF) protocols for cancer patients undergoing fertility preservation.[9] (A) COS can be started with spontaneous menses; (B) or with menses following luteolysis induced by gonadotropin-releasing hormone (GnRH) antagonist; (C) COS can also be initiated in the late follicular; (D) or luteal phase following spontaneous luteinizing hormone (LH) surge; (E) or after ovulation induction with human chorionic gonadotropin (hCG) or GnRH agonist.

Late follicular ovarian stimulation involves assessment of the ovaries for the presence or absence of dominant follicles. If the ovary contains dominant follicle more than 12 mm, further management would involve leutolysis of the dominant follicle with either GnRH antagonist or progesterone followed by stimulation for the rest of the follicles. Prior to leutolysis, stimulation of the follicle with minimal dose of follicle-stimulating hormone (FSH) until the follicle reaches 18 mm followed by triggering and aspiration of the follicle and preserving it if viable. GnRH antagonist is then administered for 4–5 days depending on the ovarian reserve of the patient, ovarian stimulation can then be started by appropriate gonadotropins based on age, ovarian reserve parameters [anti-Müllerian hormone (AMH) and antral follicular count (AFC)].

Early luteal phase is defined as the completion of spontaneous luteinizing hormone (LH) surge and presence of corpus luteum in the ovaries. Early and late luteal phase can be essentially treated in the same way. Leutolysis of the corpus luteum can be achieved by GnRH antagonist 3 mg stat or in multiple doses of 0.25 mg for 4–5 days. The objective of antagonist is to achieve estradiol levels below 60 pg/mL and not to delay the stimulation cycle until the start of new menstrual cycle. This can be followed by gonadotropin stimulation in conventional way preferably with recombinant FSH avoiding exogenous LH activity, which might prevent leutolysis. Pituitary suppression for LH surge by GnRH antagonist can be initiated in usual way when the dominant follicle reaches 14 mm and use of either human chorionic gonadotropin (hCG) or GnRH agonist for trigger of the final maturation of the oocyte.

The dose of gonadotropin should be individualized depending on age, ovarian reserve, and weight of the patient. Using higher doses of gonadotropins can be one of the strategies to increase the embryo and oocyte yield per cycle. In a study comparing a low-dose antagonist IVF protocol (150 IU FSH) and a higher-dose antagonist IVF protocol (>150 IU) in cancer patients, although the number of follicles more than 17 mm was greater in the higher-dose group, there was no difference in numbers of oocytes generated between the two groups.[10] That study suggests that the use of higher doses of gonadotropins may not necessarily result in higher oocyte/embryo yield consistent with the theory that higher doses of gonadotropins may stimulate the recruitment of chromosomally abnormal or incompetent oocytes.[11] However, in patients with decreased ovarian reserve as assessed with the use of AFC and/or AMH, higher doses of gonadotropins may be required.

The studies have suggested that these protocols have been able to provide reasonable number of mature eggs able to fertilize but the exact implantation potential and subsequent pregnancy rates of embryos and oocytes retrieved through these protocols is still unanswered. Being relatively new and being tried mainly in cases in cancer patients, these have been reported in very few studies.

Controlled ovarian stimulation leads to elevation of the serum estradiol levels up to 10–15 times higher than physiological levels. In women with estrogen sensitive breast tumors, to avoid this elevation, addition of aromatase inhibitors (letrozole) and tamoxifem is recommended. The peak of estradiol in the protocols of ovarian stimulation with tamoxifen or with letrozole is slightly higher than the levels achieved in natural cycle around 300–350 pg/mL. Letrozole (5 mg/day) or tamoxifen (20–40 mg/day) is usually administered 2–3 days prior to starting gonadotropins. Study by Oktay et al.[12] concluded that stimulation protocols using letrozole alongside with gonadotropins are currently preferred over tamoxifen protocols as treatment with letrozole results in a higher number of oocytes obtained and fertilized when compared to tamoxifen protocols.

There has been a case report by Reichmann et al.[13] of using these ovarian stimulation protocols for oocyte vitrification in prepubertal girls diagnosed with cancer that have not yet attained menarche and hence got no gonadotropin recruitable follicles. This has been reported as having successful ovarian stimulation and oocyte retrieval. This approach needs further robust evidence before it can be widely applicable to such groups of cancer affected females.

The goal of superovulation for this group of patients represents a compromise between obtaining a relatively large number of oocytes for vitrification, to maximize chances of later pregnancy, and the absolute need for avoidance of ovarian hyperstimulation in a patient who will shortly begin chemotherapy.

The patients referred for fertility preservation may not necessarily represent the typical population of subfertile patients treated in IVF units. Cancer may affect multiple tissues throughout the body and can result in a variety of complications during ovarian stimulation. Cancer may induce hypercoagulable state and when combined with increased serum estradiol levels may put cancer patients undergoing controlled ovarian stimulation at increased risk of thromboembolic events. Therefore, consideration should be given for commencement of anticoagulation therapy around the time of ovarian stimulation. The other strategy of preventing thromboembolic events is to use letrozole during ovarian stimulation as in women undergoing ovarian stimulation with estrogen sensitive malignancies to keep estradiol levels close to less than 500 pg/mL. Letrozole or GnRH antagonist should be continued even after oocyte retrieval for up to a week depending on the estradiol levels at the time of ovulation induction.

Some blood-borne malignancies may alter the hemostatic function and may create a tendency toward bleeding during oocyte retrieval owing to thrombocytopenia, platelet dysfunction, or defective coagulation factor synthesis. Collaborative team approach involving hematologist and anesthetist should be preferred to prevent complication of bleeding in these patients. Pelvic infection after oocyte retrieval can be a problem especially in neutropenic patients. In the case of neutropenia, consultation from the patient's oncologist for the use of granulocyte colony-stimulating factor to increase the neutrophil count should be obtained, and prophylactic antibiotics should be given before oocyte retrieval to decrease the risk of infection. Cancers involving tracheal compression, or large pleural effusion, may preclude safe administration of anesthesia for oocyte pick up. This should be discussed with anesthetists prior to starting ovarian stimulation.

Another aspect of ovarian stimulation, which needs further consideration, is the fact that success in vitrification has been seen in nonmalignant healthy infertile population and little information is obtained about vitrification in cancer patients though studies have shown no difference in oocytes and embryos derived from patients with cancer and in nonmalignant conditions.

Successful implementation of fertility preservation services requires establishing liaisons with reproductive specialists and oncology colleagues. Whilst survival is clearly the most important issue facing a young woman with cancer, it is clear that future fertility is also important. A rapid and efficient referral system with minimal delay can bring good results and this can be established in close collaboration and effective communication with colleagues in medical, surgical and radiation oncology.

In cancer patients, antagonist protocols should be preferred and where possible trigger for final maturation to be planned with GnRH agonist to prevent the risk of ovarian hyperstimulation syndrome (OHSS). The impact of OHSS can be profound and all measures should be taken to prevent it. In cancer patients, its effect can be more profound as it may result in delaying or complicating planned life-saving cancer therapy.

REFERENCES

1. Partridge AH, Gilbert S, Peppercorn J, et al. Web-based survey of fertility issues in young women with breast cancer. J Clin Oncol. 2004;22:4174-83.
2. Van Casteren NJ, Boellaard WP, Romijn JC, et al. Gonadal dysfunction in male cancer patients before cytotoxic treatment. Int J Androl. 2010;33:73-9.

3. Knopman JM, Noyes N, Talebian S, et al. Women with cancer undergoing ART for fertility preservation: a cohort study of their response to exogenous gonadotropins. Fertil Steril. 2009;91:1476-8.
4. Pal L, Leykin L, Schifren JL, et al. Malignancy may adversely influence the quality and behavior of oocytes. Hum Reprod. 1998;13:1837-40.
5. Quintero RB, Helmer A, Huang JQ, et al. Ovarian stimulation for fertility preservation in patients with cancer. Fertil Steril. 2010;93:865-8.
6. Friedler S, Koc O, Gidoni Y, et al. Ovarian response to stimulation for fertility preservation in women with malignant disease: a systematic review and meta-analysis. Fertil Steril. 2012;97:125-33.
7. Das M, Shehata F, Moria A, et al. Ovarian reserve, response to gonadotropins, and oocyte maturity in women with malignancy. Fertil Steril. 2011;96:122-5.
8. Oktay K, Kim JY, Barad D, et al. Association of BRCA1 mutations with occult primary ovarian insufficiency: a possible explanation for the link between infertility and breast/ovarian cancer risks. J Clin Oncol. 2010;28:240-4.
9. Cakmak H, Rosen MP. Ovarian stimulation in cancer patients. Fertil Steril. 2013;99:1476-84.
10. Lee S, Oktay K. Does higher starting dose of FSH stimulation with letrozole improve fertility preservation outcomes in women with breast cancer? Fertil Steril. 2012;98:961-4.e1.
11. Baart EB, Martini E, Eijkemans MJ, et al. Milder ovarian stimulation for in-vitro fertilization reduces aneuploidy in the human preimplantation embryo: a randomized controlled trial. Hum Reprod. 2007;22:980-8.
12. Oktay K, Buyuk E, Libertella N, et al. Fertility preservation in breast cancer patients: a prospective controlled comparison of ovarian stimulation with tamoxifen and letrozole for embryo cryopreservation. J Clin Oncol. 2005;23:4347-53.
13. Reichmann DE, Davis OK, Zaninovic N, et al. Fertility preservation utilizing controlled ovarian hyper-stimulation and oocyte cryo-preservation in a pre-menarcheal female with myelodysplastic syndrome. Fertil Steril. 2012;98:1225-8.

CHAPTER

55

Complications of Ovarian Stimulation: Prevention and Management

Julia K Bosdou, Stratis Kolibianakis

INTRODUCTION

The goal of ovarian stimulation is to induce development of multiple follicles and in the case of in vitro fertilization (IVF) to enable the retrieval of several oocytes. This approach has led to increased pregnancy rates[1,2] in infertile couples, however, it might be accompanied by complications. The most serious complications of ovarian stimulation are ovarian hyperstimulation syndrome (OHSS)[3] and multiple pregnancy.[4] In addition, ovarian stimulation has also been associated with adnexal torsion[5] and thromboembolic events.[6]

Clinicians should be familiar with these complications and understand the underlying pathophysiological mechanisms, in order to be able to adequately prevent, recognize and manage them. Although this is true for any medical intervention, it is especially important in assisted reproductive technologies (ART), since ovarian stimulation is applied to otherwise healthy women longing for parenthood.

OVARIAN HYPERSTIMULATION SYNDROME

Ovarian hyperstimulation syndrome is the most serious iatrogenic complication of ovarian stimulation that is triggered by exogenous administration of human chorionic gonadotropin (hCG), used for induction of final oocyte maturation and/or by its endogenous production in cases of pregnancy. OHSS can be early or late, based on the time of its onset. Early OHSS occurs in the early luteal phase, within 10 days from oocyte retrieval,[7] while late OHSS occurs in the late luteal phase, more than or equal to 10 days from oocyte retrieval and usually in cycles leading to pregnancy.[8]

Ovarian hyperstimulation syndrome has traditionally been classified as mild, moderate, severe or critical[9,10] (Fig. 1). Mild and moderate OHSS do not require specific treatment and patients can be treated symptomatically

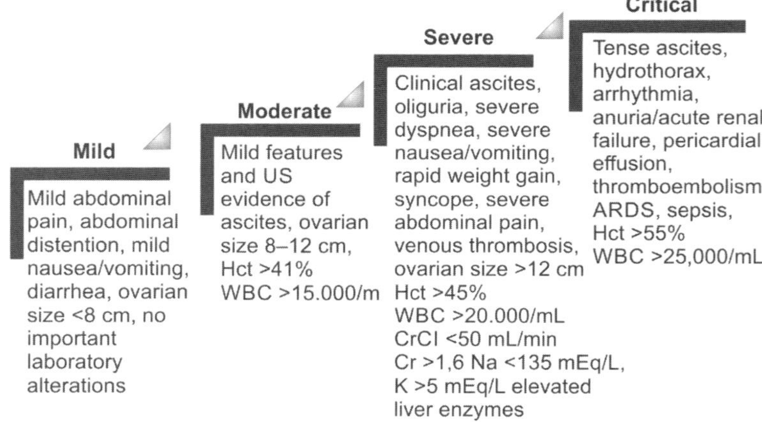

Fig. 1: Classification of ovarian hyperstimulation syndrome (OHSS): clinical symptoms and laboratory features. (Hct: hematocrit; WBC: white blood cell; CrCl: creatinine clearance; Cr: creatinine; ARDS: acute respiratory distress syndrome).

Source: Adapted from Navot D, Bergh PA, Laufer N. Ovarian hyperstimulation syndrome in novel reproductive technologies: prevention and treatment. Fertil Steril. 1992;58:249-61.

Mathur R, Jenkins J. Towards a clinically useful classification of OHSS. Reprod Biomed Online. 2009;19:434.

on an outpatient basis. On the other hand, severe OHSS requires patient hospitalization.

Although most OHSS cases will occur during ovarian stimulation for IVF, this is also possible, albeit less frequently, in patients undergoing ovulation induction or enhancement of ovulation.

Ovarian Hyperstimulation Syndrome after Ovulation Induction/Enhancement of Ovulation

In anovulatory women, such as those with polycystic ovarian syndrome (PCOS), the goal of ovarian stimulation is to induce monofollicular growth.[2] For this purpose, several approaches have been proposed, the most commonly used being clomiphene citrate (CC), aromatase inhibitors or low-dose gonadotropins.

Clomiphene citrate, the standard first-line treatment for ovulation induction, acts as an estrogen receptor blocker, leading to elevation of endogenous follicle-stimulating hormone (FSH) production, which in turn stimulates follicular development.[11] This inexpensive, simple and widely used approach is considered quite efficient since it may lead to ovulation in about 75% of patients.[12]

Letrozole is an aromatase inhibitor which has been introduced as an alternative treatment to CC for ovulation induction in women with PCOS. Even though it is still an off-label drug in many countries, it is considered an efficient treatment for ovulation induction, by inhibiting the aromatase activity and thus inducing an hypoestrogenic state that stimulates the release of FSH.[13]

Clomiphene citrate and letrozole usually lead to induction of monofollicular development [CC: 54.85%, 95% confidence interval (CI): 40.3–68.9; letrozole: 79.49%, 95% CI: 65.3–88.9].[14] Not unexpectedly, the incidence of OHSS with the use of both CC and letrozole is very rare. In a meta-analysis of randomized controlled trials (RCTs), comparing aromatase inhibitors with CC for ovulation induction in subfertile women with PCOS, no OHSS cases were reported in 1,809 patients, while no difference was present in the incidence of OHSS when letrozole was compared with CC [risk difference (RD): 0.00, 95% CI: –0.01 to 0.00][15] (Figs. 2A and B).

An alternative treatment of infertility in anovulatory women with PCOS involves the use of low-dose gonadotropins.[16] Based on the meta-analysis by Weiss et al. (2015), the incidence of OHSS in PCOS patients with the use of low-dose recombinant FSH (rFSH) is 2% (95% CI: 1–3) (Fig. 3) and is not dependent on the type of gonadotropins used.[17] However, it has to be noted that in the majority of the RCTs included in that meta-analysis, either no definition of OHSS was given or the definition was variable, while hCG was not administered in case of excessive response using variable criteria.

Clomiphene citrate, letrozole as well as low-dose gonadotropins have also been used for enhancement of ovulation in women with unexplained infertility. However, since in these patients, the target of ovarian stimulation is to allow development of two to three follicles, in order to increase the probability of conception, CC and letrozole, whose administration is associated usually with monofollicular development, are less frequently used. No cases of OHSS after CC administration for unexplained fertility were reported in meta-analyses of relevant RCTs comparing CC with letrozole[18] (Figs. 4A and B).

Based on data reported in a meta-analysis of RCTs employing ovarian stimulation with the use of low dose gonadotropins for the treatment of women with unexplained infertility, male infertility or mild endometriosis, the incidence of OHSS (for which, however, no definition was given) was 2% (95% CI: 0–3)[19] (Fig. 5).

In an attempt to reduce the risk of OHSS when an excessive follicle number has developed following ovulation induction or enhancement of ovulation, cycle cancellation by withholding hCG or conversion of the cycle to IVF/embryo transfer have been proposed. In this way, the occurrence of OHSS is largely prevented,[20-23] although it can still occur. However, it should be noted that cycle cancellation has been associated with patient's disappointment and dissatisfaction, whereas conversion to IVF might not be acceptable by the patient due to financial constraints.[22]

Ovarian Hyperstimulation Syndrome after Multifollicular Development for In Vitro Fertilization

Based on data provided by the European IVF-monitoring Consortium, the incidence of OHSS (for which, however, no definition was given) in Europe, is estimated to be 0.78% (95% CI: 0.74–0.82) of all stimulated IVF cycles.[1] Moreover, data from the USA show that the incidence of severe OHSS is 0.28% (95% CI: 0.25–0.31).[24] Based on published meta-analyses of RCTs comparing gonadotropin-releasing hormone (GnRH) agonists with antagonists[25] and recombinant daily FSH versus corifollitropin alfa,[26] the incidence of OHSS varies from 1.3% to 20.3% according to the characteristics of the patients treated and the type of IVF protocol used (Table 1).

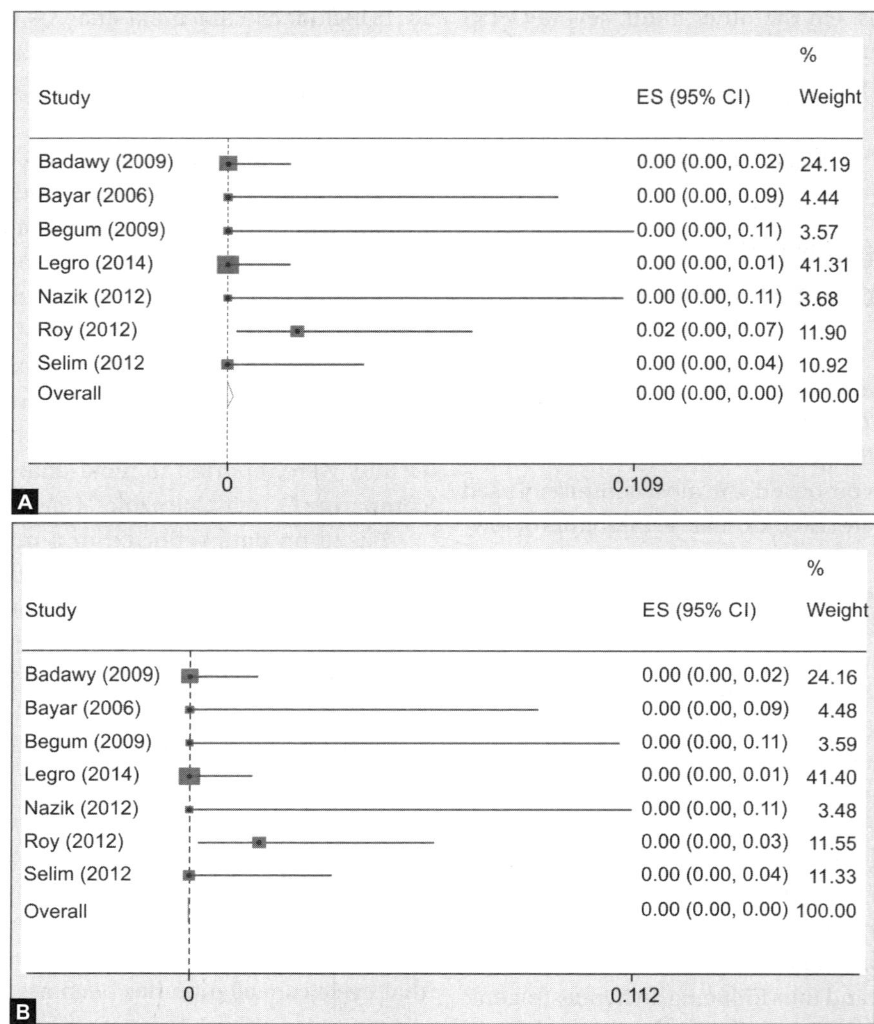

Figs. 2A and B: (A) Incidence of ovarian hyperstimulation syndrome (OHSS) with the use of clomiphene citrate (CC) in polycystic ovarian syndrome (PCOS) patients; (B) Incidence of OHSS with the use of letrozole in PCOS patients. (ES: estimate; CI: confidence interval).

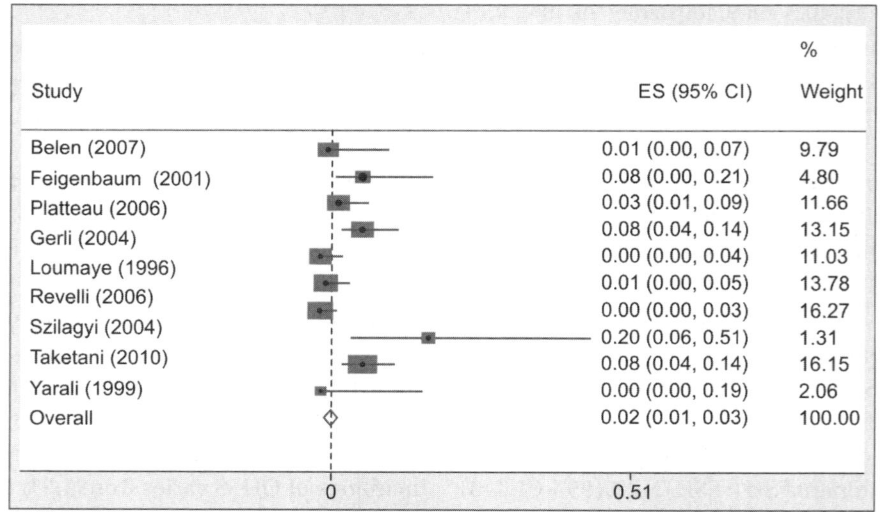

Fig. 3: Incidence of ovarian hyperstimulation syndrome (OHSS) with the use of low-dose recombinant follicle-stimulating hormone (FSH) in polycystic ovarian syndrome (PCOS) patients. (ES: estimate; CI: confidence interval).

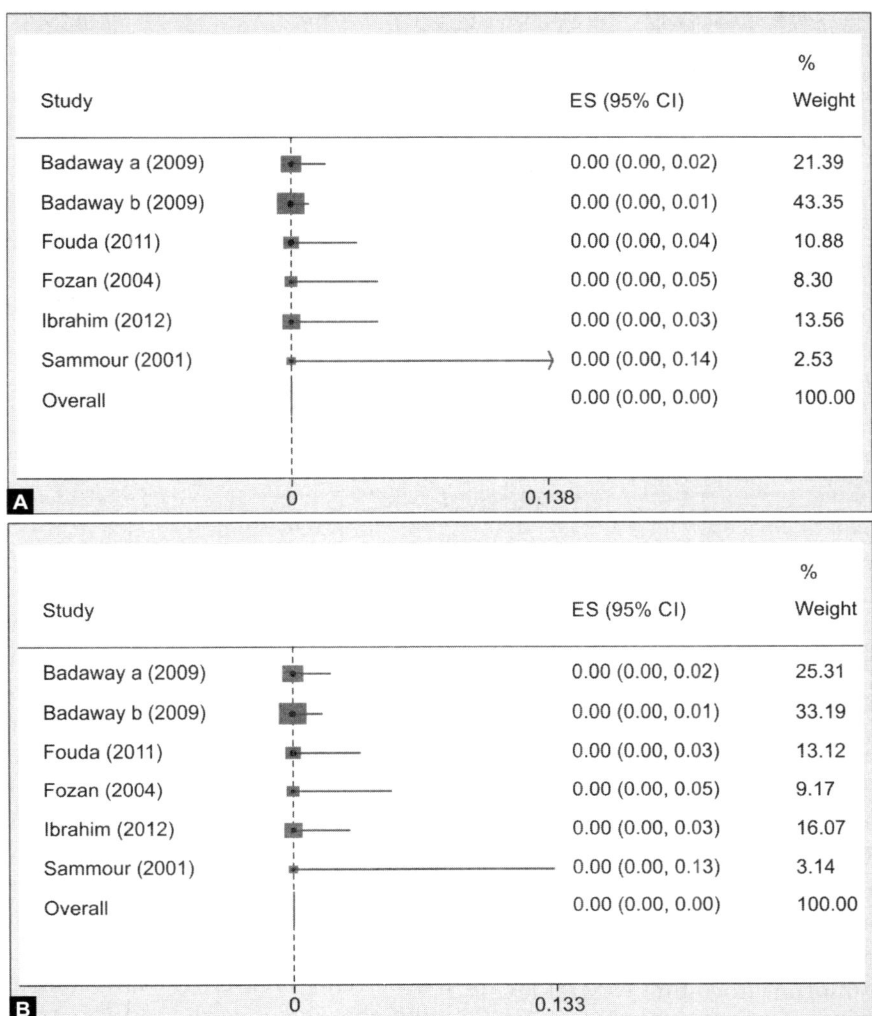

Figs. 4A and B: (A) Incidence of ovarian hyperstimulation syndrome (OHSS) with the use of clomiphene citrate (CC) in patients with unexplained fertility; (B) Incidence of OHSS with the use of letrozole in patients with unexplained fertility. (ES: estimate; CI: confidence interval).

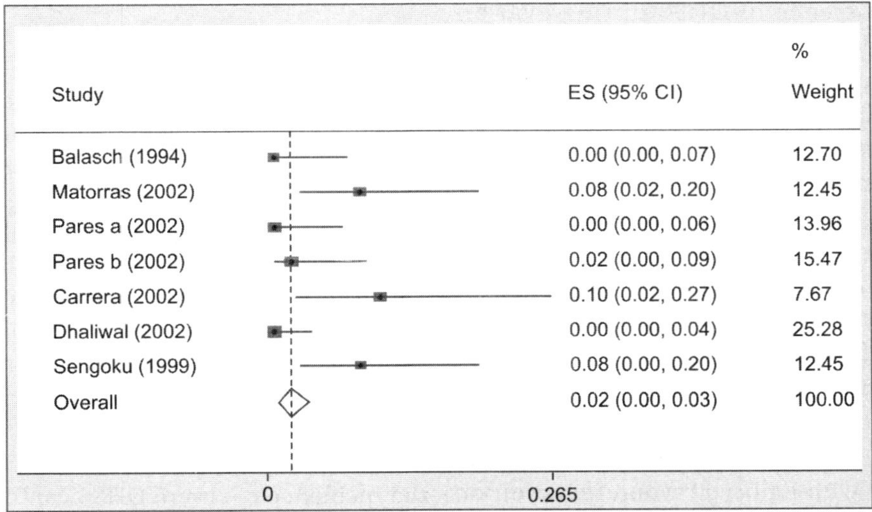

Fig. 5: Incidence of ovarian hyperstimulation syndrome (OHSS) with the use of low-dose recombinant follicle-stimulating hormone in patients with unexplained fertility, male infertility or mild endometriosis. (ES: estimate; CI: confidence interval).

Table 1: Incidence of ovarian hyperstimulation syndrome (OHSS) according to the characteristics of the patients treated and the type of in vitro fertilization (IVF) protocol used in published meta-analyses of randomized controlled trials (RCTs) comparing gonadotropin-releasing hormone (GnRH) agonists with antagonists and recombinant daily follicle-stimulating hormone (FSH) versus corifollitropin alfa.

Protocol	*Population*	*Source*	*Incidence %*	*95% CI*
GnRH agonists	All women	Al-Inany, 2011	9	7.7–10.5
GnRH agonists	PCOS	Al-Inany, 2011	20.3	16–25.5
GnRH antagonists	All women	Al-Inany, 2011	3.2	2.6–4
GnRH antagonists	PCOS	Al-Inany, 2011	4.8	2.9–7.9
Corifollitropin alfa	Normal responders	Tarlatzis, 2012	1.8	1.1–2.8
rFSH	Normal responders	Tarlatzis, 2012	1.3	0.7–2.2

(GnRH: gonadotropin-releasing hormone; PCOS: polycystic ovarian syndrome; rFSH: recombinant follicle-stimulating hormone).
Source: Adapted from Al-Inany HG, Youssef MA, Aboulghar M, et al. Gonadotrophin-releasing hormone antagonists for assisted reproductive technology. Cochrane Database Syst Rev. 2011;5:CD001750.
Tarlatzis BC, Griesinger G, Leader A, et al. Comparative incidence of ovarian hyperstimulation syndrome following ovarian stimulation with corifollitropin alfa or recombinant FSH. Reprod Biomed Online. 2012;24:410-9.

Prevention of Ovarian Hyperstimulation Syndrome

Although a substantial decrease in the incidence of severe OHSS has been observed following the introduction of GnRH antagonists, severe OHSS is still possible, especially in high risk patients, such as those with PCOS.

Prevention of OHSS can be attempted at different time points and preferably before the initiation of ovarian stimulation. This is feasible by identifying known risk factors for OHSS and classifying patients accordingly. For this purpose, important variables to consider include history of OHSS, assessment of the antral follicle count (AFC) and of anti-Müllerian hormone (AMH) levels. Following assessment of OHSS risk, selection of appropriate stimulation protocols, dose individualization and tight monitoring of ovarian stimulation are essential. Alarming signals for the occurrence of OHSS during ovarian stimulation are a rapid rise of estradiol (E2) levels, very high E2 levels or an excessive number of developing follicles. In an attempt to predict high-risk patients for developing severe OHSS, a cut-off value for more than or equal to 19 follicles of more than or equal to 11 mm on the day of hCG has been proposed, yielding a sensitivity of 74.3% and a specificity of 75.3%.[27]

Several strategies have been suggested to minimize the risk of severe OHSS after hCG administration, including co-administration of dopamine agonists, intravenous administration of albumin, hydroxyethyl starch (HES), low-dose aspirin, ketoconazole, corticosteroids, metformin, "coasting", continuation of GnRH agonist administration after hCG combined with embryo cryopreservation or reduction of the hCG dose used to trigger final oocyte maturation. However, the use of these strategies can only decrease the incidence of severe OHSS but not result in its elimination.[28]

The use of GnRH antagonists for suppressing premature luteinizing hormone(LH) surge has made feasible the substitution of hCG for final oocyte maturation with GnRH agonists. This has changed dramatically clinical practice in ART, resulting in the virtual elimination of severe OHSS, increasing in this way the safety of ovarian stimulation to the benefit of infertile couples.[29] The replacement of hCG with a GnRH agonist for triggering final oocyte maturation avoids the sustained hCG stimulation of corpora lutea for 10 days. With the use of GnRH agonist triggering, the endogenously elicited LH lasts only 24–36 hours, decreasing in this way the occurrence of severe OHSS as compared to hCG. However, the absence of corpora lutea stimulation results in low steroids levels and is associated with a decreased probability of pregnancy after fresh embryo transfer.[30]

In an effort to enhance the endogenous sex steroid production and restore the deficient luteal phase after triggering with GnRH agonist, hCG supplementation in the luteal phase has been proposed. However, severe OHSS is still present with this strategy.[31] Other alternative approaches include the luteal supplementation with recLH after triggering with GnRH agonist,[32] the dual triggering of final oocyte maturation with the combination of GnRH agonist and hCG,[33] the stimulation of endogenous LH levels with repeated GnRH agonist administration,[34] the intensive luteal phase steroid supplementation after GnRH agonist triggering[35] and the administration of GnRH antagonist in the luteal phase and cryopreservation of all embryos.[36,37] Although no severe OHSS cases were observed following these approaches, no firm conclusions regarding the incidence of severe OHSS can be drawn, due to the small number of studies performed and the participants included.[30]

A simpler approach to the problem of low pregnancy rates, due to a defective luteal phase after GnRH agonist triggering, is to avoid any attempt of enhancing either LH activity or steroid levels and instead defer embryo transfer in a subsequent cycle. In this way, embryo transfer takes place in a normally developed endometrium with optimal chances to support implantation. This is the basis for the "freeze all" approach after GnRH agonist triggering.[38] By synthesizing the results from all available studies until November 2015, prospective and retrospective,[39-50] in which GnRH agonist was used for triggering final oocyte maturation and no luteal phase support was administered,[30] the incidence of severe OHSS was 0% (95% CI: 0–0) (Fig. 6).

Management of Ovarian Hyperstimulation Syndrome

The management of OHSS depends on its severity and the presence or absence of pregnancy. The basic principles for evaluating, monitoring and managing severe OHSS are shown in Figure 7.[51,52]

Outpatient Management of Ovarian Hyperstimulation Syndrome

Women undergoing outpatient management of OHSS should be appropriately counseled and provided with information regarding fluid intake and output monitoring.

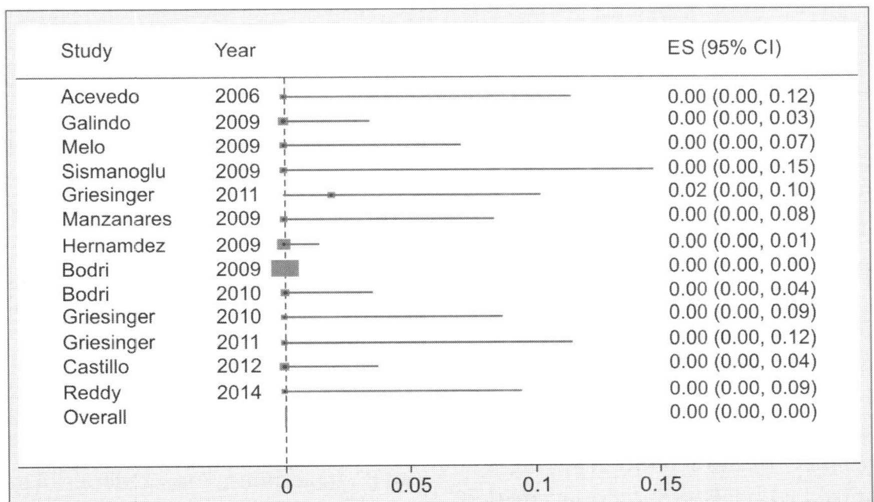

Fig. 6: Estimated probability of severe ovarian hyperstimulation syndrome (OHSS) in patients triggered by gonadotropin-releasing hormone (GnRH) agonist. (ES: estimate; CI: confidence interval).
Source: Adapted from Tarlatzis B, Bosdou J, Kolibianakis E. Elimination of OHSS by GnRH Agonist and Freezing Embryos. In: Rizk B, Gerris J (Eds). Complications and Outcomes of Assisted Reproduction. United Kingdom: Cambridge University Press; 2017. pp. 149-63.

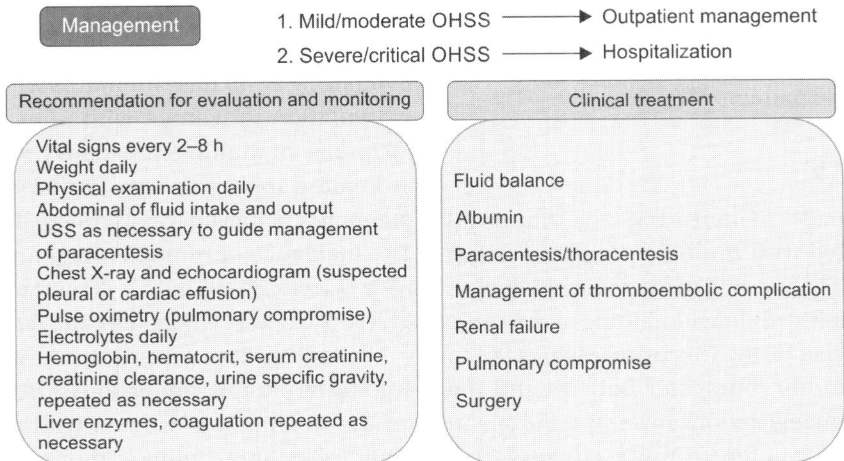

Fig. 7: Management of ovarian hyperstimulation syndrome (OHSS).

Nonsteroidal anti-inflammatory agents should be avoided, as they may compromise renal function. Women with severe OHSS being managed on an outpatient basis should receive thromboprophylaxis. In patients with severe OHSS, outpatient ultrasound-guided paracentesis has been suggested as a safe alternative to hospitalization for the management of OHSS in an outpatient setting.[51,52]

Hospitalization

Assessment of severity usually involves physical examination, recording of vital signs, body weight, abdominal circumference, ultrasound examination and laboratory tests such as hemoglobin, hematocrit, serum creatinine, electrolytes, liver enzymes and coagulation.[10] Since symptomatic moderate or severe OHSS is a hypovolemic state, the mainstay of treatment involves fluid resuscitation, supportive care, paracentesis and prophylactic anticoagulation.[52]

There are no trials on the optimum method for maintaining fluid balance in women with severe OHSS.[10] Women with hemoconcentration and dehydration may need more intensive initial rehydration and may benefit from colloids such as human albumin, HES, dextran or mannitol.

Paracentes is under ultrasound guidance should be carried out for patients with severe discomfort, abdominal pain, respiratory distress or oliguria due to the large amount of ascites.[52] Symptomatic hydrothorax persisting despite abdominal paracentesis may be drained directly.[10]

All patients hospitalized with OHSS shouldbeprovided with prophylactic anticoagulation to avoid the potentially serious effects of thromboembolism. The duration of thromboprophylaxis should be individualized according to patient risk factors and outcome of treatment.[51,52]

Since the risk of adnexal torsion or ovarian rupture appears to be increased in women with OHSS, particularly in the presence of pregnancy, surgery is indicated as a treatment option in these patients.[51,52]

Multiple Pregnancy

The increased incidence of maternal and neonatal complications associated with multiple pregnancies has been well recognized.[53,54] Thus, one of the main challenges in ART is to avoid multiples while maintaining at the same time the probability of live birth. This principle has led to significant changes in embryo transfer policies and the establishment of relevant legislations in several European countries. Moreover, it has led to more conservative approaches to ovulation induction and enhancement of ovulation which are responsible for the majority of multiple pregnancies in infertility treatment.[55-57]

Ovulation Induction/Enhancement of Ovulation

As it has already been mentioned, both the use of letrozole and CC lead to monofollicular development in the majority of women treated. Thus, the expected incidence of multiple pregnancy with their use is low. Indeed, based on data reported in the meta-analysis by Franik et al. (2014), comparing aromatase inhibitors with CC for ovulation induction in patients with PCOS, the incidence of multiple pregnancy per patient treated with the use of aromatase inhibitors was 0% (95% CI: 0–1), while that with the use of CC was 1% (95% CI: 0–2) (Figs. 8A and B). The incidence of multiple pregnancy per pregnancy achieved with the use of aromatase inhibitors was 0% (95% CI: 0–1), while that with the use of CC was 3% (95% CI: 1–6) (Figs. 9A and B). The difference in the incidence of multiple pregnancy per woman treated between these two agents used for ovulation induction was not statistically significant [odds ratio (OR): 0.41, 95% CI: 0.17–1.01].[15]

Based on data reported in the meta-analysis by Weiss et al. (2015), comparing various types of gonadotropins for ovulation induction in women with PCOS and CC resistance or CC failure, the incidence of multiple pregnancy per woman treated with low-dose rFSH was 2% (95% CI: 1–3),[17] while that per pregnancy was 7% (95% CI: 3–12), (Figs. 10A and B). In addition, the incidence of multiple pregnancy per woman treated with urinary FSH was 2% (95% CI: 1–3),[17] while that per pregnancy was 9% (95% CI: 4–15) (Figs. 11A and B). No evidence of a difference in multiple pregnancy either per woman treated (OR: 0.86, 95% CI: 0.44–1.65) or per pregnancy (OR: 0.69, 95% CI: 0.33–1.43) was present between rFSH and urinary FSH.[17]

Based on data reported in a meta-analysis of RCTs comparing aromatase inhibitors with CC for enhancement of ovulation in women with unexplained infertility, the incidence of multiple pregnancy per woman treated with aromatase inhibitors was 1% (95% CI: 0–1) and that per pregnancy achieved was 2% (95% CI: 0–5) (Figs. 12A and B). The incidence of multiple pregnancy per woman treated with CC was 2% (95% CI: 1–3) and per pregnancy achieved 6% (95% CI: 3–11) (Figs. 13A and B).[18]

Based on data reported in a meta-analysis of RCTs employing ovarian stimulation with the use of gonadotropins for the treatment of women with unexplained infertility, male infertility or mild endometriosis, the incidence of multiple pregnancy was 4% (95% CI: 3–5) per women treated

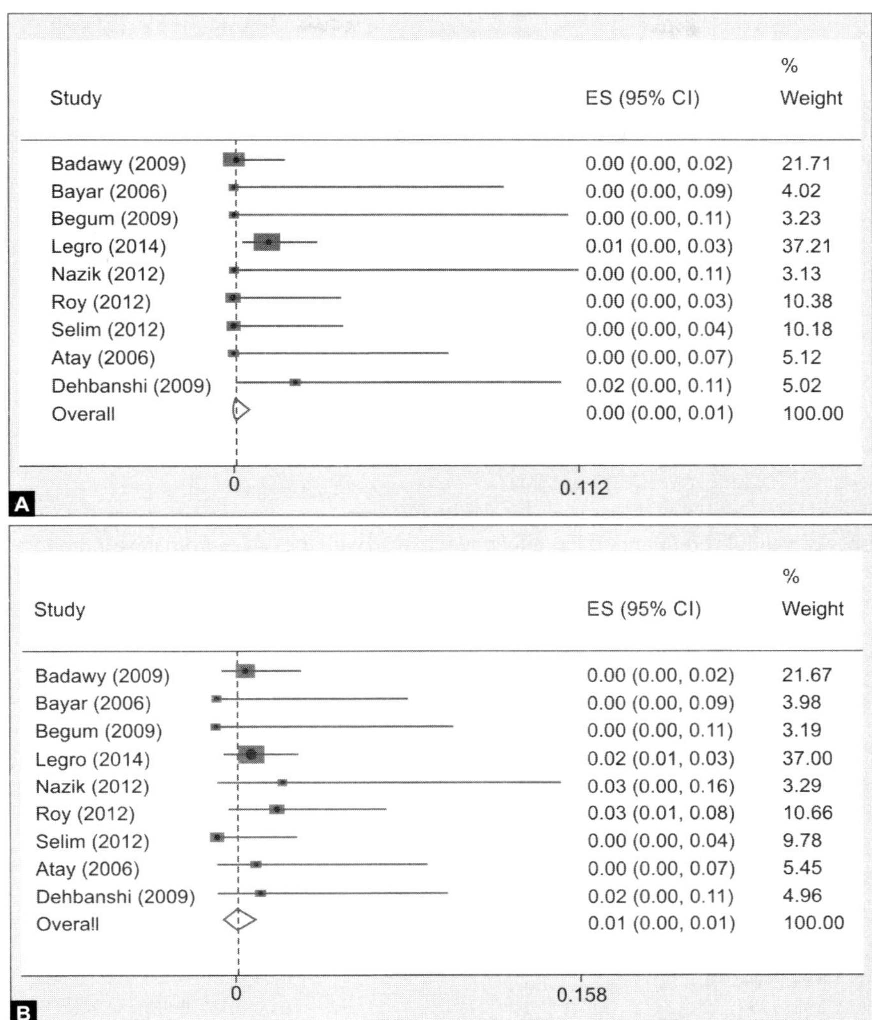

Figs. 8A and B: (A) Incidence of multiple pregnancy per patient treated with the use of aromatase inhibitors for ovulation induction in women with polycystic ovarian syndrome (PCOS); (B) Incidence of multiple pregnancy per patient treated with the use of clomiphene citrate (CC) for ovulation induction in women with PCOS. (ES: estimate; CI: confidence interval).

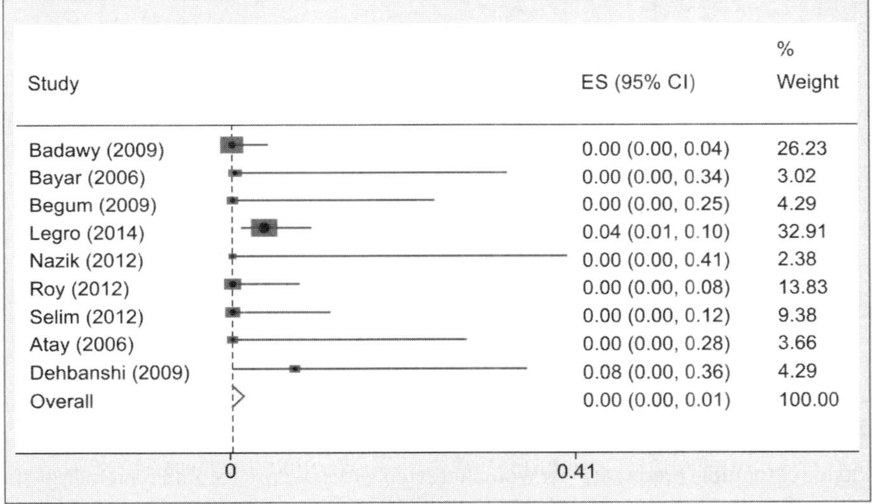

Fig. 9A

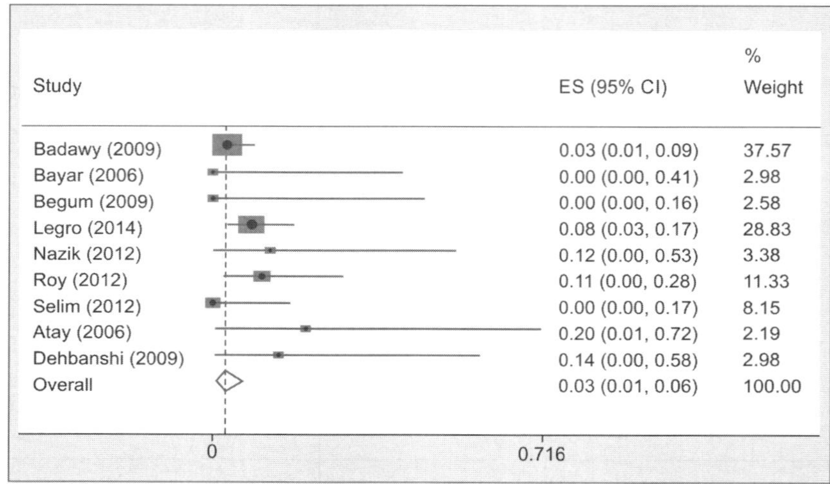

Fig. 9B

Figs. 9A and B: (A) Incidence of multiple pregnancy per pregnancy achieved with the use of aromatase inhibitors for ovulation induction in women with polycystic ovarian syndrome (PCOS); (B) Incidence of multiple pregnancy per pregnancy achieved with the use of clomiphene citrate (CC) for ovulation induction in women with PCOS. (ES: estimate; CI: confidence interval).

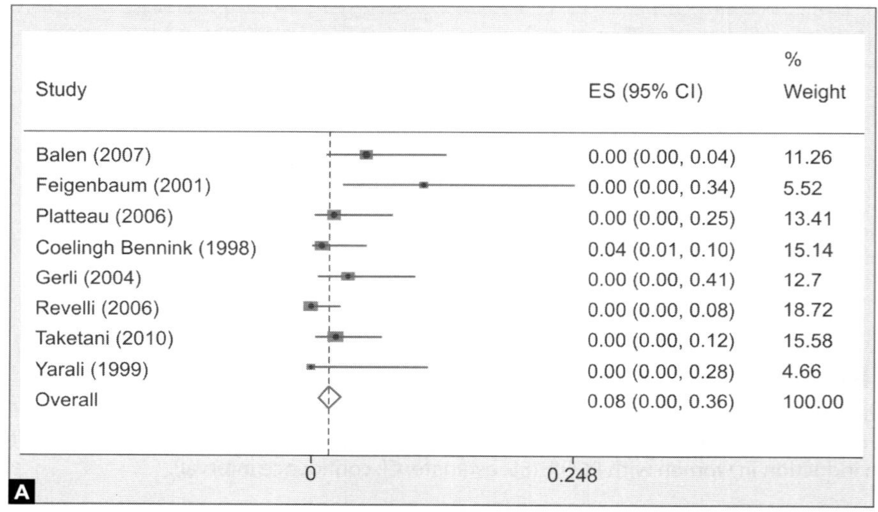

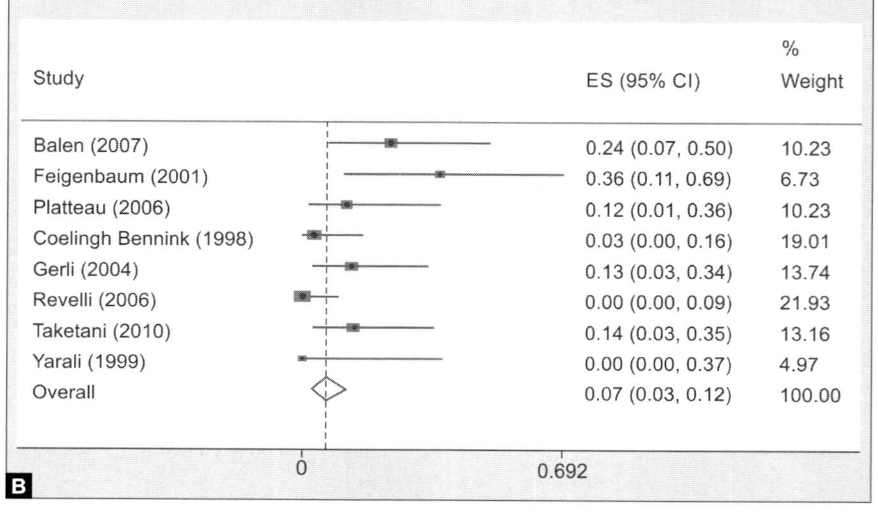

Figs. 10A and B: (A) Incidence of multiple pregnancy per woman treated with lowdose recombinant follicle-stimulating hormone (FSH) for ovulation induction in women with polycystic ovarian syndrome (PCOS); (B) Incidence of multiple pregnancy per pregnancy achieved with low-dose recombinant FSH for ovulation induction in women with PCOS. (ES: estimate; CI: confidence interval).

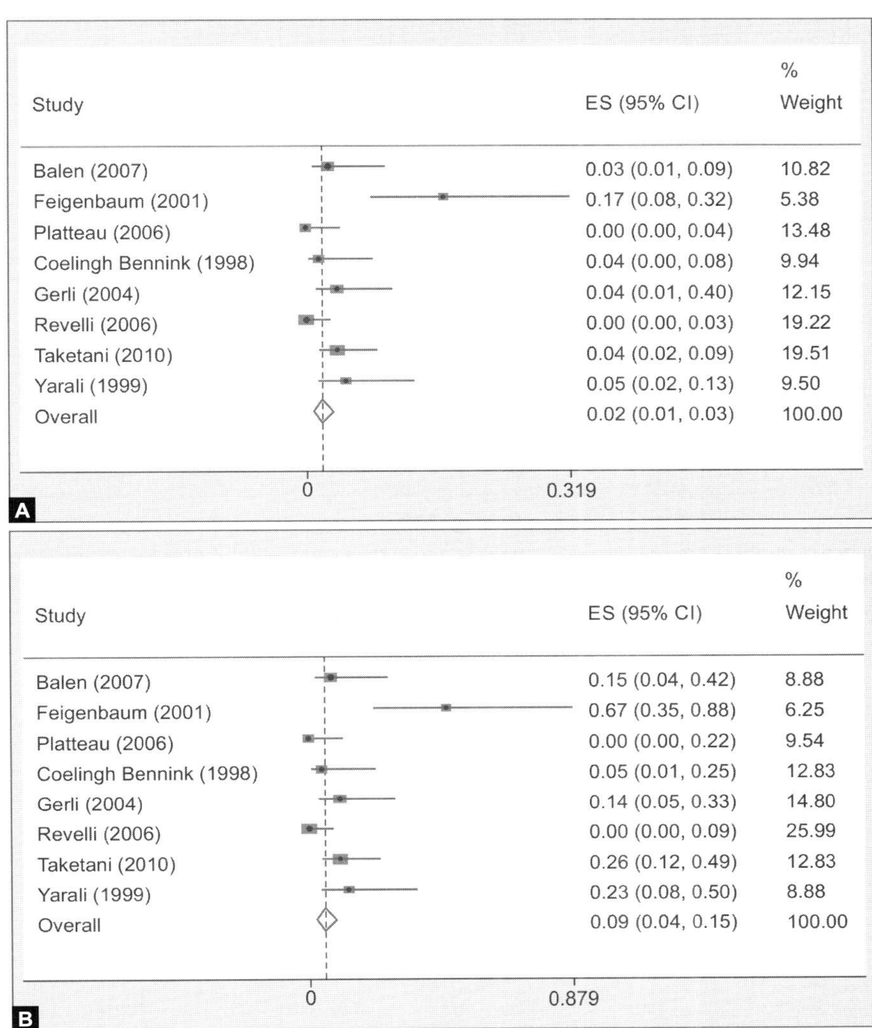

Figs. 11A and B: (A) Incidence of multiple pregnancy per woman treated with urinary follicle-stimulating hormone (FSH) for ovulation induction in women with polycystic ovarian syndrome (PCOS); (B) Incidence of multiple pregnancy per pregnancy achieved with urinary FSH for ovulation induction in women with PCOS. (ES: estimate; CI: confidence interval).

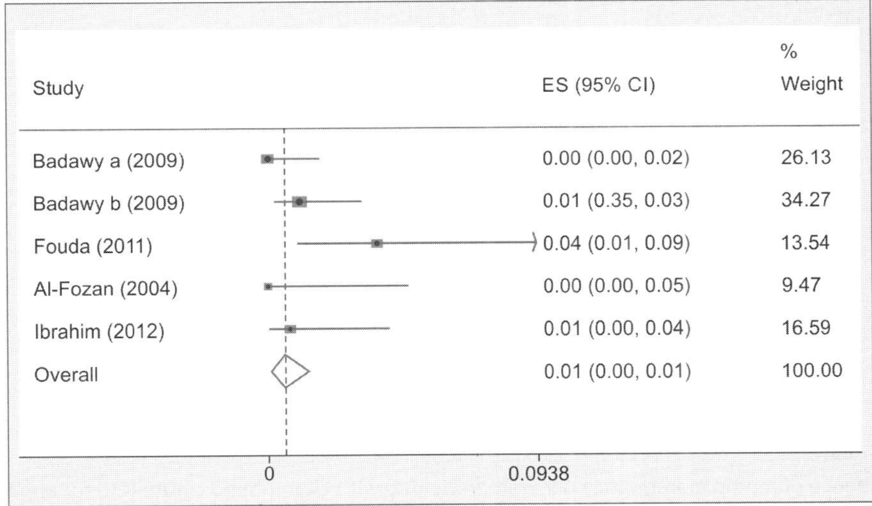

Fig. 12A

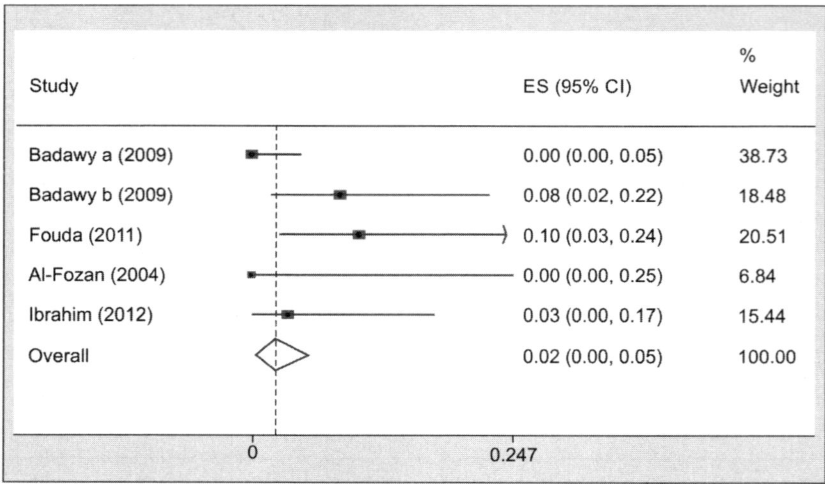

Fig. 12B

Figs. 12A and B: (A) Incidence of multiple pregnancy per woman treated with aromatase inhibitors for enhancement of ovulation in women with unexplained infertility; (B) Incidence of multiple pregnancy per pregnancy achieved with aromatase inhibitors for enhancement of ovulation in women with unexplained infertility. (ES: estimate; CI: confidence interval).

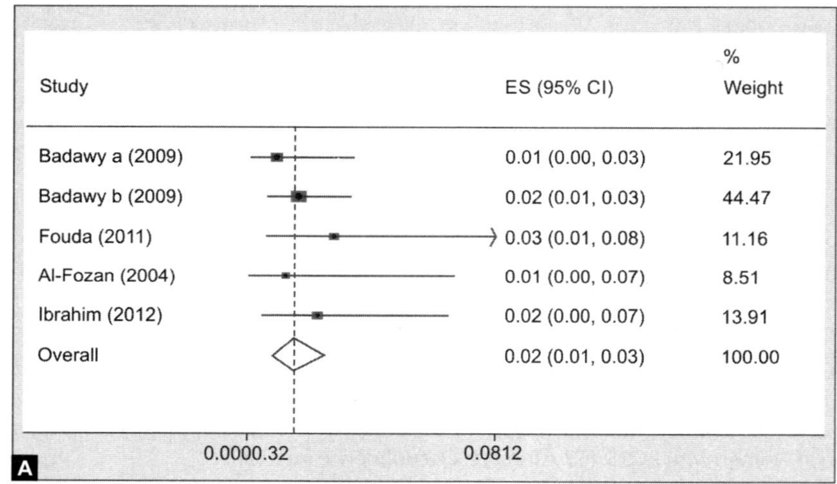

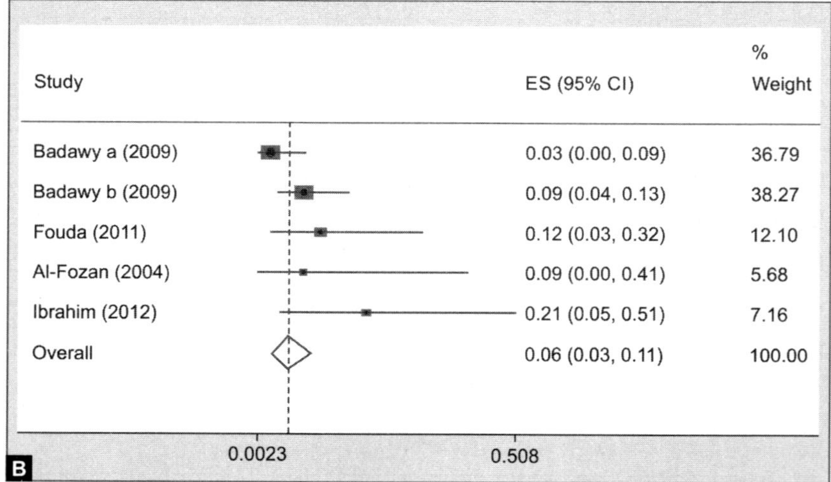

Figs. 13A and B: (A) Incidence of multiple pregnancy per woman treated with clomiphene citrate (CC) for enhancement of ovulation in women with unexplained infertility; (B) Incidence of multiple pregnancy per pregnancy achieved with CC for enhancement of ovulation in women with unexplained infertility. (ES: estimate; CI: confidence interval).

and 15% (95% CI: 11–19) per pregnancy achieved[19] (Figs. 14A and B). In the above studies, the estimated incidence of multiple pregnancy per woman treated without the use of GnRH analogs was 4% (95% CI: 3–6), while that per pregnancy achieved without the use of GnRH analogs was 13% (95% CI: 9–18) (Figs. 15A and B). In addition, the estimated incidence of multiple pregnancy per woman treated with the use of GnRH agonist for inhibition of premature LH surge was 8% (95% CI: 4–12), while that per pregnancy achieved was 40% (95% CI: 25–55) (Figs. 15A and B). The estimated incidence of multiple pregnancy per woman treated with the use of GnRH antagonist was 1% (95% CI: 0–7), while that per pregnancy achieved was 7% (95% CI: 0–22) (Figs. 15A and B).

In order to reduce the risk of multiple births when high E2 levels and/or an excessive follicle number has developed following ovulation induction or enhancement of ovulation, cycle cancellation by withholding hCG or conversion of the cycle to IVF/embryo transfer should be considered. High E2 levels and numbers of follicles (E2 ≥1,500 pg/mL or >3 mature follicles) have been considered as warning signals for multiple gestation and could be used as indications for cycle cancellation or conversion to IVF.[23,58,59]

Multiple Pregnancy after Multifollicular Development for In Vitro Fertilization

The chance of multiple pregnancy after IVF is dependent on the number of embryos transferred and their implantation potential. The transfer of fewer embryos of high implantation potential maintains the probability of pregnancy and dramatically reduces the incidence of multiple pregnancy.[55]

Elective single embryo transfer has been widely accepted as a strategy eliminating the risk of twins particularly in young, good-prognosis women.[60,61] The principle of this policy is based on selecting a single embryo of the best morphological quality for transfer and freezing any additional embryos for replacement in subsequent cycles. Such a policy, however, appears to be associated with a decreased probability of pregnancy. In a systematic

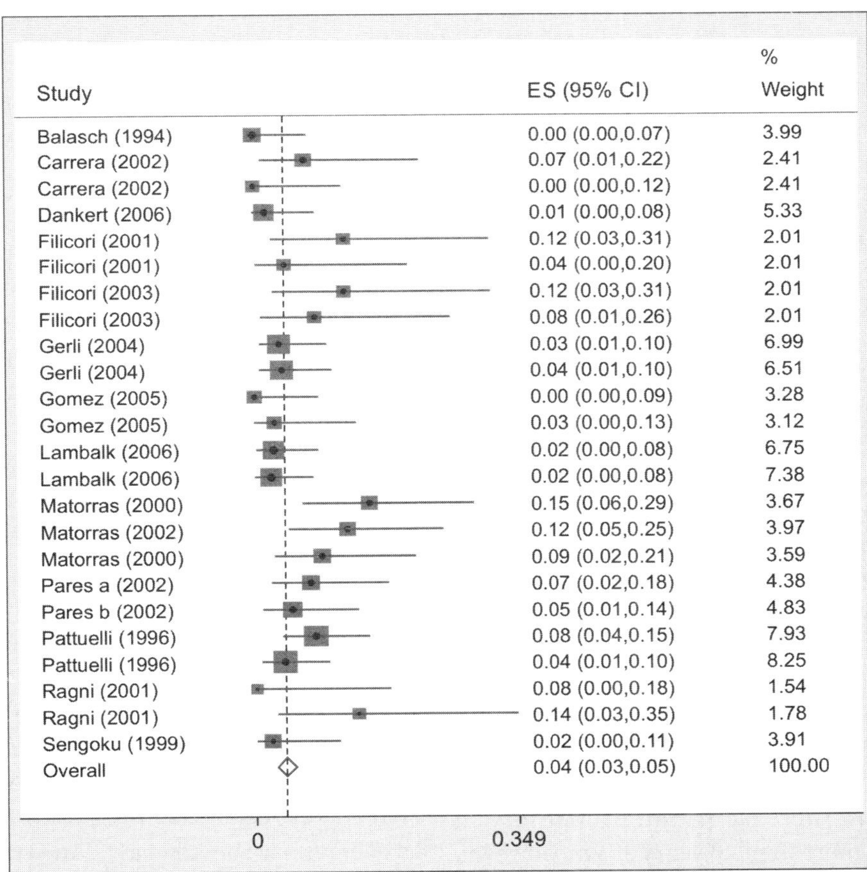

Fig. 14A: Incidence of multiple pregnancy per woman treated with the use of gonadotropins for the treatment of women with unexplained infertility.

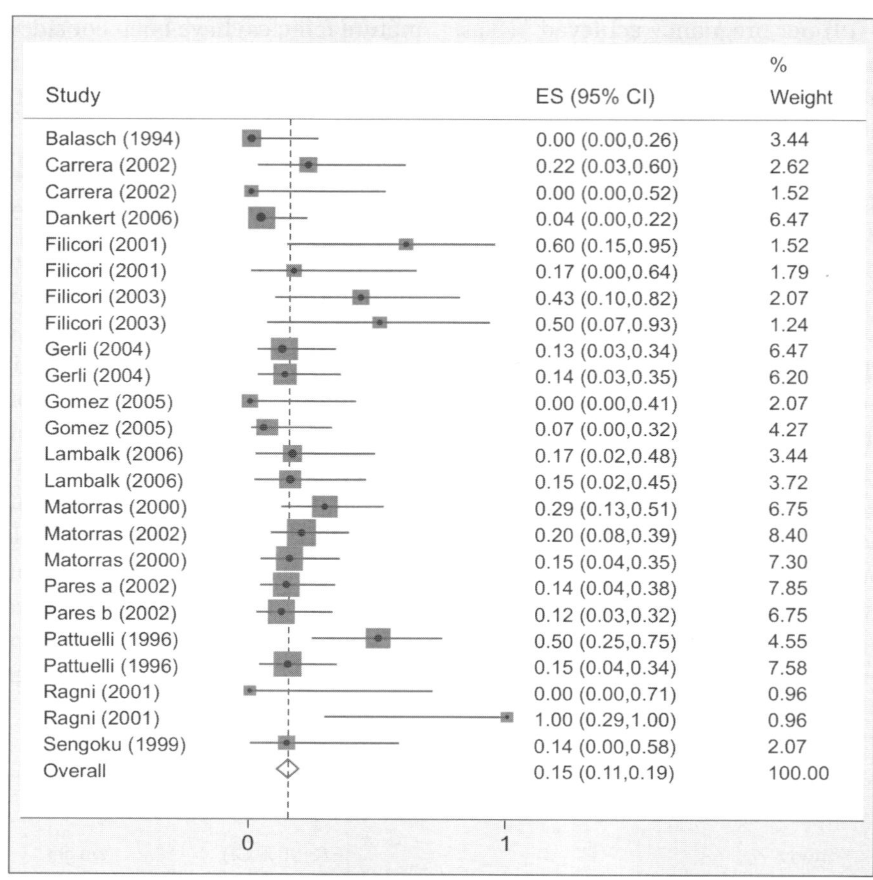

Fig. 14B: Incidence of multiple pregnancy per pregnancy achieved with the use of gonadotropins for the treatment of women with unexplained infertility. (ES: estimate; CI: confidence interval).

review and meta-analysis of studies performed in women less than 36 years old, it was shown that elective single embryo transfer compared with double embryo transfer was associated with a statistically significant reduction in the probability of live birth,[61] although the cumulative probability of live birth seems to be similar. This appears to be true even in women of advanced reproductive age.[62]

In Belgium, the application of a policy that restricts the number of embryos transferred, depending on the patient's age and treatment cycle resulted in reduction of multiple pregnancy rate from 29.1% to 9.5% in all patients and from 28.9% to 6.2% in women less than 36 years.[60] Despite the obvious advantages of single embryo transfer in eliminating multiple pregnancies, rates of single embryo transfer vary markedly across nations, with the highest reported in Sweden (69.4%) and the lowest in the USA (2.8%).[63]

It should be noted that the transfer of multiple embryos is associated with an increase in the probability of pregnancy in women more than 40 years of age, however, in this age group multiple pregnancies (twins and triplets) can still occur.[64]

The use of preimplantation genetic screening (PGS) for selecting a single euploid blastocyst for transfer has been considered an important tool for eliminating multiple pregnancies and maintaining the probability of live birth particularly in patients of advanced reproductive age.[65,66] In a recent systematic review and meta-analysis, the use of comprehensive chromosome screening after blastocyst biopsy maintained similar ongoing pregnancy rates between PGS and control groups, while sharply decreasing multiple pregnancy rates.[67]

In the unfortunate case of triplets following embryo transfer, fetal reduction is considered as an appropriate management if ethical or religious issues are not present.[68-70] Fetal reduction was first described in the 1980s as a surgical procedure of selectively reducing the number of fetuses in an attempt to improve pregnancy outcomes by reducing the high adverse sequela of multiple pregnancies.[69] Although its benefits have been clearly shown for reduction of triplets to twins, it is still debatable whether the reduction of twins to singleton is justified.[69]

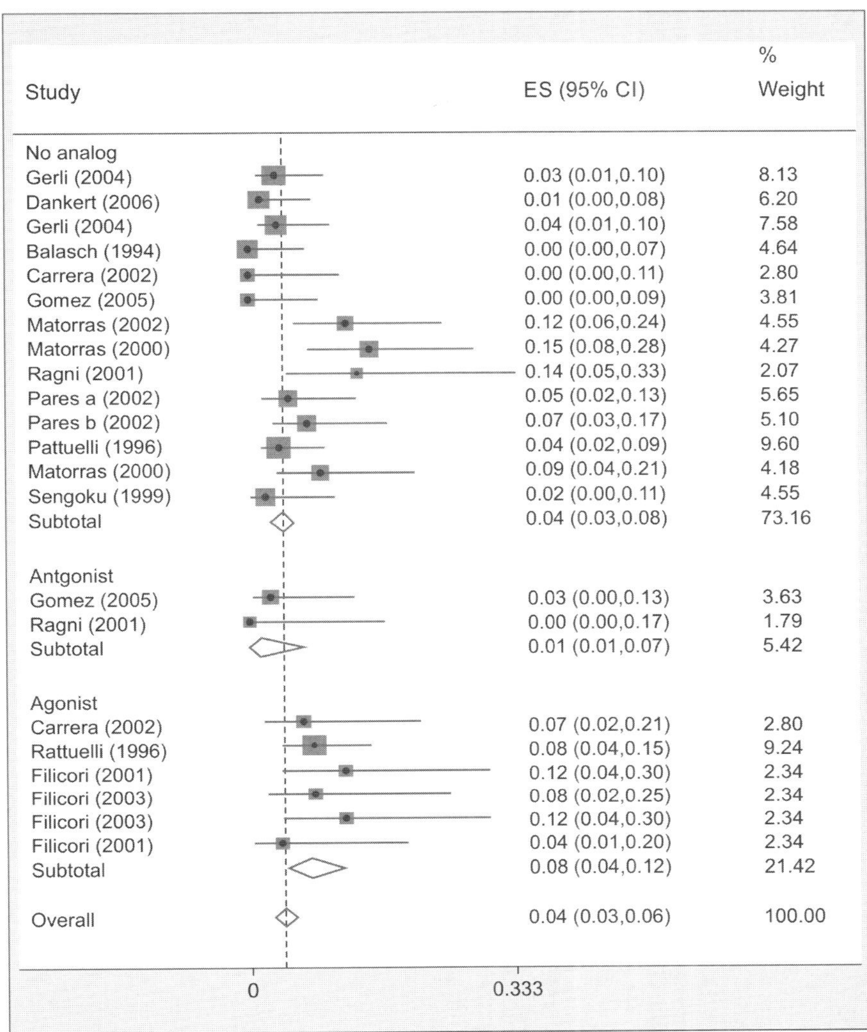

Fig. 15A: Incidence of multiple pregnancy per woman treated with follicle-stimulating hormone (FSH) without gonadotropin-releasing hormone (GnRH) analogs, with GnRH agonist or with GnRH antagonists.

ADNEXAL TORSION

Acute abdominal pain, nausea, vomiting and ovarian enlargement at ultrasound are signs indicative of adnexal torsion. Following ovarian stimulation, cystic ovaries are predisposed to torsion,[5,71] the risk of which increases when ovarian stimulation is complicated with OHSS or leads to pregnancy.[71,72] In the first trimester of gestation following IVF, adnexal torsion should be suspected in all episodes of acute abdominal pain.[73,74]

The reported incidence of adnexal torsion in women who develop OHSS and do not achieve pregnancy is 2.3% (95% CI: 0.8–6.8), whereas in women who develop OHSS and achieve pregnancy the incidence increases to 16% (95% CI: 9.4–25.9).[75] In pregnant women who develop OHSS, ovarian cysts persist and this prolongs the period of increased risk for adnexal torsion.[72] In a series of 165 pregnant women who developed OHSS, the risk ratio for adnexal torsion was 3.7 (95% CI: 1.1–12.6) in twins as compared to singletons.[76]

It should be noted that history of adnexal torsion and the presence of multiple risk factors increase the probability of subsequent adnexal torsion.[77,78] The incidence of adnexal torsion recurrence is reported to be 19.5% (95% CI: 8.8–34.9) for pregnant and 9.1% (95% CI: 3.7–17.8) for nonpregnant women.[79]

Laparoscopy is a safe and effective first-line treatment for the management of adnexal torsion in both pregnant and nonpregnant women, minimizing postoperative discomfort and leading to shorter hospitalization.[80] However, special considerations should be present in pregnant women regarding the creation of pneumoperitoneum and the insertion of the Veress needle.[74]

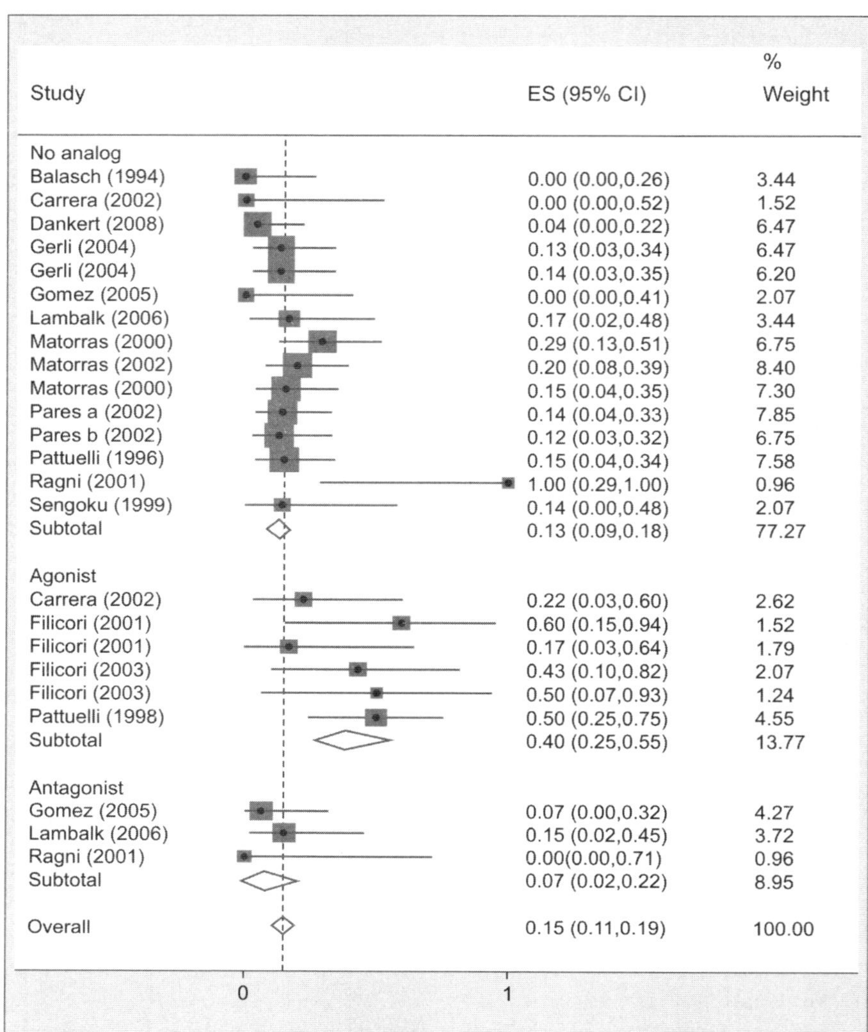

Fig. 15B: Incidence of multiple pregnancy per pregnancy achieved with the use of FSH without GnRH analogs, with GnRH agonist or with GnRH antagonists. (ES: estimate; CI: confidence interval).

Laparoscopic derotation of adnexal torsion is recommended even for ovaries which are already ischemic, since in 73% of cases it is sufficient to preserve ovarian function.[5] Unwinding of the affected adnexa is carried out by pushing the ovary contralaterally to the direction of the torsion using two blunt probes and if successful results in recoloration and disappearance of the congestion.[81] Complete absence of blood flow in the ovarian vessels has been suggested as an indication for adnexectomy.[74] Oophoropexy or shortening of utero-ovarian ligament have been advocated to avoid adnexal torsion recurrence.[5]

THROMBOEMBOLIC COMPLICATIONS

Thromboembolic complications both arterial and venous have been ascribed to the presence of OHSS, although they can also occur in its absence.[82] The exact mechanism by which OHSS creates a prothrombotic state is not clear.[83] However, high E2 concentrations, hemoconcentration after ovarian hyperstimulation as well as inherited thrombophilias are strongly hypothesized to be supportive of a hypercoagulable state, which induces the occurrence of thromboembolism.[6,84]

The development of thrombotic complications after ovarian stimulation is an infrequent event with an incidence for venous thrombosis ranging between 0.04% (95% CI: 0.01–0.11)[85] and 0.08% (95% CI: 0.01–0.29) per IVF cycle.[83] The incidence of arterial thrombosis is likely to be several times lower.[86] Women who develop arterial thrombosis are less often pregnant and have a lower rate of inherited thrombophilia, whereas those who develop venous thrombosis are more often pregnant and have underlying thrombophilic disorders.[86]

Prevention of thromboembolic complications involves administration of thromboprophylaxis in women at high risk, such as those who develop moderate-to-severe OHSS as well as in women with known thrombophilia, who undergo ovarian stimulation. For patients who develop moderate-to-severe OHSS, thromboprophylaxis should be initiated and be continued for a period of 4–8 weeks beyond resolution of OHSS.[86]

The management of thromboembolism requires appropriate therapy and adequate anticoagulation with close follow-up.[86] The use of aspirin, low molecular weight heparin (LMWH) and unfractionated heparin should be considered even when pregnancy is present and these patients would likely remain on therapeutic LMWH throughout pregnancy.[87]

REFERENCES

1. Kupka MS, D'Hooghe T, Ferraretti AP, et al. Assisted reproductive technology in Europe, 2011: results generated from European registers by ESHRE. Hum Reprod. 2016;31:233-48.
2. Birch Petersen K, Pedersen NG, Pedersen AT, et al. Mono-ovulation in women with polycystic ovary syndrome: a clinical review on ovulation induction. Reprod Biomed Online. 2016;32:563-83.
3. Abramov Y, Elchalal U, Schenker JG. Severe OHSS: An 'epidemic' of severe OHSS: a price we have to pay? Hum Reprod. 1999;14:2181-3.
4. Callahan TL, Hall JE, Ettner SL, et al. The economic impact of multiple-gestation pregnancies and the contribution of assisted-reproduction techniques to their incidence. N Engl J Med. 1994;331:244-9.
5. Spitzer D, Wirleitner B, Steiner H, et al. Adnexal torsion in pregnancy after assisted reproduction—case study and review of the literature. Geburtshilfe Frauenheilkd. 2012;72:716-20.
6. Stewart JA, Hamilton PJ, Murdoch AP. Thromboembolic disease associated with ovarian stimulation and assisted conception techniques. Hum Reprod. 1997;12:2167-73.
7. Mathur RS, Jenkins JM. Is ovarian hyperstimulation syndrome associated with a poor obstetric outcome? BJOG. 2000;107:943-6.
8. Fiedler K, Ezcurra D. Predicting and preventing ovarian hyperstimulation syndrome (OHSS): the need for individualized not standardized treatment. Reprod Biol Endocrinol. 2012;10:32.
9. Navot D, Bergh PA, Laufer N. Ovarian hyperstimulation syndrome in novel reproductive technologies: prevention and treatment. Fertil Steril. 1992;58:249-61.
10. Mathur R, Jenkins J. Towards a clinically useful classification of OHSS. Reprod Biomed Online. 2009;19:434.
11. Randall JM, Templeton A. The effects of clomiphene citrate upon ovulation and endocrinology when administered to patients with unexplained infertility. Hum Reprod. 1991;6:659-64.
12. van Santbrink EJ, Eijkemans MJ, Laven JS, et al. Patient-tailored conventional ovulation induction algorithms in anovulatory infertility. Trends Endocrinol Metab. 2005;16:381-9.
13. Palomba S. Aromatase inhibitors for ovulation induction. J Clin Endocrinol Metab. 2015;100:1742-7.
14. Kar S. Clomiphene citrate or letrozole as first-line ovulation induction drug in infertile PCOS women: a prospective randomized trial. J Hum Reprod Sci. 2012;5:262-5.
15. Franik S, Kremer JA, Nelen WL, et al. Aromatase inhibitors for subfertile women with polycystic ovary syndrome. Cochrane Database Syst Rev. 2014;2:CD010287.
16. Melo AS, Ferriani RA, Navarro PA. Treatment of infertility in women with polycystic ovary syndrome: approach to clinical practice. Clinics (Sao Paulo). 2015;70:765-9.
17. Weiss NS, Nahuis M, Bayram N, et al. Gonadotrophins for ovulation induction in women with polycystic ovarian syndrome. Cochrane Database Syst Rev. 2015;9:CD010290.
18. Liu A, Zheng C, Lang J, et al. Letrozole versus clomiphene citrate for unexplained infertility: a systematic review and meta-analysis. J Obstet Gynaecol Res. 2014;40:1205-16.
19. Cantineau AE, Cohlen BJ, Heineman MJ. Ovarian stimulation protocols (anti-oestrogens, gonadotrophins with and without GnRH agonists/antagonists) for intrauterine insemination (IUI) in women with subfertility. Cochrane Database Syst Rev. 2011;2:CD005356.
20. Nisker J, Tummon I, Daniel S, et al. Conversion of cycles involving ovarian hyperstimulation with intra-uterine insemination to in-vitro fertilization. Hum Reprod. 1994;9:406-8.
21. Pasqualotto EB, Falcone T, Goldberg JM, et al. Risk factors for multiple gestation in women undergoing intrauterine insemination with ovarian stimulation. Fertil Steril. 1999;72:613-8.
22. Olufowobi O, Sharif K, Papaioannou S, et al. Role of rescue IVF-ET treatment in the management of high response in stimulated IUI cycles. J Obstet Gynaecol. 2005;25:166-8.
23. Antman AM, Politch JA, Ginsburg ES. Conversion of high-response gonadotropin intrauterine insemination cycles to in vitro fertilization results in excellent ongoing pregnancy rates. Fertil Steril. 2002;77:715-20.
24. Kawwass JF, Kissin DM, Kulkarni AD, et al. Safety of assisted reproductive technology in the United States, 2000-2011. JAMA. 2015;313:88-90.
25. Al-Inany HG, Youssef MA, Aboulghar M, et al. Gonadotrophin-releasing hormone antagonists for assisted reproductive technology. Cochrane Database Syst Rev. 2011;5:CD001750.
26. Tarlatzis BC, Griesinger G, Leader A, et al. Comparative incidence of ovarian hyperstimulation syndrome following ovarian stimulation with corifollitropin alfa or recombinant FSH. Reprod Biomed Online. 2012;24:410-9.
27. Griesinger G, Verweij PJ, Gates D, et al. Prediction of ovarian hyperstimulation syndrome in patients treated with corifollitropin alfa or rFSH in a GnRH antagonist protocol. PLoS One. 2016;11:e0149615.
28. Aboulghar MA, Mansour RT. Ovarian hyperstimulation syndrome: classifications and critical analysis of preventive measures. Hum Reprod Update. 2003;9:275-89.
29. Devroey P, Adriaensen P. OHSS Free Clinic. Facts Views Vis Obgyn. 2011;3:43-5.
30. Tarlatzis B, Bosdou J, Kolibianakis E. Elimination of OHSS by GnRH Agonist and Freezing Embryos. In: Rizk B,

Gerris J (Eds). Complications and Outcomes of Assisted Reproduction. United Kingdom: Cambridge University Press; 2017. pp. 149-63.
31. Humaidan P, Polyzos NP, Alsbjerg B, et al. GnRHa trigger and individualized luteal phase hCG support according to ovarian response to stimulation: two prospective randomized controlled multi-centre studies in IVF patients. Hum Reprod. 2013;28:2511-21.
32. Papanikolaou EG, Verpoest W, Fatemi H, et al. A novel method of luteal supplementation with recombinant luteinizing hormone when a gonadotropin-releasing hormone agonist is used instead of human chorionic gonadotropin for ovulation triggering: a randomized prospective proof of concept study. Fertil Steril. 2011;95:1174-7.
33. Decleer W, Osmanagaoglu K, Seynhave B, et al. Comparison of hCG triggering versus hCG in combination with a GnRH agonist: a prospective randomized controlled trial. Facts Views Vis Obgyn. 2014;6:203-9.
34. Pirard C, Donnez J, Loumaye E. GnRH agonist as luteal phase support in assisted reproduction technique cycles: results of a pilot study. Hum Reprod. 2006;21:1894-900.
35. Engmann L, DiLuigi A, Schmidt D, et al. The use of gonadotropin-releasing hormone (GnRH) agonist to induce oocyte maturation after cotreatment with GnRH antagonist in high-risk patients undergoing in vitro fertilization prevents the risk of ovarian hyperstimulation syndrome: a prospective randomized controlled study. Fertil Steril. 2008;89:84-91.
36. Lainas GT, Kolibianakis EM, Sfontouris IA, et al. Pregnancy and neonatal outcomes following luteal GnRH antagonist administration in patients with severe early OHSS. Hum Reprod. 2013;28:1929-42.
37. Lainas GT, Kolibianakis EM, Sfontouris IA, et al. Outpatient management of severe early OHSS by administration of GnRH antagonist in the luteal phase: an observational cohort study. Reprod Biol Endocrinol. 2012;10:69.
38. Griesinger G, Kolibianakis EM, Papanikolaou EG, et al. Triggering of final oocyte maturation with gonadotropin-releasing hormone agonist or human chorionic gonadotropin. Live birth after frozen-thawed embryo replacement cycles. Fertil Steril. 2007;88:616-21.
39. Bodri D, Guillen JJ, Galindo A, et al. Triggering with human chorionic gonadotropin or a gonadotropin-releasing hormone agonist in gonadotropin-releasing hormone antagonist-treated oocyte donor cycles: findings of a large retrospective cohort study. Fertil Steril. 2009;91:365-71.
40. Bodri D, Guillen JJ, Trullenque M, et al. Early ovarian hyperstimulation syndrome is completely prevented by gonadotropin releasing-hormone agonist triggering in high-risk oocyte donor cycles: a prospective, luteal-phase follow-up study. Fertil Steril. 2010;93:2418-20.
41. Castillo JC, Dolz M, Moreno J, et al. Triggering with GnRH agonist in oocytedonation cycles: oestradiol monitoring is not necessary during ovarian stimulation. Reprod Biomed Online. 2012;24:247-50.
42. Hernandez ER, Gomez-Palomares JL, Ricciarelli E. No room for cancellation, coasting, or ovarian hyperstimulation syndrome in oocyte donation cycles. Fertil Steril. 2009;91:1358-61.
43. Acevedo B, Gomez-Palomares JL, Ricciarelli E, et al. Triggering ovulation with gonadotropin-releasing hormone agonists does not compromise embryo implantation rates. Fertil Steril. 2006;86:1682-7.
44. Galindo A, Bodri D, Guillen JJ, et al. Triggering with HCG or GnRH agonist in GnRH antagonist treated oocyte donation cycles: a randomised clinical trial. Gynecol Endocrinol. 2009;25:60-6.
45. Melo M, Busso CE, Bellver J, et al. GnRH agonist versus recombinant HCG in an oocyte donation programme: a randomized, prospective, controlled, assessor-blind study. Reprod Biomed Online. 2009;19:486-92.
46. Sismanoglu A, Tekin HI, Erden HF, et al. Ovulation triggering with GnRH agonist vs. hCG in the same egg donor population undergoing donor oocyte cycles with GnRH antagonist: a prospective randomized cross-over trial. J Assist Reprod Genet. 2009;26:251-6.
47. Griesinger G, Berndt H, Schultz L, et al. Intensified ovarian stimulation in a GnRH antagonist protocol with agonist triggering: a prospective, clinical feasibility study. Reprod Biomed Online. 2011;22:133-9.
48. Griesinger G, Schultz L, Bauer T, et al. Ovarian hyperstimulation syndrome prevention by gonadotropin-releasing hormone agonist triggering of final oocyte maturation in a gonadotropin-releasing hormone antagonist protocol in combination with a "freeze-all" strategy: a prospective multicentric study. Fertil Steril. 2011;95:2029-33, 33 e1.
49. Reddy J, Turan V, Bedoschi G, et al. Triggering final oocyte maturation with gonadotropin-releasing hormone agonist (GnRHa) versus human chorionic gonadotropin (hCG) in breast cancer patients undergoing fertility preservation: an extended experience. J Assist Reprod Genet. 2014;31:927-32.
50. Manzanares MA, Gomez-Palomares JL, Ricciarelli E, et al. Triggering ovulation with gonadotropin-releasing hormone agonist in in vitro fertilization patients with polycystic ovaries does not cause ovarian hyperstimulation syndrome despite very high estradiol levels. Fertil Steril. 2010;93:1215-9.
51. Practice Committee of the American Society for Reproductive Medicine. Electronic address: ASRM@asrm.org1; Practice Committee of the American Society for Reproductive Medicine. Prevention and treatment of moderate and severe ovarian hyperstimulation syndrome: a guideline. Fertil Steril. 2016;106:1634-47.
52. RCOG. (2006). The Management of Ovarian Hyperstimulation Syndrome. Green-top Guideline No. 5. [online] Available from https://www.rcog.org.uk/ globalassets/documents/ guidelines/green-top-guidelines/gtg_5_ohss.pdf [Accessed March, 2017].
53. Sebire NJ, Nicolaides KH. Screening for fetal abnormalities in multiple pregnancies. Baillieres Clin Obstet Gynaecol. 1998;12:19-36.
54. Scher AI, Petterson B, Blair E, et al. The risk of mortality or cerebral palsy in twins: a collaborative population-based study. Pediatr Res. 2002;52:671-81.
55. Fauser BC, Devroey P, Macklon NS. Multiple birth resulting from ovarian stimulation for subfertility treatment. Lancet. 2005;365:1807-16.
56. Farhi J, West C, Patel A, et al. Treatment of anovulatory infertility: the problem of multiple pregnancy. Hum Reprod. 1996;11:429-34.

57. Navot D, Goldstein N, Mor-Josef S, et al. Multiple pregnancies: risk factors and prognostic variables during induction of ovulation with human menopausal gonadotrophins. Hum Reprod. 1991;6:1152-5.
58. European Society of Human Reproduction and Embryology (ESHRE) Capri Workshop Group. Multiple gestation pregnancy. Hum Reprod. 2000;15:1856-64.
59. Dickey RP. Strategies to reduce multiple pregnancies due to ovulation stimulation. Fertil Steril. 2009;91:1-17.
60. Van Landuyt L, Verheyen G, Tournaye H, et al. New Belgian embryo transfer policy leads to sharp decrease in multiple pregnancy rate. Reprod Biomed Online. 2006;13:765-71.
61. Gelbaya TA, Tsoumpou I, Nardo LG. The likelihood of live birth and multiple birth after single versus double embryo transfer at the cleavage stage: a systematic review and meta-analysis. Fertil Steril. 2010;94:936-45.
62. Fujimoto A, Morishima K, Harada M, et al. Elective single-embryo transfer improves cumulative pregnancy outcome in young patients but not in women of advanced reproductive age. J Assist Reprod Genet. 2015;32:1773-9.
63. Maheshwari A, Griffiths S, Bhattacharya S. Global variations in the uptake of single embryo transfer. Hum Reprod Update. 2011;17:107-20.
64. Klipstein S, Regan M, Ryley DA, et al. One last chance for pregnancy: a review of 2,705 in vitro fertilization cycles initiated in women age 40 years and above. Fertil Steril. 2005;84:435-45.
65. Yang Z, Liu J, Collins GS, et al. Selection of single blastocysts for fresh transfer via standard morphology assessment alone and with array CGH for good prognosis IVF patients: results from a randomized pilot study. Mol Cytogenet. 2012;5:24.
66. Forman EJ, Hong KH, Ferry KM, et al. In vitro fertilization with single euploid blastocyst transfer: a randomized controlled trial. Fertil Steril. 2013;100:100-7.e1.
67. Dahdouh EM, Balayla J, Garcia-Velasco JA. Impact of blastocyst biopsy and comprehensive chromosome screening technology on preimplantation genetic screening: a systematic review of randomized controlled trials. Reprod Biomed Online. 2015;30:281-9.
68. Evans MI, Britt DW. Multifetal pregnancy reduction: evolution of the ethical arguments. Semin Reprod Med. 2010;28:295-302.
69. Evans MI, Andriole S, Britt DW. Fetal reduction: 25 years' experience. Fetal Diagn Ther. 2014;35:69-82.
70. Balasch J, Gratacos E. Delayed childbearing: effects on fertility and the outcome of pregnancy. Curr Opin Obstet Gynecol. 2012;24:187-93.
71. Rackow BW, Patrizio P. Successful pregnancy complicated by early and late adnexal torsion after in vitro fertilization. Fertil Steril. 2007;87:697.e9-12.
72. Gorkemli H, Camus M, Clasen K. Adnexal torsion after gonadotrophin ovulation induction for IVF or ICSI and its conservative treatment. Arch Gynecol Obstet. 2002;267:4-6.
73. Djakovic A, Honig A, Gross M, et al. Adnexal torsion in a patient with bichorial twin pregnancy in the 21st week of gestation treated by open laparoscopy: a case report. Arch Gynecol Obstet. 2006;274:248-9.
74. Arena S, Canonico S, Luzi G, et al. Ovarian torsion in in vitro fertilizationinduced twin pregnancy: combination of Doppler ultrasound and laparoscopy in diagnosis and treatment can quickly solve the case. Fertil Steril. 2009;92:1496.e9-13.
75. Mashiach S, Bider D, Moran O, et al. Adnexal torsion of hyperstimulated ovaries in pregnancies after gonadotropin therapy. Fertil Steril. 1990;53:76-80.
76. Wiser A, Levron J, Kreizer D, et al. Outcome of pregnancies complicated by severe ovarian hyperstimulation syndrome (OHSS): a follow-up beyond the second trimester. Hum Reprod. 2005;20:910-4.
77. Weitzman VN, DiLuigi AJ, Maier DB, et al. Prevention of recurrent adnexal torsion. Fertil Steril. 2008;90:2018.e1-3.
78. Djavadian D, Braendle W, Jaenicke F. Laparoscopic oophoropexy for the treatment of recurrent torsion of the adnexa in pregnancy: case report and review. Fertil Steril. 2004;82:933-6.
79. Hasson J, Tsafrir Z, Azem F, et al. Comparison of adnexal torsion between pregnant and nonpregnant women. Am J Obstet Gynecol. 2010;202:536.e1-6.
80. Ko ML, Lai TH, Chen SC. Laparoscopic management of complicated adnexal masses in the first trimester of pregnancy. Fertil Steril. 2009;92:283-7.
81. Bassil S, Steinhart U, Donnez J. Successful laparoscopic management of adnexal torsion during week 25 of a twin pregnancy. Hum Reprod. 1999;14(3):855-7.
82. Whelan JG 3rd, Vlahos NF. The ovarian hyperstimulation syndrome. Fertil Steril. 2000;73:883-96.
83. Chan WS, Ginsberg JS. A review of upper extremity deep vein thrombosis in pregnancy: unmasking the 'ART' behind the clot. J Thromb Haemost. 2006;4:1673-7.
84. Ou YC, Kao YL, Lai SL, et al. Thromboembolism after ovarian stimulation: successful management of a woman with superior sagittal sinus thrombosis after IVF and embryo transfer: case report. Hum Reprod. 2003;18:2375-81.
85. Arya R, Shehata HA, Patel RK, et al. Internal jugular vein thrombosis after assisted conception therapy. Br J Haematol. 2001;115:153-5.
86. Chan WS. The 'ART' of thrombosis: a review of arterial and venous thrombosis in assisted reproductive technology. Curr Opin Obstet Gynecol. 2009;21:207-18.
87. Bates SM, Greer IA, Hirsh J, et al. Use of antithrombotic agents during pregnancy: the Seventh ACCP Conference on Antithrombotic and Thrombolytic Therapy. Chest. 2004;126:627S-44S.

Section 6

Basic Laboratory Procedures in Assisted Reproductive Technology

CHAPTER

56

Semen Analysis and Sperm Preparation

Hetal Shukla, Deven Patel, Preeti Shah

INTRODUCTION

Semen analysis though being imperfect is an important tool in the diagnosis of male infertility.[1] Cellular and chemical components of human semen can provide information on the functional properties of the organs producing this fluid, i.e. the testis, epididymis, and accessory glands.[2]

In Table 1, we can see the historic evolution from the first semen observations to the latest guidelines published about the topic.

While semen analysis is an important tool in diagnosing male infertility, it is to be remembered that reference ranges given by the World Health Organization (WHO) manual are not diagnostic cutoff values but only results obtained out of an observation of a fertile population. Male fertility cannot be determined solely on the result of a semen analysis, as there is no evidence stating the exact number and quality of sperm required for a man to be considered fertile. As Christopher De Jonge has rightly said, semen analysis is still the subject of both commendation and condemnation.[3]

Table 1: History and milestones on the semen sample analysis.

1677	Anton van Leeuwenhoek	First observed human spermatozoa from an ejaculate, along with his student, Johan Ham. The microscope used was created by him and saw millions of small motile "animals" which he called animalcules[4] and he was the first to observe the serpentine motion of the animalcules and different shapes of spermatozoa across different species[5]
1771	Lazzaro Spallanzani	After extensive work on artificial insemination, observed spermatic animalcules in various species and documented the fertilizing capacity of the sperm[6]
1837	Rudolf Wagner	Documented his observations on spermatozoa of more than 400 species, including humans. He concluded "the motility of the sperm was greatest at the point of ejaculation and was less in sperm taken from vas deferens and even lesser or nonexistent in sperm taken from testis"[7]
1866	J Marion Sims	He made an important observation after postcoital cervical mucus test that the presence of spermatozoa indicates that the male is not barren[8]
1929	Macomber and Sanders	Quantitatively assessed spermatozoa. From the study which involved 294 males, it was deduced that a "normal" reference value of above 60 million/ mL significantly increases the chances of pregnancy. They also tried to establish a method for counting spermatozoa with the help of a blood counting chamber[9]
1951	John Macleod	After his remarkable study on 1,800 men comparing sperm characteristics between fertile and infertile populations—normal reference value was brought down to 20 million/mL[10]
1980	World Health Organization (WHO)	Published first manual on semen analysis to help establish uniformity in methods of evaluating spermatozoa worldwide. It has been updated periodically with the fifth edition currently being in use[11]
1981	Rune Eliasson	Stated that it was not justified to discriminate a semen sample with 5 million/mL sperm concentration as infertile[2]
1990s	Cell Soft, Hamilton-Thorne and SQM	Introduction of computer-assisted semen analysis (CASA)

SEMEN ANALYSIS

Semen analysis involves different steps to be followed:
- Semen sample collection
- Examining the physical characteristics of the seminal fluid
- Enumerating and classifying the morphological aspects of sperms and other cells
- Evaluating the functional status of the sperm
- Detecting perceptible immunological effects in semen
- Estimating concentrations of the various biochemical substances present in the seminal plasma to understand functional properties of the organs producing this fluid, i.e. the testis, epididymis, and accessory glands.

Semen Sample Collection and Handling

Semen ejaculate of the patient must be collected in a sterile container preferably by masturbation in a special private room provided. Hands and genitals must be washed and dried using soap and dry tissues before collection. Before sample collection, the WHO manual recommends a maximum interval of abstinence between 2 days and 7 days, but recommends that the interval should be "as constant as possible". Therefore, standardization of, "abstinence time" to 3–4 days is strongly advised.[12] As the initial portion of the semen is rich in sperm quantity, spillage if any either initial or later must be recorded.

Some men may have difficulties in producing a semen sample at the laboratory. In these cases, the man may collect a first sample at home and deliver it to the laboratory within 60 minutes.[12,13] During the transport sample container must be tightly closed and kept in polystyrene box to protect from the temperature variation. Rarely, for the man unable to ejaculate through masturbation may use a special, nonspermicidal condom to collect a sample at intercourse.

Semen sample collection container must be properly labeled with patient's name, the clinical history number if any, date of collection and task to be performed. The sample submission must be registered with the patient at the laboratory and acknowledgment signature with relevant consent must be taken duly signed.

As semen sample can show variations, semen samples with compromised semen parameters should be checked a minimum of two properly collected samples, ideally collected over two spermatogenic cycles, examined at 37°C is a good recommendation.

Safety Considerations while Performing Semen Analysis

Semen samples are potentially hazardous due to possible presence of bacteria, protozoan related to sexually transmitted diseases and infectious virus. In the andrology laboratory technicians handling, the semen sample must take utmost care to protect oneself and the semen sample and the laboratory environment.

Following precautions must be taken:
- Routine disinfection of the platform and the surfaces of the andrology laboratory
- Carry out all the procedures under the laminar air flow unit (LAFU)
- Use disposable gloves, laboratory coat and protective face mask
- Avoid sample spillage in the work area
- Disinfect all the laboratory equipment before and after the work
- Wash hands and disinfect the hands at the end of the analysis
- Careful disposal of all the waste material, segregated in different bins, i.e. biohazardous material, for sharp material and decomposable material
- Do not consume food or drinks in the work area.

Physical Examination of Semen

Coagulation and Liquefaction

Normally, semen is ejaculated in a liquid state, which gels shortly thereafter. Absence of coagulation of the sample indicates ejaculatory duct obstruction or congenital absence of vas deferens and seminal vesicles.[14]

Occasionally, samples may not liquefy, making semen evaluation difficult. In these cases, additional treatment, mechanical mixing or enzymatic digestion may be necessary. There are different approaches in those cases:
- Some samples can be induced to liquefy by the addition of an equal volume of physiological medium (e.g. Dulbecco's phosphate-buffered saline; followed by repeated pipetting)[12]
- Inhomogeneity can be reduced by repeated (6–10 times) gentle passage through a blunt gauge 18 (internal diameter 0.84 mm) or gauge 19 (internal diameter 0.69 mm) needle attached to a syringe[12]
- Digestion by bromelain/physiological medium, a broad specificity proteolytic enzyme, may help to promote liquefaction—prepare 10 IU/mL bromelain in Dulbecco's phosphate-buffered saline; it is difficult to dissolve but, with mixing, most should dissolve within 15–20 minutes. Dilute semen 1 + 1 (1:2) with the 10 IU/mL bromelain, stir with a pipette tip, and incubate at 37°C for 10 minutes. Mix the sample well before further analysis.[12]

Comment: These treatments may affect seminal plasma biochemistry, sperm motility and sperm morphology, and their use must be recorded. The 1 + 1 (1: 2) dilution of semen with bromelain must be accounted for when calculating sperm concentration.

Viscosity measures the seminal fluid's resistance to flow. High viscosity may interfere with determination of sperm motility, concentration, and antibody coating of spermatozoa. Normally, semen coagulates upon ejaculation and usually liquefies within 15–20 minutes. Semen that remains a coagulum is termed nonliquefied, whereas that which pours in thick strands instead of drops is termed hyperviscous. The clinical significance of abnormalities in liquefaction remains controversial.[15] Exact liquefaction time is of no diagnostic importance unless more than 2 hours elapse without any change. Failure to liquefy is usually a sign that there is inadequate secretion by the prostate of the proteolytic enzymes fibrinolysin, fibrinogenase, and aminopeptidase.[16] Importantly, liquefaction should be differentiated from viscosity, as abnormalities in viscosity can be the result of abnormal prostate function and/or the use of an unsuitable type of plastic container.

Color

Grayish, white, milky white with opacity is the normal color. Pathologically, seminal discoloration may be due to fresh blood, drugs, jaundice, or contamination of semen with urine (e.g. bladder neck dysfunction).

Physiologic yellowish tinge in samples with prolonged abstinence is due to carotene pigment.

Odor

Normal sample may be unpleasant to some but normally it smells spicy or musky. Abnormal semen sample with possible infection or high sperm oxidation may cause malodorous, and pungent smell. Abnormal prostate function may be the reason of odorless semen sample.

pH

Normal semen pH is in the range of 7.2–7.8 and it tends to increase with time after ejaculation as natural buffering decreases. Changes are usually due to inflammation of the prostate or seminal vesicles. In cases of acute prostatitis, vasculitis or bilateral epididymitis the pH will be more than 8 and in cases of chronic infection of these organs or in cases where only prostatic fluids are present the pH will invariably less than 7.2.

Osmolality

Osmolality can be measured by freezing point or vapor pressure osmometer. This is to be determined in the seminal plasma separating it by low speed centrifugation. Normal range of semen osmolality is 340–380 mOsmol/kg. Low osmolality is usually associated with morphologically abnormal sperms.[17]

Volume

Measuring volume should be as precise as possible to the nearest 0.1 mL in graduated centrifuge tube. Lower reference value of semen volume as per WHO manual is 1.5 mL. Volume more than 6 mL may be due to prolonged abstinence or excessive secretion from the accessory sex glands. If a laboratory weighs the semen to find the volume, semen density to be considered varies between 1.043 g/mL and 1.102 g/mL.[18,19]

Aspermia

No sperm seen in ejaculate after orgasm.

Hypospermia

Less than 1.5 mL of semen (Table 2).

Hyperspermia

More than 6 mL of semen ejaculated (Table 2).

Comment: Improper collection, hypogonadism, retrograde ejaculation, and obstruction of lower urinary tract may yield low volume.

Microscopic Evaluation of Semen

Ideally, microscopic evaluation of semen should be carried out using phase contrast microscope with 20x, 40x, and 100x objective lenses.

Motility

The first aspect of sperm function to assess is sperm motility. This assessment should begin immediately to avoid temperature drop or dehydration of the preparation. As per

Table 2: Summary of the main semen characteristics and its reference values.

Characteristics	*Normal (fertile)*	*Abnormal (subfertile)*
Coagulation	Present	Absent
Liquefaction	15–30 minutes	>60 minutes
Odor	Musky or spicy	Malodorous
Color	Greyish or white	Reddish/brown/ yellow
Volume	1.5–4.5 mL	<1.5 mL, >6 mL
pH	7.2–7.8	Variable
Osmolality	340–380 mOsmol/kg	Variable

WHO guidelines 2010,[12] the motility score is represented in percentage progressive motile sperms, percentage of nonprogressively motile sperms and percentage of nonmotile sperms. Rapid and slow progressive motility is calculated by the speed at which sperm moves with flagellar movement in a given volume as a percentage (range 0–100%) by counting 200 sperms.

The efficient passage of spermatozoa through cervical mucus is dependent on rapid progressive motility,[20,21] that is, spermatozoa with a forward progression of at least 25 μm/s. Reduced sperm motility can be a symptom of disorders related to male accessory sex gland secretion and the sequential emptying of these glands.

According to previous editions of the WHO manual motility was scored in following four grades:

1. Rapid progressive motility (i.e. >25 μm/s at 37°C and >20 μm/s at 20°C; note: 25 μm is approximately equal to five head lengths or half a tail length)
2. Slow or sluggish progressive motility
3. Nonprogressive motility (<5 μm/s)
4. Immobility.

A normal semen analysis must contain at least 50% grade A and B, progressively motile spermatozoa. If greater than 50% sperms are immotile then the sperms should be checked for viability. Persistent poor motility is a good predictor of failure in fertilization, an outcome that is actually more important when making decisions regarding a couple's treatment options.[22]

Sperm Concentration

A phase contrast microscope using volumetric dilution and hemocytometry is recommended for all examinations of unstained preparations of fresh or washed semen and is reported as millions of sperm per milliliters.

Improved Neubauer hemocytometer, Makler chamber, Cell-Vu chamber and computer-assisted semen analysis (CASA) can be used to measure sperm count. Hu Ya et al. in their comparative study of accuracy and precision of four methods including hemocytometer, Makler chamber, Cell-Vu chamber, and computer-aided semen analysis for determining sperm concentration concluded that there was not any significant difference between Cell-Vu chamber and CASA.[23] In another study by Sukcharoen et al.[24] a comparison of Makler counting chamber and improved Neubauer hemocytometer was carried out and the sperm concentration obtained with Makler counting chamber was not statistically different from those determined by improved Neubauer hemocytometer in semen samples with concentrations over 40 × 106/mL. But using Makler counting chambers caused a shift in concentration, which were overestimated significantly (p-value <0.0001) in semen samples with concentrations less than 40 × 106/mL. Overall, Makler chamber counts were 11.2% higher. Although less complicated than the improved Neubauer hemocytometer method, measurement of sperm concentration by Makler counting chamber is an inaccurate method, especially in semen samples with concentrations less than 40 × 106/mL.

Anyway, each laboratory can select its own proper method for manual or computer-aided analysis. Although use of—Makler chamber is showing subjective variations the ease of use with acceptable accuracy, it is commonly used in semen analysis to determine the sperm concentration.

Aggregation of Spermatozoa

The adherence of immotile spermatozoa to each other or of motile spermatozoa to mucus strands, either nonsperm cells or debris is considered to be nonspecific aggregation and should be recorded as such.

Agglutination of Spermatozoa

The tight junctions of sertoli cells forming the blood-testis barrier provide immunologic protection to sperm antigens. The spermatozoon evokes an immune response when exposed to the systemic immune defense system in conditions in which this barrier is disrupted, leading to the formation of antisperm antibodies (ASAs). Certain ASAs have a cytotoxic effect on the spermatozoa and can cause cell death and immobilization of sperm cells. Other effects of ASAs include creating agglutinated clumps of moving sperm in the semen sample, hampering passage of sperm through the cervical mucus, and zonal binding and passage.[25]

Agglutination specifically refers to motile spermatozoa sticking to each other, head-to-head, tail-to-tail or in a mixed way. The motility is often vigorous with a frantic shaking motion, but sometimes the spermatozoa are so agglutinated that their motion is limited. Any motile spermatozoa that stick to each other by their heads, tails or mid pieces should be noted.

Two current methods of detecting antibodies bound to the surface of motile sperm are the mixed agglutination reaction assay [MAR test; only for immunoglobulins G (IgGs)] and the immunobead-binding assay (for IgA, IgG, and IgMs).[26] A positive finding of more than 50% of motile sperm with attached beads is considered to be clinically significant, but with the advent of assisted reproductive technology (ART), ASAs testing has lost its relevance.

The major type of agglutination [reflecting the degree (grades 1–4) and the site of attachment (grades A–E)] should be recorded (Rose et al., 1976):[27]

- *Grade 1:* Isolated, less than 10 spermatozoa per agglutinate, many free spermatozoa
- *Grade 2:* Moderate, 10–50 spermatozoa per agglutinate, free spermatozoa
- *Grade 3:* Large, agglutinates of more than 50 spermatozoa, some spermatozoa still free
- *Grade 4:* Gross, all spermatozoa agglutinated and agglutinates interconnected.

Note:

- *Motile spermatozoa stuck to cells or debris or immotile spermatozoa stuck to each other (aggregation) should not be scored as agglutination*
- *The presence of agglutination is not sufficient evidence to deduce an immunological cause of infertility, but is suggestive of the presence of ASAs; further testing is required*
- *Severe agglutination can affect the assessment of sperm motility and concentration.*

Cellular Elements Other than Spermatozoa

The ejaculate contains cells other than spermatozoa, some of which may be clinically relevant (infection of the male reproductive tract can directly or indirectly cause infertility).[28] These include epithelial cells from the genitourinary tract, as well as leukocytes and immature germ cells, the latter two collectively referred to as "round cells".[29] They can be identified by examining a stained smear at 1,000X magnification. These cells can be more precisely identified and quantified by detecting peroxidase activity or the antigen CD45. Their concentration can be estimated as for spermatozoa, from wet preparations or from the ratio of these cells to the number of spermatozoa on the stained smear and the sperm concentration.

Pyospermia is a laboratory finding categorized as the abnormal presence of leukocytes in human ejaculate and may indicate genital tract inflammation.[30] To differentiate round cells from polymorphonuclear (PMN) leukocytes, which are primary sources of reactive oxygen species (ROS) generation, peroxidase staining is used. Neutrophils, polynuclear leukocytes, and macrophages are peroxidase-positive granulocytes (PMN should be 1 × 106/mL), whereas degranulated PMNs, lymphocytes, and immature germ cells are peroxidase-negative (Fig. 1 and Table 3).[31-33]

SPERM MORPHOLOGY

Historical Evolution of Sperm Morphology

Up to 1970s, only the head of the spermatozoa was considered while assessing morphology. In 1971, Rune Eliasson emphasized the importance of evaluation of the whole spermatozoon including the mid-piece and tail. Eliasson was one of the first to standardize this parameter through a classification system containing three groups—head, mid-piece, and tail.[34] Evaluation of sperm morphology has seen two approaches—liberal and strict. The liberal approach as followed by MacLeod, considered all forms to be normal except those that were highly distorted, therefore no criteria was put forth for normal spermatozoa.[35] But in the strict criteria, as described by Menkveld and Kruger, even borderline forms are to be considered abnormal.[36] A normal spermatozoa was defined on the basis of spermatozoa obtained from the internal cervical os (after coitus) and from those tightly bound to zona pellucida,[36] thereby providing guidelines which were adopted by the WHO manual. The WHO manual in its first two editions followed the liberal approach after which it implemented the stricter criteria;[34] this would explain the dramatic reduction in the normal

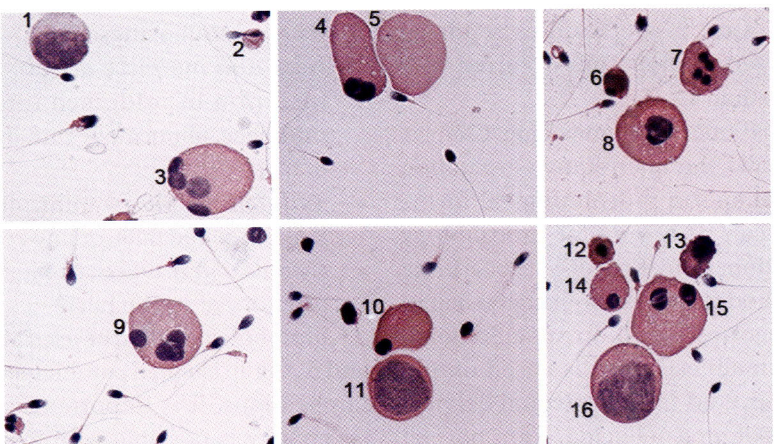

Fig. 1: Cellular elements other than spermatozoa. (1-11-16 macrophage, 2 abnormal sperm, 3 and 4 dividing spermatid, 5 cytoplasm, 6 unknown, and 7-8-9-10-12-13-14-15 degenerating spermatid).

Table 3: Nomenclature related to semen quality [World Health Organization (WHO) manual, fifth edition].

Aspermia	*No semen (no or retrograde ejaculation)*
Asthenozoospermia	Percentage of progressively motile (PR) spermatozoa below the lower reference limit [≥40% PR + nonprogressive motility (NP), or ≥32% PR]
Asthenoteratozoospermia	Percentages of both PR and morphologically normal spermatozoa below the lower reference limits
Azoospermia	No spermatozoa in the ejaculate (given as the limit of quantification for the assessment method employed)
Cryptozoospermia	Spermatozoa absent from fresh preparations but observed in a centrifuged pellet
Hemospermia (hematospermia)	Presence of erythrocytes in the ejaculate
Leukospermia (leukocytospermia, pyospermia)	Presence of leukocytes in the ejaculate above the threshold value
Necrozoospermia	Low percentage of live, and high percentage of immotile, spermatozoa in the ejaculate
Normozoospermia	Total number (or concentration, depending on outcome reported)* of spermatozoa, and percentages of PR and morphologically normal spermatozoa, equal to or above the lower reference limits
Oligoasthenozoospermia	Total number (or concentration lower reference value ≥15 million/mL or ≥39 million total sperm count, depending on outcome reported)* of spermatozoa, and PR spermatozoa, below the lower reference limits
Oligoasthenoteratozoospermia	Total number (or concentration lower reference value ≥15 million/mL or ≥39 million total sperm count, depending on outcome reported)* of spermatozoa, and percentages of both PR and morphologically normal spermatozoa, below the lower reference limits
Oligoteratozoospermia	Total number (or concentration lower reference value ≥15 million/mL or ≥39 million total sperm count, depending on outcome reported)* of spermatozoa, and percentage of morphologically normal spermatozoa, below the lower reference limits
Oligozoospermia	Total number (or concentration lower reference value ≥15 million/mL or ≥39 million total sperm count, depending on outcome reported)* of spermatozoa below the lower reference limit
Teratozoospermia	Percentage of morphologically normal spermatozoa below the lower reference limit

*Preference should always be given to total number, as this parameter takes precedence over concentration.

morphology reference value from 80% (1st edition)[11] to 4% (5th edition).[12]

The clinical implications of poor morphology scores remain highly controversial. The initial studies using rigid criteria reported that patients undergoing in vitro fertilization (IVF) who had greater than 14% normal forms had better fertilization rates.[37] Later studies reported that most impairment in fertilization rates occurred with morphology scores of less than 4% (Fig. 2).[38]

The staining of a seminal smear (Papanicolaou, Giemsa, Shorr, and Diff-Quik) allows the quantitative evaluation of normal and abnormal sperm morphological forms in an ejaculate. Smears can be scored for morphology using the WHO classification, or by Kruger's strict criteria classification.[38] WHO method classifies abnormally shaped sperm into specific categories based on specific head, tail, and midpiece abnormalities, which is based on the appearance of sperm recovered from postcoital cervical mucus or from the surface of zona pellucida (>30% normal forms). In contrast, Kruger's strict criteria classifies sperm as normal only if the sperm shape falls within strictly defined parameters of shape and all borderline forms are considered abnormal (>14% normal forms).

- *Head defects:* Large, small, tapered, pyriform, round, amorphous, vacuolated (>20% of the head area occupied by unstained vacuolar areas) heads with small acrosomal area (<40% of head area), double heads, any combination of these
- *Neck and midpiece defects:* Bent neck, asymmetrical insertion of midpiece into head, thick, irregular midpiece, abnormally thin midpiece, any combination of these
- *Tail defects:* Short, multiple, hairpin, broken, bent, kinked, coiled tails, or any combination of these
- *Cytoplasmic droplets:* Greater than one-third of the area of a normal sperm head.

Morphology should be used along with other parameters, and not as an isolated parameter, when determining clinical implications. It is important to realize that, in general, pregnancy is possible with low morphology scores and that both motility and morphology have also demonstrated prognostic value, as do combinations of parameters.[39,40]

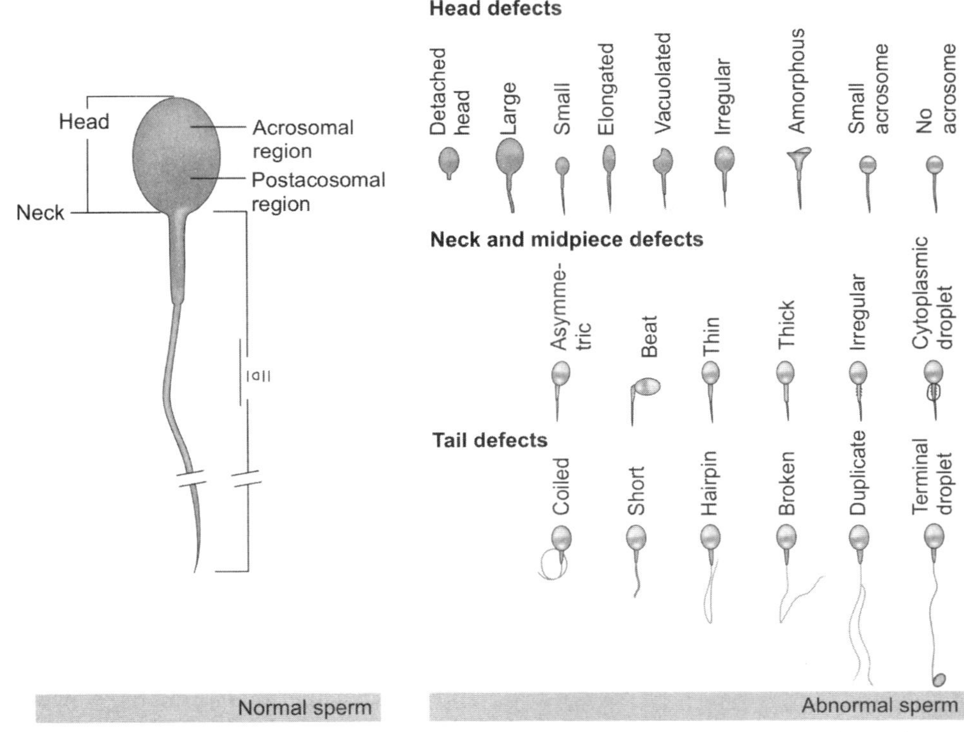

Fig. 2: There is a sperm with normal shape and on the right side the multiple defects the sperms can have; these can affect the head, neck or tail region.

BIOCHEMICAL ANALYSIS OF SEMINAL PLASMA

Biochemical analysis of seminal plasma is an important exercise to assess the impairment of epididymal, vesicular, and prostatic function and which may be clinically relevant in patients with hyperviscous semen and to understand genital fluid interactions during the semen coagulation-liquefaction process.

Fructose reflects secretory function of seminal vesicles and in cases of azoospermia absence of fructose points the congenital absence of seminal vesicles and vas deferens whereas lower or absence of concentrations of citric acid and zinc are reliable indicators of prostatic dysfunction or prostatic obstruction.[41-43]

SPERM FUNCTION TESTS

There are various sperm-function tests available; some of the most commonly used are:

- Viability test
- Sperm acrosome intactness test
- Deoxyribonucleic acid (DNA) fragmentation index test
- Assessment of ROS testing
- Mitochondrial activity index test
- Cervical mucus penetration test
- Hemizona and zona pellucida binding test
- Sperm penetration assay (SPA)/zona-free hamster oocyte penetration test/sperm capacitation test.

Viability Test

If the semen sample shows significantly low or no motility it is difficult to judge the percentage of viable sperms. Sperm viability testing is used to determine if nonmotile sperm arealiveor dead and are indicated when sperm motility is less than 5–10%. It is useful in primary ciliary dyskinesia where ultrastructural defects in sperm flagella result in absent or extremely low motility but with high viability. Also used to select sperm for intracytoplasmic sperm injection (ICSI), in surgically retrieved testicular tissue, sperms are alive but generally nonmotile, because of lack of epididymal transit.[44,45]

A functional membrane is requisite for the fertilizing ability of spermatozoa, as it plays an integral role in sperm capacitation, acrosome reaction (AR), and binding of the spermatozoon to the egg surface. Viability testing is based on the membrane permeability and it can be done by dye exclusion assays or hypo-osmotic swelling (HOS) test.

- *Dye exclusion assays:* This test relies on the ability of live sperm to resist absorption of certain dyes, whereas these dyes (Eosin Y and Nigrosin or Eosin Y and Trypan blue) penetrate and stain nonviable sperm. Trypan blue and Eosin Y stains, which do not stain live sperm, are the most commonly employed. However, as the technique requires air drying after staining, sperms are killed and not practically useful (Fig. 3)[46]

- *Hypo-osmotic swelling test:* The HOS test evaluates the functional integrity of the sperm's plasma membrane and serves as a useful indicator of fertility potential of sperm. When live cells are placed in hypo-osmotic media, water enters the cytoplasm causing the cell to swell, particularly the tail, which is calculated as a percentage. This assay does not damage or kill the sperm and is very useful for identifying viable, and nonmotile sperm for ICSI. HOS has a limited ability to predict male fertility, but an HOS result less than 50% is associated with increased miscarriage rates (Figs. 4A and B).

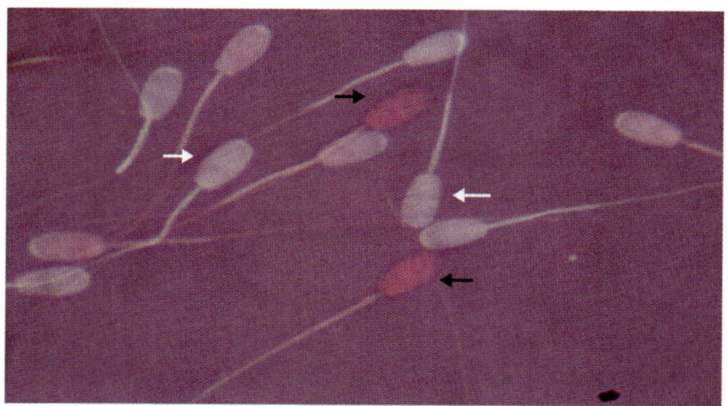

Fig. 3: Image of sperm viability test evaluated under a light microscope (1000x) following Eosin-Nigrosin staining. Sperm with an unstained head (white arrows) were regarded as the live sperm. Sperm having red head (black arrows) were deemed as dead sperm.

Sperm Acrosome Intactness Test

With the use of the ICSI the role of AR in fertilization is minimal, but the percentage value of acrosome intactness can still be of an important tool to predict the male factor, especially when it is idiopathic and repeated failures in natural conception or intrauterine insemination (IUI) with most semen parameters being normal.

Deoxyribonucleic Acid Fragmentation Index Test

Mammalian fertilization involves the direct interaction of the sperm and the oocyte, fusion of the cell membranes, and union of male and female gamete genomes. Although a small percentage of spermatozoa from fertile men also possess detectable levels of DNA damage, (which is repaired by oocyte cytoplasm), there is evidence to show that the spermatozoa of infertile men possess substantially more DNA damage and that this damage may adversely affect reproductive outcomes.[47,48] There appears to be a threshold of sperm DNA damage, which can be repaired by oocyte cytoplasm (i.e. abnormal chromatin packaging, protamine deficiency) beyond which embryo development and pregnancy are impaired.[49,50] We have different tests to assess the DNA fragmentation grade.

Deoxyribonucleic Acid Damage—Direct Tests

- Terminal deoxynucleotidyl transferase-mediated deoxyuridine triphosphate (dUTP) nick end-labeling (TUNEL) assay
- Deoxyribonucleic acid oxidation measurement.

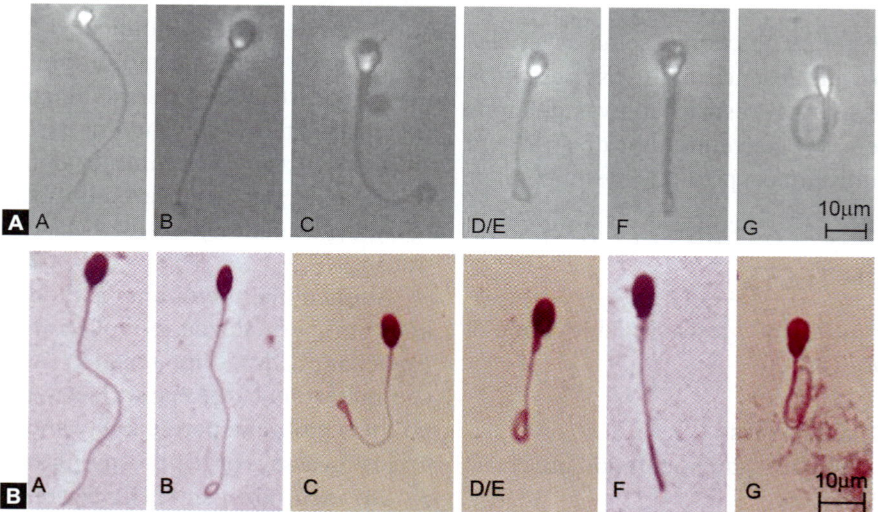

Figs. 4A and B: Microscopic observation of different grades of sperm swelling. The different sperm swelling grades (A–G) as observed using (A) Phase-contrast microscopy (1000x magnification) of fresh samples; and (B) Fixed and stained samples using normal light microscopy.

Deoxyribonucleic Acid Damage—Indirect Tests

- Sperm chromatin structure assay (SCSA)
- Sperm chromatin dispersion assay
- Sperm fluorescence in situ hybridization (FISH) analysis.

Assessment of Reactive Oxygen Species Testing

Reactive oxygen species, also referred to as free radicals, are formed as a byproduct of oxygen metabolism. Contaminating leukocytes are the predominant source of ROS in these suspensions.[51] They can be eradicated by enzymes (e.g. catalase or glutathione peroxidase) or by nonenzymatic antioxidants, such as albumin, glutathione, and hypotaurine, as well as by vitamins C and E. Small amounts of ROS may be necessary for the initiation of critical sperm functions, including capacitation and the AR. On the other hand, a high ROS level produces a state known as oxidative stress that can lead to biochemical or physiologic abnormalities with subsequent cellular dysfunction or cell death. Significant levels of ROS can be detected in the semen of 25% of infertile men, whereas fertile men do not have a detectable level of semen ROS.[52–54] Sperm ROS can also be measured by using cellular probes coupled with flow cytometry by detection of chemiluminescence.[55] Briefly, this is done by incubating fresh semen or sperm suspensions with a redox-sensitive, light-emitting probe (e.g. luminol) and by measuring the light emission over time with a light meter (luminometer).

The clinical value of semen ROS determination in predicting IVF outcome remains unproved but identifying oxidative stress as an underlying cause of sperm dysfunction has the advantage that it suggests possible therapies. Administration of antioxidants has been attempted in several trials with mixed results. But at this point there are no established semen ROS cutoff values that can be used to predict reproductive outcomes.[56,57]

Hemizona and Zona Pellucida Binding Test

The interaction between spermatozoa and the zona pellucida is a critical event leading to fertilization and reflects multiple sperm functions (i.e. completion of capacitation as manifested by the ability to bind to the zona pellucida and to undergo ligand-induced AR).[58-60]

The two most common sperm-zona pellucida binding tests currently utilized are the hemizona assay (HZA)[61] and a competitive intact-zona binding assay.[57] The HZA, which uses nonfertilized oocytes is useful in couples who have failed to fertilize during regular IVF, to determine the cause of the failure. Because the binding is species-specific,[62,63] human zona must be used, thus limiting the utility of these assays.

The induced-AR assays appear to be equally predictive of fertilization outcome and are simpler in their methodologies. The use of a calcium ionophore to induce AR is at the present time the most widely used methodology.[64,65]

Sperm Penetration Assay/Zona-free Hamster Oocyte Penetration Test/Sperm Capacitation Test

The concept of the SPA was introduced by Yanagimachi.[66] It yields information regarding the fertilizing capacity of human spermatozoa by testing capacitation, AR, sperm or oolemma fusion, sperm incorporation into the ooplasm, and the decondensation of the sperm chromatin during the process. However, penetration of the zona pellucida and normal embryonic development are not tested. The SPA utilizes the golden hamster egg, which is unusual in that removal of its zona pellucida results in loss of all species specificity to egg penetration. Thus, a positive SPA does not guarantee fertilization of intact human eggs nor their embryonic development, whereas a negative SPA has not been found to correlate with poor fertilization in human IVF.[67]

The acrosin assay an indirect measure of sperm penetrating capability measures acrosin, which may be responsible for penetration of the zona pellucida and also triggering the AR.[68] Measurement of acrosin is thought to correlate with sperm binding and penetration of the zona pellucida.[63,69]

Sperm Mitochondrial Activity Index Test

The lack of mitochondrial enzymes impairs sperm motility and may lead to subfertility. This test estimates the incidence of spermatozoa having full complement of mitochondria containing respiratory enzymes which provides energy to sperm for motility. In this test sperms are scored on the basis of the amount of nitroblue tetrazolium (NBT) precipitate. NBT precipitation is classified as standard, substandard, low, residual, or nil. Sperm mitochondrial activity index (SMAI) more than 50% is characteristics of fertile semen sample.[70]

Cervical Mucus Penetration Test

The ejaculated spermatozoa must traverse the cervical mucus—a barrier to sperms attempting entry into uterus.

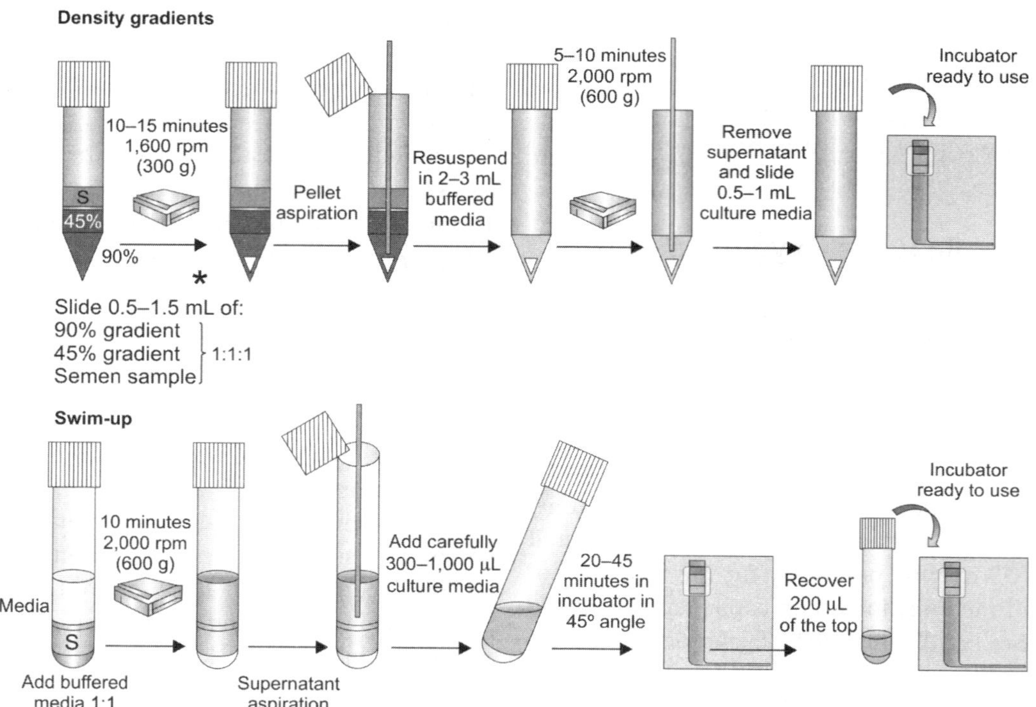

Fig. 5: Scheme of the density gradient and swim-up techniques.

It is important to determine the ability of sperms to traverse the natural barrier—mucus. The cervical mucus penetration test is an in vitro test wherein the distance traveled by sperms in a mucus filled capillary tube placed in the reservoir containing semen. The capillary is examined under microscope at different intervals of 10 minutes, 30 minutes, and 3 hours to determine linear progression, density of penetration and motility.

SPERM PREPARATION

Isolation of a sperm fraction that contains highly motile, mostly morphologically normal sperm free of other cells and debris. The importance of separating the spermatozoa from the seminal plasma is to remove decapacitating factors, reduce the concentration of ROS and to remove contaminating round cells as (leukocytes and immature sperm) responsible for the release of cytotoxic and cytostatic factors.

There are different methods to prepare a semen sample.

Pellet—Swim-up

- Liquefied semen is mixed well in a 6 mL/14 mL round-bottom tube (or in the collection jar) with fresh sperm wash medium up to 1:1 dilution, according to the initial sperm count
- Centrifuge at 600 g for 10 minutes with cap tightly closed. Remove the supernatant and layer with approximately 0.7 mL fresh sperm wash media without disturbing the pellet
- Place the tube in the conventional incubator with tight cap in a slanting position for a period of 20–45 minutes, or until a cloudy middle layer forms
- Collect the upper 0.5 mL cloudy layer and load a drop on the Makler chamber for assessing the final count.

Density Gradient

- In a 15 mL conical tube, make gradients with 1.0 mL of 90% density gradient medium, gently over-laid with 1.0 mL of 45% density gradient medium. Layer up to 2 mL of semen sample on top of the upper gradient layer*
- Spin at 300 g for 20 minutes. Cells, debris and immotile or abnormal sperm accumulate at the interfaces, and the pellet would contain functionally normal sperm
- Carefully collect the pellet, suspend in approximately 0.7 mL sperm wash medium and centrifuge in a second round at 600 g for 5 minutes to remove the remaining gradients
- Resuspend the pellet with 0.5 mL sperm wash medium
- Assess count and motility by loading on the Makler chamber.

*Volume of gradient layers can be changed according to the sperm count and debris (Fig. 5).

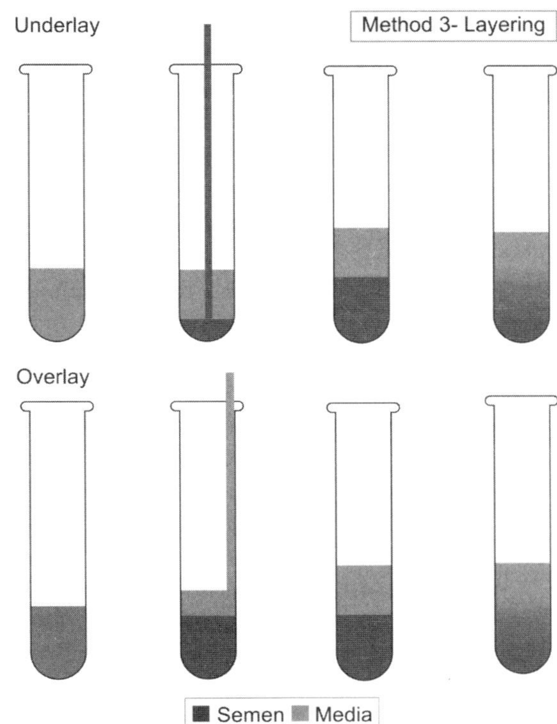

Fig. 6: Scheme of the layering technique.

Layering (Underlay and Overlay)

- 2 mL of culture medium is pipetted into a 6 mL/14 mL round-bottom tube. Approximately 1.0 mL neat semen is then gently pipetted underneath (underlay) the medium (being very careful not to disturb the interface formed between the semen and the medium) (Fig. 6)
- Alternatively 2 mL of medium is gently layered over 1.5–2 mL semen already taken in a 6 mL tube (overlay) (Fig. 6).
- Tightly cap the tube and keep it in the conventional incubator or heating block in a standing position for up to 45–60 minutes or until a cloudy middle layer forms
- Pipette 0.5 mL cloudy middle layer in a 6 mL round bottom tube and use it for the IUI/IVF/ICSI, etc.

MAGNETIC-ACTIVATED CELL SORTING

This is a novel technique that enables the immune magnetic separation of healthy spermatozoa by maintaining the structure, viability and functionality of the sperm. This technique is aimed to be used in IUI, IVF, or IVF-ICSI cycles as the sperm thus obtained can be used in real time.

Currently, selection of sperm during ICSI is mainly based on motility and morphology. In spite of correlation between sperm motility and morphology with the aforementioned sperm functional markers, invisible anomalies such as programmed cell death (apoptosis), disruption of mitochondrial membrane potential (MMP), caspase-3 activity and damaged chromatin are relatively ignored. This novel sperm selection technique has recently been implemented to ensure that the selected sperms have intact chromatin.

The DNA sperm fragmentation due to apoptosis (programmed cell death), is a regulation process of the cell cycle. This may be due to either inherent (spermatogenesis) or external factors like addiction. DNA damage represented by fragmentation and subsequent sperm apoptosis may be a cause of male infertility that standard methods of semen evaluation, sperm concentration, morphology assessment and motility analysis cannot detect. Several case studies on infertile patients show that there is a high level of apoptotic spermatozoa found in an ejaculate in comparison to a fertile male.

This means that the autoregulation process has failed or that there was a high level of damaged cells. Magnetic-activated cell sorting (MACS) helps to remove such apoptotic sperm from the cohort for fertilization which have less possibilities of survival.

Despite MACS is highly effective at removing apoptotic sperm cells, it is not able to eliminate leukocytes, immature germ cells, seminal plasma and other contaminants from the semen sample. This is the reason why MACS separation is normally performed in conjunction with density gradient centrifugation (DGC).

Mode of Action

- In the presence of physiological Ca^{2+}, phosphatidylserine (PS) has high affinity for annexin-V, which is phospholipid-binding protein showing highly selective binding to PS
- Annexin-V beads, binds to disturbed integrity of sperm membrane but do not have ability to pass the intact sperm membrane. These microbeads are biodegradable superparamagnetic beads conjugated to proteins or antibodies to label target cells (annexin V)
- Externalized PS is early sign of apoptosis
- Efficient removal of caspase in spermatozoa, which represents the main pathway of apoptosis
- High-gradient magnetic field is required to retain the labeled cells in specific columns. Based on annexin binding and subsequent magnetic separation two fractions are obtained:
  - *Annexin negative:* Unlabeled, intact membrane and nonapoptotic
  - *Annexin positive:* Labeled, altered membrane and apoptotic (Fig. 7).

PROTOCOL

- Prepare 1x binding buffer using sterile distilled water from the 10x stock binding buffer supplied in the kit and warm it to 37°C. It will act as working binding buffer
- Prepare 200 µL of capacitated sperms in a 6 mL tube (the capacitation method can be either density gradient or swim-up)
- Add 300 µL working binding buffer to the 200 µL capacitated sperm to complete a total volume of 500 µL. Mix well
- Add 100 µL of annexin-V beads (the volume of annexin V beads may be reduced to 50 µL in case of poor samples)
- Tightly close the tube, cover it with aluminum foil and incubate for 25 minutes (it can be used an autoshaker or can be shaked manually each 5 minutes)

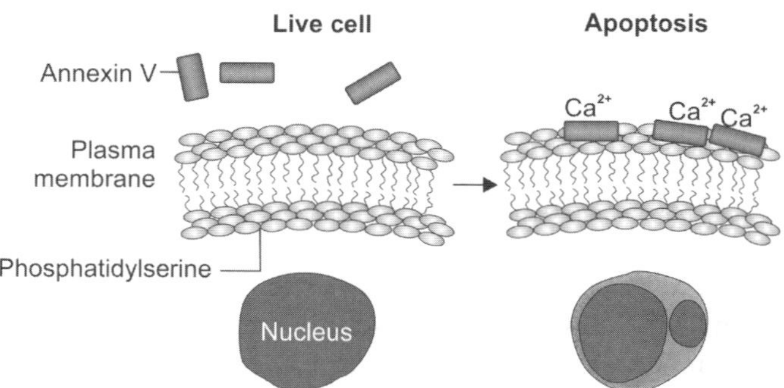

Fig. 7: Binding of annexin V beads with externalized phosphatidylserine (PS) on the plasma membrane of the apoptotic cell in the presence of Ca^{2+} in binding buffer solution whereas annexin V does not bind live cell with intact plasma membrane without PS externalization.

- 5 minutes before the incubation ends, place the MS column in the magnetic block
- Equilibrate the MS column by washing it with 1 mL binding buffer, twice
- Pour the annexin-V beads processed sample from the MS column
- Collect the eluted sperms in a clean 6 mL round-bottom tube and add 100 µL of culture medium
- Centrifuge the filtrate at 250 g for 3 minutes, remove the supernatant
- Add 0.4 mL of culture media and mix the sperm pellet. Check the sperm count and motility
- Incubate for at least 15 minutes before use.

Notes:

1. The semen samples that will be used for ICSI should have a total count post-capacitation of at least 3×10^6 sperms
2. The kit has to be put back in the refrigerator immediately after use
3. Annexin-V is light sensitive, so it is recommended to avoid the prolonged exposure of the beads to light (Fig. 8).

MACS might be indicated for:

- Previous ART failure (more than 2 cycles without achieving pregnancy)
- Repeated miscarriages
- Patients who have poor embryo quality which is not attributable to the oocytes
- Infertile patients who have a high level of DNA fragmentation in their spermatozoa

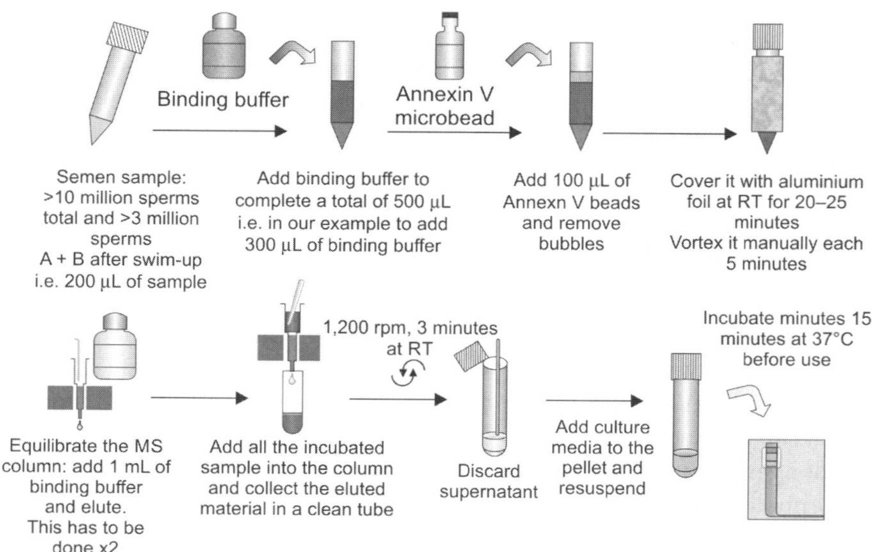

Fig. 8: Scheme of the magnetic-activated cell sorting (MACS) protocol.

- Frozen semen samples
- Addiction like smoking, tobacco chewing and alcohol
- Extensive exposure to external heat (e.g. laptop), hazardous chemicals and pollutants.

CONCLUSION

The larger point of concern with the andrology laboratories is to obtain objective and reproducible results of semen parameters like sperm count, morphology and motility. A sperm preparation is always critical in andrology laboratories. Nowadays, MACS sperm preparation technique is remedy to sperm DNA damage and the details to it in this chapter will be useful to the laboratories performing semen analysis and preparing sperm for the assisted reproduction. MACS demand more research to adopt them as a routine tool of sperm preparation for ICSI.

Computer-assisted semen analysis, microfluidic sperm sorting techniques and flow cytometry may become integral tools of objective semen analysis in near future.

ACKNOWLEDGMENTS

To Dr SS Vasan, Director, Ankur, (Bangalore, India), for his valuable contribution through the "Semen analysis and sperm function tests: How much to test?" publication in the Indian Journal of Urology, 2011. E-mail: moc.liamg@ nasavrd.

Also to Daniel R Franken, PhD (Free State University, South Africa) and his contribution to "WHO, normal abnormal sperm images and images of cellular components of semen".

REFERENCES

1. Prathima T, Ranjani S, Pandiyan N. From the pages of history: history of semen analysis. Chettinad Health City Med J. 2015;4(1):63-4.
2. Eliasson R. Analysis of semen. In: Burger H, de Kretser DM (Eds). The Testis. New York: Raven Press; 1981 pp. 381-99.
3. De Jonge C. Semen analysis: looking for an upgrade in class. Fertil Steril. 2012; 97(2):260-6.
4. Van Leeuwenhoek A. De natis è semine genital animalculis. R Soc (Lond) Philos Trans. 1678;12:1040-3.
5. Karamanou M, Poulakou-Rebelakou E, Tzetis M, et al. Anton van Leeuwenhoek (1632-1723): father of micromorphology and discoverer of spermatozoa. Rev Argent Microbiol. 2010;42(4):311-4.
6. Capanna E. Lazzaro Spallanzani. At the roots of modern biology. J Exp Zool. 1999;285(3):178-96.
7. Birkhead TR, Montgomerie R. Three centuries of sperm research. In: Birkhead TR, Hosken DJ, Pitnick SS (Eds). Sperm Biology: An Evolutionary Perspective, 1st edition. USA: Elsevier; 2008.
8. Sims JM. Clinical Notes on Uterine Surgery: With Special Reference to the Management of the Sterile Condition. New York: William Wood; 1866. p. 430.
9. Macomber D, Sanders MB. The spermatozoa count: its value in the diagnosis, prognosis and treatment of sterility. N Engl J Med. 1929;200:981-4.
10. MacLeod J. Semen quality in 1000 men of known fertility and in 800 cases of infertile marriage. Fertil Steril. 1951;2(2): 115-39.
11. World Health Organization (WHO). WHO Laboratory Manual for the Examination of Human Semen and Sperm-Cervical Mucus Interaction, 1st edition. UK: Cambridge University Press; 1980.
12. World Health Organization (WHO). WHO Laboratory Manual for the Exami nation and Processing of Human Semen, 5th edition. Geneva: WHO press; 2010.
13. The Nordic Association for Andrology (NAFA), European Society of Human Reproduction and Embryology (ESHRE) (2002). Manual on Basic Semen Analysis. [online] Available from www.slideshare.net/netopenscienart/manu al-on-basic-semen-analysis [Accessed February, 2017].
14. Gopalkrishnan K, Anand Kumar TC. Simple method to evaluate semen viscosity: model to test male contraception. Adv Cont Deliv Syst. 1990;5:355-60.
15. Keel BA. The semen analysis. In: Keel BA, Webster BW (Eds). Handbook of the Laboratory Diagnosis and Treatment of Infertility. Boca Raton: CRC Press; 1990. pp. 27-69.
16. Amelar RD. Coagulation, liquefaction and viscosity of human semen. J Urol. 1962;87:187-90.
17. Gopalkrishnan K, Hinduja IN, Anand Kumar TC. Determining the osmolality of seminal fluid aids in the rapid diagnosis of the fertilizing potential of spermatozoa. J IVF-ET. 1989;6: 119-21.
18. Huggins C, Scott WW, Heinen JH, et al. Chemical composition of human semen and of the secretions of the prostate and seminal vesicles. Am J Physiol. 1942;136:467-73.
19. Cooper TG, Brazil C, Swan SH, et al. Ejaculate volume is seriously underestimated when semen is pipetted or decanted into cylinders from the collection vessel. J Androl. 2007;28:1-4.
20. Björndahl L. The usefulness and significance of assessing rapidly progressive spermatozoa. Asian J Androl. 2010;12(1):33-5.
21. Lindholmer C. The importance of seminal plasma for human sperm motility. Biol Reprod. 1974;10(5):533-42.
22. Aitken RJ, Sutton M, Warner P, et al. Relationship between the movement characteristics of human spermatozoa and their ability to penetrate cervical mucus and zona-free hamster oocytes. J Reprod Fertil. 1985;73(2):441-9.
23. Hu YA, Lu JC, Lu NQ, et al. Comparison of four methods for sperm counting. Zhonghua Nan Ke Xue. 2006;12(3):222-4.
24. Sukcharoen N, Ngeamjirawat J, Chanprasit Y, et al. A comparison of Makler counting chamber and improved Neubauer hemocytometer in sperm concentration measurement. J Med Assoc Thai. 1994;77(9):471-6.
25. Mortimer D. Antisperm antibodies. In: Mortimer D (Ed). Practical Laboratory Andrology. Oxford: Oxford University Press; 1994. pp. 111-25.

26. Jarow JP, Sanzone JJ. Risk factors for male partner antisperm antibodies. J Urol. 1992;148(6):1805-7.
27. Rose NR, Hjort T, Rümke P, et al. Techniques for detection of isoand autoantibodies to human spermatozoa. Clin Exp Immunol. 1976;23(2):175-99.
28. Mortimer D. Semen microbiology and virology. In: Mortimer D (Ed). Practical Laboratory Andrology. Oxford: Oxford University Press; 1994. pp. 127-33.
29. Johanisson E, Campana A, Luthi R, et al. Evaluation of 'round cells' in semen analysis: a comparative study. Hum Reprod Update. 2000;6(4):404-12.
30. Anderson DJ. Should male infertility patients be tested for leukocytospermia? Fertil Steril. 1995;63(2):246-8.
31. Punab M, Lõivukene K, Kermes K, et al. The limit of leucocytospermia from the microbiological viewpoint. Andrologia. 2003;35(5):271-8.
32. Politch JA, Wolff H, Hill JA, et al. Comparison of methods to enumerate white blood cells in semen. Fertil Steril. 1993;60(2):372-5.
33. Wolff H, Panhans A, Zebhauser M, et al. Comparison of three methods to detect white blood cells in semen: leukocyte esterase dipstick test, granulocyte elastase enzymeimmunoassay, and peroxidase cytochemistry. Fertil Steril. 1992;58(6):1260-2.
34. Coetzee K, Kruge TF, Lombard CJ. Predictive value of normal sperm morphology: a structured literature review. Hum Reprod Update. 1998;4(1):73-82.
35. MacLeod J, Gold RZ. The male factor in fertility and infertility. IV. Sperm morphology in fertile and infertile marriage. Fertil Steril. 1951;2(5):394-414.
36. Menkveld R, Stander FS, Kotze TJ, et al. The evaluation of morphological characteristics of human spermatozoa according to stricter criteria. Hum Reprod. 1990;5(5):586-92.
37. Menkveld R, Holleboom CA, Rhemrev JP. Measurement and significance of sperm morphology. Asian J Androl. 2011;13(1):59-68.
38. Menkveld R, Stander FS, Kotze TJ, et al. The evaluation of morphological characteristics of human spermatozoa according to stricter criteria. Hum Reprod. 1990;5:586-92.
39. Van Waart J, Kruger TF, Lombard CJ, et al. Predictive value of normal sperm morphology in intrauterine insemination (IUI): a structured literature review. Hum Reprod Update. 2001;7(5):495-500.
40. Keegan BR, Barton S, Sanchez X, et al. Isolated teratozoospermia does not affect in vitro fertilization outcome and is not an indication for intracytoplasmic sperm injection. Fertil Steril. 2007;88(6):1583-8.
41. Johnsen O, Eliasson R. Evaluation of a commercially available kit for the colorimetric determination of zinc in human seminal plasma. Int J Androl. 1987; 10(2):435-40.
42. Cooper TG, Yeung CH, Nashan D, et al. Improvement in the assessment of human epididymal function by the use of inhibitors in the assay of alphaglucosidase in seminal plasma. Int J Androl. 1990;13(4):297-305.
43. Mortimer D. Biochemistry of spermatozoa and seminal plasma. In: Mortimer D (Ed). Practical Laboratory Andrology. Oxford: Oxford University Press; 1994. pp. 89-109.
44. Bachtell NE, Conaghan J, Turek PJ. The relative viability of human spermatozoa from the vas deferens, epididymis and testis before and after cryopreservation. Hum Reprod. 1999;14(12):3048-51.
45. Wilcox AJ, Weinberg CR, Baird DD. Timing of sexual intercourse in relation to ovulation. Effects on the probability of conception, survival of the pregnancy, and sex of the baby. N Engl J Med. 1995;333(23):1517-21.
46. Jeyendran RS, Van der Ven HH, Perez-Pelaez M, et al. Development of an assay to assess the functional integrity of the human sperm membrane and its relationship to other semen characteristics. J Reprod Fertil. 1984;70(1):219-28.
47. Evenson DP, Jost LK, Marshall D, et al. Utility of the sperm chromatin structure assay as a diagnostic and prognostic tool in the human fertility clinic. Hum Reprod. 1999;14:1039-49.
48. Zini A, Bielecki R, Phang D, et al. Correlations between two markers of sperm DNA integrity, DNA denaturation and DNA fragmentation, in fertile and infer tile men. Fertil Steril. 2001;75:674-7.
49. Ahmadi A, Ng SC. Fertilizing ability of DNA-damaged spermatozoa. J Exp Zool. 1999;284:696-704.
50. Cho C, Jung-Ha H, Willis WD, Goulding EH, Stein P, Xu Z, et al. Protamine 2 deficiency leads to sperm DNA damage and embryo death in mice. Biol Reprod. 2003;69:211-7.
51. Aitken RJ, Clarkson JS, Fishel S. Generation of reactive oxygen species, lipid peroxidation, and human sperm function. Biol Reprod. 1989;41(1):183-97.
52. Aitken RJ, Clarkson JS, Hargreave TB, et al. Analysis of the relationship between defective sperm function and the generation of reactive oxygen species in cases of oligozoospermia. J Androl. 1989;10(3):214-20.
53. Aitken RJ, Irvine DS, Wu FC. Prospective analysis of sperm-oocyte fusion and reactive oxygen species generation as criteria for the diagnosis of infertility. Am J Obstet Gynecol. 1991;164(2):542-51.
54. Agarwal A, Sharma RK, Nallella KP, et al. Reactive oxygen species as an inde pendent marker of male factor infertility. Fertil Steril. 2006;86(4):878-85.
55. Marchetti C, Obert G, Deffosez A, et al. Study of mitochondrial membrane potential, reactive oxygen species, DNA fragmentation and cell viability by flow cytometry in human sperm. Hum Reprod. 2002;17(5):1257-65.
56. Agarwal A, Allamaneni SS, Nallella KP, et al. Correlation of reactive oxygen species levels with the fertilization rate after in vitro fertilization: a qualified meta-analysis. Fertil Steril. 2005;84(1):228-31.
57. Agarwal A, Makker K, Sharma R. Clinical relevance of oxidative stress in male factor infertility: an update. Am J Reprod Immunol. 2008;59(1):2-11.
58. Oehninger S, Blackmore P, Morshedi M, et al. Defective calcium influx and acrosome reaction (spontaneous and progesterone-induced) in spermatozoa of infertile men with severe teratozoospermia. Fertil Steril. 1994;61(2):349-54.
59. Liu DY, Baker HW. Disordered zona pellucida-induced acrosome reaction and failure of in vitro fertilization in patients with unexplained infertility. Fertil Steril. 2003;79(1):74-80.
60. Consensus workshop on advanced diagnostic andrology techniques. ESHRE (European Society of Human Reproduction and Embryology) Andrology Special Interest Group. Hum Reprod. 1996;11(7):1463-79.

61. Quintero I, Ghersevich S, Caille A, et al. Effects of human oviductal in vitro secretion on spermatozoa and search of sperm-oviductal proteins interactions. Int J Androl. 2005;28(3):137-43.
62. Fénichel P, Donzeau M, Farahifar D, et al. Dynamics of human sperm acrosome reaction: relation with in vitro fertilization. Fertil Steril. 1991;55(5):994-9.
63. Cross NL, Morales P, Overstreet JW, et al. Two simple methods for detecting acrosome-reacted human sperm. Gamete Res. 1986;15(3):213-26.
64. Henkel R, Müller C, Miska W, et al. Determination of the acrosome reaction in human spermatozoa is predictive of fertilization in vitro. Hum Reprod. 1993;8(12):2128-32.
65. Katsuki T, Hara T, Ueda K, et al. Prediction of outcomes of assisted reproduction treatment using the calcium ionophore-induced acrosome reaction. Hum Reprod. 2005;20(2):469-75.
66. Yanagimachi R. Penetration of guinea-pig spermatozoa into hamster eggs in vitro. J Reprod Fertil. 1972;28:477-80.
67. Yanagimachi R, Yanagimachi H, Rogers B. The use of zona-free animal ova as a test-system for the assessment of the fertilizing capacity of human sperma tozoa. Biol Reprod. 1976;15:471-6.
68. Rogers B, Brentwood J. Capacitation, acrosome reaction and fertilization. In: Zaneveld L, Chattterton T, (Eds). Biochemistry of mammalian reproduction. 1982. p. 203.
69. Cummins JM, Pember SM, Jequier AM, et al. A test of the human sperm acrosome reaction following ionophore challenge. Relationship to fertility and other seminal parameters. J Androl. 1991;12:98-103.
70. Gopalkrishnan K, Hinduja IN, Anand Kumar TC. Assessment of mitochondrial activity of human spermatozoa: motility/viability in fertile/infertile men. Mol Androl. 1991;3:243-50.

CHAPTER

57

Cryopreservation of Semen Samples

Pallavi Menon, Carol Rubina D'Souza

INTRODUCTION

The techniques used to stabilize cells at cryogenic temperatures are referred to as cryopreservation. Advances in this field have enabled the maintenance of cell types including male and female gametes and embryos as well. The conventional obstacles to reproduction such as death, age, nonsynchronous maturation and many as such have become insignificant with the progress in the field of cryobiology. At extremely low temperatures like –196°C, there is no evident biochemical activity[1] due the lack of adequate thermal energy for the chemical reactions and the deficit of liquid water essential for metabolic processes.[2] A successful cryopreservation technique involves maintenance of the postthaw structural and functional integrity of the frozen cells. Considerable survival of frozen cells post-thaw was attained only after the finding and use of cryoprotective agents.[3] Among the mammalian cells, spermatozoa were the first to be successfully cryopreserved.[3] With a large surface area or volume ratio, human spermatozoa are relatively simple cells with a high permeability to water. This ensures rapid osmotic equilibrium when exposed to cryoprotectants (CPAs), facilitating a superior cryoresistance. The appreciable number of simple protocols have resulted in cryopreservation of spermatozoa forming an integral part of assisted reproductive technology (ART) providing the opportunity for future fertility under various circumstances. In 1953, Bunge and his group reported the first human birth which was the result of artificial insemination (AI) of cryopreserved semen.[4]

The techniques of sperm cryopreservation have gained popularity due to its varied applications including in the field of fertility preservation for cancer patients. Before the initiation of gonadotoxic chemotherapy or radiation,[5] pelvic or testicular surgeries which may lead to testicular failure or ejaculatory dysfunction, patients are advised to cryostore semen sample for future use. Patients with nonmalignant diseases such as diabetes, autoimmune disorders, multiple sclerosis, spinal cord disease or injury which lead to testicular damage can benefit from sperm cryopreservation too.[6] Also, to avoid repeated aspirations and biopsies in azoospermic patients, who have undergone percutaneous epididymal sperm aspiration (PESA) or testicular sperm aspiration (TESA), storage of sperm by cryopreservation, is favorable.[7]

Semen cryopreservation also facilitates donor samples to be quarantined to ensure prevention of transmitting infectious agents to recipients such as human immunodeficiency virus (HIV), hepatitis B virus, etc.[8] Furthermore, patients undergoing ART procedures, routinely have to cryostore the semen samples to avoid inconveniences caused due to failed ejaculation as a consequence of stress or inability to be physically present to provide semen sample on the day of oocyte retrieval.[9]

The generic steps involved in semen cryopreservation include, dilution, cryoprotection, cooling and freezing, storage and thawing.[10] The most commonly used methods for cryopreservation are vitrification and slow freezing. Literature confirms that the success of cryopreservation, despite the technique used, is strongly determined by the initial quality of the sample to be frozen.[11] During the process of cryopreservation, cells undergo transformation in their physical and chemical structures, as there is a drastic temperature drop from +37°C to –196°C. Almost 95% of cellular water content is lost, resulting in increased concentration of solutes, which could trigger an osmotic shock. The potential intracellular ice crystallization and mechanical deformation caused by extracellular ice, may contribute to the cell death. Osmotic shock could hamper the cell survival during the thawing procedure due to uncontrollable swelling and ice recrystallization.[12] Therefore, poor quality spermatozoa are more susceptible to cryoinjury.[13,14]

CRYOPROTECTANTS

Cryoprotectants (CPAs) are low-molecular weight chemical components, which provide defense to the cells from freezing damage or ice crystal formation by decreasing the freezing point of materials. CPAs are broadly classified into two groups—(1) penetrating and (2) nonpenetrating depending on their mode of action.

1. *Penetrating CPAs* function by readily permeating the spermatozoa through the plasma membrane and thereby act intracellularly and extracellularly. This class of CPAs follows the osmolarity gradient while moving across the plasma membrane. These molecules prevent ice crystal formation by forming hydrogen bonds with water. Examples include dimethyl sulfoxide (DMSO), dimethylacetaldehyde, propylene glycol, ethylene, methanol and glycerol. These CPAs stabilize the plasma membrane proteins and reduce the concentration of electrolytes.[15] In the scenario of semen freezing, glycerol is commonly used
2. *Nonpenetrating CPAs* are large molecules that remain and act only extracellularly. They create an osmolarity gradient by extracting the water content from within the cell and thereby dehydrating the intracellular space. Prolonged exposure and at high temperatures these molecules could be toxic to the cells, which is prevented by using them in combination with the penetrating CPAs. Examples include sucrose, raffinose, glycine, albumins, dextrans, egg yolk citrate, hydroxyethyl, polyethylene glycols (PEG) and polyvinylpyrrolidone (PVP). These CPAs minimize intracellular crystallization by increasing the viscosity of the sample (Table 1).

Table 1: Summary of permeating and nonpermeating cryoprotectants and their characteristics.

	Mechanism of action	*Names*
Permeating	• Permeating cryoprotectants are compounds that readily permeated the plasma membranes of cells • Their movements across the membranes follow the osmolarity gradient • These molecules form hydrogen bonds with water molecules and prevent ice crystallization	• Dimethyl sulfoxide (DMSO), propylene glycol and glycerol • Glycerol is commonly used for semen freezing
	• Nonpermeating cryoprotectants are larger molecules that remain extracellular • These create osmolarity gradient by drawing water from within the cell, thus dehydrating the intracellular space • Can be toxic to the cells at higher temperatures and after prolonged exposure • Used in combination with the penetrating cryoprotectants to prevent cytotoxicity	• Sucrose, raffinose, and glycine

TECHNIQUES FOR CRYOPRESERVATION

The common practice for routine cryopreservation of spermatozoa involves exposure of straws or vials to liquid nitrogen vapor followed by direct plunging into liquid nitrogen. This results in differences in cooling rates among different straws or vials causing a significant fall in survival and motility after thawing.[16] This procedure even after being replaced by automated cryobiology freezers, the motility of the spermatozoa after a freeze-thaw cycle is only 50–60%.[17-19] The reduction in the motility could be due to the atypical response of the spermatozoa to different cooling rates. This kind of insensitivity could be an attribution of its unique structure involving, large surface area to volume ratio, small cytoplasmic volume with high protein concentration and low water content, high cellular permeability to water and CPAs and presence of a heterogeneous mixture of sperm that vary in shape, maturation status and functional potential. The two most commonly used techniques for routine semen cryopreservation are: (1) slow freezing and (2) vitrification.

Slow Freezing

This technique allows the cells in a medium to be cooled below the freezing point, was first proposed by Behrman and Sawada.[20] There is a brief pre-equilibration of cells in CPA solution followed by slow, and gradual controlled cooling at optimized rates. The entire procedure is carried

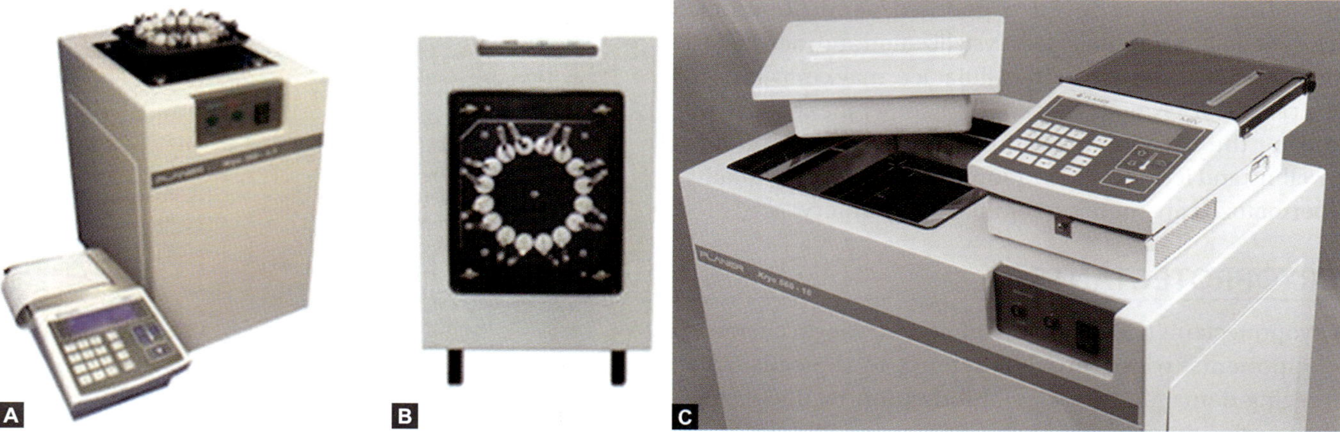

Figs. 1A to C: An example of programmable freezers from Planer (models Kryo 360-1.7, Kryo 360-3.3, and Kryo 560-16).

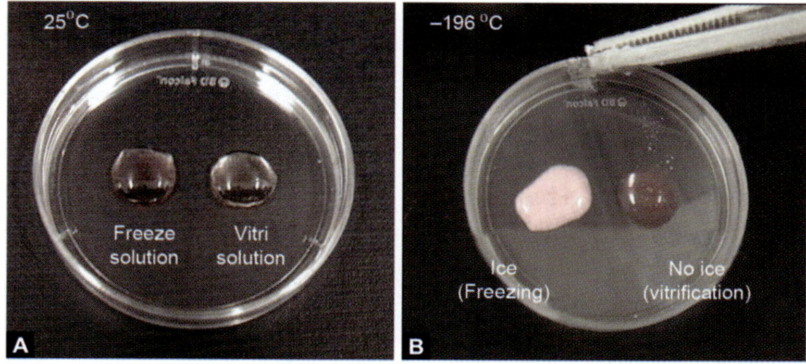

Figs. 2A and B: An example of the difference of freezing, hence forming ice and vitrification, forming glass.

out with the use of special programmable cell freezing equipments and requires about 3–6 hours for completion (Figs. 1A to C).

The temperature of the cells is reduced to a supercooled state ice crystal formation that is initiated by a process called seeding. As the size of the ice crystal increases, the water in the solution solidifies. This leads to an increase in the solute concentration in the extracellular medium which leads to the expulsion of intracellular water. The result is the dehydration of the cell, resulting in an increase in the intracellular solute concentration, which further lowers the freezing point of the cell to approximately -35°C. As the cell is devoid of any water content at this stage, freezing of the cells at this temperature has negligible ice crystal formation. The rate of cooling determines the rate at which the water exits the cell. Rapid cooling rates do not enable the complete expulsion of cellular water leading to intracellular ice crystal formation detrimental to the cells. Very slow cooling of cells leads to severe volume shrinkage resulting in high intracellular solute concentration. This has an adverse impact on the lipid-protein complexes of the cell membranes. Also these cells are prone to be affected by chilling injury. Hence optimization of the cooling rate and CPAs concentration is essential to avoid intracellular ice crystallization and high solute concentration which are the main events of cellular cryoinjury. The success of the slow cooling procedure is determined by the attainment of the optimal balance between the rate at which the water can exit the cell and the rate at which it is cooled before its conversion into ice.[21]

Vitrification

The term vitrification was first proposed by Luyet and it translates to glass formation, and transition from liquid to solid in the absence of crystallization.[22] This technique was developed in order to overcome the inadequacy of slow freezing. The solidification of a solution occurs at low temperature, not by ice crystallization but by elevation in its viscosity using high cooling rates of 15,000–30,000 C/min. During vitrification, the viscosity of the cytosol becomes much greater until the molecules are immobilized and it attains the properties of a solid (Figs. 2A and B).[23]

Vitrification involves exposure of the cells to high concentration of CPAs for a brief period at room temperature,

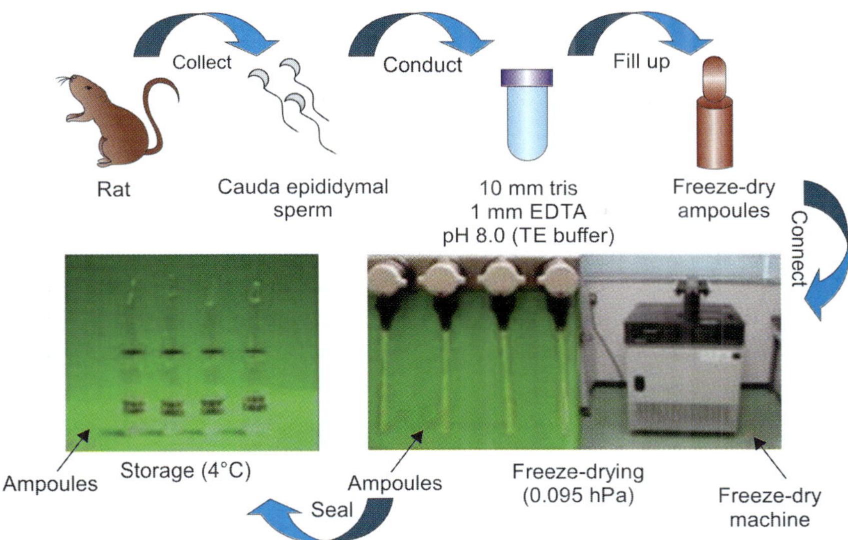

Fig. 3: Diagram of the sperm freeze-drying method in animal models. (EDTA: ethylenediaminetetraacetic acid).

followed by rapid cooling by exposure to liquid nitrogen. The initial pre-equilibration of the cells is in a CPA solution of lower concentration, leading to dehydration of the cells and permeation of CPAs. This is then followed by very short incubation in higher concentration of CPA solution followed by swift plunging into liquid nitrogen. The high osmolarity of CPAs leads to complete dehydration of the cell. By the time the cells are immersed in liquid nitrogen, they are nearly devoid of any water and hence there is no ice crystal formation. While warming, the process of vitrification is reversed. In a stepwise manner, the cells are exposed to hypotonic solutions of decreasing concentrations of nonpenetrating CPAs to remove the intracellular CPAs and gradually rehydrate. The success of vitrification depends on the rate of cooling and the concentration of CPA used. The high concentration of CPAs used in vitrification medium (30–50% when compared to slow freezing media) could have detrimental osmotic effects on the spermatozoa.[24-26] The concentrations of CPAs used in conventional freezing protocols resulted in severe toxic effects.[27] Studies have demonstrated that the spermatozoa vitrified without CPAs resulted in higher motility after thawing when compared to conventional freezing with CPAs.[28] The study also suggested that use of very rapid cooling and warming rates along with very small specimen size with different carrier systems [open pulled straw (OPS), grids, and cryoloops] support the vitrification of the spermatozoa. Evenson and his group demonstrated the integrity of sperm deoxyribonucleic acid (DNA) even at rapid cooling rate.[29]

Survival of the spermatozoa in the absence of permeable CPA could be due to the presence of large quantity of osmotically inactive water bound to the macromolecular structures like DNA, histones, and hyaluronidase.[30] The presence of high-molecular weight components in the spermatozoa could affect the viscosity and glass transition temperature of the intracellular cytosol.[31]

Freeze-drying or Lyophilization of Spermatozoa

The uninterrupted supplies of liquid nitrogen to ensure the frozen samples are maintained add to the cost factor of semen cryopreservation. Considering this, attempts were made to develop techniques to store semen samples for long-term without liquid nitrogen. Lyophilization or freeze-drying is a preservation technique which allows the sperm to be stored at suprazero temperatures by sublimation of ice (Fig. 3). The quality of the products thus acquired is not altered during the drying process and can be easily rehydrated.[32] Though the DNA of the lyophilized sperm has been shown to remain intact, the other sperm structures are irreversibly damaged.[33] Though live births in several animal species have been reported[34] by this technique, lyophilization of human sperm is still an experimental technique which is not offered to patients due to lack of supportive literature.

DETRIMENTAL EFFECT OF SEMEN CRYOPRESERVATION

When compared to other cells, spermatozoa appear to be less susceptible to cryoinjury which is attributed to the low water content and high membrane fluidity. Nevertheless, cryopreservation could still have deleterious impact on the structural and functional aspects of the sperm (Figs. 4A to C).[35]

Effect of Cryopreservation on Deoxyribonucleic Acid Integrity

There is literature to support the fact that amendment in the DNA integrity of human sperm is noted following cryopreservation.[13,36-38] However, there are also studies that challenge this concept and claim no effect is seen.[39-42] This disagreement between studies could be because of sample size, the freezing-thawing protocol in use, sperm preparation techniques before or during cryopreservation and the use of diverse tests to assess the sperm DNA integrity (Table 2).

Effect of Cryopreservation on Motility and Viability

The plasma membrane of the spermatozoa is the prime site where cryoinjury occurs.[10,43,44] The mitochondria which is essential for sperm motility, is placed along the midpiece

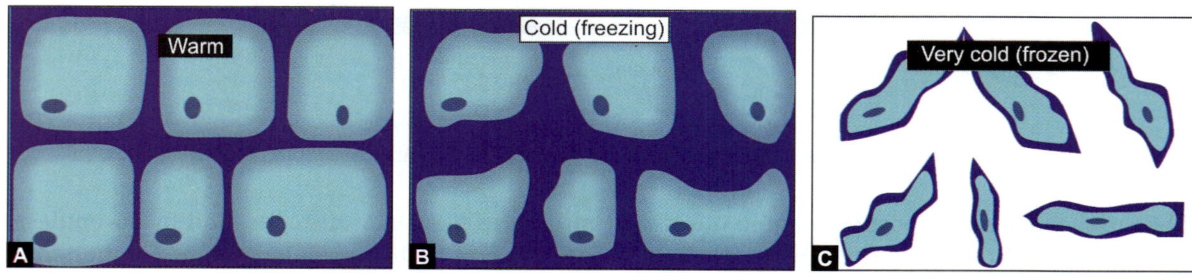

Figs. 4A to C: On a cellular scale, ice forms first outside cells, the growing extracellular ice causes cell dehydration and eventually the cells shrink. Finally cells are left damaged and squashed between ice crystals. The damage is mostly mechanical.

Table 2: Different cryopreservation methods and the DNA damage.

Authors	*Test to evaluate DNA integrity*	*Cryopreservation method*	*"Does the freezing-thawing procedure induce sperm DNA damage?"*
Hamamah et al.	Acridine orange staining and Feulgen-DNA quantitative microspectrophotometry	Unspecified	Yes
Span`o et al.	SCSA + Acridine orange staining	Equilibration at 37°C, freezing in liquid nitrogen vapor at –80°C and then storage in liquid nitrogen at –196°C	Yes
Hammadeh et al.	Acridine orange staining	Computerized slow-stage freezer + static liquid nitrogen vapor	Yes
Donnelly et al.	Comet assay	Equilibration at 37°C, freezing in liquid nitrogen vapor at –80°C and then storage in liquid nitrogen at –196°C	Yes
Gandini et al.	Acridine orange staining	Equilibration at 37°C, freezing in liquid nitrogen vapor at –80°C and then storage in liquid nitrogen at –196°C	Yes
de Paula et al.	TUNEL assay	Use of freezer at –20°C, freezing in liquid nitrogen vapor, then storage in liquid nitrogen at –196°C	Yes
Petyim and Choavaratana	Acridine orange staining	Freezing with liquid nitrogen vapor + computerized program freezer	Yes
Nagamwuttiwong and Kunathikom	Acridine orange staining	Freezing with liquid nitrogen vapor	Yes
Dejarkom and Kunathikom	Acridine orange staining	Computerized controlled rate freezing	Yes
Thomson et al.	TUNEL assay	Use of programmable freezer	Yes
Thomson et al.	TUNEL assay	Sample frozen with and without cryoprotectant by slow controlled-rate method using a programmable freezer	Yes

Contd...

Contd...

Zribi et al.	TUNEL assay	Equilibration at 37°C, freezing in liquid nitrogen vapor at –80°C, then storage in liquid nitrogen at –196°C	Yes
Donnelly et al.	Comet assay	Equilibration at 37°C, freezing in liquid nitrogen vapor at –80°C, then storage in liquid nitrogen at –196°C	Yes, but semen from fertile men appears to be more resistant to freezing damage
Kalthur et al.	Comet assay + acridine orange staining	Equilibration at 37°C, freezing in liquid nitrogen vapor at –80°C, then storage in liquid nitrogen at –196°C	Yes, but morphologically abnormal sperms seems to be less resistant to freezing damage
Ahmad et al.	Comet assay	Freezing with static phase vapor cooling procedure	Yes, but the sperm DNA integrity of frozen samples of fertile men is higher
Høst et al.	Immunoperoxidase detection of digoxigenin-labeled genomic DNA	Conventional cryopreservation	No
Steele et al.	Comet assay	Freezing in liquid nitrogen vapor	No
Duru et al.	TUNEL assay + annexin V	Equilibration at 37°C, freezing in liquid nitrogen vapor at –80°C, then storage in liquid nitrogen at –196°C	No
Isachenko et al.	Comet assay	Programmable slow freezing + vitrification	No
Paasch et al.	TUNEL assay + flow cytometric kit for apoptosis	Equilibration at 37°C, freezing in liquid nitrogen vapor at –80°C, then storage in liquid nitrogen at –196°C	No

[DNA: deoxyribonucleic acid; SCSA: sperm chromatin structure assay; TUNEL: terminal deoxynucleotidyl transferase-mediated deoxyuridine triphosphate (dUTP) nick end-labeling].

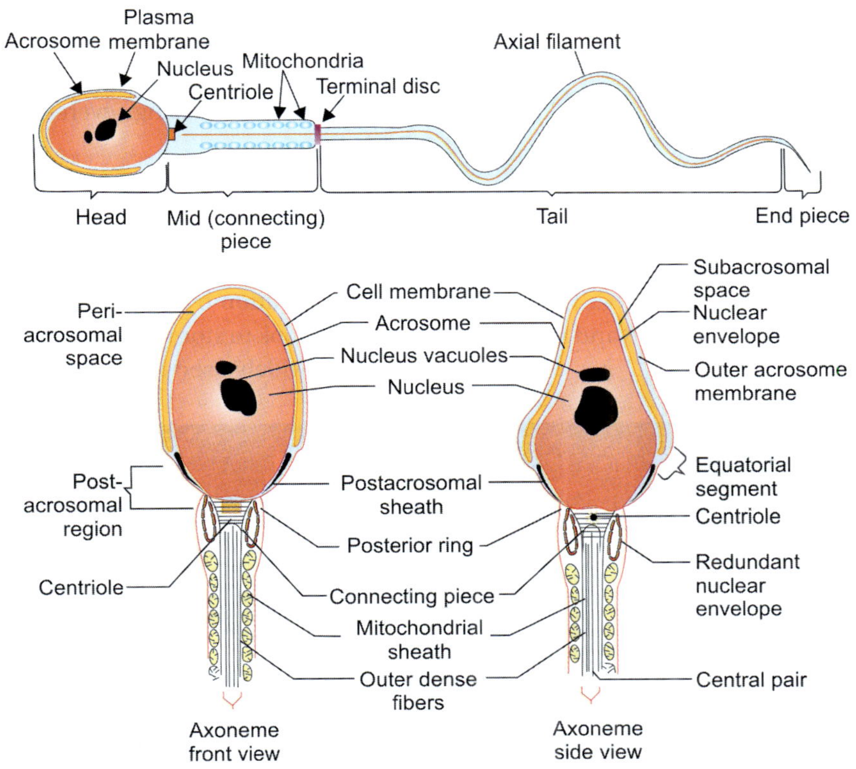

Fig. 5: Schematic representation of human spermatozoa.

between the plasma membrane and the nine fibrous columns, this is assumed to have similar vulnerability to cryoinjury as the plasma membrane (Fig. 5).[45]

The maximum energy is derived from the adenosine triphosphate (ATP) molecules which are synthesised either by glycolysis in the cytoplasm[46] or through oxidative phosphorylation in the mitochondria.[47] Therefore any damage to the plasma membrane or mitochondria may lead to decline in the motility.[45] The same study also showed a significant reduction in the number of viable sperm after cryopreservation.

Effect of Cryopreservation on Fertilizing Ability

Cryopreservation also has been shown to have adverse impact on the fertilizing ability of the spermatozoa. In a study, it was suggested that the alterations in the plasma membrane of the spermatozoa due to the process of cryopreservation made the spermatozoa more susceptible to their milieu and thereby making them partially capacitated post-thaw.[44] This cryocapacitation reduces the life span of spermatozoa in vivo and powerfully decreases the efficiency of the entire population.

DEVICES USED IN SEMEN CRYOPRESERVATION

The devices used for the storage of the frozen semen sample depend on various factors including the freezing protocol in use and the type of sperm sample to be frozen. They are broadly classified into two categories—(1) biological carriers and (2) nonbiological carriers.

1. *Biological carriers*: It include empty zonae of various species and Volvox globator algae
2. *Nonbiological carriers*: It include cryovials, straws, 5 mm copper loops, cryoloops, calcium alginate beads, intracytoplasmic sperm injection (ICSI) pipettes, microdroplets on dry ice or plastic dish and agarose gel microspheres.

Vials

The most commonly used device for semen cryopreservation is the cryovials. These are usually made of specially formulated polypropylene and commercially available in various volumes ranging from 0.5 mL up to 5 mL. These are usually provided with a white marking area for easy sample identification. Several commercially available brands have color-coding system for identification. The vials are available with either external or internal threads (Figs. 6A and B).

The sample to be frozen is exposed to the CPAs before loading into the vials. The vials are then placed on aluminium canes inside the storage tanks. The major disadvantage of vials is the possibility of liquid nitrogen entering inside as a result of improper sealing, making the sample vulnerable to cross-contamination. There is also a high probability of the vial bursting during the thawing process, if the liquid nitrogen has entered the empty space inside the vial during freezing.

Straws

Freezing of semen samples in aliquots or storages of surgically retrieved spermatozoa are preferably done using straws. The usage of straws as carriers is very simple and easily applicable. The mixture of spermatozoa and CPAs is loaded into straws, which are then sealed before freezing. This provides a sterile system for storage.

The major disadvantage in this practice is the loss of sample due to adherence to the straws making it incompatible for storing severely impaired samples (Figs. 7A to D).

Empty Zona Pellucida

With the introduction of the concept of single sperm cryopreservation by Cohen et al., usage of empty zona as a pocket book to store individually selected sperm became the most widely used technique for freezing.[48]

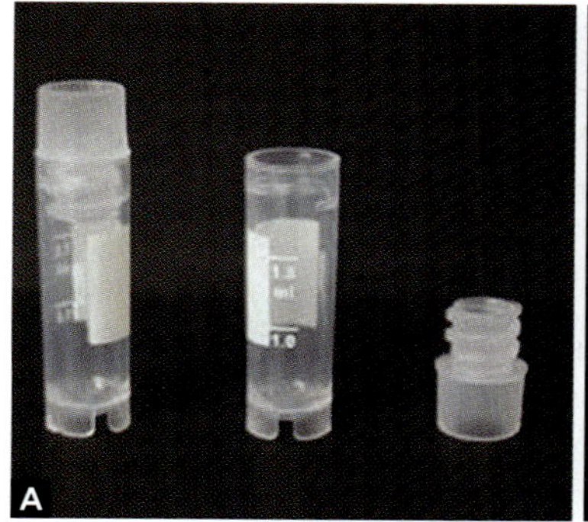

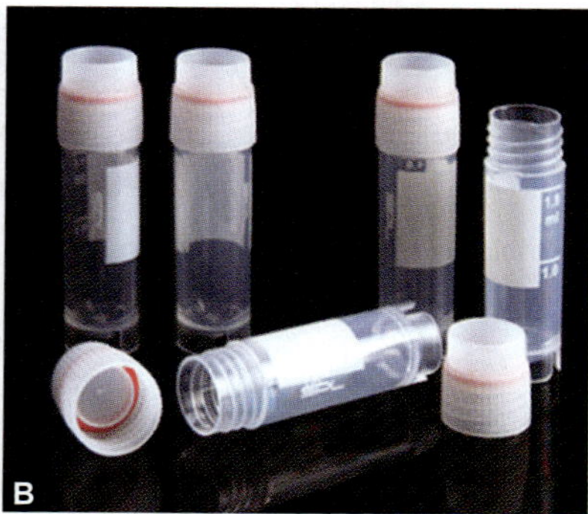

Figs. 6A and B: Different cryovials available in the market.

Individually selected sperm are deposited into an empty zona with an ICSI pipette,[48,49] and then the zona are equilibrated with CPAs prior to loading into straws. The usage of empty zonae is beneficial in cases of severe oligozoospermia or azoospermia. Also the addition and removal of CPAs without the loss of dilution of the spermatozoa enclosed within the zona can be easily achieved. The major disadvantage of this technique is the risk of biological contamination (Figs. 8A and B).

Microdroplets

To overcome the loss of sperm through adherence carriers the direct cryopreservation of sperm in microdroplets was introduced in 2000.[50,51] Aliquots of 50 or 100 μL of the spermatozoa and CPA mixture are placed on the surface of dry ice or cold stainless steel plate and then plunged into liquid nitrogen. These aliquots or pills can be removed as per requirement and thawed for use.

The major disadvantage of this practice is the risk of cross-contamination. In addition, the shape and size of the steel plate in use could cause hindrance during handling and storage in liquid nitrogen tanks or conventional freezers (Figs. 9A and B).

Intracytoplasmic Sperm Injection Pipettes

Freezing of spermatozoa can be done using ICSI pipette as a sterile carrier.[52,53] Between 5 and 50 spermatozoa, either surgically retrieved or ejaculated can be stored in each

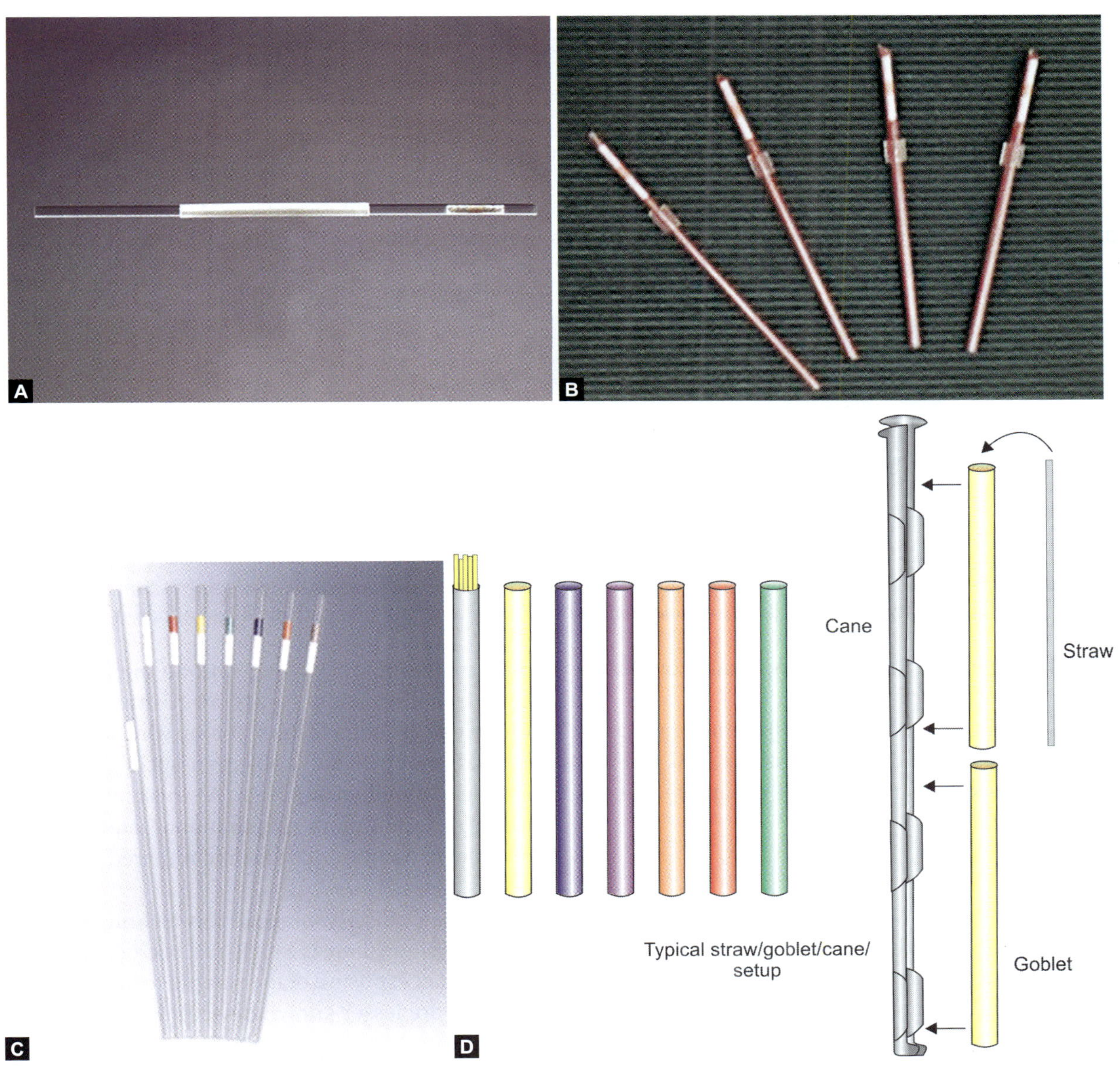

Figs. 7A to D: Different straws available in the market.

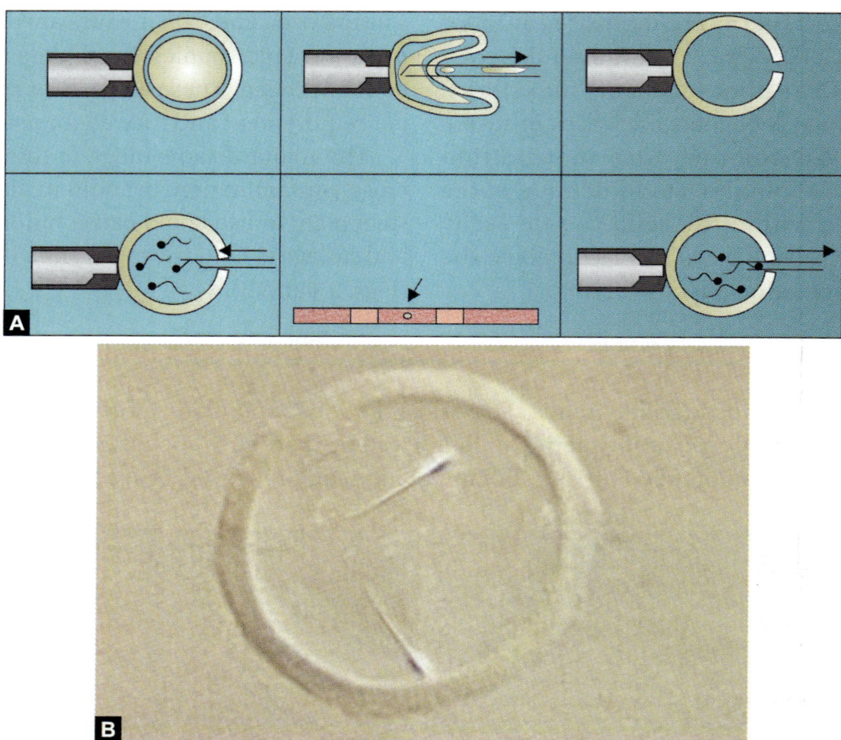

Figs. 8A and B: Empty zona pellucida and the mechanism to individually select sperms and deposit them into an empty zona with an intracytoplasmic sperm injection (ICSI) pipette.

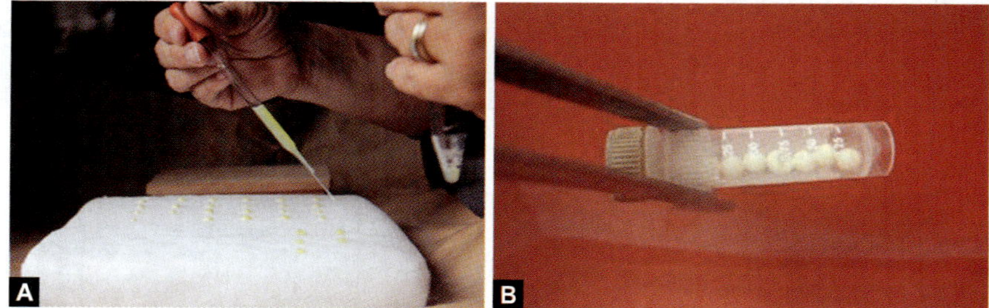

Figs. 9A and B: With the microdroplets technique, aliquots of 50 or 100 μL of the spermatozoa and cryoprotectant (CPA) mixture are placed on the surface of dry ice or cold stainless steel plate and then plunged into liquid nitrogen.

pipette. This technique is relatively simple and convenient system.

The disadvantage is that it is not a feasible practice for long-term storage. Due to the fragility of the ICSI pipettes, it can be easily broken resulting in loss of sample and risk of cross-contamination.

Cryoloop

Cryoloop was first introduced as a device for embryo freezing.[54] Later on this was used as a potential device to cryopreserve small volumes[27,40,55,56] and small numbers of spermatozoa (Figs. 10A to D).[57] Cryoloop serves as an excellent device for vitrification due to the diminutive volume of fluids (1/10–1/100th of a microliter) enabling rapid freezing rates. Apart from this, the inert, and nonbiological nature of the cryoloop which is made of nylon material helps to avoid problems associated with the usage of vessels of biological origin. As these are commercially available, no additional preparation is required. Cryoloops are easier to handle and store as compared to various other devices.

The major disadvantage of this technique is that being an open system, there is a high-risk of cross-contamination due to direct exposure of the sample to liquid nitrogen.

There are lesser known devices used for spermatozoa cryopreservation including, Volvox globator spheres, alginate beads, and agarose microspheres:

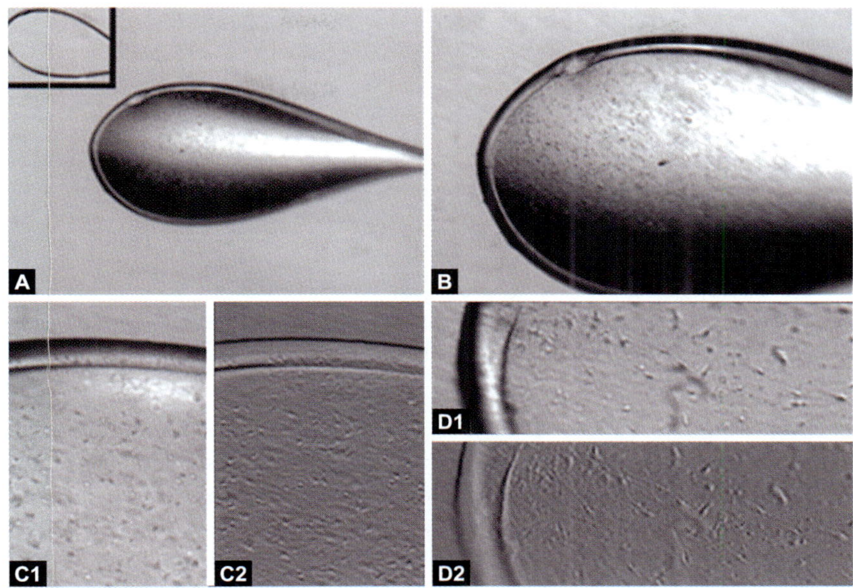

Figs. 10A to D: In this figure the empty cryoloop prior to sperm inoculation can be seen. [Inoculated cryoloops at 3100 (A), 3200 (B), 3400 (C1) and 3640 (D1)]. To enhance visualization of individual spermatozoa, embossed photographs of 3400 and 3640 are shown in C2 and D2 respectively.

Source: Schuster TG, Keller LM, Dunn RL, et al. Ultra-rapid freezing of very low numbers of sperm using cryoloops. Hum Reprod. 2003;18(4):788-95.

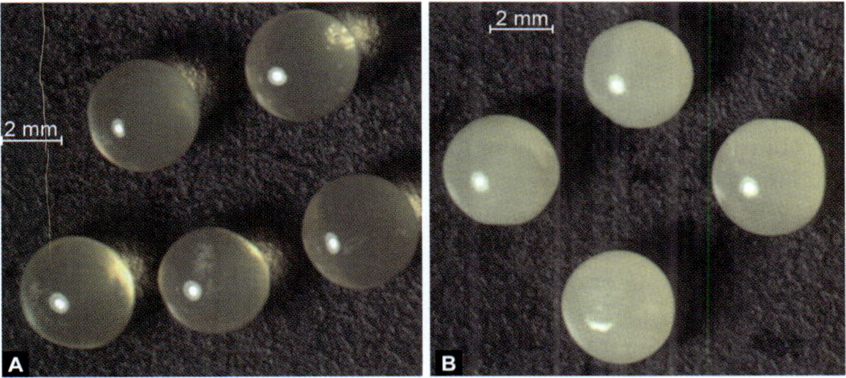

Figs. 11A and B: Alginate beads used for sperm cryopreservation.

- Volvox globator algal colonies are held tightly in a sphere-like structure into which spermatozoa are injected. The exposure of the spermatozoa to the genetic material of the algae which may be introduced to the oocyte during ICSI and the constant availability of the algal material are the concerns
- Alginate beads are prepared from a nontoxic polysaccharide derived from different species of brown seaweed. The retention of alginic acid on the sperm surface resulted in reduced motility post-thaw makes it unfavorable for use (Figs. 11A and B)
- The spermatozoa can also be stored in agarose microspheres, which is a nonbiological carrier. However, the clinical approach of this technique is not well evaluated and documented (Figs. 12A and B).

DONOR SEMEN SAMPLES

With the alarming increase in male infertility, various techniques such as testicular sperm extraction (TESE)-ICSI have evolved, which help patients with obstructive azoospermia. However, patients with nonobstructive azoospermia have no technique proven to be helpful. Studies suggest that patients with azoospermia have a genetic disposition to the condition which could be transmitted to subsequent generations. In such cases of severe male infertility, patients could be counseled for usage of donor sperm as an approach to infertility treatment.[58] Usage of fresh donor semen is almost always avoided for the fear transmitting common infectious diseases or any genetic disorders. However, in certain countries,

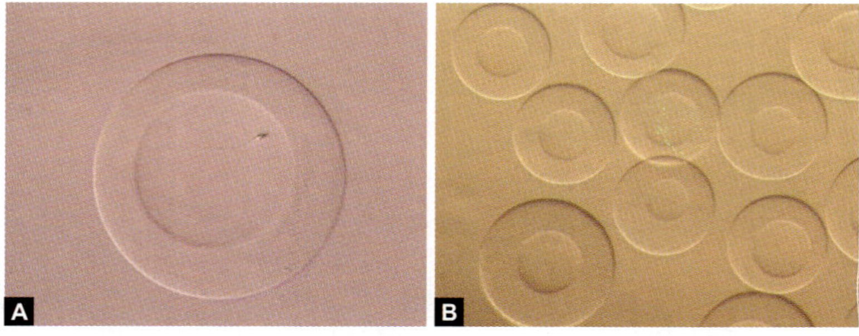

Figs. 12A and B: Solitary spermatozoa placed into agarose microsphere by similar to ICSI technique and with the same microtools can be frozen by conventional methods (DIC, 40x). (DIC: differential interference contrast; ICSI: intracytoplasmic sperm injection).

it is legitimate for the semen donor to be known to the couple or the recipient women. The screening process for donors is painstaking as it includes the acquisition of the complete medical and sexual history, psychological and physical assessment, and examination of blood, urine and semen samples to screen for pathogens, such as hepatitis B and C, HIV, venereal disease research laboratory test for syphilis, cytomegalovirus and pathogens for other sexually transmitted diseases. Also genetic screening is performed for heritable diseases depending upon the ethnicity of the donor. This screening is necessary to protect the recipient and the future offspring. Regulatory bodies such as US Food and Drug Administration (FDA) require only the anonymous donors to undergo these through screening process. Many countries have age restrictions for sperm donors. The minimum age is usually 18 years and considering the age-related genetic risks, the recommended upper age limit for the semen donor is more than 40 years.

After the recruitment and screening of donors, it is advised to retest them after a required quarantine interval, which is a minimum of 180 days. During this period, the samples are cryopreserved and stored. The samples are released for the use of recipients only after the repeated test reports indicate negative results.

The samples from potential donors are collected by masturbation. The sample is then subjected to semen analysis for the macroscopic and microscopic assessment of the sample. This is then concentrated into aliquots and frozen. The postfreezing or thawing semen parameters are assessed. Donors whose postfreeze or thaw semen parameters meet a minimum standard are selected.

CONCLUSION

Today, with the advancement in the field of cryobiology, multiple options are available for cryopreservation of human spermatozoa. This chapter briefly discusses about various techniques involved, the selection of most suitable technique depending on the semen samples, the advantages and disadvantages of diverse variants of devices available for semen cryopreservation and the various applications of semen cryopreservation. Though several studies suggest the negative impact of cryopreservation, monitoring the children born through this technique would provide a better insight to the long-term effects. As semen cryopreservation could be the only help for certain patients to have their own babies, clinics providing this service must ensure all the necessary precautions are taken to maintain the frozen samples.

REFERENCES

1. Chian RC. Cryobiology: an overview. In: Chian RC, Quinn P (Eds). Fertility Cryopreservation. Cambridge: Cambridge University Press; 2010. pp. 1-9.
2. Mazur P. Freezing of living cells: mechanisms and implications. Am J Physiol. 1984;247(3 Pt 1):C125-42.
3. Polge C, Smith AU, Parkes AS. Revival of spermatozoa after vitrification and dehydration at low temperature. Nature. 1949;164(4172):666.
4. Bunge RG, Keettel WC, Sherman JK. Clinical use of frozen semen: report of four cases. Fertil Steril. 1954;5(6):520-9.
5. Sanger WG, Olson JH, Sherman JK. Semen cryobanking for men with cancer— criteria change. Fertil Steril. 1992;58(5):1024-7.
6. Anger JT, Gilbert BR, Goldstein M. Cryopreservation of sperm: indications, methods and results. J Urol. 2003;170(4 Pt 1):1079-84.
7. Donnelly ET, McClure N, Lewis SE. Cryopreservation of human semen and prepared sperm: effects on motility parameters and DNA integrity. Fertil Steril. 2001;76(5): 892-900.
8. Morris GJ, Acton E, Avery S. A novel approach to sperm cryopreservation. Hum Reprod. 1999;14(4):1013-21.
9. Fabbri R, Ciotti P, Di Tommaso B, et al. Tecniche di crioconservazione riproduttiva. Rivista Italiana di Ostetricia e Ginecologia. 2004;3:33-41.
10. Hammerstedt RH, Graham JK, Nolan JP. Cryopreservation of mammalian sperm: what we ask them to survive. J Androl. 1990;11(1):73-88.

11. Hammadeh ME, Askari AS, Georg T, et al. Effect of freeze-thawing procedure on chromatin stability, morphological alteration and membrane integrity of human spermatozoa in fertile and subfertile men. Int J Androl.1999;22:155-62.
12. Woods EJ, Benson JD, Agca Y, et al. Fundamental cryobiology of reproductive cells and tissues. Cryobiology. 2004;48(2): 146-56.
13. Kalthur G, Adiga SK, Upadhya D, et al. Effect of cryopreservation on sperm DNA integrity in patients with teratospermia. Fertil Steril. 2008;89(6):1723-7.
14. Kopeika E, Kopeika J. Variability of sperm quality after cryopreservation in fish. In: Alavi SM, Cosson JJ, Coward K, Rafiee G (Eds). Fish Spermatology. Oxford: Alpha Science Ltd; 2008.
15. Arakawa T, Carpenter JF, Kita YA, et al. The basis for toxicity of certain cryoprotectants: a hypothesis. Cryobiology. 1990;27(4):401-15.
16. Raju GAR, Krishna KM, Prakash GJ, et al. Vitrification: an emerging technique for cryopreservation in assisted reproduction programmes. Embryo Talk. 2006; 1(4):210-27.
17. Henry MA, Noiles EE, Gao D, et al. Cryopreservation of human spermatozoa IV. The effect of cooling rate and warming rate on the maintenance of motility, plasma membrane integrity, and mitochondrial function. Fertil Steril. 1993; 60(5):911-8.
18. Mortimer D. Current and future concepts and practices in human sperm cryobanking. Reprod Biomed Online. 2004;9(2):134-51.
19. Almlid T, Hofmo PO. A brief review of frozen semen applications under Norwegian AI swine conditions. Repord Domest Anim;31:169-73.
20. Behrman SJ, Sawada Y. Heterologous and homologous inseminations with human semen frozen and stored in a liquid-nitrogen refrigerator. Fertil Steril. 1966;17(4):457-66.
21. Joshi AJ. A Review and Application of Cryoprotectant: The Science of Cryonics. PharmaTutor. 2016;4(1):12-8.
22. Luyet BJ. The vitrification of organic colloids and of protoplasm. Biodynamica. 1937;1(29):1-14.
23. Fahy GM. Vitrification: a new approach to organ cryopreservation. In: Meryman HT (Ed). Transplantation: Approaches to Graft Rejection. New York: Alan R. Liss; 1986. pp. 305-35.
24. Holt WV. Alternative strategies for the long-term preservation of spermatozoa. Reprod Fertil Dev. 1997;9(3):309-19.
25. Katkov II, Katkova N, Critser JK, et al. Mouse spermatozoa in high concentrations of glycerol: chemical toxicity vs osmotic shock at normal and reduced oxygen concentration. Cryobiology. 1998;37(4):325-38.
26. Mazur P, Katkov II, Katkova N, et al. The enhancement of the ability of mouse sperm to survive freezing and thawing by the use of high concentrations of glycerol and the presence of an Escherichia coli membrane preparation (Oxyrase) to lower the oxygen concentration. Cryobiology. 2000;40(3):187-209.
27. Nawroth F, Isachenko V, Dessole S, et al. Vitrification of human spermatozoa without cryoprotectants. Cryo Letters. 2002;23(2):93-102.
28. Isachenko E, Isachenko V, Katkov II, et al. Vitrification of human spermatozoa without cryoprotectants: review of problem and practical success. Reprod BioMed Online. 2003;6:191-200.
29. Evenson DP, Jost LK, Baer RK, et al. Individuality of DNA denaturation patterns in human sperm as measured by the sperm chromatin structure assay. Reprod Toxicol. 1991;5(2):115-25.
30. Gao D, Mazur P, Critser JK. Fundamental cryobiology of mammalian spermatozoa. In: Karow AM, Critser JK (Eds). Reproductive Tissue Banking Scientific Principles. New York: Academic Press; 1997. pp. 263-328.
31. Isachenko E, Isachenko V, Katkov II, et al. DNA integrity and motility of human spermatozoa after standard slow freezing versus cryoprotectant-free vitrification. Hum Reprod. 2004;19(4):932-9.
32. Krokida MK, Karathanos VT, Maroulis ZB. Effect of freeze-drying conditions on shrinkage and porosity of dehydrated agricultural products. J Food Eng. 1998;35(4):369-80.
33. Gianaroli L, Magli MC, Stanghellini I, et al. DNA integrity is maintained after freeze-drying of human spermatozoa. Fertil Steril. 2012;97(5):1067-73.
34. Gil L, Olaciregui M, Luño V, et al. Current status of freeze-drying technology to preserve domestic animals sperm. Reprod Domest Anim. 2014;49(Suppl 4):72-81.
35. Watson PF. The causes of reduced fertility with cryopreserved semen. Anim Reprod Sci. 2000;60-61:481-92.
36. Thomson LK, Fleming SD, Aitken RJ, et al. Cryopreservation-induced human sperm DNA damage is predominantly mediated by oxidative stress rather than apoptosis. Hum Reprod. 2009;24(9):2061-70.
37. Zribi N, Feki Chakroun N, El Euch H, et al. Effects of cryopreservation on human sperm deoxyribonucleic acid integrity. Fertil Steril. 2010;93(1):159-66.
38. Meamar M, Zribi N, Cambi M, et al. Sperm DNA fragmentation induced by cryopreservation: new insights and effect of a natural extract from Opuntia ficus-indica. Fertil Steril. 2012;98(2):326-33.
39. Duru NK, Morshedi MS, Schuffner A, et al. Cryopreservation-Thawing of fractionated human spermatozoa is associated with membrane phosphatidylserine externalization and not DNA fragmentation. J Androl. 2001;22(4): 646-51.
40. Isachenko V, Isachenko E, Katkov II, et al. Cryoprotectant-free cryopreservation of human spermatozoa by vitrification and freezing in vapor: effect on motility, DNA integrity, and fertilization ability. Biol Reprod. 2004;71(4):1167-73.
41. Kadirvel G, Kumar S, Kumaresan A. Lipid peroxidation, mitochondrial membrane potential and DNA integrity of spermatozoa in relation to intracellular reactive oxygen species in liquid and frozen-thawed buffalo semen. Anim Reprod Sci. 2009;114(1-3):125-34.
42. Vutyavanich T, Piromlertamorn W, Nunta S. Rapid freezing versus slow programmable freezing of human spermatozoa. Fertil Steril. 2010;93(6):1921-8.
43. Parks JE, Graham JK. Effects of cryopreservation procedures on sperm membranes. Theriogenology. 1992;38(2):209-22.
44. Watson PF. Recent developments and concepts in the cryopreservation of spermatozoa and the assessment of their post-thawing function. Reprod Fertil Dev. 1995;7(4):871-91.
45. O'Connell M, McClure N, Lewis SE. The effects of cryopreservation on sperm morphology, motility and mitochondrial function. Hum Reprod. 2002;17(3): 704-9.
46. Ford WC, Rees JM. The bioenergetics of mammalian sperm motility. In: Gagnon C (Ed). Controls of Sperm Motility:

Biological and Clinical aspects. Boca Raton: CRC Press; 1990. pp. 175-202.
47. Mahadevan M, Trounson AO. Effect of cooling, freezing and thawing rates and storage conditions on preservation of human spermatozoa. Andrologia. 1984; 16(1):52-60.
48. Cohen J, Garrisi GJ, Congedo-Ferrara TA, et al. Cryopreservation of single human spermatozoa. Hum Reprod. 1997;12(5):994-1001.
49. Borini A, Sereni E, Bonu MA, et al. Freezing a few testicular spermatozoa retrieved by TESA. Mol Cell Endocrinol. 2000;169(1-2):27-32.
50. Gil-Salom M, Romero J, Rubio C, et al. Intracytoplasmic sperm injection with cryopreserved testicular spermatozoa. Mol Cell Endocrinol. 2000;169(1-2):15-9.
51. Quintans CJ, Donaldson MJ, Asprea I, et al. Development of a novel approach for cryopreservation of very small numbers of spermatozoa. Hum Reprod. 2000;15:99.
52. Gvakharia M, Adamson GD. A method of successful cryopreservation of small numbers of human spermatozoa. Fertil Steril. 2001;76(3):S101.
53. Sohn JO, Jun SH, Park LS, et al. Comparison of recovery and viability of sperm in ICSI pipette after ultra rapid freezing or slow freezing. Fertil Steril. 2003;80 (Suppl 3):S128.
54. Lane M, Bavister BD, Lyons EA, et al. Containerless vitrification of mammalian oocytes and embryos. Nat Biotechnol. 1999;17(1):1234-6.
55. Schuster TG, Keller LM, Dunn RL, et al. Ultra-rapid freezing of very low numbers of sperm using cryoloops. Hum Reprod. 2003;18(4):788-95.
56. Isachenko V, Isachenko E, Montag M, et al. Clean technique for cryoprotectantfree vitrification of human spermatozoa. Reprod Biomed Online. 2005;10(3): 350-4.
57. Desai NN, Blackmon H, Goldfarb J. Single sperm cryopreservation on cryoloops: an alternative to hamster zona for freezing individual spermatozoa. Reprod Biomed Online. 2004;9(1):47-53.
58. Botchan A, Hauser R, Gamzu R, et al. Results of 6139 artificial insemination cycles with donor spermatozoa. Hum Reprod. 2001;16(11):2298-304.

CHAPTER

58

New Techniques for Sperm Selection in the Andrology Laboratory

Cristina González-Ravina, Alberto Pacheco, Irene Rubio Palacios, Javier Herrero Zapata

INTRODUCTION

Male infertility is a relatively common condition that affects approximately 30–40% of the male population. Although a majority of such patients produce sufficient numbers of spermatozoa to achieve conception, fertility is compromised because these cells are functionally deficient and could influence both the fertilizing potential of the spermatozoa and their ability to promote normal embryonic development as a consequence of high levels of deoxyribonucleic acid (DNA) damage in the paternal genome.

Semen samples consist of cellular mixtures suspended in seminal plasma composed of precursor germ cells, subpopulations of viable and nonviable spermatozoa, debris and multiple leukocyte subtypes. During the ejaculation process, the human male deposits millions of spermatozoa in the woman's vagina, near the cervical orifice, from where they begin a competitive race through the genital tract until they reach and fertilize the oocyte in the fallopian tube. Until a few years ago, it was thought that the enormous amount of sperm ejaculated in the female genital tract competed from the beginning to reach the oocyte and fertilize it. However, it is known that only a few spermatozoa are able to reach the fallopian tubes, and even fewer are able to fertilize the oocyte (Fig. 1).

When assisted reproduction techniques first appeared, sperm selection protocols were initially based on sperm separation from seminal plasma and retrieval of motile spermatozoa. However, since spermatozoa with nuclear DNA damage have the ability to fertilize the oocyte, and depending on the level of fragmentation, give rise to repeat miscarriage in the recipient woman, or to generate embryos with uncertain prognosis in future neonates, in the last years new techniques of sperm selection have been developed focusing on the isolation of functional spermatozoa. This is really important as it is recognized that the spermatozoa are more than a mere DNA delivery vehicle to the oocyte, and play a role far beyond the fertilization process by contributing paternal messenger ribonucleic acids (mRNAs), which it is believed to be crucial for normal early and late embryonic development.[1]

In order to develop new methodologies that would help to improve the currently low live birth rates achieved by assisted reproductive technologies (ARTs), it has been of great relevance to analyze how the selection of functional spermatozoa with low level of DNA fragmentation by the female organism is carried out. While it is true that some of the processes are more or less controlled, the exact mechanism by which this process is regulated in women is still unknown (Fig. 1). In any case, what is clear is that the techniques developed should be focused on selecting spermatozoa with good functional capacity and integral nuclear DNA.

The new techniques of sperm selection are based on two fundamental principles:

1. Greater precision in the morphological analysis of spermatozoa
2. An analysis focused on molecular characteristics associated with functionality and genomic integrity.

To date an ideal protocol for selection of sperm cells with high fertilizing ability should be:

- Nontoxic for spermatozoa
- Easy to perform and inexpensive
- Able to support high-throughput sample processing

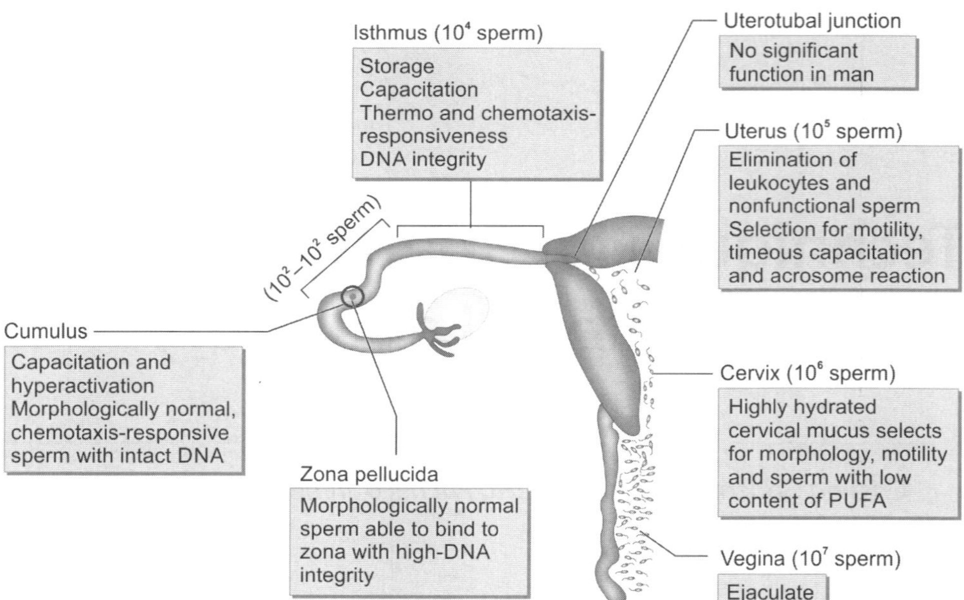

Fig. 1: Sites of sperm selection in the human female. Estimated numbers of spermatozoa in the respective sections of the female genital tract are given in brackets. Soon after deposition in the vagina, spermatozoa move out of the seminal plasma and enter the highly hydrated cervical mucus where sperm selection for morphology and motility takes place. Spermatozoa that are selected here are characterized by a low plasma membrane content of polyunsaturated fatty acid (PUFA). Subsequently, spermatozoa are transported through the uterus where male germ cells are selected for motility and timely capacitation. Dysfunctional spermatozoa are eliminated. After passing the uterotubal junction, which has in contrast to numerous animal species, no significant function in man, spermatozoa enters the isthmus of the fallopian tube. In the isthmus, spermatozoa can be stored for up to 5 days. In the isthmus and the cumulus, spermatozoa are selected for capacitation, thermo- and chemotaxis-responsiveness and DNA integrity. Finally, after passing through the cumulus, spermatozoa bind to the zona pellucida where another morphological selection takes place. Moreover, male germ cells are further selected for zonabinding ability and DNA integrity.[4] (DNA: deoxyribonucleic acid).

- Capable of selecting the best sperm subpopulation for ARTs. Unfortunately, to date no single sperm selection protocol meets all desirable characteristics mentioned earlier.[2]

Advanced sperm selection techniques are thought to improve the chance that structurally intact and mature sperm with high DNA integrity are selected for fertilization and theoretically improve ART outcomes. These procedures include selection according to surface charge, sperm apoptosis, sperm birefringence, ability to bind to hyaluronic acid (HA), and sperm morphology under ultra-high magnification.

CONVENTIONAL SPERM SELECTION TECHNIQUES: ADVANTAGES AND DISADVANTAGES

Semen preparation techniques are intended to separate sperm from seminal plasma containing decapacitating substances, prostaglandins and lymphocytes as well as to remove dead spermatozoa, leukocytes, round cells, and infectious agents. The purpose of capacitation is to make the population of spermatozoa morphologically normal and of better motility, separated from the rest of the components that often interfere with their capacity of fertilization. Adequate processing of the sample will influence the fertilizing capacity of spermatozoa, both in vivo and in vitro, and will be fundamental for the success of assisted reproduction treatments.

A variety of sperm preparation techniques have been proven to select spermatozoa that are characterized by superior motility and morphology and are capable of fertilizing the oocyte. Among them, the double density gradient centrifugation (DGC) and the swim-up procedure are currently used as standard preparation techniques.[3,4] The capacitation process is necessary so that the spermatozoon will be able to cross the layer of cumulus cells surrounding the oocyte and once there, suffer the acrosomal reaction that allows it to cross the oocyte cover and fuse with the membrane. Only small fractions of the spermatozoa (less than 10% in humans) at some point reach the capacitated state. Both the cells of the cluster and the zona pellucida are the last two barriers to selection of optimal and morphologically normal functional spermatozoa.

The sperm migration or swim-up method is easy and very cost-effective. It is the most physiological sperm selection procedure, and is based on spermatozoa self-propelled active movement from a cell pellet into an overlaying medium. The disadvantage of this method is that the immature spermatozoa and the rest of the cells remain in contact throughout the process with the mature spermatozoa and may produce adverse effects on them. In addition, many of the motile spermatozoa may be trapped at the bottom of the sediment and never reach the culture medium. Only a small fraction of total motile sperm is recovered, therefore its use is mostly restricted to ejaculates with high sperm counts and good motility.[5]

The sperm DGC method is less physiological than the swim-up procedure, and is mainly used for semen with low parameters and cryopreserved sperm samples. The density gradients currently used colloidal suspension of silica particles covalently attached to silane molecules, which are used discontinuously in isotonic solutions at different concentrations. It is recommended to use volumes of 0.5–1 mL of each concentration gradient to prepare the layers. After centrifuging, highly motile sperm cells are enriched in the soft pellet at the bottom of the tube. This method is based on the selection of spermatozoa that can overcome the difficulty of density gradients and reach the bottom of the tube, besides acting as a filter for seminal plasma, round cells, detritus, and those spermatozoa with nonprogressive motility:

- Mature spermatozoa are compacted cells and reach the highest density gradient (at the bottom of the tube)
- Seminal plasma remains floating on the lower density gradient
- Immature and dead spermatozoa are located at the interface between the two gradients.

In conclusion, conventional sperm preparation techniques, namely, swim-up and DGC, are not efficient enough to produce sperm populations free of DNA damage, because these techniques are not physiological and not modeled on the stringent sperm selection processes taking place in the female genital tract. By employing conventional sperm preparation strategies for ART, natural sperm selection processes taking place at various levels of the female genital tract (Fig. 1) are bypassed to varying extents. To improve the sperm selection, methodologies is crucial since the intracytoplasmic sperm injection (ICSI) became the gold standard procedure in ART; a single spermatozoa is selected by the technician based solely on motility and morphology parameters, and therefore, optimal selection of these gametes is mandatory. Thus, we should emphasize the need for more accurate sperm markers of fertilizing and normal developmental potential. However, while some of the advanced sperm selection methods are of value in specific clinical ART settings, further evaluation of most of them are needed before universally implement them in ART.

MAGNETIC-ACTIVATED CELL SORTING TECHNIQUE

Principle of the Technique

Magnetic-activated cell sorting (MACS, Miltenyi Biotec™) is a cell separation technique based on the use of 50 nm superparamagnetic particles that are conjugated to highly specific antibodies against a particular antigen on the cell surface that is used to discriminate the cells in which is present or not. Due to their small size, the superparamagnetic particles do not activate cells and will not saturate cell surface epitopes; besides, they are nontoxic and biodegradable, so they can be used for clinical purpose. After labeling with the specific antibody, samples must be poured into a specific column that is placed onto a very strong magnet. The column contains a matrix composed of ferromagnetic spheres that amplify the magnetic field by 10,000-fold, thus inducing a high gradient within the column, allowing the isolation of cells that are only minimally labeled, and leaving enough epitopes free for concurrent antibody staining. The space between the spheres is several times larger than sperm cells, allowing them to freely flow through the column. Moreover, magnetically labeled cells are held in suspension within the column and do not actually "bind" the column matrix. This suspension minimizes stress on the cells and allows for efficient sterile washing by avoiding cell aggregation. For that reason, MACS technology can be used to perform a positive (with cells retained into the column) or negative (with cells flowed through the column) cell selection.

Although this technique is valid for any membrane marker present in the cell (in fact, it is routinely used in hematology or immunology), in human reproduction the technique only has at present clinical application for the separation of nonapoptotic cells from a semen sample.

Magnetic-activated Cell Sorting and Apoptosis

Apoptosis is a highly regulated physiological process that is crucial to maintain testicular cell homeostasis, and to eliminate those sperm cells that have been generated with meiotic errors during spermatogenesis. This process can be deregulated by different intrinsic (alterations during spermatogenesis, meiotic errors) and/or extrinsic factors (drugs, pharmacological treatments) causing an increase of apoptotic sperm cells in the ejaculate that, if they are used in an ART treatment, can reduce the probabilities to obtain a pregnancy.

One of the early events in the apoptotic cascade is the externalization of phosphatidylserine residues of the plasma membrane, so its detection on the cell surface serves to the recognition of apoptotic cells and their separation from the other spermatozoa with higher fertilization potential. Annexin V is a calcium-dependent phospholipid binding protein (PBP) with high affinity for phosphatidylserine;[6] for that reason, this molecule has been the chosen candidate to detect apoptotic, (i.e. annexin V-positive) cells in MACS technology.[7]

Published studies showed that the use of MACS together with DGC when preparing a human sperm sample reduces the percentage of apoptotic sperm after preparation and improves sperm motility and viability.[8,9] In addition, some works have described an increase of several sperm functional parameters by using MACS selection technique, showing that annexin V-negative sperm fraction has less nucleus DNA fragmentation and is of higher morphological quality compared to the annexin V-positive sperm fraction;[10,11] other authors have shown that MACS sperm selection improves the acrosome reaction in couples with unexplained infertility.[12] Finally, an improvement of sperm motility and other functional parameters has been described when a combination of conventional sperm separation procedures plus MACS technique is used in thawed sperm samples.[13]

Magnetic-activated Cell Sorting Technique and Assisted Reproductive Technology Results

Some works have been published using this technique of cell separation in intrauterine insemination (IUI) treatments, showing that MACS technique can significantly improve the pregnancy rate in IUI.[14,15]

However, most of the published studies that use of this sperm selection technique have been performed in in vitro fertilization (IVF) or ICSI cycles. In some of them, the results showed that the technique does not offer significant improvements in reproductive outcome when unselected males were used for the cycles,[16] but it may have clinical utility when there is a male factor associated, as shown in a published meta-analysis.[17]

Indeed, it seems especially useful in cases of samples with high levels of sperm DNA fragmentation. In this sense, several publications have correlated the use of MACS with a significant decrease in both apoptotic markers and sperm DNA fragmentation in which pregnancies were obtained.[18,19] In another study performed by Lukaszuk et al. a pregnancy is described in a couple undergoing an ICSI treatment with spermatozoa isolated by testicular sperm aspiration (TESA) and further MACS selection in order to reduce sperm DNA fragmentation, suggesting that the use of MACS can be considered as valid support in cases where a high percentage of fragmented DNA is observed in the sample.[20]

It is also important to mention that a recent published article has confirmed that the use of the MACS technique has no adverse obstetric effects[21] confirming the safety use of this technique in ART.

INTRACYTOPLASMIC MORPHOLOGICALLY SELECTED SPERM INJECTION

Principle of the Technique

In a daily clinical practice, the selection of spermatozoa to perform ICSI is solely based on motility and morphology criteria carried out by optic microscopy under 400× magnification. Although it is widely described that sperm morphology is related to embryo quality and the probability of pregnancy, due to the small size of sperm cells, at this level of magnification only gross morphological defects can be observed.[22] An increase in the magnification level would allow a more detailed analysis of sperm morphology, such as the presence of vacuoles or other anomalies of sperm head or midpiece, and therefore a better selection of the best spermatozoa to be used for the ICSI cycle. In this sense, Bartoov and colleagues described in 2001 a pregnancy by using a new optic system that increased to 6,000 × the level of magnifications. It allowed also the selection of spermatozoa based on motile sperm organelle morphology examination (MSOME),[23] and then by performing an ICSI cycle using this sperm selection technique. It was called intracytoplasmic morphologically selected sperm injection (IMSI). This new optic allows the visualization of much denser specimens because the projected image is three-dimensional, describing new sperm morphological characteristics, as the number and size of vacuoles on the sperm head (Fig. 2). Thanks to this optic, new morphological classification criteria have been established, although there is no agreement in the classification system, nor in the clinical consequences that can have the new observed morphological characteristics.

On the other hand, the main disadvantages of this technique are the high cost of the equipment required and the time consuming of its application. It is important to keep in mind that the time taken to perform sperm selection

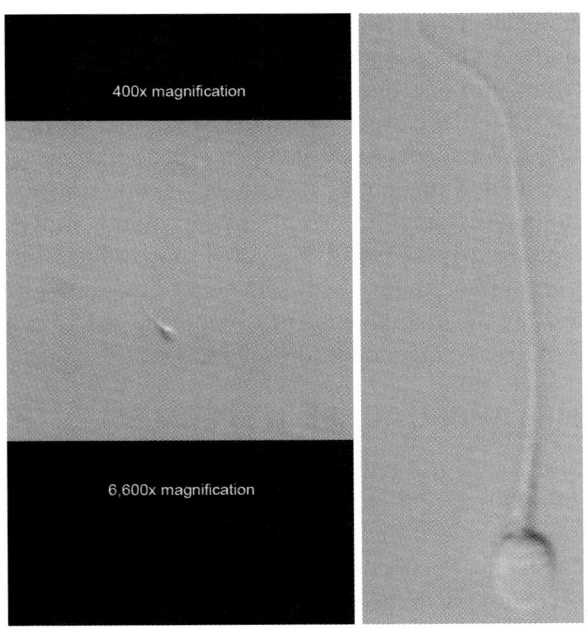

Fig. 2: Morphological differences in the observation of spermatozoa in normal optic (400 × level of magnification) and Nomarski optics used for motile sperm organelle morphology examination (6,600 × level of magnification).

through MSOME may impair sperm viability and have subsequent deleterious effects on embryo quality.

Intracytoplasmic Morphologically Selected Sperm Injection and Assisted Reproductive Technology Results

Although there have been many publications since its development that have shown results in IMSI cycles, the utility of routine use of IMSI is still under controversial.

In any case, there are many data of cycles performed with IMSI that suggest that the presence of vacuoles in the sperm nucleus adversely affects the reproductive outcome. Different works indicate that MSOME can improve clinical outcomes in assisted reproduction cycles, with an increase of fertilization rate, and also an increase of the number of good quality embryos and of the obtained blastocysts.

Some works have described that IMSI increases the implantation rate in couples with male factor infertility and in cases of advanced maternal age, and therefore should be the method of choice for these cases.[24,25] In agreement of these data, other works suggest that IMSI should have a clear role as a routine procedure in every IVF laboratory.[26]

On the contrary, others groups suggest that there are not enough randomized studies to confirm the effectiveness of IMSI and therefore its use should be limited strictly in cases of severe male factor infertility and repeated implantation failures following ICSI,[27] or when there is at least one previous failed ICSI cycle.[28]

In conclusion, IMSI may have clinical utility in selected cases, such as recurrent implantation failure following ICSI and severe male factor infertility[28] so it is crucial to select the cases to be included and that can in fact benefit from it.

PHYSIOLOGICAL INTRACYTOPLASMIC SPERM INJECTION

Principle of the Technique

The formation of HA-binding sites on the sperm plasma membrane is one of the signs of sperm maturity that has been used as a basis for a sperm binding assay.[29,30] Early studies have revealed that the percentage of sperm bound to HA reflect their maturational status and function, and therefore can be used for fertility diagnosis as well as for the selection of functional spermatozoa for ICSI. This method of sperm selection is highly specific and has minimal safety concerns.[31]

To date, there are two methods for HA binding in use, namely, the physiological ICSI (PICSI) dish (hyaluronan-coated chamber) and the hyaluronan-containing medium. Both methods are commercially ready to use systems that have received official recognition for conformity with health and safety requirements in the European Union (EU) and the United States (US).

The first of them is a PICSI dish, which consists of a petri dish with spots of immobilized HA on it (MidAtlantic Diagnostic, Mount Laurel, NJ, USA). With this selection assay, one drop of a spermatozoa suspension is placed on top of these spots of HA and incubated for 15 minutes at 37°C. Subsequently, the freely moving spermatozoa are removed by gently rinsing the HA droplet and removing the nonbound sperm. After this, the bound spermatozoa attached to the dish are picked up with an ICSI pipette (hence PICSI).

The other method consists of a viscous hyaluronan-containing medium (Sperm Slow, MediCult, Jyllinge, Denmark). In this assay, a 5 mL droplet of density gradient prepared spermatozoa is connected with a pipette tip to a 5 mL droplet of sperm slow medium by dragging the suspension into contact and incubated for 15 minutes at 37°C under oil. Afterward, spermatozoa bound to HA at the interface of the two droplets are selected with an ICSI pipette.[32]

In both cases, as HA is a natural occurring compound present in cervical mucus, cumulus cells and follicular fluid, the binding method is considered to have minimal biosafety risks for both the embryo and the patient.

Main Described Applications of Physiological ICSI Technique

As previously mentioned, the human oocyte is surrounded by HA, which acts as a natural selector of spermatozoa. For this reason, human sperm that express HA receptors and bind to HA are expected to have normal shape, minimal DNA fragmentation, better progressive motility, nonreacted acrosomes as well as lower frequency of chromosomal aneuploidies.[31,33]

Intracytoplasmic sperm injection, introduced over 25 years ago, is widely used in ART treatments;[34] however, the optimal technique for selecting the spermatozoa for insemination is yet to be determined.[35]

Current sperm selection techniques, such as DGC and swim-up, depend on sedimentation or migration of the sperm, and unfortunately important sperm characteristics, such as apoptosis, DNA integrity, membrane maturation and ultrastructure are not targeted by these techniques.[35] Current research seeks to improve ICSI outcome by isolating mature, structurally intact and nonapoptotic spermatozoa with high DNA integrity. This method (HA binding) is based on membrane maturity. It has been described that only mature spermatozoa that express receptors specific to HA can fertilize the oocyte. For this reason, this technique has been recommended in order to improve the selection of the optimal spermatozoa for ICSI and therefore obtain better clinical outcomes reducing the risks for genetic complications associated with the use of abnormal spermatozoa.[36] However, it is important to know that this added step of selection will require embryologists to invest more time into preparatory steps during ICSI.

Physiological ICSI and Assisted Reproductive Technology Results

Use of HA binding assays in PICSI cycles to improve clinical outcomes has been studied, although none of the studies had sufficient statistical power. The proportion of sperm capable of binding to HA had no correlation with fertilization, cleavage, good quality embryos, and miscarriage and pregnancy rates in couples undergoing IVF.[37] Consistently, patients with clinical pregnancies had a percentage of HA-bound sperm that was comparable to those without pregnancy.[37]

A recent systematic review and meta-analysis has been published in order to clarify if this binding selection method is beneficial in patients undergoing ART. In the selected articles, the main outcomes were fertilization rate and clinical pregnancy rate, and the secondary outcomes included cleavage rate, embryo quality, implantation rate, spontaneous abortion and live birth rate.[36] The use of HA binding sperm selection technique yielded no improvement in fertilization and pregnancy rates. Meta-analytic pooling of the data revealed no association between sperm selection technique and pregnancy rate, however, one prospective study demonstrated improved embryo quality in the HA binding group ($p = 0.005$).[38] The conclusion is that evidence does not support routine use of HA binding assays in all ICSI cycles, and the identification of patients that might benefit from this technique needs further study.

OTHER APPROACHES IN SPERM SELECTION

In addition to the techniques mentioned earlier, there are other emerging approaches for sperm selection that are currently in a development phase, such as Raman spectroscopy, electric charge-based selection method, and sperm chemotactic-based method.

Techniques Based on Deoxyribonucleic Acid Integrity (Raman Spectroscopy)

It is well-established that a high sperm DNA fragmentation index can be negatively associated with embryo quality.[39] Moreover high DNA fragmentation can be positively associated with an increase of pregnancy loss, confirming the importance of chromatin packaging in maintaining a viable pregnancy.[40]

For that reason, several test have been performed [terminal deoxynucleotidyl transferase-mediated deoxyuridine triphosphate (dUTP) nick end-labeling (TUNEL), sperm chromatin structure assay (SCSA), sperm chromatin dispersion (SCD), and Comet assay] to study the DNA integrity in a semen sample. All of them are diagnostic tools that can be only used to know the level of sperm DNA fragmentation in a specific sample, and therefore there is no possibility to use the same sample to isolate viable spermatozoa with high DNA integrity for a reproduction treatment.

In this sense, Raman microspectroscopy, the combination of Raman spectroscopy and confocal microscopy is a new technique that can solve this problem. This technique can give information of the composition and localization of different internal structures of the cell without its manipulation.[41] The study published by Sanchez V et al. showed that Raman microspectroscopy is able to identify individual spermatozoa with oxidative DNA damage to a degree comparable to the most dependable currently available technique. The utility of the technique for both clinical and andrology research is its ability to not only to identify sperm with physiologically damaged DNA but also to do this in a noninvasively and nondestructively manner,[42] permitting the use of this spermatozoa with high DNA integrity to be used or the ICSI treatment. Although Raman microspectroscopy still requires further validation, this technique may potentially provide a means of assessing the DNA status of a living sperm.[43]

Techniques Based on Electric Charge (Electrophoresis Separation)

The negative electrical charge of the spermatozoon depends largely on the expression of various glycocalyx proteins, especially gp20 or CD52, which is a sialoglycoprotein present in the sperm surface. This sialoglycoprotein is added during the passage of the spermatozoa through the epididymis and its expression levels appear to be positively correlated with the morphology, DNA integrity and functional status of the cell. Based on these characteristics of the sperm cells, several selection systems have been developed focused on the isolation and separation of those cells with higher negative charge. The most known system is the microelectrophoresis using specific devices that was firstly developed by Ainsworth et al. in 2005.[44] This device is composed of four chambers—two outer, filled with buffer, and two inner chambers (for inoculation of sample and collection, separated by a polycarbonate membrane). After application a current of 75 mA and variable voltage, the selected sperm population with high negative electric charge is collected from the inner compartment. Several works have been published by using this technique, showing that the selected populations are correlated with better morphology and with low-levels of DNA damage[44] and the first pregnancy reported by using this system was published in 2007.[45]

Techniques Based on Microgradients

One of the physiological processes of sperm selection is the attraction of the spermatozoa to the proximity of the egg mediated by chemical gradients, especially progesterone secreted by oocyte cumulus cells. As only a small proportion of capacitated spermatozoa are capable of responding to these gradients, it has been hypothesized that those spermatozoa with a greater capacity to migrate to chemoattractants will be those with better functional characteristics. Based on this principle, different devices that produce microgradients of chemoattractants have been developed.[46-48] However, the impact of using these devices to isolate chemotaxis selected sperm on ART outcomes is currently unknown.

Techniques Based on Microfluidic Sperm Sorting

Recently, different devices have been designed to sort and separate healthy normal sperm from semen sample and eliminate sperm-damaging procedures such as centrifugation and mixing. These devices contain an inlet port connected to a larger outlet collection port by a microfluidic channel. The limited depth of the channel constrains the migration of compromised sperm, permitting the selection of the most motile sperm to migrate to the outlet chamber. The inlet port is filled with unprocessed semen sample, and after a short incubation period, the sorted sperm population can be recovered from the outlet chamber for subsequent use in ICSI or IVF procedures. Recent published works using this method have shown that this selection chamber selectively isolate sperm with no double strand DNA breaks.[49] However, the impact of using these devices is still under evaluation.

CONCLUSION

Reproductive specialists are constantly looking for methods to improve treatment success rates. Considering the central role of the male gamete, finding a way to select the adequate spermatozoon is clearly warranted.

In natural reproduction, sperm selection is a necessary step to achieve a pregnancy. Conventional techniques of sperm selection (swim-up and density gradients) are based primarily on sperm motility, although other sperm parameters may be indirectly improved. On the contrary, the new techniques of sperm selection are based on the analysis of functional characteristics, trying to mimic what happens physiologically. Between them, there are techniques that improve the global sperm population, such as MACS or microgradients, while other techniques are focused on the individual selection of spermatozoa to be used in ART, such as IMSI, PICSI, or Raman spectroscopy. The data obtained so far, although sometimes conflicting, seem to indicate that these techniques may be useful in selected infertile cases, especially when there is an associated male factor, such as MACS and IMSI, or in cases of repetitive abortion, such as PICSI. Even so, although the results obtained so far are promising are still necessary more prospective and randomized studies to draw more consistent conclusions.

REFERENCES

1. Barroso G, Valdespin C, Vega E, et al. Developmental sperm contributions: fertilization and beyond. Fertil Steril. 2009;92(3):835-48.

2. Ortega NM, Bosch P. Methods for sperm selection for in vitro fertilization. In: Friedler S, (Ed). In Vitro Fertilization-innovative Clinical and Laboratory Aspects. Croatia: InTech; 2012.
3. Henkel RR, Schill WB. Sperm preparation for ART. Reprod Biol Endocrinol. 2003;1:108.
4. Henkel R. Sperm preparation: state-of-the-art—physiological aspects and application of advanced sperm preparation methods. Asian J Androl. 2012;14(2):260-9.
5. Mahadevan M, Baker G. Assessment and preparation of semen for in vitro fertilization. In: Wood C, Trounson A, (Ed). Clinical In Vitro Fertilization. Berlin: Springer-Verlag; 1984. pp. 83-97.
6. Arends MJ, Wyllie AH. Apoptosis: mechanisms and roles in pathology. Int Rev Exp Pathol. 1991;32:223-54.
7. Grunewald S, Paasch U, Glander HJ. Enrichment of non-apoptotic human spermatozoa after cryopreservation by immunomagnetic cell sorting. Cell Tissue Bank. 2001;2(3):127-33.
8. Said TM, Agarwal A, Grunewald S, et al. Evaluation of sperm recovery following annexin V magnetic-activated cell sorting separation. Reprod Biomed Online. 2006;13(3):336-9.
9. Said TM, Agarwal A, Zborowski M, et al. Utility of magnetic cell separation as a molecular sperm preparation technique. J Androl. 2008;29(2):134-42.
10. Hoogendijk CF, Kruger TF, Bouic PJ, et al. A novel approach for the selection of human sperm using annexin V-binding and flow cytometry. Fertil Steril. 2009;91(4):1285-92.
11. Bucar S, Gonçalves A, Rocha E, et al. DNA fragmentation in human sperm after magnetic-activated cell sorting. J Assist Reprod Genet. 2015;32(1):147-54.
12. Lee TH, Liu CH, Shih YT, et al. Magnetic-activated cell sorting for sperm preparation reduces spermatozoa with apoptotic markers and improves the acrosome reaction in couples with unexplained infertility. Hum Reprod. 2010;25(4):839-46.
13. Said TM, Grunewald S, Paasch U, et al. Effects of magnetic-activated cell sorting on sperm motility and cryosurvival rates. Fertil Steril. 2005;83(5):1442-6.
14. Khalid SN, Qureshi IZ. Effect of magnetic selected sperm on fertilization and embryo development: an animal model study. Fertil Steril. 2011;96(3):S169.
15. Romany L, Meseguer M, Garcia-Herrero S, et al. Magnetic activated sorting selection (MACS) of non-apoptotic sperm (NAS) improves pregnancy rates in homologous intrauterine insemination (IUI) preliminary data. Fertil Steril. 2010;94(4):S14.
16. Romany L, Garrido N, Motato Y, et al. Removal of annexin V-positive sperm cells for intracytoplasmic sperm injection in ovum donation cycles does not improve reproductive outcome: a controlled and randomized trial in unselected males. Fertil Steril. 2014;102(6):1567-75.
17. Gil M, Sar-Shalom M, Melendez Sivira Y, et al. Sperm selection using magnetic activated cell sorting (MACS) in assisted reproduction: a systematic review and meta-analysis. J Assist Reprod Genet. 2013;30(4):479-85.
18. Dirican EK, Ozgün OD, Akarsu S, et al. Clinical outcome of magnetic activated cell sorting of non-apoptotic spermatozoa before density gradient centrifugation for assisted reproduction. J Assist Reprod Genet. 2008;25(8):375-81.
19. Herrero MB, Delbes G, Chung JT, et al. Case report: the use of annexin V coupled with magnetic activated cell sorting in cryopreserved spermatozoa from a male cancer survivor: healthy twin newborns after two previous ICSI failures. J Assist Reprod Genet. 2013;30(11):1415-9.
20. Lukaszuk K, Wcislo M, Liss J, et al. First Pregnancy, Somatic and Psychological Status of a 4-Year-Old Child Born following Annexin V TESA Sperm Separation. AJP Rep. 2015;5(2):e105-8.
21. Romany L, Garrido N, Cobo A, et al. Obstetric and perinatal outcome of babies born from sperm selected by MACS from a randomized controlled trial. J Assist Reprod Genet. 2017;34(2):201-7.
22. De Vos A, Van de Velde H, Bocken G, et al. Does intracytoplasmic morphologically selected sperm injection improve embryo development? A randomized sibling-oocyte study. Hum Reprod. 2013;28(3):617-26.
23. Bartoov B, Berkovitz A, Eltes F. Selection of spermatozoa with normal nuclei to improve the pregnancy rate with intracytoplasmic sperm injection. N Engl J Med. 2001;345(14):1067-8.
24. Setti AS, Figueira RC, Braga DP, et al. Intracytoplasmic morphologically selected sperm injection is beneficial in cases of advanced maternal age: a prospective randomized study. Eur J Obstet Gynecol Reprod Biol. 2013;171(2):286-90.
25. Setti AS, Paes de Almeida Ferreira Braga D, Iaconelli A, et al. Twelve years of MSOME and IMSI: a review. Reprod Biomed Online. 2013;27(4):338-52.
26. Berkovitz A, Eltes F, Lederman H, et al. How to improve IVF-ICSI outcome by sperm selection. Reprod Biomed Online. 2006;12(5):634-8.
27. Boitrelle F, Guthauser B, Alter L, et al. High-magnification selection of spermatozoa prior to oocyte injection: confirmed and potential indications. Reprod Biomed Online. 2014;28(1):6-13.
28. Ebner T, Shebl O, Oppelt P, et al. Some reflections on intracytoplasmic morphologically selected sperm injection. Int J Fertil Steril. 2014;8(2):105-12.
29. Jakab A, Sakkas D, Delpiano E, et al. Intracytoplasmic sperm injection: a novel selection method for sperm with normal frequency of chromosomal aneuploidies. Fertil Steril. 2005;84(6):1665-73.
30. Huszar G, Sbracia M, Vigue L, et al. Sperm plasma membrane remodeling during spermiogenetic maturation in men: relationship among plasma membrane beta 1,4-galactosyltransferase, cytoplasmic creatine phosphokinase, and creatine phosphokinase isoform ratios. Biol Reprod. 1997;56(4):1020-4.
31. Huszar G, Ozenci CC, Cayli S, et al. Hyaluronic acid binding by human sperm indicates cellular maturity, viability, and unreacted acrosomal status. Fertil Steril. 2003;79 Suppl 3:1616-24.
32. Parmegiani L, Cognigni GE, Bernardi S, et al. Comparison of two ready-to-use systems designed for sperm-hyaluronic acid binding selection before intracytoplasmic sperm injection: PICSI vs. Sperm Slow: a prospective, randomized trial. Fertil Steril. 2012;98(3):632-7.
33. Ye H, Huang GN, Gao Y, et al. Relationship between human sperm-hyaluronan binding assay and fertilization rate in conventional in vitro fertilization. Hum Reprod. 2006;21(6):1545-50.

34. Mansour R, Ishihara O, Adamson GD, et al. International Committee for Monitoring Assisted Reproductive Technologies world report: Assisted Reproductive Technology 2006. Hum Reprod. 2014;29(7):1536-51.
35. Said TM, Land JA. Effects of advanced selection methods on sperm quality and ART outcome: a systematic review. Hum Reprod Update. 2011;17(6):719-33.
36. Beck-Fruchter R, Shalev E, Weiss A. Clinical benefit using sperm hyaluronic acid binding technique in ICSI cycles: a systematic review and meta-analysis. Reprod Biomed Online. 2016;32(3):286-98.
37. Tarozzi N, Nadalini M, Bizzaro D, et al. Sperm-hyaluronan-binding assay: clinical value in conventional IVF under Italian law. Reprod Biomed Online. 2009;19 Suppl 3:35-43.
38. Parmegiani L, Cognigni GE, Ciampaglia W, et al. Efficiency of hyaluronic acid (HA) sperm selection. J Assist Reprod Genet. 2010;27(1):13-6.
39. Avendaño C, Oehninger S. DNA fragmentation in morphologically normal spermatozoa: how much should we be concerned in the ICSI era? J Androl. 2011;32(4):356-63.
40. Ioannou D, Miller D, Griffin DK, et al. Impact of sperm DNA chromatin in the clinic. J Assist Reprod Genet. 2016;33(2):157-66.
41. Mallidis C, Wistuba J, Bleisteiner B, et al. In situ visualization of damaged DNA in human sperm by Raman microspectroscopy. Hum Reprod. 2011;26(7):1641-9.
42. Sánchez V, Redmann K, Wistuba J, et al. Oxidative DNA damage in human sperm can be detected by Raman microspectroscopy. Fertil Steril. 2012;98(5):1124-9.
43. Mallidis C, Sanchez V, Wistuba J, et al. Raman microspectroscopy: shining a new light on reproductive medicine. Hum Reprod Update. 2014;20(3):403-14.
44. Ainswoth C, Nixon B, Aitken RJ. Development of a novel electrophoretic system for the isolation of human spermatozoa. Hum Reprod. 2005;20(8):2261-70.
45. Ainswoth C, Nixon B, Jansen RP, et al. First recorded pregnancy and normal birth after ICSI using electrophoretically isolated spermatozoa. Hum Reprod. 2007;22(1):197-200.
46. Chung Y, Zhu X, Gu W, et al. Microscale integrated sperm sorter. Methods Mol Biol. 2006;321:227-44.
47. Xie L, Ma R, Han C, et al. Integration of sperm motility and chemotaxis screening with a microchannel-based device. Clin Chem. 2010;56(8):1270-8.
48. Gatica LV, Guidobaldi HA, Montesinos MM, et al. Picomolar gradients of progesterone select functional human sperm even in subfertile samples. Mol Hum Reprod. 2013;19(9):559-69.
49. Quin MM, Jalalian L Ribeiro S, et al. Microfluidic sorting selects sperm for clinical use with reduced DNA damage compared to density gradient centrifugation with swim-up in split semen samples. Hum Reprod. 2018;33:1388-93.

CHAPTER

59

From the Gamete to the Zygote

Alberto Tejera, Belén Aparicio, Maria J de los Santos

INTRODUCTION—THE CUMULUS-OOCYTE COMPLEX

The mature cumulus oocyte complex (COC) is composed of the secondary oocyte [which is arrested at metaphase II (MII)] surrounded by a multilayer of specialized granulosa cells called cumulus cells. They possess highly specialized transzonal cytoplasmic projections that penetrate through the zona pellucida (ZP) and form gap junctions at their tips with the oocyte.[1] The gap junctions will allow paracrine factors and low molecular weight factors to freely travel in both directions.[2,3]

Since fully-grown oocytes from late antral follicle to preovulatory follicle are meiotically competent, after stimulation and ovulation triggering, the majority of the aspirated follicles will contain nuclear mature "MII" oocytes. However, before arrival of mature oocytes to laboratories, oocytes have had to initiate a rather long journey from the arrested phase of the diplotene stage of prophase I, to MII oocytes.[4,5] Endocrinological inactive primordial follicles are capable to generate mature oocytes at ovulation process. During the last phase of follicular growth, hormones will act on the oocyte, releasing the G2 arrest and causing the oocyte to progress through a receptive configuration for fertilization.

After puberty, follicular enclosed oocytes will need to pass through a series of follicular growing phases, the first phase is not hormone-dependent and the second is dependent on them.[6] This journey lasts around 180 days and is not easy for oocytes to progressively gain oocyte competence.[4] During this long travel, different processes are triggered giving rise to the expression of a new set of genes, cytoplasmic organization, reorganization and formation of new organelles, and creation of the glycoprotein layer of the zona pellucida. For example, it has been shown that the presence of endocytic vacuoles, reorganization of organelles [like the endoplasmic reticulum-mitochondria (M-SER) aggregates] or the appearance of necrotic areas emerge in the final part of maturation.[7] Other processes such as the transformation of the Golgi apparatus into Golgi-derived vesicles called cortical granules (CG) occurs during the early stages of oocyte growth.[8] Also, ooplasma may also accumulate lipid droplets, multivesicular and crystalline bodies, which may remain until ovulation and may play a role during fertilization and further embryo development.

With Luteinizing hormone (LH) surge, a cascade of events starts, which leads to further cumulus cell (CC) proliferation and expansion by mediating the synthesis of hyaluronic acid and organization of and stable cellular matrix. The degree of expansion of the cumulus cells has been proposed as an indicator of the nuclear maturation stage of the oocytes, however objective criteria of assessment oocyte quality are lacking and do always exist a direct correlation between degree of expansion and nuclear maturity.

Generally speaking, the oocyte cumulus cells complexes can be divided into three main categories with regard to the degree of expansion and nuclear maturity of the enclosed oocytes:

- *Grade 1 (containing MII oocytes):* Cumulus cells with even distribution and a much expanded appearance
- *Grade 2 (containing MI oocytes):* Cumulus cells with a dense matrix with and an intermediate degree of expansion
- *Grade 3 oocytes (containing GV oocytes):* Cumulus cells very compacted and dark.

Once the oocytes have been stripped from the surrounded layer of cumulus cells, it becomes easy to observe the morphology of the denuded oocyte.

THE OOCYTE

From a broad general agreement, although a morphological normal MII,[9] oocyte should be in spherical form, and have a large perivitelline space, a homogenous cytoplasm with no inclusions and zona pellucida of around 15–20 μm thick, physiological variation throughout oocyte growth may cause differences in oocyte phenotypes, and consequently, in their morphologies. Some aspects occurred during follicular stimulation process and oocyte growth could affect to the different oocyte dimorphisms. For example, the hormonal follicular environment seems to be related to the incidence of specific oocyte morphological features, such as polar body fragmentation, a large perivitelline space and presence of cytoplasmic inclusions. Interestingly, one curious point is that for some authors, the so-called "normal oocyte phenotype" is actually the least recently used. As a result between 60% and 70% of the oocytes from stimulated cycles present one or more phenotypic alterations.[10,11]

Assessment of Oocyte Phenotypic Characteristics

Oocyte phenotypes can be classified by morphological categories based on the cytoplasmic and extra cytoplasmic attributes observed; van Blerkom and Alikani previously described most of them.[12] In their study, oocytes were grouped into 12 classes as follows:

1. Normal oocytes (N) with homogenous or very slightly granulated cytoplasm, a nonfragmented, normal size polar body and without an overlarge perivitelline space, a normal zona pellucida
2. Oocytes with altered necrotic bodies in the cytoplasm (NB)
3. Oocytes with refractile bodies (RB)
4. Oocytes with homogenous very granular cytoplasm (HGC)
5. Oocytes with severe centrally located granular cytoplasm (CLGC)
6. Oocytes with smooth endoplasmic reticulum (SER)
7. Oocytes with vacuoles (VAC)
8. Oocytes with multiple abnormalities (M).
9. Oocytes with a large perivitelline space (LPS)
10. Oocytes with abnormal polar bodies (PB)
11. Elongated oocytes (E)
12. Oocytes with debris in the perivitelline space (Db)

Moreover, oocytes were also grouped according to the appearance of the zona pellucida:

- Oocytes with normal zona (nZP)
- Oocytes with an elongated zona (eZP)
- Oocytes with a pigmented or dark zona (pZP)
- Oocytes with a thick zona (thckZP)
- Oocytes with a thin zona (tZP)
- Oocytes with an evident bilayered zona (bZP)
- Oocytes with a zona of irregular thickness (irZP)
- Oocytes with a rough inner zona (izrZP).

Provided below is a brief description of each of these phenotypic characteristics assessed in the oocytes.

Refractile and Necrotic Bodies

Both these kinds of phenotypes include a variety of cytoplasmic features that are considered small necrotic areas of around 10 μm in size, composed of lipid droplets that can be located isolated or in groups.[13,14]

Homogenous Granular and Located Granular Cytoplasm

In some cases, one can appreciate the granulation in the cytoplasm, which is located homogeneously or centrally. When this is the case [homogenous granular and located granular cytoplasm (CLGC)], it is diagnosed as being a larger, dark, granular area. This phenotype may correspond to the central location of organelles in the cytoplasm. Severity of granulation is based on the diameter of the granular area and depth.

Smooth Endoplasmic Reticulum

This dimorphism is the result of a massive accumulation of tubular-type smooth endoplasmic reticulum clusters.[15] Even though we do not really have a clear explanation for the mechanisms that allow to the appearance of SER aggregates, different groups have observed a positive effect between presence of SER and serum estradiol concentrations on the day of ovulation induction, as well as concentrations of anti-Müllerian hormone.[16-18]

Vacuoles

One of the most common oocyte dimorphisms is cytoplasmic vacuolization. Vacuoles are, according to Van Blerkom, membrane-bound cytoplasmic inclusions filled with fluid that is similar to perivitelline fluid. The incidence involves 5–12% of oocytes, and the size and number may vary. Appearance of vacuoles can be spontaneous or through the fusion of pre-existing vesicles which derive from the Golgi apparatus or the smooth endoplasmic reticulum.[19]

Large Perivitelline Space

This dimorphism can be clearly visualized under an inverted microscope due to an increase in the perivitelline space, and there is no contact, so the oocyte seems to float within the interior of the zona pellucida. Some authors have reported that an increase in the perivitelline space can be related to extreme oocyte maturation.[20,21]

First Polar Body

It seems that the morphology of the first polar body (PB) changes within first hours of in vitro culture and, consequently, may vary depending on the observation time.[22] Different dimorphisms are related to the first polar body such as number or fragmentation. However, apart from the very large first polar body, the impact and effect of this dimorphism on the development potential of this oocyte is not clear.

Cellular Debris in the Perivitelline Space

The presence of cellular debris in the perivitelline space is considered an extra-cytoplasmic abnormality. Even though, there is currently no scientific evidence for the influence of this dimorphism on the oocyte, and it cannot be quantified or measured, some authors have related this kind of dimorphism to internal zona pellucida deterioration, while others have observed that the presence of detritus may correspond to a sign of an "overdose" of gonadotropins used in stimulation protocols.[23]

Experts from the Istanbul consensus have expressed that given the limited knowledge and controversial topic of biological significance of the most of oocytes dimorphisms, their primary concern is focused in those oocyte phenotypes relevant to the result. In other words, those dimorphisms with greater impact on embryo development, e.g. oocytes with severe central granularity, called cluster oocytes; oocytes with a smooth endoplasmic reticulum; oocytes with vacuoles >14 μm; oocytes with big polar bodies.[24] Many articles regard to oocyte dimorphisms and their relation to adverse IVF outcomes have been published. Even though extensive reviews have been performed.[25,26] a consensus about the predictive value to consider an oocyte with poor or good quality based merely on its morphology is lacking.

This section will show the association of oocyte morphology with the fertilization and embryos cleavage event, as well as the influence of zygote score pronuclear to embryo implantation.

Oocyte Phenotype

From a study including 5,252 oocytes at the IVF lab of IVI Valencia, it was observed that the highest proportion corresponded to "normal category", as expected, (38.3%), followed by OR (25%), AC (12.1%), fPB (10%), LPS (6.6%), M (5.9%), and PB (1.6%). The zona pellucida phenotypes of the oocytes resulting from this study population were distributed as follows: 1.3% dZP, 0.6% hZP, 3% eZP, 4.5% tZP, 3.2% thZP, 2.1% irZP, 0.2% mZP, 72.7% nZP, 0.6% pZP, 0.9% blZP. In order to simplify the data, we divided the zona pellucida phenotypes into two main groups (nZP and abZP).

Fertilization and Oocyte Phenotypes

When looking at the effect of oocyte phenotype on fertilization ability, we observed that only three types of oocyte morphologies showed statistically lower fertilization ability compared to normal oocytes. These oocytes were those with multiples abnormalities (66.0%), those with vacuoles (64.3%), and the heavily granulated ones (68.15), whereas the normal oocytes had a 78.6% fertilization rate (Table 1). Fertilization was also similar regardless of type of zona pellucida (normal and abnormal).

Embryo Quality and Oocyte Phenotype

Our experience after checking the impact of oocyte phenotype on embryo quality is that embryo quality was not affected by oocyte morphological categories, obtaining similar percentages in different phenotypes (Table 1), and the same embryo quality was achieved considering the shape of zona pellucida (Table 2).

Morphokinetic and Oocyte Phenotype

Similarly when the kinetics parameters were evaluated, no discrepancies were seen among all the phenotypes analyzed (Table 3), or between the embryos originated from oocytes with normal or abnormal zona pellucida (Table 4).

Fertilization Initial Stages

After the oocytes have been inseminated by ICSI of conventional IVF, some of them will become fertilized.

Sperm Preparation

Although, the male gamete is morphologically complete, is not functional; as is not able to fertilize the egg by itself. In order to do it, the gamete needs to be prepared; this implies a number of changes or modifications aimed at increasing their motility and their ability to fertilize. In vivo, such

Table 1: Distribution of oocyte dysmorphisms, fertilization ability, and embryo quality. (*Only fertilization rates were significant different among some types of oocyte dysmosrphisms, * p <0.05*).

Oocyte phenotype	*Phenotype distribution*	*Fertilization n (5%)*	*OR IC 95%*	*GQ embryos n (%)*	*OR CI (95%)*
Normal	3,456 (66.9%)	2,715 (78.6%)*	–	1,368 (50.4 %)	
NB	91 (1.8%)	66 (72.5%)	0.72 (0.41–1.27)	39 (59.1 %)	0.43–1.26
RB	249(4.8%)	198 (79.5%)	1.06 (0.77–1.46)	100 (50.5%)	1.47–1.52
HGC	285 (5.5%)	194 (68.1%)*	0.58* (0.45–0.76)	95 (48.7%)	0.37–1.17
CLGC	266 (5.2 %)	202 (75.9%)	0.86 (0.63–1.15)	108 (53.5 %)	0.51–2.15
SER	76 (1.5 %)	57 (75.0%)	0.82 (0.48–1.39)	33 (57.9%)	0.33–1.80
VAC	42 (0.8%)	27 (64.3%)*	0.49* (0.26–0.93)	12 (44.4%)	0.38–1.39
M	53 (1.0%)	35 (66.0%)*	0.53* (0.30–0.94)	13 (36.4%)	0.41–1.35
LPS	434(6.6%)	297 (74.6%)	0.82 (0.63–1.06)	141 (47.5%)	0.23–1.47
PB	136 (2.6 %)	104 (76.5%)	0.89 (0.59–1.33)	52 (50%)	0.38–1.26
E	48 (0.9%)	35 (72.9%)	0.74 (0.39–1.40)	18 (51.4%)	0.17–1.1
A	54 (1.0%)	41 (77.4%)	0.93 (0.49–1.78)	12 (29.3%)	0.13–071
Db	62 (1.2%)	45 (72.6%)	0.72 (0.45–1.15)	20 (44.4%)	0.26–128

Table 2: Distribution of zona pellucida morphology, fertilization ability, and embryo quality. (*Regarding fertilization and embryo quality, no significant differences were observed among the groups*).

Zona pellucida phenotypes	*Zona pellucida distribution*	*Fertilization n (%)*	*OR CI 95%*	*GQ embryos N(%)*	*OR CI 95%*
nZP	4,312 (81.6%)	3,329 (77.4)%	–	1,678 (50.4%)	
eZP	152 (3.0%)	116 (76.3 %)		52 (44.8%)	0.48–6.65
tZP	172 (3.3%)	135 (78.5%)	0.74–5.65	74 (54.5%)	0.46–8.69
thZP	276 (5.3%)	221(80.1%)	0.40–4.57	101 (45.7%)	0.42–5.41
lrZP	42 (0.8%)	29 (69.0%)	0.84–6.91	16 (57.1%)	0.34–4.59
Dark ZP	16 (0.3%)	10 (62.5%)	0.61–5.36	4(40.0%)	0.54–7.63
bZP	52 (1.0%)	36 (69.2%)	0.74–6.42	19 (52.8%)	0.48–6.65
izrZP	141 (2 .7%)	106 (75.2%)	0.65–5.68	62 (57.5%)	0.46–7.70

Table 3: Kinetik timings including some early fertilization events and the most relevant cleavage morphokinetic parameters in each type of oocyte dysmorphism.

Oocyte phenotype	*tPB2*	*tPNa*	*tPNf*	*t2*	*cc2*	*s2*	*ts*
Normal	3.5 (3.4–3.6)	7.9 (7.7–8.0)	23.3 (22.8–23.6)	26.0 (25.6–26.4)	12 (11.6–12.5)	3.9 (3.6–4.2)	47.7 (46.8–48.5)
NB	3.4 (2.8–3.9)	8.2 (7.3–9.2)	24.4 (22.2–26.7)	24.4 (22.2–26.7)	11.7 (8.7–14.8)	4.2 (1.6–6.7)	43.6 (38.6–48 . 7)
RB	3.5 (3.2–3.7)	7.9 (7.2–8.6)	23.0 (21.5–24.5)	25.2 (23.8–26.5)	12.0 (10.3–13.7)	3.5 (2.2–4.8)	46.5 (42.9–50.0)
HGC	3.9 (3.3–4.6)	8.5 (7.8–9.2)	24.9 (22.8–27 .2)	25.8 (24.3–27.3)	11.8 (9.8–13.6)	4.8 (3.4–6.2)	46.8 (44.1–49.6)
CLGC	3.8 (3.5–4.0)	8.3 (7.7–8.9)	22.9 (21.4–24.3)	27.1 (25.2–28.9)	12.6 (11.1–14.1)	3.7 (2.5–4.9)	50.1 (46.7–53.3)
SER	3.9 (3.2–4.7)	7.2 (6.4–7.9)	22.5 (19.9–25.1)	25.3 (21.8–29.9)	12.3 (9.7–14.9)	6.8 (2.2–11.4)	42.1 (37.0–47.0)

Contd...

Contd...

VAC	3.4 (2.4–4.3)	9.3 (6.9–11.8)	24.5 (19.2–29.7)	27.1 (24.1–30.1)	10.8 (5.4–16.2)	4.6 (0.5–8.6)	48.0 (41.6–64.3)
M	3.1 (2.6–3.6)	8.1 (6.1–10.1)	25.1 (21.3–28.8)	28.3 (26.7–30.1)	9.4 (4.2–14.6)	8.7 (0.5–16.9)	39.1 (24.1–64.1)
LPS	3.3 (3.1–3.5)	7.8 (7.4–8.4)	22.2 (21.1–23.9)	25.9 (24.9–26.9)	11.9 (10.9–12.9)	3.7 (2.6–4.7)	47.5 (45.1–50.0)
PB	3.3 (3.0–3.7)	8.5 (7.4–9.7)	25.9 (24.2–27.7)	26.3 (24.6–28.0)	11.9 (9.6–14.2)	3.8 (2.2–5.3)	45.5 (41.4–49.6)
E	3.8 (3.1–4.4)	7.5 (6.3–8.7)	25.0 (23.7–26.3)	25.7 (22.6–28.7)	13.4 (9.9–17.0)	1.2 (0.5–3.4)	52.5 (45.4–69.4)
A	3.6 (3.0–4.3)	7.3 (5.6–9.0)	25.2 (21.4–29.1)	25.6 (22.5–28.9)	11.6 (7.9–15.2)	2.8 (1.3–4.3)	44.9 (38.8–50.9)
Db	4.4 (3.6–5.2)	6.9 (5.4–8.5)	19.7 (19.9–25.1)	25.8 (23.3–28.2)	12.4 (8.5–16.2)	3.8 (1.4–6.0)	48.4 (42.9–63.8)

Table 4: Kinetic timings in embryos with normal and abnormal zona pellucida. Values between brackets are 95% confidence interval.

Zona pellucida phenotype	*tPB2*	*tPNa*	*tPNf*	*t2*	*cc2*	*s2*	*t5*
Normal ZP	3.5 (3.4–3.6)	7.9 (7.7–8.0)	23.3 (22.8–23.6)	26.2 (25.6–26.4)	11.9 (11.6–12.5)	4.0 (3.6–4.2)	47.3 (46.8–48.5)
Abnormal ZP	3.5 (2.8–4.3)	7.9 (7.3–8.5)	22.9 (20.9–24.9)	25.4 (23.9–26.8)	12.7 (8.7–14.8)	3.1 (2.3–4.1)	47.3 (44.1–50.4)

changes take place during migration of sperm through the female genital tract and in vitro, by processing the sperm sample in the laboratory and later culture in a medium with an appropriate concentration of Ca^{2+}, HCO_3^- and other factors contributing to sperm capacitation.[27,28]

Some of the changes that occur during sperm preparation include an increase in fluidity of the plasma membrane (mainly due to loss of cholesterol and reorientation of the molecules that compose the lipid bilayer), changes in the state of tyrosine phosphorylation of certain sperm proteins, hyperpolarization of membrane potential and increased intracellular pH and Ca^{2+} levels. Aimed all to the acquisition of hyperactivity, finally the sperms acquire a fast movement in situ and a large lateral displacement of the head to facilitate their passage through the granulosa cells and penetration of the ZP.[29,30]

Interaction of Spermatozoon with the Zona Pellucida and Acrosome Reaction

Once the spermatozoon is prepared, it interacts with the oocyte ZP. This interaction is species-specific and a series of ZP glycoproteins are involved—ZP1, ZP2, ZP3 and ZP4. The initial adhesion sperm-ZP is mediated by ZP3, the receptor-ligand interaction results in an entry of Ca^{2+} through T-type channels and this increases the concentration of Ca^{2+}, which triggers the sperm acrosome reaction. This releases the contents of the acrosome vesicle, including enzymes such as acrosina, galactosyl transferase and hyaluronidase, to help the sperm to digest the ZP on its way to the plasma membrane of the oocyte to finally merge with it. ZP penetration by spermatozoon therefore occurs mechanically, facilitated by the pointed shape of the head and tail shaking and enzymatic action conducted by acrosome enzymes.[29]

Fusion between Oocyte Membrane and Sperm

A transmembrane protein located in the plasma membrane of sperm catalyzes the fusion. When the sperm fuses with the plasmatic membrane of the oocyte, it activates cell signaling pathway of inositol phospholipids in the oocyte. This activation, in turn, generates a local increase in cytosolic Ca^{2+} concentration, which as a wave spreads throughout the cell. It seems that the increase of cytosolic calcium activates to oocyte and initiates the cortical reaction, in which the cortical granules release their contents by exocytosis. The enzymes released by the cortical reaction change the structure of ZP, which become hardened, so finally that spermatozoon cannot join it longer, forming a barrier to polyspermy. Among the changes taking place in the ZP, it is noteworthy ZP2 proteolytic degradation and hydrolysis of sugar groups on ZP3.[31,32]

Oocyte Activation

Just after the sperm enters the oocyte, oocyte activation occurs, resulting in the resumption of meiosis with subsequent extrusion of the second polar body and formation of female pronuclei (PN), while at the same time the head of the spermatozoon is decondensed to form the male PN which attracts the female PN adopting both a central position.

From now on, the development of the zygote begins after the haploid pronuclei of spermatozoon and oocyte have contacted by mixing their chromosomes to form a diploid nucleus. Human embryos inherit the male centriole, whose function is the assembly of microtubules around the paternal nucleus and alignment of male PN to female PN, so that centriole defects could cause problems in the syngamy and subsequent embryonic development. The human embryo in addition to receiving the genetic heritage of the DNA nucleus, receives the genetic heritage contained in the mitochondria. This mitochondrial genome is inherited only from the mother.

Fertilization Assessment

Despite is a process requiring many steps to be successfully completed; the fertilization assessment is a simple process. Oocytes will be considered that have been successfully fertilized if they show the presence of two PN and two polar bodies (PB). The presence of PN is not an absolute evidence of normal fertilization, because it cannot be determined that one has maternal origin and the other paternal. Likewise, the evaluation of the second polar body can also be misleading, since the first polar body is often fragmented and cause misinterpretations. Despite those facts, it continues to be one of the most useful systems for the fertilization assessment when you clearly observe two polar bodies and two pronuclei centrally located, with even or similar sized, clearly defined by distinct membranes.

THE ZYGOTE

Since the zygote morphological attributes are associated with the time postfertilization, an agreement has been reached whereby zygote scoring should be carried through according to pre-fixed times postinsemination. Regarding the appearance time by the PN and CP, it has been studied that after conventional IVF, PN formation occurs between 8 and 14 hours postinsemination and after intracytoplasmic sperm microinjection (ICSI) between 3 and 13 hours postinjection.[33]

Recent data obtained by our group using the EmbryoScope confirm these time ranges, being 9.3 ± 2.3 hours the average of appearance of the PN and 24.2 ± 3.3 hours the average of disappearance of PN.[34]

Pronuclear Scoring

Regarding the predictive value of pronuclear scoring, it continues to puzzle frequently debated during the last years with articles demonstrating a positive effect[35-39] and others that found no positive predictive value.[40,41] Pronuclear scoring refers to the annotation of different features of the zygote, such as the symmetry and alignment of the PN, taking into account the number and relative position of the nucleolar precursor bodies (NPBs) located in the PN. The Istanbul consensus established the classification of the zygotes according to the NPBs into four main categories assessed 17 ± 1 hours after ICSI:

- Z1 = Zygotes having 3–7 polarized NPB
- Z2 = Zygotes with homogeneously dispersed NPB
- Z3 = All the zygotes with a NPB distribution not included in groups 1, 2, or 4 (i.e. >7 polarized NPB, one PN polarized and the other dispersed or both dispersed but not homogeneously).
- Z4 = Zygotes with only one or two NPB, as described by Gamiz et al in 2003.

Concerning to the PN symmetry, 3 classes were established—symmetry 1, 2 and 3, defined as equal size, similar size or very different size, respectively.[42]

As prescribed by the consensus,[22] there are some features of PN to note, being considered as strongly atypical—broadly separated PN, pronuclei of grossly different sizes, micronuclei and the presence of SER disks. Embryos from zygotes with different pronuclear sizes (>4 mm difference) have been related to a high rate of embryonic developmental arrest, a high rate of multinucleation on day 2 of development and a greater percentage of chromosomal abnormalities.[43,44] So, according to consensus, there should be three categories on pronuclear scoring—symmetrical (equivalent to Z1 and Z2); nonsymmetrical (other aspects, including peripheral PN) and abnormal (those pronuclei with 0 or 1 NPB, which have been associated with abnormal outcomes in animal models).[22]

Historically, it has always been believed that equality in number and distribution of NPBs was sign of good prognosis or normality, while any inequality in number or distribution of the NPBs was considered to be abnormal. Since the burgeoning growth of time-lapse systems, it suggests us to call into question this general belief. Time lapse technology provides extra information as the identification of the precise cell division timings. Focusing only on timing of early fertilization events, we can determine the extrusion of the 2nd polar body (tPB2), PN appearance (tPNa) and PN fading (tPNf), and some of the first divisions and intervals (division to 2 cells (t2), the duration of 2nd cell cycle (cc2), the synchrony of divisions from the 2-cell to 4-cell stages (s2) and the division to 5 cells (t5).[45]

Embryo Implantation Rate According to Pronuclear Score

In most cases, both pronuclei appeared simultaneously (96.4%), just in few instances (3.6%) one pronucleus appeared before the other. The analysis of the categorical fertilization events showed the following results: the

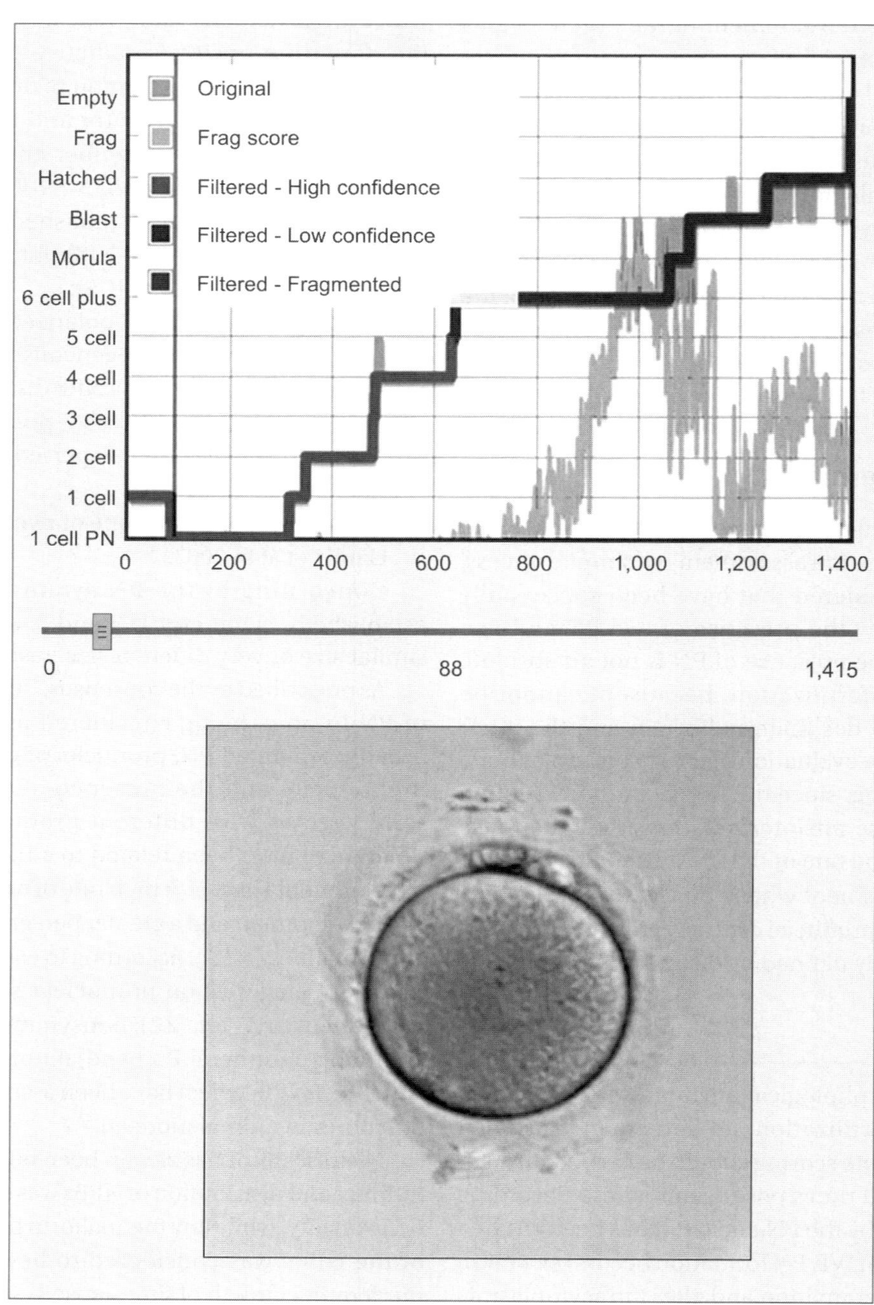

Fig. 1: Exact moment when pronuclei appear, being detected by Geri system.

distribution of the four Z-scores (Z1, Z2, Z3, and Z4) did not differ between implanted and nonimplanted embryos Z1 = 23.7%, Z2 = 28.2%, Z3 = 21.1%, and Z4 = 30.8%. Regarding score distribution Z1 and Z3 were the most majorities (41% and 40% respectively) and Z2 and Z4 were the lower proportion (18% and <1%). The percentage of implanting KID embryos according to PN symmetry (1, 2, 3) did not show significant differences; those zygotes with equal or similar size (symmetry 1 and 2) reached to 22.1% and 22.5% IR respectively, while those zygotes with different size(symmetry 3) just achieved a 13.3% of implantation rate. The symmetry distribution was 58%, 39% and 3%, respectively.[34]

NEW AUTOMATIC TIME-LAPSE SYSTEM TO DETECT PN APPEARANCE AND FADING

Lately, there is a new tendency to automate most of the processes occurred in the lab to avoid the subjectivity existing during the daily work. The new advances in the software of time-lapse systems are permitting the development of new tools to improve the PN detection

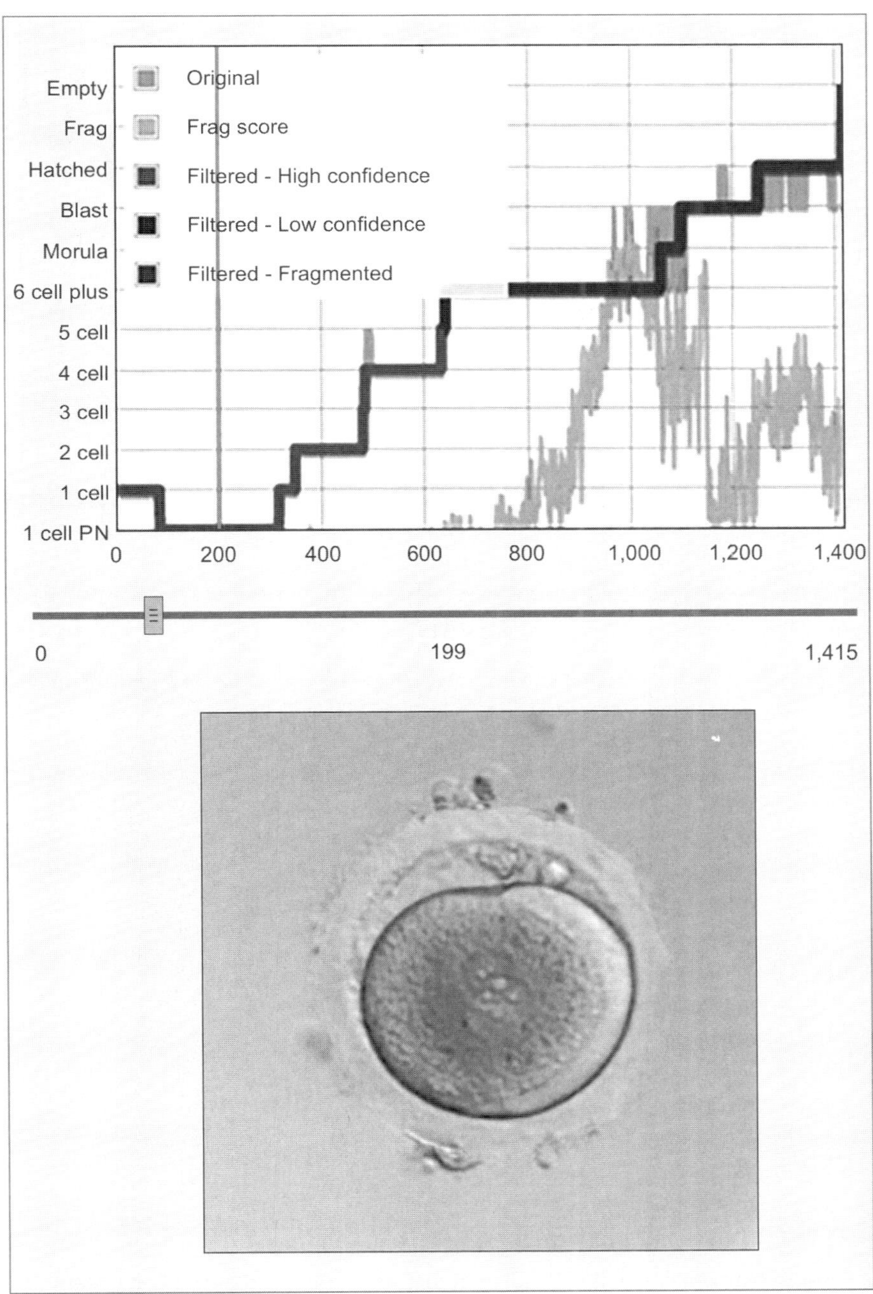

Fig. 2: PN clearly defined.

and fading automatically providing more objectivity and reliability to the identification. Two of the systems that have incorporated this new technology are Geri and EmbryoScope time-lapse. Both systems include accurate records of the PN appearance and fading moments. Even though, it has been implemented recently and is still in its infancy, the artificial intelligence is part of emerging trend and its implementation on the IVF laboratories is simply a matter of time. Both systems work similarly, first you have to teach them how to identify the different events, and when the systems have learnt to detect them properly, then they are ready for use. While Geri system consists of automatic system capable of distinguishing both events (PN appearance and fading) based on an image analysis algorithm (Figs. 1 to 3), the other system (embryoscope) incorporates a semi-automatic system through identified both events, with option to modify the indicated event if it would be moved (Figs. 4).

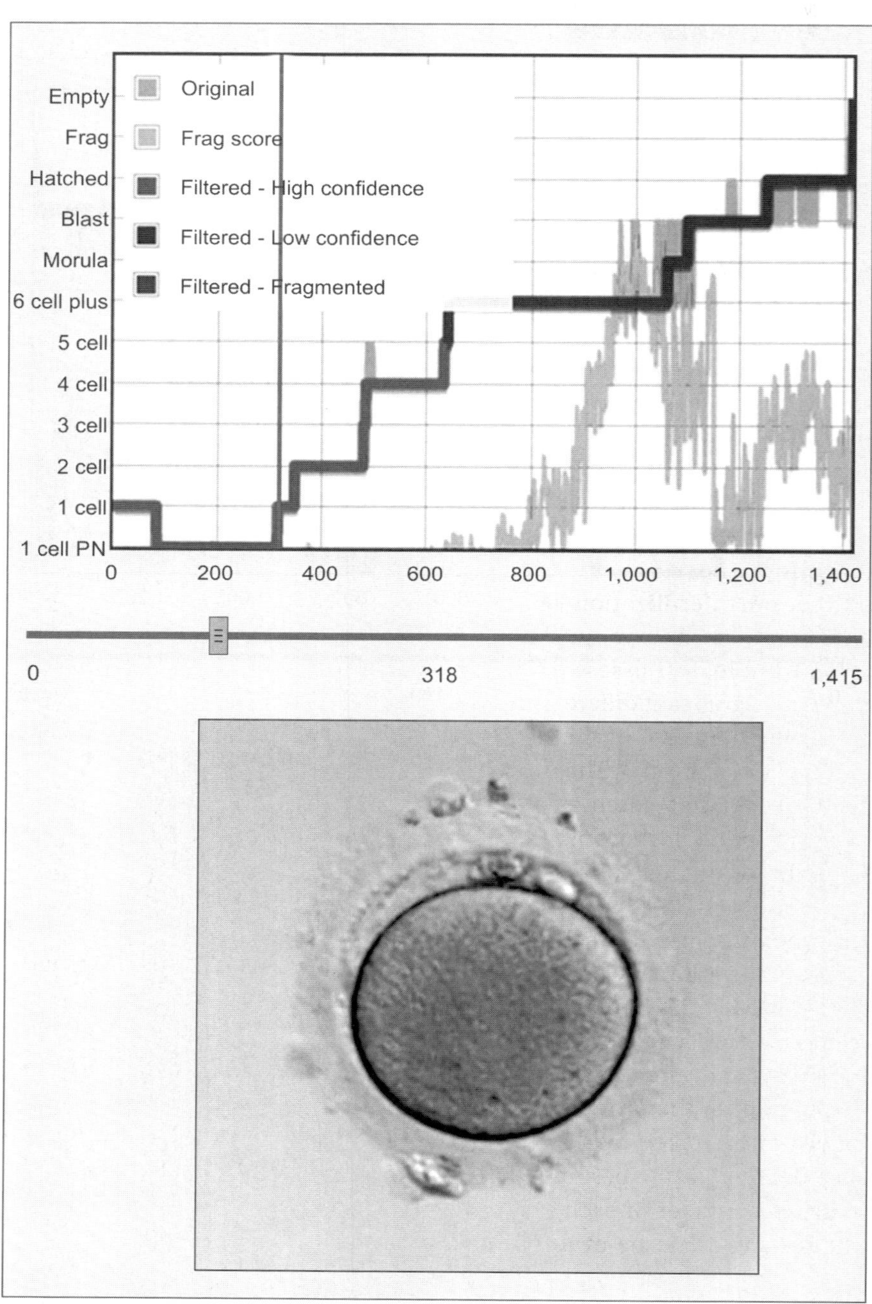

Fig. 3: Moment when the PN fading occurs and is identified by the Geri system.

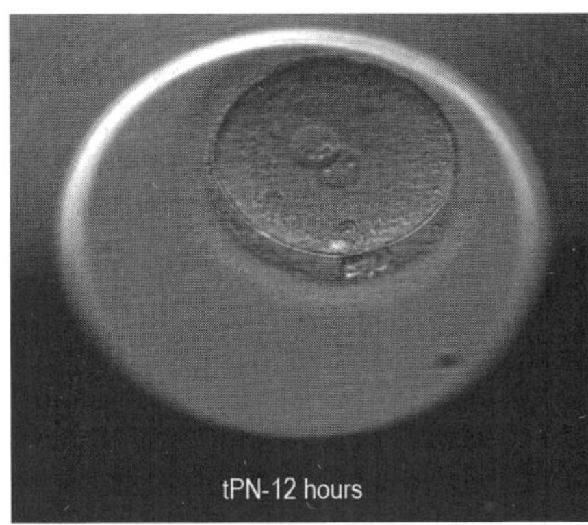

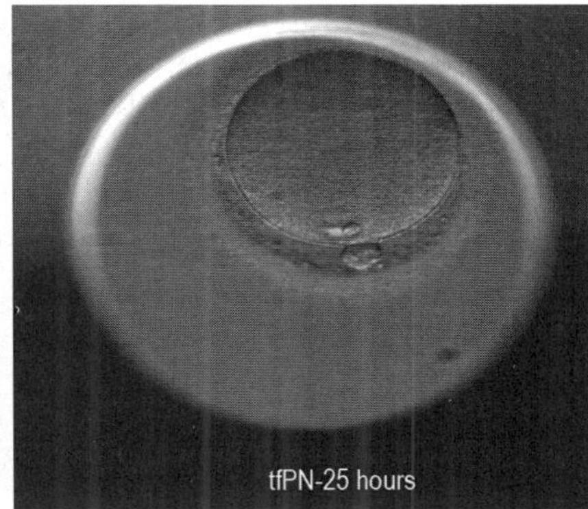

Fig. 4: Identification of PN appearance (tPN) and fading (tfPN) by embryoscope system semi-automatically.

CONCLUSION

The present chapter summarizes that specific phenotypes, such as presence of multiple abnormalities, vacuoles and heavily granulated cytoplasms, could compromise the zygotes viability. These are associated with a significant 10% decrease in fertilization ability, as described in previous chapter by our colleagues.[34] No differences were observed in the accurate timings related to fertilization events, such as second polar body extrusion (tPB), pronuclear appearance (tPNa), and pronuclear fading (tPNf), which actually occurred within the optimal ranges previously established by our team[45] and were comparable and similar to the timing undertaken by the normal oocytes.

It should be noted that once fertilization stage has passed, it is very difficult to predict embryo quality using just the simple oocyte morphological assessment; this was proven by the fact that no significant differences were observed in the kinetic evaluation data of the embryos generated from different types of oocytes.[45] The influence of other types of phenotypes studied, such as necrotic and refractile bodies, was not evident, showing the same cleavage pattern as the embryos originated from normal oocytes.

Regarding PN score, the most usual Z-score was 1, followed by 3 and 2, with Z4 being the lower pronuclear pattern achieved (1.2%). However, the implantation was not affected by Z-score. As is well known to everybody, the pronuclear morphology is a dynamic process from first PN appearance until the fading out of the pronuclei, so, we recommend the use of last image taken by a time-lapse system before pronuclear fade out as the best moment to assess the Z-score, when the diameter of each PN is the biggest and pronuclear scoring could be evaluated wit better preciseness.

All in all, the new approach to measure embryo cleavage timings of the embryos resulting from a variety of oocyte phenotypes shows that the great majority exhibit a similar pattern. Some categories of dimorphisms, such as presence of vacuoles and multiple abnormalities have been significantly related to a lower fertilization rate, but once fertilization takes place, both embryo development measurements are similar among groups, confirming that variations in oocytes morphology are not predictive of oocyte competence after ICSI.[45]

REFERENCES

1. Albertini DF, Combelles CM, Benecchi E, et al. Cellular basis for paracrine regulation of ovarian follicle development. Reproduction. 2001;121(5):647-53.
2. Canipari R. Oocyte—granulosa cell interactions. Hum Reprod Update. 2000;6(3):279-89.
3. Feuerstein P, Cadoret V, Dalbies-Tran R, et al. Oocyte-cumulus dialog. Gynecol Obstet Fertil. 2006;34(9):793-800.
4. Brewer L, Corzett M, Balhorn R. Condensation of DNA by spermatid basic nuclear proteins. J Biol Chem. 2002 11;277(41):38895-900.
5. Boissonneault G. Chromatin remodeling during spermiogenesis: a possible role for the transition proteins in DNA strand break repair. FEBS Lett. 2002 13;514(2-3):111-4.
6. Diaz I, Navarro J, Blasco L, et al. Impact of stage III-IV endometriosis on recipients of sibling oocytes: matched case-control study. Fertil Steril. 2000;74(1):31-4.
7. Jamnongjit M, Hammes SR. Oocyte maturation: the coming of age of a germ cell. Semin Reprod Med. 2005;23(3):234-241.
8. Liu DY, Baker HW. Defective sperm-zona pellucida interaction: a major cause of failure of fertilization in clinical in-vitro fertilization. Hum Reprod .2000;15(3):702-8.
9. Parks JE, Graham JK. Effects of cryopreservation procedures on sperm membranes. Theriogenology. 1992;38(2):209-22.
10. World Health Organization. Laboratory manual of the WHO for the examination of human semen and sperm-cervical mucus interaction. Ann Ist Super Sanita. 2001;37(1): I-XII, 1-123.
11. Anger JT, Gilbert BR, Goldstein M. Cryopreservation of sperm: indications, methods and results. J Urol. 2003;170(4 Pt 1):1079-84.

12. Van Blerkom J, Henry G. Oocyte dysmorphism and aneuploidy in meiotically mature human oocytes after ovarian stimulation. Hum Reprod. 1992;7(3):379-90.
13. Ombelet W, Campo R. Affordable IVF for developing countries. Reprod Biomed Online. 2007;15(3):257-65.
14. Glasier A, Gebbie A. Contraception for the older woman. Baillieres Clin Obstet Gynaecol. 1996;10(1):121-38.
15. Kably Ambe A, Carballo Mondragon E, Karchmer Krivitsky S. Gamete laboratory. Determining factors of success in in-vitro fertilization. Ginecol Obstet Mex. 2001;69:172-9.
16. Tournaye H, Camus M, Goossens A, et al. Recent concepts in the management of infertility because of non-obstructive azoospermia. Hum Reprod. 1995;10 Suppl 1:115-9.
17. Matsumiya K, Namiki M, Kondoh N,et al. New indication of testis biopsy for azoospermia: a clinical study in Japanese patients. Int J Urol. 1994;1(2):177-80.
18. Raman JD, Schlegel PN. Testicular sperm extraction with intracytoplasmic sperm injection is successful for the treatment of nonobstructive azoospermia associated with cryptorchidism. J Urol. 2003;170(4 Pt 1):1287-90.
19. McLachlan RI, Rajpert-De Meyts E, Hoei-Hansen CE,et al. Histological evaluation of the human testis--approaches to optimizing the clinical value of the assessment: mini review. Hum Reprod. 2007;22(1):2-16.
20. Larson-Cook KL, Brannian JD, Hansen KA,et al. Relationship between the outcomes of assisted reproductive techniques and sperm DNA fragmentation as measured by the sperm chromatin structure assay. Fertil Steril. 2003;80(4):895-902.
21. Benchaib M, Braun V, Lornage J, et al. Sperm DNA fragmentation decreases the pregnancy rate in an assisted reproductive technique. Hum Reprod. 2003;18(5):1023-8.
22. Chehval MJ, Purcell MH. Deterioration of semen parameters over time in men with untreated varicocele: evidence of progressive testicular damage. Fertil Steril. 1992;57(1):174-7.
23. Bloch EH, Kafig E, Meryman HT, et al. A comparison of the surfaces of human erythrocytes from health and disease by in vivo light microscopy and in vitro electron microscopy. Angiology. 1956;7(6):479-94.
24. Hall LF, Neubert AG. Obesity and pregnancy. Obstet Gynecol Surv. 2005;60(4):253-60.
25. Kruger TF, Acosta AA, Simmons KF, et al. New method of evaluating sperm morphology with predictive value for human in vitro fertilization. Urology. 1987;30(3):248-51.
26. Muldrew K, McGann LE. Mechanisms of intracellular ice formation. Biophys J. 1990;57(3):525-32.
27. Marin-Briggiler CI, Vazquez-Levin MH, Gonzalez-Echeverria F,et al. Effect of antisperm antibodies present in human follicular fluid upon the acrosome reaction and sperm-zona pellucida interaction. Am J Reprod Immunol. 2003;50(3):209-19.
28. Gadella BM, Van Gestel RA. Bicarbonate and its role in mammalian sperm function. Anim Reprod Sci. 2004; 82-83:307-19.
29. Visconti PE, Galantino-Homer H, Moore GD, et al. The molecular basis of sperm capacitation. J Androl. 1998;19(2):242-8.
30. Visconti PE, Kopf GS. Regulation of protein phosphorylation during sperm capacitation. Biol Reprod. 1998;59(1): 1-6.
31. Evans JP. The molecular basis of sperm-oocyte membrane interactions during mammalian fertilization. Hum Reprod Update. 2002;8(4):297-311.
32. Evans JP, Florman HM. The state of the union: the cell biology of fertilization. Nat Cell Biol. 2002;4:s57-63.
33. Payne D, Flaherty SP, Barry MF, et al. Preliminary observations on polar body extrusion and pronuclear formation in human oocytes using time-lapse video cinematography. Hum Reprod. 1997;12(3):532-41.
34. Aguilar J, Motato Y, Escriba MJ, et al. The human first cell cycle: impact on implantation. Reprod Biomed Online. 2014;28(4):475-84.
35. Tesarik J, Greco E. The probability of abnormal preimplantation development can be predicted by a single static observation on pronuclear stage morphology. Hum Reprod. 1999;14(5):1318-23.
36. Scott L, Alvero R, Leondires M, et al. The morphology of human pronuclear embryos is positively related to blastocyst development and implantation. Hum Reprod. 2000;15(11):2394-403.
37. Tesarik J, Junca AM, Hazout A, et al. Embryos with high implantation potential after intracytoplasmic sperm injection can be recognized by a simple, non-invasive examination of pronuclear morphology. Hum Reprod. 2000;15(6): 1396-9.
38. Balaban B, Urman B, Isiklar A, et al. The effect of pronuclear morphology on embryo quality parameters and blastocyst transfer outcome. Hum Reprod. 2001;16(11):2357-61.
39. Scott L. Pronuclear scoring as a predictor of embryo development. Reprod Biomed Online. 2003;6(2):201-14.
40. Salumets A, Hyden-Granskog C, Suikkari AM, et al. The predictive value of pronuclear morphology of zygotes in the assessment of human embryo quality. Hum Reprod. 2001;16(10):2177-81.
41. James AN, Hennessy S, Reggio B, et al. The limited importance of pronuclear scoring of human zygotes. Hum Reprod. 2006;21(6):1599-604.
42. Sadowy S, Tomkin G, Munne S, et al. Impaired development of zygotes with uneven pronuclear size. Zygote. 1998;6(2): 137-41.
43. Gamiz P, Rubio C, de los Santos MJ, et al. The effect of pronuclear morphology on early development and chromosomal abnormalities in cleavage-stage embryos. Hum Reprod. 2003;18(11):2413-9.
44. Munne S, Cohen J. Chromosome abnormalities in human embryos. Hum Reprod Update. 1998;4(6):842-55.
45. Meseguer M, Herrero J, Tejera A, et al. The use of morphokinetics as a predictor of embryo implantation. Hum Reprod. 2011;26(10):2658-71.

CHAPTER

60

Embryo Culture

Deven Patel, Preeti Shah, Aditi Kotdawala

INTRODUCTION

The ultimate goal of embryo culture in an assisted reproductive technology (ART) programme is to improve the quality of embryos developing in the laboratory and the chances of successful delivery of a healthy baby.

Culture conditions for human embryos have evolved over the past 3 decades.[1,2] In the natural environment, cleaving embryos develop in the fallopian tube, whereas the morulae and blastocysts in the uterine cavity. The success of clinical in vitro fertilization (IVF) was initially compromised by suboptimal culture conditions, resulting in impaired embryo development[3-5] and a subsequent loss of viability. There has been extensive research on the metabolism of in vitro fertilized embryos that have revealed that there are specific needs, depending on the developmental stage of the preimplantation embryo which has helped in improving the culture media system according to the oviduct and uterine milieu.[6-8] Over the last 10–15 years there have been major advancements in this area, with culture media developing from simple salt solutions into highly complex defined media, specifically designed to reduce stress to the embryo and maintain high pregnancy rates.

EVOLUTION OF EMBRYO CULTURE MEDIA

The idea introduced by Bernard in the late 1800s, that the immediate environment surrounding living tissues is an active one led, in turn, to the notion that organs and tissues could be studied outside their setting in a suitable fluid formulated to facilitate these studies.[9] It is an interesting aspect that the culture media evolved and used in the clinical setting were construed to support the development of somatic cell culture applications. The first success of fertilization of the human oocyte in vitro by Robert Edwards was accomplished in a simple, chemically defined media. These commercially available media were a modified Earle's balanced salt solution, and a modified Ham's F-10 or T6. They were supplemented with maternal serum thus converting them into biological media.[10,11] These varying compositions of culture media for clinical IVF appeared to be hardly different in their ability to support development of the human embryo in vitro for up to 48 hours or in subsequent pregnancy rates after transfer.[12] This led to a great deal of confusion concerning the formulation of embryo culture media and the role of individual components in embryo development. A culture medium is a foreign environment for the human embryo. Hence, the design of media is complicated, because the components must be selected, and their concentrations determined in order to minimize stress for the cultured embryo.[2,13,14]

An understanding of the role of culture media and their components is to some extent hampered by the routine inclusion of serum in human embryo culture media. Serum has the ability to both mask potential embryo toxins and suppress the beneficial effects of other medium components. In light of this, there has been considerable research into the development of serum-free embryo culture media. Such studies have been invaluable in the understanding of the embryo's requirements during the preimplantation period. Menezo et al.[15] broke the tradition of using balanced salt solution and produced a medium containing amino acids (AAs) without the need of a serum supplement. Another medium specifically designed for human IVF was human tubal fluid (HTF).[16] HTF, supplemented with either whole serum or with serum albumin, gained great popularity for the use of day 2 or day 3 human embryo culture, and has remained in use ever since. It also became clear that early embryos show an evolving need for energy substrates, moving from a pyruvate-lactate preference, while the embryos are under maternal genetic control—to glucose-based metabolism after activation of the embryonic genome.[17,18] Media used to culture the mammalian preimplantation embryo generally fall into one of four types.

Simple Salt Solutions with Added Energy Substrates

These media were originally formulated to support the development of zygotes from certain inbred strains of mice and their F1 hybrids.[19] Examples of this type of media used in clinical IVF are M[16,20] T6,[20] Earle's,[11] CZB,[21] and potassium simplex optimization medium (KSOM).[22] Derived from such types of media were HTF medium,[15,23] and P1.[24] Such 'simple' media are usually supplemented with either whole serum or serum albumin, and are used for the cleavage stage embryo only, i.e. pronucleate oocyte to the 8-cell stage.

Complex Tissue Culture Media

These media are commercially available and are designed to support the growth of somatic cells in culture, e.g. Ham's F-10.[25,26] Such media are far more complex, containing AAs, vitamins, nucleic acid precursors, and transitional metals, and are usually supplemented with 5–20% serum. Importantly, such media were not formulated with the specific needs of the human embryo in mind, and they contain components which are now known to be detrimental to the developing embryo.

Simplex Optimized Media

This approach to formulate culture media depending on a computer program to generate successive media formulations based on the response of mouse embryos in culture.[27,28] Once a specific medium was formulated, tested, and blastocyst development analyzed, the computer program would then generate several more media formulations for use in the next series of cultures. This procedure was performed several times to generate media that supported high rates of blastocyst development of embryos derived from the oocytes of outbred mice (CF1) crossed with the sperm of an F1 hybrid male, and were termed SOM and KSOM. Such media were subsequently modified by another laboratory to include KSOM (AA)s.[29] This last phase of medium development was based on previous studies on the mouse embryo[26] and did not involve the simplex procedure. This single medium formulation, KSOM (AA), has been used to produce human blastocysts in culture.[30] In such types of media, the embryo therefore has to adapt to its surroundings as it develops and differentiates.

Sequential Media

The approach of sequential media is a learning from the environment to which the embryos are exposed in vivo.[18,31] It helps to understand the physiology and metabolism of the embryo in culture, in order to determine what causes intracellular stress to the embryo.[8,32-35] Examples of sequential media include G1/G2,[36-38] universal IVF medium and M[3,39] and P1 together with blastocyst medium.[40] Interestingly, medium M3 is a modification of Ham's F-10 and F-12, while blastocyst medium is a modification of Ham's F-10.

PHILOSOPHIES BEHIND HUMAN EMBRYO CULTURE MEDIA

The culture media preparation of preimplantation embryos is been influenced by two fundamentally different philosophies.[2,41] The growth of in vitro embryos is inferior to that of in vivo embryos, indicating that ART procedures create cellular and metabolic stress situations. Thus, the ART embryos are forced to spend energy, so that they can adapt to this foreign environment. Moreover, the culture media is an important factor for successful in vitro interactions between gametes and subsequent embryo development.[42] All the manufacturers of human embryo culture media tend to follow either the 'back-to-nature' (sequential media) or the 'let-the-embryo-choose' (single step media) philosophy.[43]

Sequential Culture "Back-to-Nature" Principle

The "back-to-nature" hypothesis mimics the changing needs of the developing zygote and embryo in a culture media that approximates the concentration to which the embryo is physiologically exposed.[42,43] The embryo is capable of actively controlling the ionic gradients, etc. and can regulate its internal environment. Thus as per embryo physiology, the preimplantation period can be subdivided in at least two phases: (1) pre and (2) postcompaction.[42] This breakdown of the preimplantation period is crucial for considering changes to medium formulations and the time when the embryonic genome activation takes place.[42]

Monoculture "Let-the-Embryo-Choose" Principle

This culture system design involves the simultaneous use of all the concentrations in a mixture because the effects of each component in the medium may depend on the concentrations of the other components.[43] As long as concentrations are within "tolerable ranges", the embryo itself will adapt and utilize whatever it requires.[2,43,44] This includes the group of media in which all the necessary substances for early embryological development are provided, and there is no need for a media change. Single-step formulation is applied throughout the in vitro development from fertilization to the blastocyst stage of the embryo.

Four protocols can be used for the culture from fertilization to the blastocyst stage in an ART laboratory:

1. Sequential media protocol, with an interrupted culture where two media of different compositions are used sequentially, change of medium occurs on day 3 of embryo culture.
2. Sequential media protocol with fresh medium change everyday.
3. Monoculture, uninterrupted culture using one medium throughout the 5 days of embryo culture.
4. Interrupted culture where a monoculture medium is used throughout but is renewed on day 3 of embryo culture.

KEY COMPONENTS OF ASSISTED REPRODUCTIVE TECHNOLOGY CULTURE MEDIA

Studies using the development of mammalian preimplantation embryos in vitro have played a major role in the understanding of pre-embryo physiology.[42,44-50] The most widely used models for understanding the human embryo have been the mouse and the cow. The composition of embryo culture systems can be broken down into water, ion, carbohydrates, AAs, vitamins, chelators, antioxidants, antibiotics, protein or macromolecules, hormones and growth factors, and buffer system. Each component has a crucial role to play in embryo development in culture, with focus on the pre and postcompaction stages.

Water

Water is the major component of any culture medium, making up around 99% of the content. The source and purity of water used for media preparation is a major factor in assuring the quality of media. The ability of embryos to develop in culture is positively correlated to water quality. Whit-tingham[20] has reported that in vitro development of 2-cell mouse embryos to the blastocyst was enhanced when the media was prepared using triple distilled water as opposed to double or single distilled water. It is recommended to use commercially available high quality water which is endotoxin tested (less than 0.1 IU/mL).

Cell Volume Regulation: Ions and Osmolytes

Clinical IVF media vary markedly as far as ionic basis are considered. Maintenance of a constant volume in the face of extracellular and intracellular osmotic perturbations is a critical problem faced by all cells. Most cells respond to swelling or shrinkage by activating specific metabolic or membrane transport processes that return cell volume to its normal resting state. These processes are essential for the normal function and survival of cells.[51] Surprisingly, the role of ions during the preimplantation development is not well understood. The osmotic pressure of oviduct fluid is more than 360 mOsmol.[52] However, the osmolarity of most commercially available ART culture media is lower at about 250–300 mOsmol. Unfortunately, it is difficult to interpret the effects of individual ions on embryo development and viability, as there are many subtle interactions which exist between ions, carbohydrates, and AAs. When the $NaCl^-$ concentration is forced up to 290 mOsmol, the development of the embryo is severely impaired.[53] Addition of extracellular AA, such as glycine, betaine, proline, alanine and hypotaurine (which act as organic osmolytes), protects the preimplantation embryo against hypertonicity and increases embryo development.[30,53,54]

Carbohydrates

Carbohydrates are present within the luminal fluids of the female reproductive tract. Their levels vary both between the oviduct and uterus and within the cycle.[18,55] Therefore, the developing embryo is exposed to gradients of carbohydrates as it develops. The early embryo shows a rather simplistic physiology and maintains only low levels of oxidative metabolism, whereas it exhibits a somatic cell-like physiology postcompaction using wider spectrum of nutrients. The biosynthetic rates increase, along with an increase in respiratory capacity and an ability to utilize glucose.[8,48] This involves a shift in the energy requirements at the time at which the embryonic genome is activated or at the postcompaction stage. Zygotes and subsequent cleavage stages prefer pyruvate as the primary source of energy, while the 8-cell stage embryo uses glucose.[56-58] Glucose is a key anabolic precursor and is required for the synthesis of triacylglycerol and phospholipids, and as a precursor for complex sugars and glycoproteins. Glucose also metabolized by the pentose phosphate pathway (PPP) generates ribose moieties required for nucleic acid synthesis.[59]

Amino Acids

It is well accepted that all 20 naturally occurring AAs are important for regulation of mammalian preimplantation development.[8,60] On one side, oviduct and uterine fluids contain significant levels of free AAs;[31,61,62] on the other side, oocytes and embryos possess specific transport systems for AAs[63] and maintain an endogenous pool of them.[64] From various reports, the physiological role of AAs in pre and peri-implantation stages of embryonic development is now well-understood.[65] The carboxyl group acts as the energy source prior to embryonic genome activation of the embryo.[49] They have many other supportive roles in formation of biosynthetic precursor molecules,[66] osmolytes,[54] buffers of internal pH,[35] antioxidants[67] and chelators, especially for heavy metals.[68] One of the major component of culture media is AA group containing the sulphur, which helps in minimizing apoptosis, causative factor of monozygotic twinning.[69]

Chelators: Ethylenediaminetetraacetic Acid

Chelators of heavy metal ions in culture media enhance the development of preimplantation embryos. They have the ability to 'sequester' metal ions. The metal ions after binding with ethylenediaminetetraacetic acid (EDTA) remain in solution but their reactivity is diminished. EDTA helps in alleviating the 2-cell block in mice embryos.[69] It also helps in inhibiting premature utilization of glycolysis by cleavage stage embryos preventing any crabtree-like effect that can cause arrest in culture.[70] However, in postcompaction stage embryos, EDTA at a concentration of 0.1 mmol/L reduces blastocyst development and cell number.[71,72]

Impact of pH and Buffers

The pH only refers to hydrogen ion, and the pH of an aqueous solution is very dynamic. Association and dissociation of compounds and ions like sodium, potassium, magnesium, chloride, lactate and glycine regulate the balance of pH.[73,74] The culture media pH is maintained by the balance of carbon dioxide (CO_2) concentration and the concentration of bicarbonate in the media.

The intracellular pH (pHi) in human cleavage embryo cells is 7.2,[75] so an acceptable pH range for embryo culture media is usually set between pH 7.2 and 7.4. In postcompaction stage after formation of tight junctions between the cells, embryos appear to have more control over their pHi.[76,77] Hence, there is a trend to culture cleavage stage embryos in a slightly lower pH and morulae and blastocysts in a slightly higher pH (low-high paradigm).

The most commonly used buffer in commercially available culture media are [4-(2-hydroxyethyl)-1-piperazineethanesulfonic acid (HEPES) at 21 mmol/L] and 3-(N-morpholino) propanesulfonic acid (MOPS). Both buffers have a pKa value of 7.2, it is the closest of the zwitter ionic buffers to the pHi of embryos of 7.2. There is not much understanding about the impact of either of the buffers on embryo osmotic regulation.[78]

Macromolecules

Human serum albumin or synthetic serum serves as the common source of proteins in human embryo culture medium. It is usually added at 5–20% concentrations. All new generation media include synthetic serum as it has known composition. Albumin helps in maintaining cell membrane stability and chelation of toxic components of culture components and water as well as the culture dishes. It also aids in capillary membrane permeability and osmoregulation. The presence of proteins in the culture media facilitates the manipulation of gametes and embryos.[8] However, the uses of any blood products involve the risk of potential contamination and infection of preimplantation embryos.

Vitamins

All the commercially available media formulations contain vitamins. Although their effects on embryo development remain largely unknown both human[79] and mouse zygotes[19] form blastocysts in culture in the absence of vitamins. It may be postulated that the role of vitamin in the culture media is to act in synergy with AAs to prevent distress in metabolism and loss of vitality induced by suboptimal culture conditions.[8,80] The addition of vitamins as antioxidants to the culture media containing glucose and phosphate help to prevent a loss in respiration and metabolic control.[81] The B-group vitamins are integral part of carbohydrate and AA metabolism; thereby certain vitamins may have an important role to play in embryo development especially in the presence of AAs.

Growth Factors

Mammalian embryos are naturally exposed to a complex mixture of growth factors that play a key role in growth and differentiation from the time of morula to blastocyst transition. However, defining their role and potential for improving in vitro preimplantation development is complicated by factors such as gene expression of both the factors and their receptors. The blastocyst expresses ligands and receptors for several growth factors, many of which can cross-react thus making it difficult to interpret the effect of single factors added to a culture media.[82,83]

Antibiotics

Embryo culture media are routinely supplemented with antibiotics to prevent bacterial contamination.[84] Nowadays, commonly used antibiotics are penicillin (β-lactam, 100 U/mL), streptomycin (aminoglycoside, 100 µg/mL) and gentamicin (aminoglycoside, 50 µg/mL). The antibacterial effect of penicillin is attributed to its disturbance of cell wall integrity through the inhibition of the synthesis of peptidoglycan. Penicillin has no direct toxic effects on the preimplantation embryo. Streptomycin and gentamicin disturb bacterial protein synthesis. However, the aminoglycosides show more toxic effects.[84]

CULTURE SYSTEMS

For the optimum embryo development in vitro, not just the composition of the culture media used, but also the physical parameter, such as the incubation environment and gas phase play an important role (Flowchart 1).

Flowchart 1 serves to illustrate the complex and interdependent nature of human IVF treatment. For example, the stimulation regimen used not only impacts oocyte quality (hence embryo physiology and viability), but can also affect subsequent endometrial receptivity. Furthermore, the health and dietary status of the patient can have a profound effect on the subsequent developmental capacity of the oocyte and embryo. The dietary status of patients attending IVF is typically not considered as a compounding variable, but growing data would indicate otherwise. In this schematic, the laboratory has been broken down into its core components, only one of which is the culture system. The culture system has in turn been broken down into its components, only one of which is the culture media. Therefore, it would appear rather simplistic to assume that by changing only one part of the culture system (i.e. culture media), that one is going to mimic the results of a given laboratory or clinic. A major determinant of the success of a laboratory and culture system is the level of quality control (QC) and quality assurance (QA) in place. For example, one should never assume that anything coming into the laboratory that has not been pretested with a relevant bioassay (for example, mouse embryo assay) is safe merely because a previous lot has performed satisfactorily. Only a small percentage of the disposables and plastic ware used in IVF come suitably tested. Therefore, it is essential to assume that everything entering the IVF laboratory without a suitable pretest is embryo toxic until proven otherwise.[85]

Oxygen Concentration

Studies on several types of mammalian embryo have demonstrated that culture at a reduced oxygen concentration

Flowchart 1: A holistic analysis of human IVF.

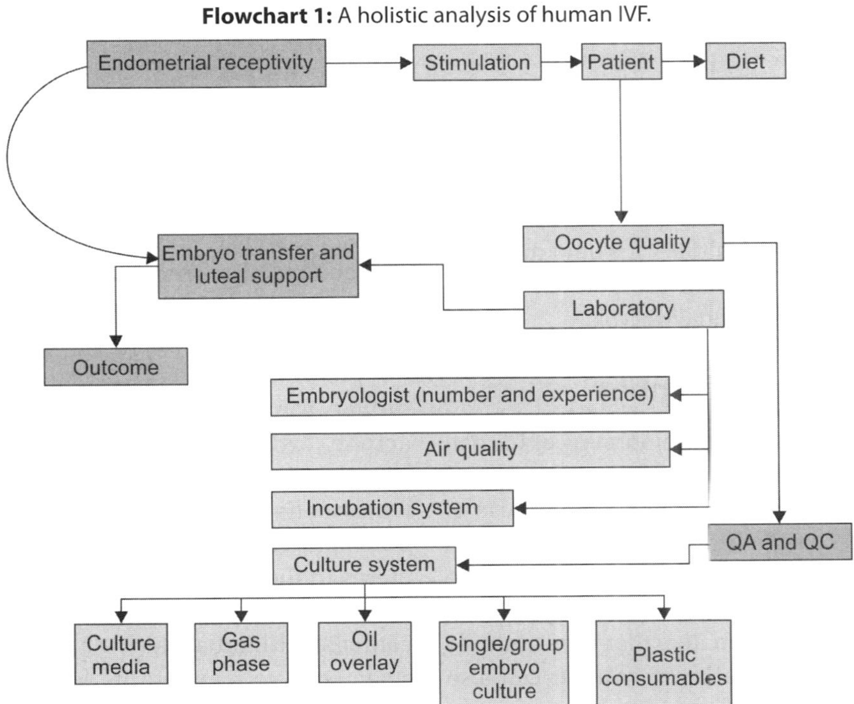

(IVF: in vitro fertilization; QC: quality control; QA: quality assurance).

results in enhanced development in vitro.[86] It has been observed that human blastocysts cultured in a low oxygen environment (5%) have significantly more cells than those cultured in a high oxygen environment (20%) (Gardner DK, unpublished data, 2006).[85] However, human and mouse embryos can grow at elevated oxygen concentrations and this has led to some confusion regarding the optimal concentration for embryo culture. The physiology of the reproductive tract and the beneficial effects of using a reduced oxygen concentrations determined in controlled studies indicate that to employ low oxygen concentrations appears prudent.

Carbon Dioxide

Carbon dioxide is not only required to maintain the pH of bicarbonate buffered medium, but is readily incorporated into protein and nucleic acids by the mouse embryo at all stages prior to implantation.[87] Culture systems for the preimplantation mammalian embryo routinely employ a CO_2 concentration of 5% coupled with a bicarbonate concentration of around 25 mm. It has been proposed that the beneficial effects of a high CO_2 concentration is due to a decrease in the pH of the medium as the beneficial effects of increased CO_2 could be replaced with a weak acid.[88] The optimal concentration of CO_2 for human embryo development has yet to be determined; however the CO_2 concentration is related to pH of the medium which also needs to be considered.

Temperature

Temperature fluctuations at the early cleavage stages have been demonstrated to decrease the subsequent development potential of embryos in vitro. Exposure of human oocytes to room temperature has been reported to induce damage to the meiotic spindle.[89] It would therefore seem advisable to maintain a constant temperature of 37°C when handling human oocytes and embryos.

Incubator or Incubation Chamber

As discussed earlier, for optimal development of human embryos in vitro it is important to maintain both the pH of the medium and temperature. The choice and use of incubators is therefore paramount for the success of an IVF program. Several studies have determined that embryo development in vitro is increased by restricting the opening of an incubator.[90] The use of incubators that have multiple chambers within the single incubator chamber can also reduce fluctuations in temperature and CO_2 levels induced by frequent door openings.

Light

Several studies have investigated the effect of exposure to visible light on the development of mammalian preimplantation embryos in vitro. In the human, implementation of an oocyte collection system employing low light at low oxygen concentration resulted in significantly increased rates of blastocyst formation of spare embryos and increased pregnancy and live birth rates when embryos were transferred on days 2–4 of culture.[91] Therefore, it would seem prudent to perform all oocyte and embryo collections and manipulations under low illumination.

Incubation Volume, Embryo Grouping and Oil Overlay

Within the lumen of the female reproductive tract, the developing embryo is exposed to microliter volumes of fluid.[92] In contrast, the embryo grown in vitro is subject to relatively larger volumes of culture medium (up to 1 mL). Consequently, any autocrine factor(s) produced by the developing embryo will be diluted and may therefore become ineffectual. Of greatest significance is the observation that decreasing the incubation volume significantly increases embryo viability[93] due to an increase in inner cell mass (ICM) development.[94,95] In order to culture in such reduced volumes (20–50 mL), an oil overlay is required. Although the use of an oil overlay is time-consuming, it prevents the evaporation of media, thereby reducing the harmful effects of increase in osmolality, and reduces changes in pH caused by a loss of CO_2 from the medium when culture dishes are taken out of the incubator for embryo examination. Furthermore, it has been proposed that an overlay of mineral oil can actually act as a trap for potential embryo toxins.[96]

As it is shown in Figure 1, as per the in vivo exposure of gradients of nutrients and environment to embryo in the female reproductive tract, culture media is tailored accordingly. During the precompaction stage, embryo has low biosynthetic activity, thus preferring pyruvate as the primary source of nutrition compared to high biosynthetic activity exhibiting postcompacting embryo preferring glucose. The AA availability also changes from primarily nonessential AA (NEAA) to essential AA (EAA), as it passes from fallopian tube during the precompaction stage to the uterus in the postcompaction stage. Female reproductive tract shows hypoxic condition in the fallopian tube compared to uterus, which may suggest that precompaction stage embryo may require lower oxygen concentration compared to postcompaction stage when embryo starts utilizing glucose as primary energy substrate.

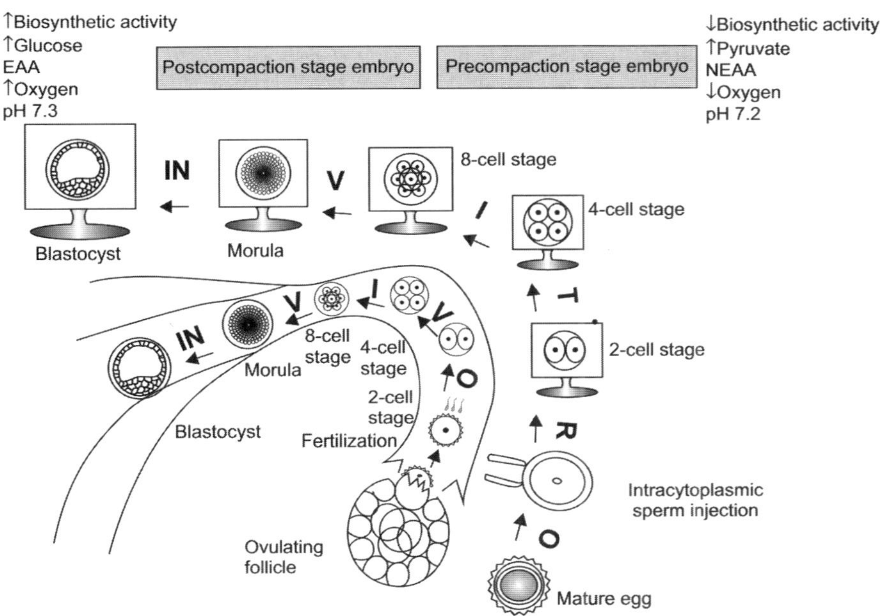

Fig. 1: Stage-specific requirements of developing preimplantation embryo. (EAA: essential amino acid; NEAA: nonessential amino acid).

QUALITY CONTROL

Mouse Bioassay

The QC of commercial media includes pH, osmolality, sterility, endotoxin tests and the mouse embryo assay (MEA). The preimplantation mouse embryo is the most widely used bioassay for medium components, culture media, and equipment used in clinical IVF. The medium can usually pass the MEA, if it supports development of more than or equal to 80% of mouse embryos to blastocyst stage. Using mice for testing media for human embryos has been the focus of discussion due to conflicting reports in the literature of its suitability as a bioassay.[97,98] The apparent contradiction of these studies can be resolved by taking into account the different stages of development used at the start of culture, the types of media used, and the supplementation of medium with protein. Furthermore, all studies used blastocyst development as the sole criterion for assessing embryo development, which is a poor indicator of embryo quality and does not reflect developmental potential.[99,100] A far more sensitive and quantitative parameter is blastocyst cell number.[77] A practical mouse embryo bioassay is to culture the zygote for 96 hours in protein-free medium. The rationale for using protein-free medium is that serum or serum albumin can chelate toxins, such as heavy metal ions, present in the medium. The presence of proteins would therefore hide any potential detrimental effects of the medium. One can readily obtain 80% blastocyst development on day 5, but it is important also to note how many embryos formed blastocysts in the afternoon of day 4 (i.e. on time development), and what is the cell number of resultant blastocysts.[85,101]

Using such an approach to testing, one can pick up subtle problems that can exist with any media, or more typically with any contact supplies. However, the mouse model should be used with caution as it presents obvious differences in reproductive physiology compared with humans[102] and there is no standardization of the day the culture should start, the mouse strain, number of embryos, etc. Efforts to increase its sensitivity include one cell as the starting point,[101,103] zona-free embryos,[104] the inclusion of positive controls,[105] accurate sample size calculations[106] and assessment of multiple endpoints and of blastocyst cell number.[85,105]

The ultimate QC on all media for IVF is their ability to support human embryo growth. It is obviously unethical to use human embryos for this purpose. A possible solution would be the use of triploid embryos as an assay of media quality, as these cannot be replaced in the prospective mother. Therefore vigilant monitoring of embryo development within the IVF laboratory is not only essential, but should be considered as part of the laboratory's overall QC system.

Sperm Bioassay

An alternative method to the mouse embryo bioassay is to use sperm motility as a method to detect potential embryo toxins. This assay utilizes both the number of motile sperm and degree of motility to determine the suitability of media to support embryo development. An advantage of this test is that it can be performed in 4–6 hours as opposed to the several days for the embryo bioassay. However, its sensitivity is very low, as human sperms are able to maintain their motility in very adverse culture conditions. Unfortunately, there is little clinical data on the applicability of such tests.

CONCLUSION

Unlike the dynamic changes in the environment of female reproductive tract, most conventional culture media systems are static in nature, where single system is used for the entire preimplantation period. Therefore, embryos have different requirements over the growing period those are reflected in the physiology and energy metabolism.[8,47,107] We also need to consider the other problems of a static culture media generation of potential toxins over the time. Thus, the change of media over the time through the development of zygote to blastocyst is required rather than using single media is necessary to support the development and differentiation. Again the recent reports support using single media throughout the growth with competitive results like sequential media.

We also need to remember that unlike the in vivo conditions, ART culture media contain only a subset of parts resulting in the continuous stressed condition for growing embryo. Any suboptimal condition forces the embryo to undergo adaptations, which may lead to lower pregnancy and higher abortion rates. It is evident that all necessary steps in ART as part of the treatment of infertility can influence the epigenetic programming during early development.[108] Thus, it is essential that the best level of QC exists in the laboratory and optimal environmental conditions are maintained for the development of the preimplantation embryo.

REFERENCES

1. Biggers JD. Pioneering mammalian embryo culture. In: Bavister BD (Ed). The Mammalian Preimplantation Embryo: Regulation of Growth and Differentiation in Vitro. New York: Plenum Press; 1987. pp. 1-22.
2. Bigger JD. Thoughts on embryo culture conditions. Reprod Biomed Online. 2002; 4(Suppl 1):30-8.
3. Bowman P, McLaren A. Cleavage rate of mouse embryos in vivo and in vitro. J Embryol Exp Morphol. 1970;24(1):203-7.
4. Harlow GM, Quinn P. Development of preimplantation mouse embryos in vivo and in vitro. Aust J Biol Sci. 1982;35(2):187-93.
5. Edwards RG. Causes of early embryonic loss in human pregnancy. Hum Reprod. 1986;1(3):185-98.
6. Biggers JD. Fundamentals of the design of culture media that support human preimplantation development. In: Van Blerkom J (Ed). Essential IVF. Norell: Kluwer Academic Press; 2003. pp. 291-332.
7. Leese HJ. The formation and function of oviduct fluid. J Reprod Fertil. 1988;82(2):843-56.
8. Gardner DK. Changes in requirements and utilization of nutrients during mammalian preimplantation embryo development and their significance in embryo culture. Theriogenology. 1998;49(1):83-102.
9. Freshney RI. Culture of Animal Cells: A Manual of Basic Technique, 4th edition. New York: Wiley-Liss; 2000. p. 600.
10. Edwards RG. Test-tube babies, 1981. Nature. 1981;293(5830):253-6.
11. Edwards RG, Purdy JM, Steptoe PC, et al. The growth of human preimplantation embryos in vitro. Am J Obstet Gynecol. 1981;141(4):408-16.
12. Staessen C, Van den Abbeel E, Janssenswillen C, et al. Controlled comparison of Earle's balanced salt solution with Ménézo B2 medium for human in-vitro fertilization performance. Hum Reprod. 1994;9(10):1915-9.
13. Barnett DK, Bavister BD. What is the relationship between the metabolism of preimplantation embryos and their developmental competence? Mol Reprod Dev. 1996;43(1):105-33.
14. Gardner DK, Lane M. Embryo culture systems. In: Trounson AO, Gardner DK (Eds). Handbook of In Vitro Fertilization, 2nd edition. Boca Raton: CRC Press; 1999. pp. 205-64.
15. Menezo Y, Testart J, Perrone D. Serum is not necessary in human in vitro fertilization, early embryo culture, and transfer. Fertil Steril. 1984;42(5):750-5.
16. Quinn P, Kerin JF, Warnes GM. Improved pregnancy rate in human in vitro fertilization with the use of a medium based on the composition of human tubal fluid. Fertil Steril. 1985;44(4):493-8.
17. Gardner DK, Lane M, Calderon I, et al. Environment of the preimplantation human embryo in vivo: metabolite analysis of oviduct and uterine fluids and metabolism of cumulus cells. Fertil Steril. 1996;65(2):349-53.
18. Leese HJ, Barton AM. Production of pyruvate by isolated mouse cumulus cells. J Exp Zool. 1985;234(2):231-6.
19. Whitten WK, Biggers JD. Complete development in vitro of the pre-implantation stages of the mouse in a simple chemically defined medium. J Reprod Fertil. 1968;17(2):399-401.
20. Whittingham DG. Culture of mouse ova. J Reprod Fertil Suppl. 1971;14:7-21.
21. Chatot CL, Ziomek CA, Bavister BD, et al. An improved culture medium supports development of random-bred 1-cell mouse embryos in vitro. J Reprod Fertil. 1989;86(2):679-88.
22. Lawitts JA, Biggers JD. Joint effects of sodium chloride, glutamine, and glucose in mouse preimplantation embryo culture media. Mol Reprod Dev. 1992;31 (3):189-94.
23. Quinn P. Enhanced results in mouse and human embryo culture using a modified human tubal fluid medium lacking glucose and phosphate. J Assist Reprod Genet. 1995;12(2):97-105.

24. Carrillo AJ, Lane B, Pridman DD, et al. Improved clinical outcomes for in vitro fertilization with delay of embryo transfer from 48 to 72 hours after oocyte retrieval: use of glucoseand phosphate-free media. Fertil Steril. 1998;69(2): 329-34.
25. Ham RG. An improved nutrient solution for diploid Chinese hamster and human cell lines. Exp Cell Res. 1963;29:515-26.
26. Gardner DK, Lane M. Amino acids and ammonium regulate mouse embryo development in culture. Biol Reprod. 1993;48(2):377-85.
27. Lawitts JA, Biggers JD. Optimization of mouse embryo culture media using simplex methods. J Reprod Fertil. 1991;91(2):543-56.
28. Lawitts JA, Biggers JD. Culture of preimplantation embryos. Methods Enzymol. 1993;225:153-64.
29. Ho Y, Wigglesworth K, Eppig JJ, et al. Preimplantation development of mouse embryos in KSOM: augmentation by amino acids and analysis of gene expression. Mol Reprod Dev. 1995;41(2):232-8.
30. Biggers JD, Racowsky C. The development of fertilized human ova to the blastocyst stage in KSOM(AA) medium: is a two-step protocol necessary? Reprod Biomed Online. 2002;5(2):133-40.
31. Gardner DK, Leese HJ. Concentrations of nutrients in mouse oviduct fluid and their effects on embryo development and metabolism in vitro. J Reprod Fertil. 1990;88(1):361-8.
32. Gardner DK, Pool TB, Lane M. Embryo nutrition and energy metabolism and its relationship to embryo growth, differentiation, and viability. Semin Reprod Med. 2000;18(2):205-18.
33. Edwards LJ, Williams DA, Gardner DK. Intracellular pH of the mouse preimplantation embryo: amino acids act as buffers of intracellular pH. Hum Reprod. 1998;13(12):3441-8.
34. Lane M, Gardner DK. Understanding cellular disruptions during early embryo development that perturb viability and fetal development. Reprod Fertil Dev. 2005;17(3):371-8.
35. Lane M. Mechanisms for managing cellular and homeostatic stress in vitro. Therio-genology. 2001;55(1):225-36.
36. Gardner DK. Mammalian embryo culture in the absence of serum or somatic cell support. Cell Biol Int. 1994;18(12):1163-79.
37. Gardner DK, Lane M. Development of viable mammalian embryos in vitro: evolution of sequential media. In: Cibelli R, Lanza K, Campbell AK, West MD (Eds). Principles of Cloning. San Diego: Academic Press; 2002. p. 187.
38. Barnes FL, Crombie A, Gardner DK, et al. Blastocyst development and birth after in-vitro maturation of human primary oocytes, intracytoplasmic sperm injection and assisted hatching. Hum Reprod. 1995;10(12):3243-7.
39. Bertheussen K, Forsdahl F, Maltau JM. In vitro fertilization. New media for embryo culture to the blastocyst stage. In: Gomel V, Leung PC (Eds). In Vitro Fertilization and Assisted Reproduction. Bologna: Monduzzi Editore; 1997. pp. 199-204.
40. Behr B, Milki AA, Giudice LC, et al. High yield blastocyst culture and transfer: a new approach using P1 and blastocyst medium in reduced O2 environment. Fertil Steril. 1998;70(3 Suppl 1):S98.
41. Biggers JD. Reflections on the culture of the preimplantation embryo. Int J Dev Biol. 1998;42(7):879-84.
42. Gardner DK, Lane M. Culture and selection of viable blastocysts: a feasible proposition for human IVF? Hum Reprod Update. 1997;3(4):367-82.
43. Summers MC, Biggers JD. Chemically defined media and the culture of mammalian preimplantation embryos: historical perspective and current issues. Hum Reprod Update. 2003;9(6):557-82.
44. Biggers JD, Summers MC. Choosing a culture medium: making informed choices. Fertil Steril. 2008;90(3):473-83.
45. Whitten WK. Culture of tubal mouse ova. Nature. 1956;177(4498):96.
46. Brinster RL. Studies on the development of mouse embryos in vitro. IV. Interaction of energy sources. J Reprod Fertil. 1965;10(2):227-40.
47. Leese HJ. Metabolism of the preimplantation mammalian embryo. Oxf Rev Reprod Biol. 1991;13:35-72.
48. Rieger D. Relationships between energy metabolism and development of early mammalian embryos. Theriogenology. 1992;37(1):75-93.
49. Bavister BD. Culture of preimplantation embryos: facts and artefacts. Hum Reprod Update. 1995;1(2):91-148.
50. Bavister BD. Glucose and culture of human embryos. Fertil Steril. 1999;72(2): 233-4.
51. McManus ML, Churchwell KB, Strange K. Regulation of cell volume in health and disease. N Engl J Med. 1995;333(19):1260-6.
52. Borland RM, Biggers JD, Lechene CP, et al. Elemental composition of fluid in the human Fallopian tube. J Reprod Fertil. 1980;58(2):479-82.
53. Biggers JD, Lawitts JA, Lechene CP. The protective action of betaine on the deleterious effects of NaCl on preimplantation mouse embryos in vitro. Mol Reprod Dev. 1993;34(4):380-90.
54. Van Winkle LJ, Haghighat N, Campione AL. Glycine protects preimplantation mouse conceptuses from a detrimental effect on development of the inorganic ions in oviductal fluid. J Exp Zool. 1990;253(2):215-9.
55. Nichol R, Hunter RH, Gardner DK, et al. Concentrations of energy substrates in oviductal fluid and blood plasma of pigs during the peri-ovulatory period. J Reprod Fertil. 1992;96(2):699-707.
56. Leese HJ, Barton AM. Pyruvate and glucose uptake by mouse ova and preimplantation embryos. J Reprod Fertil. 1984;72(1):9-13.
57. Leese HJ, Biggers JD, Mroz EA, et al. Nucleotides in a single mammalian ovum or preimplantation embryo. Anal Biochem. 1984;140(2):443-8.
58. Leese HJ, Conaghan J, Martin KL, et al. Early human embryo metabolism. Bioessays 1993;15(4):259-64.
59. Reitzer LJ, Wice BM, Kennell D. The pentose cycle. Control and essential function in HeLa cell nucleic acid synthesis. J Biol Chem. 1980;255(12):5616-26.
60. Biggers JD, McGinnis LK, Lawitts JA. One-step versus two-step culture of mouse preimplantation embryos: is there a difference? Hum Reprod. 2005;20(12):3376-84.
61. Casslén BG. Free amino acids in human uterine fluid. Possible role of high taurine concentration. J Reprod Med. 1987;32(3):181-4.
62. Miller JG, Schultz GA. Amino acid content of preimplantation rabbit embryos and fluids of the reproductive tract. Biol Reprod. 1987;36(1):125-9.

63. Van Winkle LJ. Amino acid transport in developing animal oocytes and early conceptuses. Biochim Biophys Acta. 1988;947(1):173-208.
64. Schultz GA, Kaye PL, McKay DJ, et al. Endogenous amino acid pool sizes in mouse eggs and preimplantation embryos. J Reprod Fertil. 1981;61(2):387-93.
65. Chatot CL, Tasca RJ, Ziomek CA. Glutamine uptake and utilization by preimplantation mouse embryos in CZB medium. J Reprod Fertil. 1990;89(1):335-46.
66. Crosby IM, Gandolfi F, Moor RM. Control of protein synthesis during early cleavage of sheep embryos. J Reprod Fertil. 1988;82(2):769-75.
67. Liu Z, Foote RH. Development of bovine embryos in KSOM with added superoxide dismutase and taurine and with five and twenty percent O2. Biol Reprod. 1995;53(4):786-90.
68. Lindenbaum A. A survey of natural occurring chelating ligands. Adv Exp Med Biol. 1973;40:67-77.
69. Cassuto G, Chavrier M, Menezo Y. Culture conditions and not prolonged culture time are responsible for monozygotic twinning in human in vitro fertilization. Fertil Steril. 2003;80(2):462-3.
70. Gardner DK, Lane M. The 2-cell block in CF1 mouse embryos is associated with an increase in glycolysis and a decrease in tricarboxylic acid (TCA) cycle activity: alleviation of the 2-cell block is associated with the restoration of in vivo metabolic pathway activities. Biol Reprod. 1993;49(Suppl 1):152.
71. Abramczuk J, Solter D, Koprowski H. The beneficial effect EDTA on development of mouse one-cell embryos in chemically defined medium. Dev Biol. 1977;61(2):378-83.
72. Gardner DK, Lane MW, Lane M. Bovine blastocyst cell number is increased by culture with EDTA for the first 72 h of development from the zygote. Theriogenology. 1997;47:278.
73. Bavister BD, McKiernan SH. Regulation of hamster embryo development in vitro by amino acids. In: Bavister BD (Ed). Preimplantation Embryo Development. New York: Springer-Verlag; 1992. pp. 57-72.
74. Ducibella T, Anderson E. Cell shape and membrane changes in the eight-cell mouse embryo: prerequisites for morphogenesis of the blastocyst. Dev Biol. 1975;47(1):45-58.
75. Lane M, Boatman DE, Albrecht RM, et al. Intracellular divalent cation homeostasis and developmental competence in the hamster preimplantation embryo. Mol Reprod Dev. 1998;50(4):443-50.
76. Lane M, Bavister BD. Calcium homeostasis in early hamster preimplantation embryos. Biol Reprod. 1998;59(4):1000-7.
77. Gardner DK, Lane M. Culture and selection of viable blastocysts: a feasible proposition for human IVF? Hum Reprod Update. 1997;3(4):367-82.
78. Swain JE. Optimizing the culture environment in the IVF laboratory: impact of pH and buffer capacity on gamete and embryo quality. Reprod Biomed Online. 2010;21(1):6-16.
79. Bavister BD. Preimplantation Embryo Development. New York: Springer-Verlag; 1993. p. 184.
80. Lane M, Gardner DK. Amino acids and vitamins prevent culture-induced metabolic perturbations and associated loss of viability of mouse blastocysts. Hum Reprod. 1998;13(4):991-7.
81. Lane M, Gardner DK. Embryo culture medium: which is the best? Best Pract Res Clin Obstet Gynaecol. 2007;21(1):83-100.
82. Bulgurcuoglu S, Özsait B, Attar E. Büyüme Faktörlerinin Oosit ve Embriyo Gelisimi Üzerindeki Etkisi. Artemis. 2003;4:18-26.
83. Richter KS. The importance of growth factors for preimplantation embryo development and in-vitro culture. Curr Opin Obstet Gynecol. 2008;20(3):292-304.
84. Lemeire K, Van Merris V, Cortvrindt R. The antibiotic streptomycin assessed in a battery of in vitro tests for reproductive toxicology. Toxicol In Vitro. 2007;21(7):1348-53.
85. Gardner DK. In Vitro Fertilization: A Practical Approach. New York: CRC Press; 2006. p. 528.
86. Thompson JG, Simpson AC, Pugh PA, et al. Effect of oxygen concentration on in-vitro development of preimplantation sheep and cattle embryos. J Reprod Fertil. 1990;89(2):573-8.
87. Graves CN, Biggers JD. Carbon dioxide fixation by mouse embryos prior to implantation. Science. 1970;167(3924): 1506-8.
88. Carney EW, Bavister BD. Regulation of hamster embryo development in vitro by carbon dioxide. Biol Reprod. 1987;36(5):1155-63.
89. Gardner DK, Lane M. Alleviation of the '2-cell block' and development to the blastocyst of CF1 mouse embryos: role of amino acids, EDTA and physical parameters. Hum Reprod. 1996;11(12):2703-12.
90. Pickering SJ, Braude PR, Johnson MH, et al. Transient cooling to room temperature can cause irreversible disruption of the meiotic spindle in the human oocyte. Fertil Steril. 1990;54(1):102-8.
91. Noda Y, Goto Y, Umaoka Y, et al. Culture of human embryos in alpha modification of Eagle's medium under low oxygen tension and low illumination. Fertil Steril. 1994;62(5):1022-7.
92. Leese HJ. The formation and function of oviduct fluid. J Reprod Fertil. 1988;82 (2):843-56.
93. Lane M, Gardner DK. Effect of incubation volume and embryo density on the development and viability of mouse embryos in vitro. Hum Reprod. 1992;7(4):558-62.
94. Gardner DK, Lane MW, Lane M. Development of the inner cell mass in mouse blastocyst is stimulated by reducing the embryo: incubation volume ratio. Hum Reprod. 1997;12(1):132.
95. Ahern TJ, Gardner DK. Culturing bovine embryos in groups stimulates blastocyst development and cell allocation to the inner cell mass. Theriogenology. 1998;49(1):194.
96. Miller KF, Goldberg JM, Collins RL. Covering embryo cultures with mineral oil alters embryo growth by acting as a sink for an embryotoxic substance. J Assist Reprod Genet. 1994;11(7):342-5.
97. Weiss TJ, Warnes GM, Gardner DK. Mouse embryos and quality control in human IVF. Reprod Fertil Dev. 1992;4(1):105-7.
98. Gerrity M. Mouse embryo culture bioassay. In: Wolf DP (Ed). In Vitro Fertilization and Embryo Transfer. New York: Plenum Publishers; 1988. p. 57.
99. Gardner DK, Sakkas D. Mouse embryo cleavage, metabolism and viability: role of medium composition. Hum Reprod. 1993;8(2):288-95.
100. Lane M, Gardner DK. Selection of viable mouse blastocysts prior to transfer using a metabolic criterion. Hum Reprod. 1996;11(9):1975-8.

101. Scott LF, Sundaram SG, Smith S. The relevance and use of mouse embryo bioassays for quality control in an assisted reproductive technology program. Fertil Steril. 1993;60(3):559-68.
102. Ménézo YJ, Hérubel F. Mouse and bovine models for human IVF. Reprod Biomed Online. 2002;4(2):170-5.
103. Davidson A, Vermesh M, Lobo RA, et al. Mouse embryo culture as quality control for human in vitro fertilization: the one-cell versus the two-cell model. Fertil Steril. 1988;49(3):516-21.
104. Montoro L, Subias E, Young P, et al. Detection of endotoxin in human in vitro fertilization by the zona-free mouse embryo assay. Fertil Steril. 1990;54(1):109-12.
105. Dubin NH, Bornstein DR, Gong Y. Use of endotoxin as a positive (toxic) control in the mouse embryo assay. J Assist Reprod Genet. 1995;12(2):147-52.
106. Hendriks JC, Teerenstra S, Punt-Van der Zalm JP, et al. Sample size calculations for a split-cluster, beta-binomial design in the assessment of toxicity. Stat Med. 2005;24(24):3757-72.
107. Lane M, Gardner DK. Lactate regulates pyruvate uptake and metabolism in the preimplantation mouse embryo. Biol Reprod. 2000;62(1):16-22.
108. Rivera RM, Stein P, Weaver JR, et al. Manipulation of mouse embryos prior to implantation result in aberrant expression of imprinted genes on day 9.5 of development. Hum Mol Genet. 2008;17(1):1-14.

CHAPTER 61

Embryo Selection and Transfer

Anisha Uberoi, Himani Agnihotri

INTRODUCTION

Ever since the inception of in vitro fertilization (IVF), accurate selection of embryos with high implantation potential has been an integral part of the practice. The quality of embryos and their rate of development may vary across different clinics. This may be attributed to the inherent potential of the embryo itself, the IVF method or the culture medium used.

Embryo assessment before transfer in IVF or intracytoplasmic sperm injection (ICSI) helps to select the most viable embryo during culture by evaluating the embryo at specific time points from day 1 zygote to day 3 embryos or day 5 blastocyst, thereby increasing the pregnancy rates (PRs).

Morphological parameters have been the basis of selecting the most viable embryo or blastocyst for transfer globally. The parameters influencing the selection of good quality embryos are as follows:

- Pronuclear (PN) morphology
- Polar body (PB) structure and placement
- Appearance of cytoplasm [vacuoles, necrotic bodies, smooth endoplasmic reticulum (SER), granularity, etc.] and zona pellucida (ZP)
- Number, symmetry, fragmentation and multinucleation of blastomeres on day 2 and day 3 of embryo culture
- Compaction of blastomeres and expansion of blastocoel on day 5.

MORPHOLOGICAL ASSESSMENT

Accurate selection of embryos for transfer is of paramount importance. Thus, it is highly crucial to evaluate the quality of embryo at appropriate time in the laboratory (Table 1).

Fertilization Assessment (Day 1)

Fertilization can be assessed by the presence of two PBs and two centrally located juxtaposed pronuclei (PNs) [which contains nucleolar precursor bodies (NPBs) equatorially aligned] that are even sized with distinct membranes. Ideal features shared by the zygote are illustrated in Figure 1:

Table 1: Standardized timing relative to insemination time-based on the Istanbul consensus workshop.[1]

Assessment	*Timing (hours postinsemination)*	
Fertilization (Day 1)	16–19 hpi	ICSI at 13.00: 5–8 am
Day 2	44–47 hpi	9–12 am
Day 3	67–71 hpi	8–12 am
Day 5	116–120 hpi	8–12 am
Day 6	140–144 hpi	8–12 am

(ICSI: intracytoplasmic sperm injection).

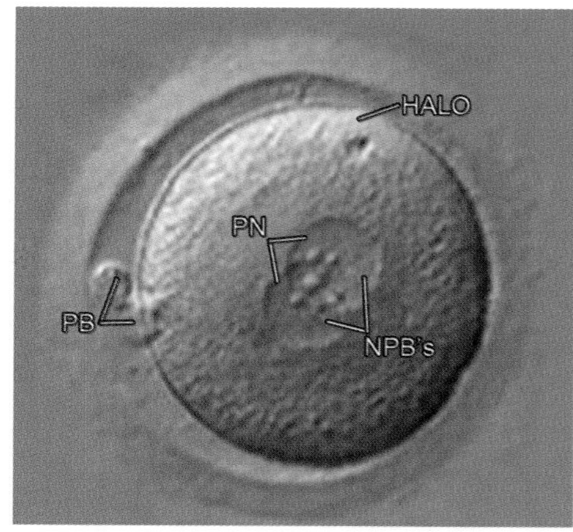

Fig. 1: Zygote showing 2 PN, 2 PB and Halo. (NPBs: nucleolar precursor bodies; PB: polar body; PN: pronucleus)

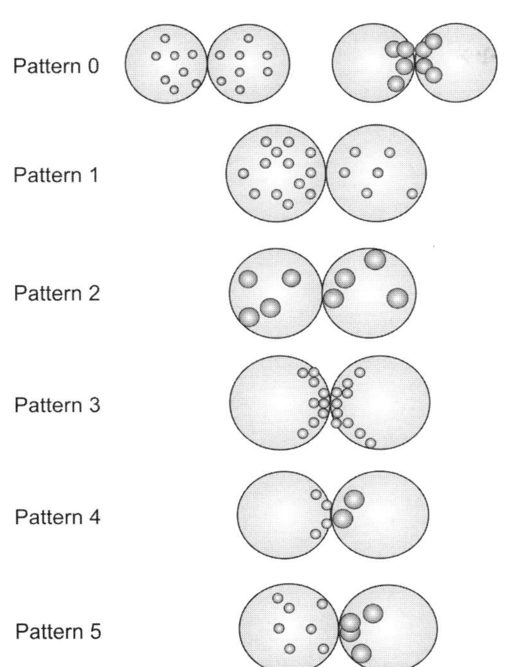

Fig. 2: Zygote classification according to Tesarik and Greco, 1999.

- The cytoplasm should be heterogeneous with a cortical halo effect on the peripheral side. Studies have reported higher quality embryos (60.9%) in zygotes with halo in comparison to zygotes without a halo (52.2%)[2,3]
- Number of NPBs in both the nuclei should not differ by three.[4]

This PN scoring should be performed 16–19 hour postinsemination.

There are numerous systems in literature which classify zygotes based on the size, number and distribution of nucleoli within the nuclei.

Garello and his colleagues established a correlation between the orientation of PNs relative to the PBs and the embryo quality, thus angle β plays a crucial role while evaluating the zygote.[5]

- *Angle β*: The angle between a line drawn through the axis of the PNs and the position of the furthest PB
- Generally, the angle β should be less than 50°.

The grading system recommended by Tesarik and Greco classifies the zygotes (day 1) based on six patterns of PN, wherein pattern 0 corresponds to normal zygotes and patterns 1–5 represent the varying irregularities in the zygote (Fig. 2).[4]

According to the model proposed by Scott and his colleagues, zygotes are classified according to PN morphology labeled with grades corresponding to their quality.[6] The Z-score describes the number, size, and position of the nucleoli and the equality between the nuclei for these characteristics (Box 1).

Box 1: Z-scoring for pronuclear (PN) zygote by Scott and his colleagues.

Definition	
Z1	Equal pronuclei. Equal number and size of nucleoli, aligned in both pronuclei at the pronuclear junction. The absolute number of nucleoli ranges between three and seven.
Z2	Equal pronuclei. Equal number and size of nucleoli, scattered in both pronuclei. The absolute number of nucleoli ranges between three and seven.
Z3	Equal pronuclei. Equal number and even or (and) uneven size of nucleoli, aligned in one pronucleus at the pronuclear junction. The other pronucleus with randomly scattered nucleoli. The absolute number of nucleoli ranges between three and seven.
Z4	Unequal or separated pronuclei.

According to Association for the Study of the Biology of Reproductive (ASEBIR) grading, zygotes are classified based on the PN symmetry and the distribution of NPB within the PN. Ideally, in a zygote the PN should be of the same size, have 3–7 polarized NPBs and a cytoplasmic halo (Tables 2 and 3).[7]

Presence of more than or equal to 3 PN or 1 PN after IVF or ICSI is the most common anomaly seen on day 1 (Fig. 3), caused by dispermy in IVF and by parthenogenetic activation of oocytes due to mechanical or chemical factors during ICSI.[8,9]

Cleavage Stage Embryos (Day 2 and Day 3)

Cleavage stage embryos range from 2-cell stage to the compacted morula composed of 8–16 cells. Ideally, on day 2 and on day 3, the number of blastomeres is assessed and each embryo is given a particular score based on the number and uniformity of blastomeres, fragmentation and presence of multinucleation. Number of blastomeres is known to have the highest predictive value.[10,11] Additionally, embryos must exhibit appropriate kinetics and synchrony of division. In normal developing embryos, cell division occurs every 18–20 hour.

Cell Number

The single cell zygote divides into 2–4 cells at 44–47 hours postinsemination (hpi) (day 2) and 7–10 cells after 67–71 hpi (day 3) (Figs. 4A to C).

Transferring a 4-cell embryo on day 2 has a higher implantation rate (IR) as compared to 2 or 5 cells, 3 or 6 cells, 1 cell or less than 6-cell embryo. Moreover, embryos

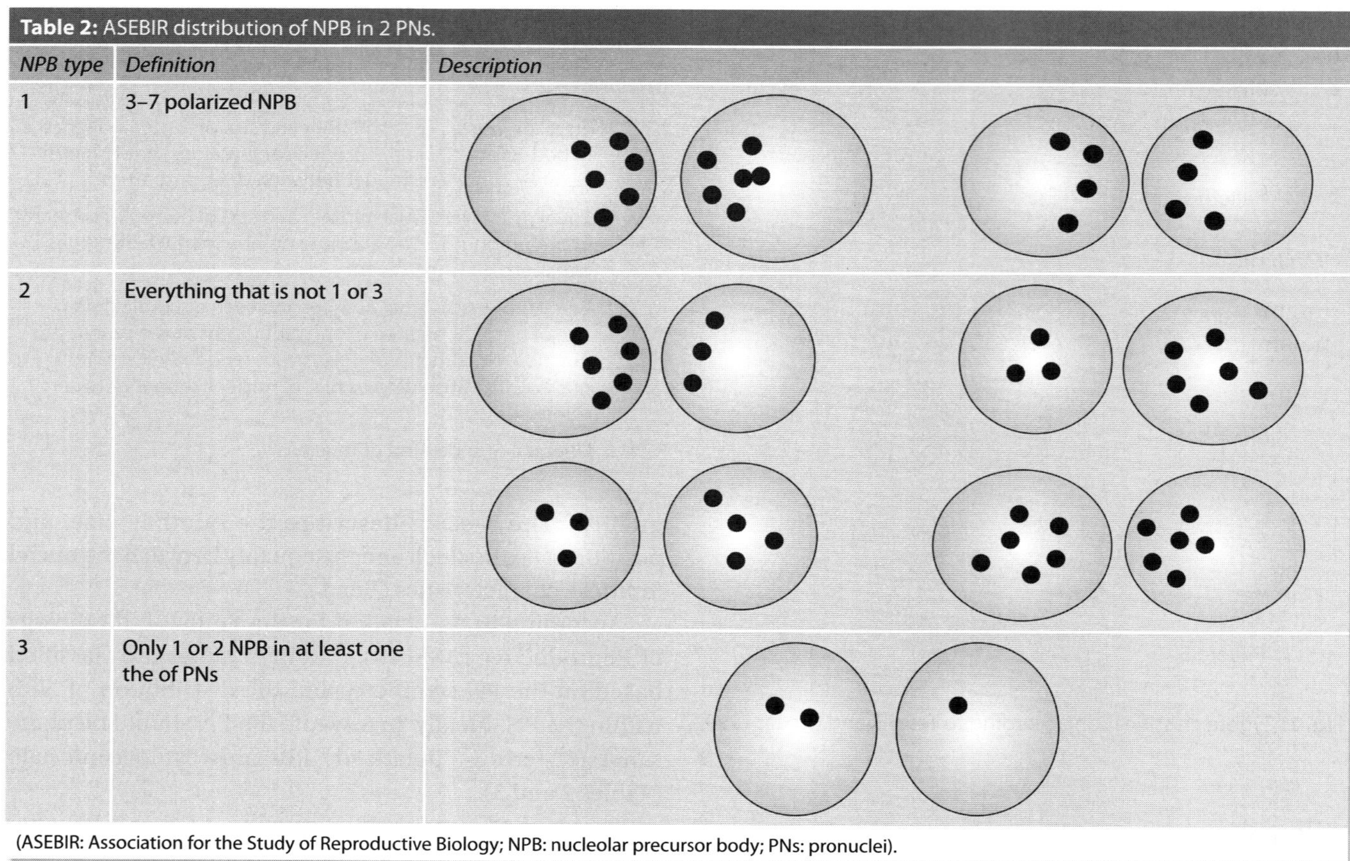

Table 2: ASEBIR distribution of NPB in 2 PNs.

NPB type	*Definition*	*Description*
1	3–7 polarized NPB	
2	Everything that is not 1 or 3	
3	Only 1 or 2 NPB in at least one the of PNs	

(ASEBIR: Association for the Study of Reproductive Biology; NPB: nucleolar precursor body; PNs: pronuclei).

on day 3 are evaluated on the basis of rate of cell division between day 2 and day 3. Thus, embryos can be categorized according to their implantation potential.

Embryos dividing either too slow or too fast may have metabolic and/or chromosomal defects.[12] Different morphological anomalies are often associated with each other, and uneven cleavage has shown to be related to multinucleation[13] and fragmentation.[14]

Size and Shape of the Blastomere

Cell regularity plays an important role in the cleavage stage embryos. Usually the blastomeres should be same or similar in size, to maximize the overall pregnancy outcome.[13,15] Irregular blastomeres may indicate cell division or a physiological alteration (Table 4).

Concordant observations were also reported wherein embryos with uneven sized blastomeres displayed a higher rate of multinucleation and aneuploidy, consequently lowering the IR.

When cell division is not synchronous, it corresponds to the fact that the cells from two different cell cycle coexist. As a result, embryos with 3, 5, 7, 9, etc. blastomeres have two

Table 3: ASEBIR classification on the basis of PN size.

Symmetry	*Definition*	*Description*
1	Same PN size	
2	Similar PN size	
3	Different PN size	

(ASEBIR: Association for the Study of Reproductive Biology; PN: pronucleus).

different sizes of cells. Positive classification of embryos with odd number of cells is as follows:

- 3 cell: 1 large blastomere and 2 small blastomere
- 5 cell: 3 large blastomere and 2 small blastomere
- 7 cell: 1 large blastomere and 6 small blastomere
- 9 cell: 2 large blastomere and 7 small blastomere.

Fragmentation

Fragmentation, also known as blebbing is portions of the embryo cell that has broken off and separated from the nucleated portion of the cell (Fig. 5). The degree of fragmentation, size of fragments and its distribution all contribute in evaluating the developmental potential of an embryo.

A good quality embryo should have no fragmentation or less fragmentation, i.e. less than or equal to 10%.[15] Numerous studies in literature have correlated a high degree of fragmentation with low IRs.[16] Moreover, fragmentation has also been related to aneuploidy.[17,18] In contrast, presence of low fragmentation has no negative or possibly even a positive impact on the developing embryo and the PRs.[19]

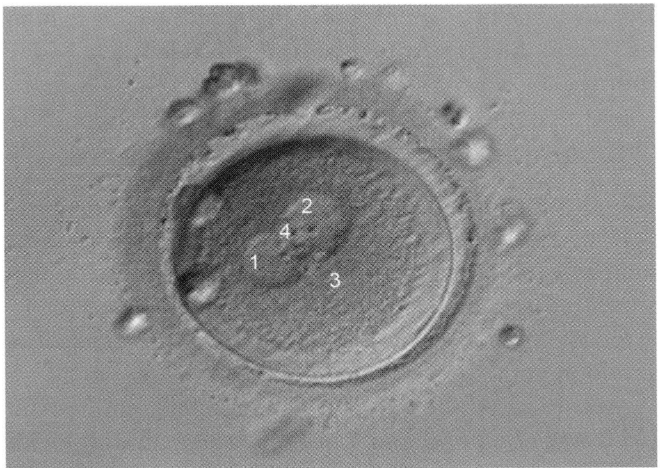

Fig. 3: Zygote showing more than 3 pronuclear (PN) on day 1.

Nucleation

Nucleation is defined as the presence of the nuclei in the blastomeres of the cleavage stage embryo. Ideally it should be one nucleus per blastomere, but no visible nuclei or multinucleation is often observed in cohort of embryos (Figs. 6A and B).

Multinucleation is the presence of more than one nucleus in each blastomere on day 2 or day 3 and has been associated with an increased rate of aneuploidy and chromosomal abnormalities.[13,20] It has been reported that multinucleated cells arise from a failure of cytokinesis, thereby leading to cleavage stage arrest in vitro.[13] Numerous other studies reported low IR and increased rate of abortions

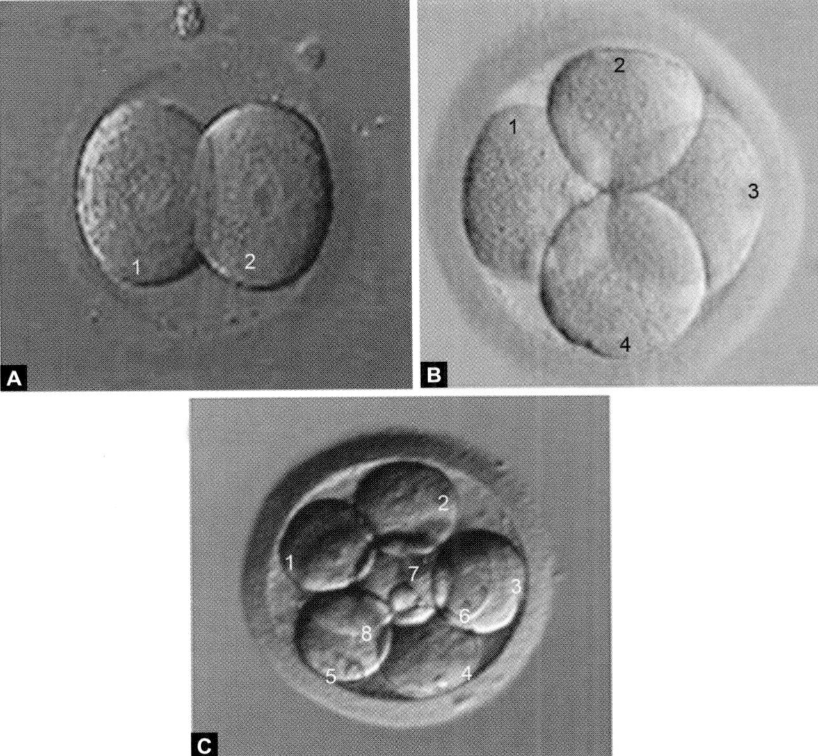

Figs. 4A to C: Embryos showing cell division. (A) 2-cell embryo at 45 hours; (B) 4-cell embryo at 47 hours; and (C) 8-celled embryo at 68 hours postinsemination.

Table 4: Cell regularity in cleavage stage embryos.

Symmetry	*Definition*	*Description*
1	Same cell size	
2	Similar cell size	
3	Different cell size	
4	One dominant cell	

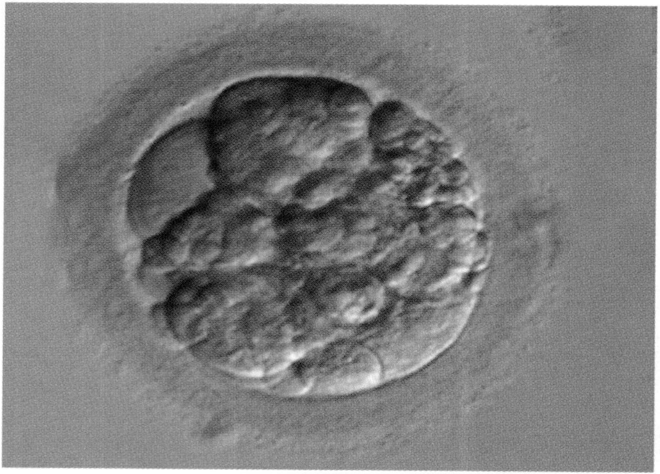

Fig. 5: Day 3 embryo exhibiting 20% of fragmentation.

due to multinucleation in cleavage stage embryos.[21] Additionally, in extended culture systems, multinucleation was associated with a lower blastocyst formation rate.[10]

Cytoplasmic Pitting

Cytoplasmic pitting is characterized by the presence of numerous small pits on the surface of the cytoplasm (Fig. 7).[22] It indicates cytoplasmic activation on day 3 and should not be misjudged with extensive vacuolization.[23]

Cytoplasmic Ring

Cytoplasmic ring is formed during contraction of the cytoplasm leaving a large translucent ring without the organelles close to the edge of the blastomere (Fig. 8). The presence of a cytoplasmic ring relates to the cellular lysis[24] and thus is detrimental to the development of the embryo.

Cytoplasmic Anomalies

The cytoplasm of the cleaving embryos is normally pale in appearance and less granular.[25] Anomalies, such as cytoplasmic granularity and vacuoles can also be scored morphologically on day 2 or day 3 (Fig. 9). Extensive vacuolization is detrimental mainly to spatial development.[24]

According to the described parameters, embryos at 4-cell stage on day 2 and 7 or 8-cell stage on day 3 with minimum fragmentation, no multinucleation and with the absence of any cytoplasmic anomalies make the most viable embryos.

Morula Stage (Day 4)

On day 4 the embryos should be assessed 92 ± 2 hpi. They are in that stage when embryos begin their transition from multi-blastomeres to compacting or compacted embryo (Table 5). A good quality morula is composed of 16–32 blastomeres showing considerable compaction on day 4 (Fig. 10).[26]

Blastocyst Scoring (Day 5 and Day 6)

Usually, 5–6 days after fertilization, embryos develop to the blastocyst stage, consisting of two cell layers: (1) the outer cells of the blastocyst, forming the blastocyst structure itself are called the trophectoderm (TE) cells and (2) the cells located inside the blastocoel, often forming a cell clump at one pole of the blastocyst are called the inner cell mass (ICM) cells.

Generally, blastocysts are graded by evaluating three separate quality scores that include:

1. *Blastocoel cavity*: A defining moment in embryonic development is when fluid starts to accumulate between

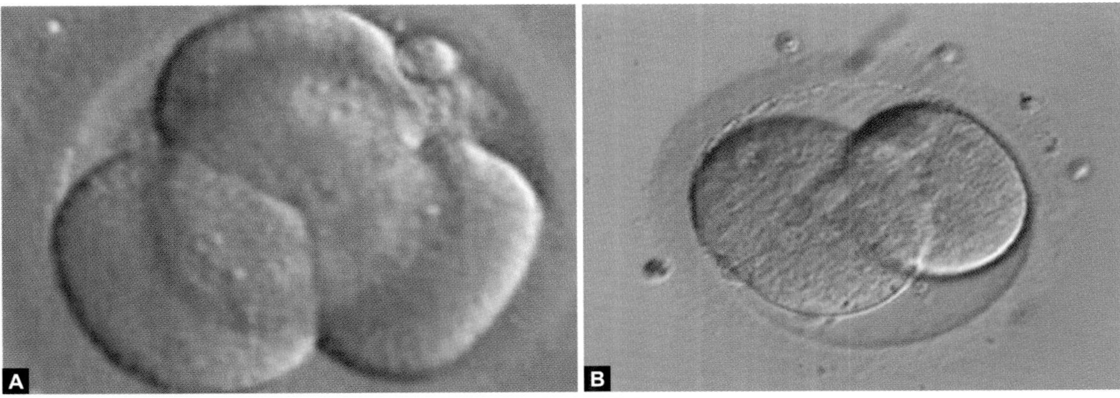

Figs. 6A and B: (A) 4-cell embryo showing distinct nuclei in each blastomere; and (B) 2-cell embryo showing multinucleation in one of the blastomere.

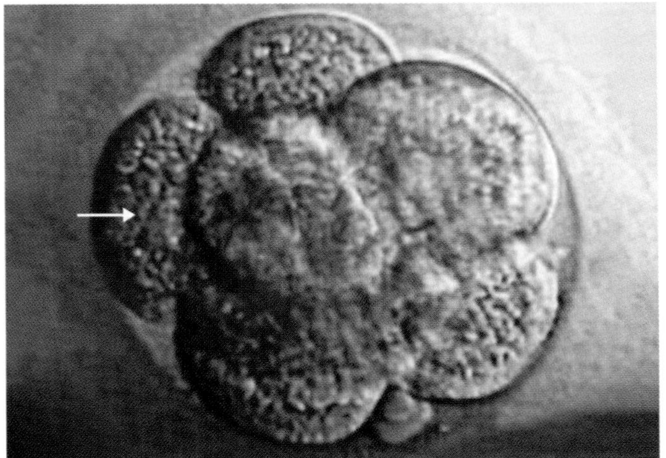

Fig. 7: Embryo showing pitting on day 3.

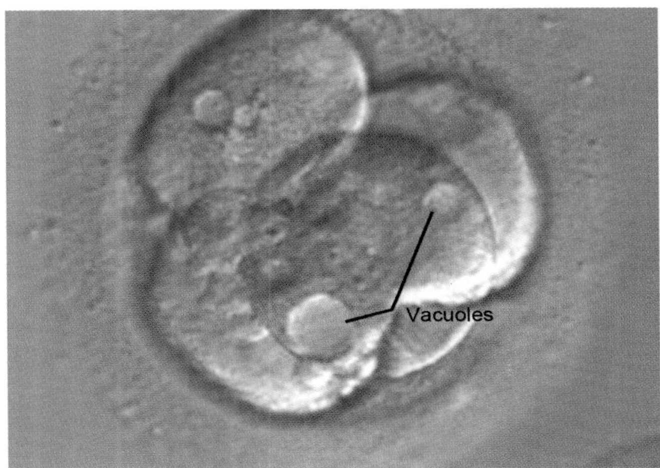

Fig. 9: 4-cell embryo exhibiting high number of small and medium vacuoles.

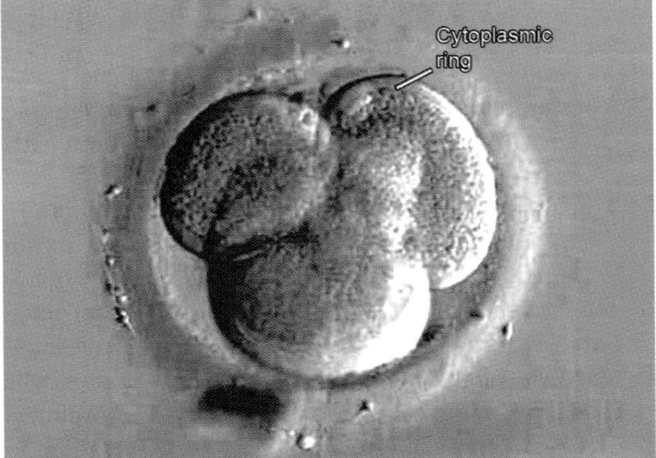

Fig. 8: Embryo showing acytoplasmic ring on day 2.

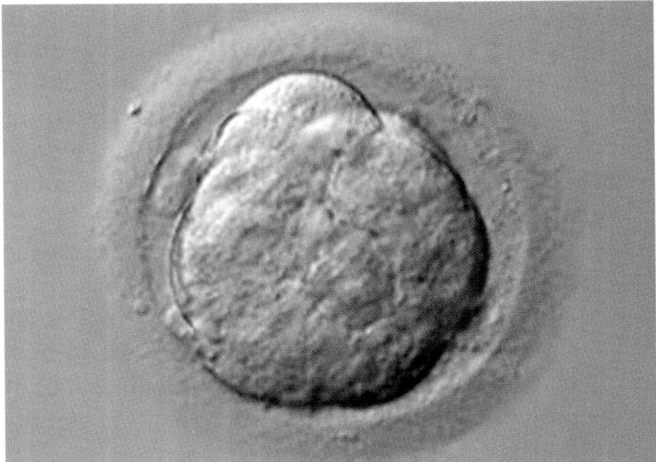

Fig. 10: A well-compacted morula on day 4.

cells at the morula stage of development. As the fluid's volume increases, a cavity appears gradually forming the blastocoel. As the development of blastocyst progresses, blastocoel increases resulting in thinning of the ZP. Finally, the blastocyst breaks free of the ZP through a process called hatching.

Table 5: Classifying day 4 embryos according to degree compaction.

Compaction	*Definition*	*Description*
0	No compaction	
1	Losing cell definition	
2	Starting compaction	
3	Very compacted	

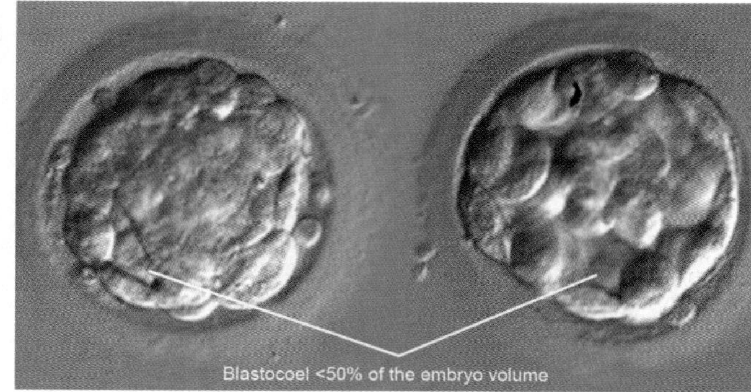

Fig. 11: Early blastocyst with fluid-filled cavity occupying less than 50% of the volume of the embryo.

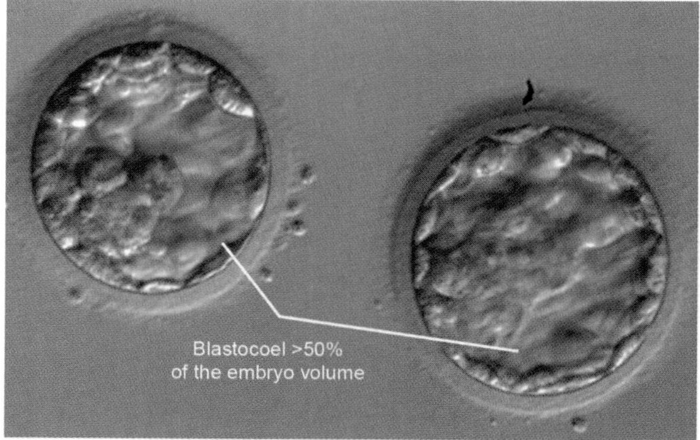

Fig. 12: Cavitating blastocyst (left) and full blastocyst (right) and with fluid-filled cavity occupying more than 50% of the total volume of the embryo.

Depending on the degree of expansion and hatching status, there has been described different system for blastocysts grading but perhaps the most complete is the system presented by Hardarson et al. in 2012,[27] as it is a compilation between the Istanbul consensus document[1] and the system described by Gardner and Schoolcraft in 1999.[28] According to this system blastocyst can be classified as:

- Grade I (early blastocyst): It is the early stage of the blastocyst formation on D5 with a cavity occupying less than 50% of the volume of the embryo (Fig. 11)
- Grade II (cavitating blastocyst): The next stage of blastulation in which the cavity occupies half or more than half of the total volume of the embryo (Fig. 12)
- Grade III (full blastocyst): These are those blastocysts in which the blastocoel cavity completely fills the embryo (Fig. 12)
- Grade IV (expanded blastocyst): It is the advanced stage of the blastocyst in which the blastocoel cavity now is greater than the original volume of the embryo and it is characterized by zona thinning (Fig. 13)
- Grade V (hatching blastocyst): The blastocoel cavity is greater than the original volume of the embryo and the TE is herniating through a natural breach in the ZP (Fig. 14)
- Grade VI (hatched blastocyst): These are those in which the blastocyst has completely escaped from a natural breach in the ZP (Fig. 15).

2. *Inner cell mass*: Cells forming the ICM are compacted and oval in shape and its size varies between 1,900 μm^2 and 3,800 μm^2. ICM can range from tightly packed cells to loosely bound cells and thus are scored accordingly. They can be graded from A–D or 3 to 1, according to different grading systems, but basically the best ICM category (A or 1) contains many cells that are tightly packed together, the middle ICM category (B or 2) is composed of several cells that are loosely grouped and the worst category (C or 3) describes an ICM that

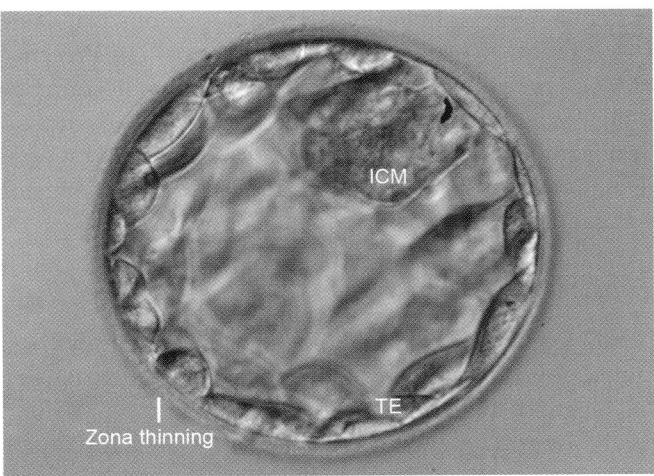

Fig. 13: Expanded blastocyst with well-compacted inner cell mass (ICM) and a cohesive trophectoderm.

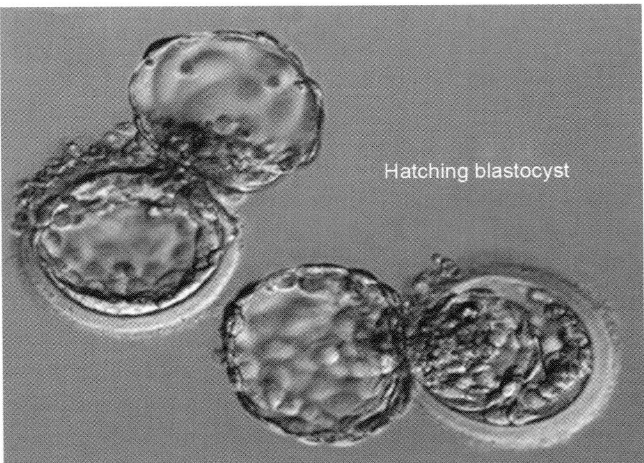

Fig. 14: Hatching blastocyst at 117 hours postinsemination.

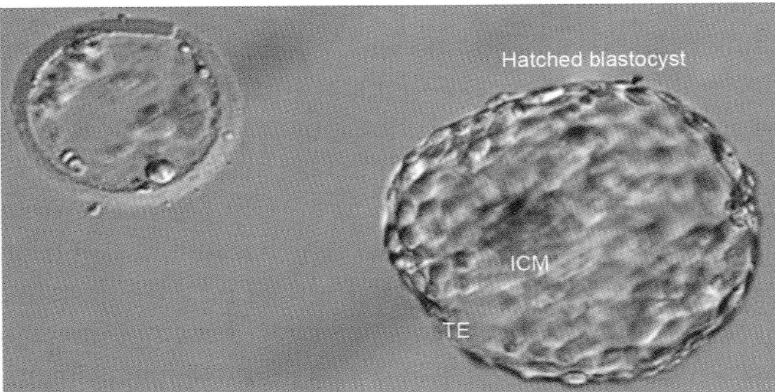

Fig. 15: Hatched blastocyst on day 6 of embryo culture. (ICM: inner cell mass; TE: trophectoderm).

contains very few cells that are loosely bound; category D would include those ICM that are degenerated or missing.[27]

3. *Trophectoderm:* Trophectoderm is a single layer of cohesive cells forming the wall of the blastocyst cavity and it is scored on the basis of number and the cohesiveness of the cells. It plays an important role in the adhesion and invasion of the endometrium enabling the embryo to implant. Similar to ICM, TE are scored by their number and cohesiveness from A–D or 3 to 1. The best TE category (A or 1) contains many cells that form a cohesive epithelium, the middle TE category (B or 2) is composed of a few cells forming a loose epithelium and the worst category (C or 3) describes a TE that contains very few, and large cells that struggle to form a cohesive epithelium; category D would include those TE that are degenerated.[27]

TIME-LAPSE MONITORING

Time-lapse monitoring (TLM) has made it easier for the embryologists to assess the embryo quality and development in real time instead of standardized time points, which only gives us a snapshot of the dynamic process. This enables us to evaluate abnormalities that may appear or disappear outside the set time range. Hence, continuous monitoring provides a complete picture of the embryo's developmental kinetics.

There are various TLM systems currently available: for instance, Embryo-Scope (FertiliTech) is an incubator with a built-in camera, whereas Primo Vision (Vitrolife) are small cameras that can be placed inside a regular incubator like Heracell. However in all these models, images are captured without removing the embryos from the incubator, thereby restricting exposure of embryos to suboptimal conditions. In addition, more detailed information on the timing of cell divisions, intervals between cell cycles and other important events including multinucleation, symmetry of blastomeres and dynamic PNs patterns can be annotated for analysis.

The aim of this technology is to maximize the chance of selecting the most viable embryo having a higher implantation potential based on morphokinetic parameters, thereby, encouraging elective single embryo transfer (eSET) and minimizing the risk of multiple pregnancies.

Numerous studies have demonstrated the predictive value of time-lapse system.[29-31] Moreover, studies have developed selection criteria and algorithms based on morphokinetic exclusion criteria to exclude morphologically normal embryos displaying aberrant cleavage patterns thus improving the PR and IR.[32]

EMBRYO TRANSFER

Embryo transfer (ET) is the final and one of the most critical procedures determining the success of an IVF cycle. Although tremendous progress has been made in the field of

Box 2: Factors contributing to a successful embryo transfer.

- Anatomical and physiological factors:
  - Uterine contractions
  - Anatomy of cervix and uterus
  - Uterine fluid
  - Position of the uterus
- Technical factors:
  - Catheter insertion and placement
  - Catheter withdrawal
  - Use of ultrasound guidance
  - Volume of transfer media transferred
  - Air or liquid combination
  - Viscosity of transferred media
- Catheter:
  - Type
  - Tip shape
  - Diameter
- Embryo selection:
  - Grading embryos

assisted reproduction, the IR has been maintained relatively low.[33] Multiple factors, such as poor embryo quality, compromised uterine receptivity and the ET technique itself has been documented to be responsible for the low IRs.[34]

Focusing on the ET technique, until recent years, ET was considered as a nondecisive factor as compared to the other procedures involved in IVF. However, numerous studies have highlighted the importance of a smooth ET to maximize the PRs.[35] ET technique can be divided into several components and we need to evaluate these components individually to optimize the technique and improve the success rates.

Various factors such as ultrasound guidance, choice of catheter, bacterial contamination of catheter, prolonged duration of ET, air bubble in the catheter, volume of media transferred, ease of the procedure and mock ET have an impact on the overall outcome (Box 2).

The ultimate aim of a successful ET is to deposit the embryos to a location in the uterus where chances of implantation increase. Disrupting the endometrium with the catheter, uterine contractions, damaging the embryo during the process of transfer or deposition of embryos in suboptimal locations are likely to cause a transfer failure.

Ease of Embryo Transfer

Numerous studies in literature have reported that difficult transfers often result in a lower PR and IR as compared to easy transfers, thereby correlating pregnancy outcomes with the overall ease of ET.[36] Despite its subjectivity, ease of transfer is considered an important determinant in successful implantation. In general, transfers that are more time consuming because of discomfort, require a stiffer catheter or involve extra manipulations like using a tenaculum are described as difficult transfers. Presence of blood on the catheter after ET is also an indication of a difficult transfer, increasing the chances of retained embryos and significantly lowering the IR.[37] Additionally, several techniques like ultrasound guidance, trial transfers or using soft catheters during ET can enable easy transfers.

Trial or Mock Transfer

A mock transfer can be done either before ovarian stimulation or just before the ET. During the mock transfer, full length of the uterine cavity and the cervix is measured using a catheter. All findings are recorded for future reference and these notes enable clinicians to take further precautions during the actual ET.

There are studies correlating mock transfers with better PR and IR in comparison to no trial transfers.[38] Moreover, mock transfers have shown to decrease chances of difficult transfers during the actual ET.

Ultrasound Guidance or Clinical Touch

To facilitate easy insertion of catheter and to ensure the embryos are deposited in the optimal location, ultrasound-guided ET is of paramount importance. Sonographic guidance can help avoid touching the uterine fundus and ensure the catheter is directed properly. In clinical conditions like the presence of fibroids in the uterus or in a severely flexed uterus, ultrasound guidance can be very helpful for the clinician. In addition, it is comforting for the patient to visualize the final step of their treatment. However, using an ultrasound during ET causes inconvenience of filling the patient's bladder, is more time consuming and will require another operator. Some investigators have suggested performing transfers by clinical touch wherein clinicians move the catheter to visualize its location. In this method, patients discomfort is used to assess fundal contact.[39] Discomfort is often indicative of uterine contraction, which results in expulsion of embryos, consequently lowering the PR.[40] An alternative approach suggested was to transfer the embryos at a fixed distance from the external os (approximately 6 cm), however, this will vary according to the size of the uterus and the cervical length.[39]

Encouraging results from a 2010 Cochrane review suggests using ultrasound over clinical touch to improve clinical PR.[41] Several other meta-analyses have also supported this conclusion.[42,43] Some studies have also reported a decrease in the incidence of ectopic pregnancy using ultrasound guidance.[44,45]

Patient Preparation

Subclinical infection is one of the potential reasons of implantation failure. Positive culture from catheter tips and cervix has been associated with lower clinical PR.[46] To avoid this, it has been recommended to clean the vagina and cervix with saline. Cervical mucus is also known to plug the catheter tip thereby interfering with the ET. Embryos tend to adhere to mucus and thus get displaced when the catheter is withdrawn.

Types of Catheter

Several types of catheters are commercially available for ET. An ideal catheter should be malleable so that it can be advanced in the uterine cavity along its contour. Furthermore, catheters should be soft to avoid causing any kind of trauma to the endometrium or cervix. Although in difficult transfers, hard catheters may facilitate placement, they are associated with trauma, more bleeding and uterine contractions. The outer sheath of soft catheters can also be bent to align the catheter and the uterine axis.

With extensive use of ultrasound-guided ET, numerous echogenic catheters are commercially available now which enables us to visualize the entire catheter or only the tip on ultrasound. Studies have demonstrated higher PR where soft catheters such as Cook, Frydman (Laboratoire CCD, France) and Wallace (Wallace Ltd., Colchester, England) were used in comparison to firm catheters like TDT (metal obturator), Tefcat (Cook Ob-Gyn, Spencer, IN, USA) and Tom Cat (Sherwood Medical, St. Louis, MO, USA).[47,48]

Embryo Loading

Among the aforementioned factors, less attention has been paid to embryo loading (EL). Different combinations of air and fluid volumes in the catheter are being used across different IVF centers. However, two catheter loading methods (air-fluid and fluid-only) have shown to improve the overall efficacy of ET (Figs. 16A and B).

General agreement in literature suggests improved clinical outcome by introducing air brackets around the embryo in the transfer media. Air column prevents premature expulsion of the embryo before transfer and also prevents embryo adhesion to the catheter during injection.[49] Furthermore, the air bubble is used as a marker to determine the embryo position in the uterus during ultrasound-guided ET.[50] On the contrary, studies supporting the fluid-only method postulate air as a nonphysiological factor having detrimental effect on the embryos, consequently affecting the IR.[51] Randomized controlled trials (RCTs) have reported no significant difference in the two loading techniques.[52]

Ideally, 20 μL of media surrounds the embryo in the catheter. Insufficient media (<10 μL) may interfere with embryo expulsion consequently affecting the IR.[53]

Embryos are vulnerable to environmental light, temperature or other agents in catheter and thus it is advised to decrease the time interval from loading the ET catheter to embryo deposition.[54]

Embryo Deposition

Randomized controlled trials have documented a higher PR when catheter tip was placed 15–20 mm from the fundus as compared to the traditional 10 mm. On the contrary, some investigators stress to take into account the length of the cavity (Table 6).[55] Despite the literature, the gold standard in practice is transferring embryos in the mid to lower midportion of the uterus. It is advisable to inject the embryos gently to avoid formation of bubbles and releasing excess media. However there is insufficient data to correlate the speed of injection with the PR.[56]

After injection, it is advisable to maintain the pressure on the plunger of the syringe to avoid retaining the embryos.[57] To minimize the negative pressure of the plunger, the catheter should be retracted slowly[58] and it is recommended to remove the outer sheath and the catheter simultaneously

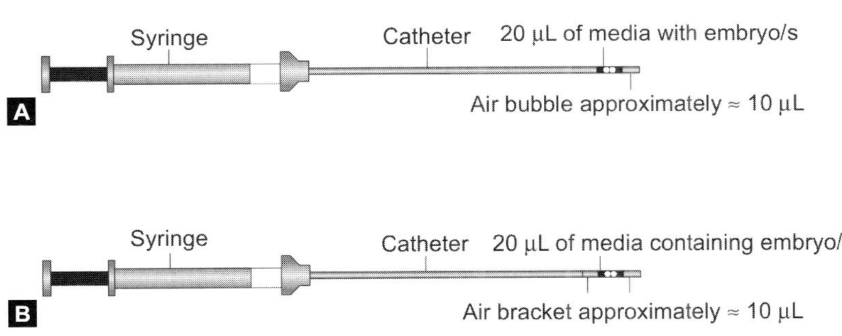

Figs. 16A and B: Embryo loading by (A) Fluid-only method; and (B) Air-fluid method.

Table 6: Distance between the catheter tip and the fundus and its impact on the pregnancy rate and implantation rate.

Pregnancy outcome	*Catheter tip (10 mm)*	*Catheter tip (15 mm)*	*Catheter tip (20 mm)*
Pregnancy rate	39.3%	49.2%	60%
Implantation rate	20.6%	31.3%	33.3%

to prevent the plunger effect. Studies show no significant increase in PR when catheters were removed after an interval as compared to immediate withdrawal.

Postembryo Transfer

After ET, the catheter should be flushed and inspected for retained embryos by the embryologist. Any retained embryo should be loaded again for transfer. There is insufficient data to support the effect of reloading and transferring the retained embryo on the pregnancy outcome.[59] Prolonged bed rest (24 h) or brief bed rest (5–30 min) have shown no benefit over immediate ambulation.[56]

LIMITING THE NUMBER OF EMBRYOS TO TRANSFER

The mechanisms underlying the implantation phenomenon are unknown and after ET, the control of the transferred embryos will be lost and we cannot distinguish which embryos reach the endometrial cavity and whether all of them have the same chance of implantation. That assumption has lead during several years to transfer of two, three or even more embryos to increase the PRs.

Nevertheless, transferring two or three embryos increases the incidence of multiple gestations. The incidence of multiple gestations after IVF in United States has been relatively high (34%) as compared to Europe (24.5%). It is well established that high-order multiple pregnancy (HOMP) leads to increase risk of low-birth weight (<2,500 g), preterm delivery (<37 weeks, gestation),[60] increased risk of neonatal morbidity and mortality, subsequently leading to long-term learning and developmental disabilities in infants.[61] Additionally, mothers are at a higher risk for pregnancy associated diabetes and hypertensive disorders, preeclampsia and postpartum hemorrhage.[62] The economic burden of multiple gestation further adds to the overall cost of the treatment.[63]

Although, multifetal reduction can be used to reduce the incidence of HOMP, the risk of pregnancy loss after fetal reduction is relatively high ranging between 4.5% and 15.4%. Moreover, the psychological, financial, ethical and religious factors can further make the whole process very stressful. To reduce the frequency of multiple gestations, there is a need to reduce the number of embryos being transferred by a better selection prior to the transfer.

Single Embryo Transfer versus Double Embryo Transfer

Several RCT have provided threshold values for the number of embryos transferred to achieve acceptable PRs and live birth rates. The most effective method to reduce occurrence of multiple pregnancy is to limit the number of embryos transferred.[64] However, it is difficult to generalize these prediction models and translate them into guidelines for every couple. Clinics that have shifted to double ET (DET) from high-order ET (three or more embryos) showed no difference in the PRs. However, a shift to single ET (SET) from DET can lower pregnancy and live birth rates.

In order to develop an effective ET policy that minimizes occurrence of multiple gestations, while maintaining the overall PRs and live birth rates, it is crucial for each IVF clinic to evaluate their own data. To determine the ideal number of embryos to be transferred, it is essential to customize the treatment according to the maternal age, the quality of embryos and the number of cycles performed for the patient.

In general, consideration should be taken to carefully select patients for eSET. Independent of age, and good prognosis patients, additional indications are:

- Morphologically assessed good quality embryos
- First IVF cycle
- Surplus embryos to necessitate cryopreservation
- Patients with successful previous IVF cycle.

There is good evidence in literature to support the following recommendations determining the number of embryos to be transferred:[65]

- Women aged less than 35 years of age with good prognosis should be offered eSET
- There are publications that defend the approach of combining eSET with a frozen ET (FET) to increase the cumulative live birth rates. The PR in such patients is equivalent to PR post-DET in young patients.[66,67] This is essential to minimize the chances of stimulating the patient again as surplus high quality embryos can be cryopreserved for subsequent attempts.
- Similarly, eSET should be strongly recommended in donor egg cycles, when the donor is less than 35 years of age.
- In women aged between 35 years and 37 years, not more than three embryos should be transferred in a fresh ET cycle. However, in patients with good prognosis

and having good quality embryos, no more than two cleavage embryos or blastocysts should be considered for transfer in the first or second cycle.

- In women aged between 38 years and 40 years, no more than three embryos should be transferred. Nevertheless, in case of extended culture only two blastocysts should be considered for transfer.
- In women aged more than 40 years, no more than three embryos or blastocysts should be transferred. There is insufficient data to recommend the number of embryos to be transferred in women aged more than 43 years.
- For FET, the number of good quality thawed embryos to be transferred should be similar in each of the above mentioned groups.

Anyway, couples should always be adequately counseled regarding chances of becoming pregnant in their particular situation and the risks involved in multifetal gestation.

Cleavage Stage Embryos versus Blastocyst Transfer

Culturing embryos to blastocyst stage is another method to promote singleton gestation. Culturing embryos till D5 has inherent advantages in comparison to D3 embryos, in terms of better synchronization between the developing endometrium and the embryo, thereby improving the overall PRs.[68] Additionally, a blastocyst transfer ensures selection of only competent embryos that have undergone the genomic activation and thus have better developmental capability.[69] Studies in literature show that selecting embryos at the blastocyst stage have a lower risk of aneuploidies, thereby improving the implantation potential considerably.[70] RCTs have reported significant increase in the IR when embryos were transferred on D5 as compared to D3 of embryo culture.[70-73]

A significant increase in the live birth rates was also reported in a meta-analysis after blastocyst transfer.[74] Thus, transferring embryos on D5 may prove to be beneficial in selecting the most viable embryos from within a cohort. Consequently, transferring fewer blastocysts than cleavage stage embryos should be taken into consideration, especially in young patients with good prognosis.

A number of studies have demonstrated that the blastulation rate in patients with severe male infertility is significantly low. This can be attributed to the fact that paternal genes in the embryo are expressed from day 3 of embryo culture. Thus, recommending a blastocyst transfer in such clinical cases.[75]

Furthermore, extended culture plays an important role in patients with recurrent implantation failure. General agreement in literature suggests culturing embryos until D5 in patients with multiple failures to improve the IR, which in turn influences the live birth rates as well.[76,77]

Another advantage of blastocyst transfer is seen in patients who have to undergo preimplantation genetic diagnosis (PGD). In addition to the natural selection of potentially competent embryos, blastocyst stage biopsy enables availability of more genetic material, thereby preventing diagnostic errors.[78]

On the other side is fair mentioning that extended culture is associated with increased incidence of cycle cancellation, wherein no embryos are available for transfer due to embryo arrest at the cleavage stage.[79] Consequently, this affects the patient both financially as well as psychologically. To overcome this situation, embryos should be cultured till D5 only when good quality embryos are available on D3 of embryo culture. This will prevent the risk of not having any embryos for transfer on D5. In addition to this, increased cost and higher risk of monozygotic twinning are few more potential disadvantages of blastocyst transfer.[80]

CONCLUSION

In vitro fertilization is a multifaceted treatment comprising various factors, each playing its role to achieve the desired endpoint of high live birth rates. Embryo selection and transfer is a crucial part of determining the success of an assisted reproductive technology (ART) cycle. One of the major concerns of ART is the occurrence of multiple gestations, which imposes considerable threat to both the maternal and fetal health. In order to minimize these risks, there is a need to limit the number of embryos transferred. Thus, it is essential to improve the current techniques of embryo selection by developing a more uniform and transferable grading system to assure selection of embryos with a higher implantation potential. In addition, optimizing the ET protocols would further help to contribute to clinical success.

REFERENCES

1. Alpha Scientists in Reproductive Medicine and ESHRE Special Interest Group of Embryology. The Istanbul consensus workshop on embryo assessment: proceedings of an expert meeting. Hum Reprod. 2011;26(6):1270-83.
2. Zollner U, Zollner KP, Hartl G, et al. The use of a detailed zygote score after IVF/ ICSI to obtain good quality blastocysts: the German experience. Hum Reprod. 2002;17(5):1327-33.
3. Balaban B, Urman B. Effect of oocyte morphology on embryo development and implantation. Reprod Biomed Online. 2006;12(5):608-15.
4. Tesarik J, Greco E. The probability of abnormal preimplantation development can be predicted by a single static

72. Margreiter M, Weghofer A, Kogosowski A, et al. A prospective randomized multicenter study to evaluate the best day for embryo transfer: does the outcome justify prolonged embryo culture? J Assist Reprod Genet. 2003;20(2):91-4.
73. Levron J, Shulman A, Bider D, et al. A prospective randomized study comparing day 3 with blastocyst-stage embryo transfer. Fertil Steril. 2002;77(6):1300-1.
74. Glujovsky D, Farquhar C, Quinteiro Retamar AM, et al. Cleavage stage versus blastocyst stage embryo transfer in assisted reproductive technology. Cochrane Database Syst Rev. 2016;(6):CD002118.
75. Shoukir Y, Chardonnens D, Campana A, et al. Blastocyst development from supernumerary embryos after intracytoplasmic sperm injection: a paternal influence? Hum Reprod. 1998;13(6):1632-7.
76. Blake DA, Farquhar C, Johnson N, et al. Cleavage stage versus blastocyst stage embryo transfer in assisted conception. Cochrane Database Syst Rev. 2007; (4):CD002118.
77. Guerif F, Bidault R, Gasnier O, et al. Efficacy of blastocyst transfer after implantation failure. Reprod Biomed Online. 2004;9(6):630-6.
78. Kahraman S, Beyazyürek C, Tac HA, et al. Recent advances in preimplantation genetic diagnosis. Adv Genom Genet. 2015;5(1):189-203.
79. Cutting R, Morroll D, Roberts SA, et al. Elective single embryo transfer: guidelines for practice British Fertility Society and Association of Clinical Embryologists. Hum Fertil (Camb). 2008;11(3):131-46.
80. Peramo B, Ricciarelli E, Cuadros-Fernández JM, et al. Blastocyst transfer and monozygotic twinning. Fertil Steril. 1999;72:1116-7.

CHAPTER

62

Oocyte and Embryo Vitrification

Ana Cobo, Aila Coello

INTRODUCTION

Vitrification is a cryopreservation procedure by which an aqueous solution is solidified into a glassy phase at low temperatures. This process is facilitated by applying high cooling rates and increasing viscosity using high concentration of cryoprotectants (CPAs).[1] These agents either permeate the cell membrane or create an osmotic gradient allowing reduced water content and, as a result, avoiding ice crystal formation. However, CPAs can be toxic at high concentration; thereby protocols have been modified in order to minimize damage. In this way, by significantly reducing the volume of the sample, the cooling rate is increased and the concentration of CPAs can be reduced while maintaining successful vitrification.

The essential role of cryopreservation in assisted reproductive technology (ART) has become obvious since the commencement of the infertility treatment, becoming a more flexible and efficient practice. Semen and embryo cryopreservation has been a successful strategy, routinely applied in in vitro fertilization (IVF) procedure for a long time. However, in spite of numerous studies conducted over the last 20 years, the reliability of oocyte cryopreservation is just being confirmed currently, thanks to vitrification.

METHODOLOGY: MEDIA AND DEVICES

The methodology used for oocyte and embryo vitrification may differ significantly between laboratories especially when different devices and solutions are used. Since the first vitrification solution was developed,[2] various CPAs have been proposed to be effective. Nowadays, a mixture of penetrating CPAs, such as ethylene glycol (EG) and dimethyl sulfoxide (DMSO) in combination with a nonpenetrating CPA, such as sucrose or trehalose, is the approach most commonly used.[3]

The basic procedure is simple and quick. Oocytes or embryos are exposed to a hypertonic solution composed of penetrating CPAs. At this point, water is removed from the cells to adjust osmolarity while CPAs begin to flow into them. The degree of permeability depends on the stage of embryo development and the type of CPA.[4] Then, oocytes or embryos are exposed briefly to a more concentrated solution composed of both penetrating and nonpenetrating CPAs which cause the proper cell dehydration. After this step, they are placed into a suitable container designed for vitrification and immediately submerged into liquid nitrogen (LN). The premise in the vitrification approach has been that the higher the cooling rate, the greater the likelihood that true vitrification can be achieved. However, high warming rate is also required as demonstrated recently.[5]

The cooling rate achieved will depend on the device and the volume of solution. Consequently, a variety of devices have been developed to facilitate rapid cooling; most of them are known as "open systems" because samples come into direct contact with LN during vitrification. Devices hermetically sealed before vitrification are known as "closed systems", which prevent samples from coming into direct contact with LN during vitrification. Obviously, the thermal isolation of samples in this way slows the cooling rate. The key to overcome this shortcoming is to find the optimal balance between the speed of cooling and warming and the necessary concentration of CPA for each step of exposure in order to reach the vitrified state without inducing osmotic swelling stress.[6]

The main drawback of using open system devices is the possibility of cross-contamination through direct contact of the vitrification sample with nonsterile LN. Although there are no documented cases of cross-contamination in the history of ART cryotransfers, it is vital that efforts be made to increase the safety of our cryopreservation methods. Hence, the design of devices that are able to prevent the risks associated with direct contact with LN during storage, while maintaining the advantages of open systems during the vitrification process, would be highly advisable. The sterilization of LN, either by filtering or by ultraviolet irradiation,[7] is also a good alternative, as is the use of vapor storage tanks, which are known to be safer than traditional ones and have proven to be very efficient in terms of preserving sample viability.[8]

OOCYTE VITRIFICATION

Nowadays the challenge of cryopreserving, storing for a long time and successfully implanting the female gamete is feasible thanks to vitrification. In spite of its great value, oocyte cryostorage has not been a valid option until relatively recently, due to the unavailability of successful methodologies. The reasons behind the long period of failures in the attempt to cryopreserve oocytes are currently well identified. Among them, the size and shape of the female gamete are two significant reasons. The female gamete is the largest cell of the human body, with a great content of water, which involves a higher probability of ice formation during the cryopreservation process. Chilling injury, defined as the irreversible damage to the cytoskeleton[9] and cell membranes[10] following exposure of cells to low temperatures (from +15°C to –5°C) before the nucleation of ice, is other major factor responsible for cell death during cryopreservation.[11] The ice crystal formation within the cytoplasm must be avoided, at all cost, in order to guarantee the survival and integrity of the oocytes when they are later thawed. Vitrification efficiently avoids chilling injury by the direct passage from room temperatures to –196°C and efficiently avoids ice formation.[12] As a result, these days we count on several efficient approaches able to provide successful outcomes comparable to those achieved with fresh oocytes.

There is a large population that is currently benefiting from oocyte vitrification technique, as cancer patients who need an option for fertility preservation (FP) before undergoing the potential sterilizing treatment,[13] or women who wish to delay their motherhood due to a variety of reasons.[14,15] Oocyte cryostorage brings additional advantages to ART programs being helpful to solve different clinical situations as in low-responder patients,[16] unpredictable unavailability of semen sample collection from the male partner, risk of suffering ovarian hyperstimulation syndrome,[17] or some other cases in which the embryo transfer is not advisable.[18] Undoubtedly, the ovum donation programs have also been major beneficiaries of egg banking.[19]

Ovum Donation Programs

Oocyte cryostorage is very useful to overcome the most common drawbacks involved with ovum donation as currently applied, such as synchronization between donors and recipients, long waiting lists subject to the availability of a suitable donor and the most important, the absence of a quarantine period. In our center, we have developed a consistent software tool that after entering parameters characteristic of the woman and her partner (as phenotypic traits, blood group, etc.) gives us a list of available donors and number of oocytes at that time on the bank, thus simplifying the process donor-recipient matching.

The first live birth after vitrification was obtained from a donated oocyte using an open system device (OPS) in 1999.[20] Since then, numerous publications using different types of devices corroborate the effectiveness of the technique (Table 1).

Our group, in 2008, published a study whose objective was to assess the impact of vitrification using donated oocytes, in terms of survival and development potential

Table 1: Key publications related to donated vitrified oocytes.

	Year	*Device*	*Survival rate (%)*	*Pregnancy rate (%)*
Kuleshova et al.	1999	OPS	64.7	33.3
Lacena et al.	2006	Cryotop	89.2	56.5
Cobo et al.	2008	Cryotop	96.9	65.2
Chang et al.	2008	Cryotop	85.4	83.3
Sher G et al.	2008	Cryoloop	96.1	81.2
Nagy et al.	2008	Cryotop	89.0	75.0
Cao et al.	2009	Cryoleaf	91.8	–
Cobo et al.	2010	Cryotop	92.5	55.4
Noyes et al.	2010	Cryotip	87.0	63.0
Trokoudes et al.	2011	Cryotop	91.4	55.6
Garcia et al.	2011	Cryolock	89.4	61.8
Stoop et al.	2012	CBS high security	90.2	50.0
Papatheodorou et al.	2013	Vitrisafe	90.9	28.0
Sole et al.	2013	Cryotop	85.6	53.5
Figueira et al.	2014	Cryotop	77.1	37.7

when compared to fresh oocytes.[21] To do this, a cohort of oocytes from a single donor was randomly divided into two groups—(1) in the first one, the oocytes were vitrified and (2) in the second one, the remaining oocytes were kept in the incubator (control fresh oocytes). Within an hour after vitrification we proceeded to devitrification and after two additional hours proceeded to simultaneous insemination of the two types of eggs—(1) fresh and (2) vitrified. The cryotop method employed for oocyte vitrification was that previously described by Kuwayama.[22] The study included 30 donors and 30 recipients (509 oocytes; 231 vitrified oocytes and 219 fresh oocytes). After a survival rate of 96.9%, we found no differences in the rate of division on day 3 (77.6% vs. 84.6% in vitrified in fresh) or the morphological quality of embryos (80.8% vs. 80.5% of good quality embryos vitrified vs. fresh). Likewise, both the blastocyst rate (48.7% vs. 47.5%) and quality of embryos (81.1% vs. 70%) were similar comparing fresh and vitrified.

We want to make special mention of the randomized, prospective, triple-blind, controlled clinical trial which included the largest sample size published to date, aimed to validate oocyte vitrification technique as a fundamental tool in running the bank of these gametes intended for ovum donation programs.[19] The study included 600 donor or recipients (300 per each branch) and 3,039 vitrified versus 3,185 fresh oocytes. In this study, we demonstrated the noninferiority of vitrified oocytes regarding ongoing pregnancy rate by intention to treat [odds ratio (OR) = 0.921, 95% confidence interval (CI) 0.667-1.274]. The overall survival rate in this study was 92.5% and ongoing pregnancy rate by intention to treat was 43.7% in the case of patients who received vitrified oocytes compared to 41.7% obtained with fresh oocytes. This study definitively confirmed our previous observations about the nonalteration of vitrified oocytes potential to develop into embryos capable of generating competent ongoing pregnancies in a similar proportion to fresh oocytes.

Because of the great potential of vitrified oocytes, and similarly to what happens with fresh donations, after embryo transfer there are often surplus viable embryos, suitable to be vitrified for future transfers. In this case, we are talking about a double round of vitrification, first at oocyte stage and later at cleavage stage (day 3) or blastocyst stage. In a publication in 2013, we showed that the double vitrification has no effect on the delivery rate or live birth.[23] This study included 796 vitrified embryos generated from vitrified oocytes (n = 471 cycles) and 4,394 vitrified embryos generated from fresh oocytes (n = 2,629 cycles). The overall survival rate was 97.2% (95% CI 95.9–98.6) versus 95.7% (95% CI 94.9–96.4) for double vitrified versus once respectively (NS). The live birth rate per warming cycle was 33.8% versus 30.6% (NS). As showed, the OR of the delivery rate, the double vitrification had no effect on embryos regardless of whether they were in early stage development (day 3) or blastocyst stage (OR = 0.867, 95% CI 0.657–1.203).

We recently published an observational study in which our experience of 6 years with the egg banking program[24] was described. The analysis included 3,610 cycles of oocyte donation where 42,152 metaphase II (MII) were warmed with a survival rate of 92.6%. The impact of storage time on the survival rate and clinical outcome was calculated by establishing different time intervals from less than 6 months to over 5 years. In any case, the storage time did not affect survival or clinical outcomes. We believe that this is very reassuring information since success after long time storage guarantees the sustainability of the approach. The clinical, ongoing pregnancy and delivery rates were 55.0%, 45.3% and 37.6% respectively, thus confirming the consistency of the results as compared to our previous findings.[13,19] The likelihood of having surplus embryos available for additional cryotransfers was very high in this series due to the mean number of oocytes donated. The possibility of further cryotransfers increased cumulative outcomes, and thus maximized the yield of a single donation cycle, which is precisely what we show herein. The cumulative delivery rate per donation cycle increased to over 70% after three cryotransfers and rose to nearly 80% after five cryotransfers. These results render the donation cycle as highly efficient.

The Kaplan–Meier analysis observed in Figure 1 provides interesting information about the number of vitrified oocytes consumed by a recipient (in either one or more cycles of ovum donation) necessary for a newborn.

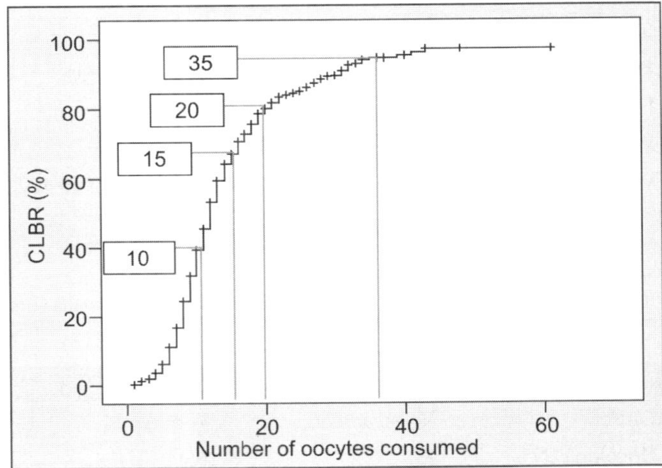

Figure 1: The Kaplan–Meier curve for the CDR of at least one baby, depending on the total number of oocytes consumed. (CDR: cumulative delivery rate; CLBR: cumulative live birth rate).

The analysis showed that the live-birth rate (LBR) increases exponentially, and the patient can achieve a baby with a probability of nearly 100% when about 3–4 cycles of egg donation (around 35–40 oocytes) are completed. This result confirms our previous findings while showing the excellent efficiency of egg banking.

Fertility Preservation

Vitrification of oocytes is currently being offered as an option for women who wish to preserve their gametes to allow them to have a chance to conceive in the future and to have their own genetic offspring.[25] The main beneficiaries of this strategy are cancer patients who must undergo chemotherapy or radiotherapy and patients with other diseases who require potentially gonadotoxic treatments.

The first reported case in Europe of a pregnancy after fertility preservation (FP) using vitrification of oocytes was from our group in a patient, whose ovarian cortex was cryopreserved first, and after grafting, four stimulation cycles were performed to accumulate and vitrify mature oocytes; a later IVF cycle successfully ended in a twin pregnancy. Since then, various studies have reported clinical out comes with cryopreserved oocytes for FP in cancer patients (Table 2).

Although FP may initially concern cancer patients, there are many other medical conditions that may compromise fertility, such as endometriosis or high-risk for early ovarian failure, where an intervention as safeguarding gametes for future use is required to uphold fertility potential. In addition, age-related decline of fertility is a very common condition in ART. Elective oocyte vitrification for nonmedical conditions is increasingly accepted as an option to postpone motherhood.[26] An updated data of FP for oncological and nononcological patients in IVI is showed in Table 3.

We have recently reported, in the largest series to date, our experience in FP in a population of women who electively decided to vitrify their gametes for future use. A

Table 2: Live birth reported after fertility preservation in cancer patients: slow freezing and vitrification of oocytes.

	Yang et al. 2007	*Porcu et al. 2008*	*Sanchez Serrano et al. 2009*	*Kim et al. 2011*	*Garcia-Velasco et al. 2013*	*Alvarez et al. 2014*	*Da Motta et al. 2014*
Type of malignancy	Hodgkin's lymphoma	Borderline ovarian tumor	Breast cancer	Chronic myeloid leukemia	Non-Hodgkin's lymphoma	Invasive ovarian carcinoma	Breast cancer
Cryopreservation technique	Slow freezing	Slow freezing	Combined OTC-SF + OV (Cryotop)	Vitrification (EMG)	Vitrification (Cryotop)	Vitrification (Cryotop)	Vitrification (Cryotip)
Age at FP	27	26	36	22	31	28	36
Number of cryopreserved oocytes	13	7	16	7	4	14	28
Storage time (years)	6	4	2	9	2	1	6
Pregnancy	Single*	Twin	Twin	Single	Single	Heterotopic	Triplet
Number of live births	1	2	2	1	1	1	1
Weeks of gestation	37	38	34	35 + 3 days	39	38	—
Weight of babies	3,062	2,100 and 2,400	1,650 and 1,830	2,410	3,440	2,651	2,970
Sex of baby	Male	Female	Male	Male	Male	Male	—

*Gestational carrier
(EMG: electron microscope grids; FP: fertility preservation; OTC-SF: ovarian tissue cryopreservation plus oocyte vitrification by cryotop).

Table 3: Clinical outcome of oncological and nononcological FP patients.

Cause	*No. of patients*	*No. of cycles*	*Clinical pregnancy (%)*	*Ongoing pregnancy (%)*	*LBR (%)*
Oncological	289	395	46.05	32.89	68
Nononcological	50	69	37.93	29.31	14
Total	339	464	44.75	32.32	82

(FP: fertility preservation; LBR: live-birth rate).

clear, and expected, effect of female age was observed in our data. Higher outcomes were achieved in women aged less than or equal to 35 years. In this group a larger number of oocytes were retrieved and finally vitrified, and the survival and clinical outcomes were equivalent to those achieved in our egg banking program for ovum donation, with the highest success rates in the youngest group of women (≤ 29 years). Otherwise, predictably fewer oocytes and worse outcomes were achieved as the age increased, resembling the results of the infertile population of similar age. There is a clear different probability of having a baby according to the number of oocytes consumed when the less than or equal to 35-year-old and more than 36-year-old groups are compared ($p < 0.05$). Obviously, the more oocytes the higher the probability, but the relationship is not linear, as shown by the curves, and is strongly related to a powerful confounder, i.e. the age of the patient (Figure 2). When we looked at our data, we observed a huge difference in cumulative live birth rate (CLBR) when using only five oocytes (15.4%) compared with using eight (40.8%), which means an 8.4% increase in CLBR per additional oocyte, if women were less than or equal to 35 years old. If they were more than 36 years old using the same number of oocytes, the increase in CLBR was considerably more modest (from CLBR of 5.1% with the use of five oocytes to 19.9% when eight oocytes were consumed, meaning an increase in CLBR of 4.9% per additional oocyte). With 15 oocytes, the CLBR continued to increase in the less than 35-year-old group, whereas with the same number of oocytes the plateau was already reached in the group of women aged more than 36 years, meaning that at this point the success is independent from the number of oocytes used up. In light of this, we suggest that at least eight to ten MII oocytes should be vitrified to obtain a reasonable success rate.

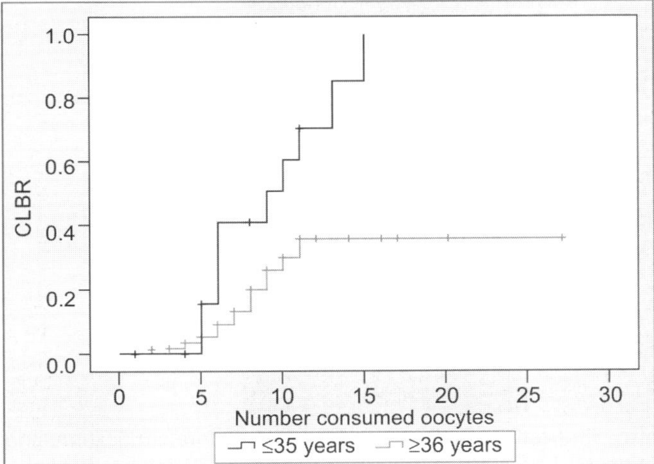

Figure 2: Kaplan–Meier plotting of the cumulative live birth rate (CLBR) of at least one baby, depending on the total number of consumed oocytes and categorized by age.

Low-responder Patients

A potential alternative to the management of low responder (LR) is to create a large stock of oocytes by accumulating vitrified MII oocytes over several stimulation cycles and inseminating them all at the same time. Theoretically, this could help to increase the chances of success by endowing patients with a "normoresponder-like" status. We reported, in 2010, a study aimed to assess the efficiency of this new strategy for managing LR that takes advantage of vitrification as a way of creating larger cohorts of oocytes.[16] This study included 242 LR patients (594 cycles) whose mature oocytes were accumulated by vitrification and inseminated simultaneously (LR-Accu-Vit) and 482 patients (588 cycles) undergoing IVF or embryo transfer with fresh oocytes in each stimulation cycle (LR-fresh). The embryo transfer cancelation per patient was significantly lower in the LR-Accu-Vit group (9.1%) than the LR-fresh group (34.0%). This result showed that this strategy is useful to avoid patients abandoning treatment due to negative results that impair their ability to cope with the situation. Live birth rate per patient was higher in the LR-Accu-Vit group (30.2%) than the LR-fresh group (22.4%) which confirmed the efficiency of this method for managing LR patients. The positive effects of this strategy are even more evident when cumulative outcome is considered, which endorses the treatment as a successful alternative for LR patients.

Other authors also reported the evaluation of this form of vitrification in the context of standard infertile patients. Rienzi et al.[27] conducted a prospective randomized sibling-oocyte study that included 120 fresh and 124 vitrified sibling oocytes from 40 infertile patients (mean age 35.5 ± 4.8 years). The survival rate was 97%, with a fertilization rate after intracytoplasmic sperm injection (ICSI) of 77% (95/124) per warmed oocyte and 79% (95/120) per warmed or inseminated oocyte. Moreover, the proportions of excellent quality embryos were the same in each group.

In another study, the cumulative outcome after the transfer of embryos derived from fresh and vitrified oocytes from a single ovarian stimulation cycle was calculated. The study included 182 ICSI cycles in which oocyte vitrification was also performed. The cumulative pregnancy rate (CPR) was calculated when after failing a fresh embryo transfer the patient underwent a second embryo transfer using embryos derived from the vitrified oocytes. Implantation rates in fresh and vitrification cycles were not significantly different for women less than or equal to 34 years.[28]

All these evidences suggest that vitrified oocytes are functionally similar to fresh oocytes in terms of fertilization, development and implantation potential.

EMBRYO VITRIFICATION

Vitrification was first applied in embryology with the use of mouse embryos almost 30 years ago,[2] with successful vitrification in 1991 by Kono et al.[29] The first human pregnancy and delivery of a baby as a result of blastocyst vitrification was published in 2001.[30] Since these landmark publications, vitrification of human embryos has played an important role in assisted reproduction treatment. It allows increasing cumulative outcomes since several pregnancies can be achieved after only one ovum retrieval. Furthermore, it has been suggested that controlled ovarian stimulation with exogenous gonadotropins adversely affects endometrial receptivity in ART cycles.[31,32] Thus, there is

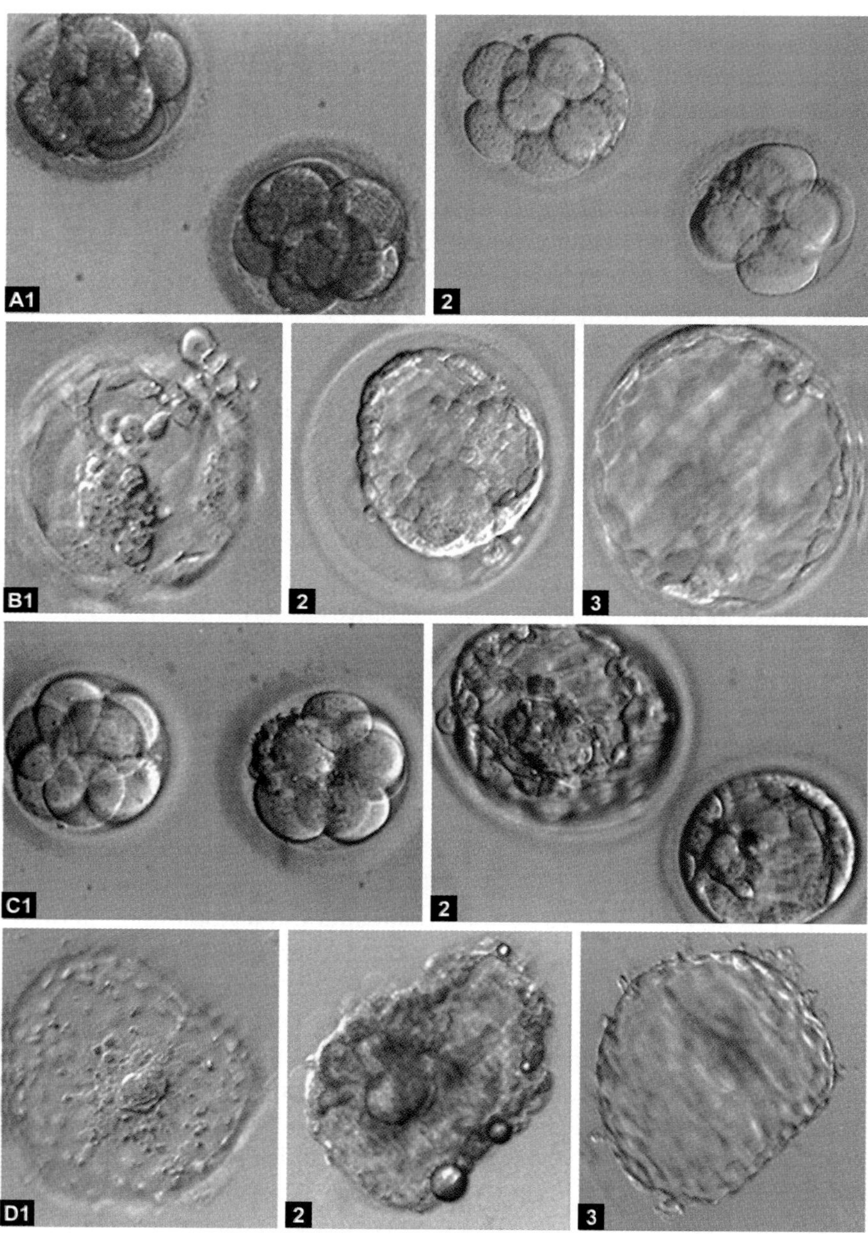

Figs. 3A to D: Cleavage stage embryos and blastocysts before and after vitrification. (A) Day 3 embryos [(1) Before vitrification, and (2) immediatly after warming]; (B) [Day 5 blastocyst [(1) Before vitrification, (2) 1 hour after vitrification (the re-expansion has not been completed), and (3) Fully re-expanded 3 hours after warming]; (C) [(1) Day 3 embryos before vitrification, and (2) Day 5 blastocyst developed from the day 3 warmed embryos]; and (D) Hatched day 6 blastocyst [(1) Before vitrification, (2) 1 hour after vitrification (the re-expansion has not been completed), and (3) Fully reexpanded blastocyst 5 hours after warming].

Table 4: Effect of blastocyst development on survival and live birth rates.

	Survival rate	*95% CI (%)*	*p value*	*LBR/warming cycle*	*95% CI (%)*	*p value*
Days 5 blastocysts (n = 1,079 warned embryos)						
Early blastocyst	432/458 (94.3%)	(91.7–96.7)	0.039	92/285 (32.3%)	(26.7–37.7)	0.21
Expanded blastocyst	537/549 (97.9%)	(96.7–99.0)[a]	–	155/349 (44.4%)	(39.2–49.6)[a]	–
Hatching-hatched blastocyst	64/72 (88.8%)	(81.5–96.6)	–	14/41 (34.1%)	(19.6–48.6)	–
Day 6 blastocyst (n = 952 warmed embryos)						
Early blastocyst	46/47 (97.9%)	(93.8–100)	0.107	6/35 (17.1%)	(4.6–29.6)[b]	0.201
Hatching-hatched blastocyst	328/335 (95.5%)	(95.8–98.8)	–	100/292 (34.2%)	(28.8–39.6)	–
Expanded blastocyst	556/570 (97.5%)	(93.0–96.9)	–	96/276 (34.7%)	(29.1–40.3)	–

[a,b]Different superscripts in the same column indicate statistical difference ($p < 0.05$) (CI: confidence interval; LBR: live birth rate).
Source: Cobo A, de los Santos MJ, Castellò D, et al. Outcomes of vitrified early cleavage-stage and blastocyst-stage embryos in a cryopreservation program: evaluation of 3,150 warming cycles. Fertil Steril. 2012;98(5):1138-46.

a trend toward cryopreservation of all viable embryos in a fresh IVF cycle followed by transfer of frozen thawed embryos in a subsequent cycle. This policy leads to place embryos in a more physiologic environment resulting in a better embryo-endometrium synchrony.

In addition, cryopreservation programs are crucial for patients at risk of ovarian hyperstimulation syndrome as well as to allow time for the testing of embryos for genetic anomalies before transfer.[33]

Currently, vitrification is being increasingly applied to both early cleavage and blastocyst stage embryos. In 2013, we reported our experience with the application of vitrification with Cryotop system to our embryo cryopreservation program.[34] Based on 3,150 warming cycles (6,019 embryos), the overall survival rate was 95%, with 93% (95% CI 90.1-95.3) of day 2 and 95% (95% CI 94.3-95.7) of day 3 embryos fully intact upon warming. Figures 1A to D show cleavage stage embryos and blastocysts before and after vitrification. Similarly to what happened to early stages, our overall blastocyst survival rate involving almost 2,000 blastocysts was considerably high (Table 4).

Other authors have published similar outcomes using the Cryotop system.[35-37] In the past, other devices have been used for blastocyst vitrification. For example, Balaban et al. reported approximately 95% survival (234 blastocysts warmed) with the use of the cryoloop, and a larger study of 1,129 vitrified blastocysts reported a 85.7% survival rate.[38] Similar outcomes were published by others involving 250-700 embryos.[30,39,40] Studies of the use of electron microscope (EM) grid, reporting data from 90-300 warmed blastocysts, have shown survival rates of approximately 50%.[41,42]

According to our data, expanded blastocysts on day 5 or day 6 achieved the highest survival rate. This finding contrasts with reports by other groups[43,44] suggesting that the likelihood of ice formation is higher in expanded blastocysts than in early blastocysts, in which the volume of the blastocoel cavity is much smaller. In fact, this is the rationale for provoking an artificial collapse of blastocysts before vitrification in some cases.[43,45,46] This is not a strategy we apply routinely, except in isolated cases of hatching blastocysts. It is possible that the high survival rate of our expanded blastocysts was due to the open system we use (Cryotop), because it ensures a very high cooling rate and, most importantly, an extremely high warming rate, which impedes the formation of ice (recrystallization) during warming.[5,47-52]

The delivery rate per warming cycle we obtained was 32.5% (95% CI 30.9-34.2). Overall implantation, clinical pregnancy, ongoing pregnancy, and LBRs per warming cycle were 35.5% (95% CI 33.5-38.5%), 41.7% (95% CI 39.9-43.4%), 32.6% (95% CI 31.0-34.2%), and 38.1% (95% CI 36.4-39.8%) respectively.

Other important aspect, it was the absence of variability in the before and after morphologic evaluation of early cleavage stages, thus confirming the safety of the cryopreservation method we employed.[53,54] These data confirmed that an efficient embryo cryopreservation program could be carried out with the help of the vitrification technique.[55]

REFERENCES

1. Yavin S, Arav A. Measurement of essential physical properties of vitrification solutions. Theriogenology. 2007;67(1):81-9.
2. Rall WF, Fahy GM. Ice-free cryopreservation of mouse embryos at -196 degrees C by vitrification. Nature. 1985;313(6003):573-5.
3. Coello A, Campos P, Remohi J, et al. A combination of hydroxypropyl cellulose and trehalose as supplementation

for vitrification of human oocytes: a retrospective cohort study. J Assist Reprod Genet. 2016;33(3):413-21.
4. Alpha Scientists In Reproductive Medicine. The Alpha consensus meeting on cryopreservation key performance indicators and benchmarks: proceedings of an expert meeting. Reprod Biomed Online. 2012;25(2):146-67.
5. Seki S, Mazur P. The dominance of warming rate over cooling rate in the survival of mouse oocytes subjected to a vitrification procedure. Cryobiology. 2009;59(1):75-82.
6. Papatheodorou A, Vanderzwalmen P, Panagiotidis Y, et al. Open versus closed oocyte vitrification system: a prospective randomized sibling-oocyte study. Reprod Biomed Online. 2013;26(6):595-602.
7. Parmegiani L, Cognigni GE, Filicori M. Efficacy of ultraviolet sterilization of liquid nitrogen. Reprod Biomed Online. 2011;22(5):501.
8. Cobo A, Romero JL, Pérez S, et al. Storage of human oocytes in the vapor phase of nitrogen. Fertil Steril. 2010;94(5):1903-7.
9. Pickering SJ, Braude PR, Johnson MH, et al. Transient cooling to room temperature can cause irreversible disruption of the meiotic spindle in the human oocyte. Fertil Steril. 1990;54(1):102-8.
10. Ghetler Y, Yavin S, Shalgi R, et al. The effect of chilling on membrane lipid phase transition in human oocytes and zygotes. Hum Reprod. 2005;20(12):3385-9.
11. Watson PF, Morris GJ. Cold shock injury in animal cells. Symp Soc Exp Biol. 1987;41:311-40.
12. Liebermann J, Dietl J, Vanderzwalmen P, et al. Recent developments in human oocyte, embryo and blastocyst vitrification: where are we now? Reprod Biomed Online. 2003;7(6):623-33.
13. Cobo A, Domingo J, Pérez S, et al. Vitrification: an effective new approach to oocyte banking and preserving fertility in cancer patients. Clin Transl Oncol. 2008;10(5):268-73.
14. Dondorp WJ, De Wert GM. Fertility preservation for healthy women: ethical aspects. Hum Reprod. 2009;24(8):1779-85.
15. Garcia-Velasco JA, Domingo J, Cobo A, et al. Five years' experience using oocyte vitrification to preserve fertility for medical and nonmedical indications. Fertil Steril. 2013;99(7):1994-9.
16. Cobo A, Garrido N, Crespo J, et al. Accumulation of oocytes: a new strategy for managing low-responder patients. Reprod Biomed Online. 2012;24(4):424-32.
17. Herrero L, Pareja S, Losada C, et al. Avoiding the use of human chorionic gonadotropin combined with oocyte vitrification and GnRH agonist triggering versus coasting: a new strategy to avoid ovarian hyperstimulation syndrome. Fertil Steril. 2011;95(3):1137-40.
18. Herrero L, Pareja S, Aragonés M, et al. Oocyte versus embryo vitrification for delayed embryo transfer: an observational study. Reprod Biomed Online. 2014;29(5):567-72.
19. Cobo A, Meseguer M, Remohi J, et al. Use of cryo-banked oocytes in an ovum donation programme: a prospective, randomized, controlled, clinical trial. Hum Reprod. 2010;25(9):2239-46.
20. Kuleshova L, Gianaroli L, Magli C, et al. Birth following vitrification of a small number of human oocytes: case report. Hum Reprod. 1999;14(12):3077-9.
21. Cobo A, Kuwayama M, Pérez S, et al. Comparison of concomitant outcome achieved with fresh and cryopreserved donor oocytes vitrified by the Cryotop method. Fertil Steril. 2008;89(6):1657-64.
22. Kuwayama M, Vajta G, Kato O, et al. Highly efficient vitrification method for cryopreservation of human oocytes. Reprod Biomed Online. 2005;11(3):300-8.
23. Cobo A, Castellò D, Vallejo B, et al. Outcome of cryotransfer of embryos developed from vitrified oocytes: double vitrification has no impact on delivery rates. Fertil Steril. 2013;99(6):1623-30.
24. Cobo A, Garrido N, Pellicer A, et al. Six years' experience in ovum donation using vitrified oocytes: report of cumulative outcomes, impact of storage time, and development of a predictive model for oocyte survival rate. Fertil Steril. 2015;104(6):1426-34.
25. Cobo A, Garcia-Velasco JA, Domingo J, et al. Is vitrification of oocytes useful for fertility preservation for age-related fertility decline and in cancer patients? Fertil Steril. 2013;99(6):1485-95.
26. Cobo A, Garcia-Velasco JA, Coello A, et al. Oocyte vitrification as an efficient option for elective fertility preservation. Fertil Steril. 2016;105(3):755-64.
27. Rienzi L, Romano S, Albricci L, et al. Embryo development of fresh 'versus' vitrified metaphase II oocytes after ICSI: a prospective randomized sibling-oocyte study. Hum Reprod. 2010;25(1):66-73.
28. Ubaldi F, Anniballo R, Romano S, et al. Cumulative ongoing pregnancy rate achieved with oocyte vitrification and cleavage stage transfer without embryo selection in a standard infertility program. Hum Reprod. 2010;25(5):1199-205.
29. Kono T, Kwon OY, Nakahara T. Development of vitrified mouse oocytes after in vitro fertilization. Cryobiology. 1991;28(1):50-4.
30. Mukaida T, Nakamura S, Tomiyama T, et al. Successful birth after transfer of vitrified human blastocysts with use of a cryoloop containerless technique. Fertil Steril. 2001;76(3):618-20.
31. Bourgain C, Devroey P. The endometrium in stimulated cycles for IVF. Hum Reprod Update. 2003;9(6):515-22.
32. Kolibianakis E, Bourgain C, Albano C, et al. Effect of ovarian stimulation with recombinant follicle-stimulating hormone, gonadotropin releasing hormone antagonists, and human chorionic gonadotropin on endometrial maturation on the day of oocyte pick-up. Fertil Steril. 2002;78(5):1025-9.
33. Roy TK, Bradley CK, Bowman MC, et al. Single-embryo transfer of vitrified-warmed blastocysts yields equivalent live-birth rates and improved neonatal outcomes compared with fresh transfers. Fertil Steril. 2014;101(5):1294-301.
34. Cobo A, de los Santos MJ, Castellò D, et al. Outcomes of vitrified early cleavage-stage and blastocyst-stage embryos in a cryopreservation program: evaluation of 3,150 warming cycles. Fertil Steril. 2012;98(5):1138-46.
35. Hiraoka K, Hiraoka K, Kinutani M, et al. Blastocoele collapse by micropipetting prior to vitrification gives excellent survival and pregnancy outcomes for human day 5 and 6 expanded blastocysts. Hum Reprod. 2004;19(12):2884-8.

36. Stehlik E, Stehlik J, Katayama KP, et al. Vitrification demonstrates significant improvement versus slow freezing of human blastocysts. Reprod Biomed Online. 2005;11(1): 53-7.
37. Kuwayama M, Vajta G, Ieda S, et al. Comparison of open and closed methods for vitrification of human embryos and the elimination of potential contamination. Reprod Biomed Online. 2005;11(5):608-14.
38. Takahashi K, Mukaida T, Goto T, et al. Perinatal outcome of blastocyst transfer with vitrification using cryoloop: a 4-year follow-up study. Fertil Steril. 2005;84(1):88-92.
39. Mukaida T, Nakamura S, Tomiyama T, et al. Vitrification of human blastocysts using cryoloops: clinical outcome of 223 cycles. Hum Reprod. 2003;18(2):384-91.
40. Huang CC, Lee TH, Chen SU, et al. Successful pregnancy following blastocyst cryopreservation using super-cooling ultra-rapid vitrification. Hum Reprod. 2005;20(1): 122-8.
41. Cho HJ, Son WY, Yoon SH, et al. An improved protocol for dilution of cryoprotectants from vitrified human blastocysts. Hum Reprod. 2002;17(9):2419-22.
42. Choi DH, Chung HM, Lim JM, et al. Pregnancy and delivery of healthy infants developed from vitrified blastocysts in an IVF-ET program. Fertil Steril. 2000; 74(4):838-9.
43. Vanderzwalmen P, Bertin G, Debauche Ch, et al. Births after vitrification at morula and blastocyst stages: effect of artificial reduction of the blastocoelic cavity before vitrification. Hum Reprod. 2002;17(3):744-51.
44. Van Landuyt L, Stoop D, Verheyen G, et al. Outcome of closed blastocyst vitrification in relation to blastocyst quality: evaluation of 759 warming cycles in a single-embryo transfer policy. Hum Reprod. 2011;26(3):527-34.
45. Lucena E, Bernal DP, Lucena C, et al. Successful ongoing pregnancies after vitrification of oocytes. Fertil Steril. 2006;85(1):108-11.
46. Chang CC, Shapiro DB, Bernal DP, et al. Two successful pregnancies obtained following oocyte vitrification and embryo re-vitrification. Reprod Biomed Online. 2008;16(3):346-9.
47. Sher G, Keskintepe L, Mukaida T, et al. Selective vitrification of euploid oocytes markedly improves survival, fertilization and pregnancy-generating potential. Reprod Biomed Online. 2008;17(4):524-9.
48. Nagy ZP, Chang CC, Shapiro DB, et al. The efficacy and safety of human oocyte vitrification. Semin Reprod Med. 2009;27(6):450-5.
49. Cao YX, Xing Q, Li L, et al. Comparison of survival and embryonic development in human oocytes cryopreserved by slow-freezing and vitrification. Fertil Steril. 2009;92(4):1306-11.
50. Noyes N, Knopman J, Labella P, et al. Oocyte cryopreservation outcomes including pre-cryopreservation and post-thaw meiotic spindle evaluation following slow cooling and vitrification of human oocytes. Fertil Steril. 2010;94(6): 2078-82.
51. Trokoudes KM, Pavlides C, Zhang X. Comparison outcome of fresh and vitrified donor oocytes in an egg-sharing donation program. Fertil Steril. 2011;95 (6):1996-2000.
52. Garcia JI, Noriega-Portella L, Noriega-Hoces L. Efficacy of oocyte vitrification combined with blastocyst stage transfer in an egg donation program. Hum Reprod. 2011;26(4):782-90.
53. Stoop D, De Munck N, Jansen E, et al. Clinical validation of a closed vitrification system in an oocyte-donation programme. Reprod Biomed Online. 2012;24 (2):180-5.
54. Solé M, Santaló J, Boada M, et al. How does vitrification affect oocyte viability in oocyte donation cycles? A prospective study to compare outcomes achieved with fresh versus vitrified sibling oocytes. Hum Reprod. 2013;28(8):2087-92.
55. Figueira Rde C, Setti AS, Braga DP, et al. The efficiency of a donor-recipient program using infertile donors' egg cryo-banking: a Brazilian reality. J Assist Reprod Genet. 2014;31(8):1053-7.

CHAPTER

63

Embryo Biopsy and Tubing

Rishina Bansal, Shridutt Gaitonde, Navin Desai

INTRODUCTION

Preimplantation genetic diagnosis (PGD) in humans was developed in late 1980s in the United Kingdom. Initially, PGD revolved around determination of gender as an indirect means of avoiding an X-linked disorder. In 1989 in London, Handyside and Scott reported the first unaffected child born following PGD performed for an X-linked disorder.[1,2]

It is an increasingly common adjunct to in vitro fertilization (IVF) and it is used to identify genetic defects in embryos created through IVF before pregnancy. To undergo a PGD cycle, the patients have to start an IVF cycle in order to retrieve oocytes that will be fertilized and result into zygotes; those zygotes will develop into embryos progressing across different stages until being transferred to the patient's uterus. It is during this procedure when the biopsy has to be done in order to obtain cells and analyze the chromosomal status. That will allow the embryologist to discriminate those embryos considered as candidates to be transferred into the patient.

The PGD along with the polymerase chain reaction (PCR) allow us to identify inheritable diseases in the embryos as this technique amplifies a fragment of deoxyribonucleic acid (DNA) and facilitates the screening to identify monogenic diseases. Therefore, we can distinguish between:

- *Preimplantation genetic diagnosis:* It refers specifically to when one or both genetic parents has a known genetic abnormality and testing is performed on an embryo to determine, if it also carries a genetic abnormality
- *Preimplantation genetic screening (PGS):* It refers to techniques where embryos from presumed chromosomally normal genetic parents are screened for aneuploidy.

Preimplantation genetic diagnosis and PGS are presently the only options available for avoiding a high-risk of having a child affected with a genetic disease prior to implantation. Preimplantation genetic testing provides an alternative to current postconception diagnostic procedures, which are frequently followed by the difficult decision of pregnancy termination, if results are unfavorable.

In order to perform preimplantation genetic testing, it can be done at different stages of the embryo development, from the first polar body (PB1) of the oocyte, in which it is still not fertilized, the second PB (PB2), that appears after the fertilization, one or two blastomeres on day 3 of development to several cells from the blastocyst's trophectoderm (TE). The technique will imply in any of the cases the breaching of the zona pellucida (ZP) to create an artificial orifice and the extraction of the sample [polar body (PB)/blastomere/TE] for further analysis. In this chapter it will be detailed the available techniques for each of those procedures.

BREACHING OF THE ZONA PELLUCIDA

The ZP of mammalian oocytes and embryos is an acellular matrix composed of sulfated glycoproteins with different roles during fertilization and embryo development, and its main function is the protection of the embryo and the maintenance of its integrity.[3]

Sampling of genetic material from oocytes and embryos relies on creating a hole in the ZP large enough for polar bodies (PBs) or blastomeres to be extruded, or TE cells to herniate out.[4] The hole size is critical, if too large several blastomeres can be dragged out with the one biopsied. If the hole is too small, stress on the blastomere may be excessive, leading to cell lysis.[5] The suggested opening diameter should be around 20–30 µm.[6]

Several methods can be used to rupture the ZP:

- Mechanical
- Chemical
- Laser
- Piezo-mediated devices.

Mechanical

This approach is simple and efficient but requires correct positioning of oocyte or embryo. Embryos denuded of corona cells are micromanipulated in microdrops of 4-(2-hydroxyethyl)-1-piperazineethanesulfonic acid (HEPES) buffered medium under paraffin oil. The procedure is performed at 37°C, under an inverted microscope. The embryo is held with a holding pipette, and the ZP is tangentially pierced with a microneedle from the 1- to the 11-o'clock position. The embryo is released from the holding pipette, and the part of the ZP between the two points is rubbed against the holding pipette until this area is completely dislodged from the rest of the oocyte or embryo.[3,7] Groups performing polar body biopsy (PBB) favor this method.[4]

Chemical

The human ZP can be dissolved using a controlled, directed stream of a low pH solution as the acid Tyrode's (AT) solution (pH of AT = 2.2–2.6).[3] One advantage of AT drilling compared with the mechanical rupture is the possibility of increasing the size of the hole in the ZP.

In order to perform chemical zona drilling, the embryo is held with a holding pipette in such a way that the micropipette containing AT (internal diameter 3–5 mm) and located at the 3-o'clock position faces a large perivitelline space to avoid damaging the blastomeres. The acid solution is gently delivered with the help of a microinjector over a small area of the ZP, with the tip of the pipette positioned very close to the zona and gently scratching it. The hole should be between 15–20 µm, never more than 30 µm. As soon as a hole in the ZP is created, suction is applied to avoid excess AT entering the perivitelline space. If the inner region of the ZP is difficult to breach, creation of the hole can be facilitated by pushing the AT micropipette against the ZP. It is necessary to rinse the embryo several times in fresh culture medium immediately after the assisted hatching (AH) and biopsy procedure, prior to returning it back into the culture dish, to avoid detrimental effects of the acid solution on the blastomeres.

This was the preferred choice for cleavage stage biopsy.[8,9] It has advantages over mechanical zona dissection in terms of speed of safety. However, the safety and the ideal size of the hole is difficult to standardize and depends on the amount of acid used and skill of the personnel (Figs 1A to D).[4]

Laser

The application of a laser on the ZP for AH results in photoablation of the ZP. The drilling mechanism is explained by a thermal effect induced at the focal point by absorption of the laser energy by water and/or ZP macromolecules, leading to thermolysis of the ZP. The effect on the ZP is greatly localized, and the holes obtained are cylindrical and precise.[3]

The preferred model of laser is the near-infrared (NIR) solid-state compact diode 1.48 mm laser. The advantage of using light as a cutting tool is that it removes the need for a double tool holder and either disposable or reusable cutting tools. It is extremely precise and, if used appropriately, provides consistent, reproducible, and rapid results.[10] Furthermore, the likelihood of introducing contamination or pH changes in the medium surrounding the embryo is greatly reduced as neither microtools nor reagents are required to dissect the zona.[11] The 1.48 mm diode laser is small but, at the appropriate pulse duration, can emit light at power levels sufficient to cause selective thermal disruption of the ZP glycoproteins and is not absorbed by water.[11] This noncontact laser can be inserted into the body of the microscope on which the manipulations take place or be integrated in a special objective and the beam delivered to the target through the dish.[12]

A culture dish with several 10 µL drops of HEPES buffered culture medium and overlaid with prewarmed mineral oil has to be prepared shortly before the procedure. Embryos selected for transfer are placed individually in separate drops, and the dish is placed on the heated

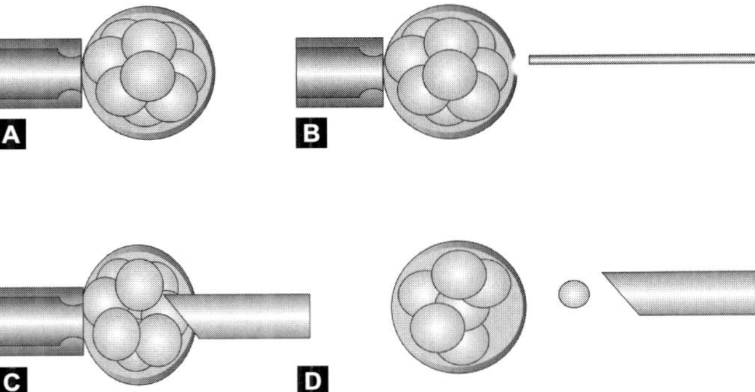

Figs. 1A to D: Schematic representation of zona drilling using acid Tyrode's.

Table 1: Cleavage stage embryo biopsy methods—benefits, limitations and critical factors to success.

Method	*Benefits*	*Limitations*	*Critical factors*
Mechanical	Less invasive to embryo Improved survival after freezing- thawing Inexpensive	Difficult to learn Operator dependent Time-consuming	Operator skill essential Appropriate tools needed
Chemical	Relatively inexpensive Widespread clinical experience	Operator dependent Difficult to limit aperture size Effect on cryopreservation Double tool holder optimal	Acidified Tyrode's pH sensitive control of acid Rinse acid from embryos
Laser	Rapid and reproducible Simple to use Software	Capital cost Not all systems portable Invisible thermal damage or stress	Laser alignment and calibration Pulse duration and number Distance between laser and zona pellucida (ZP)
Piezo	Precise movement Minimize damage to oocytes	Operator dependent Delicate technique Piezo pulse displaces Microinjection needle tip	Additional tools required Pressure to open zona operator skill essential

stage of the inverted microscope equipped with the laser technology. It is recommended to stabilize the embryo with a holding micropipette. An area between two blastomeres with a large perivitelline space has to be chosen for laser drilling. Routinely, a single opening of approximately 30 μm (about 10% of the ZP circumference) is created by dissecting the full thickness of the ZP.[3]

Piezo-mediated Devices

Piezo-actuated micromanipulation was developed by Yoshida and colleagues, and its application as a biological research tool.[13] These devices harness the piezoelectric effect to transmit a small crystal lattice distortion to the tip of a pipette, driving it forward in controlled and precise manner.[14] The embryo or oocyte is held in position using a holding pipette.[15] The injection pipette is advanced to contact the surface of the ZP. The piezo micromanipulator (PMM) is activated with foot switch as pipette is pushed through the zona. It introduces a small negative pressure within the microinjection pipette and apply piezo pulses (start with intensity = 3, frequency = 6) while gently pushing the microinjection pipette toward the holding pipette. The tip should rapidly pass through the zona, emerging into the perivitelline space. Stop pushing as soon as you see this. Failure to control the tip risks subjecting the plasma membrane to high-intensity piezo, resulting in rapid cell lysis. The piezo impact force is applied until the ZP is almost penetrated (Table 1).[13]

BIOPSY PROCEDURES

Theoretically, PGD can be accomplished at any developmental stage between the mature oocyte and blastocyst, but to date, only three discrete stages have been proposed: (1) PB, (2) cleavage stage, and (3) blastocyst.

Polar Body Biopsy

Polar bodies are by-products of meiotic division of the oocyte. PB1 is the by-product of the first meiotic division and contains the counterpart of the oocyte chromosomes, which are diploid at this stage. This is why it is an indirect approach to infer the genetic or chromosomal status of the oocyte without losing its reproductive capability.[16] As the information obtained through this PB1 refers only to the maternal inheritance, it is not possible to detect the chromosomal abnormalities that occur after fertilization. The PB2 is extruded after fertilization, so by extruding the extra 23 chromosome set the number of chromosomes in the oocyte is reduced by half.[17] This can be also biopsied and analyzed.

Polar body biopsy was first proposed in 1990s by Verlinsky and collaborators.[18] Since then, several groups have applied PBB to a variety of diagnostic applications like detection of single gene disorders, translocation analysis, human leukocyte antigen (HLA) typing and detection of X-linked disorders.[12] However, most cases of PB diagnosis are performed for aneuploidy screening, but PBs provide information only on the female part, which is critical in the case of certain monogenetic diseases. In a recessive disease, PB analysis will only distinguish whether the oocyte carries the normal or the affected allele but the state of the corresponding embryo will be determined by the paternal allele and can be normal, unaffected (carrier), or affected.[16] There is ongoing discussion on the need to biopsy and analyze both PBs. A recent study showed that in younger women, PB1 is more prone than PB2 to meiotic errors causing aneuploidies, whereas the opposite holds true in older women.[19,20]

Technical Aspects of Polar Body Biopsy

Recent investigations using polarization microscopy have shown that some oocytes presenting a PB1 may still be in telophase I owing to the presence of a connective spindle strand between the PB1 and the oocyte.[18] Such a spindle bridge is a remnant of the meiotic division and occurs during formation of PB1 as well as at the completion of the second meiotic division after extrusion of the PB2. The spindle bridge is present for only a limited time period, which is usually 1–2 hours after extrusion of the PB1 or PB2. In view of this, PBB should not be performed within too short time after their formation. As long as chromosomal material from the oocyte is still attached to these spindle fibers there is a risk of pulling this material out during biopsy, which may result in enucleating the oocyte.[16,17]

Chronology

- *Day 0:* Follicle retrieval, oocyte denudation and biopsy of the PB1 of the metaphase II (MII) oocytes after 2–4 hours. Perform the intracytoplasmic sperm injection (ICSI) 1–4 hours after the biopsy
- *Day 1:* Fertilization assessment after 17–20 hours and biopsy of the PB2 within 24 hours from the ICSI.

The removal of the PB1 and PB2 can be done at separate times (sequential approach) or at the same time (simultaneous approach). Simultaneous biopsy of the PB1 and PB2 requires only one manipulation and helps to reduce stress to the oocyte. It is best accomplished in a time window of 8–14 hours after fertilization. Too early biopsy bears the risk of spindle remnants in the PB2, and too late biopsy may result in a PB1 that already started disintegration or degeneration. The latter problem is especially important, if the analysis is based on fluorescence in situ hybridization (FISH), because it may contribute to diagnostic failures.[21,22] For simultaneous biopsy it can sometimes be difficult to distinguish PB1 and PB2 or to accurately separate PB1 and PB2 in case of fragmentation. Single-nucleotide polymorphism (SNP)-based analysis of heterozygosity could help to identify and distinguish them.[18] Otherwise, sequential biopsy may be preferred, if a fragmented PB1 is already present at the time of injection.

Steps to Follow

Zona opening to remove the PBs can be done by any one of the above mentioned techniques (mechanical, chemical, laser or piezo-mediated devices).

A 60 mm petri dish with three 50 μL drops of HEPES buffered culture medium to wash the oocytes and purge the biopsy pipette, one 25 μL drop to place the oocyte and another 25 μL drop on its side to release the PB once biopsied, and overlaid with prewarmed mineral oil, has to be prepared shortly before the procedure. Prepare one dish per oocyte to be analyzed. Once the selected oocytes are placed in the drops, place the dish on the heated stage of the inverted microscope equipped with the laser technology. The PBB is best accomplished when the oocyte is affixed to the holding capillary with the PB1 at the 6- or 12-o'clock position and the PB2 located right of the first one but in the same focal plane. An opening of 15–18 μm of diameter is drilled at 2–3-o'clock, and by pushing the biopsy capillary into the perivitelline space, both PBs can be removed simultaneously and be deposited in the clean drop for further analysis by PCR or FISH. The positioning of the PB2 next to the aspiration capillary allows pushing the PB2 far to the left side toward the holding capillary, and this stretching movement usually is enough to break the cytoplasmic bridge between the PB2 and the oocyte.

Due to the use of a blunt-ended capillary, even manipulation in direct vicinity to the oolemma does not damage the oocyte (Figs. 2A to D).

The gold standard is the use of laser for the AH, as the main benefit is that laser drilling and subsequent biopsy can be performed without changing the culture dish or the pipettes (in contrast to using AT for example) and thereby preventing contamination during diagnosing the sample with PCR.[23,24]

Genetic Screening

- *Analysis by fluorescence in situ hybridization (FISH):* Immediately after the biopsy of an oocyte, the corresponding PBs are placed in a neighboring droplet of HEPES medium until all oocytes are biopsied. For

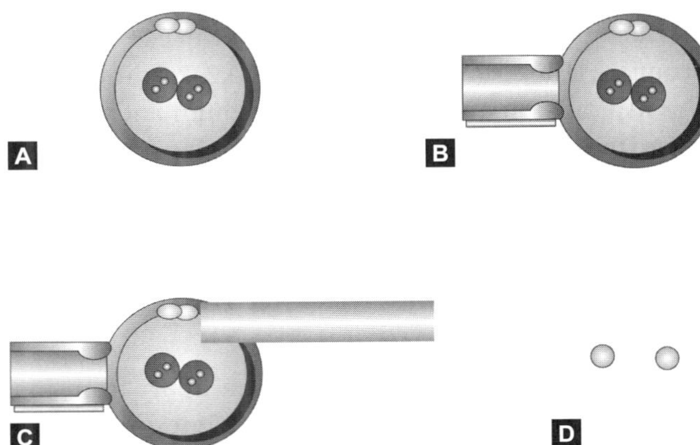

Figs. 8.2A to D: Schematic representation of polar body biopsy.

FISH, it is not essential to place the PB1 and PB2 in different droplets, as they can be visually distinguished during fluorescence evaluation. Due to the small cytoplasmic content of PBs, a special pretreatment like hypoosmotic swelling or proteinase/pronase treatment prior FISH is not necessary. For transfer onto the glass slide, PBs of one oocyte are removed from their drop and transferred into a tiny drop (0.2 mL) of water placed on a clean glass slide. The small volume guarantees that the PB will attach to the slide within a small area and that the fluid will dry out very fast, which reduces the risk of a dislocation of the PB on the slide. It is recommended to use for this transfer the biopsy capillary and to perform the complete procedure under visual control at the microscope. Placing the PBs directly at the bottom of the slide will prevent floating and rupture of the PBs. The drying process must be observed under a stereomicroscope, and the final location of the PB after air-drying should be marked on top of the slide by encircling with a diamond marker. With some experience, PBs from 6 oocytes to 10 oocytes can be placed within a round area of 10 mm, each encircled with the marker. Subsequent fixation can be performed with 2–3 drops of 10 mL methanol or acetic acid (3:1, ice-cold –20°C) followed by another fixation after air-drying using methanol at room temperature for 5 minutes.[25]

- *Analysis by polymerase chain reaction or array comparative genomic hybridization (array CGH):* In contrast to the isolation for FISH, the differentiation of the PB1 and PB2 is crucial for any PCR-based evaluation, either for monogenetic diseases or for array CGH. Therefore, the PB1 and PB2 are released after biopsy in different droplets with medium in a dish covered with mineral oil. These droplets should be rather large (approximately 10 mL) as this will facilitate to aspirate the PBs without sucking up some mineral oil. For PCR, the PBs need to be transferred into a PCR tube. This can be easily done by preloading the PCR tube with 1.6 mL buffer [phosphate buffered saline (PBS) or cell extraction buffer]. Using a low-volume pipette (0.2–2.0 mL), one PB is aspirated in a total of 0.4 mL medium and released into the buffer in the PCR tube by pipetting several times up and down. This process must be done in a laminar air flow in order to avoid any contamination with other cells or genetic material.[12]

Pitfalls

A major problem of the PB approach apart from just accounting for maternal genome is the interpretation of the results with FISH, especially for PB1. Whereas PB2 formation and aging can be precisely controlled because the time point of injection initiates the course of PB2 extrusion, the situation is different for PB1. At the time of ovum pickup the majority of oocytes are already in MII, but it is unknown at what time PB1 has been extruded and how long the chromatin of PB1 is already prone to an aging process. This aging process affects the quality of the DNA, the coherence of the chromatids, its dispersion after isolation on a slide, and, therefore, hybridization efficiency. In contrast, isolation and amplification of PB1 DNA for array CGH can be accomplished with more than 90% success rates, even from PBs that show signs of degeneration.[16]

In view of the costs of array CGH, the economic impact of PBB has to be considered as well. Because both PBs need to be separately analyzed, costs are doubled. Bearing in mind the fact that not all oocytes develop into viable embryos is another drawback of PBB.[16]

If the biopsy of both PBs is done at different time points, one should avoid drilling another opening. If PBs were retrieved through separate openings, problems may arise at the time of hatching because the embryo could hatch through both openings simultaneously and therefore may get trapped within the zona.[12]

Blastomere Biopsy

Cleavage stage or blastomere biopsy has remained the most widely practiced form of embryo biopsy worldwide according to the European Society of Human Reproduction and Embryology (ESHRE) PGD Consortium, accounting for approximately 90% of all reported PGD cycles to date.[26] Currently, this embryo biopsy strategy requires the removal of one or more cells from each embryo on day 3 of development.

The biopsy is performed when the embryo is typically composed of 6–8 blastomere cells to avoid compromising its development. Despite this, there is currently no consensus between clinics as to how many blastomeres should be removed for the genetic analysis. Some groups advocate the removal of a single blastomere, while others recommend that two blastomeres be biopsied in order to obtain a conclusive PGD result.[26]

Technical Aspects of Blastomere Biopsy

Intracytoplasmic sperm injection is the recommended technique for all PGD cases involving DNA amplification to reduce the chance of paternal contamination from extraneous sperm attached to the ZP or nondecondensed sperm within blastomeres. Similarly, as far as is practically and safely possible, all cumulus cells should be removed before biopsy as these cells can contaminate both FISH, array CGH and PCR-based diagnoses.

The use of standard IVF culture medium during biopsy is acceptable but its effectiveness may be highly dependent upon the developmental stage of the embryo biopsied with compacting 8-cell embryos proving more difficult to biopsy. Thereby, it is better to use commercially produced calcium and magnesium-free (Ca^{2+}–Mg^{2+}–free) medium which temporarily reverses calcium-dependent cell-cell adhesion, it is widely available and is used by many centers for routine clinical biopsy with the benefit of reducing the frequency of cell lysis[27] combined with a shorter time needed to perform the biopsy procedure.

Embryos are graded and selected for biopsy, however, it is "acceptable" to exclude very poor quality embryos from the embryo biopsy procedure.[28] Biopsy at cleavage stages is based on the principle that at these stages, the blastomeres remain totipotent and equivalent, such that the removal of a single blastomere will (a) provide a representative sample of the entire embryo and (b) compromise the embryo only to the extent of one-eighth of the embryo mass rather than removal of a developmentally crucial blastomere. The importance of selecting a blastomere with a single visible interphase nucleus cannot be stressed enough. Aside from the increased diagnostic efficiency observed in mononucleated blastomeres,[29] mononucleation is a marker for and directly correlates with implantation potential. Nevertheless, embryos containing blastomeres, all of which have no visible nucleus, should still be considered for biopsy as nuclear material is likely to be present and should yield results in molecular tests.[29] Time spent in careful examination of the embryo and orientation to selectively remove specific blastomeres is essential to attain the high diagnostic efficiencies required for clinical effectiveness. The following criteria can be used to select embryos for biopsy:[30,31]

- *Cell number:* More than 5 cells
- *Fragmentation:* Less than 20%
- *Multinucleate:* Less than 50%
- *Nucleus:* Present.

Chronology

- *Day 0:* Follicle retrieval, oocyte denudation and ICSI 3–5 hours after the ovum pickup
- *Day 1:* Fertilization assessment after 16–19 hours
- *Day 2:* Embryo development assessment after 44–47 hours
- *Day 3:* Embryo development assessment after 72 hours and cell biopsy and genetic analysis by array CGH or PCR
- *Day 5:* Selection of the normal or nonaffected embryos available for transfer. Day 3 biopsy provides the diagnostic laboratory 2–3 days to run the test. Given that most IVF programs do not have their own genetic laboratories, this would still allow time for the biopsied samples to be shipped to a reference laboratory, the analysis to be done, and the result reported back to the clinical program in time for a fresh transfer.[32]

Steps to Follow

Zona opening to remove the PBs can be done by any one of the above mentioned techniques (mechanical, chemical, laser or piezo-mediated devices). Once done the opening of the ZP, there are three different approaches to retrieve the blastomeres: (1) aspiration, (2) fluid displacement and (3) mechanical displacement, but the most widely used method of removal of cells is aspiration. The advantage with the aspiration method is the capability to select the cell to be removed and with an appropriate training, the risk of cell lysis is very low.

The aspiration pipette is approximated to the hole and then introduced very carefully; once it is in the same focal plane as the desired blastomere it is gently aspirated while avoiding contact or disruption of the remaining cells of the embryo (under 40x magnification). Remove the aspiration pipette with the blastomere attached and leave the cell close by the embryo. If it is required to biopsy a second cell, the aspiration pipette has to be entered again into the embryo through the same hole to repeat the operation. Release the embryo from the holding pipette carefully to avoid it aspirating the biopsied cells (under 20x magnification) (Figs. 3A to D). Push up the pipettes and place them into the next biopsy drop. Once the biopsy is concluded, the biopsied embryos should be thoroughly rinsed postbiopsy to remove traces of biopsy medium and shifted to the culture dishes. The biopsied blastomeres will remain in the biopsy dishes till further processing for the genetic analysis.

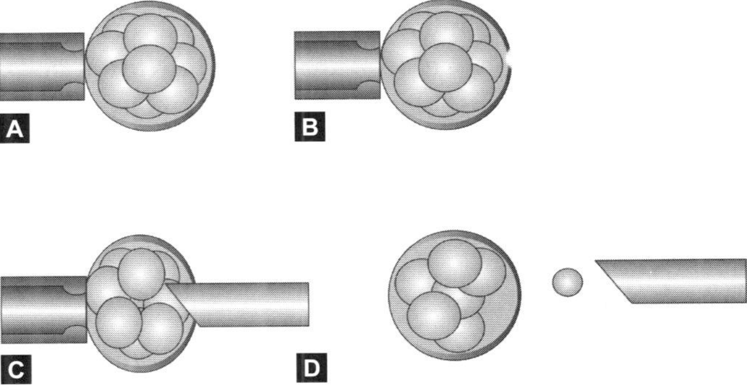

Figs. 8.3A to D: Schematic representation of blastomere biopsy.

Biopsied embryos must be cultured singly in individual wells or dishes with a clear identification system to ensure tracking of blastomeres removed and easy identification of embryos postdiagnosis.[27]

Genetic Screening

- *Analysis by fluorescence in situ hybridization:* For a successful FISH, the blastomeres fixation is crucial. The purpose of the process is not only to fix the nuclei of each single cell eliminating the remaining cytoplasm but also to do it in a way in which the nuclei integrity and its characteristics remain preserved.
  There are different methods to fix the blastomeres, being the most common Tarkowski method that uses a hypotonic solution and Carnoy fixative.[33]
  Embryos are considered normal or balanced for the autosomal chromosomes when two signals are present for each of the probes used. Embryos are considered normal or balanced for the sex chromosomes when two signals are present for X chromosome probes and no signals are present for Y chromosome probes, or when one signal was present for each of the X and Y chromosome probes. Extra or missing signals are considered to represent an unbalanced chromosome complement, which renders the embryo not suitable for transfer. Signals are considered split, if the signals are less than two domains apart and hence counted as one signal. For embryos that underwent biopsy of two blastomeres, the embryo is considered mosaic, if one blastomere is defined as normal or balanced and the other blastomere as unbalanced. The overall result for these embryos is recorded as unbalanced and not suitable for transfer. Two blastomeres are considered to be concordant if both blastomeres gave the same result of either normal or balanced or unbalanced.[26] FISH is no longer used as the preferred method and has been replaced by array CGH.
- *Analysis by polymerase chain reaction or array CGH:* Blastomere or TE cells are placed inside PCR tubes containing PBS solution with the help of glass capillaries (new capillary to be used for each individual cell). After releasing the cell the remaining fluid is released in a separate PCR tube to create a blank. The PCR tube is closed and shipped to the genetics laboratory for analysis.

Trophectoderm Biopsy

On day 5 and 6 of development the embryo has until 300 cells distributed between an inner cell mass (ICM) and the TE or outer cell mass. The main advantage is that the amount of genetic material available for analysis increases because instead of having a single blastomere (maximum two) as with the day 3 biopsy, it is possible to obtain several blastomeres from the TE. The general recommendation is to obtain 4–5 nuclei.[34] Moreover, it is considered a less invasive technique, as the ICM remains intact. Another advantage is that, as mentioned, only the embryos that reach the blastocyst stage are biopsied, so there is a prior developmental selection.

Technical Aspects of Trophectoderm Biopsy

Before undergoing the TE biopsy on day 5 it is advisable to do AH for ZP breaking on day 3 to facilitate the controlled extrusion of TE.

Chronology

- *Day 0:* Follicle retrieval, oocyte denudation and ICSI 3–5 hours after the ovum pickup
- *Day 1:* Fertilization assessment after 16–19 hours
- *Day 2:* Embryo development assessment after 44–47 hours
- *Day 3:* Embryo development assessment after 72 hours and AH
- *Day 5:* Embryo assessment, TE biopsy and genetic analysis by array CGH, vitrification of the analyzed embryos
- *Day 6:* Embryo assessment, TE biopsy and genetic analysis by array CGH, vitrification of the analyzed embryos.

In a further cycle with endometrial preparation, selection of the normal or nonaffected embryos available, thawing and transfer.

Steps to Follow

Usually, the ZP breaking is done on day 3 of development. On days 5 and 6 (and on rare occasions day 7), the embryos have to be assessed and in case of having any fully differentiated good quality blastocyst will be biopsied. Once the blastocyst is placed in the biopsy dish, attached it to the holding pipette with the suction, identifying the ICM and keeping it at 12- or 6-o'clock. The aspiration pipette is approximated to the hole, where the TE cells extruding from the expanded blastocyst are gently pulled (around 5–7 cells are enough). To change from the 40x objective to the laser objective and then make a few pulses of the laser at cell junctions in order to safely remove the cells without disrupting the ICM. Release the blastocyst from the holding pipette and move quickly the biopsy pipette over the holding to separate the blastocyst from the TE cells by friction. Release the blastocyst and the biopsied TE cells and pull up the pipettes to avoid aspirating any of them by mistake. Once finished the biopsy, shift the blastocyst to the culture dish after gently washing. The TE biopsied remains on the biopsy dish until their further processing for either array CGH or PCR. Following TE biopsy, the blastocysts will be vitrified using vitrification kits according to the manufacturer's instructions (Figs. 4A to C).[35,36]

Genetic Screening

- *Analysis by fluorescence in situ hybridization:* Trophectoderm samples are spread onto microscope slides, using a modified version of the methanol or acetic acid fixation method.[37] The isolated cells are individually washed once in 1% sodium citrate and transferred onto a glass slide and fixed using 3:1 methanol: acetic acid solution. The preparations is air dried, washed in PBS for 5 minute and dehydrated in 70, 85 and 100% ethanol. Fixed nuclei are then viewed using a phase contrast microscope and their location is marked with a diamond pen. Standard two round 9 chromosomes FISH (MultiVysion PB probe panel and the 4CC custom probe panel) are performed using a commercial ready-to-use probe mix.[38]
- *Trophectoderm cell analysis using array CGH:* Biopsied samples obtained during the study are washed in sterile PBS solution in a laminar flow cabinet to avoid any contamination of the sample, placed in microcentrifuge tubes containing 2 μL of PBS and then processed for array CGH analysis according to the protocol using a commercial genetic laboratory.[38]

  Clearly, each of these stages is biologically different, and thus, the strategic considerations have both advantages and disadvantages (Table 2).[1]

  Looking at the various technical aspects, day 5 biopsy looks like a better choice for biopsy: (I) extended culture enables selection of embryos with a greater chance of implantation and live delivery, (II) embryos reaching blastocyst stage enriches for euploid embryos, and (III) extended culture does not lead to a significant loss of euploid embryos capable of implantation.

  However, we need to apply powerful study design and come up with more evidence.[19,22,26,28,39-42]

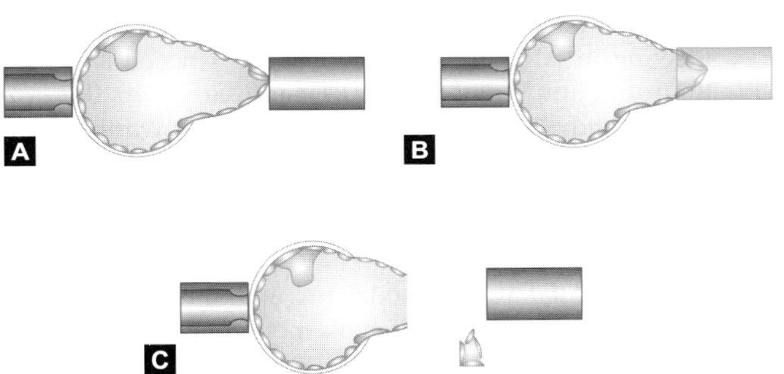

Figs. 4A to C: Schematic representation of trophectoderm biopsy.

SAFETY OF EMBRYOS

As with any micromanipulation procedure involving human gametes or embryo, every reasonable precaution should be taken to minimize cellular damage and stress during the procedure. General precautions include correct installation, calibration and maintenance of all micromanipulation equipment (particularly the laser). Biopsy and cell preparation should be performed by a suitably qualified

Table 2: Comparison between different types of biopsies and their indication.

Method	*Day performed*	*Type of cells removed*	*Indications*	*Zona drilling*	*Cell removal*	*Limitations*
Polar body	1st PB D0 2nd PB D1 or simultaneously both on D1	1st and 2nd PB	PGS monogenics carried by mother	Laser Mechanical Beveled pipette	Aspiration	Only maternal chromosomes
Cleavage stage	D3	Blastomeres	PGS monogenics, sexing, chromosome abnormalities	Laser Mechanical Tyrode's acid	Aspiration Displacement	Postzygotic mosaicism
Blastocyst	D5	Trophectoderm	PGS monogenics, sexing, chromosome abnormalities	Laser Mechanical Tyrode's acid	Herniation	Postzygotic mosaicism Arrest prior to biopsy Vitrification program

(PB: polar body; PGS: preimplantation genetic screening)

and trained person.[1] Utmost care should be taken to ensure that no harm is done to the human embryo. One must be careful not to violate the principal percept of medical science—"primum non nocere"— "first do no harm".

VITRIFICATION

A major challenge at present is to develop an effective standardized method for cryopreservation of biopsied embryos. With the high rate of multiple pregnancies reported after PGD, it is imperative to develop effective methods of cryopreservation that will:

- Allow storage of unaffected embryos for later transfer, so that the numbers transferred can be limited to two or even single embryo transfer
- Provide additional time to perform more diagnostic tests.[1,25]

CONCLUSION

Preimplantation genetic screening is a testing tool which gives us more information about the embryo apart from morphology assessment. It would help in selecting genetically normal embryos for transfer enabling higher pregnancy and implantation rates. Looking at the comparison and various technical aspects, day 5 biopsy looks like a better choice for biopsy as it gives us more information and rules out mosaicism.

REFERENCES

1. Harper JC. Introduction. Harper JC, Delhanty JDA, Handyside AH (Eds). Preimplantation Genetic Diagnosis. London, UK: John Wiley & Sons; 2001, pp. 3-12.
2. Scott RT, Upham KM, Forman EJ, et al. Cleavage-stage biopsy significantly impairs human embryonic implantation potential while blastocyst biopsy does not: a randomized and paired clinical trial. Fertil Steril. 2013;100(3):624-30.
3. Nagy ZP, Varghese AC, Agarwal A. Practical Manual of In Vitro Fertilization: Advanced Methods and Novel Devices, 1st edition. New York: Springer-Verlag; 2012. p. 703.
4. Griffiths T. Embryo biopsy. In: Coward K, Wells D (Eds). Textbook of Clinical Embryology. Cambridge: Cambridge University Press; 2013. pp. 286-99.
5. Cohen J, Feldberg D. Effects of the size and number of zona pellucida openings on hatching and trophoblast outgrowth in the mouse embryo. Mol Reprod Dev. 1991;30(1):70-8.
6. Montag M. A Practical Guide to Selecting Gametes and Embryos. New York: CRC Press; 2014. p. 328.
7. Selva J. Assisted hatching. Hum Reprod. 2000;15(Suppl 4): 65-7.
8. El-Toukhy T, Braude P. Preimplantation Genetic Diagnosis in Clinical Practice, 1st edition. London: Springer-Verlag; 2014. p. 228.
9. Geber S, Bossi R, Lisboa CB, et al. Laser confers less embryo exposure than acid tyrode for embryo biopsy in preimplantation genetic diagnosis cycles: a randomized study. Reprod Biol Endocrinol. 2011;9:58.
10. Modern Times Group (MTG). Octax laser and software. [online] Available from www.mtg.com. [Accessed March, 2017].
11. Han TS, Sagoskin AW, Graham JR, et al. Laser-assisted human embryo biopsy on the third day of development for preimplantation genetic diagnosis: two successful case reports. Fertil Steril. 2003;80(2):453-5.
12. Montag M, Köster M, van der Ven K, et al. Polar body biopsy. In: Nagy ZP, Varghese AC, Agarwal A (Eds). Practical Manual of In Vitro Fertilization: Advanced Methods and Novel Devices, 1st edition. New York: Springer-Verlag; 2012. pp. 455-9.
13. Yoshida N, Perry AC. Piezo-actuated mouse intracytoplasmic sperm injection (ICSI). Nat Protoc. 2007;2(2):296-304.
14. Huang T, Kimura Y, Yanagimachi R. The use of piezo micromanipulation for intra- cytoplasmic sperm injection of human oocytes. J Assist Reprod Genet. 1996;13 (4):320-8.
15. Prime Tech Ltd. Prime Tech Piezo PMM4G and ICSI. [online] Available from www.primetech-jp.com/en/03support/images/p-icsi.pdf. [Accessed March, 2017].
16. Montag M, Köster M, Strowitzki T, et al. Polar body biopsy. Fertil Steril. 2013;100 (3):603-7.
17. Vayena E, Rowe PJ, Griffin PD. Current Practices and Controversies in Assisted Reproduction: Report of a meeting on "Medical, Ethical and Social Aspects of Assisted Reproduction" held at WHO Headquarters in Geneva, Switzerland 17-21 September 2001. Geneva: World Health Organization; 2002. p. 381.
18. Verlinsky Y, Ginsberg N, Lifchez A, et al. Analysis of the first polar body: preconception genetic diagnosis. Hum Reprod. 1990;5(7):826-9.
19. Fragouli E, Alfarawati S, Goodall NN, et al. The cytogenetics of polar bodies: insights into female meiosis and the diagnosis of aneuploidy. Mol Hum Reprod. 2011;17(5):286-95.
20. van der Ven K, Montag M, van der Ven H. Polar body diagnosis - a step in the right direction? Dtsch Arztebl Int. 2008;105(11):190-6.
21. Munné S, Dailey T, Sultan KM, et al. The use of first polar bodies for preimplantation diagnosis of aneuploidy. Hum Reprod. 1995;10(4):1014-20.
22. Magli MC, Montag M, Köster M, et al. Implementing polar body biopsy and chromosome copy number analysis by array comparative genomic hybridisation: technical experiences from the ESHRE PGS Task Force pilot study. Hum Reprod. 2011;26(1):3181-4.
23. Montag M, van der Ven K, van der Ven H. Erste klinische Erfahrungen mit der Polkörperdiagnostik in Deutschland. J Fertil Reprod. 2002;4(1):7-12.
24. Montag M, Schimming T, van der Ven H. Spindle imaging in human oocytes: the impact of the meiotic cell cycle. Reprod Biomed Online. 2006;12(4):442-6.
25. Montag M, van der Ven K, van der Ven H. Polar body biopsy. In: Gardner DK, Weissman A, Howles CM, Shoham Z (Eds). Textbook of Assisted Reproductive Techniques: Laboratory

and Clinical Perspectives, 3rd edition. New York: Informa Healthcare; 2008. pp. 357-70.
26. Brodie D, Beyer CE, Osborne E, et al. Preimplantation genetic diagnosis for chromosome rearrangements - one blastomere biopsy versus two blastomere biopsy. J Assist Reprod Genet. 2012;29(8):821-7.
27. Harton GL, Magli MC, Lundin K, et al. ESHRE PGD Consortium/Embryology Special Interest Group—best practice guidelines for polar body and embryo biopsy for preimplantation genetic diagnosis/screening (PGD/PGS). Hum Reprod. 2011;26(1):41-6.
28. Magli MC, Gianaroli L, Ferraretti AP, et al. Embryo morphology and development are dependent on the chromosomal complement. Fertil Steril. 2007;87(1): 534-40.
29. Cui KH, Matthews CD. Nuclear structural conditions and PCR amplification in human preimplantation diagnosis. Mol Hum Reprod. 1996;2(1):63-71.
30. Igenomix: Pioneers in reproductive genetics. Advanced Reproductive Genetic Testing Services. [online] Available from www.igenomix.us. [Accessed March, 2017].
31. McArthur SJ, Leigh D, Marshall JT, et al. Pregnancies and live births after trophectoderm biopsy and preimplantation genetic testing of human blastocysts. Fertil Steril. 2005;84(6):1628-36.
32. Scott KL, Hong KH, Scott RT. Selecting the optimal time to perform biopsy for preimplantation genetic testing. Fertil Steril. 2013;100(3):608-14.
33. Tarkowski AK. An air-drying method for chromosome preparations from mouse eggs. Cytogenetics. 1966;5(6): 394-400.
34. De Boer KA, Catt JW, Jansen RP, et al. Moving to blastocyst biopsy for preimplantation genetic diagnosis and single embryo transfer at Sydney IVF. Fertil Steril. 2004;82(2):295-8.
35. Lathi RB, Massie JA, Gilani M, et al. Outcomes of trophectoderm biopsy on cryopreserved blastocysts: a case series. Reprod Biomed Online. 2012;25(5): 504-7.
36. Adler A, Lee HL, McCulloh DH, et al. Blastocyst culture selects for euploid embryos: comparison of blastomere and trophectoderm biopsies. Reprod Biomed Online. 2014;28(4):485-91.
37. Velilla E, Escudero T, Munné S. Blastomere fixation techniques and risk of misdiagnosis for preimplantation genetic diagnosis of aneuploidy. Reprod Biomed Online. 2002;4(1):210-7.
38. Capalbo A, Wright G, Elliott T, et al. FISH reanalysis of inner cell mass and trophectoderm samples of previously array-CGH screened blastocysts shows high accuracy of diagnosis and no major diagnostic impact of mosaicism at the blastocyst stage. Hum Reprod. 2013;28(8): 2298-307.
39. Braude P, Pickering S, Flinter F, et al. Preimplantation genetic diagnosis. Nat Rev Genet. 2002;3(12):941-53.
40. Verlinsky Y, Cohen J, Munne S, et al. Over a decade of experience with pre-implantation genetic diagnosis: a multicenter report. Fertil Steril. 2004;82(2): 292-4.
41. Harper JC, Sengupta SB. Preimplantation genetic diagnosis: state of the art 2011. Hum Genet. 2012;131(2):175-86.
42. Yan L, Wei Y, Huang J, et al. Advances in preimplantation genetic diagnosis/screening. Sci China Life Sci. 2014;57(7): 665-71.

CHAPTER

64

Time-lapse Imaging: A New Technology for Embryo Development

Carmela Albert, Pilar Gámiz, Natalia Basile, Marcos Meseguer

INTRODUCTION

In classical in vitro fertilization (IVF), embryo assessment is based on time-point evaluation during embryo development, and a clear correlation between embryo morphology and viability has been well established. The final decision for embryo transfer is based primarily on developmental stage, blastomere symmetry and the quality of the inner cell mass (ICM) and trophectoderm (TE) at the day of transfer.

Even though great knowledge has been achieved through this approach it has been demonstrated that embryo status can markedly change within a few hours.[1-4] In addition, inter and intraobserver variability is a commonly described problem[5] probably due to the subjective nature surrounding traditional morphological assessment.[3,6-10] In theory, increasing the number of observations could provide better information of the development of the embryo and therefore improve its assessment.[3,11,12] However, increased handling and higher evaluation frequency will expose the embryo to undesirable changes in temperature, humidity and gas composition.[11-13]

Time-lapse systems (TMSs) represent a solution to this problem. In 1997, Payne et al.[14] developed time-lapse cinematography to manage an intermittent observation of the process of oocyte fertilization. Later on, the observation period was augmented while maintaining optimal culture conditions[2] and nowadays TMSs increases the number of morphologic observation for assess embryo quality and allow the complete observation of the entire process of embryo development in the IVF laboratory. In addition to that, the TMS reduces the handling of samples and hence the human risk, implies a minimization of culture media, mineral oil and gas consumption, facilitates the detection of abnormal events that would normally occur between observations, reduce inter and intraobserver variations and decrease the number of hours needed by the embryologist in the laboratory.[15]

Morphokinetics, defined as the combination of the embryo appearance (morphology) and the timing in which cellular events occur, has been introduced as a new concept to improve embryo selection. TMS allows the precise determinations of the onset, and duration of an interval between cell divisions. The use of this strategy could allow single embryo transfers (SETs) without jeopardizing the overall IVF success,[16] becoming very attractive especially in European countries in which legislation is stricter about the number of embryo transferred.[15]

MODELS IN MARKET

There are different available options of TMS in the market. Some of them present all the items integrated in one single equipment, e.g. EmbryoScope® (Vitrolife), Geri (Genea Biomedx) and Miri® TL (Esco Medical). Others offer the option of introducing a microscope inside an available incubator, e.g. Primo Vision (Vitrolife) and the Eeva™ Test (Merck Serono). Tables 1 and 2 describe the clinical and technical features of all the TMS available in the market.

KINETIC PARAMETERS (INDIVIDUAL + CALCULATED)

As described at the proposed guidelines on the nomenclature and annotation of dynamic human embryo monitoring by a time-lapse user group, we can define the following morphokinetic individual variables:[17]

Table 1: Technical features compared between the time-lapse systems available in the market.

Technical features	*EmbryoScope®*	*Primo Vision®*	*Eeva™ test*	*Geri*	*Miri® TL*
Microscopy	Phase contrast	Phase contrast	Dark field	Phase contrast	Phase contrast
Image capture frequency	Every 10 minutes	Every 10 minutes	Every 10 minutes	Every 10 minutes	Every 10 minutes
Focusing levels	7	Several	1	Several	Several
Patients per system	6	1	1	6	6
Embryos per dish	12	16	12	16	14
Integrated incubator	Yes	No	No	Yes	Yes
Data analysis	Manual	Manual	Manual	Manual	Manual

Table 2: Clinical features compared between the time-lapse systems available in the market.

Clinical features	*EmbryoScope®*	*Primo Vision™*	*Eeva™ test*	*Geri*	*Miri® TL*
Automatic assessment	No	No	Yes	No	No
Worker dependent	Yes	Yes	No	Yes	Yes
Time consuming	Yes	Yes	No/automatic	Yes	Yes
Selection algorithm	Set by the user	Set by the user	Present	Set by the user	Set by the user
Blastocyst formation prediction by day 3	No	No	Yes	No	No
Implantation prediction by day 3	Yes	Yes	Yes	No	No
Prospective validated	Yes	No	Yes	No	No

- *t0:* Time of IVF or midtime of microinjection [intracytoplasmic sperm injection (ICSI) or intracytoplasmic morphologically selected sperm injection (IMSI)]
- *tPB2:* The second polar body completely detached from the oolemma
- *tPN:* Fertilization is confirmed
- *tPNa:* Appearance of individual pronuclei (PN); tPN1a, tPN2a, and tPN3a
- *tPNf:* Time of PN disappearance; tPN1f, and tPN2f
- *tZ:* Time of PN scoring
- *t2 to t9:* Time to two to nine discrete cells
- *tSC:* First evidence of compaction
- *tMf/p:* End of compaction
  - "f" corresponds to fully compacted
  - "p" corresponds to partial compaction.
- *tSB:* Initiation of blastulation
- *tByz:* Full blastocyst
  - "y" corresponds to morphology of ICM
  - "z" corresponds to morphology of TE cells.
- *tEyz:* Initiation of expansion; first frame of zona thinning
- *tHNyz:* Herniation; end of expansion phase and initiation of hatching
- *tHDyz:* Fully hatched blastocyst.

Additionally we can define calculated variables that represent a certain cell stage or cycle duration (Fig. 1):

Pronuclei duration	VP = tPNf–tPNa
Duration of first cell cycle	ECC1 = t2–tPB2
Duration of second cell cycle	ECC2 = t4–t2
Duration of single blastomere cell cycle	cc2a = t3–t2
	cc2b = t4–t2
Duration of third cell cycle	ECC3 = t8–t4
Duration of single blastomere cell cycle	cc3a = t5–t4
	cc3b = t6–t4
	cc3c = t7–t4
	cc3d = t8–t4

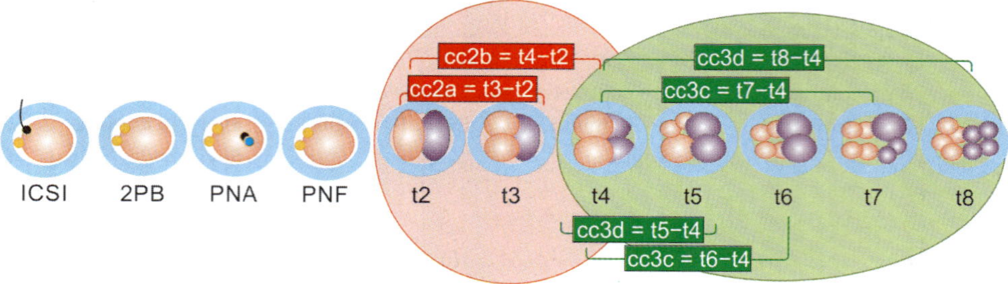

Fig. 1: Graphical representation of kinetic variables up to the eight-cell stage. (Intracytoplasmic sperm injection; PB: polar body)

Synchronization of cell divisions	s2 = t4–t3
Synchronization of cleavage pattern	s3 = t8–t5
Duration of compaction (dcom)	tMf–tSC (full compaction)
	tMp–tSC (partial compaction)
Duration of blastulation (dB)	tB–tSB
Duration of blastocyst expansion (dexp)	tHN–tE
Duration of blastocyst collapse (dcol)	tBCend(n)–tBCi(n)
"n" is number of episodes of collapse and re-expansion	
Duration of reexpansion (dreexp)	treexpend(n)–treexpi(n)
Duration of herniation (8dHN)	tHN–tHD

BLASTOCYST DEVELOPMENT STUDIES

Kinetic markers have been associated with good quality embryos and with the prediction of blastocyst formation (Table 3).

In 2010, Wong et al.[18] analyzed kinetic parameters of 100 embryos that were cultured up to day 5 or 6 of development.[18] Three parameters were founded as predictors of blastocyst formation: (1) P1: duration of the first cytokinesis (14.3 ± 6.0 min), (2) P2: interval between the end of the first mitosis and the initiation of the second mitosis (11.1 ± 2.2 h) and (3) P3: the synchrony between the second and third mitosis (1.0 ± 1.6 h). The authors concluded that embryo development to the blastocyst stage could be predicted with 94% of sensitivity and 93% of specificity after using those parameters. Embryos with one or more values outside these ranges were expected to arrest. The time of completion of the second and third mitosis was also analyzed by Hashimoto et al.[19] who observed that high-scoring blastocysts took significantly shorter times for these divisions.

Hlinka et al.[20] analyzed 180 embryos that resulted in 28 pregnancies. After calculating the average duration of the interphases and cleavages of a subset of implanting embryos, the author established a uniform time pattern of cleavage clusters (c) and interphases (i); most specifically: i2 = 11 ± 1, i3 = 15 ± 1, i4 = 23 ± 1 h/c2 = 15 ± 5, c3 = 40 ± 10, c4 = 55 ± 15. Embryos falling within these values showed a higher rate of blastocyst development than those falling outside this range (88.2% vs. 13.3%). In addition, higher morphological abnormality rates were observed in embryos falling outside the optimal ranges.

In a retrospective cohort study, Cruz et al.[21] monitored 834 embryos. Mean timings for the variables t2, t3, t4, t5, tM, cc2 and s2 were calculated for embryos that developed to blastocyst and for those that did not. Quartiles were defined for each parameter in association with the proportion of good and poor morphology blastocysts. Finally, optimal ranges were proposed as follows: t2, 24.3–27.9 hour; t3, 35.4–40.3 hour; t5, 48.8–56.6 hours; s2, less than 0.76 hours; and cc2, less than 11.9 hours. The following deselection criteria were also recorded: uneven blastomere size at the 2-cell stage and abrupt division from zygote to 3-blastomere embryo. In general, it was observed that embryos performing earlier cleavages had significantly higher developmental potential to day 5. Therefore, the capability to reach blastocyst stage seemed to be related to early embryo division kinetics.

In 2013, Chamayou et al.[22] reported time intervals of morphokinetic parameters identified as predictors of embryo competence. In this retrospective study, embryos were divided into three groups: (1) implanted (72), (2) nonimplanted (106), and (3) arrested (66). Each kinetic parameter for every single embryo was compared and significant differences were found. The authors concluded that day 3 embryos develop into viable blastocysts when their kinetic parameters met the following ranges: t1 [18.4–30.9 hours postinsemination (hpi)], t2 (21.4–34.8 hpi), t4 (33.1–57.2 hpi), t7 (46.1–82.5 hpi), t8 (46.4–97.8 hpi), tC – tF (7.7–22.9 hpi) and s3 (0.7–30.8 hpi).

A couple of prospective studies were performed in 2013; Kirkegaard et al.[23] analyzed 571 embryos from good prognosis patients and reported three markers linked to

Table 3: Kinetic markers associated to the prediction of blastocyst formation.

Author	*Study design*	*N embryos*	*Embryo origin*	*Time-lapse system*	*Predictive marker identified*
Wong et al. 2010	Retrospective Study	100	Supernumerary frozen 2PN	Modified Olympus IX-70/71; CKK- 40/41	1st cytokinesis, P2 and P3
Hashimoto et al. 2012	Experimetal study	80	Donated human embryos for research	Biostation CT	Duration of 2nd (t4–t3) and 3rd mitotic division (t8–t5)
Hlinka et al. 2012	Retrospective study	180	Clinical IVF routine	Primo Vision	c2, c3 and c4; i2, i3, and i4
Cruz et al. 2012	Retrospective cohort study	834	Oocyte donation cycles	Embryoscope	t4, s2, DC 3 sells, tM; UN 2 cells
Chamayou et al. 2013	Retrospective study	224	Fresh oocyte ICSI treatments	Embryoscope	t1, t2, t4, t7, t8, tC–tF and s3
Kirkegaard et al. 2013	Prospective multicenter cohort	571	Fresh oocyte ICSI treatments	Embryoscope	1st cytokinesis, t3, DC 3 cells
Conhagan et al. 2013	Prospective multicenter cohort study	233	Fresh oocyte ICSI treatments	Eeva	P2 and P3
Kirkegaard et al. 2014	Retrospective multicenter study	1,519	Fresh oocyte ICSI treatments	Embryoscope	P2 and P3
Cetinkaya et al. 2014	Retrospective observational cohort study	3,354	Clinical IVF routine	Embryoscope	CS2
Yang et al. 2015	Prospective observational study	345	Metaphase I donated for research	Primo Vision	Cleavage patterns
Milewsky et al. 2015	Retrospective observational study	432	Fresh oocyte ICSI treatments	Embryoscope	t2, t5, cc2, SC
Storr et al. 2015	Prospective cohort study	380	Fresh oocyte ICSI treatment	Embryoscope	s3, t8, tEB
Motato et al. 2016	Retrospective study	7,483	Clinical IVF routine	Embryoscope	tM; t8–t5

(DC: direct cleavage; ICSI: intracytoplasmic sperm injection; IVF: in vitro fertilization; PN: pronuclei)

high-quality blastocysts: duration of the first cytokinesis, duration of 3-cell stage and direct cleavage to 3-cell, all of them with comparable predictive value but with no connection to implantation results. Conaghan et al.[24] accomplished a two phase multicenter study to develop and validate an algorithm to predict blastocyst formation. A total of 1,727 embryos were monitored by an automatic cell tracking software. The time between cytokinesis 1 and 2 (P2) and the time between cytokinesis 2 and 3 (P3) turned out to be the strongest parameters in the prediction model. The results indicated a higher probability of usable blastocyst formation when both P2 and P3 were within specific cell division timing ranges (P2, 9.33–11.45 h; and P3, 0–1.73 h) and a low probability when either P2 or P3 were outside the specific cell timing ranges. Through this model, the authors observed that usable blastocysts could be predicted with a specificity of 84.2% [95% confidence interval (CI) = 78.7–88.5%], sensitivity of 58.8% (95% CI = 47.0– 69.7%), positive predictive value (PPV) of 54.1% (95% CI = 42.8–64.9%), and negative predictive value (NPV) of 86.6% (95% CI = 81.3–90.6%). By comparison, the same prediction based on morphology alone was achieved with a specificity of 52.1% (95% CI = 39.7–64.6%), sensitivity of 81.8% (95% CI = 70.6–92.9%), PPV of 34.5% (95% CI = 31.5–37.5%), and NPV of 90.9% (95% CI = 87.3–94.5%). The authors concluded that the use of this algorithm significantly improved the specificity (84.2% vs. 52.1%; p <0.0001) and PPV (54.1% vs. 34.5%; p <0.01) of usable blastocyst predictions enabling embryologists to better discriminate which embryos would be unlikely to develop to blastocyst. Therefore, they recommend the adjunctive use of this algorithm to improved embryo selection.

The Conaghan model was tested retrospectively by a different group using a set of 1,519 transferred embryos with known clinical outcome.[25] According to the algorithm, embryos were classified into usable and nonusable. The difference in implantation rate (IR) between the usable group and the whole cohort was 30% indicating that IRs could increase using this model. In addition, the percentage of nonusable embryos that resulted in implantation was 50.6%

causing alert regarding the discard of viable embryos. Even though the Conaghan model was developed for blastocyst formation and the endpoint of this study was clinical outcome, the authors expressed that implanted embryos should derive from the usable embryo group and not from the nonusable group (or at least not in such high proportion). The possible explanation, according to the authors, could be that the model is based on narrow time intervals.

In 2015, Cetinkaya et al.[26] studied 17 kinetic markers on 3,354 embryos cultured up to day 5. The parameters: t8–t5, cleavage synchronicity from 4 to 8 cells (CS4–8) and cleavage synchronicity from 2 to 8 cells (CS2–8) were found as good indicators. In particular, CS2–8 defined as: CS2–8 = [(t3–t2) + (t5–t4)]/(t8–t2) was selected as the best predictor on day 3 for blastocyst formation and quality [area under the curve (AUC): 0.786]. The authors concluded that relative timings (time intervals and relative ratios) were better indicators of development than absolute time points that cannot be standardized for general applicability in different laboratories.

Yang et al.[27] took a different approach and developed a study to describe different types of abnormal divisions and how they may affect the developmental potential of the embryo. Seven types of divisions within two categories were defined according to the impact caused on blastocyst development. Category 1 included divisions with low impact on the development potential—normal division, uneven blastomere formation and appearance of big fragments.

Category 2 included divisions with high impact on embryo development— direct cleavage, fragmentation, developmental arrest and disordered division. Taking this in consideration a hierarchical classification model was developed based on the division patterns during the three initial embryo cleavages rather than on morphokinetic parameters as in previous studies. Day 3 embryos were then classified into six categories "A" to "F" according to the number and category of the abnormal cleavages they had presented. More specifically: (A) embryos that had normal cleavage in the initial three cleavages, (B) embryos that had category 1 behaviors in all three cleavages, (C) embryos undergoing category 1 behaviors in the initial two cleavages and category 2 behaviors in the third cleavage, (D) embryos that showed category 1 behaviors in the first cleavage and one of the two blastomeres (partial) showed category 2 behaviors in the second cleavage, (E) embryos that showed category 1 behaviors in the first cleavage and two blastomeres (all) showed category 2 behaviors in the second cleavage, and (F) embryos that showed category 2 behaviors in the first cleavage. The model was validated in a prospective observational study in which images from 345 embryos were acquired. The study revealed that 72.2% of the embryos presented at least one abnormal division. According to the model, blastocyst formation rate decreases from 94.8% to 21.2%, good quality blastocyst formation rate decreases from 70.8% to 3.8% and IR (for those that were transferred) decreases from 67% to 0% as we move on from "A" to "F".

In a study by Milewski et al. the parameters t2, t3, t4, t5, cc2 and s2 were measured and differences were observed between embryos that reached the blastocyst stage and embryos that arrested. A total of 432 embryos were analyzed. The resultant data for each parameter was divided into four intervals (C1–C4) and score values were assigned in order to find out which parameter values corresponded to the highest blastocyst development rate. The highest ones generally belonged to compartments C3 and C2. The extreme compartments, C1 and C4, had the lowest rates. The univariate logistic regression analysis concluded that all the studied parameters were significantly associated with blastocyst development. However, after multivariate logistic regression only t2, t5 and cc2 parameters were taken into account and combined into a new parameter (SC) defined as predictor of development to blastocyst.[28]

Storr et al. recorded the timings of 380 blastocysts and found eight significant prediction markers of top-quality blastocyst: s3, t6, t7, t8, tM, tSB, tB and tEB. Out of these potential predictors, s3 was identified as the one with the best individual discriminatory capacity before compaction (area under the curve—AUC 0.585, 95% CI 0.534–0.635), and tEB was identified as the best predictor regardless of embryo stage (AUC 0.727, 95% CI 0.675–0.775). By combining ts3, tEB and t8, a model with higher discriminatory capacity for predicting top-quality embryos was proposed.[29]

Diamond et al.[30] found that, adjunctive use of Eeva test is highly informative and allow embryologist to consistently improve the selection of embryos with high developmental potential.

Motato et al.[31] in 2016 published a three-phase observational, retrospective, single-center clinical study, in which the author described the events associated with blastocyst formation and implantation based on the largest sample size ever described with time-lapse monitoring:

- *Phase 1:* Embryo scoring based on a classification tree to select embryos with higher blastocyst formation probabilities. The observed correlations between morphokinetic parameters and blastocyst formation are the basis for a proposed hierarchical classification procedure to select viable embryos with a high blastocyst formation potential. A detailed retrospective analysis of cleavage times was made for 7,483 zygotes. A total of 17 parameters were studied and several were significantly correlated with blastocyst formation and implantation. The most predictive parameters for blastocyst formation were: time of morula formation, tM (81.28–96.0 h after ICSI), and t8–t5 (≤8.78 h) or time of transition of 5-blastomere embryos to 8-blastomere embryos with a receiver operating characteristic (ROC) curve value = 0.849 (95% CI, 0.835–0.854). These parameters were less predictive of implantation, with a ROC value = 0.546 (95% CI, 0.507–0.585).

- *Phase 2:* Blastocyst transferred and IR. Owing to the lack of a relationship between the previously described variables with implantation potential, the authors identified new variables by comparing transferred blastocysts (n = 383) that implanted with those that did not implant (n = 449). Once again they analyzed 17 morphokinetic parameters and identified the variables: time for expansion blastocyst, tEB (107.9–112.9 h after ICSI), and t8–t5 (5.67 h after ICSI) to predict blastocyst implantation, with a ROC curve value = 0.591 (95% CI, 0.552–0.630). Using these data, a hierarchical model representing a classification tree was proposed. The model subdivided blastocysts into four categories from A to D with higher or lower IR (i.e. from 72.2% in category A to 39.7% in category D).
- *Phase 3:* Validation of the implantation model. After the conclusion of phase 2, the created model was validated on an independent data set composed of 257 embryos and 123 blastocysts with known implantation data (KID) embryos, giving a ROC of 0.596 (95% CI, 0.526–0.666; p = 0.008).

The authors concluded that the inclusion of kinetic parameters into score evaluation could improve blastocyst selection criteria as well as predict blastocyst formation with high accuracy. In addition, the proposed models classify embryos according to their probabilities of blastocyst stage and implantation.

The most recent study on blastocyst prediction was published by Aparicio et al.[32] in 2016 the authors founded that there is a direct correlation between blastocyst rate and percentage of optimal blastocyst according to each of the categories: high, medium and low. A total of 3,002 embryos were automatically classified by means of the Eeva system according to the timing of P2 and P3. These embryos were also classified with the use of Association for the Study of Reproductive Biology (ASEBIR) morphology classification. The results suggest that the automated embryo diagnostic test provided extra information to the embryologist to select the best embryos, independently from clinical features of the patient or day of transfer.

IMPLANTATION STUDIES

In addition to blastocyst formation, the scientific community has also correlated kinetic markers to embryo implantation as an endpoint (Table 4).

Starting in 2008, Lemmen et al.[33] retrospectively compared time lapse recordings of a small group of

Table 4: Kinetic markers associated to the embryo implantation as an endpoint.

Author	*Study design*	*Total number of embryos*	*Embryo origin*	*Time-lapse system*	*Predictive marker identified/utilized*
Lemen et al. 2008	Retrospective study	19	IVF/ICSI cycles	Nikon Diaphot 300 microscope with camera in a closed system	Nuclei apperance in the first blastomere
Meseguer et al. 2011	Retrospective study	247	ICSI cycles	EmbryoScope	t5, s2, cc2, UN 2 cell, MN 4 cell, DC 1–3 cells
Arazello et al. 2012	Prospective study	159	ICSI cycles	EmbryoScope	PN breakdown
Hlinka et al. 2012	Retrospective study	114	ICSI cycles	Primovision	c2, c3 and c4; i2, i3 and i4
Rubio et al. 2012	Multicenter retrospective study	5,225 (1,659 transferred)	IVF cycles from donated and autologous oocytes	EmbryoScope	DC 2–3 cells
Freour et al. 2013	Retrospective analysis and prospectively collected database	191	ICSI cycles	EmbryoScope	t4 and s3
Chamayou et al. 2013	Retrospective study	178	ICSI cycles	EmbryoScope	cc3
Kirkegaard et al. 2013a	Prospective cohort study	84	ICSI cycles	EmbryoScope	None

Contd...

Contd...

Rubio et al. 2014	Prospective randomized control trial	2,638	ICSI cycles from donated oocytes	EmbryoScope	T5; s2; cc2; UN 2 cell; MN 4 cell; DC 1–3 cells
Aguilar et al. 2012	Retrospective cohort study	1,448	ICSI cycles from donated oocytes	EmbryoScope	Time to 2PB; PF; length of S-phase
Basile et al. 2012	Retrospective multicentric study	1122	ICSI cycles from donated and autologous oocytes	EmbryoScope	Cc2, t3, t5, UN 2 cell, MN 4 cells DC 1–3 cell
Vermilea et al. 2014	Retrospective multicentric study	331	IVF/ICSI cycles	Evea	P2 and P3
Freour et al. 2015	Retrospective study	528	ICSI cycles	EmbryoScope	t5, s2, cc2, UN 2 cell, MN 4 cells DC 1–3 cell
Dominguez et al. 2015	Retrospective cohort study	28	ICSI cycles from donated oocytes	EmbryoScope	Cc2
Adamson et al. 2016	Prospective concurrent cohort study		ICSI and IVF cycles from autologous oocytes	Eeva	P2 and P3
Goodman et al. 2016	Prospective randomized controlled trial	2092	ICSI and IVF cycles from autologous oocytes	Embryo Scope	Cc2, s2, t5, s3, tSB, MN, irregular division

(DC: direct cleavage; ICSI: intracytoplasmic sperm injection; IVF: in vitro fertilization; MN: multinucleation; PB: polar body; PN: pronuclei)

Flowchart 1: Algorithm by Meseguer et al. (2011).

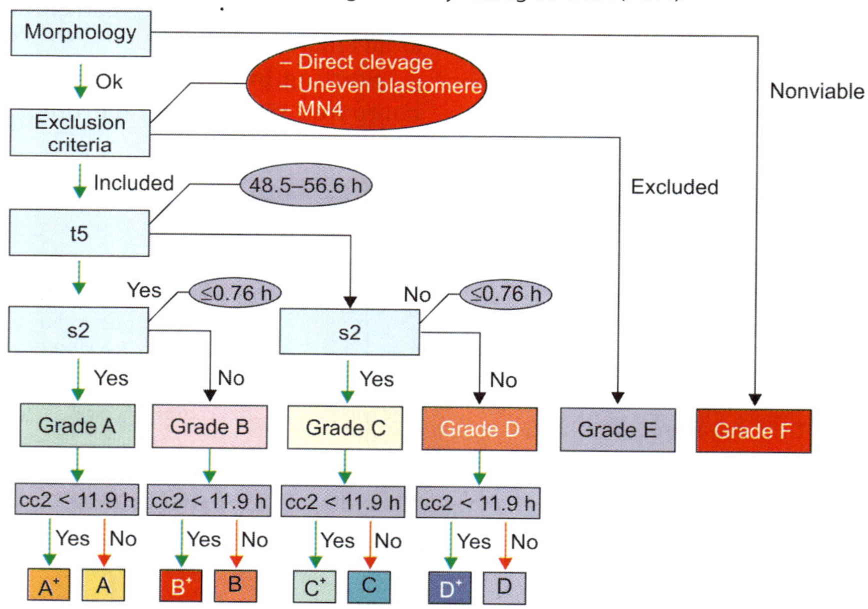

embryos transferred at the 4-cell stage that resulted in eight pregnancies. In this case, the author observed that nuclei appearance in the first blastomere following the first cleavage was faster in embryos that implanted versus those that did not, and that the nuclei appearance in the first two blastomeres was significantly more synchronous ($p < 0.05$).

Three years later, Meseguer et al.[1] published a study were explaining several parameters were correlated with embryo implantation. The study was based on 247 KID embryos and it developed a hierarchical model that subdivided embryos into six categories from A to F. Four of these categories (A–D) were further subdivided into two subcategories (+) or (–) (Flowchart 1). The hierarchical classification procedure starts with a morphological screening of all embryos in a cohort to eliminate those embryos that are clearly not viable (i.e. highly abnormal, atresia or clearly arrested embryos).

Those embryos that are clearly not viable are discarded and not considered for transfer (category F). Next step in the model is to exclude embryos that fulfill any of the three exclusion criteria: (1) uneven blastomere size at the 2-cell stage, (2) abrupt division from one to three or more cells or (3) multinucleation at the 4-cell stage (category E). The subsequent levels in the model follow a strict hierarchy based on the binary timing variables t5, s2 and cc2. First, if the value of t5 falls inside the optimal range (48.8–56.6 h), the embryo is categorized as A or B. If the value of t5 falls outside the optimal range (or if t5 has not yet been observed at 64 h), the embryo is categorized as C or D. If the value of s2 falls inside the optimal range (≤0.76 h) the embryo is categorized as A or C depending on t5; similarly, if the value of s2 falls outside the optimal range, the embryo is categorized as B or D depending on t5. Finally, the embryo is categorized with the extra plus (+), if the value for cc2 is inside the optimal range (≤ 11.9 h) (A+/B+/C+/D+) and is categorized with a minus (–) (as A-/B-/C-/D-), if the value for cc2 is outside the optimal range.

In 2012, Azzarello et al.[34] performed a prospective study transferring 159 embryos and proposed the variable 'time of pronuclear breakdown' as a predictor of pregnancy. In this study, the pronuclear breakdown of embryos resulting in live birth occurred significantly later than those that did not. In fact, the author proposed the limit of 20 hours 45 minutes and recommended to avoid transferring embryos presenting pronuclear breakdowns at earlier times.

The same year, Hlinka et al.,[20] proposed a novel method to predict implantation. The model relied on cleavage ratings of the embryos; more specifically time pattering of cleavage clusters and interphases were used to select the highest quality embryos. Diagnostic relation between blastocyst implantation and cleavage success was 100% specific for all the embryos analyzed (180) and all the pregnancies resulted from timely cleaved embryos.

Direct cleavage is another parameter that has been correlated with implantation. Meseguer et al.[1] initially observed this phenomenon based on 247 KID embryos. Later on, these findings were confirmed by a multicenter retrospective study performed by Rubio et al.[35] In this case the number of embryos analyzed was much higher (5,225) and embryo implantation for embryos presenting direct cleavage from two to three cells (DC 2 to 3 <5 h) was statistically lower than for those with normal cleavage pattern. Only 1 out of 109 embryos with DC 2–3 cells resulted in clinical pregnancy.

The impact of extrinsic factors on embryo kinetics and its relation with implantation has been studied as well. In 2013, Freour et al.[36] focused on smoking women observing that embryo divisions occurred later in smokers than in nonsmokers, resulting in worst outcome for the first group. The author analyzed 191 embryos indicating t4 and s3 as the most relevant kinetic parameters with respect to implantation. According to the distribution of these two variables, implantation was significantly higher in the first two quartiles. Embryos were graded as A or B depending on the optimal range defined for t4 (A = inside the range and B = outside the range). In addition, embryos were given a "+" or "–" value according to the optimal range of s3 (+ = inside the range and – = outside the range). The authors validated this classification model in a database including all transferred embryos observing IRs of 38.7%, 33.3%, 30.7% and 15.3% for A+, A–, B+ and B– categories, respectively. The proportion of A+ and A– embryos was higher in nonsmoker patients.

Chamayou et al.[22] retrospectively compared morphokinetic parameters of 72 implanted and 106 nonimplanted embryos. No differences were found for PN appearance, PN disappearance, t1, t2, t4, t7, t8, tC–tF and s3 parameters. The authors concluded that these markers were not predictors of implantation but that they could predict embryo development to the blastocyst stage. In this study, the only predictor marker of implantation and production of a viable pregnancy was cc3. Embryos with cc3 between 9.7 and 21 hours seemed to have the highest probability of implantation and clinical pregnancy.

As opposed to many authors, Kirkegaard et al.,[23] showed no differences in the timings of cellular division or embryonic stage between implanted and nonimplanted embryos. The study was based on the observation of 84 SETs. The author defined the duration of first cytokinesis, duration of the 3-cell stage and direct cleavage to three cells as predictors of high quality embryo development but not of implantation or pregnancy. Therefore, this group concluded that a universal algorithm for optimal timing might not be feasible. Validation of Meseguer's algorithm from 2001[1] came along with a triple-blind randomized prospective controlled trial published by Rubio et al. in 2014.[37] In this study, 405 patients were included in the control group in which embryos were selected based purely on morphology and 438 patients were included in the study group in which embryos were selected based on the algorithm. IRs were significantly higher in the study group (44.9%; 95% CI, 41.4–48.4) versus the control group (37.1%; 95% CI, 33.6–40.7). In addition, the ongoing pregnancy rate was also higher in the study group versus the control group (54.5%; 95% CI, 49.6–59.2 vs. 45.3%; 95 CI, 40.3–50.4). The authors concluded that morphokinetic variables allow us to reject embryos with lower implantation while distinguishing those with higher implantation probabilities. Selecting embryos through kinetic markers may therefore improve reproductive outcomes.[37]

A second randomized controlled trial published by a different group reached similar results although they were not able to achieve statistical significance.[38] As opposed to Rubio's study, in which both study groups had different culture conditions (standard incubator vs. EmbryoScope), one of the strengths of this study was that it was the first one to evaluate all embryos cultured within identical culture conditions and to demonstrate whether the addition of continuously monitored morphokinetic parameters improve clinical outcomes compared with conventional once daily morphologic assessment. The study anticipated a 10% increase and although it did not reach statistical significance, there were increased clinical pregnancy and IRs with the use of the additional parameters. In addition, the time of the start of blastulation, the absence of multinucleation, and the use of a score based on morphology and kinetics were significant predictors of implantation. The authors concluded that in this dynamic and evolving field, larger studies were needed to confirm their findings.

In 2014, Aguilar et al.[39] studied the human's first cell cycle and its impact on implantation based on morphokinetics. For this aim the author did a retrospective analysis of 1,448 transferred embryos and compared the timings of second polar extrusion, first and second pronuclear appearance, pronuclear abuttal, pronuclear fading and length of S-phase between implanted and nonimplanted embryos. The time ranges successfully linked to implantation were: 3.3–10.6-hour for second polar body extrusion, 22.2–25.9-hour for pronuclear fading and 5.7–13.8-hour for the length of S-phase.

The same year, Basile et al.[40] continued the study by Meseguer et al.[1] and published an improved version of the algorithm by studying a larger data set of embryos from four different IVF clinics (Flowchart 2). For that aim a sequential approach was adopted by the author. During phase 1 of the study, an algorithm was developed taking in consideration morphokinetic data of 754 KID embryos that were selected for transfer based only on conventional morphological criteria. The new algorithm included the variables t3, cc2 and t5 in combination with morphology and exclusion criteria [direct cleavage (DC), uneven blastomere size(UBS) and multinucleation(MN)] and classified embryos from A to E according to their implantation potential. Subsequently, during phase 2 of the study, the predictive ability of this new algorithm was tested by applying it for embryo classification in a different group of IVF patients (885 cycles). Considering only cycles with known implantation (100% or 0% implantation, n = 1,137), a significant decrease in IR was observed as embryo categories decreased from A to E. More specifically: "A" 32%, "B" 28%, "C" 26.25%, "D" 20.19% and "E" the lowest 17% $p < 0.001$.

Another study by VerMilyea et al.[41] established the relationship between implantation and three embryo categories derived from a computer automated TMS. The system classified embryos into the categories: high, medium or low based on the variables P2 and P3. According to this multicenter study (205 patients) IRs were significantly linked to the three categories; more specifically: 37%, 35% and 15% for high, medium and low respectively. In addition, clinical pregnancy rate for patients that had one

Flowchart 2: Algorithm by Basile et al. (2015).

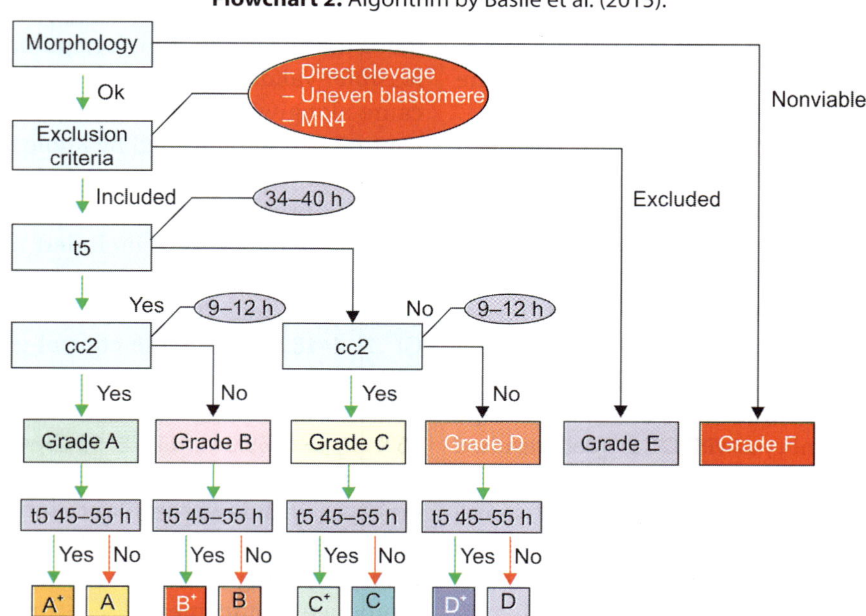

or more "high" embryos transferred was significantly higher (51% vs. 34%; p = 0.02).

A most recent study published by Adamson et al. in 2016,[42] tested the same technology in a prospective way. The aim of the study was to prove if an automatic time-lapse test (TL-test) combined with traditional morphology improves day 3 IRs compared with morphology alone. Two concurrently collected groups of patients were compared: those who received a day 3 transfer with the use of the TL test together with morphology (test group), and those who received a day 3 transfer with the use of morphology alone (control group). To further assess the impact of the automated TL-test score, the authors evaluated the implantation potential of embryos assigned by the TL-test as category TL-high versus TL-low among all transferred embryos (TL-high: duration of 2-cell stage within 9.33–11.45 h and duration of 3-cell stage within 0–1.73 h; TL-low: outside the TL-high ranges) and among those with only good morphology. Analysis of the study's primary endpoint, IR showed a significantly higher IR for day 3 transfer among the test group (30.2%, 58/192) than the control group (19.0%, 84/442; p = 0.003); clinical pregnancy rate was also significantly higher among the test group (46.0%, 45/98) than the control group (32.1%, 71/221; p = 0.02). Within the test group, patients receiving at least one TL-high embryo had significantly higher IRs than patients receiving only TL-low embryos (36.8% vs. 20.6%). TL-high compared with TL-low embryos had significantly higher IRs (44.7% vs. 20.5%). Among morphologically good embryos, TL-high embryos were more likely to implant than TL-low embryos (44.1% vs. 20.6%). The authors concluded that the noninvasive TL-test adds valuable information to traditional morphologic grading and that it should be used to increase clinician's confidence in recommending elective SET (eSET) with day 3 transfer, and that we would expect higher IRs and higher clinical pregnancy rates, as well as reduced multiple pregnancy rates, compared with patients with embryos not assessed by the TL-test.

Limitations on the external performance and the universal use of published algorithms have been addressed.[12] In a study published by Freour et al.[36] an external validation of Meseguer's algorithm[1] was performed in an unselected patient population. The model was applied showing a heterogeneous distribution of IRs in the resultant categories. In addition, correlation coefficients were significantly lower than the ones in the original study. However, a simplified version from the model (in which only the two main morphokinetic variables, t5 and s2, were consider and not cc2) performed acceptably. The author explained that the differences could be the result of differences in oxygen culture conditions, oocyte source (donor cycles versus autologous cycles), restrictions in the studied population and/or the stimulation protocols used. The conclusion was that a hierarchical prediction model should not be used universally in an unselected population; it should be center specific.

The combination of technologies may be the key for improving results in the future. Dominguez et al.,[44] combined proteomics and time-lapse analysis of implanted[16] and nonimplanted[12] embryos. After logistic regression analysis the model identified the presence or absence of protein interleukin-6 (IL-6) and the duration of cc2 as the most relevant embryo features. Based on these results, the author developed a hierarchical model (*see* Flowchart 3) based on

Flowchart 3: Algorithm by Dominguez et al. (2015).

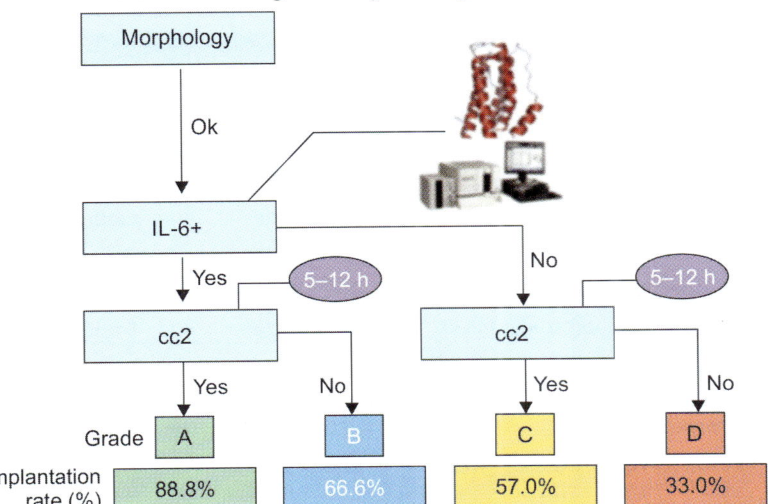

(IL-6: interleukin-6)

these two variables classifying embryos in four categories "A–D". IRs are expected to decrease as we move on from A to D as observed in this study (A = 88.8%, B = 66.6%, C = 57% and D = 33%).[40]

ANEUPLOIDY STUDIES

The correlation between euploidy and embryo kinetics has been studied as well (Table 5).

In 2010 Wong et al.,[18] collected single embryos for gene expression analysis and revealed that embryos with P1, P2, and P3 outside of the optimal ranges exhibited abnormal ribonucleic acid (RNA) patterns for embryo cytokinesis, microRNA (miRNA) biogenesis, and maternal messenger RNA (mRNA) reserve, suggesting that embryo fate may be predetermined and inherited very early in development (by the 4-cell stage).

Chavez et al.[44] subsequently observed that euploid embryos clustered tightly in the P1, P2, or P3 window that was predictive of blastocyst formation according to Wong's study. Performing further molecular analysis, the authors discovered that fragmentation dynamics, together with P1, P2 and P3, could potentially distinguish euploid from aneuploid embryos at the 4-cell stage considering that the fragments contained nuclear deoxyribonucleic acid (DNA), kinetochore proteins, and whole chromosomes as detected by fluorescence in situ hybridization (FISH).

In 2013, Campbell et al.[46] elaborated an aneuploidy risk model based on the differences of tSB and tB between euploid and aneuploid embryos that had undergone TE biopsy. The model includes three categories: (1) low-risk, tB less than 122.9 hpi and tSB less than 96.2 hpi, (2) medium-risk, tB less than 122.9 hpi and tSB 96.2 hpi, and (3) high-risk, tB 122.9 hpi.[36] The same group in a different study[46] applied this model to evaluate its effectiveness and potential clinical impact for unselected IVF patients without undergoing preimplantation genetic screening (PGS) after analyzing KID embryos. The study revealed significant differences in fetal heart rate (72.7; 25.5; 0) and live-birth rate (61.1; 19.2; 0) between the three categories low, medium and high respectively. This demonstrates that time-lapse imaging using defined morphokinetic data can be used to classify human preimplantation embryos according to their risk of aneuploidy, without performing biopsy and PGS, and that this correlates well with clinical outcomes.

The following year Basile et al.[47] also correlated morphokinetics with embryo aneuploidy based on 77 patients undergoing genetic screening due to recurrent miscarriage or implantation failure. In this case embryo biopsy was performed on day 3 of development and the total number of embryos analyzed was 504. A logistic regression analysis was used to select and organize which observed timing events (expressed as binary variables inside or outside the optimal range) were most relevant to select embryos with higher probability of being chromosomally normal. The model identified t5–t2 odds ratio (OR) = 2.853 (95% CI 1.763–4.616) followed by cc3 OR = 2.095 (95% CI 1.356–3.238) as the most relevant variables related to normal chromosomal content. An algorithm for embryo selection based on these two variables classifies embryos from A to D (Flowchart 4) with significant differences in the percentage of normal embryos as we move on from A to D. More specifically: A: 35.9%, B: 26.4%, C: 12.1%, and D: 9.8% ($p < 0.001$).

As opposed to the previous studies, Rienzi et al.[49] reported no correlation at all between 16 commonly detected morphokinetic parameters and embryo ploidy. This was a longitudinal cohort study conducted using 455

Table 5: Studies analyzing the correlation between euploidy and embryo kinetics.

Author	*Study design*	*Number of embryos*	*Embryo origin*	*Time-lapse system*	*Predictive marker identified*
Chavez et al. 2012	Research study	75	Freezed zygotes	Custom-built miniature microscope system	4 cells stage
Campbell et al. 2013	Retrospective study	98	PGD cycles	Embryoscope	tSB, tB
Campbell et al. 2013	Retrospective study	88	PGD cycles	Embryoscope	FHB, LB
Basile et al. 2014	Retrospective study	504	PGD cycles	Embryoscope	t5–t2, cc3
Rienzi et al. 2015	Longitudinal cohort study	455	PGD cycles	Embryoscope	No correlation
Chawla et al. 2015	Retrospective study	460	PGD cycles	Embryoscope	tPNf, t2, t5, cc2, cc3 and t5–t2
Vera-Rodriguez et al. 2015	Retrospective study	85	PCR and PGD cycles	Embryoscope	PNd
Minasi et al. 2016	Retrospectively study	1,730	PGD cycles	Embryoscope	t4, t4–t3, tSB, tB, tEB, tHB

(PCR: polymerase chain reaction; PGD: preimplantation genetic diagnosis)

Flowchart 4: Algorithm by Basile et al. (2014).

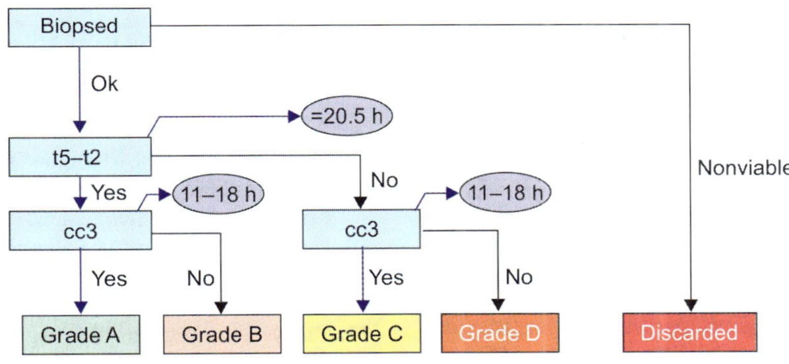

blastocysts from 138 patients at increased risk of aneuploidy because of advance maternal age, history of unsuccessful IVF treatments or both. The analyzed parameters included: t2, t3, t4, t5, t8, cc1, cc2, s2, s3, cc3, cc3 or cc2, t5–t2, syngamy, tSB, tSC and tB.

In 2015 two studies observed correlations between embryo kinetics and euploidy. The first one, reported by Chawla et al.,[49] identified tPNf, t2, t5, cc2, cc3 and t5-t2 as parameters that significantly differed between chromosomally normal and abnormal embryos. The second one by Vera-Rodriguez et al.[50] combined chromosomal assessment and single cell quantitative reverse transcription polymerase chain reaction (RT-qPCR) to simultaneously obtain information from all the blastomeres of human embryos until approximately the 8-cell stage (n = 85). According to their results, the chromosomal status of aneuploid embryos (n = 26) correlates with significant differences in the duration of the first mitotic phase when compared with euploid embryos (n = 28). Moreover, gene expression profiling in this study suggested that a subset of genes is differentially expressed in aneuploid embryos during the first 30-hour of development.

In 2016 Minasi et al.[51] in a retrospective study analyzed the morphology and morphokinetic of 1,730 blastocysts, obtained in 530 preimplantation genetic diagnosis (PGD) cycle. They found that the euploid blastocyst started to form, reached the full stage, expanded and hatched significantly faster, compared to aneuploid ones. Although there seems to be a relationship between the ploidy status and blastocyst morphology or development dynamic, the evaluation of morphological and morphokinetic parameters cannot currently be improved upon, and therefore replace, PGS.

However, time-lapse monitoring could be used in conjunction with PGS to analyze the blastocysts or select the one that should be transferred.

RESEARCH STUDIES

We can use also kinetic markers and cleavage pattern to learn the behavior of the embryos until blastocyst stage.

Regarding ploidy, Grau et al.[52] described that half tripronucleated (TPN) ICSI-derived embryos became diploid during early in vitro development, whereas the other TPN embryos remained triploid. Regarding morphokinetics, Escrich et al.[53] reported that TPN embryos showed a delay at all the timings that cells cleaved at, except the cleavage timing to five cells, and significantly prolonged second and third cell cycles (cc2 and cc3, respectively) when compared to bipronucleated (BPN) embryos. However, once the ploidy of the TPN embryos was known, the TPN population was not homogeneous in most morphokinetic variables.

Taking this information into account, Grau et al.[54] showed that TPN embryos displayed different morphokinetic behavior according to ploidy; TPN self-corrected to diploidy were morphokinetically closer to correctly fertilized embryos, and morphokinetic variable t5 can predict their ploidy.

CONCLUSION

Static observations obtained from standard microscopes have contributed significantly to the knowledge of embryo development; however it is becoming more challenging to identify embryos with the highest implantation potential due to the static and notoriously subjective character of this type of morphological evaluation. The study of embryo kinetics through time-lapse technology has given rise to new markers for embryo selection representing a new and exciting powerful tool for viewing cellular activity and embryogenesis in a coherent and uninterrupted manner, otherwise not available through standard microscopy.

The present chapter presents an overview of the most recent studies that describe the use of this new technology in the IVF laboratory. It is our opinion that standard morphological assessment should remain the gold standard to initiate embryo evaluation; however, if possible, it should be complemented with the detection of kinetic markers known to improve clinical results. This new approach will allow the embryologist to perform a more accurate and objective embryo selection and therefore the goal of a SET slowly becomes more tangible.

REFERENCES

1. Meseguer M, Herrero J, Tejera A, et al. The use of morphokinetics as a predictor of embryo implantation. Hum Reprod. 2011;26(10):2658-71.
2. Mio Y, Maeda K. Time-lapse cinematography of dynamic changes occurring during in vitro development of human embryos. Am J Obstet Gynecol. 2008;199(6):660.e1-5.
3. Gardner DK, Meseguer M, Rubio C, et al. Diagnosis of human preimplantation embryo viability. Hum Reprod Update. 2015;21(6):727-47.
4. Alpha Scientists in Reproductive Medicine and ESHRE Special Interest Group of Embryology. The Istanbul consensus workshop on embryo assessment: proceedings of an expert meeting. Hum Reprod. 2011;26(6):1270-83.
5. Baxter Bendus AE, Mayer JF, Shipley SK, et al. Interobserver and intraobserver variation in day 3 embryo grading. Fertil Steril. 2006;86(6):1608-15.
6. Kaser DJ, Racowsky C. Clinical outcomes following selection of human preimplantation embryos with time-lapse monitoring: a systematic review. Hum Reprod Update. 2014;20(5):617-31.
7. Paternot G, Wetzels AM, Thonon F, et al. Intraand interobserver analysis in the morphological assessment of early stage embryos during an IVF procedure: a multicentre study. Reprod Biol Endocrinol. 2011;9:127.
8. Sundvall L, Ingerslev HJ, Breth Knudsen U, et al. Interand intra-observer variability of time-lapse annotations. Hum Reprod. 2013;28(12):3215-21.
9. Arce JC, Ziebe S, Lundin K, et al Interobserver agreement and intraobserver reproducibility of embryo quality assessments. Hum Reprod. 2006;21(8):2141-8.
10. Scott L. The biological basis of non-invasive strategies for selection of human oocytes and embryos. Hum Reprod Update. 2003;9(3):237-49.
11. Meseguer M, Rubio I, Cruz M, et al Embryo incubation and selection in a time-lapse monitoring system improves pregnancy outcome compared with a standard incubator: a retrospective cohort study. Fertil Steril. 2012;98(6):1481-9.e10.
12. Kirkegaard K, Ahlström A, Ingerslev HJ, et al. Choosing the best embryo by time lapse versus standard morphology. Fertil Steril. 2015;103(2):323-32.
13. Zhang JQ, Li XL, Peng Y, et al. Reduction in exposure of human embryos outside the incubator enhances embryo quality and blastulation rate. Reprod Biomed Online. 2010;20(4):510-5.
14. Payne D, Flaherty SP, Barry MF, et al. Preliminary observations on polar body extrusion and pronuclear formation in human oocytes using time-lapse video cinematography. Hum Reprod. 1997;12(3):532-41.
15. Basile N, Caiazzo M, Meseguer M. What does morphokinetics add to embryo selection and in-vitro fertilization outcomes? Curr Opin Obstet Gynecol. 2015;27(3):193-200.
16. Herrero J, Meseguer M. Selection of high potential embryos using time-lapse imaging: the era of morphokinetics. Fertil Steril. 2013;99(4):1030-4.
17. Ciray HN, Campbell A, Agerholm IE, et al. Proposed guidelines on the nomenclature and annotation of dynamic human embryo monitoring by a time-lapse user group. Hum Reprod. 2014;29(12):2650-60.
18. Wong CC, Loewke KE, Bossert NL, et al. Non-invasive imaging of human embryos before embryonic genome activation predicts development to the blastocyst stage. Nat Biotechnol. 2010;28(10):1115-21.
19. Hashimoto S, Kato N, Saeki K, et al. Selection of high-potential embryos by culture in poly(dimethylsiloxane) microwells and time-lapse imaging. Fertil Steril. 2012;97(2):332-7.
20. Hlinka D, Kalatová B, Uhrinová I, et al. Time-lapse cleavage rating predicts human embryo viability. Physiol Res. 2012;61(5):513-25.
21. Cruz M, Garrido N, Herrero J, et al. Timing of cell division in human cleavage-stage embryos is linked with blastocyst formation and quality. Reprod Biomed Online. 2012;25(4):371-81.
22. Chamayou S, Patrizio P, Storaci G, et al. The use of morphokinetic parameters to select all embryos with full capacity to implant. J Assist Reprod Genet. 2013;30(5):703-10.
23. Kirkegaard K, Kesmodel US, Hindkjaer JJ, et al. Time-lapse parameters as predictors of blastocyst development and pregnancy outcome in embryos from good prognosis patients: a prospective cohort study. Hum Reprod. 2013;28(10):2643-51.
24. Conaghan J, Chen AA, Willman SP, et al. Improving embryo selection using a computer-automated time-lapse image analysis test plus day 3 morphology: results from a prospective multicenter trial. Fertil Steril. 2013;100(2):412-9.e5.
25. Kirkegaard K, Campbell A, Agerholm I, et al. Limitations of a time-lapse blastocyst prediction model: a large multicentre outcome analysis. Reprod Biomed Online. 2014;29(2):156-8.
26. Cetinkaya M, Pirkevi C, Yelke H, et al. Relative kinetic expressions defining cleavage synchronicity are better predictors of blastocyst formation and quality than absolute time points. J Assist Reprod Genet. 2015;32(1):27-35.
27. Yang ST, Shi JX, Gong F, et al. Cleavage pattern predicts developmental potential of day 3 human embryos produced by IVF. Reprod Biomed Online. 2015;30(6):625-34.
28. Milewski R, Kuć P, Kuczyńska A, et al. A predictive model for blastocyst formation based on morphokinetic parameters in time-lapse monitoring of embryo development. J Assist Reprod Genet. 2015;32(4):571-9.
29. Storr A, Venetis CA, Cooke S, et al. Morphokinetic parameters using time-lapse technology and day 5 embryo

quality: a prospective cohort study. J Assist Reprod Genet. 2015;32(7):1151-60.
30. Diamond MP, Suraj V, Behnke EJ, et al. Using the Eeva TestTM adjunctively to traditional day 3 morphology is informative for consistent embryo assessment within a panel of embryologists with diverse experience. J Assist Reprod Genet. 2015;32(1):61-8.
31. Motato Y, de los Santos MJ, Escriba MJ, et al. Morphokinetic analysis and embryonic prediction for blastocyst formation through an integrated timelapse system. Fertil Steril. 2016;105(2):376-84.e9.
32. Aparicio-Ruiz B, Basile N, Pérez Albalá S, et al. Automatic time-lapse instrument is superior to single-point morphology observation for selecting viable embryos: retrospective study in oocyte donation. Fertil Steril. 2016;106(6):1379- 85.e10.
33. Lemmen JG, Agerholm I, Ziebe S. Kinetic markers of human embryo quality using time-lapse recordings of IVF/ICSI-fertilized oocytes. Reprod Biomed Online. 2008; 17(3):385-91.
34. Azzarello A, Hoest T, Mikkelsen AL. The impact of pronuclei morphology and dynamicity on live birth outcome after time-lapse culture. Hum Reprod. 2012;27(9):2649-57.
35. Rubio I, Kuhlmann R, Agerholm I, et al. Limited implantation success of directcleaved human zygotes: a time-lapse study. Fertil Steril. 2012;98(6):1458-63.
36. Fréour T, Dessolle L, Lammers J, et al. Comparison of embryo morphokinetics after in vitro fertilization-intracytoplasmic sperm injection in smoking and nonsmoking women. Fertil Steril. 2013;99(7):1944-50.
37. Rubio I, Galán A, Larreategui Z, et al. Clinical validation of embryo culture and selection by morphokinetic analysis: a randomized, controlled trial of the EmbryoScope. Fertil Steril. 2014;102(5):1287-94.e5.
38. Goodman LR, Goldberg J, Falcone T, et al. Does the addition of time-lapse morphokinetics in the selection of embryos for transfer improve pregnancy rates? A randomized controlled trial. Fertil Steril. 2016;105(2):275-85.e10.
39. Aguilar J, Motato Y, Escribá MJ, et al. The human first cell cycle: impact on implantation. Reprod Biomed Online. 2014;28(4):475-84.
40. Basile N, Vime P, Florensa M, et al. The use of morphokinetics as a predictor of implantation: a multicentric study to define and validate an algorithm for embryo selection. Hum Reprod. 2015;30(2):276-83.
41. VerMilyea MD, Tan L, Anthony JT, et al. Computer-automated time-lapse analysis results correlate with embryo implantation and clinical pregnancy: a blinded, multi-centre study. Reprod Biomed Online. 2014;29(6):729-36.
42. Adamson GD, Abusief ME, Palao L, et al. Improved implantation rates of day 3 embryo transfers with the use of an automated time-lapse-enabled test to aid in embryo selection. Fertil Steril. 2016;105(2):369-75.e6.
43. Dominguez F, Meseguer M, Aparicio-Ruiz B, et al. New strategy for diagnosing embryo implantation potential by combining proteomics and time-lapse technologies. Fertil Steril. 2015;104(4):908-14.
44. Chavez SL, Loewke KE, Han J, et al. Dynamic blastomere behaviour reflects human embryo ploidy by the four-cell stage. Nat Commun. 2012;3:1251.
45. Campbell A, Fishel S, Bowman N, et al. Modelling a risk classification of aneuploidy in human embryos using non-invasive morphokinetics. Reprod Biomed Online. 2013;26(5):477-85.
46. Campbell A, Fishel S, Bowman N, et al. Retrospective analysis of outcomes after IVF using an aneuploidy risk model derived from time-lapse imaging without PGS. Reprod Biomed Online. 2013;27(2):140-6.
47. Basile N, Nogales Mdel C, Bronet F, et al. Increasing the probability of selecting chromosomally normal embryos by time-lapse morphokinetics analysis. Fertil Steril. 2014;101(3):699-704.
48. Rienzi L, Capalbo A, Stoppa M, et al. No evidence of association between blastocyst aneuploidy and morphokinetic assessment in a selected population of poor-prognosis patients: a longitudinal cohort study. Reprod Biomed Online. 2015;30(1):57-66.
49. Chawla M, Fakih M, Shunnar A, et al. Morphokinetic analysis of cleavage stage embryos and its relationship to aneuploidy in a retrospective time-lapse imaging study. J Assist Reprod Genet. 2015;32(1):69-75.
50. Vera-Rodriguez M, Chavez SL, Rubio C, et al. Prediction model for aneuploidy in early human embryo development revealed by single-cell analysis. Nat Commun. 2015;6:7601.
51. Minasi MG, Colasante A, Riccio T, et al. Correlation between aneuploidy, standard morphology evaluation and morphokinetic development in 1730 biopsied blastocysts: a consecutive case series study. Hum Reprod. 2016;31(10):2245-54.
52. Grau N, Escrich L, Martín J, et al. Self-correction in tripronucleated human embryos. Fertil Steril. 2011;96(4): 951-6.
53. Escrich L, Grau N, Meseguer M, et al. Detailed kinetics and morphology analysis of human triplonucleated embryos: a comparison with correctly fertilized transferred embryos. Fertil Steril. 2013;28:171.
54. Grau N, Escrich L, Galiana Y, et al. Morphokinetics as a predictor of self-correction to diploidy in tripronucleated intracytoplasmic sperm injection-derived human embryos. Fertil Steril. 2015;104(3):728-35.

CHAPTER

65

Design, Equipment, and Personnel Management

Irene Rubio Palacios, Javier Herrero Zapata

INTRODUCTION

The purpose of this chapter is to provide key aspects for the design of the assisted reproductive technology (ART) unit, the necessary equipment and personnel management in terms of requirements and safety, based on the specific procedures that an ART unit can offer.

Designing an ART laboratory involves the consideration of many aspects, which can be encompassed into two groups. On the one hand, recommendations and obligations applicable at the time of designing the lab and providing proper facilities and equipment, on the other hand, the setting of specific objectives for the service being offered.[1] On the first group, laboratory set-up providing ART services would have to be setup as per the guidelines of the reproductive medicine societies of the respective nations.[2] Success of any ART unit mainly depends on the infrastructure of the laboratories and the formation of the personnel working. In this sense, a detailed layout and assessment of all laboratory furniture and equipment is essential prior to construction and can drastically improve the cost-benefit ratio. Regarding the personnel, authorized technical staff with a good theoretic background and proved experience and competence in the concerned specialty is critical for the well functioning of the unit.

LABORATORY

Laboratory Design

As described in the "European Society of Human Reproduction and Embryology (ESHRE) guidelines for good practice in in vitro fertilization (IVF) laboratories", a laboratory should have adequate space to follow good laboratory practice.[3] There are different key points that should be taken into account. The first step is to determine the estimated number of cycles the laboratory is expected to perform in a given time period. The second point to consider should be the design and organization of the laboratories, where the most recent developments in facilities, equipment and procedures should be considered. Immediately after, attention should be payed to embryologist or andrologist comfort in order to minimize risks to gametes by means of maximizing the efficiency and use of space.[4] To ensure an optimal handling of gametes during the treatment, there should be a dedicated andrology laboratory, an IVF laboratory with a different area dedicated to cryopreservation, and a separate area for the administrative work, such as record keeping and data entry. In those cases in which preimplantation genetic diagnosis (PGD) treatments are offered also, a separate laboratory should be included in the design.

Another important point is the location of each of the laboratories with respect to the other areas. The semen collection room, if possible, should be located adjacent to the andrology laboratory to facilitate the handling of the collected specimen. In fact, the ideal location of the andrology laboratory is between the semen collection room and the insemination room. The IVF laboratory must be adjacent to the operating room where the clinical procedures are performed. The cryopreservation area should be included in the core of the IVF but separated by walls to ensure proper isolation from the nitrogen sources and with visible access to the interior (via a window or camera). The cryostorage units should be continuously monitored and equipped with alarm systems detecting any out of range temperature and/or levels of liquid nitrogen

(LN). All the staff dealing with LN should be trained in safety aspects of its use, and protection devices as glasses, cryogloves, etc. should be used during LN handling. The PGD laboratory, if any, should be also in a separated isolated room. It should be provided with a safety fume hood for analysis using fixatives and other toxic reagents. In addition, its isolation is crucial to prevent contamination during the tubing processes.

Regarding the laboratory building, the walls and ceiling should have absolute minimum number of penetrations. The materials used in laboratory construction, painting, flooring and furniture should be appropriate for clean room standards, minimizing volatile organic compounds (VOCs) release and embryo toxicity. The walls should reach the roof and be made of joint free stainless steel; covered with epoxy paint (no interior paint should contain materials like formaldehyde, acetaldehyde, benzene, etc.). Avoid false ceiling construction. Floor should be dust, crevices, and crack free. It should be covered with large marble tiles, or granite tiles; alternatively, with vitrified tiles. Bench surfaces should be resistant to acid, alkali, solvent and heat. Door will require seals and sweeps, and should be lockable. Another important issue is that electrical wearing should be concealed. Continuous power supply with power protection is essential. It is very important also to take into account that ducts and equipment must be laid out in such a way that routine and emergency maintenance and repair work can be performed outside the laboratory with minimum disruption.[5] Consideration should also be given to local health and safety requirements.

The location of storage areas and equipment, such as incubators, centrifuges and cryoequipment should be logically planned for efficiency and safety within each working area. It should have enough space to store LN cylinders and tanks, disposables, media, and other supplies. The laboratories design should ensure optimal workflow over minimal distances while handling reproductive cells during all treatment phases.

Laboratory designer must keep in mind that laboratory personnel has to work for long hours. It is essential to take into account aspects related to ergonomics, such as bench height, adjustable chairs, microscope eye height, efficient use of space and surfaces, sufficient air condition and the amount of daylight, all contribute to a working environment that minimizes distraction and fatigue.[4]

Laboratory Air Quality

During the in vitro culture of both gametes and embryos they are under a wide variety of artificial and stressful conditions such as temperature and light variations, or changes in the percentage of oxygen (O_2) or carbon dioxide (CO_2) that could ultimately affect their viability. In addition to that, they are exposed also to substances that circumstantially will be present in their environment such as dust particles, glass powder, plastic shavings, VOCs, and disinfectants. All those conditions that potentially may affect the development of gametes and embryos can be minimized by the laboratory transformation into white rooms.

The maintenance of cleanliness is an uncompromising issue in a white room. Air should be clean, free of dust, smoke, gases and microbes. For that purpose, the clinic and hence the laboratories should be located away from traffic, dust and fumes. The air supply in the laboratory should be equipped with filters, preferably high efficiency particulate air (HEPA) filters to minimize the airborne contamination, and VOC control.[4] To create a positive pressure is recommended also to minimize air contamination.

The access to the laboratories should be restricted to authorized personnel. All the individuals handling samples in the laboratory should change into clean clothes made up of cotton preferably, and wear slippers and nonpowdered gloves while working in the laboratory (and the rooms for changing clothes should be separate from the laboratory).[4]

A water source is also required for hand washing, ideally it should be located in a corner and deep enough to avoid splashing.[6]

As mentioned in the previous point, attention should be given to the operator comfort. In this sense, humidity and temperature should be completely controlled according to climate and seasonal variation. As a reference, the temperature of airflow within the laboratory should be around 20–24°C and at less than 40% relative humidity.

EQUIPMENT

A detailed layout and assessment of all laboratory furniture is essential prior to construction in order to reach the best space achievement and create a distribution as more comfortable and functional as possible. Equipment should be suitably located in the laboratory to allow accessibility and sequential utilization, thus minimizing the need for frequent movement of specimens or reagents.

A detailed list of equipment should be prepared out and checked against the planned location of each item, and should be of adequate capacity to meet workload requirement and easy to disinfect and keep clean to avoid contamination. Also an automatic emergency backup power system must be in place for all critical equipment.

All the equipment must be validated as fit for its purpose, and the performance verified by calibrated instruments. Equipment should be in good working condition at all times; for this purpose, periodic inspection and cleaning

Table 1: Parameters and verification frequency for the supervision of the laboratory equipment.

Equipment	*Type of external measurement*	*Measurement frequency*
Incubators	Carbon dioxide (CO_2) and Temperature	Daily
Heating surfaces	Temperature	Daily
Heating blocks	Temperature	Daily
Freezers and refrigerators	Temperature	Daily
Automatic pipettes	Volume	Annual
Cryotanks	Temperature	Daily

should be done (the frequency will depend on the type of equipment); also a calibration check for all equipment using reference standards or reference material (Table 1). In fact, all the tasks related to equipment validation, calibration, maintenance and repair must be documented and records retained. Accepted ranges of use for all measured parameters should be determined and recorded. If measurements are out of range, corrections should be made and their effectiveness verified.[4]

For every item of equipment, the instruction manual and simplified instructions where needed, should be available. Laboratories should have necessary instructions for operation and maintenance of equipment in the form of standard operating procedures (SOPs) that should include also troubleshooting measures to be adopted for preventing equipment malfunction. In this sense, a copy of SOP should be readily available for the staff.[7]

Incubators

The incubator number is critical and should be based on the number of cycles and embryo culture duration. As a general rule, gametes, and embryos should be conveniently distributed across incubators to minimize door openings, hence to maintain stable culture conditions.

- *Working incubators:* Adjusted to 35–37°C and 5–6% CO_2; to be used for the storage of bicarbonate-based media and as working incubators when handling gametes and embryos. The number will depend on the workload but it is advisable to have at least one in the IVF laboratory, one in the cryoroom and one in the andrology laboratory. There is a high variety of models available in the market, i.e. Penguin from Astec, Heracell from Thermo Fisher Scientific™, LabX from Sanyo, Cell Culture™ from ESCO, Galaxy from Eppendorf, etc.
- *Culture incubators:* Adjusted to 35–37°C and 5–6% CO_2 or those designed to work in hypoxia at 6%; to be used for the culture of gametes and embryos. Any of the previous mentioned could be used for this purpose but there are other incubators with different characteristics that could be included in this group. Those adjusted to low-oxygen culture conditions could be either because of the Tri-gas use (i.e. MINC from COOK) or the N_2 use (miriESCO from ESCO) (Figs. 1A to F). There is another group of culture incubators that include time-lapse technology—the possibility of recording the development of the gametes or embryos. Part of them are devices to be included in regular incubators, hence the culture conditions (hypoxia or normoxia) will depend on the "external" incubator (i.e. Primo Vision™ from Vitrolife or Eeva from Auxogyn). The other type includes independent incubators with in-built cameras in which the culture conditions are autonomously decided (i.e. EmbryoScope from Vitrolife or Geri from Genea Biomedx).

Heating Devices

Those should be installed to maintain the temperature of media and reproductive cells during handling (Figs. 2A to D).

- *Laboratory ovens:* Adjusted to 35–37°C without CO_2 for liquefaction of semen samples and warming of buffered media and mineral oil (this can be used in both the IVF and andrology laboratories) (i.e. Thermo Scientific™ Precision™ from Thermo Fisher Scientific or the High Temperature Laboratory Oven from Bio Technics India).
- *Block heaters or dry bath incubators with heating blocks:* Adjusted to 35–37°C; to be used during the oocyte pick up (OPU) to maintain the temperature of the follicular fluid before the oocyte cumulus complex screening. Usually those are present inside the operating theater (OT) and in the pass box that ideally communicates it with the IVF laboratory (i.e. G73 Dry Bath Incubator from K-systems or the Tube Warmer from IVF Tech).

Gas Cylinders

Those should be located outside of the laboratory. There should be an automatic change-over system and sufficient cylinders stocked for immediate replacement. High-purity gas and inline HEPA and VOC filters are highly recommended.

Microscopes and Stereomicroscopes

- Binocular phase contrast microscope with 20x, 40x, and 100x objectives and 10x eyepiece for the andrology laboratory (semen analysis—sperm count, motility, and morphology). Oil immersion lens should be available,

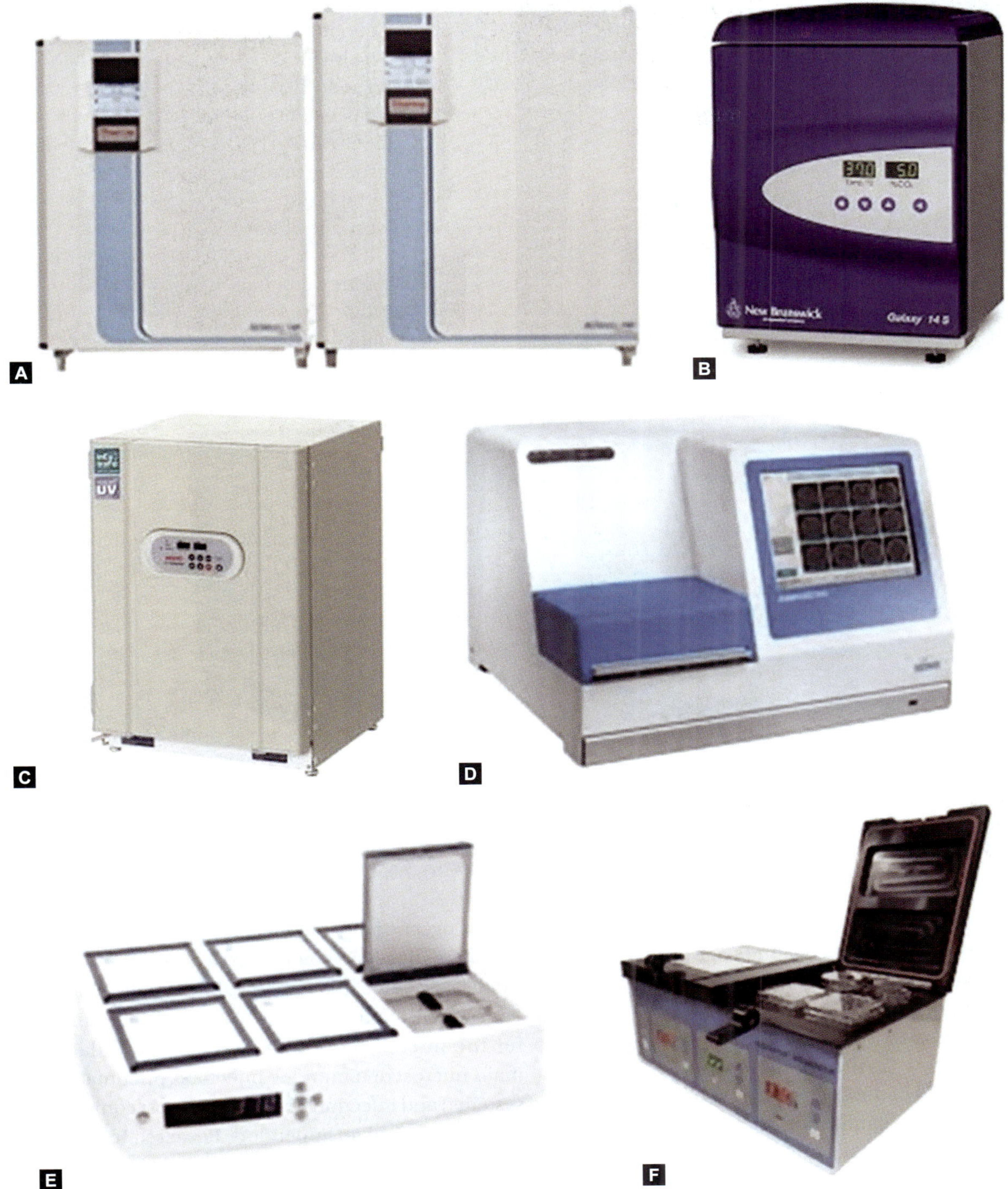

Figs. 1A to F: Different types of incubators used in an assisted reproductive technology laboratory. (A) Heracell from Thermo Fisher Scientific; (B) Galaxy from Eppendorf; (C) LabX from Sanyo; (D) EmbryoScope from Vitrolife; (E) MiriESCO from ESCO; and (F) MINC from COOK.

and if possible, also photography or video camera attached if training is desired, i.e. Olympus CX21 or Nikon Eclipse E200

- Inverted microscope with 4x, 10x, 20x, and 40x objectives and heating stage for the IVF laboratory (for oocyte and embryo assessment, microinjection and biopsy), i.e.

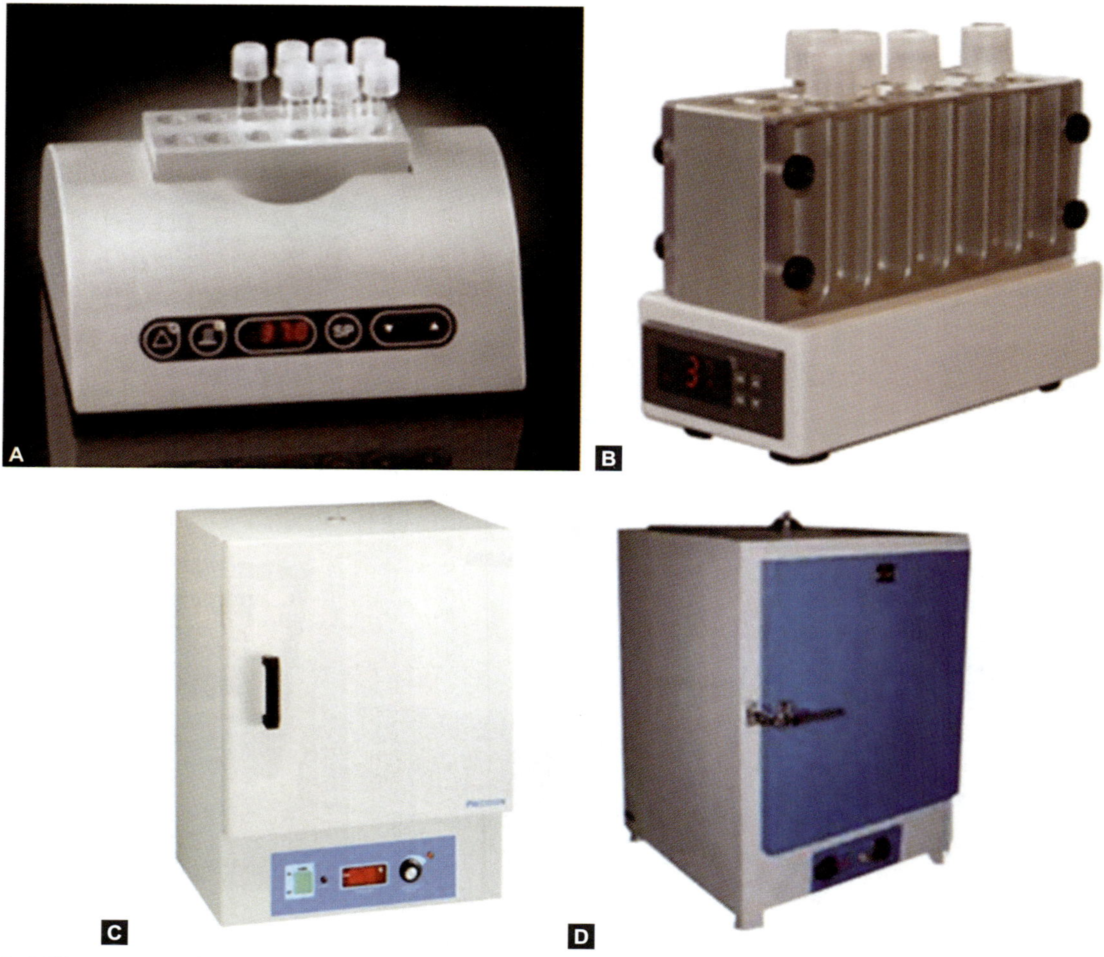

Figs. 2A to D: Different types of heating devices used in an assisted reproductive technology (ART) laboratory. (A) G73 Dry Bath Incubator from K-systems; (B) Tube Warmer from IVF Tech; (C) Thermo Scientific™ PrecisionTM from Thermo Fisher Scientific; and (D) High Temperature Laboratory Oven from Bio Technics India.

Eclipse Ti-U from Nikon or IX73 from Olympus (Figs. 3A to D). It is required to add a heating stage to maintain the temperature constant at 35–37°C (i.e. glass or metallic Tokai heating stage)

- *Stereomicroscopes:* These have to be installed in the laminar air flow (LAF) hoods of the IVF and PGD laboratories and in the cryoroom to handle the oocytes or embryos. The magnification and other specifications will depend on the laboratory designer discretion. There are different models available in the market as for example SZX10, SZ61 from Olympus or SMZ-745T, SMZ-1270 from Nikon.

Injection System

The injection system has to be installed in the inverted microscope and it is highly recommended placing the whole station over an antivibration table to provide stability during the microinjection or biopsy procedures. There are different models available in the market but mainly all consist into: Four-axis Hanging Joystick Micromanipulators, adaptor for the microscope (usually they are available for the main microscope brands), injectors (pneumatic/air or oil systems) and injection holders. The most common systems are from Narishige, Eppendorf, Research Instrument (RI), etc. (Fig. 4).

If PGD procedures are performed in the IVF laboratory, the micromanipulation system will require the attachment of a laser for the embryo biopsy. Basically laser systems can be fixed or portable. There are different fixed systems, being the most commonly used Laser Shot or NaviLase from Octax, regarding portable laser probably the most commonly used is the one from Hamilton Thorne.

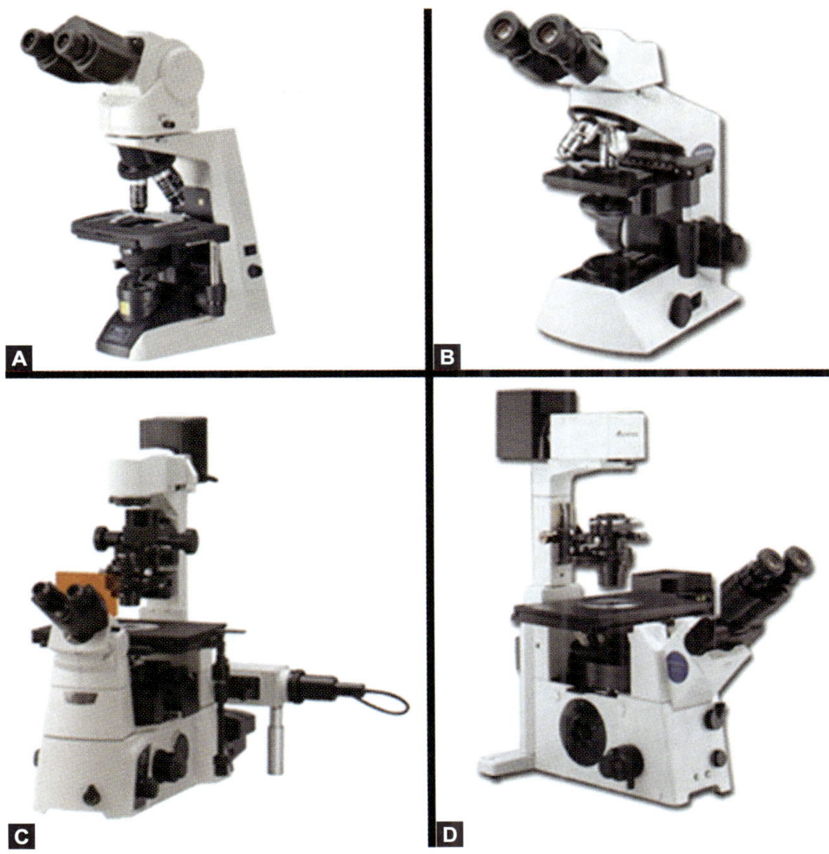

Figs. 3A to D: Different types of microscopes used in an assisted reproductive technology (ART) laboratory. (A) Nikon Eclipse E200; (B) Olympus CX21; (C) Eclipse Ti-U from Nikon; and (D) IX73 from Olympus.

Laminar Air Flow Hoods

A laminar flow hood is recommended. The hood reduces contamination of the samples as well as offering protection to laboratory personnel. A laminar flow hood can be either a vertical or a horizontal flow. Vertical flow is less harmful to the laboratory workers as the airflow is not directly aimed at their faces. On the other hand, a horizontal flow is more effective in reducing contamination. In any case, they should include HEPA filters to provide a particle free work environment and should have a heated stage to maintain the temperature of the samples handled constant at 37°C. The only LAF hoods that do not need to be with heated stage are those destined to vitrification or thawing procedures, media preparation and tubing after embryo biopsy. The desired stereomicroscopes have to be built-in as under them will happen the manipulation of samples (Figs. 5A to C).

Fridges and Freezers

Laboratory refrigerators and freezers are generally used for storing culture and buffer media, and nonvolatile biological specimens with temperature ranges from +2°C to +15°C (in case of refrigerators) and from –10°C to –40°C (in case of freezers).

Nitrogen Tanks

There are several items related with the cryopreservation procedures that should be present in both the cryopreservation area of the IVF laboratory and the andrology laboratory.

- *Liquid nitrogen storage containers:* Specific tanks to storage the nitrogen in liquid phase for the vitrification procedures. There are different brands and sizes available (depending on the nitrogen volume to storage), and can be complemented with semi-automatic or manual bombs and dispensers
- *Frozen sample containers:* Specific tanks to store the samples once frozen or vitrified. There are containers in which the samples are stored in LN and others (called dry containers) in which they are immersed in nitrogen in vapor phase. The choice should be based on each laboratory necessities, capacities, and expected use. It is strongly advised to provide each tank with a nitrogen level or temperature sensor. The first one measures the level of nitrogen and the alarm is activated when the level

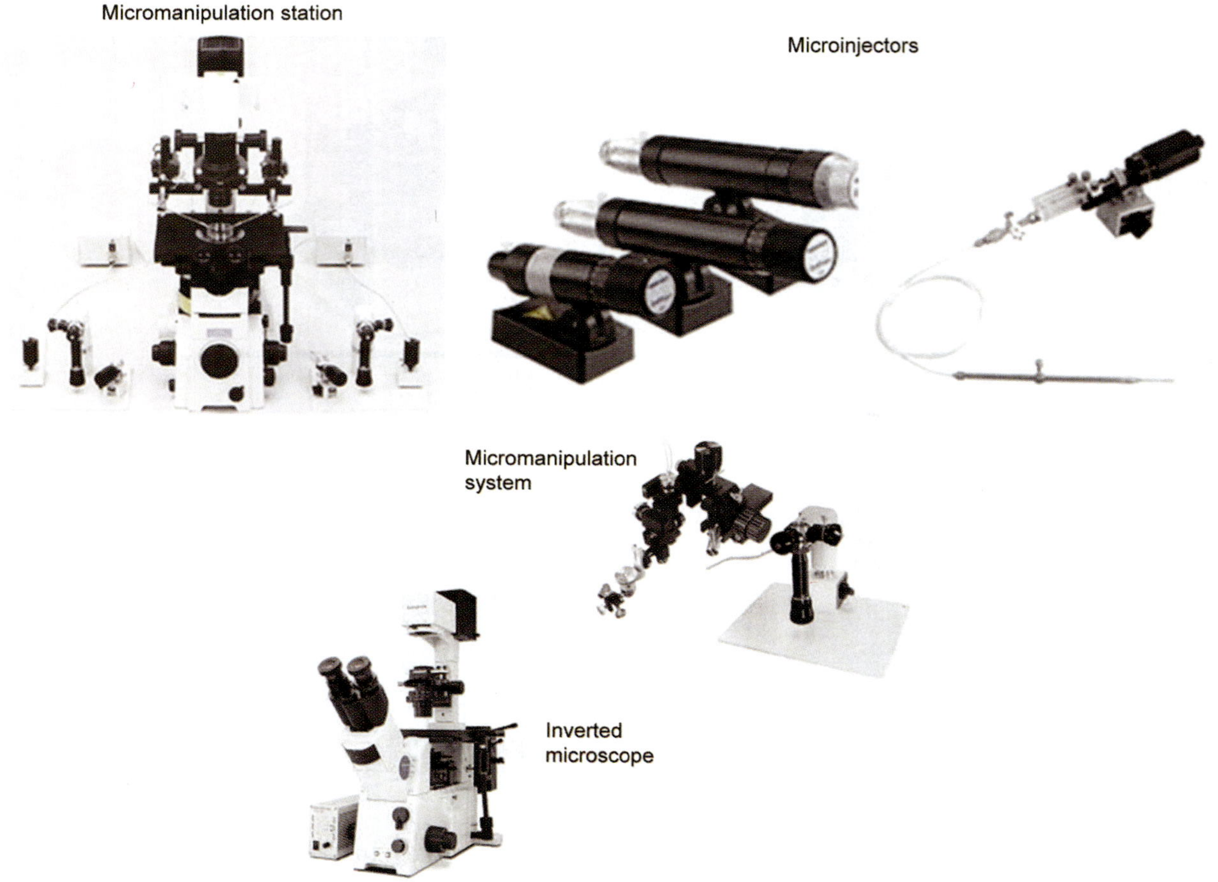

Fig. 4: Different components of a micromanipulation station.

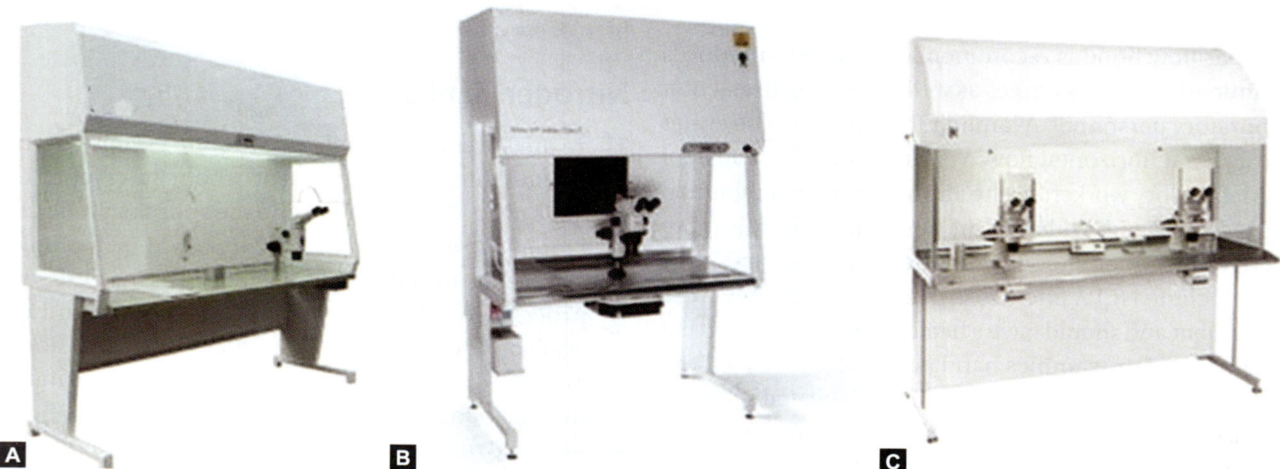

Figs. 5A to C: Different types of laminar air flow (LAF) hoods available in the market. (A) IVF Tech Sterile Cabinet, from IVF Tech; (B) Fortuna Clean Air from Origio; and (C) L125 IVF workstation from K-systems.

decreases below a certain preset level; the temperature sensor detects the decrease of temperature below a certain preset level also so ultimately both ensure the triggering of the alarm when the samples are under risk

- *Oxygen alarm:* The physical properties of the nitrogen in vapor phase facilitate the removal of the oxygen present in the environment, so an alarm system is strongly recommended to avoid accidents

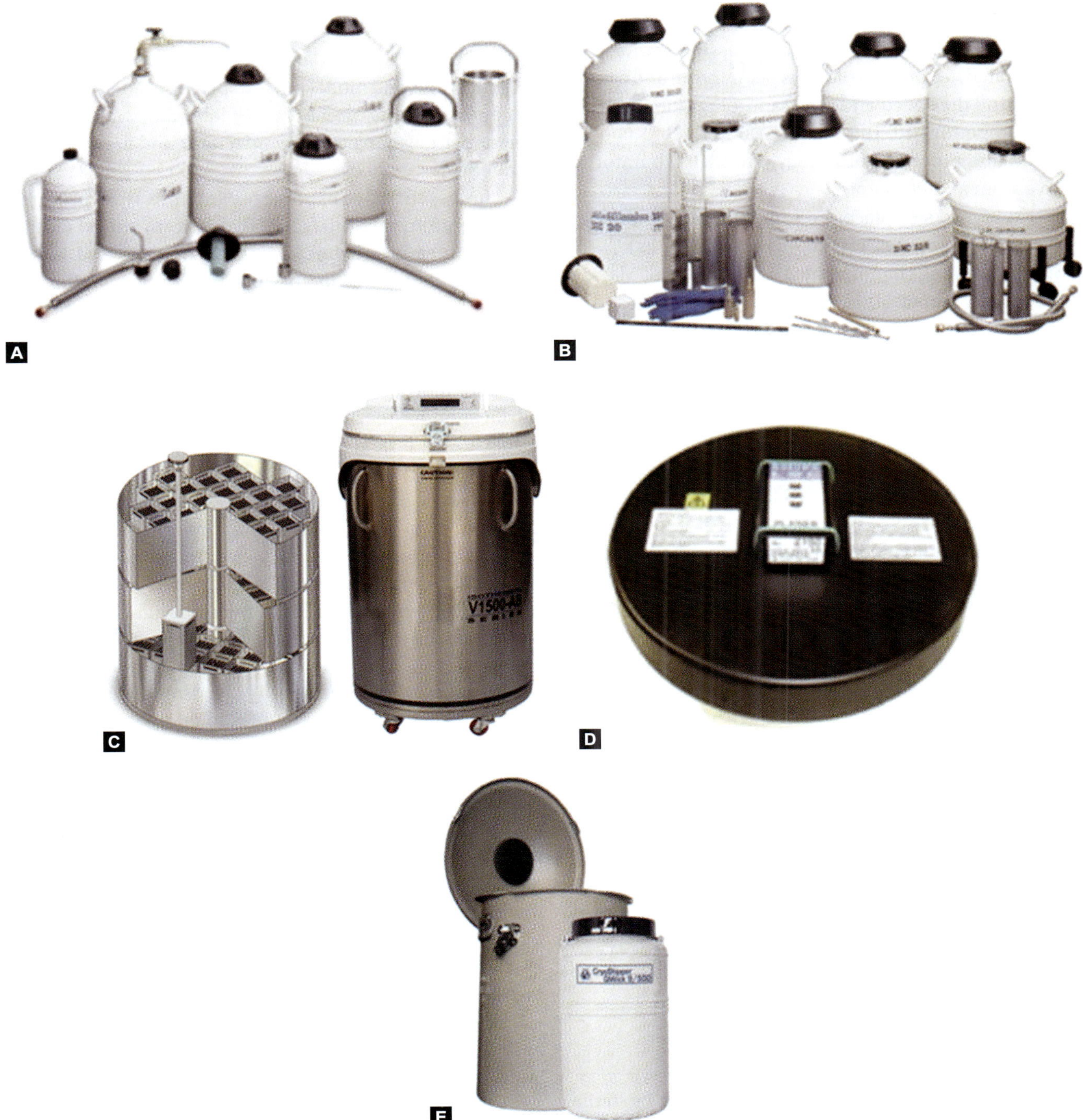

Figs. 6A to E: Different items available for a cryopreservation unit. (A) Liquid Nitrogen Storage Dewars, from LabIVF; (B) Cryogenic Dewars for storing samples from LabIVF; (C) Isothermal Straw Freezer, from Custom BioGenic systems; (D) Data Logger for Vapor Shipper, from LabIVF; and (E) MVE CryoShipper QWick, from LabIVF.

- *Shippers:* It is very frequent to send and receive frozen or vitrified samples from other clinics or banks, so every unit should have at least one shipper (vapor nitrogen is the best option). It is advisable also to provide the shipper with a data logger to record the temperature variations during the shipment and ensure that they have been properly maintained (Figs. 6A to E).

Small Items

- A bench centrifuge for sperm processing with a rotor (calibrated in g or in revolutions per minute) and a timer, to control the speed and time (andrology laboratory)
- Micropipettors 10–100 µL, 20–200 µL, 100–1,000 µL, automatic pipettor (andrology, and IVF laboratories, cryoroom and PGD units)
- Test tube racks to place the sample tubes (andrology, and IVF laboratories, cryoroom and PGD units)
- Sperm counting chamber, such as Neubauer or Mackler (andrology laboratory)
- Spirit burners (andrology and IVF laboratories)
- Laboratory counter, to make easier the counting of the semen samples moreover in laboratories with a large volume of work (andrology laboratory)
- Calculator
- Thermometers for both incubators or heater and fridges or freezer (andrology, and IVF laboratories, cryoroom and PGD units)
- *Timer:* It is used for control the time incubation of the sample, indicating the end of the processing. It is used also during the freezing or vitrification procedures (andrology laboratory and cryoroom)
- Protective gloves and glasses for the nitrogen related activities (cryoroom and andrology laboratory)
- Dustbins for the safe disposal of biological and laboratory materials; they can be recipients made of paperboard, plastic sharped containers or waste plastic bags, always with the international "biohazard" symbol. If possible, glassware should be omitted in the laboratory, otherwise the Pasteur pipettes and broken glassware should be discarded in special containers (andrology, and IVF laboratories, cryoroom and PGD units)
- Computer, preferably networked, to introduce all the date referred to the patient's sample.[5,6,8]

CONSUMABLES AND MEDIA

In the laboratory, all supplies and materials should be sterile single-use and disposable, and must be tested also by the supplier as being nontoxic to gametes and embryos. This aspect is fundamental to prevent contamination and makes the whole process as safe as possible minimizing the risks. If appropriate quality control testing for IVF purposes is not provided, this must be performed by the laboratory itself or by a designated company. In addition, packaging integrity and appropriate delivery conditions must be checked. Documentation of quality control testing must be supplied for any commercial media and this must correspond with the delivered batch.[4]

Most consumables and media have more than one manufacturer and model but the specific branch to be used depends on costs, preference of laboratory and medical personnel, location of the manufacturer, and the availability of after-sales service.

The essential consumables include tips, pipettes, round bottom test tubes, conical bottom tubes, culture dishes, injection dishes, injection, holding and biopsy pipettes, denudation tips, pH test paper, slides and coverslips, intrauterine insemination (IUI) catheters, embryo transfer (ET) catheters, OPU needles, BD syringes and semen containers; also stains and jars to stain the slides for morphology assessment. Specific disposables for vitrification or freezing procedures have to be considered also. Gloves to be used in the IVF unit should ideally be powder-free.

With respect to media, the best option for IVF laboratories is to purchase buffer solutions and media that are sterile and already cell culture tested. Today it is uncommon for each laboratory prepares their own media, as the commercial ones offer all the necessary guarantees and are optimized to the maximum. These are easily available, nontoxic, tested for quality control and have consistent performance. The commonly used media are simple balanced salt solutions or complex solutions supplemented with proteins, vitamins, glucose and antibiotics, but can be supplemented with two different types of buffer. It can be supplemented with 4-(2-hydroxyethyl)-1-piperazineethanesulfonic acid (HEPES) buffer (when exposed to atmosphere, it maintains the pH between 7.2 and 7.4, so these media do not require CO_2 incubation to maintain pH) or bicarbonate buffer (it requires a 5% CO_2 atmosphere to maintain the pH between 7.2 and 7.4).[6]

Cryopreservation requires a ready supply of LN and its own special supplies and media.

The size of the bottles and other packaging must be appropriate to minimize openings and time between first and last use.[4]

Appropriate refrigeration facilities must be available for storage of media and reagents. The correct temperature during their shipment to the clinic should be verified. Repeated shifts of temperature should be avoided while handling in the laboratory.[4]

An appropriate stock management system for media, oil and consumables, including the batch number, date of entry and expiration date should be available.[4] Each batch of culture media should be tested before use for osmolarity. Media pH testing should be performed following

Table 2: Recommended staff according to volume.

Number of cycles	*Minimum number of embryologists*
1–150	2
151–300	3
301–600	4
>600	1 additional embryologist per additional 200 cycles

equilibration with CO_2 at concentrations used for ART procedures. All lots of media and media components should be recorded and traceable to each patient procedure.[9]

Reagents, media and consumables should always be used prior to the manufacturer's expiry date.[4]

PERSONNEL MANAGEMENT

Personnel are one of the most important parts of an IVF laboratory. Staff resources shall be adequate to carry out all the procedures and functions in the laboratory according to the level of facility and the workload. The ESHRE recommends that clinics that perform up to 150 retrievals and/or cryopreservation cycles per year should have always a minimum number of two qualified clinical embryologists. This initial number will increase depending not only on the number of treatments, but also on the complexity of the procedures, techniques and tasks undertaken within the laboratory. Other duties such as administration, training, education, quality management and communication also need consideration.[4] The American Society for Reproductive Medicine (ASRM) coincides on the same ratios: always a minimum of two qualified clinical embryologists and increasing according to the number of cycles (Table 2).[9]

Appropriate human resources should provide an adequate climate to perform all laboratory tasks in a timely manner, to ensure patient safety and quality care. Sufficient qualified personnel should be available to provide backup for the laboratory staff.[4]

The hierarchical laboratory organization depends on staff size (larger facilities will need to delegate responsibilities to different levels). A person with officially recognized qualifications and expertise in clinical embryology and biological or medical sciences should direct the laboratory. According to the Guidelines for Good Clinical Laboratory Practices (GCLP) from the Indian Council of Medical Research (ICMR) each laboratory should designate a Head of the laboratory who should be overall incharge of the daily functioning of the laboratory including administration.[7] A quality manager should be designated for monitoring and maintaining of day-to-day quality management system (QMS). This laboratory manager shall have an organizational plan, personnel policies and job descriptions to define responsibility and authority of all personnel. Clinical embryologists represent the first line of participation in daily clinical practice. Their responsibilities include execution of SOPs, participation in daily practice, communication and organization, contribution to laboratory clinical decisions and training of staff members and students.[4]

A program for technical training and updating of skills on a regular basis should be in place. Laboratory management should be committed for providing continuing professional development and training opportunities to staff. Action plan for improvement in the laboratory should be determined and revised according to the feedback received from previous trainings and experiences, as reflected in the International Organization for Standardization (ISO) 15189:2007 and document 112 of National Accreditation Board for Testing and Calibration Laboratories (NABL).[2]

Qualification level and experience required of the staff are also specified in the latter document.

The roles and responsibilities of the staff should be also clearly outlined, even more, policies defining the competency of each person to perform tasks such as using the computer system, access to patient data, enter and charge patient results or correct billing shall be established. However, all personnel shall maintain confidentiality of information and data regarding patients.

Laboratory should organize or conduct periodic staff evaluation, preferably, once a year, but the frequency and method of evaluation should be decided by the laboratory.

LABORATORY SAFETY AND INFECTION CONTROL

As a general rule, procedures and policies on laboratory safety must be available to all laboratory personnel and should be reviewed annually by the laboratory director. The following guidelines are recommended:

- All patient worksheets should have clear patient identifying information as well as laboratory accession numbers that uniquely identify the patient during related procedures. All disposable material used during the preparation of the sample should be properly labeled or identified.
- Disposable, and nontoxic (nonpowdered) gloves should be worn when handling fresh or frozen semen samples or any material that has come in contact with them. Gloves should be removed and discarded when leaving the laboratory or handling the telephone. Gloves should never be reused.

- Hands should be washed after removing gowns and gloves and immediately if they become contaminated with body fluids. All hand washing should be done with disinfectant soap and hot water or alcohol-based solutions.
- A laboratory coat or appropriate gown should be worn in the laboratory and removed upon leaving the laboratory.
- Safety glasses or goggles are suggested where appropriated.
- Disposable laboratory supplies must be used whenever possible.
- All discarded body fluid samples and disposable laboratory supplies should be disposed off properly in a container marked "biological hazard" and disposed off accordingly.
- Protocols should be available for fire and electrical safety and internal and external disaster preparedness (including provisions for equipment backup in the event of equipment failure).
- Mechanical pipetting devices should be used for the manipulation of liquids in the laboratory. Mouth pipetting is never permitted.
- Eating, drinking, and smoking are not permitted in the laboratory.
- Use of cosmetics should be minimized and perfumes should be avoided.

Infectious Agents

All ARTs involve handling of biological material, and pose a potential hazard of transmitting diseases to personnel and to other patient's biological material (cross-contamination).

- Vaccination of all personnel against hepatitis B or other viral diseases, for which vaccine is available, is recommended.
- All patients must be screened for infectious diseases according to national and international regulations.
- Staff must be informed when a viral-positive patient is to be treated and be aware of the risks of handling infected biological material.
- Extraordinary precautions should be taken to avoid accidental wounds from sharp instruments contaminated with body fluids. Accident/incident/injuries record of laboratory personnel should be maintained and reported to the designated authority. The report should include description of the event, factors contributing to the event and information on first aid or other health care provided. This information can be analyzed periodically toward effectively controlling and preventing future events.
- Contaminated laboratory equipment and/or work surfaces should be disinfected and sterilized after a spill.[9]
- To ensure adequate safety measures, the treatment of viral-positive patients should be only performed in IVF laboratories with dedicated areas and equipment. Alternatively, such patient treatments could be allocated to specific time slots provided processing of their biological material is followed by a thorough disinfection of the allocated areas and equipment.

RECORD MAINTENANCE

Records may include but are not limited to request forms, report results, staff training, quality control records, audit records, examination procedures, instruments printout, interlaboratory comparison or management reviews and SOPs.

The laboratory shall establish and implement policies and procedures for identification, indexing, access, storage, and overall control of the registers. Records shall be legible and stored in a suitable environment to prevent damage, loss or unauthorized access but they should be retrievable in any moment.

The laboratory shall decide the retention time of records as per the national, regional and local regulations. However, NABL requires following minimum retention time for ensuring the quality service and patient care. The minimum period for retention of IUI related test reports issued shall be 1 year.[2]

QUALITY MANAGEMENT SYSTEM

Working in compliance with a QMS is mandatory and it is the mechanism to review the quality of all factors involved in laboratory functioning. It is recommended that a clinical embryologist is made responsible for quality management within the laboratory.

The requirements cover the organization, management personnel, equipment and materials, facilities or premises, documentation, records and quality review. This includes:

- Defining responsibilities and ensuring all personnel are qualified and competent.
- Having validated, and written instructions for each process (SOP) in order to optimize outcomes, including management of adverse events. The laboratory director or designated supervisory personnel should review and update all procedures on at least an annual basis. Any changes must be approved, signed, and dated by the laboratory director or by designated proxy.

- Ensuring full traceability of cells and tissues, materials, equipment and personnel involved in specific laboratory activities, with records maintained accordingly.
- Ensuring proper and periodic equipment maintenance, service and calibration. It should include aspects referred to equipment maintenance and calibration, validation and documentation of new protocols, vendor certification of media batch, safety laboratory procedures and record maintenance. Moreover, a written procedure manual must be readily available and followed by laboratory personnel.
- Taking corrective action to keep procedures under conformity.
- All relevant data concerning laboratory work must be recorded in a database that allows key performance indicator (KPI) extraction and statistical analysis. Corrections, either written or electronic, should be traceable. Data should include:
  - Morphological characteristics of gamete and embryos.
  - Detailed information of the procedures, including timing and staff involved.
  - All information needed to comply with the requirements of national and international data registries.
  - Every relevant communication with the patients should be recorded in the patient's files or in the informatics system.
- Key performance indicators should be objective and relevant, regularly checked and discussed, and communicated to all staff. For each indicator incorporated, a threshold needs to be established for setting the critical level of quality laboratory performance. These markers may concern a wide variety of parameters such as technical aspects of the laboratory (e.g. temperature of working surfaces, percentage of CO_2 in incubators or pH in culture media) or clinical variables (e.g. concerning percentage of progressive motile spermatozoa recovered per sample or gestational rates by group of analysis).
- In addition to laboratory and clinical performance, operator performance should be checked regularly to ensure competence, compliance and consistency, via direct observation of procedural skills (DOPSs) and/or individual KPIs. If necessary, retraining should be implemented.
- Participation in internal quality control (IQC) and external quality assurance (EQA) programs, either commercial or in collaboration with other laboratories, is highly recommended. IQC records should be maintained and reviewed, including documentation of results and any corrective action.
- An audit system, both internal and external, must be in place. An independent, competent auditor should verify compliance of all procedures with SOPs and requirements. Any findings, corrective actions and their effectiveness must be documented.[2,4]

CONCLUSION

The important components that make a laboratory great are the people, procedure, equipment and the laboratory design. All those aspects are fundamental to providing a service catalogued as excellent to fullfill patients' expectations.

REFERENCES

1. Pai RD. Pai's Textbook of Intrauterine Insemination. New Delhi: Jaypee Brothers Medical Publishers (P) Ltd; 2011. pp. 39-54.
2. National Accreditation Board for Testing and Calibration Laboratories (NABL). Specific Criteria for Accreditation of Medical Laboratories., 2012 [online] Available from www.nabl-india.org/nabl/file_download.php?filename=201210170522-NABL-112-doc.pdf. [Accessed March, 2017].
3. Gianaroli L, Plachot M, van Kooij R, et al. ESHRE guidelines for good practice in IVF laboratories. Committee of the Special Interest Group on Embryology of the European Society of Human Reproduction and Embryology. Hum Reprod. 2000;15(10):2241-6.
4. De los Santos MJ, Apter S, Coticchio G, et al. Revised guidelines for good practice in IVF laboratories (2015). The ESHRE Guideline Group on Good Practice in IVF Labs. Hum Reprod. 2016;31(4):685-6.
5. Mahmud N, Malhotra N, Malhotra J. Manual on IUI. What, When and Why. New Delhi: Jaypee Brothers Medical Publishers (P) Ltd; 2013. pp. 12-23.
6. Mukherjee GG, Chakravarty BN. Intrauterine Insemination. New Delhi: Jaypee Brothers Medical Publishers (P) Ltd; 2012. pp. 62-75.
7. Indian Council of Medical Research (ICMR). Guidelines for Good Clinical Laboratory Practices (GCLP), 2008. [online] Available from www.icmr.nic.in/ guidelines/GCLP.pdf [Accessed March, 2017].
8. Mukherjee GG, Chakravarty BN. Intrauterine insemination. In: Shah R (Ed). Infertility Management Series. New Delhi: Jaypee Brothers Medical Publishers (P) Ltd; 2015. pp. 115-34.
9. Practice Committee of American Society for Reproductive Medicine, Practice Committee of Society for Assisted Reproductive Technology. Revised guidelines for human embryology and andrology laboratories. Fertil Steril. 2008;90 (5 Suppl):S45-59.

CHAPTER

66

Future Perspectives: Developing Gametes from Stem Cells

José V Medrano, Carlos Simón

INTRODUCTION

Regenerative medicine is an emerging multidisciplinary field that comprises knowledge from cellular biology, developmental biology, genetics, molecular biology and tissue engineering, aiming to the study of stem cells and their potential clinical application to regenerate tissues and organs.

Among the multiple translational applications of regenerative medicine, the study of stem cells for their use in reproductive medicine has achieved significant progress in the last years. In particular, the use of animal models for the study of germ cell development, together with a significant improvement of current knowledge of human germ cell biology, recently achieved thanks to the access to early human embryos for research purposes, has allowed an important step forward in the possibility of obtaining human functional gametes from different cell sources that convert this promise in a reality that is closer than ever (Flowchart 1).

Here, we will discuss the different approaches and applications that regenerative medicine is currently developing in order to offer a solution to infertile patients aiming to have genetically matched children.

PLURIPOTENT STEM CELLS (ESCs AND iPSCs) AS A SOURCE OF HUMAN FUNCTIONAL GAMETES

The potential use of mouse embryonic stem cells (mESCs) as a source of gametes was first reported in 2003 when some oocyte-like structures able to achieve parthenogenetic activation and form pseudoblastocysts were spontaneously formed upon culture of mESCs without feeders nor leukemia inhibitory factor (LIF).[1] Upon this first probe of concept, a variety of strategies have been reported to achieve the formation of both male and female gametes from mESCs and induced pluripotent stem cells (iPSCs) with disparaging results.[2-7]

However, the real functionality of these in vitro generated gametes was not demonstrated until very recently when a Japanese group achieved for the first time the generation of viable offspring from sperm and oocytes derived from mESCs and iPSCs.[8,9] In their experiments, authors based in the unique potential of epiblastic cells to give rise to primordial germ cells (PGCs) in response to bone morphogenetic proteins 4 (BMPs4) and BMP8b secreted from the adjacent extraembryonic ectoderm (ExE) at embryonic day 6.25 (E6.25) in vivo.[10,11] Based on this, they designed an in vitro induction protocol to induce naive mESCs and iPSCs cultured in 2i + LIF conditions into epiblast-like cells (EpiLCs) resembling their in vivo counterparts by treating them with activin A and basic fibroblast growth factor (bFGF). Subsequently, in a second induction step, EpiLCs were exposed to LIF, stem cell factor (SCF), epidermal growth factor (EGF) and BMP4 or 8b to trigger the acquisition of a PGC-like cell (PGCLC). Resulting PGCLCs showed a phenotype resembling in vivo mouse PGCs, including the expression of key PGC markers, but also signs of epigenetic reprogramming including genome-wide demethylation, loss of H3K9me2 and gain of H3K27me3, as their in vivo counterparts. Moreover, PGCLCs were able to differentiate either into sperm or germinal vesicle oocytes when transplanted into the mouse testicular lumen or under the ovarian bursa in reconstituted mouse ovaries that produced healthy and fertile offspring

Flowchart 1: Schematic diagram of the circuitry of different approaches that regenerative medicine offers for the development of gametes.

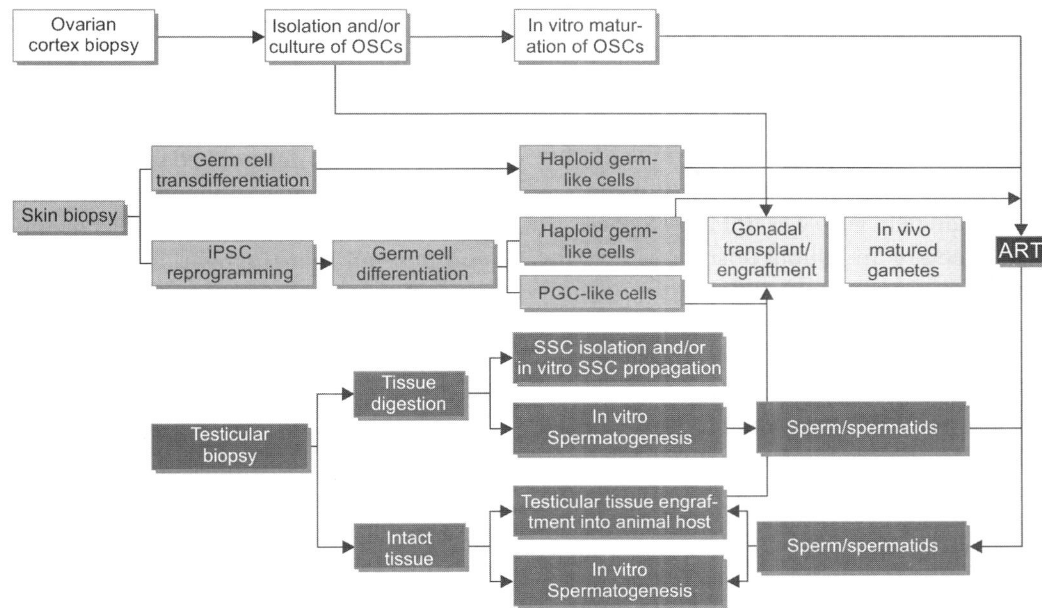

(ART: Assisted reproductive technology; iPSC: induced pluripotent stem cell; OSCs: ovarian stem cells; PGC: primordial germ cell; SSC: spermatogonial stem cell).

upon intracytoplasmic sperm injection (ICSI). These works were complemented by a third report of the same group showing that the ectopic expression of the key transcription factors downstream of BMP signaling Prdm1, Prdm14 and Tfap2c over preinduced mouse EpiLCs resulted also in a PGCLC phenotype that formed sperm and gave rise to healthy offspring after transplantation into mouse testes.[12] In summary, these three complementary reports demonstrated for the first time the possibility to create functional gametes from pluripotent cells. At the same time, they described the regulatory signaling network of mouse PGC specification, where Prdm1, Prdm14 and AP2g together constitute a transcriptional network necessary to enable the repression of somatic genes by Prdm1 and Prdm14 blocking of Hox enhancers, the expression of pluri-potency and PGC-specific genes (executed mainly by Prdm14 and AP2γ) and the induction of epigenetic reprogramming by Prdm14 and Prdm1 repression of the de novo deoxyribonucleic acid (DNA) methyltransferase Dnmt3b and its cofactor Uhrf1; at the same time Prdm14 recruits 10-11 topoisomerases TET1 and TET2 to activate active hydroxylation of 5-methylcytosines and induce methylation marks erasure.

Following this approach, an interesting report has recently demonstrated the BMP independent function of Nanog as a master regulator of PGCLC specification from EpiLCs in vitro.[13] In this study, ectopic expression of Nanog over EpiLCs resulted in the activation of Prdm1 and Prdm14 as well as the acquisition of a PGCLC phenotype in vitro. Thus, this new study highlighted the plasticity of PGC specification with the context-dependent role of a pluripotency-related transcription factor, such as Nanog, acting as a member of the core pluripotency network in mESCs and iPSCs, but inducing PGCLC formation in EpiLCs.

Although there exist several reports on differentiation of human pluripotent stem cells into germ cells using different approaches,[14-21] the success of the reports described earlier in the mouse model inspired another recent works that adopted a very similar approach on human ESCs (hESCs) and iPSCs, demonstrating its reliability.[22-24] With slight differences in the cocktails employed to induce a mesodermic epiblast state from hESCs and human iPSCs (hiPSCs), in all three studies authors achieved the formation of a human PGCLC (hPGCLC) phenotype upon exposure of preinduced cells to BMPs, LIF, SCF and EGF. With similar conclusions, these works highlighted the mesodermic origin of hPGCLCs based on the need of creating a mesodermic epiblast phenotype expressing T (Brachyury) for their efficient derivation. Also, resulting human PGCLCs from all three studies displayed several differences compared to the ones obtained in mouse, such as null activation of SOX2, a delayed expression of PRDM14 and an upregulation of SOX17 and GATA4. Results from one of the studies also concluded that in contrast with mouse PGC specification, SOX17 might play an essential role in human germ line specification by acting upstream and synergistically with BLIMP1 or PRDM1 as the master regulators of PGC specification, at the same time that BLIMP or PRDM1 acts as a repressor of the somatic program in human PGCLCs.[22] However, compared with mouse studies where PGCLCs were matured into functional gametes by transplanting them into mouse gonadal hosts, further maturation of human PGCLCs obtained in vitro was not investigated.

Related to the need of an animal host to achieve the complete maturation of human PGCLCs, it has recently been reported a new mouse study that based in the same approach has overcome this need and achieved the formation of functional gametes totally in vitro.[25] In this report, authors also followed the two-step induction of PGCLCs from EpiLCs. However, instead of transplanting them into a mouse gonad recipient, they used testicular somatic cells from KITW or KITW-V mice lacking germ cells to coculture with PGCLCs. After 2 weeks of PGCLC or testicular cells coculture with follicle-stimulating hormone (FSH), testosterone and bovine pituitary extract, around 14% of PGCLCs matured into spermatid-like haploid cells that were able to generate healthy offspring upon ICSI. This new achievement has supposed a new landmark since avoids totally the need of an animal host to generate gametes from pluripotent cells, offering an exceptional tool for the study of germ cell development and paves the way to its translation to humans.

Compared to the current knowledge of murine germ cell development, data regarding this process in humans has been scarce and based on classical histological studies.[26] However, the use of in vitro models of human germ cell derivation from pluripotent cells, together with very recent reports focused on the study of the germ cells development in early human embryos from a molecular point of view have supposed a new landmark.[27-29] Thanks to these last reports, now we have a better knowledge of the transcriptomic and epigenetic dynamics of human germ cells and indeed, the recent discovery of some evolutionary young transposable elements such as SINE-variable number of tandem repeats-Alu elements (SVAs) to resist epigenetic reprogramming of germ cell development in vivo opens new lines of study of the possibility of epigenetic inheritance with hPGCLCs obtained in vitro.[27]

MILLION-DOLLAR QUESTION: ARE THERE STEM CELLS IN THE HUMAN OVARY?

It is generally accepted that follicular regeneration occurs in most nonvertebrate animals[30] and in some vertebrates.[31] However, one of the central dogmas in reproductive medicine is that female mammals are born with a finite number of germ cells (follicular reserve) that decreases along individual's lifespan until become completely depleted at the start of menopause.[32] However, this view was questioned a few years ago when John Tilly's group at Harvard University postulated the existence of ovarian stem cells in postnatal mammalian ovaries.[33] After counting the amount of atretic follicles in mouse ovaries, Tilly's group hypothesized that the ovarian reserve should become depleted at a much faster rate than what actually occurs, suggesting the presence of some kind of germinal stem cells within mammalian ovaries that replace atretic follicles by neofolliculogenesis. In order to test this hypothesis, ovarian fragments from wild-type mice were transplanted into the ovarian bursal cavity of transgenic green fluorescent protein (GFP) mice, resulting in the appearance of newly formed chimeric follicles with GFP positive oocytes surrounded by non-GFP expressing granulosa cells.[33] This first report on neofolliculogenesis caused great criticism since many argued against the methods employed to calculate follicle atresia and the ovarian graft results.[34,35]

In response to these criticisms, only 1 year later, based on the observation that stage-specific embryonic antigen-1 (SSEA-1) positive cells isolated from either disassociated mouse ovaries or bone marrow shared the expression of early germ line markers, Tilly's group suggested the bone marrow as the putative source of germ stem cells for adult neofolliculogenesis in mammals.[36] Supporting this idea, transplantations of both bone marrow and peripheral blood from GFP transgenic mice into chemotherapy-ablated wild-type females resulted in the formation of new chimeric follicles with GFP-positive oocytes.

In response to the intense discussion derived to these reports,[37] a new study comprising parabiosis experiments in which the circulatory systems of wild-type and GFP transgenic female mice were joined for up to 6 months demonstrated the presence of some GFP-positive granulosa cells associated with ovulated oocytes in wild-type mice, but no evidence of GFP-positive oocytes derived from GFP donors in wild-type females. In contrast to Tilly's results, transplantation of bone marrow from a GFP donor into wild-type females treated with cyclophosphamide or busulfan also failed to demonstrate the presence of oocyte chimerism, suggesting that the recovery of ovulation in chemically sterilized mice could be explained by incomplete depletion of endogenous follicles by the alquilant drugs, whereas the presence of some GFP-positive cells within the granulosa cell layer could be a consequence of the infiltration of white cells from the GFP donor.

After the publication of several reports supporting[38-42] or arguing against[43-45] the neofolliculogenesis hypothesis in mammalian ovaries, a new report in 2009[46] established germ stem cell lines in vitro from mouse vasa homolog (Mvh)-positive cells isolated from mouse ovaries. In vitro cultured Mvh cells expressed pluripotency-associated markers as well as early germ cell markers. Since Mvh is a ribonucleic acid (RNA) helicase that localizes in the cytoplasm of all germ cells, the use of an antibody for Mvh to isolate germ cells based on its surface membrane localization generated scepticism about these results.

More recently, Tilly's group published a new report in 2012 describing a similar approach to isolate Mvh or VASA germ cells from both mouse and human ovaries and establish germ cell line cultures in vitro.[47] Additionally, this report also demonstrated the spontaneous formation of oocyte-like cells (OLCs) able to complete meiosis in ovarian germ cell cultures. As a functional assay, in vitro cultures were labeled with GFP and either transplanted into mouse ovaries or co-cultured with disassociated adult human cortical tissues and transplanted into immunosuppressed mice, resulting in the formation of GFP-positive oocytes that were able to form healthy embryos upon ICSI fertilization in the case of mouse oocytes. However, another recent report from a consortium of independent groups replicating the same experimental approach did not support the presence of VASA positive cells in the human ovary.[48]

With the exciting controversy upon the existence of neofolliculogenesis in the mammalian ovaries, some authors proposed an ovarian cell dedifferentiation process that, under specific in vitro conditions or stress may produce cells with certain potential to develop into germ-like cells in the same way as previously described for other cell types,[49-52] as one possible explanation for the existence of germinal stem cells in mammalian ovaries. Related to this hypothesis, some authors have even postulated a possible relationship between the existence of stem cells in the ovarian surface epithelium (OSE) and the origin of ovarian cancer of epithelial cells.[53] Alternatively, others also propose the presence of very small embryonic-like (VSEL) stem cells resident in the ovaries which have the potential to differentiate into both germ and somatic cells.[54]

Besides the great interests on demonstrating the existence of germ stem cells in the mammalian ovary that may lead to neofolliculogenesis and thus the design of strategies to restore the fertility of infertile women without follicular reserve, as can be the case of patients suffering premature follicular reserve depletion due to cancer treatments, their existence is not fully supported and further research is needed in order to solve this scientific debate. Nevertheless, with independence of the existence of stem cells in the ovary, other methods for fertility preservation, such as oocyte or embryo vitrification currently offered to this kind of patients is a worldwide employed technique with excellent results. Alternatively, in prepubertal patients or patients without possibility of obtaining oocytes before the initiation of their oncological treatment, ovarian cortex cryopreservation for its reimplantation after the disease has been overpassed is an experimental technique that has already probed its efficiency to restore fertility of oncological patients.[55]

SPERMATOGONIAL STEM CELLS: TAKING ADVANTAGE OF PLASTICITY OF SPERMATOGENESIS FOR FERTILITY PRESERVATION

Spermatogonial stem cells (SSCs) are the resident stem cells in the mammalian testes and the origin of the process of spermatogenesis during adult-hood. The SSC pool is comprised by a subset of spermatogonia attached to the basal layer of the seminiferous tubules.[56] SSCs were first described in 1994 by Brinster's laboratory using a murine germ cell transplant model, and were defined as "the spermatogonial subpopulation of spermatogenic stem cells with the ability to colonize the seminiferous epithelium and fully reconstitute spermatogenesis".[57,58]

Due to their ability to potentially restore full spermatogenesis, there is great interest in the study and use of SSCs as a tool for fertility restoration. Specifically, patients unable to generate sperm such as prepubertal boys in risk of acquired permanent azoospermia due to the gonadotoxic effect of oncologic treatments can be potential beneficiaries from biotechnology derived of the study of SSCs.[59] Indeed, having in mind the use of SSCs to restore spermatogenesis, based in the Oncofertility Consortium of North-western University database, there are currently more than 120 health centers around the world offering the cryopreservation of testicular biopsies to prepubertal oncological patients in risk of permanent azoospermia as a consequence of their oncologic treatment.[60-65]

Among the strategies designed to restore spermatogenesis in azoospermic patients, the SSC transplantation (SSCT) is probably the most interesting.[66,67] Described for the first time by Brinster's laboratory in mice, transplantation of testicular cell suspensions containing spermatogonial cells into the germ cell depleted seminiferous lumen of mice results in its colonization and fully restoration of spermatogenesis, producing sperm able to give rise to healthy offspring.[57,58] Moreover, this technique has been applied to other animal models including nonhuman primates with successful results.[68] However, despite these encouraging results, there are three main issues to solve before the use of SSCT in humans. First, since transplantation of human SSCs (hSSCs) into germ cell depleted mouse testes results in colonization of the seminiferous epithelium, but fails to restore spermatogenesis because of phylogenetic discrepancies,[69] there is a need for appropriate models for spermatogenic restoration in humans beyond the technical trials performed in human cadaveric testes.[70] Second, the lack of appropriate markers to isolate SSCs has hampered their study, leaving their ability to colonize mouse testes is the best approach to identify them. By using this approach as a read out, several surface markers, such as GFRA1,[71] CD9,[72] fibroblast growth factor receptor 3 (FGFR3),[73,74] epithelial cell adhesion molecule (EpCAM),75 integrin alpha 6 (ITGA6)[75-77] and THY-1,[76] as well as intracellular markers, such as PLZF, Sal-like protein 4 (SALL4), UTF1 and UCHL176 have been identified as putative hSSCs markers. The isolation of pure SSC populations is not only necessary for their study, but also as a technique to prevent the transplantation of malignant cells back into the testes of cancer survivors.[75] Finally, due to the limited size of testicular biopsies, in vitro propagation to increase the number of SSCs to transplant is a necessary step prior to perform SSCT in humans. However, although long-term in vitro propagation of mouse SSCs was first reported in 2003,[77] in vitro propagation of hSSCs[78,79] has been difficult to replicate.[80-83]

An alternative promising strategy to restore spermatogenesis is the testicular tissue grafting.[84] This approach consists of the engraftment of small pieces of immature (prepubertal) testicular tissue under the skin of immunosuppressed mice previously castrated in order to prevent the feedback inhibition of gonadotropins by their own testes. In this way, the host animals serve as bioreactors that activate spermatogenesis of engrafted tissue after few weeks, producing sperm that can be retrieved for ICSI and production of healthy offspring. As happened with the SSCT, this technique has also demonstrated its feasibility in other donor species, using always mice as hosts,[85,86] as well as slight improvement of results by modifying the engraftment in the scrotum[60] or even in intratesticular orthotopic grafts.[87] However, xenografts from other species with higher than average daily sperm production such as pig, goat and human donors show limited survival of the engrafted tissues and fibrosis probably due to insufficient vascularization causing ischemia.[60,61,85,88,89] Thus although data suggests that grafts from immature tissue show better resistance to ischemia due to the quiescent nature of tissue, so far human grafts designed to preserve spermatogenesis have not been able to develop beyond the spermatocyte stage,[61] highlighting once again that probably the mice are not the most appropriate hosts for human testicular grafts. Thus, despite its success in other animal models, this approach still needs further research to prevent ischemia of engrafted tissue as well as improvements to the technique to support full maturation of sperm cells before an eventual possible clinical application to produce functional human sperm in azoospermic patients.

In vitro spermatogenesis is a third approach that has gained interest in the last years as a possible source of sperm from SSCs. Despite the achievement of a recent report describing the production of haploid human spermatids able to fertilize mouse oocytes from SSCs obtained from cryptorchid patients and treated with SCF and retinoic acid (RA),[90] due to the three-dimensional (3D) structure of the spermatogenesis with several maturation stages of germ cells tightly dependent of sertoli cells regulation, most efficient strategies to achieve the production of sperm from mouse SSCs comprise 3D co-cultures of both somatic and immature germ cells.[91] In a similar way to these 3D models of in vitro spermatogenesis, in 2011 a Japanese group obtained for the first time sperm able to be used in ICSI in a model of mouse 3D testis tissue culture.[92,93] In their work, authors used immature testicular pieces from newborn mice carrying *GFP* gene expression under the control of the postmeiotic markers Gsg2 (haspin) and acrosin, and placed them in a liquid-gas interphase onto agarose rafts soaked in a medium containing knockout serum replacement that were placed at 34°C to mimic in vivo testicular conditions. After around 3 weeks, GFP spermatids and sperm were retrieved and used for ICSI, giving rise to healthy offspring. Although this technique has been reproduced in further reports,[94,95] no data regarding the feasibility of this technique with human tissue has been reported so far. However, the use of cytocompatible scaffolds from decellularized human testicular tissue may be an interesting approach to test the potential of hSSCs to mature in vitro.[96]

With an experience of more than 15 years of cryopreserving immature testicular biopsies from prepubertal patients, it seems a matter of time that the first reports on fertility restoration in azoospermic men appear.[97] However, even the success of different techniques of spermatogenesis restoration in animal models, as described earlier, there are still important issues to solve before the application of SSCs as a clinical cell therapy in the next years, making this possibility still an experimental procedure that should be offered only to patients with a high-risk of acquired azoospermia as the unique via to preserve their fertility.

ANSWER OF REGENERATIVE MEDICINE TO REPRODUCTIVE NEEDS: THE PROMISE MAY NOT BE SO FAR TO BE ACCOMPLISHED

Apart from the important advances of regenerative medicine about the potential use of stem cells as a source of functional gametes for human reproduction, their study itself has provided key insights for the better understanding of gamete-related diseases, as well as the design of new strategies to help patients affected by them.

Based on the expression of germ cell markers such as DAZL in hESCs, suggesting that this pluripotent stem cell stage could be formed by a heterogeneous population in which some cells may be primed toward a germ cell fate,[14] further investigation on the role of evolutionary conserved germ cell RNA-binding proteins such as the DAZL family[17,18] or VASA[21] suggested their role in the initiation of meiosis of in vitro differentiated germ cells from hESCs upon their exogenous expression. In the same line, another report demonstrated that DAZL may function in limiting pluripotency as well as differentiation to control apoptosis in PGCs through a robust interactive network. If this network is broken or DAZL expression is lost, the consequence is teratoma formation.[98] Moreover, by the employment of xenotransplantation of in vitro derived human germ cell-like cells into seminiferous tubules of immunosuppressed mice, one study demonstrated that ectopic expression of VASA in hiPSCs improved their colonization efficiency, highlighting the role that VASA plays in controlling the pluripotency state in a combined in vitro or in vivo model.[99] In the same line, recent reports have also designed a potential cell therapy for azoospermic men with microdeletions of the Y chromosome (AZFa), demonstrating the decreased ability of iPSCs derived from this kind of patients to colonize the seminiferous tubules of mice, and how the complementation via ectopic expression of DDX3Y can be a potential genetic therapy to rescue their ability to colonize this niche and form germ cell-like cells in vivo.[100,101] This same approach has also been used recently to demonstrate that germ cell-like cells can be formed in vivo independently of X chromosomes genetic profile.[102] In this case, hiPSCs from infertile Turner syndrome patients (46, XO) were derived and xenotransplanted into mice testes, resulting in proper colonization and demonstrating that the presence of a second X chromosome is not required for human germ cell formation, although is necessary for their maintenance until adulthood.

Finally, a recent study performed by our group opened a new interesting strategy for the obtention of human gametes by direct reprogramming of somatic cells.[103] Based in the success of direct transdifferentiation of somatic cells into other somatic cell fates,[104-108] human male somatic cells were directly transdifferentiated into a meiotic germ cell-like phenotype by the ectopic expression of PRDM1, PRDM14, LIN28A, DAZL, VASA and SYCP3 in vitro. Induced germ cell-like cells were able to colonize the seminiferous tubules of germ cell depleted mouse testes, showed their ability to form haploid cells and evidences of epigenetic reprograming toward an oocytelike expected epigenetic profile. Despite the low efficiency of the germ cell-like transdifferentiation, it can represent a step forward to the creation of human functional gametes and serve as an in vitro model to test the role of critical key factors in human germ cell development.

CONCLUSION

The study of germ cells is critical for our society not only because of their potential use in human reproduction but because they have the extremely important task of transmitting genetic and epigenetic information to the next generation. In summary, all the advances discussed earlier represent significant improvements to our current knowledge of germ cell biology. Those may have important implications in reproductive medicine from the point of view of the future clinical use of the in vitro obtained gametes, but also for the information that they provide about germ cell biology for the design of new strategies to offer to infertile patients. Ultimately, with the proper ethical precautions, the combination of the study of germ cells with the new molecular techniques of gene editing can even be the next scientific landmark for the eradication of genetic diseases, as demonstrated by some preliminary reports.[109-111]

Taking together, for the first time in recent history it seems that the promise of regenerative medicine as a tool for treating all kind of diseases, including reproductive diseases, may not be so far to be accomplished.

ACKNOWLEDGMENT

This work was supported by a private donation of the Villarreal CF to Hospital Universitario y Politécnico La Fe intended to promote the scientific research on fertility preservation in child with cancer.

AUTHOR CONTRIBUTIONS

José V Medrano and Carlos Simón conceived this work and José V Medrano wrote the manuscript.

REFERENCES

1. Hübner K, Fuhrmann G, Christenson LK, et al. Derivation of oocytes from mouse embryonic stem cells. Science. 2003;300(5623):1251-6.
2. Toyooka Y, Tsunekawa N, Akasu R, et al. Embryonic stem cells can form germ cells in vitro. Proc Natl Acad Sci U S A. 2003;100(20):11457-62.
3. Geijsen N, Horoschak M, Kim K, et al. Derivation of embryonic germ cells and male gametes from embryonic stem cells. Nature. 2004;427(6970):148-54.
4. Novak I, Lightfoot DA, Wang H, et al. Mouse embryonic stem cells form follicle-like ovarian structures but do not progress through meiosis. Stem Cells. 2006;24(8):1931-6.
5. West JA, Viswanathan SR, Yabuuchi A, et al. A role for Lin28 in primordial germ- cell development and germ-cell malignancy. Nature. 2009;460(7257):909-13.
6. Nicholas CR, Haston KM, Grewall AK, et al. Transplantation directs oocyte maturation from embryonic stem cells and provides a therapeutic strategy for female infertility. Hum Mol Genet. 2009;18(22):4376-89.
7. Hayashi K, Surani MA. Self-renewing epiblast stem cells exhibit continual delineation of germ cells with epigenetic reprogramming in vitro. Development. 2009;136(21):3549-56.
8. Hayashi K, Ohta H, Kurimoto K, et al. Reconstitution of the mouse germ cell specification pathway in culture by pluripotent stem cells. Cell. 2011;146(4): 519-32.
9. Hayashi K, Ogushi S, Kurimoto K, et al. Offspring from oocytes derived from in vitro primordial germ cell-like cells in mice. Science. 2012;338(6109):971-5.
10. Okamura D, Hayashi K, Matsui Y. Mouse epiblasts change responsiveness to BMP4 signal required for PGC formation through functions of extraembryonic ectoderm. Mol Reprod Dev. 2005;70(1):20-9.
11. Günesdogan U, Magnúsdóttir E, Surani MA. Primoridal germ cell specification: a context-dependent cellular differentiation event. Philos Trans R Soc Lond B Biol Sci. 2014;369(1657).
12. Nakaki F, Hayashi K, Ohta H, et al. Induction of mouse germ-cell fate by transcription factors in vitro. Nature. 2013;501(7466):222-6.
13. Murakami K, Günesdogan U, Zylicz JJ, et al. NANOG alone induces germ cells in primed epiblast in vitro by activation of enhancers. Nature. 2016;529(7586): 403-7.
14. Clark AT, Bodnar MS, Fox M, et al. Spontaneous differentiation of germ cells from human embryonic stem cells in vitro. Hum Mol Genet. 2004;13(7):727-39.
15. Kee K, Gonsalves JM, Clark AT, et al. Bone morphogenetic proteins induce germ cell differentiation from human embryonic stem cells. Stem Cells Dev. 2006;15 (6):831-7.
16. Tilgner K, Atkinson SP, Golebiewska A, et al. Isolation of primordial germ cells from differentiating human embryonic stem cells. Stem Cells. 2008;26(12): 3075-85.
17. Kee K, Angeles VT, Flores M, et al. Human DAZL, DAZ and BOULE genes modulate primordial germ-cell and haploid gamete formation. Nature. 2009;462 (7270):222-5.
18. Panula S, Medrano JV, Kee K, et al. Human germ cell differentiation from fetal- and adult-derived induced pluripotent stem cells. Hum Mol Genet. 2011;20 (4):752-62.
19. Park TS, Galic Z, Conway AE, et al. Derivation of primordial germ cells from human embryonic and induced pluripotent stem cells is significantly improved by coculture with human fetal gonadal cells. Stem Cells. 2009;27(4):783-95.
20. Easley CA, Phillips BT, McGuire MM, et al. Direct differentiation of human pluripotent stem cells into haploid spermatogenic cells. Cell Rep. 2012;2(3):440-6.
21. Medrano JV, Ramathal C, Nguyen HN, et al. Divergent RNA-binding proteins, DAZL and VASA, induce meiotic progression in human germ cells derived in vitro. Stem Cells. 2012;30(3):441-51.
22. Irie N, Weinberger L, Tang WW, et al. SOX17 is a critical specifier of human primordial germ cell fate. Cell. 2015;160 (1-2):253-68.
23. Sasaki K, Yokobayashi S, Nakamura T, et al. Robust In Vitro Induction of Human Germ Cell Fate from Pluripotent Stem Cells. Cell Stem Cell. 2015;17(2):178-94.
24. Sugawa F, Araúzo-Bravo MJ, Yoon J, et al. Human primordial germ cell commitment in vitro associates with a unique PRDM14 expression profile. EMBO J. 2015;34(8):1009-24.
25. Zhou Q, Wang M, Yuan Y, et al. Complete Meiosis from Embryonic Stem Cell-Derived Germ Cells In Vitro. Cell Stem Cell. 2016;18(3):330-40.
26. Napalkov P, Felici DM, Chu LK, et al. Incidence of catheter-related complications in patients with central venous or hemodialysis catheters: a health care claims database analysis. BMC Cardiovasc Disord. 2013;13:86.
27. Tang WW, Dietmann S, Irie N, et al. A Unique Gene Regulatory Network Resets the Human Germline Epigenome for Development. Cell. 2015;161(6): 1453-67.
28. Gkountela S, Zhang KX, Shafiq TA, et al. DNA Demethylation Dynamics in the Human Prenatal Germline. Cell. 2015;161(6):1425-36.
29. Guo F, Yan L, Guo H, et al. The Transcriptome and DNA Methylome Landscapes of Human Primordial Germ Cells. Cell. 2015;161(6):1437-52.
30. Lin H. The stem-cell niche theory: lessons from flies. Nat Rev Genet. 2002;3 (12):931-40.
31. Nakamura S, Kobayashi K, Nishimura T, et al. Identification of germline stem cells in the ovary of the teleost medaka. Science. 2010;328(5985):1561-3.
32. Green SH, Zuckerman S. The number of oocytes in the mature rhesus monkey (Macaca mulatta). J Endocrinol. 1951;7(2):194-202.
33. Johnson J, Canning J, Kaneko T, et al. Germline stem cells and follicular renewal in the postnatal mammalian ovary. Nature. 2004;428(6979):145-50.
34. Gosden RG. Germline stem cells in the postnatal ovary: is the ovary more like a testis? Hum Reprod Update. 2004;10(3): 193-5.
35. Bristol-Gould SK, Kreeger PK, Selkirk CG, et al. Fate of the initial follicle pool: empirical and mathematical evidence

supporting its sufficiency for adult fertility. Dev Biol. 2006;298(1):149-54.
36. Johnson J, Bagley J, Skaznik-Wikiel M, et al. Oocyte generation in adult mammalian ovaries by putative germ cells in bone marrow and peripheral blood. Cell. 2005;122(2):303-15.
37. Eggan K, Jurga S, Gosden R, et al. Ovulated oocytes in adult mice derive from non-circulating germ cells. Nature. 2006;441(7097):1109-14.
38. Lee HJ, Selesniemi K, Niikura Y, et al. Bone marrow transplantation generates immature oocytes and rescues long-term fertility in a preclinical mouse model of chemotherapy-induced premature ovarian failure. J Clin Oncol. 2007;25 (22):3198-204.
39. Bukovsky A, Caudle MR, Svetlikova M, et al. Origin of germ cells and formation of new primary follicles in adult human ovaries. Reprod Biol Endocrinol. 2004;2:20.
40. Bukovsky A, Svetlikova M, Caudle MR. Oogenesis in cultures derived from adult human ovaries. Reprod Biol Endocrinol. 2005;3:17.
41. Virant-Klun I, Zech N, Rozman P, et al. Putative stem cells with an embryonic character isolated from the ovarian surface epithelium of women with no naturally present follicles and oocytes. Differentiation. 2008;76(8):843-56.
42. Szotek PP, Chang HL, Brennand K, et al. Normal ovarian surface epithelial label-retaining cells exhibit stem/progenitor cell characteristics. Proc Natl Acad Sci U S A. 2008;105(34):12469-73.
43. Liu Y, Wu C, Lyu Q, et al. Germline stem cells and neo-oogenesis in the adult human ovary. Dev Biol. 2007;306(1):112-20.
44. Begum S, Papaioannou VE, Gosden RG. The oocyte population is not renewed in transplanted or irradiated adult ovaries. Hum Reprod. 2008;23(10):2326-30.
45. Veitia RA, Gluckman E, Fellous M, et al. Recovery of female fertility after chemotherapy, irradiation, and bone marrow allograft: further evidence against massive oocyte regeneration by bone marrow-derived germline stem cells. Stem Cells. 2007;25(5):1334-5.
46. Zou K, Yuan Z, Yang Z, et al. Production of offspring from a germline stem cell line derived from neonatal ovaries. Nat Cell Biol. 2009;11(5):631-6.
47. White YA, Woods DC, Takai Y, et al. Oocyte formation by mitotically active germ cells purified from ovaries of reproductive-age women. Nat Med. 2012;18(3): 413-21.
48. Zhang H, Panula S, Petropoulos S, et al. Adult human and mouse ovaries lack DDX4-expressing functional oogonial stem cells. Nat Med. 2015;21(10):1116-8.
49. Lei L, Spradling AC. Female mice lack adult germ-line stem cells but sustain oogenesis using stable primordial follicles. Proc Natl Acad Sci U S A. 2013;110 (21):8585-90.
50. Wei S, Zan L, Hausman GJ, et al. Dedifferentiated adipocyte-derived progeny cells (DFAT cells): Potential stem cells of adipose tissue. Adipocyte. 2013;2 (3):122-7.
51. Herreros-Villanueva M, Zhang JS, Koenig A, et al. SOX2 promotes dedifferentiation and imparts stem cell-like features to pancreatic cancer cells. Oncogenesis. 2013;2:e61.
52. Lee ST, Gong SP, Yum KE, et al. Transformation of somatic cells into stem cell-like cells under a stromal niche. FASEB J. 2013;27(7):2644-56.
53. Bowen NJ, Walker LD, Matyunina LV, et al. Gene expression profiling supports the hypothesis that human ovarian surface epithelia are multipotent and capable of serving as ovarian cancer initiating cells. BMC Med Genomics. 2009; 2:71.
54. Bhartiya D, Unni S, Parte S, et al. Very small embryonic-like stem cells: implications in reproductive biology. Biomed Res Int. 2013;2013:682326.
55. Donnez J, Dolmans MM, Pellicer A, et al. Restoration of ovarian activity and pregnancy after transplantation of cryopreserved ovarian tissue: a review of 60 cases of reimplantation. Fertil Steril. 2013;99(6):1503-13.
56. de Rooij DG. The spermatogonial stem cell niche. Microsc Res Tech. 2009;72 (8):580-5.
57. Brinster RL, Avarbock MR. Germline transmission of donor haplotype following spermatogonial transplantation. Proc Natl Acad Sci U S A. 1994;91(24):11303-7.
58. Brinster RL, Zimmermann JW. Spermatogenesis following male germ-cell transplantation. Proc Natl Acad Sci U S A. 1994;91(24):11298-302.
59. Geens M, Goossens E, De Block G, et al. Autologous spermatogonial stem cell transplantation in man: current obstacles for a future clinical application. Hum Reprod Update. 2008;14(2):121-30.
60. Wyns C, Curaba M, Martinez-Madrid B, et al. Spermatogonial survival after cryopreservation and short-term orthotopic immature human cryptorchid testicular tissue grafting to immunodeficient mice. Hum Reprod. 2007;22 (6):1603-11.
61. Wyns C, Van Langendonckt A, Wese FX, et al. Long-term spermatogonial survival in cryopreserved and xenografted immature human testicular tissue. Hum Reprod. 2008;23(11):2402-14.
62. Baert Y, Van Saen D, Haentjens P, et al. What is the best cryopreservation protocol for human testicular tissue banking? Hum Reprod. 2013;28(7):1816-26.
63. Goossens E, Van Saen D, Tournaye H. Spermatogonial stem cell preservation and transplantation: from research to clinic. Hum Reprod. 2013;28(4):897-907.
64. Poels J, Van Langendonckt A, Many MC, et al. Vitrification preserves proliferation capacity in human spermatogonia. Hum Reprod. 2013;28(3):578-89.
65. Gassei K, Orwig KE. Experimental methods to preserve male fertility and treat male factor infertility. Fertil Steril. 2016;105(2):256-66.
66. Medrano JV, Martinez-Arroyo AM, Sukhwani M, et al. Germ cell transplantation into mouse testes procedure. Fertil Steril. 2014;102(4):e11-2.
67. Ogawa T, Aréchaga JM, Avarbock MR, et al. Transplantation of testis germinal cells into mouse seminiferous tubules. Int J Dev Biol. 1997;41(1):111-22.
68. Hermann BP, Sukhwani M, Winkler F, et al. Spermatogonial stem cell transplantation into rhesus testes regenerates spermatogenesis producing functional sperm. Cell Stem Cell. 2012;11(5):715-26.
69. Nagano M, Patrizio P, Brinster RL. Long-term survival of human spermatogonial stem cells in mouse testes. Fertil Steril. 2002;78(6):1225-33.
70. Faes K, Tournaye H, Goethals L, et al. Testicular cell transplantation into the human testes. Fertil Steril. 2013;100(4):981-8.

71. von Schönfeldt V, Wistuba J, Schlatt S. Notch-1, c-kit and GFRalpha-1 are developmentally regulated markers for premeiotic germ cells. Cytogenet Genome Res. 2004;105 (2-4):235-9.
72. Kanatsu-Shinohara M, Toyokuni S, Shinohara T. CD9 is a surface marker on mouse and rat male germline stem cells. Biol Reprod. 2004;70(1):70-5.
73. von Kopylow K, Schulze W, Salzbrunn A, et al. Isolation and gene expression analysis of single potential human spermatogonial stem cells. Mol Hum Reprod. 2016;22(4): 229-39.
74. von Kopylow K, Staege H, Schulze W, et al. Fibroblast growth factor receptor 3 is highly expressed in rarely dividing human type A spermatogonia. Histochem Cell Biol. 2012;138(5): 759-72.
75. Dovey SL, Valli H, Hermann BP, et al. Eliminating malignant contamination from therapeutic human spermatogonial stem cells. J Clin Invest. 2013;123(4): 1833-43.
76. Valli H, Sukhwani M, Dovey SL, et al. Fluorescence- and magnetic-activated cell sorting strategies to isolate and enrich human spermatogonial stem cells. Fertil Steril. 2014;102(2):566-80.e7.
77. Kanatsu-Shinohara M, Ogonuki N, Inoue K, et al. Long-term proliferation in culture and germline transmission of mouse male germline stem cells. Biol Reprod. 2003;69(2):612-6.
78. Sadri-Ardekani H, Mizrak SC, van Daalen SK, et al. Propagation of human spermatogonial stem cells in vitro. JAMA. 2009;302(19):2127-34.
79. Sadri-Ardekani H, Akhondi MA, van der Veen F, et al. In vitro propagation of human prepubertal spermatogonial stem cells. JAMA. 2011;305(23):2416-8.
80. Chikhovskaya JV, Jonker MJ, Meissner A, et al. Human testis-derived embryonic stem cell-like cells are not pluripotent, but possess potential of mesenchymal progenitors. Hum Reprod. 2012;27(1):210-21.
81. Chikhovskaya JV, van Daalen SK, Korver CM, et al. Mesenchymal origin of multipotent human testis-derived stem cells in human testicular cell cultures. Mol Hum Reprod. 2014;20(2):155-67.
82. Eildermann K, Gromoll J, Behr R. Misleading and reliable markers to differentiate between primate testis-derived multipotent stromal cells and spermatogonia in culture. Hum Reprod. 2012;27(6):1754-67.
83. Baert Y, Braye A, Struijk RB, et al. Cryopreservation of testicular tissue before long-term testicular cell culture does not alter in vitro cell dynamics. Fertil Steril. 2015;104(5):1244-52.e1-4.
84. Honaramooz A, Snedaker A, Boiani M, et al. Sperm from neonatal mammalian testes grafted in mice. Nature. 2002;418(6899):778-81.
85. Arregui L, Rathi R, Zeng W, et al. Xenografting of adult mammalian testis tissue. Anim Reprod Sci. 2008;106(1-2):65-76.
86. Shinohara T, Inoue K, Ogonuki N, et al. Birth of offspring following transplantation of cryopreserved immature testicular pieces and in-vitro microinsemination. Hum Reprod. 2002;17(12):3039-45.
87. Van Saen D, Goossens E, Bourgain C, et al. Meiotic activity in orthotopic xenografts derived from human postpubertal testicular tissue. Hum Reprod. 2011; 26(2):282-93.
88. Geens M, De Block G, Goossens E, et al. Spermatogonial survival after grafting human testicular tissue to immunodeficient mice. Hum Reprod. 2006;21(2): 390-6.
89. Schlatt S, Honaramooz A, Ehmcke J, et al. Limited survival of adult human testicular tissue as ectopic xenograft. Hum Reprod. 2006;21(2):384-9.
90. Yang S, Ping P, Ma M, et al. Generation of haploid spermatids with fertilization and development capacity from human spermatogonial stem cells of cryptorchid patients. Stem Cell Reports. 2014;3(4):663-75.
91. Stukenborg JB, Wistuba J, Luetjens CM, et al. Coculture of spermatogonia with somatic cells in a novel three-dimensional soft-agar-culture-system. J Androl. 2008;29(3):312-29.
92. Sato T, Katagiri K, Gohbara A, et al. In vitro production of functional sperm in cultured neonatal mouse testes. Nature. 2011;471(7339):504-7.
93. Sato T, Katagiri K, Kubota Y, et al. In vitro sperm production from mouse spermatogonial stem cell lines using an organ culture method. Nat Protoc. 2013;8 (11):2098-104.
94. Sato T, Yokonishi T, Komeya M, et al. Testis tissue explantation cures spermatogenic failure in c-Kit ligand mutant mice. Proc Natl Acad Sci U S A. 2012;109 (42):16934-8.
95. Yokonishi T, Sato T, Komeya M, et al. Offspring production with sperm grown in vitro from cryopreserved testis tissues. Nat Commun. 2014;5:4320.
96. Baert Y, Stukenborg JB, Landreh M, et al. Derivation and characterization of a cytocompatible scaffold from human testis. Hum Reprod. 2015;30(2):256-67.
97. Picton HM, Wyns C, Anderson RA, et al. A European perspective on testicular tissue cryopreservation for fertility preservation in prepubertal and adolescent boys. Hum Reprod. 2015;30(11):2463-75.
98. Chen HH, Welling M, Bloch DB, et al. DAZL limits pluripotency, differentiation, and apoptosis in developing primordial germ cells. Stem Cell Reports. 2014;3(5):892-904.
99. Durruthy Durruthy J, Ramathal C, Sukhwani M, et al. Fate of induced pluripotent stem cells following transplantation to murine seminiferous tubules. Hum Mol Genet. 2014;23(12):3071-84.
100. Ramathal C, Angulo B, Sukhwani M, et al. DDX3Y gene rescue of a Y chromo-some AZFa deletion restores germ cell formation and transcriptional programs. Sci Rep. 2015;5:15041.
101. Ramathal C, Durruthy-Durruthy J, Sukhwani M, et al. Fate of iPSCs derived from azoospermic and fertile men following xenotransplantation to murine seminiferous tubules. Cell Rep. 2014;7(4):1284-97.
102. Dominguez AA, Chiang HR, Sukhwani M,et al. Human germ cell formation in xenotransplants of induced pluripotent stem cells carrying X chromosome aneuploidies. Sci Rep. 2014;4:6432.
103. Medrano JV, Martinez-Arroyo AM, Miguez JM, et al. Human somatic cells subjected to genetic induction with six germ line-related factors display meiotic germ cell-like features. Sci Rep. 2016;6:24956.
104. Kim J, Efe JA, Zhu S, et al. Direct reprogramming of mouse fibroblasts to neural progenitors. Proc Natl Acad Sci U S A. 2011;108(19):7838-43.

105. Vierbuchen T, Ostermeier A, Pang ZP, et al. Direct conversion of fibroblasts to functional neurons by defined factors. Nature. 2010;463(7284):1035-41.
106. Szabo E, Rampalli S, Risueño RM, et al. Direct conversion of human fibroblasts to multilineage blood progenitors. Nature. 2010;468(7323):521-6.
107. Ieda M, Fu JD, Delgado-Olguin P, et al. Direct reprogramming of fibroblasts into functional cardiomyocytes by defined factors. Cell. 2010;142(3):375-86.
108. Buganim Y, Itskovich E, Hu YC, et al. Direct reprogramming of fibroblasts into embryonic Sertoli-like cells by defined factors. Cell Stem Cell. 2012;11(3): 373-86.
109. Chapman KM, Medrano GA, Jaichander P, et al. Targeted Germline Modifications in Rats Using CRISPR/Cas9 and Spermatogonial Stem Cells. Cell Rep. 2015;10(11): 1828-35.
110. Sato T, Sakuma T, Yokonishi T, et al. Genome Editing in Mouse Spermatogonial Stem Cell Lines Using TALEN and Double-Nicking CRISPR/Cas9. Stem Cell Reports. 2015;5(1):75-82.
111. Vassena R, Heindryckx B, Peco R, et al. Genome engineering through CRISPR/ Cas9 technology in the human germline and pluripotent stem cells. Hum Reprod Update. 2016;22(4):411-9.

CHAPTER

67

Assisted Hatching

Jayesh Shinde, Supreet Pal Singh

INTRODUCTION

The zona pellucida (ZP) is a specialized extracellular matrix composed of sulfated glycoproteins which encapsulate the mammalian eggs and early preimplantation embryos. The envelope is synthesized by the oocyte during folliculogenesis and is post-translationally modified by glycosylation. Human ZP is composed of four intermediate filament proteins ZP1, ZP2, ZP3, and ZP4. The ZP averages 15–20 µm in width.

This covering plays diverse roles in events ranging from fertilization to the preimplantation embryonic development. Postovulation, the ZP acts as a barrier for the sperm. The capacitated sperm have to bind to zona proteins during the process of fertilization and then undergo zona-mediated acrosomal exocytosis, somewhere suggesting that ZP can indirectly have a role in sperm selection. Moreover, biochemical changes have been observed postfertilization, which cause conformational changes in ZP proteins advocating that it helps in preventing polyspermic fertilization. Postfertilization the zona helps in maintenance of blastomere integrity during embryo's trip through the oviduct. Several studies have also looked into the protective effect of the zona against various hostile uterine factors and immune responses as well.

Although the ZP is a product of the oocyte, it is a prerequisite for the mammalian embryo to hatch out of the envelope, so that implantation can ensue. Hatching from the ZP in vivo is controlled by the various proteolytic factors synthesized by the embryo and the female reproductive tract. Preceding hatching, phases of repeated contraction and expansion have also been documented by time-lapse video recording of mammalian blastocysts in in vitro culture. But now there is sufficient data in the literature that suggest that it is the proteolysins, such as "strypsin", secreted by the embryonic trophectodermal cells, and other uterolysins, which are the key mechanisms behind hatching and not the blastocyst expansion-contraction cycles. This suggests that hatching in vitro will not be quite physiological as the uterolysins in this case remain absent.

ROLE OF ASSISTED HATCHING IN ASSISTED REPRODUCTIVE TECHNOLOGY

Hatching of the blastocyst is a climacteric phase in the series of events cresting to implantation. Failure in doing so might be one of numerous dynamics which restrain human reproductive competence. In present day, in vitro fertilization (IVF) laboratories, culture conditions support blastocysts till hatching, but studies show that the incidence, timing, and mechanism might be affected.[1] The fact that only a small fraction of human embryos undergo spontaneous hatching in vitro, following long culture can be due to the culture conditions itself but also because of the embryo quality which in turn represents the patient characteristics.[2] Morphological ZP anomalies, such as disproportionate and excessive thickness, can interfere with hatching and thus negatively affect the implantation potential of the embryo.[3] Zona thickness appears to be influenced by the maternal age and follicle-stimulating hormone (FSH) levels and negatively influences embryo implantation rates.[4] Moreover, studies suggest that surplus ZP hardening can occur in mammalian embryos as a consequence of in vitro culture.[5] Commonly, cryopreserved-thawed embryos, in spite of recommencing mitosis and being morphologically intact, might fail to implant following an embryo transfer (ET).

This can be due to the cryopreservation-thawing procedure affecting the embryos by hardening of the zona. In all the mentioned cases, hatching could be inhibited in these in vitro manipulated human embryos due to the failure of the blastocysts to escape from a copious or hardened ZP.[2] The trophectoderm of some embryos may not be able to synthesize the lysins required for hatching. The production of these factors can be influenced by the patient's age.[6] Moreover, some studies have also shown that the uterolysin action could also be compromised in some patients or might be influenced negatively during assisted reproductive technology (ART) cycles.[7]

In the year 1990, during a randomized controlled trial (RCT), Cohen and his colleagues subjected human embryos to a mechanical breach in the zona using micromanipulation and reported improved implantation rates in a selected cohort of patients. These patients had "poor prognosis" based on zona thickness, blastomere number, fragmentation rates, and maternal age.[8] Similar study by the same group, conducted a couple of years later, also showed that the procedure was not effective in good prognosis patients.[2] The procedure was thus termed "assisted hatching (AH)" and involved the artificial thinning or breaching of the ZP. Since then, it has been applied clinically by many ART programs in an effort to improve clinical outcomes.

The method by which AH improves embryo implantation remains uncertain. Precise synchronization between the embryo and the endometrium is essential. Moreover, even though the ZP is porous in nature and facilitates transport of certain growth factors or metabolites across, this rate of exchange might be diminished if the ZP is too thick or stiff. The breach in ZP might be helpful in facilitating the transport of these molecules, which might be important for the crosstalk between the endometrium and embryonic cells in order to establish a successful implantation.[2] This can be supported by a study where it has been shown that the AH embryos implant a little earlier than their counterparts, which might be due to their better response to the "implantation window" owing to improved molecular communication.[9]

Going by the existing literature, which is not sufficient to reach any conclusion, it is indicated that AH may or may not be of help to only a small subgroup of patients, such as the following:

- Patients undergoing day 3 transfers with cleavage stage embryos exhibiting a thick or uneven ZP
- Patients with advanced maternal age, as their embryonic or uterine cells may have defective lysine production necessary for hatching
- Female patients with raised FSH levels in proliferative phase
- While transferring vitrified-thawed embryos during a frozen-thawed ET (FET) cycle.
- Patients with recurrent implantation failures due to idiopathic causes.

However, there is no significant or conclusive high-quality evidence on AH improving implantation and live birth rates (LBRs) in all these groups. But, however, the clinics offering AH to their patients otherwise should have a patient selection criterion to justify the use of AH. This way it will be helpful in counseling of patients that randomly request the technique versus in identifying those who might actually need it.

METHODS

There are different micromanipulation techniques available to perform AH in routine clinical practice, but it is crucial to note that the ideal AH technique should require minimum exposure of the embryos outside the incubator, so that they undergo minimal pH and temperature fluctuations to avoid any detrimental impact on the embryo development.

To combat these variations, the manipulation should be performed at a heated microscopic stage at 37°C, and media used should be independent of carbon dioxide for maintaining its buffering mechanism. It should be overlaid with oil for further minimizing impact of any changes in the embryo's surroundings. To make the manipulation quicker, it is always better to have a contrast system. After the procedure, the ZP-manipulated embryos can be incubated for some time before an ET is performed carefully, to avoid any damage to the embryo's structural integrity.

CHEMICAL ZONA DRILLING

Chemically, AH can be performed using the Acid Tyrode's (AT) solution. It has been used in embryology since 1986,[10] but it was used clinically for the first time in the year 1992.[2] The solution is commercially available (MediCult or Vitrolife) or can also be prepared in-house using standardized existing protocols. The pH of the solution should be between 2.2 and 2.5. Limiting embryo exposure to AT by precise and rapid manipulation is indispensable to avoid its harmful effects on embryo development.[11]

To perform AH using chemical zona drilling, the embryo is held with a holding pipette and another micropipette containing AT is brought near the site of the embryo, which has a large perivitelline space or cytoplasmic fragments. The solution is then delivered with the help of a microinjector. The moment an opening becomes visible on the ZP, it is necessary to rinse the embryo several times in fresh culture medium.

The main drawback of using AT is its toxicity and cytoplasmic acidification, which changes the intracellular pH, leading to cytoplasmic degeneration.[12] In addition, exposure of four-cell human embryos to AT has also been suggested to reduce their viability and preimplantation development.[13]

MECHANICAL ZONA DISSECTION

This method involves the use of a sharpened micropipette to mechanically pierce the zona and make a hole or a slit. First reported in 1990, this method has showed to improve implantation rate.[8] Mechanical zona dissection can be done by partial zona dissection (PZD), three-dimensional (3D)-PZD (3D-PZD), and controlled zona dissection (CZD).

In PZD, the embryo is held with a holding pipette, and a microneedle is inserted tangentially in the envelope. After this, the embryo is rubbed against the holding pipette, so that the portion of the ZP between the two points gets scrubbed off, and a slit is produced in the ZP. For the 3D-PZD, the shape of a cross is made on the zona. The procedure begins as a regular PZD, but in the end, a second slit is also made just beneath the previous one. This method allows the formation of greater openings. For CZD, the embryo is held and a microinjection needle is inserted at 5 o'clock position, which is then navigated to insert deeply into the holding pipette. It is then pressed against the bottom of the dish to cut the pierced ZP. With this technique, we can get a large slit in the zona in a single go.

Cohen et al. had suggested that mechanical zona dissection was nontraumatic as compared to the zona drilling by AT treatment.[14] Other advantages of mechanical drilling are that there are no effects of chemicals or heat during the procedure. In addition, reports indicate that the further embryonic development is not compromised in these embryos.[15]

However, the precision in positioning the hole is jeopardized when compared to AT. Also, it has been suggested that with PZD openings can be very constricted in comparison to the spherical apertures in the zona which can be prepared by using other drilling methods. This can subsequently induce more trauma to the cells during blastocyst hatching.

ENZYMATIC ZONA DIGESTION

By the end of the 20th century, the first healthy baby after the transfer of enzymatically treated embryos was born.[16] This enzyme was a proteolytic enzyme called pronase. The ZP can be softened or totally dissolved after exposure of embryos to 10 IU/mL pronase concentrations for 60–90 seconds. Blastocyst transfer, after pronase treatment of the ZP, has shown to improve pregnancy and implantation rates in patients with previous implantation failures.[17] However, there are some evidence that pronase treatment in embryos for longer than 90 seconds can cause adverse effects on the trophectoderm and inner cell mass (ICM).[18]

LASER-ASSISTED HATCHING

The application of a laser on the ZP results in its thermolysis. The first use of a laser for ZP drilling was reported in 1991.[19] But it was done by using an irradiation spectrum, which was later felt unsuitable for clinical applications.

Problems included possible damage to the DNA and other cellular macromolecules due to the absorption of ultraviolet light and the need for a complex setup that delivers laser energy directly to the target (i.e. contact mode). The necessity of sterile micropipettes and optical fibers restricted their widespread use.

Later the 1.48 μm, diode, noncontact infrared (IR) laser emerged as the most acceptable for use on human embryos as they have longer wavelengths of the IR range which cannot cause mutagenic effect on the embryo, as it is not absorbed by the DNA.[20] The drilling takes place as the ZP macromolecules at a focal point absorb the laser energy, ultimately leading to photoablation. It can be delivered directly from a specialized microscope objective. The size of the hole created can be controlled. Drilling can start at the outer edge of the zona and, using multiple shots, the embryologist can gradually move inward keeping the firing position a safe distance from the adjacent blastomeres. It is important to understand that the laser actually creates a 3D furrow in the ZP, which spreads beyond the apparent hole.

It is recommended to do laser AH (LAH) setup on an antivibration table; if that is not available, the embryo can be stabilized with a holding micropipette as the diode laser beam produces a temperature of 200°C on its axis, and it must be strictly limited to the ZP. The potential to damage adjacent blastomeres can be minimized by using short pulse durations and mild laser power at a safe distance.

LASER-ASSISTED HATCHING AND PREIMPLANTATION GENETIC DIAGNOSIS

The safety and usefulness of the system has been demonstrated in mice and human. LAH is preferred to drill the ZP of human embryos since it is simple, quick, and easy to use. Its application extends beyond AH. To perform preimplantation genetic diagnosis (PGD)/preimplantation genetic screening (PGS) for oocytes, cleavage stage embryos, and blastocysts, the zona has to be breached for a smooth or atraumatic entry of the blunt biopsy needle to collect genetic samples. Hence, LAH is the ideal technique for that. The ZP can be hatched with the laser just at the time of biopsy (for oocytes and cleavage stage embryos), or for blastocysts, it is recommended to give laser shots at day 3 which in turn induces early hatching at day 5. Protruding trophectoderm cells on day 5 thus make the manipulation easier for the embryologists and also give them more hatching blastocysts to choose from. In a study, LAH was used in the blastocyst biopsy of 231 patients. After 119 fresh ETs, the IR was 41%, and after 24 thaw ETs, IR was 26%. Therefore, it was concluded that blastocyst biopsy can be routinely carried out with good outcomes.[21]

Other applications of LAH are to use it to collapse hatching or expanded blastocysts as many studies have compared the survival rates and pregnancy rates after vitrification of noncollapsed versus collapsed blastocysts. But, however, it has shown no statistical difference in embryological or clinical results.[22]

ASSISTED HATCHING TIMING: CLEAVAGE VERSUS BLASTOCYST STAGE

Although zona can be breached at any stage of the embryonic growth, but most of the studies available on AH have performed the micromanipulation on cleavage stage embryos and not blastocysts. The rationale behind this choice can be the simple fact that in the earlier days of IVF, extended cultures were rare, and most laboratories were performing cleavage stage ETs.

Technically, hatching cleavage stage embryos should be much safer and easier than blastocysts, as they have large perivitelline space, so it becomes easier to identify sites for hatching. But the concept of hatching a blastocyst before ET should be more physiological theoretically as in vivo hatching occurs just before implantation. There are studies to validate that AH performed at the blastocyst stage appears to improve implantation potential of the embryos. To make the process safer, AH techniques, such as LAH, can be applied to early blastocysts, rather than blastocysts with expanded blastocoel.

CLINICAL CONSIDERATIONS

Clinical Pregnancy Rates

A meta-analysis looked into 31 RCTs from Cochrane (CENTRAL), MEDLINE, and EMBASE for clinical pregnancy rates (CPRs) in 2,933 women who had undergone AH before ET, from a total of 5,728 women who were undergoing ART treatment. The study concluded that CPRs in women who underwent AH were slightly improved, but the level only just reached statistical significance [odds ratio (OR) 1.13, 95% confidence interval (CI)]. Interestingly, the heterogeneity for this combined analysis for CPRs was also statistically significant ($p = 0.001$).[23] This suggests that combining multiple trials may not be the best approach.

In single trials, the study with the largest subject size published and assessed CPRs in fresh and FET cycles after AH. A total of 760 fresh ETs and 200 FET cycles were randomly assigned to AH or the non-AH group. They reported a CPR of 39% versus 37% in AH group versus no-hatching group (189/487 vs. 173/473; OR 1.10; 95% CI) which was nonsignificant statistically.[24]

Live Birth Rates

In a comprehensive Cochrane review analyzing the existing studies on AH, it was observed that "take home baby" rate had been assessed by only 33% of the studies in literature.[23] This is quite disappointing considering the fact that AH has been in clinical use since the 1990s. However, the meta-analysis looked into nine studies with a total of 1,921 participants and reported the live birth in 311 women in AH group versus 305 in non-AH group per 1,000 women undergoing ART cycles. Again the difference remained nonsignificant (OR 1.03, 95% CI).[23] Owing to the limited quantity of studies available in the existing literature, there is an insufficient evidence that subjecting human embryos to AH increases LBRs.

CONCERNS

Assisted Hatching and Monozygotic Twinning

Breaching of zona in vitro for the purpose of AH has been linked to an increased risk of monozygotic twinning (MZT).[25,26] One such study assessed data from the Society for ART (SART) for 35,503 IVF cycles. After adjustment of variables, such as patient age and number of embryos transferred, MZT was threefolds more likely to take place after AH were done when compared to multiple gestation or singleton IVF pregnancies.[26] One of the factors behind the relation of AH and MZT can be the diameter of breach created in zona during AH. A constricted or narrow passage may cause mechanical trauma to the blastocyst, causing its ICM to split, resulting in monozygotic twin pregnancies.

However, other studies have not shown an increase in MZT with AH in patients undergoing either fresh or frozen transfer cycles. Overall, the risk of multiple pregnancies appears to be higher in women who undergo AH based on the results from 14 RCTs.[27] Most of these were dizygotic gestations, and only a few studies have reported a spike in MZT. A Cochrane review summarized results from six clinical trials and showed an insignificant difference in MZT after AH (0.8% vs. 0%).[23] Another retrospective study where data from last one decade was analyzed by an IVF unit found no association between MZT and AH or intracytoplasmic sperm injection, which also breaches the integrity of the ZP.[28]

Therefore, there is an evidence that AH is associated with multiple pregnancy, but the evidence is insufficient that it is related to MZT.

CONCLUSION

Although as discussed previously in the chapter, there are different methods available to perform AH, all of them require manipulation of the embryos outside the incubator which can induce iatrogenic damage and affect embryonic development negatively. Each AH technique has the potential to cause lethal damage to the embryo or individual blastomeres, if not performed carefully. This can eventually lead to reduction of embryo viability thereby defeating the whole purpose of the treatment. However, as compared to the other methods, LAH appears to be the safest method when performed under controlled conditions for embryo biopsy before PGS/PGD. But applying LAH at the blastocyst stage to improve implantation rate should be reconsidered, as a study has shown that the blastocysts collapse and re-expand after approximately 4 hours of AH. Embryos which were not subjected to LAH in this experiment started hatching early as compared to hatched ones.[28] This delayed hatching in AH blastocysts might cause an asynchrony between the embryos coming out of the envelope for implantation and the "implantation window".

Also, the Practice Committee of the American Society for Reproductive Medicine in collaboration with the SART,[27] as a service to its members and other practicing clinicians has concluded that AH should not be recommended routinely for all the IVF patients as the use of AH is not justified, because there is lack of evidence in the existing literature.

Therefore, charging IVF patients for adjunct add-on treatments, such as AH, where they are told that this might improve the chances of LBR despite no sufficient clinical evidence supporting its efficacy should be reconsidered. More RCTs need to be done to provide high-quality evidence that AH as a procedure is safe and effective and can actually help to improve the LBRs in patients.

REFERENCES

1. Edwards RG, Mettler L, Walters DE. Identical twins and in vitro fertilization. J In Vitro Fert Embryo Transf. 1986;3(2):114-7.
2. Cohen J, Alikani M, Trowbridge J, et al. Implantation enhancement by selective assisted hatching using zona drilling of human embryos with poor prognosis. Hum Reprod. 1992;7(5):685-91.
3. Gabrielsen A, Lindenberg S, Peterson K. The impact of the zona pellucida thickness variation of human embryos on pregnancy outcome in relation to suboptimal embryo development. A prospective randomized controlled study. Hum Reprod. 2001;16:2166-70.
4. Loret De Mola JR, Garside WT, Bucci J, et al. Analysis of the human zona pellucida during culture: correlation with diagnosis and the preovulatory hormonal environment. J Assist Reprod Genet. 1997;14:332-7.
5. De Felici M, Siracusa G. Spontaneous hardening of the zona pellucida of mouse oocytes during in vitro culture. Gamete Res. 1982;6:107-13.
6. Schiewe MC, Hazeleger NL, Sclimenti C, et al. Physiological characterization of blastocyst hatching mechanisms by use of a mouse antihatching model. Fertil Steril. 1995;63:288-94.
7. Mandelbaum J. The effects of assisted hatching on the hatching process and implantation. Hum Reprod. 1996;11:43-50.
8. Cohen J, Elsner C, Kort H, et al. Impairment of the hatching process following IVF in the human and improvement of implantation by assisting hatching using micromanipulation. Hum Reprod. 1990;5(1):7-13.
9. Liu HC, Cohen J, Alikani M, et al. Assisted hatching facilitates earlier implantation. Fertil Steril. 1993;60:871-5.
10. Gordon JW, Talansky BE. Assisted fertilization by zona drilling: a mouse model for correction of oligospermia. J Exp Zool A Ecol Genet Physiol. 1986;239(3):347-54.
11. Hogan B, Costantini F, Lacy E. Manipulating the mouse embryo: a laboratory manual. Cold Spring Harbor, NY: Cold Spring Harbor Laboratory; 1986.
12. Depypere HT, Leybaert L. Intracellular pH changes during zona drilling. Fertil Steril. 1994;61(2):319-23.
13. Garrisi GJ, Talansky BE, Grunfeld L, et al. Clinical evaluation of three approaches to micromanipulation-assisted fertilization. Fertil Steril. 1990;54(4):671-7.
14. Malter HE, Cohen J. Partial zona dissection of the human oocyte: a nontraumatic method using micromanipulation to assist zona pellucida penetration. Fertil Steril. 1989;51(1): 139-48.
15. Fong CY, Bongso A, Ng SC, et al. Ongoing normal pregnancy after transfer of zona-free blastocysts: implications for embryo transfer in the human. Hum Reprod. 1997;12:557-60.
16. Fong CY, Bongso A, Ng SC, et al. Blastocyst transfer after enzymatic treatment of the zona pellucida: improving in-vitro fertilization and understanding implantation. Hum Reprod. 1998;13:2926-32.
17. Fong CY, Bongso A, Sathananthan H, et al. Ultrastructural observations of enzymatically treated human blastocyst: zona-free blastocyst transfer and rescue of blastocyst with hatching difficulties. Hum Reprod. 2001;16:540-6.

18. Palanker D, Ohad S, Lewis A, et al. Technique for cellular microsurgery using the 193 nm excimer laser. Laser Surg Med. 1991;11:589-6.
19. Veiga A, Boiso I, Belil I. Assisted hatching. In: Gardner DK, Weissman A, Howles CM, Shoham Z (Eds). Textbook of assisted reproductive technologies. 3rd edition. London: Informa Healthcare; 2009. pp. 181-90.
20. McArthur SJ, Leigh D, Marshall JT, et al. Pregnancies and live births after trophectoderm biopsy and preimplantation genetic testing of human blastocysts. Fertil Steril. 2005;84(6):1628-36.
21. Mukaida T, Oka C, Goto T, et al. Artificial shrinkage of blastocoeles using either a micro-needle or a laser pulse prior to the cooling steps of vitrification improves survival rate and pregnancy outcome of vitrified human blastocysts. Hum Reprod. 2006;21(12):3246-52.
22. Carney SK, Das S, Blake D, et al. Assisted hatching on assisted conception (in vitro fertilisation (IVF) and intracytoplasmic sperm injection (ICSI)). Cochrane Database Syst Rev. 2012;12:CD001894.
23. Ge HS, Zhou W, Zhang W, et al. Impact of assisted hatching on fresh and frozen-thawed embryo transfer cycles: a prospective, randomized study. Reprod Biomed Online. 2008;16(4):589-96.
24. Practice Committee of the American Society for Reproductive Medicine, Practice Committee of the Society for Assisted Reproductive Technology. Role of assisted hatching in in vitro fertilization: a guideline. Fertil Steril. 2014;102(2): 348-51.
25. Schieve LA, Meikle SF, Peterson HB, et al. Does assisted hatching pose a risk for monozygotic twinning in pregnancies conceived through in vitro fertilization? Fertil Steril. 2000;74:288-94.
26. Valojerdi MR, Eftekhari-Yazdi P, Karimian L, et al. Effect of laser zona pellucida opening on clinical outcome of assisted reproduction technology in patients with advanced female age, recurrent implantation failure, or frozen-thawed embryos. Fertil Steril. 2008;90:84-91.
27. Hershlag A, Paine T, Cooper GW, et al. Monozygotic twinning associated with mechanical assisted hatching. Fertil Steril. 1999;71:144-6.
28. Montag M, van der Ven H. Laser-assisted hatching in assisted reproduction. Laser. 1999;40(3):398-403.

CHAPTER

68

In Vitro Maturation

Mona Shroff

INTRODUCTION

The term in vitro maturation (IVM) refers to recovering immature oocytes from follicles that may or may not have been exposed to exogenous follicle-stimulating hormone (FSH), not exposed to exogenous luteinizing hormone (LH) or human chorionic gonadotropin (hCG) prior to retrieval and maturing them in culture to induce meiotic resumption. During IVM, such immature oocytes progress from prophase I stage [i.e. from the germinal vesicle (GV)] through meiosis I to reach metaphase II. The use of exogenous LH or hCG prior to retrieval ("follicular priming") has been introduced in order to increase the probability of obtaining more usable oocytes.

The history of IVM dates back to 1935 when Pincus and Enzmann first reported its use in mammals.[1] The primary reason for the advent of IVM was to avoid ovarian hyperstimulation syndrome (OHSS) and reduce the cost associated with ovarian stimulation in conventional in vitro fertilization (IVF). But it has not become a routinely adopted procedure, and the American Society for Reproductive Medicine defines it as an "Experimental Technique."[2] The reason being its lower implantation rate (IR) compared to conventional IVF due to asynchrony between nuclear and cytoplasmic maturation, leading to lower developmental competence even after morphological maturity, and suboptimal culture conditions. Research so far has been directed toward improving culture conditions and oocyte quality. Benefits in non-polycystic ovarian (PCO) are doubtful due to lower number of oocytes available. In recent years with advances in cancer diagnostics and therapeutics, life expectancy of treated patients in reproductive age group is improving thus increasing need of IVM in oncofertility (Table 1).

Table 1: Historical landmarks.

1935	Used in rabbit	Pincus and Enzmann
1960	Clinical use in humans	Edwards and Edwards
1969	Use of chemically defined media, need of cumulus for oocyte maturation in vitro	Kennedy and Donnahue
1991	Used unstimulated oocytes in egg donation program	Cha KY
1994	First successful IVM-IVF pregnancy in PCO	Trounson
1998	FSH priming	Wynn P
1999	HCG priming	Chian RC
2012	First embryo transfer after ex-vivo collection of immature oocytes	Fadini R

(FSH: follicle-stimulating hormone; hCG: human chorionic gonadotropin; IVF: in vitro fertilization; IVM: in vitro maturation; PCO: Polycystic ovaries)

INDICATIONS

- Polycystic ovary syndrome (PCOS): To avoid OHSS caused by controlled ovarian hyperstimulation (COH) in conventional IVF procedure. With the use of antagonist protocol, agonist trigger, and "Freeze-all" policy, the risk is much lower than before but a few cases have been reported worldwide even after agonist trigger. IVM prevents early- and late-onset OHSS. Symptoms related to high estradiol levels are avoided along with IVM being simpler, gentler, cheaper, and of shorter duration than conventional IVF.
- Fertility preservation (FP) (oncofertility): COH delays cancer treatment by an average of 30 days, with increased risk in estrogen-sensitive breast and ovarian cancer along with added cost. IVM can be used alone, or in combination with other FP techniques as per

feasibility (ovarian tissue cryopreservation, mature oocyte cryopreservation, and embryo vitrification). Ovarian function may decline due to malignant disease process; hence, quality and quantity of oocytes remain questionable.

- Salvage of immature oocytes in conventional IVF: Rescue IVM.
- Repeated conventional IVF failures, poor embryo quality, repeated retrieval of germinal vesicles (GVs), empty follicular syndrome, recurrent fertilization failures, and recurrent pregnancy loss (due to need for multiple attempts).
- Natural cycle IVF/IVM: It has been demonstrated that atresia does not occur in the nondominant follicles even after the dominant follicle is selected in the ovary during folliculogenesis, because immature oocytes retrieved from nondominant follicles have been successfully matured in vitro, fertilized, and have resulted in several pregnancies and healthy live births. Thus IVM can be used to enhance the success of natural cycle of IVF treatment in combination with immature oocyte retrieval. The clinical pregnancy rate has been reported to reach up to as high as 45% per embryo transfer following natural cycle IVF/IVM in a selected group of patients.[3-6]
- Oocyte donors: To avoid risk of OHSS and unknown long-term side effects.

PATIENT PREPARATION IMAGE

Role of Follicle-stimulating Hormone Priming

Conventionally the target follicles for IVM are 5–10 mm. Due to poor IR after IVM in unstimulated PCO patients, further studies used FSH priming before retrieval. Mild stimulation can increase size up to 13 mm and enhance oocyte pickup (OPU) procedure and possibly improve oocyte quality.

Theoretically, the use of FSH priming at the beginning of follicular or luteal phases may enhance more follicular development and the maturational competence of immature oocytes in vivo but results are conflicting on the benefits of using FSH priming in women with regular menstrual ovaries versus irregular menstrual cycles of PCOS.[7-13] Most studies showed no differences in the rates of oocyte maturation, fertilization, cleavage, or IR with FSH pretreatment.

Follicular size may be important for the subsequent embryonic development, but the developmental competence of oocytes derived from the small antral follicles seems not to be adversely affected by the presence of a dominant follicle.[14,15] Contrary to this theory, there is a possibility of accelerating folliculogenesis in turn leading to some atresia in erratic manner and dilemma regarding optimal OPU timing.

Role of Human Chorionic Gonadotropin Priming

It has been demonstrated that by priming with 10,000 IU hCG for 36 hours before retrieval of immature oocytes from women with PCOS, the time course of oocyte maturation in vitro is hastened, and the rate of oocyte maturation is increased.[16,17] The hCG priming not only promotes some oocytes to initiate the maturation process to metaphase I stage from the relatively bigger size of follicles (>10 mm in diameter) but also enhances some GV stage oocytes from the small follicles to acquire maturational and developmental competence in vivo.[13] This hypothesis may be controversial as LH receptors are not proven to exist in immature oocytes. Multiple studies showed mixed results with FSH and hCG priming with some benefits only in PCO patients. Metformin pretreatment in PCOS before IVM was found to have favorable clinical outcome by improving intrafollicular milieu and oocyte quality plus beneficial effect on endometrial receptivity.[18]

Oocyte Retrieval, Culture, and Fertilization

There are no established criteria to identify the ideal timing or method for oocyte retrieval. The lead follicular diameter used in most studies was 10 mm.[19,20] Lead-follicle diameters greater than 13 mm have been associated with reduced numbers of oocytes collected and matured,[21] possibly related to subsequent atresia of the nondominant follicles from withdrawal of endogenous FSH support. Some protocols require an endometrial thickness of more than 5 mm, while others do not include endometrial thickness as a criterion. With "Freeze-all" policy for better embryonal–endometrial synchrony, endometrial thickness in primary cycle may no longer be relevant.

The aspiration technique also differs for immature oocytes compared to traditional IVF. The optimal aspiration pressure and needle design have yet to be determined with negative pressures ranging between 40 mm Hg and 300 mm Hg and needles ranging from 16 gauge (ga) to 21 ga described. Double-lumen needles to flush the follicles and double needles (IVF Osaka IVM needle), outer (17 ga) for holding the ovary and inner (21 ga) for aspirating, have been described. Extremely high aspiration pressure has been shown to negatively impact development.[22] Careful ultrasound of follicles and locating large vessels

Table 2: In vitro maturation in PCOS and PCO-like patients.[2]

Reference	*N*	*Priming*	*Mean no. oocytes*	*Mean no. ET*	*PR/ET (%)*	*IR (%)*	*MC (%)*
Cha et al.[25]	203	None	15.5	5.0	21.9	5.5	37
Chian et al.[17]	13	hCG	7.8	2.8	38.5	16.6	40
	11	None	7.4	2.5	27.3	14.8	0
Child et al.[26]	107	hCG	10.3	2.5	21.5	9.5	26
Mikkelsen et al.[10]	12	None	6.8	1.7	0	0	0
	24	FSH	6.5	1.8	33.0	21.6	63
Le Du et al.[19]	45	hCG	11.4	2.5	22.5	10.9	40
Lin et al.[13]	35	FSH/hCG	21.9	3.8	31.4	9.7	–
	33	hCG	23.1	3.8	36.4	11.3	–

(ET: Embryos transferred; FSH: Follicle-stimulating hormone; hCG: Human chorionic gonadotropin; IR: Implantation rate; MC: Miscarriage rate; PR/ET: Pregnancies per embryo transfer procedure)

by Doppler is recommended. There is no consensus on which formulation is best suited for the purpose of in vitro oocyte culture. Media are frequently supplemented with pyruvic acid along with essential and nonessential amino acids, such as tissue culture media.[23] Addition of hCG to IVM medium has also not shown to improve results and needs further studies. Maturation rate reported in PCO has been in the range of 50–80% and lower in FP 30–60%. Albuz et al. proposed a novel IVM method called stimulated physiological oocyte maturation in animal biology to improve oocyte quality by improved cytoplasmic maturation (Fig. 1, Table 2).[24]

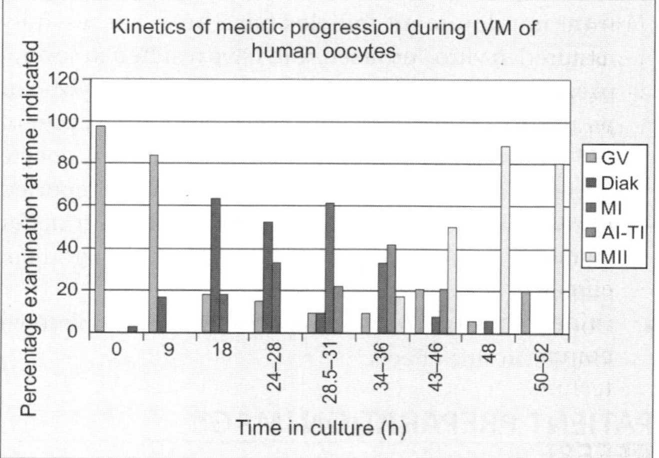

Fig. 1: Kinetics of meiotic progression during in vitro maturation of human oocytes. (AI-TI: Anaphase I to Telophase I; Diak: Diakinesis; GV: germinal vesicle; MI: metaphase I; MII: metaphase II)
Source: The Practice Committees of the American Society for Reproductive Medicine and the Society for Assisted Reproductive Technology. In vitro maturation: a committee opinion. Fertil Steril. 2013; 99:663-666.[2]

Clinical Outcomes and Safety

Over 5,000 live births have been reported so far with no increase in fetal anomalies or perinatal health issues and no difference in birth weight,[27] although some alteration in methylation process of maternally expressed genes during IVM is possible and there are concerns for epigenetic disorders (Table 3). Chian et al. have reported a clinical pregnancy rate of 35–45% and implantation rate of 10–15% in PCO women, which seems promising.[28]

SUMMARY

- Available data indicate that IVM results in lower IR and success rates compared to conventional IVF/ intracytoplasmic sperm injection, limiting more universal utilization.
- Asynchrony between nuclear and cytoplasmic maturation, leading to lower developmental competence even after morphological maturity is the prime concern.
- Candidates for this technology include those at risk for OHSS (PCOS or PCO-like ovaries), women with estrogen-sensitive cancers, or those with limited time prior to initiating potentially gonadotoxic treatments for FP.
- Priming with hCG and/or FSH appears to improve implantation and pregnancy rates in PCO, compared to no priming in a few studies but needs further large-scale data and less heterogeneity (e.g. number of embryos transferred).
- Application of frozen cycle in IVM improves clinical outcome because of improved uterine receptivity.
- Although IVM has been proven to be safe, considering the lower number of children born so far, information on its safety with regard to malformation and long-term developmental outcomes cannot be assessed accurately.

Table 3: Obstetric outcomes and congenital abnormalities in infants conceived with oocytes matured in vitro.[27]

Characteristics from 1,187 pregnancies	*Singleton pregnancies (n = 960)*	*Twin gestation pregnancies (n = 221)*	*Triplet gestation pregnancies (n = 5)*	*Quadruplet gestation pregnancies (n = 1)*
Mean gestational age at delivery (weeks + days)	37 + 4	36 + 5	35 + 2	29 + 0
No. of deliveries at >37 weeks (%)	855 (89)	60 (27)	0 (0)	0 (0)
No. of deliveries at 34–37 weeks (%)	82 (9)	132 (60)	5 (100)	0 (0)
No. of deliveries at <34 weeks (%)	23 (2)	29 (13)	0 (0)	1 (100)
Total of 1,421 newborns	*Singleton newborns (n = 960)*	*Twin newborns (n = 442)*	*Triplet newborns (n = 15)*	*Quadruplet newborns (n = 4)*
Birth weight (mean ± SD) (g)	2,965 ± 532	2,434 ± 365	1,968 ± 472	1,330 ± 84
No. of LBW (%)	35 (4)	59 (13)	12 (80)	0 (0)
No. of VLBW (%)	5 (1)	12 (3)	2 (13)	4 (100)
Median Apgar score at 1 min (interquartile range)	9 (7–9)	8 (7–9)	8 (8–9)	–
No. of Apgar score at 1 min less than 7 (%)	133 (14)	31 (14)	0 (0)	–
Median Apgar score at 5 min (interquartile range)	10 (9–10)	10 (9–10)	8 (8–9)	–
No. of Apgar score at 5 min less than 7 (%)	25 (3)	5 (2)	0 (0)	–
Incidence of congenital anomalies (%)	15 (2)	3 (1)	0 (0)	0 (0)

(LBW: low birth weight; SD: standard deviation; VLBW: very low birth weight)

- In vitro maturation should be performed in specialized centers for carefully selected patients evaluating both efficacy and safety. Informed consent must include information regarding pregnancy rates of IVM in comparison to conventional assisted reproductive technology and alternative options, if any.

REFERENCES

1. Pincus G, Enzmann EV. The comparative behaviour of mammalian eggs in vivo and in vitro: I. The activation of ovarian eggs. J Exp Med. 1935;62:665-75.
2. The Practice Committees of the American Society for Reproductive Medicine and the Society for Assisted Reproductive Technology. In vitro maturation: a committee opinion. Fertil Steril. 2013;99:663-6.
3. Chian RC, Buckett WM, Abdul-Jalil AK, et al. Natural cycle in vitro fertilization combined with in vitro maturation of immature oocytes is an alternative approach in infertility treatment. Fertil Steril. 2004;84:1675-8.
4. Lim JH, Yang SH, Chian RC. New alternative to infertility treatment for women without ovarian stimulation. Reprod Biomed Online. 2007;14:547-9.
5. Lim JH, Yang SH, Xu Y, et al. Selection of patients for natural cycle in vitro fertilization combined with in vitro maturation of immature oocytes. Fertil Steril. 2009;91:1050-5.
6. Janssens RM, Lambalk CB, Vermeiden JP, et al. In-vitro fertilization in a spontaneous cycle: easy, cheap and realistic. Hum Reprod. 2000;15:314-8.
7. Liu J, Katz E, Garcia JE, et al. Successful in vitro maturation of human oocytes not exposed to human chorionic gonadotropin during ovulation induction, resulting in pregnancy. Fertil Steril. 1997;67:566-8.
8. Mikkelsen AL, Smith SD, Lindenberg S. In-vitro maturation of human oocytes from regularly menstruating women may be successful without follicle stimulating hormone priming. Hum Reprod. 1999;14:1847-51.
9. Suikkari AM, Tulppala M, Tuuri T, et al. Luteal phase start of low-dose FSH of follicles results in an efficient recovery, maturation and fertilization of immature human oocytes. Hum Reprod. 2000;15:747-51.
10. Mikkelsen AL, Lindenberg S. Benefit of FSH priming of women with PCOS to the in vitro maturation procedure and the outcome: a randomized prospective study. Reproduction. 2001;122:587-92.
11. Mikkelsen AL, Host E, Blaabjerg J, et al. Time interval between FSH priming and aspiration of immature human oocytes for in-vitro maturation: a prospective randomized study. Reprod Biomed Online. 2003;6:416-20.
12. Hreinsson J, Rosenlund B, Friden B, et al. Recombinant LH is equally effective as recombinant hCG in promoting oocyte maturation in a clinical in-vitro maturation programme: a randomized study. Hum Reprod. 2003;18:2131-6.
13. Lin YH, Hwang JL, Huang LW, et al. Combination of FSH priming and hCG priming for in-vitro maturation of human oocytes. Hum Reprod. 2003;18:1632-6.
14. Smith LC, Olivera-Angel M, Groome NP, et al. Oocyte quality in small antral follicles in the presence or absence of a large dominant follicle in cattle. J Reprod Fertil. 1996;106:193-9.
15. Chian RC, Chung JT, Downey BR, et al. Maturational and developmental competence of immature oocytes retrieved from bovine ovaries at different phases of folliculogenesis. Reprod Biomed Online. 2002;4:127-32.

16. Chian RC, Gulekli B, Buckett WM, et al. Priming with human chorionic gonadotropin before retrieval of immature oocytes in women with infertility due to the polycystic ovary syndrome. N Engl J Med. 1999;341:1624-6.
17. Chian RC, Buckett WM, Tulandi T, et al. Prospective randomized study of human chorionic gonadotrophin priming before immature oocyte retrieval from unstimulated women with polycystic ovarian syndrome. Hum Reprod. 2000;15:165-70.
18. Fukuda AI, Kanaya H, Oku H, et al. Pretreatment of polycystic ovarian syndrome (PCOS) patients with Metformin optimizes results from the clinical appli-cation of in vitro maturation, in vitro fertilization and embryo transfer (IVM–IVF). Fertil Steril. 2004;82:S49-50.
19. Le Du A, Kadoch IJ, Bourcigaux N, et al. In vitro maturation for the treatment of infertility associated with polycystic ovarian syndrome: the French experience. Hum Reprod. 2005;20:420-4.
20. Cobo AC, Requena A, Neuspiller F, et al. Maturation in vitro of human oocytes from unstimulated cycles: selection of the optimal day for ovum retrieval based on follicular size. Hum Reprod. 1999;14:1864-8.
21. Jurema M, Noguiera D. In vitro maturation of human oocytes for assisted reproduction. Fertil Steril. 2006;86:1277-91.
22. Hashimoto S, Fukuda A, Murata Y, et al. Effect of aspiration vacuum on the developmental competence of immature human oocytes retrieved using a 20-gauge needle. Reprod Biomed Online. 2007;14:444-9.
23. Kennedy JF, Donahue RP. Human oocytes: maturation in chemically defined media. Science. 1969;164:1292-3.
24. Albuz FK, Sasseville M, Lane M, et al. Simulated physiological oocyte maturation (SPOM): A novel in vitro maturation system that substantially improves embryo yield and pregnancy outcomes. Hum Reprod. 2010;25:2999-3011.
25. Cha KY, Chung HM, Lee DR, et al. Obstetric outcome of patients with polycystic ovary syndrome treated by in vitro maturation and in vitro fertilization-embryo transfer. Fertil Steril. 2005;83:1461-5.
26. Child TJ, Phillips SJ, Abdul-Jalil AK, et al. A comparison of in vitro maturation and in vitro fertilization for women with polycystic ovaries. Obstet Gynecol. 2002;100:665-70.
27. Chian RC, Xu CL, Huang JY, et al. Obstetric outcomes and congenital abnormalities in infants conceived with oocytes matured in vitro. Facts Views Vis Obgyn. 2014;6:15-8.
28. Chian RC, Lim JH, Tan SL. State of the art in in-vitro oocyte maturation. Curr Opin Obstet Gynecol. 2004;16:211-9.

Section 7

Abnormalities of Pelvis

CHAPTER

69

Fibroids and Infertility: Evidence-based Approach to Management

Javier Martínez-Salazar, Carlos Iglesias

EPIDEMIOLOGY AND ETIOLOGY

Uterine fibroids are the most common pelvic tumors in women, appearing in approximately 70% of women over 30 years of age. Although the growth of fibroids responds to sexual steroids, these hormones are not exclusively responsible for the genesis of the tumor.

Current research on the basic mechanism of the origin of fibroids has confirmed that they are a clonal disease[1] since they come from a single smooth muscle cell and their formation is linked to the function, proliferation, and differentiation of a specific subgroup of human myometrial cells, which have characteristics of somatic stem cells (SSCs) that are influenced by different genetic and hormonal factors.

It has been reported that approximately 40–50% of fibroid cells present chromosomal alterations detectable by a karyotype. The recent emergence of mass gene sequencing technologies has confirmed that most of the SSC in fibroids show a high presence of mutations of the *MED12* gene (subunit 12 of the complement mediator) located on the X chromosome.[2]

Evidence of the differences in incidence and symptomatology of fibroids according to ethnicity (more common in women of African origin) seems to support the idea of the role of genetic factors in the formation and development of fibroids.[1]

In addition to genetic factors, other known risk factors for fibroids are those that produce a long high exposure to estrogen and/or progesterone, such as an early menarche, polycystic ovarian syndrome, obesity, and pregnancy in advanced maternal age.[1]

The role of the combined action of estrogen and progesterone in the growth of fibroids is well known. Estrogens act primarily through their alpha receptor [estrogen receptor alpha (ERα)] and progesterone through the two isoforms of their nuclear receptor, progesterone receptor A (PRA) and progesterone receptor B (PRB).[3] The action of estradiol is to induce the expression of progesterone receptors that control the proliferation of smooth muscle cells and extracellular matrix.[4] However, while growth of fibroids seems to depend on sex steroids; ERα, PRA, and PRB receptors are not found in all fibroid cells, suggesting the presence of paracrine mechanisms acting through growth factors, such as cytokines and chemokines; however, the mechanisms are still unknown.[3]

The most common age group for the appearance of symptoms is 30–40 years and only in rare occasions have fibroids been diagnosed in adolescents. Fibroids are found in pathological specimens of approximately 80% of hysterectomies.[5] During menopause, a reduction in size of fibroids is noted.[6]

CLINICAL MANIFESTATIONS

Fibroids are commonly asymptomatic but can have an impact on the woman's health, depending on their location and size. Traditionally, symptoms related to uterine fibroids are classified into three categories: abnormal uterine bleeding, pelvic pain or pressure, and impaired reproductive function.

More than 50% of fibroids are small and asymptomatic.[7] When symptoms are present, it is difficult to ascertain whether they are related to fibroids or to concomitant pathologies in the endometrial cavity.

Many classifications have been reported according to the location of the fibroids. The one proposed by the International Federation of Gynecology and Obstetrics

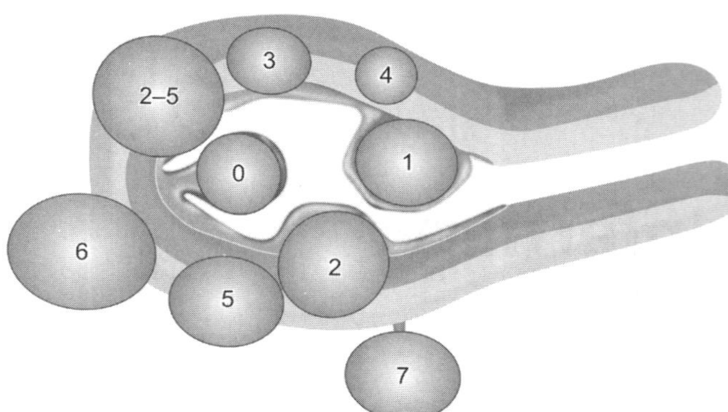

Fig. 1: The FIGO classification of uterine fibroids. Fibroid types range from 0 to 8. 0 = Pedunculated, intracavitary; 1 = Submucosal, <50% intramural; 2 = Submucosal, >50% intramural; 3 = Contact with endometrium, 100% intramural; 4 = Intramural; 5 = Subserosal, >50% intramural; 6 = Subserosal, <50% intramural; 7 = Subserosal, pedunculated; 8 = Other (e.g. cervical, parasitic). Where two numbers are given (e.g. 2–5), the first number refers to the relationship with the endometrium, while the second number refers to the relationship with the serosa, e.g. 2–5 = Submucosal and subserosal, each with less than half the diameter in the endometrial and peritoneal cavities, respectively.[8] (FIGO: International Federation of Gynecology and Obstetrics)

(FIGO)[8] describes eight types of fibroids, including a hybrid class (association of two types of fibroids) (Fig. 1).

Abnormal uterine bleeding is the most common symptom and may show a pattern of heavy and/or prolonged menstrual bleeding.[9] Excessive uterine bleeding may be responsible for anemia with iron deficiency, asthenia, and loss of productivity at work. Intermenstrual and postmenopausal bleeding is not characteristic of fibroids and should be evaluated for an endometrial cause. The presence and degree of bleeding are mainly determined by the location of the fibroid, and size is a secondary issue. Submucous fibroids that protrude into the cavity (FIGO types 0–2) are most frequently associated with bleeding.

Other less frequent symptoms are more related to tumor size than to location. They compress adjacent organs, such as the genitourinary and rectal organs, producing pelvic pain, dyspareunia, and urinary symptoms, such as dysuria and polyuria.

The relationship between fibroids and fertility is controversial. However, a review of literature reports a general decreased conception compared to women with unexplained infertility. In general terms, myomectomy increases the pregnancy rate.[10] Large submucous or intramural fibroids may distort the uterine cavity and thereby cause difficulties in pregnancy due to difficult sperm migration, oocyte transport, and embryo implantation. The local endometrial inflammation and endometrial vascular alterations increase the risk of miscarriage. However, there is no randomized study to confirm this theory. Fibroids may also be associated with adverse obstetric outcomes, such as placental abruption, intrauterine growth restriction, and preterm labor.

DIAGNOSIS

Ultrasonography

Ultrasound is the gold standard test for uterine fibroids. It is easily available and enables an easy and inexpensive confirmation in almost all cases. Three-dimensional imaging technology is a useful tool for the investigation of myometrial pathology due to its ability to analyze the coronal visualization of the uterus.

Hysteroscopy

Hysteroscopy is usually performed in an outpatient setting and does not require any anesthesia. It is useful to differentiate intracavitary myomas from large endometrial polyps.

Magnetic Resonance Imaging

Magnetic resonance imaging (MRI) can provide information on the number, size, and vascularity of the fibroids and also their relationship with the endometrial cavity and the serosal surface. Magnetic resonance imaging findings can help to diagnose a sarcoma, which remains a very infrequent condition (1/1,500 in women aged <40 years and 1/1,100 in women aged 40–44 years).[11]

CURRENT MANAGEMENT OF FIBROIDS

Many women with fibroids do not have any symptoms, and fibroids are an incidental finding in approximately 50% of affected women. Since histologic confirmation is rarely needed, women with asymptomatic fibroids can be followed up without any therapeutic intervention.[12] Prophylactic therapy is also not recommended just to avoid future complications.[13]

In symptomatic cases, treatment is required. The most common treatment for symptomatic fibroids is surgery, and medical pharmacological options have been limited so far. However, the radical nature of surgery, coupled with the morbidity and complications that may occur, has forced the need to develop new medical approaches in order to avoid or reduce the need for surgery, or as presurgical treatments to reduce the potential risks of surgery.

In the last few years, different medical treatments have been evaluated for their role in the amelioration of symptoms. Treatment aim should be resolution of symptoms[14] and therefore restoration of fertility and/or improvement of reproductive prognosis.

MEDICAL TREATMENT

Nowadays, women wish to avoid surgical treatment for fibroids, especially hysterectomy, in order to preserve their maternity desire. Surgery can be avoided if there is a medical option that can control heavy menstrual bleeding, improve symptoms related to anemia, and improve quality of life.

As far as medical treatment is concerned, it is important to note that all medical approaches to reduce fibroid size induce anovulation or cannot be given to pregnant women or to women trying to conceive. Most current medical treatments are based on the close relationship between ovarian sex steroids and fibroids. Fibroids have a high concentration of estrogen and progesterone receptors compared to normal myometrium,[15] and it has been reported that progesterone plays a key role in the growth of fibroids.

At present, available medical treatments are used as short-term therapies, due to the absence of evidence of their benefits and long-term safety, and are usually given to improve the patient's symptoms, or preoperatively to reduce the size of fibroids and improve anemia, or within clinical trials.

Gonadotropin-releasing Hormone Agonists

Gonadotropin-releasing hormone (GnRH) agonists have been used extensively in the expectant management of fibroids since 1995 when they were authorized for preoperative use.[16] Until now, they were considered the most effective medical treatment for fibroids.

Most women on GnRH agonists become amenorrheic with resultant improvement in their anemia, and uterine size is reduced from 35 to 60% in the first 3 months of treatment.[17] The myoma regression, however, is reversible, with fibroids returning to their original size after stopping treatment. In addition, the hypoestrogenism associated with GnRH agonist use can lead to distressing symptoms, such as hot flashes, insomnia, vaginal dryness, myalgia, and arthralgia. Osteoporosis is a serious adverse effect after prolonged treatment and is usually the limiting factor for the use of GnRH agonists.

Due to the side effects and the quick reappearance of symptoms after stopping treatment, GnRH agonists are used only as preoperative treatment. They are approved to be used for preoperative management for 3–6 months, along with iron supplements, to facilitate surgery and improve anemia before surgery.[18]

In addition, the use of GnRH analogs has been shown to be a risk factor for myoma relapse after surgery[19] presumably because small fibroids are reduced and go unnoticed in surgery, increasing in size upon cessation of treatment. A cost-benefit study[20] of the preoperative use of analogs shows that the costs outweigh the benefits. For all this, GnRH analogs are recommended only for preoperative use in infertile patients with anemia and/or myoma more than 3 cm.[21]

Selective Estrogen Receptor Modulator

Any molecule that blocks estrogen receptors should have effects on fibroids, but selective estrogen receptor modulator, such as raloxifene, has no clear indication. Preclinical studies in animals and postmenopausal women have been positive, but studies in women of reproductive age are less convincing.[22] Among its side effects are the presence of hot flashes, increased appetite, weight gain, gastritis, and dry skin. And the most serious adverse effect is the increased risk of venous thromboembolism.

Selective Progesterone Receptor Modulator

Progesterone has been shown to be an important factor in the development and growth of fibroids, so it was thought to use antiprogestogens, such as selective progesterone receptor modulator (SPRM) for the control of fibroids symptoms.

These are a family of progesterone receptor ligands with mixed agonist-antagonist properties. The results of small controlled studies with SPRM [asoprisnil, mifepristone, telapristone, ulipristal acetate (UPA)] support the idea that these agents may be useful for the treatment of fibroids.[23,24]

In vitro cultures of human fibrocytes have resulted in decreased cell proliferation and an induction of the proapoptotic pathway.[25] In contrast, these effects did not occur in normal myometrial cells.

The activity of the ligands at the progesterone receptor can range from pure agonists, such as progesterone to pure antagonists, such as mifepristone. Of all the SPRMs, only UPA has been approved for use in the treatment of fibroids, the others have been abandoned due to problems of liver toxicity or harmful effects on the endometrium.[23,26]

Ulipristal acetate is a synthetic steroid which reversibly blocks the progesterone receptor in target tissues and acts as a potent selective modulator. In fibroids with progesterone receptors, it exerts this action inducing a quick cessation of bleeding and subsequent amenorrhea as well as decreased fibroid size.

Ulipristal acetate is the first SPRM to have completed phase III[27] trials and has received approval by the European Medicines Agency (EMA) for use as a treatment for myoma.

An important aspect of medium- and long-term (3–6 months) administration of SPRM is that they induce characteristic nonphysiological endometrial changes, such as hyperplasia.[28] These benign endometrial changes represent a new morphological category that has been called "SPRM-associated endometrial change" and is characterized by the presence of an inactive and weakly proliferative epithelium associated with an asymmetry of stromal and epithelial growth that results in prominent cystically dilated glands. In any case, these changes are reversed after cessation of SPRM administration, and the endometrium recovers its usual histology, in most cases after 6 months without treatment.[29] It is important that pathologists know about this entity and make sure they do not get confused with endometrial polyps or endometrial hyperplasia.

Ulipristal acetate acts directly on the endometrium maintaining its glandular proliferation and stroma at very low levels, and therefore, producing amenorrhea in the majority of patients. It inhibits ovulation but with little impact on serum estrogen levels, thus avoiding the hypoestrogenic side effects characteristic of GnRH analogs.

Randomized phase III clinical trials of UPA (doses of 5 and 10 mg/day) versus placebo and GnRH analogs in symptomatic women with fibroids [PGL4001 (UPA) Efficacy Assessment in Reduction of symptoms due to uterine Leiomyomata (PEARL) I and II] have shown that treatment for 13 weeks with UPA is effective for the control of excessive menstrual bleeding and reduction of fibroid size.[30,31]

The results of long-term treatment (18 months) with UPA, 10 mg daily administered as four 3-month courses, immediately followed by 10-day double-blind treatment with norethisterone acetate or placebo (PEARL III), confirmed a high rate of amenorrhea, as well as reduction in the size of fibroids. All endometrial biopsies showed benign histology without hyperplasia or carcinoma. The resolution of menorrhagia was faster in the ulipristal treated group (6 days on average, compared to 30 days in the analog), leading to rapid improvement of preoperative anemia if iron supplements are added.

Unlike the analogs, UPA treatment does not induce an initial flare-up, which is an additional advantage for women with menorrhagia. In addition, women treated with UPA had fewer side effects, such as moderate or severe hot flashes (10% with UPA vs. 40% with analogs). There was no statistically significant difference in the reduction in myoma size, although it was numerically somewhat lower in the ulipristal treated groups (35.4% in those treated with 5 mg, 42.08% in those treated with 10 mg, and 53.5% with leuprolide).

As far as tumor size was concerned, unlike leuprolide acetate, reduction of myoma size appeared to be maintained for 6 months after the end of treatment in patients treated with UPA.

Recently, a review of Esmya (UPA) was carried out by EMA's Pharmacovigilance Risk Assessment Committee (PRAC) following reports of serious liver injury, including liver failure leading to transplantation. The PRAC concluded that UPA may have contributed to the development of some cases of serious liver injury.

The EMA has recommended that several measures be put in place to minimize the risk of rare but serious liver injury with UPA. Certain women may start treatment with UPA once the new measures are implemented.

The measures include—contraindication in women with known liver problems; liver tests before, during, and after stopping treatment; a card for patients to inform them about the need for liver monitoring; and to contact their doctor should they develop symptoms of liver injury. In addition, use of the medicine for more than one treatment course has been restricted to women who are not eligible for surgery.

The PRAC therefore recommended that use of the medicine should be restricted. It also recommended that studies should be performed to determine the effects of UPA on the liver and whether the new measures are effective in minimizing the risks.

This data supports that ulipristal acetate is clinically effective and has a better safety profile, making it very useful to modify the current protocols of surgical intervention in the treatment of fibroids,[32] by using UPA either as pre-surgical therapy or as medical treatment to avoid surgery. Its indication should be re-evaluated in infertile patients in the time to come.

SURGICAL TREATMENT

Until the 1990s, the only option for the treatment of fibroids was hysterectomy or abdominal myomectomy. Hysterectomy leads to definitive cure of all symptoms, while myomectomy was reserved for patients with unfulfilled pregnancy desires. Myomectomy is a major surgery associated with possible morbidity and may also alter fertility due to the development of adhesions. In addition, myomectomy does not protect from the possible recurrence of the disease.

Advances in instrumentation and surgical technique have made it possible to perform hysteroscopic and laparoscopic myomectomy which have become the standards for minimally invasive fibroid surgery. The surgical approach depends on the location, number, and size of fibroids.

Submucous or Intracavitary Myomas

Submucosal or intracavitary fibroids (types 0, 1, and 2 of the FIGO) are usually symptomatic and significantly reduce pregnancy rates in in vitro fertilization cycles.[10] Hence, it is recommended to remove them before planning a pregnancy.

Hysteroscopic Myomectomy

Hysteroscopic myomectomy is indicated in symptomatic and/or infertile patients with submucous fibroids.

For submucous fibroids more than 3 cm in size, UPA can be used preoperatively to reduce the size of the fibroid and to decrease bleeding during the intervention.[33]

Resectoscopes with bipolar high-frequency current and loop-shaped electrodes are used with saline as distending medium, reducing the risk of fluid overload, hyponatremia, and ammonia toxicity that may occur when glycine is used for distention.

For fibroids with a large intramural component, the procedure can be performed in two steps. First, a myomatous resection where the portion of the fibroid protruding into the cavity is removed, which allows myometrial contractility and leads to migration of the residual intramural component of the myoma into the cavity for a second intervention for complete removal.

For submucosal fibroids larger than 5 cm and with a larger intramural component than intracavitary (FIGO 3–5 types), the laparoscopic route is preferred.

Studies have not shown clear benefit from postoperative placement of intrauterine contraceptive device or with oral contraceptive pills (OCPs) for prevention of adhesions.[34] However, in patients with bleeding postsurgery, OCPs can reduce the intensity and duration of postsurgical bleeding by forcing endometrial epithelialization.[34]

The results of the hysteroscopic myomectomy in experienced hands are excellent, especially in the cases of single intracavitary fibroids, obtaining in most cases a practically normal endometrial cavity.

Subserous Myomas

Subserous fibroids do not compromise the endometrial cavity and therefore are not usually symptomatic and do not affect the reproductive capacity of a woman. However, large fibroids may produce some anatomical distortion and therefore symptoms secondary to the compression of neighboring organs.

Therefore, surgery for asymptomatic subserous fibroids is not the first line of treatment. For subserous fibroids that produce clinical symptoms by the compression of neighboring organs, the indication of myomectomy is clear and the mode of surgery, whether laparoscopy or laparotomy, depends on the size of the fibroid/s and the extent of intramural component. For fibroids larger than 10–12 cm, minilaparotomy route seems to be indicated.

Intramural Myomas

Intramural fibroids are the ones that create dilemma regarding surgery. For symptomatic patients, surgical treatment is offered. However, in the cases of infertility, the indication is less evident.[35] Studies seem to support the idea that the fibroids that do not distort the endometrial cavity do not seem to affect pregnancy rates but do increase miscarriage rates.[36]

A recent meta-analysis associates poor pregnancy outcomes in patients with intramural or submucous fibroids that distort the cavity, but also those that do not distort the cavity.[15]

On the other hand, our group performed a study comparing clinical and endometrial gene expression results in patients with intramural myoma more than 5 or less than 5 cm that did not distort the endometrial cavity in egg donation cycles.[37] Clinical results in both groups did not show significant differences in the rates of implantation, pregnancy, spontaneous embryo reduction, clinical abortion, and ongoing pregnancy. We also excluded a global alteration of gene expression relevant to endometrial receptivity in patients with fibroids.

Laparoscopic Myomectomy

Laparoscopic myomectomy in well-selected patients and in the hands of expert surgeons is a less invasive alternative to abdominal laparotomy myomectomy and with good results. Moreover, although perceived by gynecologists as more difficult, laparoscopic myomectomy is associated with less severe postoperative morbidity (less blood loss, fever, and pain), shorter hospitalization, and rapid recovery. To avoid uterine rupture after laparoscopic myomectomy, correct closure of myometrial defect is required. It is necessary to have an extensive experience in this technique.

It is important to emphasize that the presence of anemia is a relative contraindication for the performance of surgery, since it has been demonstrated to increase the postoperative morbidity.[38] Thus contraindications for laparoscopic myomectomy include fibroids more than 12 cm, more than four fibroids, and significant anemia.[32]

The recurrence of fibroids seems to be more frequent after the laparoscopic approach than after laparotomy, although in a randomized study, no differences were found in the rates of recurrences at 40 months between laparoscopic (23%) and laparotomy patients (27%).[39]

The use of analogs prior to laparoscopic myomectomy is discouraged because it increases the rate of conversion to laparotomy.

As compared to abdominal myomectomy, laparoscopic myomectomy needs longer surgical time but is associated with a lower overall rate of complications, shorter recovery time, and lower risk of adhesions.[40]

In general, pregnancy and miscarriage rates after laparoscopic myomectomy are comparable to those after abdominal myomectomy, even for patients who required laparoscopic repair of the endometrial cavity.

In very few cases, surgery for suspected malignancy should be considered. Confirmation of benignity of myoma should not be an indication for surgery, except for very fast-growing fibroids or MRI/ultrasound images that are suspicious of smooth muscle tumor of uncertain malignant potential or a sarcoma.[41]

In April 2014, the Food and Drug Administration put forward a notice advising against the use of laparoscopic electrical morcellation during myomectomy or hysterectomy in women with uterine fibroids due to the risk of dissemination of possible neoplastic tissue, especially in patients with uterine sarcomas unidentified as such initially.[42]

At present, there are no effective tools to diagnose a sarcoma with certainty in a benign-appearing myoma. However, it is necessary to take into account suspicious cases according to their presentation, evolution, and characteristics in the imaging studies to determine whether or not to use the morcellator in each case.

Uterine morcellation is clearly contraindicated in the cases where malignancy is suspected or confirmed. In Spain, although no incidents related to this problem have been reported, it is recommended to take all precautions in the preoperative evaluation of each particular case and to carry out morcellation in isolation bags for later extraction of the pieces.

As previously mentioned, a confirmation of the effectiveness and lower side effect profile of UPA in the medical treatment of fibroids has led some authors to propose a review of the current indications for myoma surgery in infertile patients[32,33] that we collect in the algorithm of action in the management of fibroids (Flowchart 1).

Flowchart 1: Myomas and sterility algorithm.

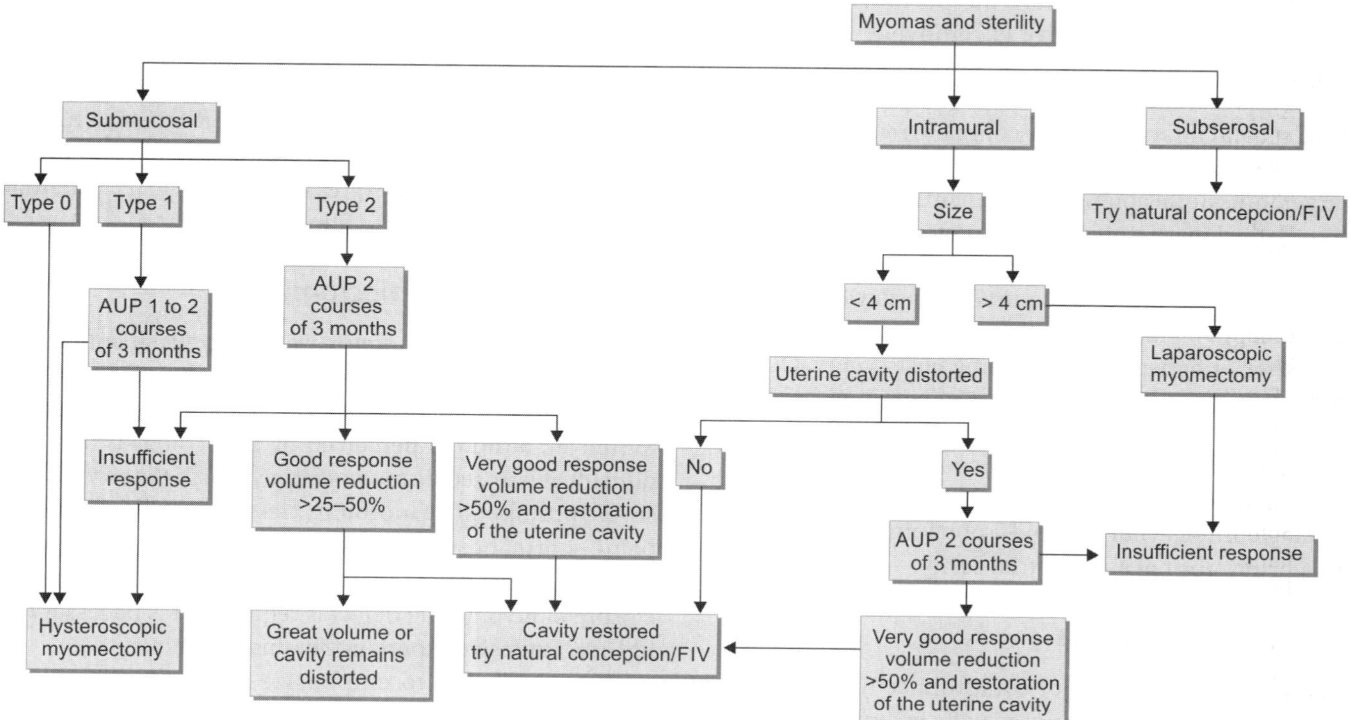

KEY POINTS

- Fibroids are very common in women of reproductive age, and their origin is unknown
- Diagnosis is made primarily by transvaginal ultrasound and in the case of multiple fibroids, MRI is very valuable.
- Surgery (myomectomy) is the definitive treatment for symptomatic fibroids
- Infertile patients with fibroids affecting the endometrial cavity should undergo myomectomy using the hysteroscopic or laparoscopic approach
- Selective progesterone receptor modulators may be useful but must still demonstrate their efficacy and safety in the case of infertile patients. For symptomatic patients who have not yet completed their family, SPRM (UPA) has become a first therapeutic option that can prevent surgery once we have ruled out liver function problems.

REFERENCES

1. Mas A, Cervello I, Gil-Sanchis C, et al. Current understanding of somatic stem cells in leiomyoma formation. Fertil Steril. 2014;102(3):613-20.
2. Makinen N, Mehine M, Tolvanen J, et al. MED12, the mediator complex subunit 12 gene, is mutated at high frequency in uterine leiomyomas. Science. 2011;334(6053):252-5.
3. Islam MS, Protic O, Stortoni P, et al. Complex networks of multiple factors in the pathogenesis of uterine leiomyoma. Fertil Steril. 2013;100(1):178-93.
4. Ishikawa H, Ishi K, Serna VA, et al. Progesterone is essential for maintenance and growth of uterine leiomyoma. Endocrinology. 2010;151(6):2433-42.
5. Cramer SF, Patel A. The frequency of uterine leiomyomas. Am J Clin Pathol. 1990;94(4):435-8.
6. Al-Inany HG, Youssef MA, Aboulghar M, et al. Gonadotrophin-releasing hormone antagonists for assisted reproductive technology. Cochrane Database Syst Rev. 2011(5):CD001750.
7. Gupta S, Jose J, Manyonda I. Clinical presentation of fibroids. Best Pract Res Clin Obstet Gynaecol. 2008;22(4):615-26.
8. Munro MG, Critchley HO, Fraser IS; FIGO Menstrual Disorders Working Group. The FIGO classification of causes of abnormal uterine bleeding in the reproductive years. Fertil Steril. 2011;95(7):2204-8, 2208.e1-3.
9. Fraser IS, Critchley HO, Munro MG, et al. Writing Group for This Menstrual Agreement Process. A process designed to lead to international agreement on terminologies and definitions used to describe abnormalities of menstrual bleeding. Fertil Steril. 2007;87(3):466-76.
10. Somigliana E, Vercellini P, Daguati R, et al. Fibroids and female reproduction: a critical analysis of the evidence. Hum Reprod Update. 2007;13(5):465-76.
11. Wright JD, Tergas AI, Burke WM, et al. Uterine pathology in women undergoing minimally invasive hysterectomy using morcellation. JAMA. 2014;312(12):1253-5.
12. Parker WH. Uterine myomas: management. Fertil Steril. 2007;88(2):255-71.
13. Lefebvre G, Vilos G, Allaire C, et al. The management of uterine leiomyomas. J Obstet Gynaecol Can. 2003;25(5):396-418; quiz 419-22.
14. American College of Obstetricians and Gynecologists. ACOG practice bulletin. Alternatives to hysterectomy in the management of leiomyomas. Obstet Gynecol. 2008;112(2 Pt 1):387-400.
15. Sunkara SK, Khairy M, El-Toukhy T, et al. The effect of intramural fibroids without uterine cavity involvement on the outcome of IVF treatment: a systematic review and meta-analysis. Hum Reprod. 2010;25(2):418-29.
16. Lethaby A, Vollenhoven B, Sowter M. Pre-operative GnRH analogue therapy before hysterectomy or myomectomy for uterine fibroids. Cochrane Database Syst Rev. 2001;(2):CD000547.
17. Minaguchi H, Wong JM, Snabes MC. Clinical use of nafarelin in the treatment of leiomyomas. A review of the literature. J Reprod Med. 2000;45(6):481-9.
18. Lethaby A, Vollenhoven B, Sowter M. Efficacy of pre-operative gonadotrophin hormone releasing analogues for women with uterine fibroids undergoing hysterectomy or myomectomy: a systematic review. BJOG. 2002;109(10):1097-108.
19. Vercellini P, Trespidi L, Zaina B, et al. Gonadotropin-releasing hormone agonist treatment before abdominal myomectomy: a controlled trial. Fertil Steril. 2003;79(6):1390-5.
20. Farquhar C, Brown PM, Furness S. Cost effectiveness of pre-operative gonadotrophin releasing analogues for women with uterine fibroids undergoing hysterectomy or myomectomy. BJOG. 2002;109(11):1273-80.
21. Sankaran S, Manyonda IT. Medical management of fibroids. Best Pract Res Clin Obstet Gynaecol. 2008;22(4):655-76.
22. Palomba S, Sammartino A, Di Carlo C, et al. Effects of raloxifene treatment on uterine leiomyomas in postmenopausal women. Fertil Steril. 2001;76(1):38-43.
23. Carbonell Esteve JL, Acosta R, Heredia B, et al. Mifepristone for the treatment of uterine leiomyomas: a randomized controlled trial. Obstet Gynecol. 2008;112(5):1029-36.
24. Nieman LK, Blocker W, Nansel T, et al. Efficacy and tolerability of CDB-2914 treatment for symptomatic uterine fibroids: a randomized, double-blind, placebo-controlled, phase IIb study. Fertil Steril. 2011;95(2):767-72.e1-2.
25. Chen W, Ohara N, Wang J, et al. A novel selective progesterone receptor modulator asoprisnil (J867) inhibits proliferation and induces apoptosis in cultured human uterine leiomyoma cells in the absence of comparable effects on myometrial cells. J Clin Endocrinol Metab. 2006;91(4):1296-304.
26. Wilkens J, Chwalisz K, Han C, et al. Effects of the selective progesterone receptor modulator asoprisnil on uterine artery blood flow, ovarian activity, and clinical symptoms in patients with uterine leiomyomata scheduled for hysterectomy. J Clin Endocrinol Metab. 2008;93(12):4664-71.
27. Donnez J, Vazquez F, Tomaszewski J, et al. Long-term treatment of uterine fibroids with ulipristal acetate. Fertil Steril. 2014;101(6):1565-73.e1-18.
28. Mutter GL, Bergeron C, Deligdisch L, et al. The spectrum of endometrial pathology induced by progesterone receptor modulators. Mod Pathol. 2008;21(5):591-8.

29. Williams AR, Bergeron C, Barlow DH, et al. Endometrial morphology after treatment of uterine fibroids with the selective progesterone receptor modulator, ulipristal acetate. Int J Gynecol Pathol. 2012;31(6):556-69.
30. Donnez J, Tomaszewski J, Vazquez F, et al. Ulipristal acetate versus leuprolide acetate for uterine fibroids. N Engl J Med. 2012;366(5):421-32.
31. Donnez J, Tatarchuk TF, Bouchard P, et al. Ulipristal acetate versus placebo for fibroid treatment before surgery. N Engl J Med. 2012;366(5):409-20.
32. Donnez J, Donnez O, Dolmans MM. With the advent of selective progesterone receptor modulators, what is the place of myoma surgery in current practice? Fertil Steril. 2014;102(3):640-8.
33. Donnez J, Dolmans MM. Uterine fibroid management: from the present to the future. Hum Reprod Update. 2016;22(6):665-86.
34. Surgery AEG. AAGL practice report: practice guidelines on intrauterine adhesions developed in collaboration with the European Society of Gynaecological Endoscopy (ESGE). Gynecol Surg. 2017;14(1):6.
35. Crosignani PG, Somigliana E. Effect of GnRH antagonists in FSH mildly stimulated intrauterine insemination cycles: a multicentre randomized trial. Hum Reprod. 2007;22(2):500-5.
36. Pritts EA, Parker WH, Olive DL. Fibroids and infertility: an updated systematic review of the evidence. Fertil Steril. 2009;91(4):1215-23.
37. Horcajadas JA, Goyri E, Higon MA, et al. Endometrial receptivity and implantation are not affected by the presence of uterine intramural leiomyomas: a clinical and functional genomics analysis. J Clin Endocrinol Metab. 2008;93(9):3490-8.
38. Kim YH, Chung HH, Kang SB, et al. Safety and usefulness of intravenous iron sucrose in the management of preoperative anemia in patients with menorrhagia: a phase IV, open-label, prospective, randomized study. Acta Haematol. 2009;121(1):37-41.
39. Rossetti A, Sizzi O, Soranna L, et al. Long-term results of laparoscopic myomectomy: recurrence rate in comparison with abdominal myomectomy. Hum Reprod. 2001;16(4):770-4.
40. Wen KC, Chen YJ, Sung PL, et al. Comparing uterine fibroids treated by myomectomy through traditional laparotomy and 2 modified approaches: ultraminilaparotomy and laparoscopically assisted ultraminilaparotomy. Am J Obstet Gynecol. 2010;202(2):144.e1-8.
41. Pritts EA, Parker WH, Brown J, et al. Outcome of occult uterine leiomyosarcoma after surgery for presumed uterine fibroids: a systematic review. J Minim Invasive Gynecol. 2015;22(1):26-33.
42. Brolmann H, Tanos V, Grimbizis G, et al. Options on fibroid morcellation: a literature review. Gynecol Surg. 2015;12(1):3-15.

CHAPTER

70

Management Options for Endometrioma Associated with Infertility

Parul Katiyar

INTRODUCTION

Endometriosis is a benign, estrogen-dependent gynecological condition characterized by presence of endometrial tissue outside the uterus. Endometriosis affects approximately 5–10% of women of reproductive age group and symptoms include chronic pelvic pain, dysmenorrhea, dyspareunia, and/or infertility.[1] Endometrioma is a distinct presentation of endometriosis and may manifest in isolation or in association with other features of endometriosis and its association with infertility or reduced ovarian reserve remains controversial. Ovarian endometrioma is seen in approximately 17–44% of women with endometriosis and over 40% of women having ovarian endometrioma have accompanying deeply infiltrating endometriosis.[2]

PATHOGEN

The exact pathogenesis of formation of ovarian endometrioma is not yet known. The three main theories to explain formation of endometrioma are:

1. Invagination of ovarian cortex secondary to bleeding of a superficial implant
2. Invagination of ovarian cortex secondary to metaplasia of coelomic epithelium in cortical inclusion cyst
3. Endometriotic transformation of functional cyst.

EFFECTS OF OVARIAN ENDOMETRIOSIS ON FERTILITY

Endometrioma has been found to be present in approximately 17% of cases with clinical infertility and approximately 20–40% women who undergo assisted reproductive technology (ART) have endometriosis. Visualization of endometrioma may be an isolated finding or may be a manifestation of underlying endometriosis. Endometriosis has been associated with pain and infertility. Although the relationship between endometriosis and pain is well proven, the link between endometriosis and infertility is less well defined.

The exact mechanism by which endometrioma causes infertility is also not known, though a number of mechanisms have been suggested. The probable mechanisms for endometriosis-related infertility include distorted pelvic anatomy, inflammation, endocrine and immunologic abnormalities, poor ovarian reserve and ovulatory dysfunction.

DIAGNOSIS OF ENDOMETRIOMA

Endometriosis often presents with pain in abdomen and pelvis, which is associated with dyspareunia, dysmenorrhea, menorrhagia, and other nonspecific IBS/PID-like symptoms. Endometrioma is a distinctly visualized cyst in the ovary. The diagnosis of endometriosis is traditionally based on laparoscopy, which is also the gold standard for diagnosis.

However, endometrioma can be easily diagnosed using a traditional transvaginal ultrasound (TVS) also because of its characteristic ultrasonographic appearance—unilocular cyst with homogeneous ground-glass echoes and thick walls resulting from hemorrhagic debris. This appearance occurs in 50% of cases. In some cases, the endometrioma may be multiloculated with presence of hyperechoic wall foci.[3]

TREATMENT OF INFERTILE WOMEN WITH ENDOMETRIOMA

Objective of Treatment

The ultimate goal of treatment in these patients is to achieve pregnancy, either spontaneously or using IVF.

Surgical Options for Management of Endometrioma

Effective and lasting treatment of endometriosis is a big challenge for gynecologists. Laparoscopy is generally considered an effective and proven treatment option for endometriosis due to its good tolerance and low morbidity.[4] However, there is limited clinical evidence and consensus to support its direct role in treating endometrioma. The high recurrence rate of ovarian endometrioma and its concurrent symptoms represents one of the less satisfactory aspects of the surgical treatment of endometriosis.[5]

Options for Surgical Management

- *Laparoscopic cystectomy*: It is a surgical procedure, which strips the entire cyst wall from the ovary and removes the entire endometrioma from the ovary. The procedure was initially considered a standard treatment care for women with endometriomas because of a reduced recurrence rate. The advantages of cystectomy are an increase in spontaneous pregnancy rates (ranging from 14% up to 54%), reduced pelvic pain and also reduced recurrence rates. In an observational study, Barri et al. compared the pregnancy outcome in patients with endometriosis who underwent surgical intervention with the ones who underwent expectant management. They found that up to 54% women in the surgical intervention group became pregnant over a 7-year follow-up, whereas only about 12% women from the expectant management group conceived.[6]
  However, laparoscopic cystectomy has its own disadvantages. Since the cyst does not have an actual cyst wall, cystectomy leads to removal of healthy ovarian cortex and follicles leading to reduced ovarian reserve and, even, ovarian failure in some cases. There is also a potential risk of scarring of the ovaries as well as inflammation which may lead to even poor outcomes. Therefore, in view of potential complications, laparoscopic cystectomy should be performed by experienced surgeons only. Laparoscopic cystectomy has been found to have a recurrence rate of 45%.[7]
- *Laparoscopic cyst aspiration and ablation of the cyst wall*: In this procedure, the cyst is first drained and then followed by ablation of the cyst wall using either electrosurgical current or laser energy. Ablating the cyst wall reduces the chances of recurrence, and spares the removal of healthy ovarian tissue that is associated with cystectomy. While both electrocautery and laser have been used for ablation, laser ablation (CO_2 or KTP) is considered to be better due to its tissue sparing effect. Laser ablation does not have the adverse effect on ovarian reserve, which could result from use of electrocautery.
  A Cochrane review that compared the clinical outcomes of cystectomy and ablative surgery in women with endometrioma concluded that excisional surgery for endometrioma had more favorable clinical outcome than drainage and ablation in form of lesser cyst recurrence rate, lesser recurrence of pain symptoms, and better subsequent spontaneous pregnancy rate in previously subfertile women. However, women planning subsequent IVF should avoid surgical intervention.[8]
- *Cyst aspiration*: This is a procedure in which the endometriotic fluid is aspirated from the transvaginal route with a needle under ultrasound visualization. This is a simple procedure yet is not popular because of a high chance of recurrence with a recurrence rate of up to 91% after a single aspiration; therefore, the patient may need to undergo multiple aspirations, with up to six aspirations reported to have a 5.4% recurrence rate.[9] The other potential risks are infection leading to ovarian abscess formation and adhesion formation. Cyst aspiration has also been tried in conjunction with sclerotherapy using 95% ethanol or methotrexate, in order to reduce the risk of recurrence after aspiration. The sclerosing agent chemically destroys the cyst wall, thereby preventing recurrence. This method, however, is not routinely practiced.
- *Other options*: Other surgical options for the management of anendometrioma include cystectomy with vasopressin injection into the cyst wall, cystectomy with ablation, cystectomy with gelatin matrix seal, and a three staged technique combining laparoscopic cyst drainage followed by gonadotropin-releasing hormone (GnRH) agonist treatment for 3 months followed by a second laparoscopic surgery for vaporization of the cyst wall using CO_2 laser. These methods also attempt to reduce the recurrence rates of endometrioma without adversely affecting the ovarian reserve.

Surgical management of endometriosis has been under considerable investigation due to high incidence of recurrence and because of the potential damage to the ovary. Many studies have analyzed the recurrence rate of endometriomas after laparoscopic surgery, and found it to be between 11.0% and 30% after more than or equal to 2 years of observation.[10-15]

Medical Management of Patients with Endometrioma

There is minimal role of medical management of endometrioma in improving pregnancy rates, as most of the medications like birth control pills are counterproductive to pregnancy. In one of the early studies on this subject, Donnez et al. compared effectiveness of GnRH with that of placebo in reducing size of the cyst and found that GnRH group had 25% higher reduction in diameter of the cyst as compared to the placebo group.[16] GnRH analogs have also been tried in conjunction with surgery in which GnRH analog is given for 3–6 months following either a laparoscopic cyst drainage or partial cystectomy to reduce the cyst size. This approach could have an advantage for selected group of patients, as this approach minimizes the loss of ovarian volume during surgery and preserves maximum ovarian reserve. However, it is a time taking approach and, therefore, is not suitable for many women.

A recent meta-analysis showed that using GnRH analogs for a 3–6 months period prior to an IVF cycle improved the odds of clinical pregnancy in women with endometriosis by four times. However, we need to be careful while extrapolating the results from this analysis to wider patient population as the study population was rather short, and also the study included three studies on patients with endometriosis and not specifically endometrioma.[7]

Medical management, however, is moderately effective in alleviating pain associated with endometriosis.

Expectant Management of Patients with Endometrioma

This entails no surgical or medical intervention in women presenting with endometrioma. The disadvantages of expectant management include:

- Missing out on an early stage malignancy (very low probability)
- Progression of endometriosis
- Rupture of the endometrioma
- Worsening of associated symptoms like pain
- Further decline in ovarian reserve, thereby further reduction in fertility potential.

While prescribing expectant management to these patients, one should counsel them for the potential pitfalls of nonintervention and recommend a repeat consultation in case the symptoms deteriorate.

In Vitro Fertilization

A significant number of women with moderate to severe endometriosis seeking treatment for infertility need ART. Intrauterine insemination (IUI) may be useful only for women with mild endometriosis. Therefore, IVF or ICSI (intracytoplasmic sperm injection) is the preferred treatment for women with endometrioma. Long and ultra-long GnRH agonist protocols are considered the most effective stimulation protocols for such patients. However, a prospective randomized trial on women with minimal to mild endometriosis and endometrioma comparing the results of GnRH antagonist and GnRH agonist protocols for IVF concluded that the implantation rate and clinical pregnancy rate with antagonist protocol were not any inferior to those for the agonist protocol.[17]

A recent meta-analysis of impact of endometrioma on outcome of IVF concluded that women with endometrioma had similar reproductive outcomes as women without the disease, although cycle cancellation rate was significantly higher in the affected women. Also prior surgical intervention had no beneficial effect on the IVF outcome.[18] Women with endometrioma undergoing IVF have higher cancellation rate, higher total gonadotropin requirement, and lower oocyte yield as compared to women undergoing IVF for other indications. However, these women have similar fertilization rate, implantation rate, and pregnancy rate to those without endometrioma.

Impact of Ovarian Endometrioma on IVF Outcome

Endometriosis and specially endometrioma has been implicated to adversely impact oocyte quality and ovarian reserve, which lead to reduced ovarian responsiveness and poor pregnancy rate.[19]

- *Impact of an ovarian endometrioma on oocyte quality*: The effect of endometrioma on oocyte quality is controversial. Early histological studies by Maneschi et al., Muzii et al., and Schubert et al. indicated toward a significant detrimental effect of presence of ovarian endometrioma on the ovary.[20-22] Matsuzaki S attributed this detrimental effect on affected ovaries to the oxidative stress resulting from presence of the ovarian endometrioma.[23] They found that the amount of oxidative stress and ROS production in the ovarian cortex surrounding ovarian endometrioma was much higher than in other kinds of ovarian cysts. However, more recent clinical studies have found that the endometrioma has less dramatic impact on the clinical outcome of IVF and pregnancy. Kumbak et al. found that the number of oocytes retrieved in women with endometrioma was significantly lesser in comparison to women with simple ovarian cysts.[24] However, the number of mature oocytes and fertilization rates were not significantly different between the two groups, though the implantation rates were lower for women with endometriomas. Fillipi et al. compared ovarian responsiveness and oocyte quality between the affected and contralateral intact ovary in women with unoperated unilateral endometrioma who underwent IVF.[25] They did not find any statistically significant difference between ovarian responsiveness and oocyte quality between the two sides. They also did not find any significant difference in fertilization rate, cleavage rate, and the percentage good quality embryos on two sides, thereby concluding that the presence of ovarian endometrioma does not affect oocyte developmental competence. Bongioanni et al. compared the outcome of IVF in women with previous or present diagnosis of ovarian endometriosis with that in patients with tubal factor infertility in a retrospective analysis.[26] While women with ovarian endometriosis were found to have significantly higher cycle cancellation rate and women with history of laparoscopic ovarian cystectomy prior to IVF had reduced ovarian responsiveness to gonadotropins, the authors found similar pregnancy, implantation, and delivery rate across the two groups.

- *Impact of an ovarian endometrioma on ovarian reserve*: Ovarian reserve, defined as a woman's total ovarian follicle pool which includes both primordial and growing follicles, is most commonly measured using the antral follicular count (AFC) on ultrasound, serum AMH (anti-Müllerian hormone) levels, and day 3 FSH (follicle-stimulating hormone) levels. Barri et al. compared AFC in women undergoing IVF for ovarian endometrioma with those undergoing IVF for male factor infertility and found that women in the endometrioma group has significantly lower AFC than the other group.[6] Almog et al. found that in women with unilateral endometrioma, the AFC was significantly lower in the affected ovary than in the unaffected contralateral ovary. However, the difference in AFC count between two ovaries was not found to be significant in cases with unilateral benign cysts.[27]
- *Impact of an ovarian endometrioma on ovarian responsiveness*: The evidence on this point is contradictory. Filippi et al. in a prospective cohort study did not find any significant difference between ovarian responsiveness and oocyte quality between the affected (ovary with endometrioma) and the intact ovary.[25] They also did not find any statistically significant difference in the number of viable embryos and number of high quality embryos between the two groups. Thus, they concluded that in women undergoing IVF, the presence of ovarian endometriomas does not affect the oocyte development. These findings are in line with similar studies conducted by Almog et al., and Benaglia et al.[27,28] However, findings from most studies on this subject are not in agreement with the above-mentioned findings. In a meta-analysis of five studies by Gupta et al., fewer oocytes were retrieved from women with endometriomas as compared to women without endometriomas.[29] Several other researchers have verified that endometrioma does have a negative effect on the ovarian responsiveness.[24,30,31] This result is also supported by a recent histological study by Kuroda et al. They studied the ovarian tissue adjacent to the ovarian endometrioma cysts in women under the age of 35 years and found that these women had 33% to 66% fewer follicles as compared to the ovarian tissue adjacent to other benign ovarian cysts.[32] The difference in number of follicles in the ovarian tissue adjacent to the endometrioma is most likely an outcome of oxidative stress led inflammatory response, which causes fibrosis of the surrounding normal ovarian cortex.[23,33,34]

Practical Approach to Management of Infertility Associated with Endometrioma

Following should serve as the guiding principles for treatment in this group of patients:

- Points to consider while evaluating patient for treatment:
  - *Age of the patient*: Age is a major determinant in selection of treatment for an infertile woman with endometrioma. Ovarian reserve and the chance of conception falls with age. Presence of ovarian endometrioma further reduces the ovarian reserve. The result of laparoscopic cystectomy is also related to patient's age.[35] Barri et al. in an observational study concluded that women over 35 years of age had significantly lower chance of spontaneous pregnancy as compared to younger women after undergoing laparoscopic cystectomy for endometrioma. The older women were also found to be at a higher risk of ovarian failure, although loss of ovarian reserve was observed in all women.[6]
  - *Duration of infertility*: Young women with short duration infertility associated with endometrioma have close to 30% probability of spontaneous pregnancy. On the other hand, women with longer duration infertility achieve better pregnancy rates

with IVF treatment. There is no added advantage of doing a surgery prior to IVF in such women.

- *Ovarian reserve*: Since women with endometrioma are at higher risk of reduced ovarian reserve and responsiveness, these women are not recommended for expectant management for prolonged periods. They should proceed to IVF early enough in order to maximize their chances of conception.
- *Nature of endometriotic cyst*:
  - *Number and size of endometrioma*: There is no correlation between size of the endometrioma and its effect on the ovarian reserve or outcome of IVF. Similarly, the number of endometriotic cysts in the affected ovary also does not impact the number of oocytes retrieved, and hence has no effect on outcome of treatment. So, the clinician should not get worried on finding large or multiple cysts in women with unilateral endometrioma.[27]
  - *Location of cyst within ovary*: Endometriomas can technically hinder oocyte retrieval because of their location, and can also cause oocyte contamination, if they get punctured. This is often cited as one of the major indications for surgical intervention prior to IVF.[27] However, there is not enough evidence to support that IVF outcome actually improves after cystectomy in such patients.
  - *Laterality of cyst:* As previously mentioned, the ovarian reserveis often found to be reduced in the ovary affected by the endometriotic cyst. This problem gets further aggravated in women with bilateral endometriomas. Therefore, operative procedures like cystectomy are not suitable for such women, as the surgery could further reduce the already reduced ovarian reserve, potentially even causing ovarian failure. This is in line with conclusions from retrospective study by Busacca et al. who found that two out of six patients with bilateral endometrioma who underwent cystectomy eventually had ovarian failure.[36]
  - *Prior surgical treatment*: Since the recurrence rate of endomerioma after laparoscopic cystectomy is rather high, IVF is a more plausible treatment option in patients with recurrent cysts, as compared to repeated cystectomy.[37]

CONCLUSION

- Surgical treatment for endometrioma in infertile patients should be reserved for a small section of young women only, as it improves spontaneous pregnancy rate among young women. However, surgical treatment has no definitive advantage over expectant management in majority of women with endometrioma.
- Many different surgical methods have been described and tried for improving fertility among women with endometrioma. However, none of these is conclusively superior to the others.
- Some of the other indications of surgical intervention in infertile women with endometrioma include cysts blocking access to ovary for egg retrieval, to treat concomitant pain symptoms, or in cases where malignancy cannot otherwise be ruled out with reasonable accuracy.
- Women with endometrioma generally have lower ovarian reserve than their age matched control group. Therefore, we recommend proceeding directly to IVF in order to reduce time to pregnancy.
- Despite of a negative impact on ovarian reserve and ovarian responsiveness, the results of IVF treatment in women with infertility associated with endometrioma are comparable to overall results of IVF in women with tubal factor infertility.

REFERENCES

1. Giudice LC, Kao LC. Endometriosis. Lancet. 2004;364 (9447):789-99.
2. Santulli P, Lamau MC, Marcellin L. et al. Endometriosis-related infertility: ovarian endometrioma per se is not associated with presentation for infertility. Hum Reprod. 2016;31(8):1765-75.
3. Van Holsbeke C, Van Calster B, Guerriero S, et al. Endometriomas: their ultrasound characteristics. Ultrasound Obstet Gynecol. 2010;35(6):730-40.
4. Porpora MG, Pallante D, Ferro A, et al. Pain and ovarian endometrioma recurrence after laparoscopic treatment of endometriosis: a long-term prospective study. Fertil Steril. 2010;93(3):716-21.
5. Busacca M, Marana R, Caruana P, et al. Recurrence of ovarian endometrioma after laparoscopic excision. Am J Obstet Gynecol. 1999;180(3 Pt 1):519-23.
6. Barri PN, Coroleu B, Tur R, et al. Endometriosis-associated infertility: surgery and IVF, a comprehensive therapeutic approach. Reprod Biomed Online. 2010;21(2):179-85.
7. Hayasaka S, Ugajin T, Fujii O, et al. Risk factors for recurrence and re-recurrence of ovarian endometriomas after laparoscopic excision. J Obstet Gynaecol Res. 2011;37(6): 581-5.
8. Hart RJ, Hickey M, Maouris P, et al. Excisional surgery versus ablative surgery for ovarian endometriomata. Cochrane Database Syst. Rev. 2008;2:CD004992.
9. Zhu W, Tan Z, Fu Z, et al. Repeat transvaginal ultrasound-guided aspiration of ovarian endometrioma in infertile women with endometriosis. Am J Obstet Gynecol. 2011;204(1):61.e1-61.e6.

10. Koga K, Takemura Y, Osuga Y, et al. Recurrence of ovarian endometrioma after laparoscopic excision. Hum Reprod. 2006;21(8):2171-4.
11. Kikuchi I, Takeuchi H, Kitade M, et al. Recurrence rate of endometriomas following a laparoscopic cystectomy. Acta Obstet Gynecol Scand. 2006;85(9):1120-4.
12. Liu X, Yuan L, Shen F, et al. Patterns of and risk factors for recurrence in women with ovarian endometriomas. Obstet Gynecol. 2007;109(6):1411-20.
13. Vercellini P, Fedele L, Aimi G, et al. Reproductive performance, pain recurrence and disease relapse after conservative surgical treatment for endometriosis: the predictive value of the current classification system. Hum Reprod. 2006;21(10):2679-85.
14. Busacca M, Chiaffarino F, Candiani M, et al. Determinants of long-term clinically detected recurrence rates of deep, ovarian, and pelvic endometriosis. Am J Obstet Gynecol. 2006;195(2):426-32.
15. Maul LV, Morrision JE, Schollmeyer T, et al. Surgical therapy of ovarian endometrioma: recurrence and pregnancy rates. J Soc Laparoendoscopic Surg. 2014;18(3):1-8.
16. Donnez J, Nisolle-Pochet M, Clerckx-Brawn F, et al. Administration of nasal buseralin as compared with subcutaneous buseralin implant for endometriosis. Fertil Steril. 1989;171:1601-5.
17. Pabuccu R, Onalan G, Kaya C. GnRH agonist and antagonist protocols for stage I-II endometriosis and endometrioma in in vitro fertilization/intracytoplasmic sperm injection cycles. Fertil Steril. 2007;88:832-9.
18. Hamdan M, Dunselman G, Li TC, et al. The impact of endometrioma on IVF/ICSI outcomes: a systematic review and meta-analysis. Hum Reprod Update. 2015;21(6):809-25.
19. Yanushpolsky EH, Best CL, Jackson KV, et al. Effects of endometriosis on oocyte quality, embryo quality, and pregnancy rates in in vitro fertilization cycles: a prospective, case-controlled study. J Assist Reprod Genet. 1998;15:193-7.
20. Maneschi F, Marasa L, Incandela S, et al. Ovarian cortex surrounding benign neoplasms: a histologic study. Am J Obstet Gynecol. 1993;169:388-93.
21. Muzii L, Bianchi A, Croce C, et al. Laparoscopic excision of ovarian cysts: is the stripping technique a tissue-sparing procedure? Fertil Steril. 2002;77:609-14.
22. Schubert B, Canis M, Darcha C, et al. Human ovarian tissue from cortex surrounding benign cysts: a model to study ovarian tissue cryopreservation. Hum Reprod. 2005;20:1786-92.
23. Matsuzaki S, Schubert B. Oxidative stress status in normal ovarian cortex surrounding ovarian endometriosis. Fertil Steril. 2010;93(7):2431-2.
24. Kumbak B, Kahraman S, Karlikaya G, et al. In vitro fertilization in normoresponder patients with endometriomas: comparison with basal simple ovarian cysts. Gynecol Obstet Invest. 2008;65(3):212-6.
25. Filippi F, Benaglia L, Paffoni A, et al. Ovarian endometriomas and oocyte quality: insights from in vitro fertilization cycles. Fertil Steril. 2014;101(4):988-94.
26. Bongioanni F, Revelli A, Gennarelli G, et al. Ovarian endometriomas and IVF: a retrospective case-control study. Reprod Biol Endocrinol. 2011;9:81.
27. Almog B, Shehata F, Sheizaf B, et al. Effects of ovarian endometrioma on the number of oocytes retrieved for in vitro fertilization. Fertil Steril. 2011;95(2):525-7.
28. Somigliana E, Benaglia L, Paffoni A, et al. Risks of conservative management in women with ovarian endometriomas undergoing IVF. Hum Reprod Update. 2015;21(4):486-99.
29. Gupta S, Agarwal A, Agarwal R, et al. Impact of ovarian endometrioma on assisted reproduction outcomes. Reprod Biomed Online. 2006;13(3):349-60.
30. Esinler I, Bozdag G, Aybar F, et al. Outcome of in vitro fertilization/intracytoplasmic sperm injection after laparoscopic cystectomy for endometriomas. Fertil Steril. 2006;85:1730-5.
31. Somigliana E, Infantino M, Benedetti F, et al. The presence of ovarian endometriomas is associated with a reduced responsiveness to gonadotropins. Fertil Steril. 2006;86(1): 192-6.
32. Kuroda M, Kuroda K, Arakawa A, et al. Histological assessment of impact of ovarian endometrioma and laparoscopic cystectomy on ovarian reserve. J Obstet Gynaecol Res. 2012;38(9):1187-93.
33. Kitajima M, Defrère S, Dolmans MM, et al. Endometriomas as a possible cause of reduced ovarian reserve in women with endometriosis. Fertil Steril. 2011;96(3):685-91.
34. Zhang X, Li XH, Ma X, et al. Redox-induced apoptosis of human oocytes in resting follicles in vitro. J Soc Gynecol Investig. 2006;13(6):451-8.
35. Carnahan M, Fedor J, Agarwal A, et al. Ovarian endometrioma: guidelines for selection of cases for surgical treatment or expectant management. Expert Rev Obstet Gynecol. 2013;8(1):29-55.
36. Busacca M, Riparini J, Somigliana E, et al. Postsurgical ovarian failure after laparoscopic excision of bilateral endometriomas. Am J Obstet Gynecol. 2006;195(2):421-5.
37. Sallam H, Garcia-Velasco JA, Dias S, et al. Long-term pituitary down-regulation before in vitro fertilization (IVF) for women with endometriosis. Cochrane Database Syst Rev. 2006;CD004635.

CHAPTER

71

Pelvic Extraovarian Endometriosis: Diagnosis and Management in the Infertile Patient

Graciela Kohls Ilgner

INTRODUCTION

Pelvic extraovarian endometriosis (PEOE) is diagnosed when endometriotic lesions infiltrate the uterosacral ligaments, rectovaginal pouch, posterior vaginal fornix or the muscularis propria of bladder, intestine or ureter. It is also called deep endometriosis and causes chronic pain which is characteristically cyclical (catamenial) and may be related to the location of the lesions. Lesions extending <5 mm of the peritoneal surface are called superficial endometriosis. Typical symptoms of PEOE include dyspareunia, dyschezia, and dysuria. In most advanced cases, it may disrupt organ function causing in particular intestinal obstruction, rectorrhagia, hematuria, ureteral obstruction, and renal failure.[1] Women with PEOE may also be infertile.[2]

Treatment includes hormonal agents and surgical excision and is aimed at alleviating symptoms or preventing imminent complications. Progestins are effective because they create a pseudopregnant state characterized by a steady hormonal condition without the physiological fluctuations in sex steroids, which are ultimately responsible for the endometriosis-related symptoms. Remarkable benefits may be obtained in most women but drugs have to be continued in the long term because symptoms typically and rapidly recur once treatment is discontinued.[3] Surgery is also highly effective and typically recommended if medical therapy fails or if it cannot be ruled out that the endometriotic nodules may soon compromise the function of the adjacent organs.[4] In some cases, surgery may definitely cure the woman. However, surgery can be demanding, requires utmost expertise and skill, and is associated with risks.[5] Removal of the lesions may cause organic or functional harm to the adjacent organs. Ureteral, bladder, and intestinal injury may occur during the intervention and can cause demanding short-term conditions, such as peritonitis, hemorrhage and ureteral damage, and long-term complications, such as fistulae, ureteral or rectal stenosis, or neurologic impairment of bladder or rectal function. Frequency of these complications varies from 1% to 10%.[5] In addition, surgery does not protect from recurrences. At least one in two operated women experiences recurrence within 5 years.[6,7]

DIAGNOSIS

Pelvic extraovarian endometriosis should be suspected in all women with unremitting hypogastric pain, especially dysmenorrhea, deep dyspareunia, severe chronic pain, dysuria, and dyschezia. Most pathognomonic signs are severe dyschezia, menstrual blood in stools, menstrual diarrhea, severe menstrual dysuria, and radiation of pain to the perineum. Although solid data linking these symptoms to size and location of PEOE are lacking, clinical symptoms remain key to suspecting deep endometriosis and deciding to perform surgery.[8]

The sensitivity and specificity of ultrasonography in the diagnosis of deep endometriosis remain unclear, although it has been reported to be >85% and even close to 100%.[9] Data linking sensitivity and specificity to the diameter and location of the endometriotic nodules are lacking. Most important, however, is that the accuracy of ultrasonography varies according to the expertise of the ultrasonographer. Answers to important questions, such as sensitivity and specificity in the absence of clinical suspicion, or after a negative clinical exam, are missing.

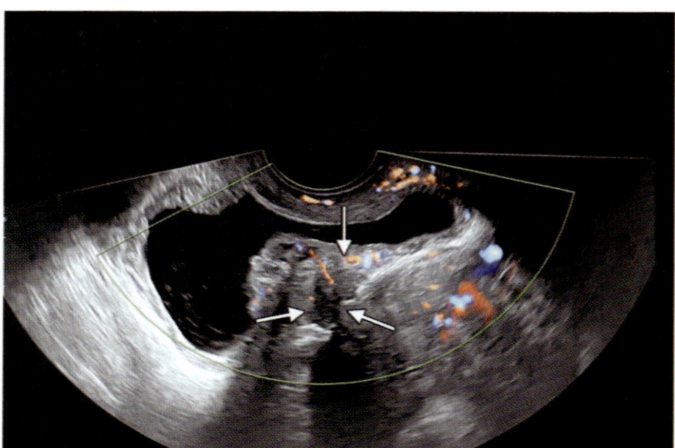

Fig. 1: Ultrasound scan in a patient with bladder endometriosis.

Clinical suspicion can be confirmed by magnetic resonance imaging (MRI). Magnetic resonance imaging might be less operator dependent and can also provide information about lesions at the level of the sigmoid, but the conclusions reached are similar to those of ultrasonographic examination.[10-13]

In conclusion, PEOE is suspected or diagnosed clinically, and the clinical suspicion can be confirmed by ultrasonography (Fig. 1) or MRI.

PELVIC EXTRAOVARIAN ENDOMETRIOSIS AND INFERTILITY

The pathogenesis and treatment of endometriosis remain debated. The relation between PEOE and infertility and the beneficial effects of available treatments is a particularly intricate question. A definite conclusion is actually not at hand.[2,4]

Interpretation of the available evidence linking PEOE to infertility is challenging. A crucial point is the association between deep endometriosis and other forms of endometriosis that may affect fertility on their own. The presence of superficial endometriotic implants, endometriomas, and pelvic adhesions was documented in 61%, 50%, and 74% of patients with deep endometriotic nodules, respectively. Overall, deep peritoneal endometriosis was isolated in only 6% of patients.[14] Similar findings were observed when considering specifically deep nodules of the bladder.[15] It is noteworthy that even though specific data on the independent impact of all the different forms of endometriosis on fertility are lacking and cannot be obtained, deep endometriosis by itself is less likely to affect fertility. Superficial implants may release inflammatory mediators in the peritoneal fluid (PF) that may be detrimental to the released oocyte and its fertilization in the distal part of the tube.[16] Adhesions may distort pelvic anatomy interfering with tubal function.[17] Endometriomas may affect folliculogenesis and oocyte quality.[18] In contrast, deep peritoneal lesions are generally buried under adhesions and the associated local inflammation is thus unlikely to reach the peritoneal cavity to interfere with the conception process. On theoretical basis, one may thus question whether these lesions independently have any impact on fertility.[19] On the other hand, there is evidence for an indirect effect mediated by the reduction in sexual function consequent to deep endometriosis-related dyspareunia.[20] The scenario is even more intricate if we consider the well-known association between endometriosis and adenomyosis[21-23] and the possible relationship between the latter and infertility.[24,25] Of particular interest is the growing evidence that adenomyosis is more frequently diagnosed in women with deep endometriosis compared with other forms of the disease.[21,22,26,27] Based on a large series of 1,618 women with endometriosis, Di Donato et al.[27] highlighted that the most significant factor associated with adenomyosis was the presence of deep lesions. The adjusted odds ratio (OR) was 3.1 [95% confidence interval (CI) 2.4–4.1]. In a systematic review of literature, Vercellini et al.[28] showed that the chances of pregnancy after surgery for deep endometriosis are markedly lower if concomitant adenomyosis is diagnosed. The common relative risk of pregnancy in women with adenomyosis was 0.3 (95% CI 0.2–0.7).

THE IMPACT OF PELVIC EXTRAOVARIAN ENDOMETRIOSIS ON NATURAL FERTILITY AND THE BENEFITS OF SURGERY

Endometriosis can cause infertility but the magnitude of this effect and the independent role of the different forms of the disease remain uncertain. In addition, as the main symptom of deep endometriosis is pain, the wish for a child only emerges once pain has been reduced, and it is obviously very intricate to dissect how many women with asymptomatic deep endometriosis are fertile or the percentage of infertile women not seeking pregnancy as they have pelvic pain or dyspareunia. Studies reporting on natural fecundity in unoperated women with endometriosis are scanty and tend to support the view that, even if subfertile, affected women can conceive naturally, even without surgery. In the control arm of two randomized controlled trials investigating the benefits of surgery in infertile women with endometriosis stages I–II,[29,30] the pregnancy rate (PR) was 18%, thus significantly lower but not markedly different from 26% observed in operated women.[7] Recently, Leone Roberti Maggiore et al.[31] observed that the 6-month cumulative PR in a large cohort (n = 244) of women with unoperated unilateral endometriomas and who did not previously seek pregnancy was 43% (95% CI 37–50%), thus lower than the expected theoretical 74% rate for fertile women,[32] but still relevant from a clinical perspective. In the subgroup of women who were diagnosed with concomitant deep endometriosis (n = 184), 76 conceived (41%, 95% CI 34–49%).[31]

Vercellini et al.[33] compared the chances of pregnancy in infertile women with rectovaginal endometriosis who did and did not undergo surgery. A total of 150 infertile women with this form of the disease but without other concomitant factors of infertility were given the possibility to choose between expectant management and surgery after an in-depth discussion of the pros and cons of the two options. At 24-month follow-up, 22 of the 61 women opting for expectant management (36%) and 15 of the 44 women choosing surgery (34%) became pregnant [p = not significant (NS)]. The study was not randomized, and the results were inevitably exposed to confounders, but at present, this evidence represents the unique available comparative study on the role of surgery.

Results of the study from Vercellini et al.[33] are in contrast with several recent opinions and reviews that advocate surgery for infertile women with deep endometriosis.[8,34-36] The main reason used to claim for surgery is the relatively good PR observed after the intervention. According to three independent systematic reviews of literature, PR after excisional surgery for rectovaginal endometriosis is 42–44%, a suboptimal but somehow satisfying result.[7,16,37] In this regard, it has to be emphasized that these results are an overestimation of the benefits of surgery and that attributing this rate of success entirely to surgery is problematic.[7,19] In fact, it has been shown that extensive surgery in women with deep and intraperitoneal endometriosis, when compared with intraperitoneal surgery only, does not modify global fertility outcome (24-month cumulative PR, 25%, and 23%, respectively; p = NS).[38] Interestingly, Vercellini et al.[19] repeated a systematic review of the literature on this topic but included only studies reporting the chances of pregnancy in infertile women with deep endometriosis and exclusively focusing on natural pregnancy. Emerging results were less optimistic with a common estimation of the rate of success of 24% (95% CI 20–28%).

THE IMPACT OF PELVIC EXTRAOVARIAN ENDOMETRIOSIS ON IN VITRO FERTILIZATION AND THE BENEFITS OF SURGERY

Available data suggest that in vitro fertilization (IVF) is a good option for PEOE. Six studies specifically informed IVF success in affected women.[39-44] Pregnancy rate per patient was reported in four of these studies[41-44] and varied between 29% and 68%, yielding an aggregated rate of 51% (95% CI 45–56%) (160/314). It is noteworthy that, case series of IVF are more informative than case series of surgery because all observed pregnancies can actually be attributed to the procedure. A main issue in the present review is disentangling whether deep endometriosis negatively impacts IVF success and whether pre-IVF surgery has some benefits. Randomized controlled trials are unavailable but four of these six studies included a control group.[39-41,44] The most informative of them was published by Bianchi et al.[39] in 2009. In that prospective study, women with deep endometriosis were given the option to choose between IVF directly or extensive laparoscopic excision of endometriotic lesions, followed by IVF. A total of 105 women opted for conservative management, whereas the remaining 64 chose surgery. The PR per cycle was significantly lower in the former group (24%) compared with the latter one (41%) (p = 0.004). The two groups differed in some characteristics, but these baseline differences were modest and are unlikely to explain the observed difference in PR. At present, this is the only evidence on the possible beneficial effect of pre-IVF surgery and indirectly supports a detrimental effect of deep endometriosis on IVF. In fact, a negative impact on IVF was also supported by Ballester et al.[41] who focused on women with ovarian endometriomas at the time of IVF and compared those women with (n = 73) and without (n = 30) deep endometriosis. They observed a lower PR in the former group (48% vs. 77%, p = 0.01). In contrast, the other two controlled studies[42,43] failed to detect a significant impact of deep endometriosis on IVF. Mathieu d'Argent et al.[40] compared women with colorectal endometriosis (n = 29), tubal factor infertility (n = 157) and male factor infertility (n = 340), and reported delivery rates of 27%, 23%, and 26%, respectively (p = NS). Papaleo et al.[44] identified women previously operated on for unilateral endometriomas and who were diagnosed with ovarian recurrences. The investigators then compared the women who did (n = 24) and did not (n = 27) have deep endometriosis but also failed to document any difference in PR (29% vs. 30%, respectively).

Reasons to explain the benefits of IVF for PEOE probably overlap with those of endometriosis in general. As mentioned previously, pelvic lesions are seldom isolated. The most plausible explanation for the benefit of IVF is the capacity of the procedure to circumvent the anatomical distortion and the possible detrimental pelvic milieu (gametes and embryos are not directly exposed to the PF). Albeit scanty and contrasting, there is some evidence that PEOE may be associated with lower chances of success. A direct causal effect is difficult to explain as the procedure overcomes the pelvic milieu but cannot be ruled out given the results reported by Bianchi et al.[39] Lower success rate could also be explained by the association with endometriosis in general, and with adenomyosis. The most recent meta-analysis[45] of the impact of endometriosis in general on IVF showed a statistically significant reduction in clinical PR (OR = 0.8, 95% CI 0.6–0.9) but it failed to document a statistically significant impact on live birth rate (OR = 0.9, 95% CI 0.8–1.1). Based on a meta-analysis[25] of the studies focusing on the impact of adenomyosis on IVF, the relative risk of clinical pregnancy and miscarriage in affected women were 0.7 (95% CI 0.5–1.0; $p = 0.01$) and 2.1 (95% CI 1.2–3.8), respectively. In addition, it is also worth noting that previous surgical excision of ovarian endometriomas is commonly reported in women with deep endometriosis undergoing IVF[41,43] and that a past history of surgery for endometriomas may affect ovarian responsiveness and IVF outcome because of the surgical-related injury to ovarian reserve.[46]

RISK FROM IN VITRO FERTILIZATION AND PREGNANCY IN WOMEN WITH PELVIC EXTRAOVARIAN ENDOMETRIOSIS

Opting for IVF rather than surgery to cure infertility in women with PEOE may expose affected women to risks. In particular, the ovarian stimulation that is generally required for IVF and/or the pregnancy itself have been suggested to stimulate the growth and progression of the lesions, ultimately increasing the risk of severe complications. To our knowledge, eight cases of deep endometriosis progression possibly linked to ovarian stimulation have been described.[47-50] Most of them were associated with clinically relevant ureteral and intestinal complications and required prompt and demanding surgery. Available controlled studies or case series[51-55] investigating the effects of ovarian stimulation on endometriosis progression failed to document significant effects, suggesting that the case reports may be exceptional events. Similar to what has been observed for ovarian endometriomas, extraovarian endometriosis may also undergo decidualization causing diagnostic troubles and possibly clinically relevant complications.

Albeit also presumably rare, intestinal perforation[50,56,57] (Figs. 2 and 3), pneumothorax,[58] and pelvic vessel rupture[59] have been reported. A crucial point is the estimation of the magnitude of these risks. Given the risks of surgery, a strategy of systematic removal of deep lesions before IVF or pregnancy would be justified only if these complications are relatively common. A precise estimate of their frequency is unfortunately lacking in literature. However, the fact that these events are reported as isolated case reports tends to support the view that they are very rare. A related but distinct issue is the rate of obstetric complications in women with deep endometriosis. Intestinal perforation, pneumothorax, or vessel perforation can be directly linked to the presence of the deep lesions, whereas classic obstetric complications, such as miscarriage, hypertensive disorders, prematurity, and placental disorders, cannot.

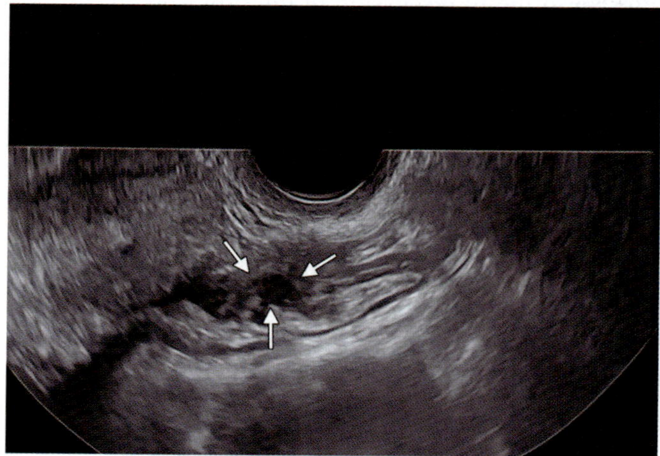

Fig. 2: Ultrasound scan in a patient with digestive endometriosis.

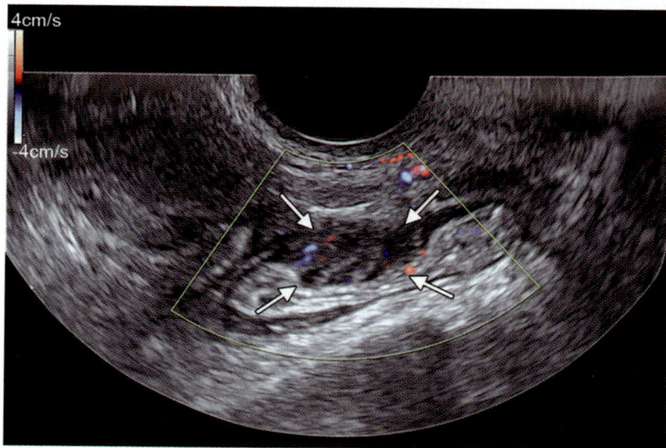

Fig. 3: Doppler ultrasound scan in the same patient with digestive endometriosis.

A specific study[60] comparing the rate of these complications in women with endometriosis according to the forms of the disease showed a higher risk of placenta previa in women previously operated for deep rectovaginal endometriosis. Compared with women with endometriomas or superficial implants, women with deep lesions had an almost sixfold increased risk (OR = 5.8, 95% CI 1.5–22.0). Interpretation of this result is difficult but a causal relationship is unlikely. The most plausible explanation is the association between endometriosis and adenomyosis, and the uterine peristalsis associated with the disease (and possibly causative of the disease) that interferes with the implantation of the embryo.[61] Finally, the mode of delivery in women with deep endometriosis is a neglected but potentially relevant issue. To bypass a challenging and risky surgery and then perform a cesarean section is somehow contradictory. There is thus a need for a thorough evaluation of the patient taking into consideration this aspect before initiating fertility treatment. For instance, performing a cesarean section in a woman with placenta previa and previous bowel resection, ureteral reimplantation with a bladder-psoas hitch, segmental bladder resection, or extensive abdominal–pelvic adhesions may be very demanding, and, if an emergency postpartum hysterectomy is needed, the woman's life may be at risk.[1]

Pregnancy rates after surgery appear to be approximately half when the case series criteria are more controlled (about one of four), thus more or less similar to the chances of pregnancy that can be achieved with a single IVF attempt. We also have to acknowledge the quality impact of the surgeons who have different training, methodology, and skills.[62] Data on IVF are also not robust. Comparative studies investigating IVF outcome based on the presence and absence of PEOE are scanty, weak, and contrasting. Disentangling the independent impact of deep endometriosis from that mediated by endometriosis in general, adenomyosis and previous surgery for endometriomas is currently unfeasible. Overall, informative literature is not available and, consequently, dealing with infertile women with deep endometriosis is a complex task. Physicians must make important decisions without robust bases. In such a scenario of uncertainty, a cautious attitude should be envisaged (primum non nocere). In asymptomatic infertile women or in those whose pain symptoms can be effectively managed with medical treatment, surgery without deep lesions removal or straight IVF may be considered. The scenario is different if surgery is required for pain symptoms because medical therapy is ineffective, if clinically relevant intestinal or ureteral stenosis is detected, or if medical therapy cannot be prescribed because of unbearable side effects, intolerance, or risks. Surgery might also be considered in young women who have had repeated IVF failures despite adequate responsiveness to ovarian stimulation. Interestingly, a recent review[4] on colorectal deep endometriosis reached similar clinical conclusions even though the investigators did not contemplate medical therapy and advocated direct surgery in infertile women in the presence of severe dyspareunia or dyschezia that impair quality of life. We partly disagree on this view as we estimate that medical therapy may play a role in women seeking pregnancy. Even if medical treatment hampers natural conception, it can improve pain and quality of life,[2] and it is not incompatible with IVF. Medical therapy may be transiently discontinued during the IVF attempts. It is noteworthy that prolonged medical therapy before IVF may even increase success rates.[63,64] Last but not least, once properly and realistically informed of the possible options and related benefits, the woman's wishes should play the central role. When favoring surgery, women should receive a complete and realistic view of the benefits and risks. Data rather than published literature should be favored because of the crucial role of expertise and skill. When opting for IVF, women should be informed about the risks of ovarian stimulation related to disease progression and pregnancy-related complications but at the same time reassured that these events are presumably extremely rare, and the magnitude of these risks do not justify prophylactic surgery. A pre-IVF evaluation should include an accurate investigation of the urinary system and bowel patency to exclude clinically relevant stenosis. Transvaginal and transabdominal sonography should be performed and, when required in specific cases, computed tomography/MRI, barium enema, rectosigmoidoscopy, colonoscopy, or intravenous pyelography. Prolonged downregulation with either gonadotropin-releasing hormone agonists[63,65] or estroprogestins[64] might be considered to overcome the detrimental effects of adenomyosis. Finally, regardless of the therapeutic approach, we advocate a more comprehensive evaluation of the affected women, taking into consideration that the ultimate aim is delivering a live birth at term in a safe situation. Women should be informed that they face an increased risk of placenta previa and prematurity. They should also be informed that the time of delivery may be demanding. If a cesarean section is needed in a woman with a history of several and complex surgeries, the intervention may be extremely risky, in particular if required in an urgent and unqualified setting. Counseling should not be limited to mere information. In an IVF setting, single embryo transfer is mandatory considering that multiple pregnancy can independently increase all reported risks (i.e. prematurity, placenta previa, and cesarean section).[66,67] In most severe situations, such as women with a history of several surgeries, including colorectal resection, one may even consider to refrain from fertility treatments. In this regard, it is worth noting that women with utmost severe endometriosis who underwent several demanding surgeries have actually scanty chances of pregnancy with IVF because most are not young and they may have had concomitant frequent severe injury to the ovarian reserve. However, the advent of oocyte donation programs is changing the scenario, and physicians are thus called to thoroughly counsel these women.

CONCLUSION

Extreme caution is warranted in drawing inferences on a causal relation between deep endometriosis and infertility. Women with PEOE may be infertile but deep lesions may not cause the infertility. Definitely disentangling this issue is of critical clinical relevance as it may have a therapeutic impact. At present, however, evidence is insufficient to definitely support a causal relationship or to claim benefit of surgery. Exposing women to the considerable risks of a demanding intervention for the removal of deep nodules to exclusively enhance fertility is debatable.

REFERENCES

1. Somigliana E, Garcia-Velasco JA. Treatment of infertility associated with deep endometriosis: definition of therapeutic balances. Fertil Steril. 2015;104(4):764-70.
2. Vercellini P, Viganò P, Somigliana E, et al. Endometriosis: pathogenesis and treatment. Nat Rev Endocrinol. 2014;10(5):261-75.
3. Vercellini P, Crosignani PG, Somigliana E, et al. Medical treatment for rectovaginal endometriosis: What is the evidence? Hum Reprod. 2009;24(10):2504-14.
4. Abrão MS, Petraglia F, Falcone T, et al. Deep endometriosis infiltrating the recto-sigmoid: critical factors to consider before management. Hum Reprod Update. 2015;21(3):329-39.
5. Vercellini P, Crosignani PG, Abbiati A, et al. The effect of surgery for symptomatic endometriosis: the other side of the story. Hum Reprod Update. 2009;15(2):177-88.
6. Guo SW. Recurrence of endometriosis and its control. Hum Reprod Update. 2009;15(4):441-61.
7. Vercellini P, Somigliana E, Viganò P, et al. Surgery for endometriosis-associated infertility: a pragmatic approach. Hum Reprod. 2009;24:254-69.
8. Koninckx PR, Ussia A, Adamyan L, et al. Deep endometriosis: definition, diagnosis, and treatment. Fertil Steril. 2012;98(3):564-71.
9. Hudelist G, English J, Thomas AE, et al. Diagnostic accuracy of transvaginal ultrasound for non-invasive diagnosis of bowel endometriosis: systematic review and meta-analysis. Ultrasound Obstet Gynecol. 2011;37(3):257-63.
10. Saba L, Guerriero S, Sulcis R, et al. MRI and "tenderness guided" transvaginal ultrasonography in the diagnosis of recto-sigmoid endometriosis. J Magn Reson Imaging. 2012;35(2):352-60.
11. Bazot M, Gasner A, Lafont C, et al. Deep pelvic endometriosis: limited additional diagnostic value of postcontrast in comparison with conventional MR images. Eur J Radiol. 2011;80(3):e331-9.
12. Bazot M, Darai E. Value of transvaginal sonography in assessing severe pelvic endometriosis. Ultrasound Obstet Gynecol. 2010;36(2):134-5.
13. Bazot M, Lafont C, Rouzier R, et al. Diagnostic accuracy of physical examination, transvaginal sonography, rectal endoscopic sonography, and magnetic resonance imaging to diagnose deep infiltrating endometriosis. Fertil Steril. 2009;92(6):1825-33.
14. Somigliana E, Infantino M, Candiani M, et al. Association rate between deep peritoneal endometriosis and other forms of the disease: pathogenetic implications. Hum Reprod. 2004;19(1):168-71.
15. Somigliana E, Vercellini P, Gattei U, et al. Bladder endometriosis: getting closer and closer to the unifying metastatic hypothesis. Fertil Steril. 2007;87(6):1287-90.
16. de Ziegler D, Borghese B, Chapron C. Endometriosis and infertility: pathophysiology and management. Lancet. 2010;376(9742):730-8.
17. Somigliana E, Viganò P, Benaglia L, et al. Adhesion prevention in endometriosis: a neglected critical challenge. J Minim Invasive Gynecol. 2015;19(4):415-21.
18. Sanchez AM, Viganò P, Somigliana E, et al. The distinguishing cellular and molecular features of the endometriotic ovarian cyst: from pathophysiology to the potential endometrioma-mediated damage to the ovary. Hum Reprod Update. 2014;20(2):217-30.
19. Vercellini P, Barbara G, Buggio L, et al. Effect of patient selection on estimate of reproductive success after surgery for rectovaginal endometriosis: literature review. Reprod Biomed Online. 2012;24(4):389-95.
20. Meulem C, Tomassetti C, Wolthuis A, et al. Increasing the quality of surgery for deep endometriosis should be based on homogenous clinical patient phenotype, surgical experience and standardized outcome reporting in multicenter multisurgeon prospective trials. Ann Surg. 2015;262(1):e26-8.
21. Kunz G, Beil D, Huppert P, et al. Adenomyosis in endometriosis—prevalence and impact on fertility. Evidence from magnetic resonance imaging. Hum Reprod. 2005;20(8):2309-16.
22. Larsen SB, Lundorf E, Forman A, et al. Adenomyosis and junctional zone changes in patients with endometriosis. Eur J Obstet Gynecol Reprod Biol. 2011;157(2):206-11.
23. Naftalin J, Hoo W, Pateman K, et al. How common is adenomyosis? A prospective study of prevalence using transvaginal ultrasound in a gynaecology clinic. Hum Reprod. 2012;27(12):3432-9.
24. Tomassetti C, Meuleman C, Timmerman D, et al. Adenomyosis and subfertility: evidence of association and causation. Semin Reprod Med. 2013;31(2):101-8.
25. Vercellini P, Consonni D, Dridi D, et al. Uterine adenomyosis and in vitro fertilization outcome: a systematic review and meta-analysis. Hum Reprod. 2014;29(5):964-77.

26. Lazzeri L, Di Giovanni A, Exacoustos C, et al. Preoperative and postoperative clinical and transvaginal ultrasound findings of adenomyosis in patients with deep infiltrating endometriosis. Reprod Sci. 2014;21(8):1027-33.
27. Di Donato N, Montanari G, Benfenati A, et al. Prevalence of adenomyosis in women undergoing surgery for endometriosis. Eur J Obstet Gynecol Reprod Biol. 2014;181:289-93.
28. Vercellini P, Consonni D, Barbara G, et al. Adenomyosis and reproductive performance after surgery for rectovaginal and colorectal endometriosis: a systematic review and meta-analysis. Reprod Biomed Online. 2014;28(6):704-13.
29. Marcoux S, Maheux R, Bérubé S. Laparoscopic surgery in infertile women with minimal or mild endometriosis. N Engl J Med. 1997;337(4):217-22.
30. Parazzini F, Cintio E Di, Chatenoud L, et al. Ablation of lesions or no treatment in minimal-mild endometriosis in infertile women: a randomized trial. Hum Reprod. 1999;14(5):1332-4.
31. Leone Roberti Maggiore U, Scala C, Venturini PL, et al. Endometriotic ovarian cysts do not negatively affect the rate of spontaneous ovulation. Hum Reprod. 2015;30(2):299-307.
32. Evers JL. Female subfertility. Lancet. 2002;360(9327):151-9.
33. Vercellini P, Pietropaolo G, De Giorgi O, et al. Reproductive performance in infertile women with rectovaginal endometriosis: is surgery worthwhile? Am J Obstet Gynecol. 2006;195(5):1303-10.
34. Moawad NS, Caplin A. Diagnosis, management, and long-term outcomes of rectovaginal endometriosis. Int J Women's Health. 2013;5:753-63.
35. Cohen J, Thomin A, D'argent EM, et al. Fertility before and after surgery for deep infiltrating endometriosis with and without bowel involvement: a literature review. Minerva Ginecol. 2014;66(6):575-87.
36. Roman H. Colorectal endometriosis and pregnancy wish: why doing primary surgery. Front Biosci (Schol Ed). 2015;7:83-93.
37. Meuleman C, Tomassetti C, D'Hoore A, et al. Surgical treatment of deeply infiltrating endometriosis with colorectal involvement. Hum Reprod Update. 2011;17(3):311-26.
38. Douay-Hauser N, Yazbeck C, Walker F, et al. Infertile women with deep and intraperitoneal endometriosis: comparison of fertility outcome according to the extent of surgery. J Minim Invasive Gynecol. 2011;18(5):622-8.
39. Bianchi PHM, Pereira RMA, Zanatta A, et al. Extensive excision of deep infiltrative endometriosis before in vitro fertilization significantly improves pregnancy rates. J Minim Invasive Gynecol. 2009;16(2):174-80.
40. Mathieu d'Argent E, Coutant C, Ballester M, et al. Results of first in vitro fertilization cycle in women with colorectal endometriosis compared with those with tubal or male factor infertility. Fertil Steril. 2010;94(6):2441-3.
41. Ballester M, Oppenheimer A, Mathieu d'Argent E, et al. Deep infiltrating endometriosis is a determinant factor of cumulative pregnancy rate after intracytoplasmic sperm injection/in vitro fertilization cycles in patients with endometriomas. Fertil Steril. 2012;97(2):367-72.
42. Ballester M, Oppenheimer A, D'Argent EM, et al. Nomogram to predict pregnancy rate after ICSI–IVF cycle in patients with endometriosis. Hum Reprod. 2012;27(2):451-6.
43. Ballester M, d'Argent EM, Morcel K, et al. Cumulative pregnancy rate after ICSI–IVF in patients with colorectal endometriosis: results of a multicentre study. Hum Reprod. 2012;27(4):1043-9.
44. Papaleo E, Ottolina J, Vigana P, et al. Deep pelvic endometriosis negatively affects ovarian reserve and the number of oocytes retrieved for in vitro fertilization. Acta Obstet Gynecol Scand. 2011;90(8):878-84.
45. Hamdan M, Omar SZ, Dunselman G, et al. Influence of endometriosis on assisted reproductive technology outcomes: a systematic review and meta-analysis. Obstet Gynecol. 2015;125(1):79-88.
46. Yang C, Geng Y, Li Y, et al. Impact of ovarian endometrioma on ovarian responsiveness and IVF: a systematic review and meta-analysis. Reprod Biomed Online. 2015;31(1):9-19.
47. Renier M, Verheyden B, Termote L. An unusual coincidence of endometriosis and ovarian stimulation. Eur J Obstet Gynecol. 1995;63(2):187-9.
48. Govaerts I, Devreker F, Delbaere A, et al. Short-term medical complications of 1500 oocyte retrievals for in vitro fertilization and embryo transfer. Eur J Obstet Gynecol Reprod Biol. 1998;77(2):239-43.
49. Anaf V, El Nakadi I, Simon P, et al. Sigmoid endometriosis and ovarian stimulation. Hum Reprod. 2000;15(4):790-4.
50. Setúbal A, Sidiropoulou Z, Torgal M, et al. Bowel complications of deep endometriosis during pregnancy or in vitro fertilization. Fertil Steril. 2014;101(2):442-6.
51. D'Hooghe TM, Denys B, Spiessens C, et al. Is the endometriosis recurrence rate increased after ovarian hyperstimulation? Fertil Steril. 2006;86(2):283-90.
52. Coccia ME, Rizzello F, Palagiano A, et al. The effect of the hormonal milieu of pregnancy on deep infiltrating endometriosis: serial ultrasound assessment of changes in size and pattern of deep endometriotic lesions. Eur J Obstet Gynecol Reprod Biol. 2012;160(1):35-9.
53. Benaglia L, Somigliana E, Vercellini P, et al. The impact of IVF procedures on endometriosis recurrence. Eur J Obstet Gynecol Reprod Biol. 2010;148(1):49-52.
54. Benaglia L, Somigliana E, Santi G, et al. IVF and endometriosis-related symptom progression: insights from a prospective study. Hum Reprod. 2011;26(9):2368-72.
55. van der Houwen LEE, Mijatovic V, Leemhuis E, et al. Efficacy and safety of IVF/ICSI in patients with severe endometriosis after long-term pituitary down-regulation. Reprod Biomed Online. 2014;28(1):39-46.
56. Lebastchi AH, Prieto PA, Chen C, et al. Appendiceal endometriosis in a pregnant woman presenting with acute perforated appendicitis. J Surg Case Rep. 2013;2013(12):rjt104.
57. Costa A, Sartini A, Garibaldi S, et al. Deep endometriosis induced spontaneous colon rectal perforation in pregnancy: laparoscopy is advanced tool to confirm diagnosis. Case Rep Obstet Gynecol. 2014;2014:907150.
58. Kim YD, Min KO, Moon SW. Thoracoscopic treatment of recurrent pneumothorax in a pregnant woman: a case of ectopic deciduosis. Thorac Cardiovasc Surg. 2010;58(7):429-30.
59. Brosens IA, Fusi L, Brosens JJ. Endometriosis is a risk factor for spontaneous hemoperitoneum during pregnancy. Fertil Steril. 2009;92(4):1243-5.

60. Vercellini P, Parazzini F, Pietropaolo G, et al. Pregnancy outcome in women with peritoneal, ovarian and rectovaginal endometriosis: a retrospective cohort study. BJOG. 2012;119(12):1538-43.
61. Kunz G, Beil D, Huppert P, Leyendecker G. Structural abnormalities of the uterine wall in women with endometriosis and infertility visualized by vaginal sonography and magnetic resonance imaging. Hum Reprod. 2000;15(1):76-82.
62. Pluchino N, Petignat P, Wenger JM. Laparoscopic "successful" excision of deep endometriosis: a fertility-enhancing surgery. Ann Surg. 2015;262(1):e26.
63. Sallam HN, Garcia-Velasco JA, Dias S, et al. Long-term pituitary down-regulation before in vitro fertilization (IVF) for women with endometriosis. Cochrane Database Syst Rev. 2006;(1):CD004635.
64. de Ziegler D, Gayet V, Aubriot FX, et al. Use of oral contraceptives in women with endometriosis before assisted reproduction treatment improves outcomes. Fertil Steril. 2010;94:2796-9.
65. Niu Z, Chen Q, Sun Y, et al. Long-term pituitary downregulation before frozen embryo transfer could improve pregnancy outcomes in women with adenomyosis. Gynecol Endocrinol. 2013;29(12):1026-30.
66. Grady R, Alavi N, Vale R, et al. Elective single embryo transfer and perinatal outcomes: a systematic review and meta-analysis. Fertil Steril. 2012;97(2):324-31.
67. Weis MA, Harper LM, Roehl KA, et al. Natural history of placenta previa in twins. Obstet Gynecol. 2012;120(4):753-8.

CHAPTER

72

Adenomyosis and Infertility: What are the Options?

Abha Bhat

INTRODUCTION

Adenomyosis is defined as the presence of ectopic endometrial glands and stroma in the myometrium, accompanied by a variable degree of hypertrophy and hyperplasia of the smooth muscle cells, causing either focal or diffuse enlargement of the uterus.[1] This pathology was first described by Karl Freiherr von Rokitansky in 1860 who described it as fibrous tumors in the uterus with gland-like structures that resemble endometrial glands, and with roots deep within the uterine muscle wall such that it is hard to distinguish the border of these tumors.[2] Frankl was the first to use the term "adenomyosis interna" in 1925.[3]

Adenomyosis remains an enigma in terms of its pathophysiology. Initially, it was thought to affect multiparous women in their third or fourth decades and until relatively recently was only diagnosed after hysterectomy. With the advent of high-resolution imaging technology such as magnetic resonance imaging (MRI) and high-resolution two- and three-dimensional (2D and 3D) transvaginal ultrasound (TVS), it is now being diagnosed more commonly and in younger women, often in infertility clinics. Although findings of studies are inconsistent, evidence of its negative impact on fertility is mounting. It is likely that the impact on fertility is through alteration in the anatomy and physiology of the junctional zone (JZ)—the site of implantation. Removal of adenomyotic lesions may reverse or alleviate the symptoms, improve the outcome of assisted reproductive technology (ART), and normalize risk of miscarriage. Advances in minimal access surgery have made this increasingly feasible. However, the consequences of the inevitable damage to normal myometrium adjacent to the lesion and thus affecting the future pregnancies cannot be overlooked.

With no agreement on diagnostic criteria, an incomplete understanding of the pathophysiology, and a lack of well-designed studies of adequate power to evaluate the different management strategies, dealing with a subfertile patient with symptomatic adenomyosis is tricky. Adequate but honest counseling of the patient is therefore essential.

CLINICAL FEATURES

The symptoms that women with adenomyosis experience are menorrhagia (50%), dysmenorrhea (30%), metrorrhagia (20%), and occasionally dyspareunia.[4] As many as one-third women may be completely asymptomatic.[5] Adenomyosis was traditionally thought to affect women in their fourth or fifth decade. However, newer studies that have used MRI criteria for diagnosis of adenomyosis suggest that this disease may affect adolescents and women of younger reproductive age than previously appreciated.[6,7] It is possible that early stage adenomyosis may have a different clinical phenotype compared to late stage disease.

As the symptoms described are not exclusive to adenomyosis, it cannot be diagnosed without further investigations. It has therefore not been possible to accurately determine its incidence or prevalence in the general population.[8] Various studies quote the prevalence to be from 5% to 70% with many quoting a figure of 30–35%.[9-12] The study group often consisted of patients presenting in the gynecology clinic or infertility clinics and so a selection bias is expected. There is no consensus on the diagnostic criteria and these vary from center to center making the prevalence difficult to ascertain.

MYOMETRIUM: NORMAL ANATOMY AND PHYSIOLOGY

During the reproductive years, three distinct layers of uterus can be identified on T2 weighted images on MRI—the high intensity endometrium, the low signal intensity inner myometrium, and the medium signal intensity outer myometrium. The inner myometrium, also called the JZ, archimyometrium or stratum subvasculare, consists of predominantly circular smooth muscle fibers with little interstitial tissue.[13] The JZ is a hormonally sensitive layer and its thickness undergoes cyclical changes in its thickness like the endometrium.[14] However, some other studies did not find a significant difference in the thickness of the JZ between phases of the menstrual cycle.[15,16] The outer myometrium, also called neomyometrium or stratum vascular, has criss-cross muscle fibers and a rich vascular supply. The demarcation of myometrium into inner and outer is lost after menopause, under suppression of ovarian activity with hormonal contraception, and following administration of GnRH agonists. The layers re-appear with hormone replacement therapy.[17]

The myocytes of the JZ or archimetra have an important physiological function—transport of sperm toward the peritoneal opening of the tube on the side of the dominant follicle. Peristaltic waves start from near the internal os and move in the fundal direction, the strongest power is exerted at the upper part of the uterine cavity.[18] After ovulation, the myometrial waves become short and asymmetrical. This change possibly enables local supply of nutrients and oxygen thus aiding implantation.[19] The trophoblast invasion involves JZ but not the outer myometrium. It has also been reported that during a conception cycle, functional disruption of the JZ occurs 7 days postovulation.[20]

Contractions of the myocytes present in the outer myometrium predominantly occur in the menstrual phase and the fundus-to-cervix direction of waves ensure orthograde efflux of menstrual debris and may also prevent retrograde flow through occlusion of the intramural part of the Fallopian tubes.[21] These contractions are primarily regulated by estrogen and progesterone but are also regulated by prostaglandins, oxytocin, vasopressin, and neurotransmitters such as acetylcholine through their receptors.[21-24] The most potent among these seems to be oxytocin. Oxytocin receptors are stimulated by follicular estrogen and the subsequent rise in progesterone.[25] The maximum mass of myocytes is in the fundus and the concentration of oxytocin receptors is also highest in the fundus.[26] As such it is suggested that the strongest contractions are in the fundal neomyometrium. It is these myometrial contractions which are perceived as dysmenorrhea.

PATHOGENESIS

The pathogenesis of adenomyosis remains elusive despite continuous efforts. Many theories have been proposed to explain the development of adenomyosis.

The most widely accepted theory is that adenomyosis results from the down-growth of basal endometrium into the myometrium during periods of regeneration and repair especially after mechanical damage such as repeated sharp curettage during pregnancy.[27] Uterus may be vulnerable to this pathology due to a natural absence of basal membrane and submucosa. Intramyometrial lymphatics may be a possible route for invagination of basal endometrium.[28] Adenomyosis may also develop de novo from metaplastic transformation of pluripotent Müllerian remains.[29]

Leyendecker et al. have proposed a theory of uterine auto-traumatization and mechanism of tissue injury and repair (TIAR) as primary events that predispose to adenomyosis. Physiological contractions of the archimetrium and neometrium put an enormous strain on the subendometrial stromal cells. The authors estimated that approximately 30 million peristaltic waves occur in the archimetra and 0.5 million contractions in the neometra during the reproductive period of a woman.[30]

It has been suggested that the healing following auto-traumatization due to the chronic mechanical strain leads to the production of interleukin-1 (IL-1). IL-1 causes activation of cyclooxygenase-2 (COX-2) enzyme which in turn causes the production of prostaglandin E2 (PGE2). PGE2 induces the activation of steroidogenic acute regulatory protein (StAR) and cytochrome p450 aromatase which leads to local hyperestrogenemia.[31] This leads to increased peristaltic activity of the subendometrial myometrium, which further compounds the mechanical strain on the cells near the fundo-cornual raphe. Thus, starts a process of sustained injury and an ever-increasing number of foci of injury. This primes multiple areas of basal endometrium to secrete estrogen and lead to hyperperistalsis presumably through endometrial oxytocin creating an auto-perpetuating cycle. Hyperperistalsis and increased intrauterine pressure eventually lead to myometrial dehiscences and proliferation of the basal endometrium into the inner myometrium. Hyperestrogenism may also account for the hypertrophy and hyperplasia of the surrounding myometrium that is a feature of adenomyosis. Once the adenomyotic lesion forms, the myometrial disorganization leads to additional mechanical strain causing further expansion of the lesion in unpredictable directions.[32-34]

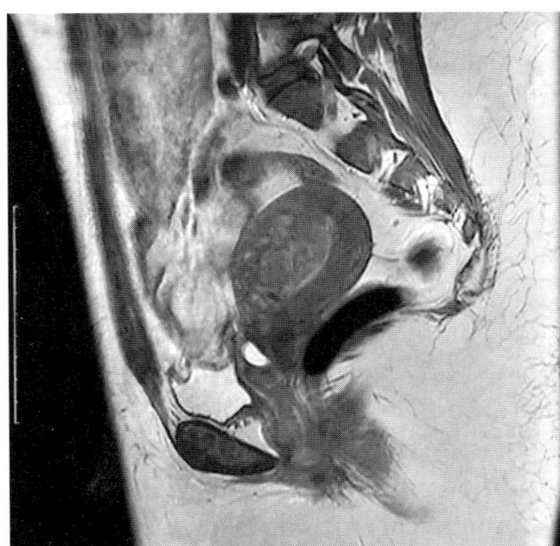

Fig. 1: MRI: Diffuse anterior wall adenomyosis.
Courtesy: Dr Deepak Patkar.

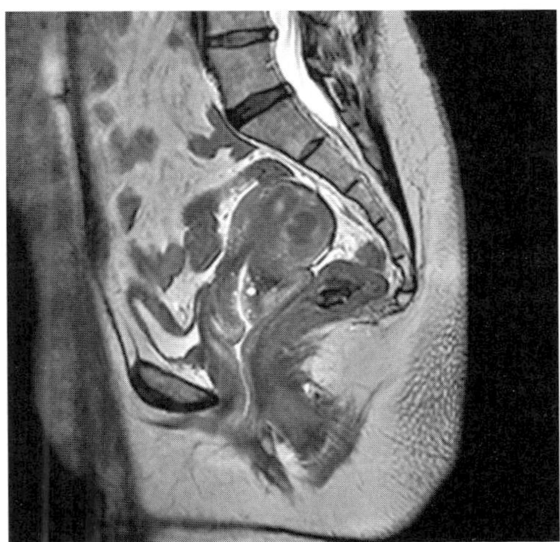

Fig. 2: MRI: Focal adenomyoma.
Courtesy: Dr Deepak Patkar.

Immune system has also been stipulated to play a role in the pathogenesis of adenomyosis.[35]

CLASSIFICATION

Several classification systems have been proposed but no system is universally accepted. Appropriate categorization of adenomyotic lesions is important, not only to plan the management but also to evaluate the results of surgical treatment. Grimbizis et al. have proposed the following comprehensive classification based on the histological characteristics and the extent of myometrial invasion:[36]

- *Diffuse adenomyosis*: Extensive disease, characterized by foci of endometrial mucosa scattered throughout the uterine musculature (Fig. 1)
- *Focal adenomyosis*: Hypertrophic and distorted endometrium and myometrium embedded within the myometrium. This is subdivided to:
  - *Adenomyoma*: A circumscribed adenomyotic mass
  - *Cystic adenomyosis*: Single cystic lesion within the myometrium (Fig. 2).
- *Polypoid adenomyomas*: Circumscribed endometrial masses of endometrioid glands and a stromal component predominantly of smooth muscle. This is subdivided into:
  - *Typical polypoid adenomyomas*: Without architectural or cellular atypia
  - *Atypical polypoid adenomyomas*: Characterized by atypical endometrial glands, often squamous metaplasia, and a cellular smooth muscle stroma.
- *Other forms*:
  - *Adenomyomas of the endocervical type*: Rare forms of adenomyomatous polyps in the uterine cervix that contain epithelial component of endocervical type
  - *Retroperitoneal adenomyomas*: Adenomyotic nodules that are thought to arise from metaplasia of Müllerian remnants beneath the peritoneum and in upper rectovaginal septum.

ABNORMALITIES IN ADENOMYOSIS

The eutopic and ectopic endometrium of women with adenomyosis exhibit many metabolic and molecular abnormalities which may play a role in the pathogenesis of the disease as well as in its symptoms including dysmenorrhea and subfertility.

Adenomyosis and endometriosis quite often coexist. Larsen et al. have found that 34.6% of patients with endometriosis had adenomyosis compared with 19.4% in the reference group and as many as 39.9% of women with endometriosis had an irregular JZ compared to 22.5% in the reference group.[37]

Hormonal Alterations

Local hyperestrogenism, induced by an increased PGE2 and an over expression of cytochrome p450 aromatase, is an important characteristic of eutopic and ectopic endometrial tissues in women with adenomyosis.[30,32-34] Increased estrogen may enhance the growth of ectopic tissue. In their study published in 1993, Lei et al. have demonstrated on hysterectomy specimens that invading endometrial gland cells expressed more human chorionic gonadotrophin/luteinizing hormone receptor mRNA and immunoreactive receptor protein than noninvading glands.[38]

Nuclear factor κB (NF-κB) is a transcription factor that seems to play a pivotal role in progesterone resistance, proinflammation, prosurvival, resistance to apoptosis, proangiogenesis, and invasion in adenomyosis and endometriosis. NF-κB activation leads to an increased expression of COX-2, tissue factor (TF), and vascular endothelial growth factor (VEGF). TF is a member of cytokine receptor superfamily and functions in many biological processes such as hemostasis, thrombosis, inflammation, angiogenesis, and tumor growth. VEGF is involved in the cyclical endometrial growth and angiogenesis. IκBα is a protein complex that functions to inhibit NF-κB by keeping it sequestered in the cytoplasm thus preventing it from migrating to the nucleus. Progesterone receptors may serve an anti-inflammatory role by antagonizing NF-κB activation and COX-2 expression.[39-41]

When compared to normal endometrium, PR-B and IκBα have been shown to be significantly reduced and NF-κB is activated in eutopic as well as ectopic endometrium from women with adenomyosis. Downregulation of PR-B and NF-κB activation may explain the lack of efficacy of progesterone therapy in women with adenomyosis.[40,41]

Angiogenesis

During the menstrual cycle, endometrium exhibits waves of angiogenesis with development of arterioles and capillary network. This is under the influence of many factors such as matrix metalloproteinases (MMPs) and VEGF, a major mediator of angiogenesis and vascular permeability. MMPs are expressed in the human endometrium and play a role in extracellular matrix remodeling.[42] Bruner et al. developed an experimental animal model and demonstrated that treatment with estrogen maintains the secretion of MMPs while use of progesterone or metalloproteinase inhibitors stopped the formation of ectopic lesions of adenomyosis.[43] MMP-2, MMP-3, and tissue inhibitor of metalloproteinase-2 (TIMP-2) expressions have been found to be similar in endometrium of women with and without adenomyosis but was significantly higher in ectopic endometrium.[44] Li et al. found a significantly higher expression of MMP-2 and MMP-9 as well as VEGF in eutopic and ectopic endometrium in women with adenomyosis in comparison to normal endometrium. They also found a higher microvessel density (MVD) in ectopic than in eutopic endometrium.[45] It is therefore likely that metalloproteinases and VEGF may contribute to the development of adenomyotic lesions through invasion and angiogenesis in the implants.

Immunological Alterations

Hyperestrogenism stimulates the production of IL-10 which is an immunomodulatory cytokine produced by eutopic and ectopic endometrium in women with adenomyosis. Since IL-10 has been demonstrated to induce HLA-G expression while downregulating the expression of classical class I and class II antigens, it was postulated that the expression of IL-10 may play a role in the establishment and maintenance of immunosuppression and thus prevents the ectopic adenomyotic foci from elimination by the immune system of the host.[46] Many changes occur in cellular and humoral immunity in women with adenomyosis. Strong expression of cell surface antigens or adhesion molecules, increased number of macrophages, deposition of immunoglobulins, and complement components have been reported. Autoantibodies are frequently exhibited in peripheral blood and in endometrium and endometrial cells seem to be under immunological stress as evidenced by the presence of heat shock proteins.[47]

Ota et al. have published their study on T cell subsets including δγT cells, HLA antigens, and adhesion molecules expressed in eutopic and ectopic endometria of women with adenomyosis. They observed a significantly increased number of δγT cells in the stroma and increased expression of HLA antigens and adhesion molecules on the glandular cells.[48] Chiang and Hill from their study on immune response elements in eutopic and ectopic endometria obtained at hysterectomy concluded that the increased numbers of T-cells, higher expression of interferon-γ (IFN-γ), and an enhanced antigen presentation in ectopic compared to eutopic endometrium is suggestive of cellular immune activation in adenomyosis.[49] The expression of very late antigens, VLA-2,3 and E-cadherin have been found to be significantly increased, while VLA-4 was significantly decreased in endometrial samples from women with adenomyosis. Based on their findings, Ota and Tanaka have suggested the presence of a defective microenvironment in the eutopic endometrium of adenomyosis patients.[50] Granulocyte macrophage-colony stimulating factor, related to macrophage recruitment and activation has also been shown to be overexpressed in adenomyosis compared with normal premenopausal women.[51]

Free Radicals

Low oxygen environment needs to be maintained in the uterus as free radicals have a negative influence on sperm transport, fertilized eggs, early embryonic development, and implantation.[52,53] To maintain homeostasis, enzymes that produce and eliminate free radicals are present throughout the body. In the endometria of normal women, nitric oxide synthase, xanthine oxidase, superoxide dismutase, and glutathione peroxidase are low during proliferative phase and increase during early or mid-secretory phase while catalase is lowest in the proliferative phase and peaks during late secretory phase. Studies have revealed that levels of these enzymes are overexpressed and do not fluctuate during the menstrual cycle and may contribute to low pregnancy rate or miscarriage in women with adenomyosis.[53-57]

Impaired Implantation

In women with adenomyosis, *HOXA10* gene expression is significantly lower during the mid-secretory phase compared with fertile controls.[58] This diminished expression may be a potential mechanism to explain the decreased implantation observed in these women. In addition, leukemia inhibitory factor (LIF) is expressed in the glandular and luminal epithelium in the mid-late secretory phase.[59] LIF expression has been shown to be decreased in the endometrium in the mid-secretory phase in a study by Xiao et al.[60]

IMPACT ON FERTILITY AND PREGNANCY

Adenomyosis was thought to be associated with multiparity. It was only after current imaging modalities that revolutionized its diagnosis, the role of adenomyosis in infertility and miscarriage was recognized. An increasing number of women are delaying their first pregnancy and consequently more women attending the infertility clinics are being diagnosed with adenomyosis. Of interest is a case-control study done in baboons which found that adenomyosis was strongly associated with lifelong infertility. Piver et al. in their study published in 2005 concluded that MRI evaluation of JZ thickness was the best negative predictive factor of implantation failure. Implantation failure was high when the average JZ was greater than 7 mm.[61]

In their meta-analysis published in 2014, Vercellini et al. found that adenomyosis was associated with a 28% (95% CI, 5–45%) reduction in the likelihood of clinical pregnancy in infertile women who underwent IVF/ ICSI with autologous oocytes. Adenomyosis was also associated with a more than double risk of miscarriage thus suggesting a causal relation. The authors found that the detrimental effect of adenomyosis on IVF/ICSI outcome appeared to be related to both reduced probability of clinical pregnancy and an increased risk of early pregnancy loss.[62] Many mechanisms have been proposed for infertility, lower pregnancy rates after IVF/ICSI, and increased risk of miscarriage in women with adenomyosis.

Myometrial architecture and function is aberrant in adenomyosis. The myocytes of the adenomyotic uteri exhibit cellular hypertrophy to the point that the smooth muscle cells are ultrastructurally different from smooth muscle cells of normal uteri. The JZ shows cellular and nuclear hypertrophy, abnormal nuclear and mitochondrial shape, and many other abnormalities that may cause a disturbance in the normal calcium cycling in the affected myocytes with a subsequent loss of normal rhythmic contractions.[63] Women with adenomyosis also show a reduced uterotubal transport capacity that progressively worsens with the severity of the disease.[64] A fundal adenomyoma may cause distortion or occlusion of one or both ostia thereby contributing to subfertility (Figs. 3 and 4).

Altered endometrial function and receptivity may also contribute to infertility and miscarriage. Abnormal levels of free radicals in the endometrium may damage the fertilized egg and inhibit embryo development.[52,53] The embryo may be attacked by activated macrophages or T cells, or be exposed to excessive levels of nitric oxide

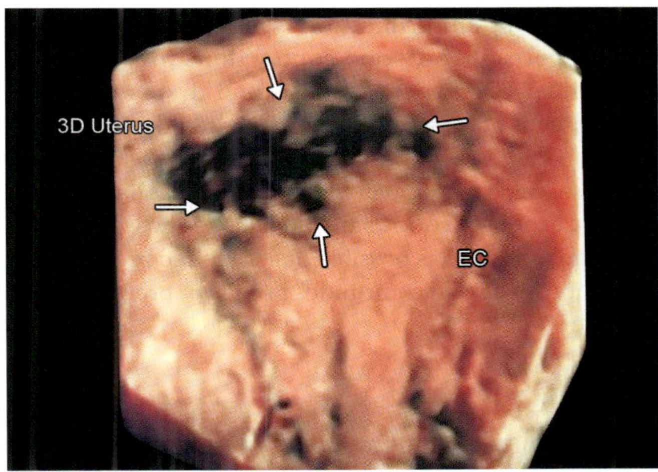

Fig. 3: Fundal adenomyoma: 3D ultrasound.

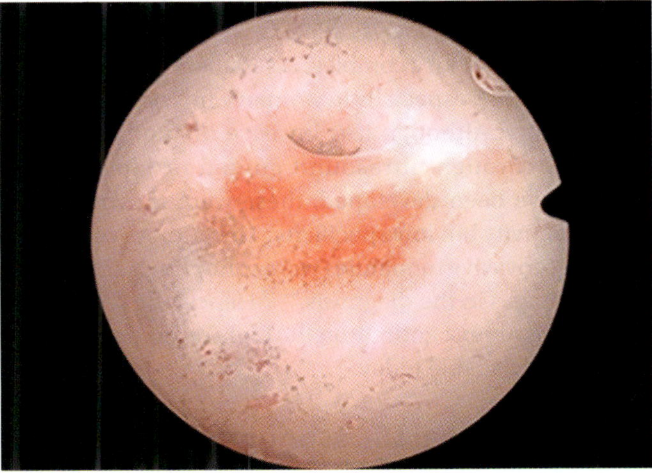

Fig. 4: Fundal adenomyoma: Hysteroscopy showing distorted and displaced ostium.

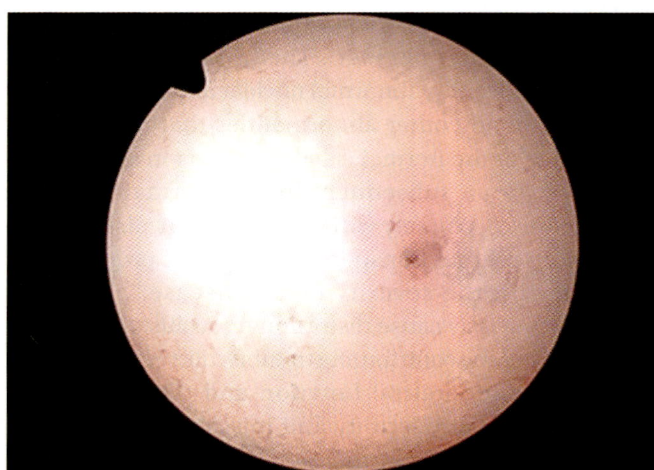

Fig. 5: Fundal adenomyoma: Post excision hysteroscopy (same patient as Fig. 4).

which may cause a miscarriage.[47] Free radicals may also increase fetal abnormalities.[65] Nitric oxide may also disturb peristaltic uterine contractions in a paracrine fashion causing hyperperistalsis and dysperistalsis. In women with adenomyosis, there is altered endometrial vascularization secondary to an abnormal inflammatory response which may impair nidation.[45] Studies have found a reduced expression of implantation markers in women with adenomyosis and it is possible that impaired implantation in adenomyosis also contributes to a lower pregnancy rate in these women.[58-60]

DIAGNOSIS

With few physical findings and symptoms that are not specific to adenomyosis, histology was once considered the only method of diagnosis. Even this is not simple as there is still no consensus on the depth of myometrial invasion to categorize the pathology as adenomyosis.[66] Performance of hysterectomy just for a complete assessment of myometrium is unacceptable, especially in women who wish to preserve their fertility. Although less invasive methods assessing histology through ultrasound guided or laparoscopic biopsy have been developed, these were shown to have high sensitivity but low specificity. The authors concluded that these invasive modalities were suboptimal and offered no advantages in the diagnosis.[67,68] Hence, the reliance for diagnosis is almost entirely on the high-resolution imaging modalities available today.

Transabdominal Ultrasonography

Transabdominal scan can pick up enlargement of uterus and asymmetric thickening of anterior or posterior wall which are features of adenomyosis. In a study of 80 patients, Siedler et al. reported a sensitivity of 63% and a specificity of 97% for diagnosing adenomyosis.[69] However, image resolution is insufficient to visualize the myometrium adequately to differentiate an adenomyoma from a leiomyoma in the presence of adiposity, scar tissue, or uterine retroversion.

Transvaginal Ultrasonography

High-resolution TVS should be preferred as a diagnostic tool for women with clinically suspected adenomyosis. A recent consensus statement was published by the MUSA group detailing the terms, definitions, and measurements that may be used for description of sonographic features of myometrium and uterine masses including adenomyosis. Typical signs of adenomyosis are asymmetric thickening, intramyometrial cysts, hyperechoic islands, fan-shaped shadowing, echogenic subendometrial lines and buds, translesional vascularity, irregular JZ, and interrupted JZ.[70] With the improvement in technology, TVS has proved to have a high diagnostic accuracy. The most specific feature of adenomyosis was the presence of intramyometrial cysts (specificity: 98%, accuracy: 78%) while the most sensitive feature of adenomyosis was identified as the finding of a heterogeneous myometrium (sensitivity: 88%, accuracy 75%).[71] The probability of adenomyosis with a normal TVU was 9.1% (95% CI, 7.3–11.1).

Three-dimensional TVS enables assessment of the lateral and fundal aspects of the JZ and enables clearer visualization of the endometrial invasion into the myometrium. Findings of JZ max of 8 mm or greater, myometrial asymmetry, and hypoechoic striations have been linked to adenomyosis. When at least two of the ultrasound features are present, the accuracy is reported to be 90% (sensitivity: 92%, specificity: 83%, positive predictive value: 99%, negative predictive value: 71%).[72] It has also been indicated that 3D TVS may be more accurate during luteal phase.

Magnetic Resonance Imaging

Magnetic resonance imaging (MRI) enables the accurate identification of inner myometrium or JZ with distinct signal density on T2-weighted images although no identifiable JZ may be seen in as many as 20% of premenopausal normal women.[73] The minimal required diagnostic width is still debated but the consensus is that when maximal JZ thickness (JZmax) is ≥12 mm, adenomyosis should be considered.[74] Even when JZ is between 8 mm and 12 mm, adenomyosis can be suspected in the presence of other signs such as relative thickening of JZ in a localized area, poorly defined JZ borders, or high signal myometrial spots.[75] The difference between the maximum and minimum thickness which measures the irregularity of JZ with a value of 5 mm or more may be a better diagnostic marker than JZmax in premenopausal women.[76]

As compared to TVS, MRI is less operator dependent and may be more accurate even in the presence of fibroids. A meta-analysis published in 2010 by Champaneria et al. concluded that both MRI and TVS have high accuracy for noninvasive diagnosis of adenomyosis. The pooled sensitivity of ultrasound was 72% and specificity was 81% whereas the sensitivity of MRI was 77% and specificity was 89%.[76] Dueholm et al. in an earlier study published in 2001 also reported that both MRI and TVS were equally good at identifying patients though MRI was superior to exclude the diagnosis of adenomyosis with an equal sensitivity but higher specificity. The combination of TVS and MRI had the highest sensitivity, but, surprisingly, it also had the lowest specificity.[77]

Hysteroscopy

Diagnostic hysteroscopy does not reveal the pathognomonic signs of adenomyosis. Findings at hysteroscopy include an abnormal vascularization, irregular endometrium, irregular distribution of vessels and thick, dilated and/or reticular vessels.[78,79] Submucous cystic adenomyoma and cystic polypoid adenomyoma may also be diagnosed and opportunistically treated at hysteroscopy.

MANAGEMENT

Management of adenomyosis should be individualized depending on the symptoms such as heavy menstrual bleeding and dysmenorrhea that can severely impact the quality of life of the patient, the extent and type of adenomyosis, the age of the patient, her fertility aspirations, and the expertise available. Hysterectomy is the gold standard for adenomyosis in those who have completed their family. Management becomes difficult when patients are symptomatic but have a strong desire to preserve their uterus. There is no consensus, and although publications on the available options are increasing, most of these are case series or retrospective studies. Counseling of patient on the options including the risks and side effects and an informed consent are crucial before planning treatment.

Medical Treatment

Medical treatments are usually aimed at symptom relief and include GnRH analogs, oral contraceptive pills (OCP), oral progestogens, levonorgestrel- releasing intrauterine device, danazol, aromatase inhibitors (AI), selective estrogen receptor modulators, and selective progesterone receptor modulators. These create a hypoestrogenic (GnRH agonists, AIs), hyperandrogenic (danazol), or hyperprogestogenic (OCPs, progestins) environment with suppression of endometrial cell proliferation. Medical therapies are symptomatic but not cytoreductive. Adenomyotic lesions survive the use of any drug, at any dose, for any length of time and resume their activity at the cessation of treatment.[80] Therefore, none of these can be recommended except in the short-term for patients actively desiring fertility.

The GnRH agonists (GnRHa) deserve special mention as these are commonly used either alone or in conjunction with surgery. There are no randomized controlled trials on the efficacy though this strategy has resulted in a few reports of successful pregnancy.[81,82] GnRHa decrease the expression of cytochrome p450 aromatase and of nitric oxide synthases. Suppression of concurrent endometriosis that may be present is likely via central downregulation. It has also been reported that GnRHa significantly reduce inflammatory reaction and angiogenesis, and induce a remarkable degree of apoptosis in endometriotic tissue and eutopic endometrium. The authors did not find any significant differences in the markers between the samples derived from women treated with GnRHa for 3–4 months and women treated for 6 months.[83] Though very effective against adenomyosis-related pain, GnRHa are costly and cause frequent and intolerant side effects such as vasomotor symptoms, headaches, genital atrophy, and mood swings.

Aromatase inhibitors have also been suggested as an alternative therapy for adenomyosis. Badawy et al. in a prospective randomized trial compared the efficacy of oral letrozole (2.5 mg/day) and subcutaneous goserelin (3.6 mg) for 12 weeks. They found no significant difference in total uterine size posttreatment between the two groups and concluded that AIs were as effective in reducing adenomyoma volume. Two of the patients on letrozole became pregnant while on treatment and delivered healthy babies without congenital anomalies.[84] AIs cannot however be recommended except in association with another hormonal treatment and in women in whom all surgical and medical treatments have failed.[85]

Surgical Treatment

In centers with surgical expertise, cytoreductive surgery is an option for patients who wish to preserve their fertility. There are many problems with offering conservative surgery. The first difficulty is in the selection of patients who would benefit. True extent of adenomyosis may be difficult to be determined and the defect after excision is difficult to repair resulting in poor healing. The uterine scan might not return to normal tensile strength due to inadequate excision of adenomyotic tissue or due to inadequate repair. This can prove dangerous in a future pregnancy as the decreased tensile strength can lead to an increased risk of uterine rupture during pregnancy or labor. In addition, postoperative pelvic adhesions, uterine deformities, intrauterine adhesions, and reduced uterine capacity may also follow. Hence, decision to use conservative uterine sparing surgery in women with adenomyosis should be taken very carefully and after appropriate patient counseling.[86,87]

Types of Uterine Sparing Surgeries

In their excellent review on uterine sparing operative treatment, Grimbizis et al. have proposed a classification based on the extent of removal of adjacent healthy myometrium and the preservation of the integrity of the uterine wall:[36]

- *Complete excision of adenomyosis*: Done in cases of adenomyoma, adenomyotic cyst and in cases with diffuse adenomyosis where all clinically recognizable lesions are completely removed and functional integrity of uterine wall is maintained
- *Cytoreductive surgery/partial adenomyomectomy*: Done in cases of diffuse adenomyosis, where only partial removal of the clinically recognizable non-microscopic lesions is possible because complete removal of the lesion would lead to the concomitant excision of critical amount of healthy myometrium, which could lead to "functional" hysterectomy
- *Nonexcisional techniques*:
  - Laparoscopic techniques including laparoscopic electrocoagulation of the myometrium and laparoscopic uterine artery ligation
  - Hysteroscopic techniques including operative hysteroscopy, rollerball endometrial ablation, transcervical resection of the endometrium, and endo-myometrial resection
  - *Other techniques*: High-frequency ultrasound (HIFU), alcohol instillation under ultrasound guidance, radiofrequency ablation of focal adenomyosis, microwave endometrial ablation, and balloon thermoablation for diffuse adenomyosis.

Surgical Techniques

For complete excision, technique is similar to myomectomy except for the differentiation of the margins from the surrounding normal myometrium. After careful recognition of adenomyotic foci by inspection and palpation (which is possible only at laparotomy), a longitudinal incision is made on the uterine wall along the lesion and the adenomyoma is dissected from the surrounding normal myometrium, taking care to preserve the maximal residual serosa or serosa-muscular layer. This is followed by reconstruction of uterine cavity using 4-0 absorbable suture if the endometrial cavity was opened and closure of the uterine wall with 1-0 absorbable sutures in layers or in the manner of a triple flap.[88] Separate closure of serosa with 4-0 or 5-0 absorbable sutures is done if possible.

It is feasible to perform this surgery through laparoscopy with excellent outcomes.[89] Various modifications in closure have been suggested including U-shaped suturing, overlapping flaps to enable reconstruction and to counter lost muscle.[90,91]

Cytoreductive surgery is more complicated and many modifications have been suggested. In the classic technique for cytoreductive surgery for adenomyosis a vertical or transverse incision is applied in the middle of the anterior or the posterior uterine wall. In this, myometrium of the subserous layer is preserved up to 10 mm and the adenomyotic lesion is excised piece by piece preserving as much of normal myometrium as possible. Closure is then done in one or more layers. Serosa is finally closed in one layer with interrupted sutures.[92]

Fujishita et al. used a transverse H-incision for excision of the lesion. A vertical incision is made in the uterine wall, and two transverse incisions are applied perpendicularly to the initial incision along the upper and lower edges of the uterus. The uterine serosa is opened bilaterally at the area under the incision and the slices of adenomyotic tissue are removed by serial resection using manual palpation to demarcate the borders of normal myometrium. Repeated chromopertubation test is done to minimize the risk of entering uterine cavity. Closure is done as usual, avoiding tension and hematoma formation.[92]

Hysteroscopic Excision

Operative hysteroscopy can be an alternative for diagnosis and treatment of adenomyosis using mechanical dissection and ablative bipolar current. Cystic adenomyosis, polypoid adenomyomas, and endocervical adenomyomas would be most suited for this approach. It has been suggested that for cystic adenomyomas that are present in the inner third of the myometrium or submucosally, a minimally invasive hysteroscopic approach is possible. On the other hand, if larger, cystic adenomyotic structures are localized in the outer intramural third, a laparoscopic approach is preferable.[93]

Robot-assisted Laparoscopic Adenomyomectomy

Robot-assisted laparoscopic surgery could be an ideal choice for adenomyomectomy as it has the advantages of open surgery and minimally invasive surgery. The effectiveness and safety of robot-assisted adenomyomectomy have not been fully evaluated yet and there is little data on the pregnancy rate and outcomes of patients.[94]

Radiologic or Sonographic Interventions

For patients who decline or are not suitable for surgical procedures, radiological procedures may be an option. These include uterine artery embolization (UAE) and MRI-guided focused ultrasound ablation. The evidence on these new techniques as a treatment of adenomyosis is limited and in the form of clinical reports. A systematic review of 15 studies on UAE as a treatment modality for adenomyosis was published in 2011. Pooled short-term results of 102 patients showed improvement of symptoms in 83.3% with minimal complications.[95] A recent review of MRI-guided focused ultrasound ablation concluded that it is a well-tolerated and effective alternative in well selected patients.[96]

Preoperative and Postoperative Use of GnRH Agonist Therapy

The GnRHa have been used either preoperatively before uterine sparing surgery or postoperatively. It is hypothesized that the GnRH agonists have a synergistic effect after cytoreductive surgery, since the affected tissues with relatively poor blood supply are removed and the response of the remaining adenomyosis to hormone treatment is enhanced. Advantages with preoperative use include the reduction of uterine vascularity, correction of anemia preoperatively, and reduction of operative bleeding. However, their use also makes recognizing adenomyotic tissues more difficult and increase the duration of surgery.[94] Hence, it may be preferable to use GnRHa postoperatively for 3–4 months at the end of which the patient is advised ART to optimize chances of pregnancy.

Therapeutic Effects of Surgical Treatment

In the meta-analysis of 1,049 women with adenomyosis, the symptom control after uterine sparing surgery was reported to be promising. In the women who had complete excision, reduction of dysmenorrhea was 82% and mean reduction of bleeding was 68.8%. In the category of patients who had partial excision of adenomyosis (n = 83), the mean reduction of pain was 81.8% and mean reduction of bleeding was 50%. In the women who underwent nonexcisional techniques, there was 84.6% reduction of pain.[36]

The conception rates after conservative surgery did not appear to be statistically significantly different between partial and complete excision of adenomyosis (46.8% vs. 60.5%, respectively, p = 0.22). As the studies included were not designed to address the fertility outcomes after surgery, the authors concluded that though there was a trend for increased fertility after surgery, more data are needed to elicit safe results for clinical practice.[36]

Kishi et al. in their study published in 2014 concluded that age is an important determinant and the uterine sparing surgery could be a beneficial treatment in women aged less than or equal to 39 years but not in the women more than or equal to 40 years. The total clinical pregnancy rate (CPR) seen in his series was 31.3%. The CPR was 41.4% and 3.7% in less than or equal to 39 years and more than or equal to 40 years age group, respectively.[97]

Pregnancy after Uterine-sparing Surgery

In most of the studies, attempts for conception were permitted after at least 3 months of surgery. It was reported that ART methods showed increased pregnancy rates compared to natural cycles. A single-embryo transfer policy was recommended to limit the risk of uterine rupture. The results did not support any technique to increase conception rates after ART.[36]

Spontaneous uterine rupture has been recorded in gravid uteri in isolated case reports even in the absence of history of cytoreductive surgery. It is speculated that decreased tensile strength of the uterus may be the consequence of dense residual adenomyotic foci concealed in the subsequent uterine scars.[98] Wang et al. have quantified the risk of uterine rupture in pregnancy/labor after cytoreductive surgery to be as high as one in eight women.[99] In addition, sporadic reports of severe atonic postpartum hemorrhage necessitating hysterectomy have also been published. For patient safety, it is therefore reasonable caution to perform elective cesarean delivery in women who have previously undergone uterine sparing surgery for adenomyosis.

KEY POINTS

- The TVS by well-trained sonographer is equal in diagnostic accuracy to MRI and therefore should be a natural choice. MRI should be done in case of difficult cases or indefinite findings
- Adenomyosis causes a 28% reduction in pregnancy and increases the risk of miscarriage by double

- ART is preferable to natural conception in women with adenomyosis who are anxious to conceive
- GnRH agonist may be used for suppression for 3–6 months followed by ART in case of low ovarian reserve or other contributory causes for infertility
- Conservative uterine sparing surgery requires a high degree of skill. In patients desiring fertility and suffering from severe dysmenorrhea, surgery may be one of the few options open to patients
- Risk of uterine rupture in pregnancy following uterine sparing surgery may be as high as 1:8.

REFERENCES

1. Bird CC, McElin TW, Manalo-Estrella P. The elusive adenomyosis of the uterus— revisited. Am J Obstet Gynecol. 1972;112:583-93.
2. Rokitansky C. Uber uterusdrusen-neubildungen in uterus- und ovarial- sarcomen. Zeitschrift der Kaiserlich Koenigl Gesellschaft der Aerzte zu Wien. 1860;37:577-81 [in German].
3. Frankl O. Adenomyosis uteri. Am J Obstet Gynecol. 1925;10:680-84.
4. Benson RC, Sneeden VD. Adenomyosis: a reappraisal of symptomatology. Am J Obstet Gynecol. 1958;76:1044-57; discussion 1057-61.
5. Azziz R. Adenomyosis: current perspectives. Obstet Gynecol Clin North Am. 1989;16:221-35.
6. Parker JD, Leondires M, Sinaii N, et al. Persistence of dysmenorrhea and non- menstrual pain after optimal endometriosis surgery may indicate adenomyosis. Fertil Steril. 2006;86:711-5.
7. Ryan GL, Stolpen A, Van Voorhis BJ. An unusual cause of adolescent dysmenorrhea. Obstet Gynecol. 2006;108:1017-22.
8. Garcia L, Isaacson K. Adenomyosis: review of the literature. J Minim Invasive Gynecol. 2011;18:428-37.
9. Bergholt T, Eriksen L, Berendt N, et al. Prevalence and risk factors of adenomyosis at hysterectomy. Hum Reprod. 2001;16(11):2418-21.
10. Vercellini P, Parazzini F, Oldani S, et al. Adenomyosis at hysterectomy: a study on frequency distribution and patient characteristics. Hum Reprod. 1995;10(5):1160-62.
11. Di Donato N, Montanari G, Benfenati A, et al. Prevalence of adenomyosis in women undergoing surgery for endometriosis. Eur J Obstetrics Gynecol Reprod Biol. 2014;181:289-93.
12. Yeniel O, Cirpan T, Ulukus M, et al. Adenomyosis: prevalence, risk factors, symptoms and clinical findings. Clin Exp Obstetrics Gynecol. 2007;34(3):163-7.
13. Tamai, K, Koyama, T, Umeoka S, et al. Spectrum of MR features in adenomyosis. Pract Res Clin Obstet Gynaecol. 2006;20:583-602.
14. Hoad CL, Raine-Fenning NJ, Fulford J, et al. Uterine tissue development in healthy women during the normal menstrual cycle and investigations with magnetic resonance imaging. Am J Obstet Gynecol. 2005;192:648-54.
15. Hauth EA, Jaeger HJ, Libera H, et al. MR imaging of the uterus and cervix in healthy women: determination of normal values. Eur Radiol. 2007;17:734-42.
16. Meylaerts LJ, Wijmem L, Grieten M, et al. Junctional zone thickness in young nulliparous women according to menstrual cycle and hormonal contraception use. Reprod Biomed Online. 2017;34:212-20.
17. McCarthy S, Tauber C, Gore J. Female pelvic anatomy: MR assessment of variations during the menstrual cycle and with use of oral contraceptives. Radiology. 1986;160:119-23.
18. Kunz G, Beil D, Deininger H, et al. The dynamics of rapid sperm transport through the female genital tract: Evidence from vaginal sonography of uterine peristalsis and hysterosalpingoscintigraphy. Hum Reprod. 1996;11:627-32.
19. Ijland MM, Evers JL, Dunselman GA, et al. Relation between endometrial wavelike activity and fecundability in spontaneous cycles. Fertil Steril. 1997;67:492-6.
20. de Ziegler D, Bulletti C, Fanchin R, et al. Contractility of the non-pregnant uterus: the follicular phase. Ann NY Acad Sci. 2001;943:172-84.
21. Hauksson A, Akerlund M, Melin P. Uterine blood flow and myometrial activity at menstruation, and the action of vasopressin and a synthetic antagonist. Br J Obstet Gynaecol. 1988;95:898-904.
22. Roth-Brandel U, Bygdeman M, Wiqvist N. Effect of intravenous administration of prostaglandin E1, and F2 on the contractility of the non-pregnant human uterus in vivo. Acta Obstet Gynecol Scand Suppl. 1970;5:19-25.
23. Akerlund M, Melin P, Maggi M. Potential use of oxytocin and vasopressin V1a antagonists in the treatment of preterm labour and primary dysmenorrhoea. Adv Exp Med Biol. 1995;395:595-600.
24. Abdalla FM, Marostica E, Picarelli ZP, et al. Effect of estrogen on muscarinic acetylcholine receptor expression in rat myometrium. Mol Cell Endocrinol. 2004;213:139-48.
25. Maggi M, Magini A, Fiscella A, et al. Sex steroid modulation of neurohypophysial hormone receptors in human nonpregnant myometrium. J Clin Endocrinol Metab. 1992;74:385-92.
26. Fuchs AR, Behrens O, Maschek H, et al. Oxytocin and vasopressin receptors in human nonpregnant endometrium, myometrium and uterine myomas during menstrual cycle and early pregnancy: characterisation, cellular localisation and comparison with rhesus monkey. Hum Reprod Update. 1998;4:594-604.
27. Curtis KM, Hillis SD, Marchbanks PA, et al. Disruption of the endometrial- myometrial border during pregnancy as a risk factor for adenomyosis. Am J Obstet Gynecol. 2002;187: 543-4.
28. Sahin AA, Silva EG, Landon G, et al. Endometrial tissue in myometrial vessels not associated with menstruation. Int J Gynecol Pathol. 1989;8:139-46.
29. Mai KT, Yazdi HM, Perkins DG, et al. Pathogenetic role of the stromal cells in endometriosis and adenomyosis. Histopathology. 1997;30:430-42.
30. Leyendecker G, Bilgicyildirim A, Inacker M, et al. Adenomyosis and endometriosis. Re-visiting their association and further insights into the mechanisms of auto-traumatisation. An MRI study. Arch Gynecol Obstet. 2015;291:917-32.
31. Yang G, Im HJ, Wang JH. Repetitive mechanical stretching modulates IL-1 beta induced COX-2, MMP-1 expression, and PGE2 production in human patellar tendon fibroblasts. Gene. 2005;363:166-72.

32. Leyendecker G, Wildt L. A new concept of endometriosis and adenomyosis: tissue injury and repair (TIAR). Hum Mol Biol Clin Invest. 2011;5:125-42.
33. Leyendecker G, Wildt L, Mall G. The pathophysiology of endometriosis and adenomyosis: tissue injury and repair. Arch Gynecol Obstet. 2009;280:529-38.
34. Kunz G, Beil D, Huppert P, et al. Adenomyosis in endometriosis—prevalence and impact on fertility. Evidence from magnetic resonance imaging. Hum Reprod. 2005;20:2309-16.
35. Ota H, Igarashi S, Hatazawa J, et al. Is adenomyosis an immune disease? Hum Reprod Update. 1998;4(4):360-67.
36. Grimbizis GF, Mikos T, Tarlatzis B. Uterus-sparing operative treatment for adenomyosis. Fertil Steril. 2014;101(2):472-87.
37. Larsen SB, Lundorf E, Forman A, et al. Adenomyosis and junctional zone changes in patients with endometriosis. Eur J Obstet Gynecol Reprod Biol. 2011;157:206-11.
38. Lei ZM, Rao CV, Lincoln SR, et al. Increased expression of human chorionic gonadotropin/human luteinizing hormone receptors in adenomyosis. J Clin Endocrinol Metab. 1993;76:763-8.
39. Benagiano G, Brosens I. The endometrium in adenomyosis. Womens Health (Lond). 2012;8(3):301-12.
40. Nie J, Lu Y, Liu X, et al. Immunoreactivity of progesterone receptor isoform B, nuclear factor κB, and IκBα in adenomyosis. Fertil Steril. 2009;92:886-9.
41. Li B, Chen M, Liu X, et al. Constitutive and tumor necrosis factor-α-induced activation of nuclear factor κB in adenomyosis and its inhibition by andrographolide. Fertil Steril. 2013;100(2):568-77.
42. Tokyol C, Aktepe F, Dilek FH, et al. Expression of cyclooxygenase-2- and matrix metalloproteinase-2 in adenomyosis and endometrial polyps and its correlation with angiogenesis. Int J Gynecol Pathol. 2009;28:148-56.
43. Bruner KL, Martisian LM, Rodgers WH, et al. Suppression of matrix metalloproteinases inhibits establishment of ectopic lesions by human endometrium in nude mice. J Clin Invest. 1997;99:2851-7.
44. Qiu F, Gao XM, Luo GL, et al. Expression of matrix metalloproteinase and tissue inhibitor of metalloproteinase in adenomyosis. Sichuan Da Xue Bao Yi Xue Ban. 2006;37:118-22.
45. Li T, Li YG, Pu DM. Matrix metalloproteinase-2 and -9 expression correlated with angiogenesis in human adenomyosis. Gynecol Obstet Invest. 2006;62:229-35.
46. Wang F, Li H, Yang Z, et al. Expression of interleukin-10 in patients with adenomyosis. Fertil Steril. 2009;91:1681-5.
47. Ota H, Igarashi S, Hatazawa J, et al. Is adenomyosis an immune disease? Hum Reprod Update. 1998;4:360-67.
48. Ota H, Igarashi S, Tanaka T. Expression of γδT cells and adhesion molecules in endometriotic tissue in patients with endometriosis and adenomyosis. Am J Reprod Immunol. 1996;35:477-82.
49. Chiang CM, Hill JA. Localization of T cells, interferon-γ and HLA-DR in eutopic and ectopic human endometrium. Gynecol Obstet Invest. 1997;43:245-50.
50. Ota H, Tanaka T. Integrin, adhesion molecules in the endometrial glandular epithelium in patients with endometriosis and adenomyosis. J Obstet Gynaecol Res. 1997;23:485-91.
51. Propst M, Quade BJ, Nowak RA, et al. Granulocyte macrophage colony stimulating factor in adenomyosis and autologous endometrium. J Soc Gynecol Invest. 2002;9:93-7.
52. Noda Y, Matsumoto H, Umaoka Y, et al. Involvement of superoxide radicals in the mouse two-cell block. Mol Reprod Dev. 1991;28:356-60.
53. Barroso RP, Osuamkpe C, Nagamani M, et al. Nitric oxide inhibits development of embryos and implantation in mice. Mol Hum Reprod. 1998;4:503-7.
54. Ota H, Igarashi S, Kato N, et al. Aberrant expression of glutathione peroxidase in eutopic and ectopic endometrium in endometriosis and adenomyosis. Fertil Steril. 200;74:313-8.
55. Ota H, Igarashi S, Tanaka T. Xanthine oxidase in eutopic and ectopic endometrium in endometriosis and adenomyosis. Fertil Steril. 2001;75:785-90.
56. Ota H, Igarashi S, Hatazawa J, et al. Immunohistochemical assessment of superoxide dismutase expression in the endometrium in endometriosis and adenomyosis. Fertil Steril. 1999;72:129-34.
57. Ota H, Igarashi S, Sato N, et al. Involvement of catalase in the endometrium of patients with endometriosis and adenomyosis. Fertil Steril. 2002;78:804-9.
58. Satokata I, Benson G, Maas R. Sexually dimorphic sterility phenotypes in Hoxa10-deficient mice. Nature 1995;374:460-3.
59. Fischer CP, Kayisili U, Taylor HS. HOXA10 expression is decreased in endometrium of women with adenomyosis. Fertil Steril. 2011;95:1133-6.
60. Xiao Y, Sun X, Yang X, et al. Leukemia inhibitory factor is dysregulated in the endometrium and uterine flushing fluid of patients with adenomyosis during implantation window. Fertil Steril. 2010;94:85-9.
61. Piver P. Uterine factors limiting ART coverage. J Gynecol Obstet Biol Reprod (Paris). 2005;34:5S30-5S33.
62. Vercellini P, Consonni D, Dridi D, et al. Uterine adenomyosis and in vitro fertilization outcome: a systematic review and meta-analysis. Hum Reprod. 2014;29(5):964-77.
63. Mehasseb MK, Bell SC, Pringle JH, et al. Uterine adenomyosis is associated with ultrastructural features of altered contractility in the inner myometrium. Fertil Steril. 2010;93(7):2130-6.
64. Kissler S, Hamscho N, Zangos S, et al. Uterotubal transport disorder in adenomyosisandendometriosis—acause-forinfertility. BJOG. 2006;113(8):902-8.
65. Jenkinson PC, Anderson D, Gangolli SD. Malformations induced in cultured rat embryos by enzimically generated active oxygen species. Teratog Carinog Mutagen. 1986;6:547-54.
66. Abbott J. Adenomyosis and abnormal uterine bleeding (AUB-A) – Pathogenesis, diagnosis, and management. Best Pract Res Clin Obstet Gynaecol. 2017;40:68-81.
67. Brosens JJ, Barker FG. The role of myometrial needle biopsies in the diagnosis of adenomyosis. Fertil Steril. 1995;63(6):1347-9.
68. Vercellini P, Cortesi I, De Giorgi O, et al. Transvaginal ultrasonography versus uterine needle biopsy in the diagnosis of diffuse adenomyosis. Hum Reprod. 1998;13(10):2884-7.
69. Siedler D, Laing FC, Jeffrey RB Jr, et al. Uterine adenomyosis: a difficult sonographic diagnosis. J Ultrasound Med. 1987;6:34-9.

70. Van den Bosch T, Dueholm M, Leone FP, et al. Terms, definitions and measurements to describe sonographic features of myometrium and uterine masses: a consensus opinion from the Morphological Uterus Sonographic Assessment (MUSA) group. Ultrasound Obstet Gynecol. 2015;46(3):284-98.
71. Meredith SM, Sanchez-Ramos L, Kaunitz AM. Diagnostic accuracy of transvaginal sonography for the diagnosis of adenomyosis: systematic review and meta-analysis. Am J Obstet Gynecol. 2009;201:107.e1-6.
72. Luciano DE, Exacoustos C, Albrecht L, et al. Three-dimensional ultrasound in diagnosis of adenomyosis: histologic correlation with ultrasound targeted biopsies of the uterus. J Minim Invasive Gynecol. 2013;20:803-10.
73. de Souza NM, Brosens JJ, Schwieso JE, et al. The potential value of magnetic resonance imaging in infertility. Clin Radiol. 1995;50:75-9.
74. Novellas S, Chassang M, Delotte J, et al. MRI characteristics of the uterine junctional zone: from normal to the diagnosis of adenomyosis. Am J Roentgenol. 2011;196:1206-13.
75. Reinhold C, Tafazoli F, Wang L. Imaging features of adenomyosis. Hum Reprod Update. 1998;4:337-49.
76. Champaneria R, Abedin P, Daniels J, et al. Ultrasound scan and magnetic resonance imaging for the diagnosis of adenomyosis: systematic review comparing test accuracy. Acta Obstetricia Gynecologica Scand. 2010;89(11):1374-84.
77. Dueholm M, Lundorf E, Hansen ES, et al. Magnetic resonance imaging and transvaginal ultrasonography for the diagnosis of adenomyosis. Fertil Steril. 2001;76:588-94.
78. Brosens I, Derwig I, Brosens J, et al. The enigmatic uterine junctional zone: the missing link between reproductive disorders and major obstetrical disorders? Hum Reprod. 2010;25:569-74.
79. Molinas CR, Campo R. Office hysteroscopy and adenomyosis. Best Pract Res Clin Obstet Gynaecol. 2006;20(4):557-67.
80. Vercellini P, Vigano P, Somigliana E, et al. Endometriosis: pathogenesis and treatment. Nat Rev Endocrinol. 2013;10:261-75.
81. Ozaki T, Takahashi K, Okada M, et al. Live birth after conservative surgery for severe adenomyosis following magnetic resonance imaging and gonadotropin- releasing hormone agonist therapy. Int J Fertil Womens Med. 1999;44:260-64.
82. Huang BS, Seow KM, Tsui KH, et al. Fertility outcome of infertile women with adenomyosis treated with the combination of a conservative microsurgical technique and GnRH agonist: long-term follow-up in a series of nine patients. Taiwan J Obstet Gynecol. 2012;51(2):212-6.
83. Khan KN, Kitajima M, Hiraki K, et al. Changes in tissue inflammation, angiogenesis and apoptosis in endometriosis, adenomyosis and uterine myoma after GnRH agonist therapy. Hum Reprod. 2010;25(3):642-53.
84. Badawy AM, Elnashar AM, Mosbah AA. Aromatase inhibitors or gonadotropin- releasing hormone agonists for the management of uterine adenomyosis: a randomised controlled trial. Acta Obstet Gynecol Scand. 2012;91: 489-95.
85. Dunselman GA, Vermeulen N, Becker C, et al. ESHRE guideline: management of women with endometriosis. Hum Reprod. 2014;29(11):400-12.
86. Yen MS, Yang TS, Yu KJ, et al. Comments on laparoscopic excision of myometrial adenomyomas in patients with adenomyosis uteri and main symptoms of severe dysmenorrhea and hypermenorrhea. J Am Assoc Gynecol Laparosc. 2004;11:441.
87. Sun HD, Su WH, Chang WH, et al. Rupture of a pregnant unscarred uterus in an early secondary trimester: a case report and brief review. J Obstet Gynaecol Res. 2012;38:442-5.
88. Osada H, Silber S, Kakinuma T, et al. Surgical procedure to conserve the uterus for future pregnancy in patients suffering from massive adenomyosis. Reprod Biomed Online. 2011;22:94-9.
89. Morita M, Asakawa Y, Nakakuma M, et al. Laparoscopic excision of myometrial adenomyomas in patients with adenomyosis uteri and main symptoms of severe dysmenorrhea and hypermenorrhea. J Am Assoc Gynecol Laparosc. 2004;11:86-9.
90. Sun AJ, Luo M, Wang W, et al. Characteristics and efficacy of modified adenomyomectomy in the treatment of uterine adenomyoma. Chin Med J (Engl). 2011;124:1322-6.
91. Takeuchi H, Kitade M, Kikuchi I, et al. Laparoscopic adenomyomectomy and hysteroplasty: a novel method. J Minim Invasive Gynecol. 2006;13:150-4.
92. Fujishita A, Masuzaki H, Khan KN, et al. Modified reduction surgery for adenomyosis. A preliminary report of the transverse H incision technique. Gynecol Obstet Invest. 2004;57:132-8.
93. Gordts S, Campo R, Brosens I. Hysteroscopic diagnosis and excision of myometrial cystic adenomyosis. Gynecol Surg. 2014;11:273-8.
94. Wang PH, Yang TS, Lee WL, et al. Treatment of infertilewomen with adenomyosis with a conservative microsurgical technique and a gonadotropin-releasing hormone agonist. Fertil Steril. 2000;73:1061-2.
95. Popovic M, Puchner S, Berzaczy D, et al. Uterine artery embolization for the treatment of adenomyosis: a review. J Vasc Interv Radiol. 2011;22:901-9.
96. Dong X, Yang Z. High-intensity focused ultrasound ablation of uterine localized adenomyosis. Curr Opin Obstet Gynecol. 2010;22:326-30.
97. Kishi Y, Yabuta M, Taniguchi F. Who will benefit from uterus-sparing surgery in adenomyosis-associated subfertility? Fertil Steril. 2014;102(3):802-7.e1.
98. Levgur M. Therapeutic options for adenomyosis: a review. Arch Gynecol Obstet. 2007;276:1-15.
99. Wang CJ, Yuen LT, Chang SD, et al. Use of laparoscopic cytoreductive surgery to treat infertile women with localized adenomyosis. Fertil Steril. 2006;86:462.e5-8.

CHAPTER

73

Genital Tuberculosis

Sandeep Shah, Reena Gupta

INTRODUCTION

Tuberculosis (TB) is a major health problem worldwide, despite a declining trend in mortality because of effective chemotherapy. Nearly one-third of world's population is infected with TB of which only 10% are known to progress to clinical disease.[1] It is the ninth leading cause of death in the world and the leading cause from a single infectious agent, ranking even above human immunodeficiency virus/acquired immunodeficiency syndrome (HIV/AIDS). There were an estimated 10.4 million new cases detected of TB in year 2016 (90% adults; 65% male; 10% people living with HIV). About 45% of the new cases in 2016 occurred in the WHO South-East Asia region. Five countries accounted for the 56% of new cases and India is top amongst them.[1]

Drug-resistant TB is another persistent threat, with 4,90,000 million cases of multidrug-resistant TB (MDR-TB) emerging in 2016 and an additional 1,10,000 cases that were susceptible to isoniazid but resistant to rifampicin (RR-TB), the most effective first-line anti-TB drug. The countries with the largest numbers of MDR/RR-TB cases (47% of the global total) are China, India, and Russia.[1]

India accounts for a quarter of the world's annual incidence of TB. Every year around 2 million people develop TB in India and 3,00,000 die of TB.[2] Over 15 million patients have been treated and 3 million additional lives have been saved by the Revised National TB Control Programme (RNTCP) over the last decade. Cure rates have consistently been above 85%.[2] However, it still continues to be a major health problem in the country.

PREVALENCE OF FEMALE GENITAL TUBERCULOSIS

Genitourinary TB is a common form of extrapulmonary TB (EPTB) worldwide accounting for approximately 27% of all EPTB cases. Genital TB alone accounts for 9% of all EPTB cases.[3] However, the burden of genital TB in females is underestimated as most of the patients are asymptomatic and usually diagnosed during evaluation for infertility.

The existing literature on the prevalence of genital TB among women with infertility is highly variable, ranging from 3% to 26%.[4-10] The prevalence is as high as 48.5% if only cases of tubal factor infertility are considered.[6] Conception rates (spontaneous or assisted) have ranged from 12% to 23% in different studies.[4,5,7,10] The difference in prevalence rates in different studies is due to different study populations, with a few studies being done at tertiary care centers where patients are referred from all over the country.

ETIOPATHOGENESIS

Female genital TB is almost always secondary to TB elsewhere in the patient's body usually pulmonary but sometimes it can be gastrointestinal, renal, bone or rarely as a part of miliary TB. It is caused most commonly by *Mycobacterium tuberculosis* and rarely by *Mycobacterium bovis*. Just like any other TB infection, predisposing factors include poverty, overcrowding, malnutrition, smoking, alcohol, drug abuse, diabetes, end-stage renal disease, cancer patients, and now more importantly HIV.

Table 1: Involvement of various structures in female genital tuberculosis.

Structure	*Involvement*
Fallopian tubes	85–100%
Uterus	50–70%
Ovaries	20–30%
Cervix	5–15%
Vagina and vulva	1–2%

The tubercle bacilli reach the genital tract by three main routes. Most common is hematogenous, then lymphatic, and rarely a direct spread from intra-abdominal or peritoneal focus. However, primary genital TB can rarely occur in women whose male partners have active genitourinary TB (e.g. TB epididymitis) by transmission through infected semen.[11] The site of involvement in these cases can be cervix, vagina or vulva.

Once the patient gets infected with tuberculous bacilli, the future course of disease depends upon the virulence of the organism and immunity of the host. If the immunity is good or virulence of organism is low, the patient remains asymptomatic and the infection remains latent for years. On the other hand, if the organism is highly virulent or the immune system of the host is weak, the infection spreads by either hematogenous or lymphatic route.

The most common genital organ involved in genital TB is fallopian tubes and 85–100% of these cases have bilateral involvement.[11,12] Uterus is the second most common genital organ to be involved, and is affected in 50–70% of cases, predominantly affecting the endometrium and occasionally myometrium.[11] Ovaries are affected in up to 20–30% of cases.[11] Cervical TB may occur in 5–15% cases of genital TB and it may masquerade cervical cancer necessitating biopsy for confirmation of diagnosis.[13] TB of vagina and vulva is very rare (1–2%), presenting as a hypertrophic lesion or a nonhealing ulcer mimicking malignancy, and requires biopsy and histopathological examination to confirm the diagnosis (Table 1).

Genital TB can also manifest as a disseminated form of peritoneal TB with tubercles all over the peritoneum, intestines, and omentum, and ascites with abdominal mass. CA-125 may be raised, and CT/MRI picture may also look similar to ovarian cancer.[14,15] Ascitic fluid tapping for biochemical analysis (elevated adenosine deaminase level in ascitic fluid in peritoneal TB) is useful in diagnosis.[16] Laparoscopic biopsy with frozen section evaluation has also been suggested to avoid laparotomy in such cases.[15,16]

CLINICAL PRESENTATION

Symptoms

Genital tract TB often presents with low-grade symptomatology and very few specific complaints. Hence, clinical diagnosis requires a high index of suspicion. The following history should arouse a suspicion of genital TB:

- Women with family history of TB
- Past history of TB
- Chronic pelvic pain associated with infertility
- Secondary amenorrhea alone or associated with infertility
- Women with adnexal mass
- Unexplained infertility more than 5 years duration
- Puberty menorrhagia not responding to usual treatment
- Primary amenorrhea
- Chronic pelvic inflammatory disease (PID) in adolescent
- Poor general health persisting over months or years.

The above cases should be investigated thoroughly for genital tuberculosis (GTB). About 80–90% of women diagnosed with TB are of age group 20–40 years and they are generally diagnosed during workup of subfertility.

The following are the common symptoms in GTB:

- *General symptoms*: Low-grade fever with evening rise in temperature, loss of appetite, and loss of weight
- *Infertility*: It is the most common initial symptom. Furthermore, the prevalence of genital TB among infertile patients has been found to be as high as 24.2% in a systematic review.[17]

  Infertility can be due to damage to the fallopian tubes (both anatomical and functional), endometrial damage leading to Asherman's syndrome, and rarely due to anovulation resulting from poor ovarian reserve
- *Pain abdomen*: Lower abdominal pain or chronic pelvic pain is seen in approximately 25–50% of patients. Pain can be because of the following reasons:
  - Peritoneal, gastrointestinal, urinary, and tubercular salpingitis can cause pain in abdomen. This pain is usually dull in nature
  - Chronic pelvic pain can occur due to chronic pelvic inflammation. It can present with repeated PID
  - Dysmenorrhea: Patients can have congestive dysmenorrhea due to chronic pelvic inflammation
  - Rarely, rupture of TO mass can cause acute abdomen
  - Pain in abdomen in TB may be aggravated by hysterosalpingogram (HSG) as well as dilatation and curettage.

- *Menstrual disturbances:* Abnormal uterine bleeding has been reported in 10–40% of patients with genital TB. Patients may present with any of the following patterns:
  - Heavy menstrual bleeding
  - *Polymenorrhea*: Seen in earlier stages of infection where there is pelvic congestion secondary to pelvic inflammation
  - Hypomenorrhea
  - *Amenorrhea*: Can be there due to chronic endometrial inflammation, atrophy, and synechiae formation (Asherman's syndrome)
  - Puberty menorrhagia
  - Postmenopausal bleeding.
- Other symptoms seen less frequently are:
  - Discharge per vagina (due to pelvic inflammation)
  - Mass per abdomen
  - Recurrent PID not responding to treatment
  - *TO mass*: Genital TB can mimic ovarian carcinoma, presenting as adnexal mass with ascites
  - Symptoms associated with urinary and bowel fistulae.

Signs

Physical examination may be normal in up to 50% of cases.

General Examination

Signs which may be found are:

- Poorly nourished
- Fever
- Cervical lymph node enlargement
- Signs of pulmonary TB.

Abdominal Examination

On palpation, abdomen may feel doughy suggestive of peritoneal TB. Abdomen may be distended due to ascites. Sometimes there are encysted ascites due to adhesions, characterized by a mass which is tympanic on percussion (due to the bowel loops adherent on the mass).

Pelvic Examination

Mobility of uterus may be restricted due to adhesions (frozen pelvis). Cervical movements can be tender. There may be a nontender adnexal mass (tubo-ovarian mass, hydrosalpinx). Uterus may be enlarged rarely due to pyometra.

Lower genital tract TB is rare. It may present with:

- Hypertrophic/ulcerative lesions in cervix, vagina or vulva
- Labial mass
- *Fistula*: Vesical, rectovaginal, tubovesical, utero-cutaneous, etc.

WORKING CASE DEFINITIONS

The recent EPTB index TB guidelines released by the Ministry of Health and Family Welfare (MoHFW), India, have provided case definitions for EPTB as below:[18]

Presumptive case: A patient with symptoms and signs of EPTB who needs to be investigated.

Bacteriologically confirmed case: A patient who has a microbiological diagnosis of EPTB, based on positive microscopy, culture or a validated PCR-based test.

Clinically diagnosed case: A patient with negative microbiological tests for TB (microscopy, culture, and validated PCR-based tests), but with strong clinical suspicion and other evidence of EPTB, such as compatible imaging findings, histological findings, ancillary diagnostic tests or response to anti-TB treatment.

A presumptive case started on ATT (antitubercular therapy) empirically, without microbiological testing, should also be considered a clinically diagnosed case (empirically treated). A clinically diagnosed case subsequently found to be bacteriologically positive (before or after starting treatment) should be reclassified as bacteriologically confirmed.

Non-EPTB case: A patient who has been investigated for EPTB and has been diagnosed with a different condition, with no microbiological evidence of EPTB found.

Presumptive relapse: A patient who was declared successfully treated at the end of ATT and now presents again with symptoms and signs of any form of TB.

Bacteriologically confirmed relapse: A patient with presumptive relapse who has microbiological evidence of persisting MTB infection on repeat diagnostic sampling.

Clinically diagnosed relapse: A patient with presumptive relapse who does not have microbiological evidence of persisting MTB infection on repeat diagnostic sampling, and has no evidence of another disease process.

A patient with presumptive relapse who is started on ATT empirically without repeat microbiological tests should also be considered a clinically diagnosed relapse (empirically treated). A clinically diagnosed relapse subsequently found to be bacteriologically positive (before or after starting treatment) should be reclassified as bacteriologically confirmed relapse.

Treatment failures have also been similarly classified to make it easier for clinicians to identify successful/unsuccessful treatment.

DIAGNOSTIC TESTS

In a presumptive case of TB, the purpose of various investigations are to directly isolate the organism, or indirectly look at the effects on the tissues and organs by hematological, histopathological or microbiological methods. However, being a paucibacillary disease, demonstration of MTB is not possible in all cases of genital TB requiring a high index of suspicion.

The diagnostic tests can be broadly classified into direct and indirect tests.

Direct tests: Direct visualization of the organism in the tissues. This includes microscopy, culture, histopathology and molecular tests such as PCR.

Indirect tests: Specific recognizable changes brought about by the disease in the tissues. These include tuberculin test, chest X-ray, QuantiFERON gold, and endoscopy findings.

Direct Tests

Traditionally, the laboratory diagnosis of TB depends on demonstration of the causative organism, MTB, by acid-fast staining and/or growth of the organism on Löwenstein-Jensen (LJ) medium. However, a substantial number of TB lesions of the genital tract are paucibacillary and hence demonstration of the Mycobacterium is not possible in all cases. Endometrial biopsy, curettage or aspiration in the premenstrual phase is the most commonly used test for the diagnosis of genital TB. Menstrual blood within 12 hours is also used for the purpose. In addition, biopsy from TO masses, peritoneal fluid/biopsy, cervical/vaginal secretions may also be subjected to smear and cultures for diagnosis.

It is important to send the specimen in normal saline for the smear and culture tests and in formalin for the histopathological examination.

Mycobacterial Staining

Staining methods include Ziehl-Neelsen (Z-N) staining (conventional staining method) and Fluorochrome-Auramine-Rhodamine staining (fluorescent staining). Microscopic examination of acid-fast bacilli (AFB) requires the presence of at least 5,000–10,000 organisms/mL in the sample to be positive. Sensitivity is very low and is rarely positive in genital TB because of its paucibacillary nature.

AFB Culture

The bacteria need to be more than 1,000 in number in order to grow in culture. At present, mycobacterial culture can be performed on conventional egg-based solid medium such as LJ medium, agar-based media such as Middlebrook 7H10 or 7H11, and liquid media such as Kirschner or Middlebrook 7H9 broth. The major constraint of culturing mycobacteria in conventional media is its slow growth which necessitates a mean incubation period of at least 4–6 weeks. The drug susceptibility tests to anti-TB drugs require additional 4 weeks. The new culture methods like the BACTEC Radiometric Culture and the MGIT (mycobacteria growth indicator tube) 960 system give results in a 7–14 day time.

Endometrial Histology

Endometrial tissue for histopathology is obtained by dilatation and curretage or hysteroscopy-directed biopsy. Demonstration of granuloma with or without Langerhans giant cells on histopathology is diagnostic of genital TB. A negative biopsy however does not rule out genital TB.

In a study by Jindal et al., the detection rates for AFB smear, MGIT culture, LJ culture, and HPE were found to be 50%, 46.7%, 3.3% and 33.3%, respectively. A combination of smear examination for AFB, MGIT 960 culture, and histopathological examination was able to detect all the positive cases. A combination of MGIT and LJ media provided no added advantage over MGIT alone since the only case where LJ culture was positive had been detected by positive MGIT culture.[19]

Molecular Test—Polymerase Chain Reaction

The PCR is a rapid, sensitive, and specific molecular biological method for detecting mycobacterial DNA in both pulmonary and extrapulmonary samples from suspected TB patients.

Sensitivity is so high that it can detect even less than 10 microorganisms in clinical specimens to achieve a positive report and this is an important feature since genital TB is paucibacillary. Results are available within 1–2 days. False negative result may be due to contamination. False positive is also possible as it cannot distinguish between live and killed bacilli. Hence this test cannot be used alone to start or stop ATT. However, Jindal et al.[20] observed high pregnancy rate after treating infertility with positive PCR alone with ATT.

The latest innovation that is recommended by WHO for rapid testing is cartridge-based nucleic acid amplification test (CB-NAAT), also known as Xpert MTB/RIF, based on the GeneXpert multi-disease platform. It is a PCR cartridge-based test which reports growth in 2 hours and drug sensitivity in another day. It has very high specificity (around 98%). The sensitivity for EPTB has been reported to be 95% for smear positive and 69% for smear negative samples.[21] International Standard for TB Care (ISTC) and Standard of TB Care in India (STCI) now recommend Xpert MTB/RIF assay for both PTB and EPTB as this allows for rapid detection of MTB DNA. Thus, Xpert MTB/RIF should be considered a central test in the workup of EPTB and should be used along with microscopy, liquid cultures, and histopathology. The limitations of this test are its sensitivity to high temperature and humid conditions. Blood contamination in endometrial biopsy can also inhibit GeneXpert making it negative. Other disadvantage is that it can only detect rifampicin resistance and not resistance to other antitubercular drugs. In comparison, linear probe assay (LPA), another molecular technique, detects resistance to both rifampicin and isoniazid. Under RNTCP, either CBNAAT or LPA should be used for diagnosis of drug-resistant TB (DR-TB).

Indirect Tests

Routine Blood Tests

Routine laboratory studies are of little value as they are mostly nonspecific. Anemia and leukocytosis with a tendency to lymphocytosis and a raised ESR may be seen.

Chest X-ray

It may be of value in excluding concurrent pulmonary TB, which is rare, but signs of previous TB may be present.

Tuberculin Sensitivity Test

The test is based on the fact that infection with MTB produces sensitivity to certain antigenic components of the organism that are contained in culture extracts called tuberculin. It is done by injecting 0.1 mL of purified protein derivative (PPD) intracutaneously into the dorsal or volar surface of the forearm. Limitation of tuberculin sensitivity test (TST) is that the antigens used are not specific to MTB. A local reaction therefore does not differentiate between an existing immune response elicited by previous Bacillus Calmette-Guérin (BCG) vaccination, exposure to nontubercular mycobacteria (NTM), or MTB.

Further, false negative results may be seen in recent TB, recent viral infections, coexisting HIV infection, chronic renal failure and people with typhoid fever, typhus, brucellosis, leprosy or pertussis. Abdelrub et al.[10] showed that TST was positive in 42.6% of patients with genital TB. Raut et al.[22] reported sensitivity and specificity of TST as 55% and 80%, respectively, in women with laparoscopically diagnosed TB.

Serological Tests

Serological tests for diagnosis of TB are not recommended for the diagnosis of TB and are banned by the government of India.

Interferon-gamma Release Assay

Interferon-gamma release assay (IGRA) (for example, the TB Gold test) is an indirect enzyme-linked immunosorbent assay (ELISA)-based test for MTB complex which includes *M. tuberculosis, M. bovis, M. africanum, M. microti,* and *M. canetti* infection.

Although it is rapid and not affected by BCG vaccination, it cannot differentiate between active TB disease and latent infection. As a result, in a high burden setting like India, where almost 40% of the population carries a latent infection, the advantage of these tests is not yet clear. Hence these tests are not recommended by the Government of India.

Role of Ultrasound

The following findings can be seen on ultrasound in genital TB:

- An adnexal mass
- Hydrosalpinx
- Irregular endometrium/adhesions in endometrium
- Calcification in the uterus
- Failure of cavity to distend on sonohysterogram.

Hysterosalpingogram

Hysterosalpingogram is a simple imaging technique to diagnose tubal and uterine pathologies. HSG is contraindicated in active genital TB. However, if performed, the following tubal findings can be seen:

- Nonspecific findings like hydrosalpinx
- Multiple constrictions along the whole length of the tube giving a beaded appearance
- Tubal occlusion either at the isthmus or ampulla
- Multiple occlusions and scarring making the tube rigid and giving a pipe-stem appearance
- Cobblestone appearance
- Leopard skin appearance
- Tubal calcifications
- *Golf club appearance*: Bilateral distal isthmic obstruction

- Decreased tubal motility or fixed tubes, resulting from scarring around the tubes and peritubal adhesions, as a part of healing process
- Caseous ulceration of the mucosa of the tube giving it an irregular contour and diverticular outpouching around the ampulla giving a tufted appearance
- Same process in the isthmic region gives the typical appearance of salpingitis isthmica nodosa (SIN).

Uterine changes that may be appreciated on HSG in genital TB are:

- *Endometritis, intrauterine adhesions, and asymmetrical cavity*: All nonspecific
- *Collar-stud abscess*: Specific
- *T-shaped uterus*: Tubercular scarring causes triangular uterine cavity and gives a T-shape or septate appearance
- *Pseudo-unicornuate uterus*: Unilateral obliteration followed by unilateral scarring in uterine cavity
- Complete obstruction of uterine cavity with glove finger appearance.

CT and MRI Scan

Peritoneal TB and tubo-ovarian lesions have usually minimal findings at CT and are frequently misdiagnosed with peritoneal carcinomatosis. MRI is useful for the diagnosis of tubo-ovarian lesions. Regular pattern of small nodularities along the peritoneum at MRI is helpful finding.

Role of Endoscopy

Laparoscopic findings include (Wadia syndrome):[23]

- High colored copious peritoneal fluid (tending to become encysted)
- Periuteritis (nonglistening uterine surface), with lepra patches or a thrush appearance
- Blue uterus on injecting methylene blue
- Perisalpingitis, SIN, beaded tubes, rosary appearance, thick tubes, and hydrosalpinx
- Tubercles, micro and macrocaseation (on tube, pouch of Douglas, and posterior part of broad ligament)
- Flimsy adhesions in iliac fossa, pouch of Douglas, and the liver area. Adhesions in the liver bed are named as Fitz-Hugh-Curtis syndrome
- Omental adhesions are fibrous and dense, if formed after surgery
- Fibrosis in posterior part of broad ligament, mimicking endometriosis because of breaking of fibrosis typically by anteverting the uterus
- Small and fibrosed uterus
- Synechiae in pouch of Douglas.

Hysteroscopy can reveal:[23]

- Microcaseation
- Hypoplasia of endometrium with no bleeding on touch with hysteroscope
- Exudation smeared in the uterine cavity
- Funnel-shaped entrance to tubal ostium is distorted or completely lost
- Non-breathing tubal ostium, suggestive of a blocked tube
- Cannulation of ostial area releases flaky caseous material
- Irregular and ulcerated endocervical canal
- Fleshy and hyperplastic cervical erosion not bleeding on touch, and placed anteriorly
- Synechiae and fibrosis in the uterine cavity, especially precipitated after a curettage.

The final diagnosis of genital TB requires a high suspicion, good history, careful systemic and gynecological examination, and combination of diagnostic modalities like endometrial biopsy for AFB, culture and GeneXpert, in conjunction with imaging methods and endoscopic visualization, especially with laparoscopy.

CLASSIFICATION OF PATIENTS

According to RNTCP 2016, microbiologically confirmed or clinically diagnosed TB cases are classified based on the following criteria:[24]

Classification Based on Anatomical Site of Disease: Pulmonary or Extrapulmonary

Pulmonary TB (PTB) refers to any bacteriologically confirmed or clinically diagnosed case of TB involving the lung parenchyma or the tracheobronchial tree. Miliary TB is classified as PTB because there are lesions in the lungs. Tuberculous intrathoracic lymphadenopathy (mediastinal and/or hilar) or tuberculous pleural effusion, without radiographic abnormalities in the lungs, constitutes a case of extrapulmonary TB. A patient with both pulmonary and extrapulmonary TB should be classified as a case of PTB. Extrapulmonary TB (EPTB) refers to any bacteriologically confirmed or clinically diagnosed case of TB involving organs other than the lungs, e.g. pleura, lymph nodes, abdomen, genitourinary tract, skin, joints and bones, meninges.

Classification Based on History of Previous Treatment

- *New case*: A TB patient who has never taken TB treatment or has taken ATT for less than 1 month

- Previously treated patient—who has received ATT for more than a month. Previously treated patients are further subclassified into:
  - Recurrent TB case—TB patient who has been successfully treated previously and is subsequently found to be microbiologically positive again
  - Treatment after failure—who have been previously treated for TB and whose treatment failed at the end of their most recent course of treatment
  - Treatment after loss to follow-up—previously treated for TB for 1 month or more and was declared lost to follow-up in their recent course of treatment and subsequently found microbiologically confirmed TB case
  - Other previously treated patients—are those who have been previously treated but whose outcome after their recent course of treatment is unknown or undocumented.

Classification Based on Drug Resistance

- *Mono-resistance (MR)*: A TB patient who is resistant to one first-line anti-TB drug
- *Poly-drug resistance (PDR)*: A TB patient who is resistant to more than one first-line anti-TB drug, other than both isoniazid and rifampicin
- *Multidrug resistance*: A TB patient who is resistant to both isoniazid and rifampicin with or without resistance to other first-line drugs
- *Rifampicin resistance (RR)*: Patients with rifampicin resistance only, these patients should also be managed as if they are an MDR TB case
- *Extensive drug resistance (XDR)*: A MDR TB case whose biological specimen is additionally resistant to a fluoroquinolone (ofloxacin, levofloxacin or moxifloxacin) and a second-line injectable anti-TB drug (Kanamycin, amikacin, or capreomycin).

TREATMENT

Medical Treatment

Multiple drug therapy in adequate doses and for sufficient duration is the main stay in the treatment of genital TB.

Table 2: Regimen for drug sensitive patients.

Type of TB case	*Regimen in intensive phase*	*Regimen in continuation phase*
New	HRZE × 2 months	HRE × 4 months
Previously treated	HRZES × 2 months + HRZE × 1 month	HRE × 5 months

(E: ethambutol; H: isoniazid; R: rifampicin; S: streptomycin; Z: pyrazinamide)

In the era before rifampicin, the ATT was given for 18–24 months with significant side effects and poor compliance. Now, short-course chemotherapy for 6–9 months has been found to be equally effective.

The following is the treatment regimen for various groups of patients:[24]

- *Drug-sensitive patients*: The RNTCP advised thrice weekly regimen for treatment of drug-sensitive patients. Daily treatment regimen can also be given especially in HIV-positive patients (Table 2)
- *Mono drug-resistant TB*: Treatment comprises of injectable second-line drug+ fluoroquinolone+ rifampicin + two of the first-line drugs (from H, E, and Z) to which the patient is sensitive to, to make a total of five effective drugs given daily. The total duration of treatment should be 9–12 months, with intensive phase of 3–6 months and continuation phase of 6 months
- *Poly-drug resistance:* The regimen is an injectable second-line drug + fluoroquinolone + rifampicin + any first-line drug to which patient is sensitive + one of the remaining group four drugs (ethionamide, cycloserine, PAS). The total duration of treatment should be 9–12 months, with intensive phase of 3–6 months, and continuation phase of 6 months
- *MDR/RR TB cases*: These patients are treated with 6–9 months of intensive phase with kanamycin, levofloxacin, ethambutol, pyrazinamide, ethionamide and cycloserine, and 18 months of continuation phase of levofloxacin, ethambutol, ethionamide, and cycloserine. All MDR TB patients should be subjected to drug sensitivity at baseline for kanamycin and levofloxacin and appropriate modifications should be done in the treatment accordingly
- *XDR-TB*: These cases are treated with standardized treatment regimen for XDR TB comprising of injection capreomycin, moxifloxacin, linezolid, PAS, clofazimine, high dose INH, and amoxicillin-clavulanate. The intensive phase is of 6–12 months and only the injectable antibiotics are stopped in continuation phase. The remaining medicines are continued for another 18 months.

All drug-resistant TB treatment should be given on daily basis under supervision. Whenever drug sensitivity pattern of extended panel of drugs is available from a quality assured culture and drug susceptibility testing (CDST) laboratory, management protocol will change according to the sensitivity of drugs, and patient should be referred to DR TB center.

Surgical Treatment

The need for surgical intervention is limited as the medical therapy is highly effective in the treatment of FGTB. Indications for surgical intervention are as follows:

- Drainage of large residual pelvic or tubo-ovarian abscesses
- Hydrosalpinx or pyosalpinx
- Presence of fistulae
- Asherman's syndrome
- Fertility evaluation after medical treatment.

The surgical intervention required may be laparoscopy, laparotomy or hysteroscopy. The chances of complications such as hemorrhage and injury to bowel, bladder, and other pelvic structures during surgery are higher due to the presence of dense adhesions and matted bowel loops. The uterus and adnexae may be buried underneath the dense adhesions making the access very difficult. In such cases biopsy must be taken from representative areas and the abdomen closed, instead of trying a difficult pelvic adhesiolysis which may carry the risk of fistula or sinus formation. In younger women, ovarian conservation should be tried. In cases of advanced TB, the prognosis for fertility is generally poor. Even if these women conceive, the risks of ectopic pregnancy and miscarriage are high.

Assisted Reproductive Techniques in Genital TB

Most women with genital TB present with infertility and have poor prognosis for fertility in spite of ATT. The prevalence of genital TB in tubal factor infertility in India is reported to be as high as 50%.[6,11] Limited evidence suggests that GTB may also affect ovarian reserve adversely.[25,26] A recent prospective study compared 431 infertile women diagnosed with latent GTB (Group I) to 453 infertile women without latent GTB, and found that women with latent GTB had significantly lower AMH (Median AMH value of 2.0 ng/mL vs. 2.8 ng/mL; $p = 0.01$) and AFC (Median AFC of 7 vs. 8; $p < 0.001$] as compared to infertile women without TB.[27] Whether ATT improves this ovarian function is not yet known, but a small prospective study stated that after ATT treatment, the ovarian function (AMH and AFC) and ovarian blood flow improved significantly in women with FGTB.[28]

The conception rate is low (19.2%), and the live birth rate is further low (7%).[4] In vitro fertilization (IVF) with embryo transfer (ET) is the only hope for some of these women whose endometrium is not damaged with reported pregnancy rates of 16.6% to 31.2% per transfer.[5,11] Latent genital TB has also been found to be responsible for repeated IVF failures in young patients presenting with unexplained infertility with apparently normal pelvis.[29] If after ATT, tubes are still damaged but the endometrium is receptive (no adhesions or mild adhesions which can be hysteroscopically resected), IVF is recommended. However, if endometrial TB has damaged the endometrium with shrunken small uterine cavity with Asherman's syndrome, adoption or gestational surrogacy should be advised.

Counseling of Genital TB Patients

Before initiating the treatment, all TB patients should be counseled and educated about the disease and treatment. Ideally, all TB patients should be screened for HIV, especially drug-resistant TB. It is important to make the patients understand that ATT should be taken very regularly to avoid drug resistance. As multiple drugs are used for the treatment, patients should be warned about possible side effects. Patients should also be advised to take high protein diet during the treatment.

CONCLUSION

Genital TB is a major cause of infertility in women and is often underdiagnosed because of its paucibacillary nature. A high index of suspicion along with direct and indirect tests are required to diagnose it, as most cases are asymptomatic. Treatment is usually medical by chemotherapy which should be taken in adequate dosage and duration to prevent the development of multidrug resistance. Prognosis for fertility is poor. However, for tubal disease in the absence of endometrial disease, ART, especially IVF–ET, may give good results. In cases of endometrial disease with shrunken cavity, prognosis for fertility is very poor even with IVF-ET.

REFERENCES

1. World Health Organization. (2017). Global tuberculosis report 2017. Available from http://apps.who.int [Last Accessed February 2019].
2. New Delhi: World Health Organization Country Office for India. (2014). Standards for TB care in India. [online]. Available from https://tbcindia.gov.in [Last Accessed February 2019].
3. Golden MP, Vikram HR. Extrapulmonary tuberculosis: an overview. Am Fam Physician. 2005;72(9):1761-8.
4. Tripathy SN, Tripathy SN. Infertility and pregnancy outcome in female genital tuberculosis. Int J Gynaecol Obstet. 2002;76(2):159-63.
5. Jindal UN. An algorithmic approach to female genital tuberculosis causing infertility. Int J Tuberc Lung Dis. 2006;10(9):1045-50.
6. Singh N, Sumana G, Mittal S. Genital tuberculosis: a leading cause for infertility in women seeking assisted conception in North India. Arch Gynecol Obstet. 2008;278(4):325-7.

7. Shaheen R, Subhan F, Tahir F. Epidemiology of genital tuberculosis in infertile population. J Pak Med Assoc. 2006;56(7):306-9.
8. Khanna A, Agrawal A. Markers of genital tuberculosis in infertility. Singapore Med J. 2011;52(12):864-7.
9. Shahzad S. Investigation of the prevalence of female genital tract tuberculosis and its relation to female infertility: An observational analytical study. Iran J Reprod Med. 2012;10(6):581-8.
10. Al eryani AA, Abdelrub AS, Al Harazi AH. Genital tuberculosis is common among females with tubal factor infertility: Observational study. Alexandria J Med. 2015;51(4):321-4.
11. Parikh FR, Nadkarni SG, Kamat SA, et al. Genital tuberculosis--a major pelvic factor causing infertility in Indian women. Fertil Steril. 1997;67(3):497-500.
12. Agarwal J, Gupta JK. Female genital tuberculosis--a retrospective clinico-pathologic study of 501 cases. Indian J Pathol Microbiol. 1993;36(4):389-97.
13. Agrawal S, Madan M, Leekha N, et al. A rare case of cervical tuberculosis simulating carcinoma cervix: a case report. Cases J. 2009;2:161.
14. Sharma JB, Jain SK, Pushparaj M, et al. Abdomino-peritoneal tuberculosis masquerading as ovarian cancer: a retrospective study of 26 cases. Arch Gynecol Obstet. 2010;282(6):643-8.
15. Koc S, Beydilli G, Tulunay G, et al. Peritoneal tuberculosis mimicking advanced ovarian cancer: a retrospective review of 22 cases. Gynecol Oncol. 2006;103(2):565-9.
16. Dwivedi M, Misra SP, Misra V, et al. Value of adenosine deaminase estimation in the diagnosis of tuberculous ascites. Am J Gastroenterol. 1990;85(9):1123-5.
17. Chaman-Ara K, Bahrami MA, Bahrami E, et al. Prevalence of genital tuberculosis among infertile women: a systematic review and meta-analysis. IJMRHS. 2016;5(4):208-15.
18. Central TB Division, Ministry of Health and Family Welfare, Government of India. (2016). Index-TB guidelines: Guidelines on extra-pulmonary tuberculosis India. [online] Available from https://tbcindia.gov.in/showfile.php?lid=3245 [Last Accessed February 2019].
19. Jindal UN, Verma S, Bala Y. Favorable infertility outcomes following anti-tubercular treatment prescribed on the sole basis of a positive polymerase chain reaction test for endometrial tuberculosis. Hum Reprod. 2012;27(5):1368-74.
20. Maynard-Smith L, Larke N, Peters JA, et al. Diagnostic accuracy of the Xpert MTB/RIF assay for extrapulmonary and pulmonary tuberculosis when testing non-respiratory samples: a systematic review. BMC Infect Dis. 2014;14:709.
21. Raut VS, Mahashur AA, Sheth SS. The Mantoux test in the diagnosis of genital tuberculosis in women. Int J Gynaecol Obstet. 2001;72(2):165-9.
22. Wadia BJ. "Wadia Syndrome" correlation of laparoscopic findings in the tuberculosis abdomen. J Am Assoc Gynecol Laparosc. 1994;1(4, Part 2):S39.
23. New Delhi: Central TB Division, Directorate of Health Services, Ministry of Health & Family Welfare (MoHFW), Government of India. (2016). Technical and Operational Guidelines for TB Control in India 2016. [online]. Available from https://tbcindia.gov.in [Last Accessed February 2019].
24. Gurgan T, Urman B, Yarali H. Results of in vitro fertilization and embryo transfer in women with infertility due to genital tuberculosis. Fertil Steril. 1996;65(2):367-70.
25. Malhotra N, Sharma V, Bahadur A, et al. The effect of tuberculosis on ovarian reserve among women undergoing IVF in India. Int J Gynaecol Obstet. 2012;117(1):40-4.
26. Jirge PR, Chougule SM, Keni A, et al. Latent genital tuberculosis adversely affects the ovarian reserve in infertile women. Hum Reprod. 2018;33(7):1262-9.
27. Jindal N, Gainder S, Dhaliwal LK, et al. The role of MGIT 960 culture medium in resolving the diagnostic dilemma for genital tuberculosis patients presenting with infertility. J Obstet Gynaecol India. 2018;68(2):123-8.
28. Sharma JB, Sneha J, Singh UB, et al. Effect of antitubercular treatment on ovarian function in female genital tuberculosis with infertility. J Hum Reprod Sci. 2016;9(3):145-50.
29. Dam P, Shirazee HH, Goswami SK, et al. Role of latent genital tuberculosis in repeated IVF failure in the Indian clinical setting. Gynecol Obstet Invest. 2006;61(4):223-7.

CHAPTER

74

Hydrosalpinx and Assisted Reproductive Technology

Pallavi Prasad

DEFINITION

A hydrosalpinx results from an accumulation of secretions when the tube is occluded at its distal end. It is usually the end result of pyosalpinx. Hydrosalpinx can also result from nontubal infection, such as adjacent appendicitis, causing distal tubal occlusion.

TYPES OF HYDROSALPINX

- Hydrosalpinx simplex—distended thinned out tube with widely separated fewer plicae
- Hydrosalpinx follicularis—tubal plicae fused resulting in compartmentalizing of lumen
- Sactosalpinx—dilatation of the inflamed uterine tube by retained secretions (saktos—stuffed).

METHODS OF DIAGNOSIS

Hysterosalpingogram: It shows a dilated fallopian tube, filling with contrast and with absence of free spillage (Fig. 1).

Ultrasound: Hydrosalpinx is seen as sausage-like structure filled with moderately echogenic fluid. It is seen as follows (Fig. 2):

- Thin or thick walled (in chronic cases)
- Elongated or folded, tubular, C-shaped, or S-shaped fluid-filled structure
- Distinct from the uterus and ovary.

Ultrasound Features of Hydrosalpinx

Cogwheel appearance—pathognomonic of hydrosalpinx. Small round nodules less than 3 mm in size seen in cross section that represent endosalpingeal folds (Figs. 3 to 6).

"Beads on a string" sign—incomplete septae give beads-on-string appearance.

"Waist sign" (indentations on opposite sides).

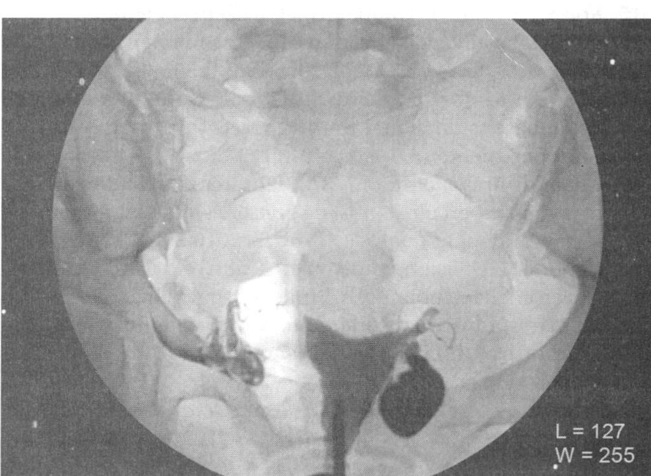

Fig. 1: Hysterosalpingogram appearance of left side hydrosalpinx.

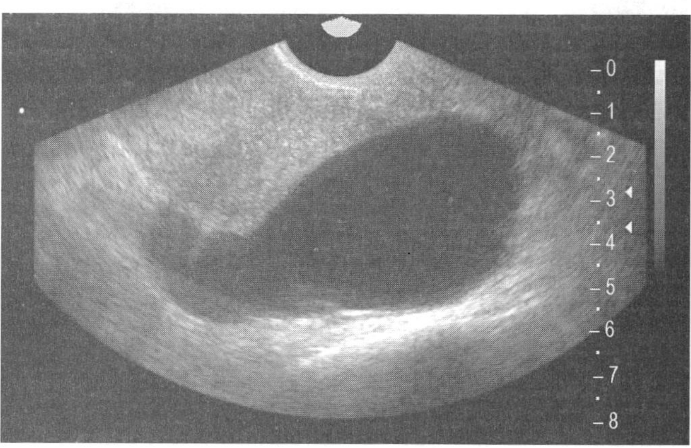

Fig. 2: Ultrasound appearance of sausage-shaped hydrosalpinx.

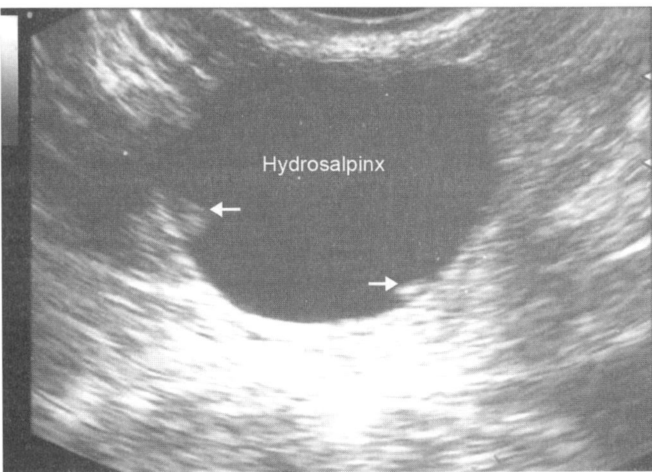

Fig. 3: "Cogwheel appearance" of hydrosalpinx on ultrasound.

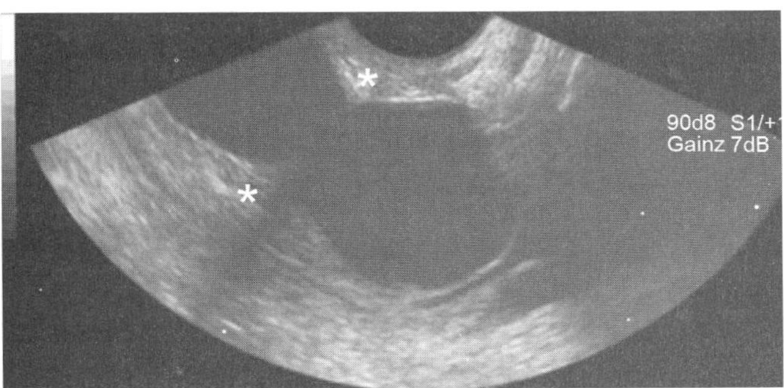

Fig. 4: "Waist sign" of hydrosalpinx on ultrasound.

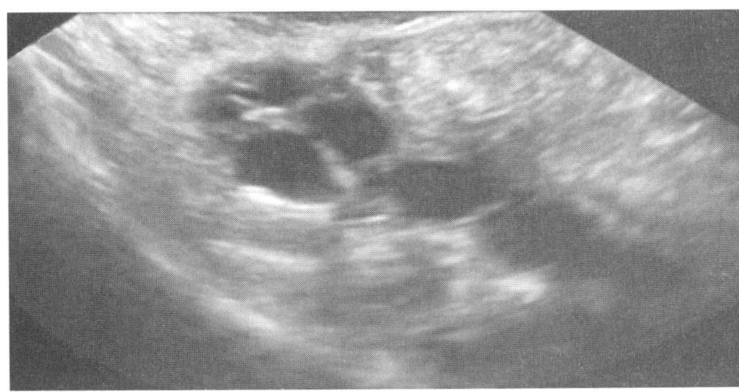

Fig. 5: "Beads-on-string sign" of hydrosalpinx on ultrasound.

"Spikes in lumen"—folds of the tubal wall in a distended hydrosalpinx depicted as typical spikes into the lumen.

Laparoscopy—diagnostic as well as therapeutic modality.

PATHOPHYSIOLOGY OF HYDROSALPINX

Hydrosalpinx can affect the pregnancy rates in in vitro fertilization (IVF).

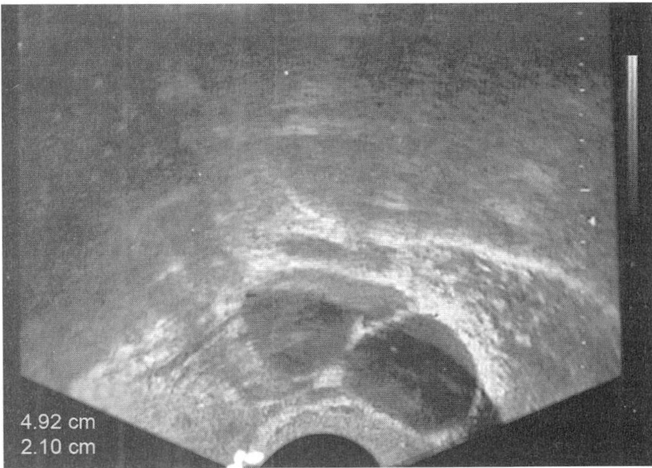

Fig. 6: "Spikes-in-lumen sign" of hydrosalpinx.

The various mechanisms by which hydrosalpinx can affect pregnancy outcomes in assisted reproductive technology are as follows:[1]

- Mechanical flushing of embryos from the uterine cavity[2-4]
- Hydrosalpinx fluid film on endometrial surface which can hinder implantation[3,5]
- Decreased endometrial receptivity because of the presence of *Chlamydia trachomatis* heat-shock proteins in hydrosalpinx fluid,[6,7] and also because of impaired endometrial and subendometrial blood flow among hydrosalpinx patients[8]
- Direct embryotoxic effect of hydrosalpingeal fluid either because of a common potent factor deleterious to embryo development or because of lack of essential substrates needed for embryo development.

Pregnancy, implantation, and delivery rates are reported to be approximately 50% lower and spontaneous abortion rates higher in the presence of hydrosalpinx.[9,10] Patients with hydrosalpinx visible on ultrasound are more significantly affected.[11,12]

SURGICAL INTERVENTION FOR HYDROSALPINX

Surgical treatment should be considered for all women with hydrosalpinx, prior to IVF treatment. The decision to repair or remove fallopian tubes is usually based on intraoperative assessment (Figs. 7A and B).

Intraoperative assessment can divide hydrosalpinx into either good prognosis for intrauterine pregnancy or poor prognosis for intrauterine pregnancy.

Good prognosis hydrosalpinx:[13]

- Limited filmy adnexal adhesions
- Mildly dilated tubes (<3 cm) with thin and pliable walls

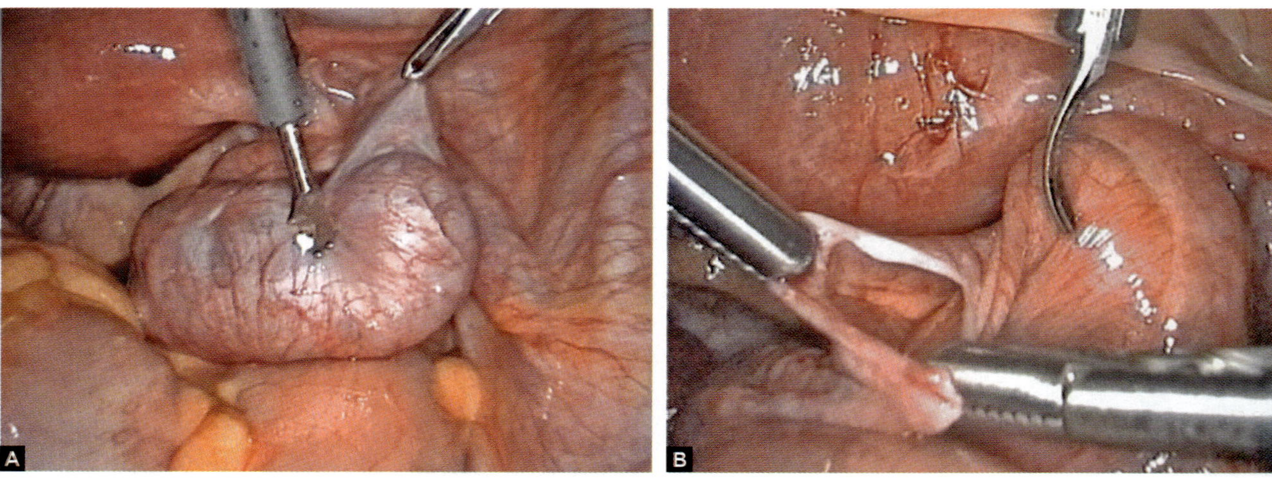

Figs. 7A and B: Surgical intervention for hydrosalpinx.

- Lush endosalpinx with preservation of the mucosal folds.

Poor prognosis hydrosalpinx:[13]

- Extensive dense peritubal adhesions
- Massively dilated tubes with thick fibrotic walls
- Sparse or absent luminal mucosa.

Neosalpingostomy

The good prognosis patients can be offered laparoscopic neosalpingostomy, which is carried out by opening a hydrosalpinx. The fimbria are then everted and secured to the tubal serosa with sutures or electrosurgery (Bruhat procedure). Neosalpingostomy is naturally the method of choice if the tube is suitable for reconstructive surgery. Tubes with more than half of the mucosa in a good condition have a fair chance of spontaneous conception (Fig. 8).[14]

Pregnancy outcomes after neosalpingostomy for mild hydrosalpinges are as follows:[15]

- Intrauterine pregnancy rates: 58–77%
- Ectopic pregnancy rates: 2–8%.

Laparoscopic Salpingectomy

Indications:[16]

- Poor prognosis hydrosalpinges
- When there is both proximal and distal occlusion
- When the fallopian tube is damaged beyond repair by infection, endometriosis, or ectopic pregnancy.

Rules for laparoscopic salpingectomy:

- Cautious use of electrocautery
- Resection very close to the actual tube to avoid damage to the medial tubal artery which also supplies the ovary
- Preferable to leave portion of adherent tube on the ovary rather than perform an excessively radical salpingectomy

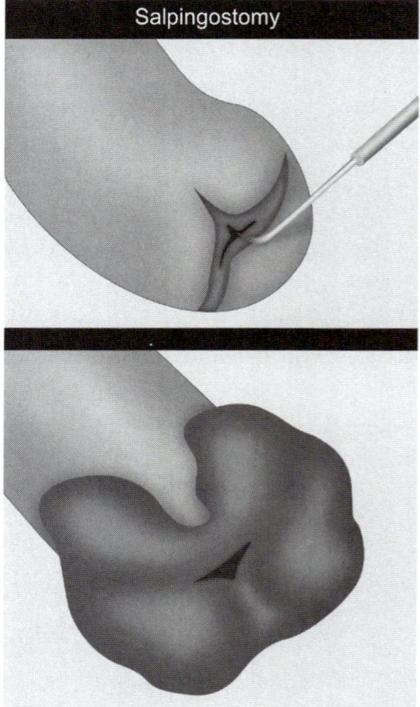

Fig. 8: Pregnancy outcomes after neosalpingostomy for mild hydrosalpinges.

- Resection not too close to the uterus because of the risk of dehiscence in the uterine wall and subsequent protrusion of the fetus.[17]

Randomized controlled trials (RCTs) report that salpingectomy restores the rates of pregnancy and live birth to levels similar to those of women without hydrosalpinx.[11,18,19] Salpingectomy of a unilateral hydrosalpinx increases the chance of spontaneous conception also.[20-22]

Patients should be counseled preoperatively for both salpingostomy as well as salpingectomy, so that the most appropriate procedure can be performed based on the extent of tubal disease. Even if a patient is scheduled for a laparoscopic salpingectomy, it is necessary to open the distally occluded tube for evaluation of the mucosa before a final decision of salpingectomy is taken. If it is appropriate to perform a salpingostomy, time for spontaneous conception should be given instead of immediate IVF.

Proximal Tubal Ligation with Distal Fenestration

This procedure is considered an alternative to laparoscopic salpingectomy in patients with extensive pelvic adhesions where salpingectomy is technically difficult.[23] For proximal tubal occlusion, mechanical clips are the preferred method.[16]

Hysteroscopic Proximal Tubal Occlusion

Hysteroscopic proximal tubal occlusion with Essure coil inserts or Adiana device can be an option in patients, where laparoscopy is contraindicated, such as in frozen pelvis. One RCT concluded that hysteroscopic proximal tubal occlusion by intratubal device is inferior to laparoscopic salpingectomy in the treatment of hydrosalpinges with respect to ongoing pregnancy rates.[24] The trailing coils of Essure device within the endometrial cavity may act as intrauterine contraceptive device, limiting embryo implantation. Adiana, a device for hysteroscopic proximal tubal occlusion, uses radiofrequency energy to stimulate interstitial scarring, followed by insertion of a small silicone elastomer matrix. The theoretical advantage of Adiana is the ability to maintain a uterine cavity free of any foreign matter.[25]

Aspiration of Hydrosalpinx

Ultrasound-guided aspiration of hydrosalpinx at the time of oocyte retrieval[26-28] leads to rapid reaccumulation of fluid by the time of transfer in many cases, which most likely compromises any beneficial effect of drainage.[29]

SUMMARY AND CONCLUSION

- In patients with severe tubal disease presenting as a hydrosalpinx on ultrasound and with a destroyed mucosa upon endoscopic inspection, IVF is the method of choice
- In the cases of extensive adhesions, rendering the salpingectomy is difficult, and bearing a risk of complications, proximal ligation, and distal fenestration is the preferred method
- Psychological aspects of removing or interrupting the tubes are very important and always have to be considered
- Patients with a preserved mucosa in the hydrosalpinx may have a good chance of spontaneous conception, if salpingostomy is performed
- In the presence of a unilateral hydrosalpinx and a contralateral healthy tube, a unilateral salpingectomy can be recommended, followed by sufficient time to await spontaneous conception, before proceeding to IVF.

REFERENCES

1. Practice Committee of the American Society for Reproductive Medicine. Salpingectomy for hydrosalpinx prior to in vitro fertilization. Fertil Steril. 2008;90:S66-8.
2. Mansour RT, Aboulghar MA, Serrour GI, et al. Fluid accumulation of the uterine cavity before embryo transfer: a possible hindrance for implantation. J In Vitro Fert Embryo Transf. 1991;8:157-9.
3. Andersen AN, Lindhard A, Loft A, et al. The infertile patient with hydrosalpinges—IVF with or without salpingectomy? Hum Reprod. 1996;11:2081-4.
4. Bloeche M, Schreiner T, Lisse K. Recurrence of hydrosalpinges after transvaginal aspiration of tubal fluid in an IVF cycle with development of serometra. Hum Reprod. 1997;12:703-5.
5. Sharara FI. The role of hydrosalpinx in IVF: simply mechanical? Hum Reprod. 1999;14:577-8.
6. Spandorfer SD, Neuer A, LaVerda D, et al. Previously undetected Chlamydia trachomatis infection, immunity to heat shock proteins and tubal occlusion in women undergoing in-vitro fertilization. Hum Reprod. 1999;14:60-4.
7. Ajonuma LC, Ng EH, Chan HC. New insights into the mechanisms underlying hydrosalpinx fluid formation and its adverse effect on IVF outcome. Hum Reprod Update. 2002;8:255-64.
8. Ng EH, Chan CC, Tang OS, et al. Comparison of endometrial and subendometrial blood flows among patients with and without hydrosalpinx shown on scanning during in vitro fertilization treatment. Fertil Steril. 2006;85:333-8.
9. Zeyneloglu HB, Arici A, Olive D. Adverse effects of hydrosalpinx on pregnancy rates after in vitro fertilization-embryo transfer. Fertil Steril. 1998;70:492-9.
10. Camus E, Poncelet C, Goffinet F, et al. Pregnancy rates after in-vitro fertilization in cases of tubal infertility with and without hydrosalpinx: a meta-analysis of published comparative studies. Hum Reprod. 1999;14:1243-9.
11. Strandell A, Lindhard A, Waldenstrom U, et al. Hydrosalpinx and IVF outcome: a prospective, randomized multicentre trial in Scandinavia on salpingectomy prior to IVF. Hum Reprod. 1999;14:2762-9.
12. de Wit W, Gowrising CJ, Kuik DJ, et al. Only hydrosalpinges visible on ultrasound are associated with reduced implantation and pregnancy rates after in-vitro fertilization. Hum Reprod. 1998;13:1696-701.

13. American Fertility Society. The American Fertility Society classifications of adnexal adhesions, distal tubal occlusion, tubal occlusion secondary to tubal ligation, tubal pregnancies, Mullerian anomalies and intrauterine adhesions. Fertil Steril. 1988;49:944-55.
14. Vasquez G, Boeckx W, Brosens I. Prospective study of tubal mucosal lesions and fertility in hydrosalpinges. Hum Reprod. 1995;10:1075-8.
15. Nackley AC, Muasher SJ. The significance of hydrosalpinx in in vitro fertilization. Fertil Steril. 1998;69:373-84.
16. Practice Committee of the American Society for Reproductive Medicine. Role of tubal surgery in the era of assisted reproductive technology. Fertil Steril. 2012;97:S39-45.
17. Inovay J, Marton T, Urbancsek J, et al. Spontaneous bilateral cornual uterine dehiscence early in the second trimester after bilateral laparoscopic salpingectomy and in-vitro fertilization. Hum Reprod. 1999;14:2471-3.
18. Dechaud H, Daures JP, Arnal F, et al. Does previous salpingectomy improve implantation and pregnancy rates in patients with severe tubal factor infertility who are undergoing in vitro fertilization? A pilot prospective randomized study. Fertil Steril. 1998;69:1020-5.
19. Kontoravdis A, Makrakis E, Pantos K, et al. Proximal tubal occlusion and salpingectomy result in similar improvement in in vitro fertilization outcome in patients with hydrosalpinx. Fertil Steril. 2006;86:1642-9.
20. Choe J, Check JH. Salpingectomy for unilateral hydrosalpinx may improve in vivo fecundity. Gynecol Obstet Invest. 1999;48:285-7.
21. Kiefer DG, Check JH. Salpingectomy improves outcome in the presence of a unilateral hydrosalpinx in a donor oocyte recipient: a case report. Clin Exp Obstet Gynecol. 2001;28:71-2.
22. Aboulghar MA, Mansour RT, Serour GI. Spontaneous intrauterine pregnancy following salpingectomy for a unilateral hydrosalpinx. Hum Reprod. 2000;17:1099-100.
23. Johnson N, van VS, Sowter MC, et al. Surgical treatment for tubal disease in women due to undergo in vitro fertilisation. Cochrane Database Syst Rev. 2010;1:CD002125.
24. Dreyer K, Lier MCI, Emanuel MH, et al. Hysteroscopic proximal tubal occlusion versus laparoscopic salpingectomy as a treatment for hydrosalpinges prior to IVF or ICSI: an RCT. Hum Reprod. 2016;31:2005-16.
25. Legendre G, Gallot V, Levaillant JM, et al. Adiana hysteroscopic tubal occlusion device for the treatment of hydrosalpinx prior to in vitro fertilization: a case report. J Gynecol Obstet Biol Reprod (Paris). 2013;42(4):401-4.
26. Sowter MC, Akande VA, Williams JA, et al. Is the outcome of in-vitro fertilization and embryo transfer treatment improved by spontaneous or surgical drainage of a hydrosalpinx? Hum Reprod. 1997;12:2147-50.
27. Van Voorhis BJ, Sparks AE, Syrop CH, et al. Ultrasound-guided aspiration of hydrosalpinges is associated with improved pregnancy and implantation rates after in-vitro fertilization cycles. Hum Reprod. 1998;13:736-9.
28. Hammadieh N, Coomarasamy A, Ola B, et al. Ultrasound-guided hydrosalpinx aspiration during oocyte collection improves pregnancy outcome in IVF: a randomized controlled trial. Hum Reprod. 2008;23:1113-7.
29. Sharar FI, McClamrock HD. Endometrial fluid collection in women with hydrosalpinx after human chorionic gonadotrophin administration: a report of two cases and implications for management. Hum Reprod. 1997;12:2816-9.

CHAPTER

75

A Silent Disease: Pelvic Inflammatory Disease and its Consequences

Nameeta Mokashi Bhalerao

INTRODUCTION

The term pelvic inflammatory disease (PID) usually refers to infection that ascends from the cervix or vagina to involve the upper genital tract involving the uterine cavity, fallopian tubes, and/or ovaries.[1] PID comprises a spectrum of inflammatory disorders of upper female genital tract, including any combination of endometritis, salpingitis, tubo-ovarian abscess, and pelvic peritonitis.

The most common cause of PID in 60–75% cases is sexually transmitted diseases (STD).[2] Intrauterine infection can be primary (spontaneously occurring and usually sexually transmitted) or secondary to postabortal and postdelivery (puerperal) events such as sepsis, invasive intrauterine surgical procedures [e.g. dilatation and curettage, termination of pregnancy, insertion of an intrauterine device (IUD), or hysterosalpingography].[1]

Infection can extend beyond the reproductive tract to cause pelvic peritonitis, generalized peritonitis, perihepatitis, perisplenitis, or pelvic abscess.[1] Rarely, in young women, infection not related to STD extends secondarily to the pelvic genital organs.[1] These secondary sources are:

- From adjacent foci of inflammation (e.g. appendicitis, regional ileitis, or diverticulitis)
- As a result of hematogenous dissemination (e.g. tuberculosis)
- As a complication of certain tropical diseases (e.g. schistosomiasis).

NATURAL BARRIERS TO PELVIC INFLAMMATORY DISEASE

Normally, several natural barriers to the ascent of pathogenic organisms from the vagina to the fallopian tubes exist. Intact hymen prevents ascending infection. When a virgin girl presents with PID, it is usually tubercular in nature. The acidity of the vaginal secretion inhibits the growth of bacteria; the cervical canal has relatively small lumen and is normally filled with a plug of alkaline mucus. The ciliary movement of endometrial lining in the uterus and the cervical canal is directed downward and discourages the upward spread of nonmotile organisms to the cavity of the uterus.[3]

VULNERABILITY TO PELVIC INFLAMMATORY DISEASE

The natural protective mechanism is impaired during menstruation, after abortion, and delivery, because the cervical canal becomes dilated, the protecting epithelium of the endometrium is shed and raw surfaces are present in the cavity of the uterus. The vaginal pH is increased, rendering the genital tract more vulnerable to infection. In addition to these factors, intrauterine manipulations such as curettage for evacuation in abortion and manual removal of placenta favor entry and spread of pathogenic organisms. Intrauterine contraceptive device (IUCD) is also a source of infection, particularly when it is not introduced under aseptic conditions or introduced in the presence of vaginal infection.[3]

Risk Factors for Pelvic Inflammatory Disease

The risk factors include presence of endocervical infection or bacterial vaginosis, a history of salpingitis or of recent vaginal douching and the use of an IUD (especially among nulliparous women, during the first few months after IUD insertion and among women with multiple sex partners). Certain other iatrogenic factors, such as dilatation and curettage or cesarean section can increase the risk of PID, especially among women with endocervical gonococcal or chlamydial infection or bacterial vaginosis.

Pelvic inflammatory disease is a disease of young women, who are sexually and reproductively active. The increased promiscuity and frequent change of sex partners are mainly responsible for PID in developed countries, so much so that almost 75% of PID are sexually transmitted. Septic abortions and puerperal sepsis are the important etiological factors in developing countries.[3,4]

In developing countries, home deliveries by untrained midwives, criminal abortions leading to postabortal and puerperal sepsis cause PID.

Minor surgical procedures such as curettage and hysterosalpingography can cause ascending infection. Manual removal of placenta and evacuation of products of conception are important sources of infection.

Tuberculosis is blood-borne mostly, rarely ascending. Pelvic peritonitis due to appendicitis and diverticulitis may spread to involve fallopian tube.

Westrom (1975) reported that women with one previous attack of PID are predisposed to another attack in 12% of the cases; two attacks of PID increase the risk to 35%, and three attacks to as much as 75%.[5]

ETIOLOGY OF PELVIC INFLAMMATORY DISEASE

The agents most often implicated in acute PID include the primary causes of endocervicitis (e.g. *Neisseria gonorrhoeae* and *Chlamydia trachomatis*)[6] and organisms that can be regarded as components of an altered vaginal flora.[1,6] In general, PID is most often caused by *N. gonorrhoeae* where there is a high incidence of gonorrhea, e.g. in developing countries.[1,7]

The microenvironment changes produced by bacterial vaginosis (BV) may aid ascension of the causative organisms of PID.[8] However, Ness and colleagues have shown that bacterial vaginosis is not a risk factor for PID development.[9,10]

In recent studies, *Mycoplasma genitalium* has also been associated with histopathologic diagnoses of endometritis and with salpingitis.[1,9]

Anaerobic and facultative organisms (especially *Prevotella* species, Peptostreptococci, *Escherichia coli*, *Haemophilus influenzae*, and Group B streptococci) as well as genital mycoplasmas have been isolated from the peritoneal fluid or fallopian tubes in a varying proportion.[11] The infection by anaerobic organisms is greatly favored by blood loss, anemia, and tissue damage.

PATHOLOGY AND THE RESULTING CONSEQUENCES OF PELVIC INFLAMMATORY DISEASE

Acute Pelvic Inflammatory Disease

The spectrum of acute PID ranges from mild-to-moderate to severe. Depending upon the severity of tubal damage, Gainesville has described five stages of PID (Table 1).[3]

The salpingitis component of acute PID can either be exosalpingitis (infection of the exterior surface of the tube) or endosalpingitis (infection of the interior mucosa of the fallopian tubes).

Exosalpingitis

The fallopian tube is swollen, edematous, and congested or hyperemic with dilated vessels on the serosal surface. Serous exudation is usually seen around the tube. Seropurulent discharge from the fimbrial end is the strongest feature in favor of salpingitis. Peritoneal surface may be congested in the pelvis.[3]

Endosalpingitis

In ascending infection, the mucosa is the first one to be affected.[3] The mucous membrane inflammation with edema, redness, and deciliation takes place in the initial stage of salpingitis. Submucosa is infiltrated with leukocytes and plasma cells. The inflammatory exudates are discharged into the lumen. Possible breach/ulceration of mucosal surface leads to adhesions between mucosal folds of the tube. This leads to narrowing and finally blockage of the tube resulting in infertility or ectopic pregnancy. In later stages, the inflammation extends to the serosal surface.[12] Depending upon the severity of tubal damage, five stages of PID have been described (Table 1).

In early part of this inflammatory process, fimbrial end remains open, and allows the seropurulent secretions to be discharged into the peritoneal cavity. The collection of this pus may lead to creation of a pelvic abscess. In later stages of the disease, fimbria get adherent to each other by

Table 1: Five stages of pelvic inflammatory disease (PID).

Stage	*Involvement*
I	Acute salpingitis without peritonitis—no adhesions
II	Acute salpingitis with peritonitis—purulent discharge
III	Acute salpingitis with superimposed tubal occlusion or tubo-ovarian complex
IV	Ruptured tubo-ovarian abscess
V	Tubercular salpingitis

fibrinous adhesions and fimbriae are drawn into the tube leading to closure of fimbrial opening.[9] With continuous secretion of such exudates the ampullary portion of the tube is distended. The formation of retort shape pyosalpinx follows. Once the ovaries are involved with tube, a tubo-ovarian mass (TOM) is formed where both tube and ovary are entangled in adhesions. The pyosalpinx or TOM becomes adherent to posterior surface of the uterus or broad ligament involving ovaries, sigmoid colon, and loops of small intestine. Tubal wall appears thickened and tense. In advanced stages and in untreated cases of PID, pelvic and general peritonitis may occur associated with paralytic ileus and rarely subdiaphragmatic and/or perinephric abscess and even septicemia. Septic thrombophlebitis, bacteremia, and metastatic abscess are rare today, because of prompt and effective antibiotic therapy.[3]

In PID following postabortal and puerperal infection, the pathogenesis is different. The infection spreads through the cervix via lymphatics to the cellular tissue in the broad ligament, causing cellulitis. The fallopian tube is affected from the outside and the mucosal as to fall. The wall of the tube is thickened considerably with hardly any distension of the lumen. Eventual involvement of mucosa ends up in blockage of the fallopian tube by multiple adhesions.[3]

Subacute PID results from inadequate treatment or from reinfection by the infected partner, if it has been sexually transmitted. Tuberculosis also manifests in the form of recurrent pelvic infection due to secondary infection.[3]

Usually, infection through cervix and endometrium causes endosalpingitis affecting inner lumen of tube and fimbriae, leading to hydrosalpinx. In some women, after abortion or vaginal delivery, infection through cervix spreads via lymphatics to parametrium and broad ligament causing parametritis.

This reaches the outer aspect of tube to cause exosalpingitis.

Chronic Pelvic Inflammatory Disease

This form of disease is the continuation of the acute form, if the infection fails to resolve completely due to inadequate antibiotic treatment or reinfection. This may result in TOM formation which may present as:

- Hydrosalpinx
- Chronic pyosalpinx
- Tubo-ovarian mass
- Chronic interstitial salpingitis.

Hydrosalpinx

If a pyosalpinx or TOM responds to antibiotics, the pus contained therein becomes sterile within 6 weeks of the initial attack, but the damage to the tube remains as chronic pyosalpinx or hydrosalpinx.

A hydrosalpinx represents the end result of a previous acute salpingitis, and is often bilateral. It is retort shaped due to enormous dilatation of the ampullary region filled with clear fluid. Fimbrial end is closed and fimbriae are drawn into the tube. The interstitial end is patent as seen by the dye visualized in the lumen during hysterosalpingogram. Outer surface appears smooth, wall is thin and translucent. Commonly, it is adherent to surrounding structures. Occasionally, if it is mobile, it may undergo torsion causing acute pain in abdomen. Histology reveals flattening of the tubal plicae and exfoliation of the lining epithelium.[2,3]

Chronic Pyosalpinx

A chronic pyosalpinx is thick walled and surrounded by dense adhesions and filled with pus. The inner wall is replaced by a granulation tissue. Usually, it is fixed to the pouch of Douglas (POD), posterior surface of the broad ligament or uterus by dense adhesions.

Tubo-ovarian Mass

In this condition, the inflamed tube and ovary are matted together to form a mass, which may lead to an ovarian abscess.

Chronic Interstitial Salpingitis

The wall of fallopian tube is thickened and fibrotic, but there is no dilatation of tube due to pus or fluid. Involvement of the ovary in adhesions results in chronic salpingo-oophoritis. Usually, adhesions are present in the pelvis.

CLINICAL MANIFESTATIONS OF PELVIC INFLAMMATORY DISEASE

Symptoms of *N. gonorrhoeae*-associated and *C. trachomatis*-associated PID often begin during or soon after the menstrual period; this timing suggests that menstruation is a risk factor for ascending infection from the cervix and vagina.[6] Experimental inoculation of the fallopian tubes of lower primates has shown that repeated exposure to *C. trachomatis* leads to the greatest degree of tissue inflammation and damage; thus, immunopathology probably contributes to the pathogenesis of chlamydial salpingitis. Women using oral contraceptives appear to be at a decreased risk of symptomatic PID and tubal sterilization reduces the risk of salpingitis by preventing intraluminal spread of infection into the tubes.[1]

Acute Pelvic Inflammatory Disease

Symptoms[1-3,9]

- The most common symptom is acute lower abdominal pain which is difficult to pinpoint. In peritonitis, pain spreads to upper abdomen.
- High temperature and vomiting may be present.
- In STD cases, dyspareunia and vaginal discharge may accompany.
- Endometritis and pelvic congestion causes menstrual problems such as intermenstrual bleeding or menorrhagia.
- Rectal irritation by pelvic abscess may cause diarrhea.
- Associated urinary tract infection produces increased frequency of micturition and dysuria.

Signs[1-3,9]

- Patient may appear ill with fever ranging between 38°C and 40°C
- Tachycardia and tachypnea may accompany
- Dehydration with tongue being dry and coated
- Abdominal examination may reveal distension, tenderness—direct or rebound, and rigidity. A tender fixed mass arising from pelvis may be palpable as tenderness reduces.
- *On speculum examination*: Purulent discharge from cervical canal or a torn cervix as in criminal abortion may be observed.
- *Bimanual pelvic examination* may reveal tender fornices and cervical movements, tender pelvic mass with restricted mobility, fluctuating tender swelling in POD in abscesses.

There being wide variations in symptoms and signs of acute PID difficulties in the diagnosis, may be faced. Subtle or mild symptoms may contribute to delay in diagnosis and therapy predisposing to late sequelae such as infertility, ectopic pregnancy, and chronic pelvic pain.

Differential diagnosis[1-3]and the various differentiating points include:

- *Acute appendicitis*
  - Pain is central/periumbilical/radiating to right iliac fossa
  - Vomiting is severe but temperature is not so high
  - Lower margin of appendicular mass can be reached (not in PID)
  - Absence of vaginal discharge or menstrual irregularities.
- *Ectopic pregnancy*
  - Irregular uterine bleed and pain.
- *Diverticulitis*:
  - Usually after age 50 (PID disease of young and sexually active)
  - Signs more on left iliac fossa.
- *Twisted ovarian cyst/paraovarian cyst*: Pain and vomiting with minimal pyrexia
  - No menstrual symptoms or leukorrhea.
- *Ruptured endometriotic cyst*:
  - History of dysmenorrhea, menorrhagia, and pelvic pain.
- *Afebrile* and no vaginal discharge
- *Septic abortion*: Amenorrhea and abdominal pain are present
- Cholecystitis
- Degenerated fibroids.

Chronic Pelvic Inflammatory Disease

Symptoms[1-3,9]

- The overall health is debilitated and exhausted.
- Constant lower abdominal pain which worsens prior to and during menstruation
- Lower backache and dyspareunia due to pelvic adhesions/mass in POD
- Vaginal discharge due to cervicitis
- Menstrual problems such as menorrhagia, polymenorrhagia, and congestive dysmenorrhea may occur due to pelvic congestion
- Infertility due to blocked tubes/pelvic adhesions
- Rectal irritation and diarrhea in cases of pelvic abscesses.

Signs

- Cervical discharge with tender cervical movements.
- *Adnexa and fornices*: Tender, thickened and fixed
- *Uterus*: Retroverted and fixed
- *Frozen pelvis*: Difficult to define uterus separately from adnexa.

Differential Diagnosis[1-3]

- *Ectopic gestation*: Pregnancy test, ultrasound, laparoscopy to differentiate
- *Uterine fibroids*: Irregular enlarged uterus, no fixity or tenderness
- *Pelvic endometriosis*: Ultrasound or laparoscopy to confirm
- *Ovarian tumor*: No menstrual problems or tenderness.

Fine needle aspiration cytology (FNAC) and ultrasound to confirm:

- Tubercular TOM PCR, histology, culture, and laparoscopy to confirm.

INVESTIGATIONS

Clinical diagnosis is accurate in only 65–70% cases and specific investigations are required to confirm the diagnosis and identify the offending organism.[3]

- Blood-hemoglobin (Hb), packed cell volume (PCV), total leukocyte count (TLC), differential leukocyte count (DLC), erythrocyte sedimentation rate (ESR), C-reactive protein, renal function tests, and serum electrolytes.
- *Wet smear microscopy*: Cervical, high vaginal, and urethral swab
  - For aerobic and anaerobic organisms and gonorrhea.
- *For chlamydial infection:*
  - Along wire swab tipped with calcium alginate is used to collect the specimen and inoculated on cycloheximide treated McCoy cells for culture
  - Serological microfluorescence test for IgM and IgG antibodies
  - Polymerase chain reaction (PCR) staining.
- Blood culture for septicemia
- *Culdocentesis*: To rule out ectopic pregnancy and diagnose pelvic abscess
- Laparoscopy
- *C-reactive protein*: An acute phase reactant distinguishes infective from noninfective mass
- *Ultrasound, computed tomography, and MRI*: To diagnose hydrosalpinx
- TOM or abscess in pelvis.[1,9,13]
- MRI of the tube scan also show increased tubal diameter, intratubal fluid, or tubal wall thickening in case of salpingitis.[1]
- *Testing for human immunodeficiency virus (HIV) and other STD*: Of sexual partner.

TREATMENT

The 2006 Centers for Disease Control and Prevention (CDC) guidelines recommend initiation of empirical treatment for PID in sexually active young women and other women at risk for PID if they are experiencing pelvic or lower abdominal pain, if no other cause for the pain can be identified and if pelvic examination reveals one or more of the criteria of cervical motion tenderness, uterine tenderness, and adnexal tenderness.[1] Box 1 illustrates the diagnostic criteria for PID. Box 2 illustrates the recommendations for antibiotic treatment of PID.

Women with suspected PID can be treated as either outpatients or inpatients.

Box 1: CDC diagnostic criteria for PID.[14]

PID should be suspected and treatment initiated if:
Patient is at risk of PID and patient has uterine, adnexal, or cervical motion tenderness with no other apparent cause
Findings that support the diagnosis
Cervical or vaginal mucopurulent (green or yellow) discharge, elevated erythrocyte sedimentation rate, or C-reactive protein, laboratory confirmation of gonorrheal or chlamydial infection, oral temperature of 101°F (38°C) or greater
White blood cells on vaginal secretion saline wet mount
Most specific criteria for the diagnosis
Endometritis on endometrial biopsy
Laparoscopic abnormalities consistent with PID
Thickened, fluid-filled tubes apparent on transvaginal ultrasound or magnetic resonance imaging

(CDC: Centers for Disease Control and Prevention; PID: pelvic inflammatory disease)
Source: Centers for Disease Control and Prevention. Sexually transmitted diseases treatment guidelines 2002.

Box 2: CDC recommendations for antibiotic treatment of PID.[14]

Parenteral regimen:*
Cefotetan (Cefotan) 2 g IV every 12 hours or cefoxitin (Mefoxin) 2 g IV every 6 hours†; plus doxycycline (Vibramycin) 100 mg orally or IV every 12 hours‡
Alternatives:
- Clindamycin (Cleocin) 900 mg IV every 8 hours§; plus gentamicin loading dose IV or IM (2 mg per kg) followed by a maintenance dose (1.5 mg per kg) every 8 hours (single daily dosing may be substituted)
- Ofloxacin (Floxin) 400 mg IV every 12 hours or levofloxacin (Levaquin) 500 mg IV once daily; with or without metronidazole (Flagyl) 500 mg IV every 8 hours Ampicillin/subactam (Unasyn) 3 g IV every 6 hours; plus doxycycline 100 mg orally or IV every 12 hours

Oral regimen
Ofloxacin 400 mg orally twice daily for 14 days or levofloxacin 500 mg orally once daily for 14 days‖; with or without metronidazole 500 mg orally twice daily for 14 days
Alternative:
Ceftriaxone (Rocephin) 250 mg IM in a single dose or cefoxitin 2 g IM in a single dose with concurrent probenecid (Benemid) 1 g orally in single dose or other parenteral third-generation cephalosporin; plus doxycycline 100 mg orally twice daily for 14 days with or without metronidazole 500 mg orally twice daily for 14 days

* Parenteral therapy generally can be discontinued 24 hours after clinical improvement.
† Cefotetan and cefoxitin have greater anaerobic activity than other third-generation cephalosporins.
‡ Doxycycline should be given orally whenever possible because of pain with infusion. Doxycycline 100 mg orally twice daily should be continued to complete 14 days of therapy. If tubo-ovarian abscess is present, the addition of clindamycin or metronidazole for continued therapy should be considered.
§ Continued oral therapy may consist of clindamycin 450 mg four times daily or doxycycline 100 mg twice daily.
‖ Consider possibility of fluoroquinolone-resistant *Neisseria gonorrhoeae*.
(CDC: Centers for Disease Control and Prevention; IM: intramuscular; IV: intravenous; PID: pelvic inflammatory disease)
Source: Centers for Disease Control and Prevention. Sexually transmitted diseases treatment guidelines 2002.

Indications of Hospitalization or Inpatient Care[1]

- Diagnosis is uncertain and surgical emergencies such as appendicitis and ectopic pregnancy cannot be excluded.
- The patient is pregnant.
- Pelvic abscess is suspected.
- Severe illness or nausea and vomiting preclude outpatient management.
- Patient has HIV infection.
- The patient is assessed as unable to follow or tolerate an outpatient regimen, or
- The patient has failed to respond to outpatient therapy.
- Some experts also prefer to hospitalize adolescents with PID for initial therapy.

Surgical Treatment of Pelvic Inflammatory Disease

Failure of medical therapy suggests the need for surgical exploration and drainage of abscess.[15]

- Drainage of pelvic abscess by colpotomy or colpocentesis.
- Dilatation and evacuation of septic products of conception.
- *Laparotomy:*
  - To drain peritoneal pus
  - To correct intestinal obstruction
  - In ruptured and twisted TO masses or abscesses
- *Laparoscopy to drain TO abscess:*
  - Size of abscess is less than 10 cm.
  - No response to antibiotic treatment in 42–72 hours
  - Abscess ruptures
  - Pyoperitoneum
- Ultrasound-guided abscess aspiration can be done vaginally, but success is limited.

LONG-TERM COMPLICATIONS

Although mortality has come down considerably in recent years with effective antibiotics, PID remains the source of considerable morbidity in the form of chronic pelvic pain, menorrhagia, ectopic pregnancy, and infertility, which would in turn require further surgical procedures, both investigatory and therapeutic. Other symptoms are backache, dyspareunia, vaginal discharge, and recurrent PID.

In advanced stages and in untreated cases of PID, pelvic and general peritonitis may occur associated with paralytic ileus and rarely subdiaphragmatic and/or perinephric abscess and even septicemia. Septic thrombophlebitis, bacteremia, and metastatic abscess are rare today, because of prompt and effective antibiotic therapy.[3]

Apart from endometriosis, PID is said to be the most important etiology of nonsurgical adhesions in women and intra-abdominal adhesions is an important contributor of infertility and dyspareunia.[16]

It has been stated that despite adequate treatment, 15% of patients fail to respond to chemotherapy, 20–25% have at least one recurrence, and 20% develop chronic pelvic pain. About 15% suffer from infertility and 8% of those who conceive will have an ectopic pregnancy.[3]

UNCOMMON COMPLICATIONS OF CHLAMYDIA AND GONORRHEA

Both these infections may spread into the abdominal cavity and cause periappendicitis and perihepatitis.

- *Fitz-Hugh-Curtis syndrome*: PID with perihepatitis has been known as Fitz-Hugh-Curtis syndrome. These women present with right hypochondrial pain, tenderness, and hyperpyrexia. Can be confused with cholecystitis. On laparoscopy, fine violin string adhesions are seen between the liver capsule and visceral peritoneum. For many years, it was specifically attributed to gonococcal salpingitis, most cases are now attributed to chlamydial salpingitis.[1]
- *Sexually acquired reactive arthritis (SARA)*: Occurs due to dissemination of *Chlamydia* to joints. Seen in less than 1% of PID women.[2] There is usually an asymmetrical oligoarthritis, affecting large joints of the lower limb.[3]
- *Reiter's syndrome*: In this condition, chlamydial arthritis is accompanied by uveitis and a rash which if florid, may be similar to psoriasis.
- *Gonococcal arthritis*: Disseminated gonococcal infection occurs rarely and presents as a septic oligoarthritis, usually affecting the small joints of the hand or wrist, with a scanty popular rash.

REFERENCES

1. Holmes KK. Sexually transmitted infections: Overview and clinical approach. In: Fauci AS, Kasper DL, Longo DL, et al (Eds). Harrison's Principles of Internal Medicine, 17th edition. USA: McGraw Hill; 2008. pp. 821-35.
2. Sharma S, Kumar P. Pelvic inflammatory disease. In: Arul Kumaran S, Sivanesaratnam V, Chatterjee A (Eds). Essentials of Gynaecology, 2nd edition. New Delhi: Jaypee Brothers Medical Publishers; 2010. pp. 121-8.
3. Padubidri VG, Daftary SN (Eds). Pelvic inflammatory disease. In: Howkins and Bourne Shaw's Textbook of Gynaecology, 16th edition; New Delhi: Elsevier; 2015; pp. 177-86.
4. Cunnigham FG, Leveno KJ, Bloom SL (Eds). Sexually transmitted infections. In: Williams Obstetrics, 24th edition. New York: McGraw Hill Education; 2014.

5. Westrom L. Effect of acute pelvic inflammatory disease on fertility. Am J Obstet Gynecol. 1975;121:707.
6. Schachter J, Stephens R. Infections caused by *Chlamydia trachomatis*. In: Morse S, Ballard RC, Holmes KK, et al. (Eds). Atlas of Sexually Transmitted Diseases, 3rd edition. Edinburgh: Mosby; 2003. p. 80.
7. Soper DE, Brockwell NJ, Dalton HP, et al. Observations concerning the microbial etiology of acute salpingitis. Am J Obstet Gynecol. 1994;170:1008-17.
8. Soper DE. Pelvic inflammatory disease. Obstet Gynecol. 2010;116(2Pt1):419.
9. Hoffman BL, Schorge JO, Bradshaw KD, et al (Eds). Gynecologic infection. In: Williams Textbook of Gynaecology, 3rd edition. McGraw Hill Education; 2016. pp. 50-85.
10. Ness RB, Hillier SL, Kip KE, et al. Bacterial vaginosis and risk of pelvic inflammatory disease. Obstet Gynecol. 2004;104:761.
11. Landers DV, Sweet RL. Tubo-ovarian abscess: Contemporary approach to management. Rev Infect Dis. 1983;5(5):876.
12. Patton DL, Moore DE, Spadoni LR, et al. A comparison of the fallopian tubes' response to overt and silent salpingitis. Obstet Gynecol. 1989;73:622.
13. Timor Tritsch IE, Lerner JP, Monteagudo A, et al. Transvaginal sonographic markers of tubal inflammatory disease. Ultrasound Obstet Gynecol. 1998;12(1):56.
14. Centers for Disease Control and Prevention. Sexually transmitted diseases treatment guidelines 2002. MMWR Recomm Rep. 2002;51(RR-6):1-78.
15. Reed SD, Landers DV, Sweet RL. Antibiotic treatment of tubo-ovarian abscesses: Comparison of broad spectrum beta lactum agents versus clindamycin-containing regimens. Am J Obstet Gynecol. 1991;164:1556-62.
16. Tabibian N, Swehli E, Boyd A. Abdominal adhesions: A practical review of an often overlooked entity. Ann Med Surg. 2017;15:9-13.

CHAPTER

76

The Patient with Congenital Uterine Anomalies

Nozer Sheriar, Rajneet Bhatia

INTRODUCTION

Though the uterus is vital for conception and a home to every fetus, however conceived, for 38 important weeks, the role of uterine factors in the etiology of infertility and reproductive wastage is often difficult to define. It is important to make a distinction between the failure to conceive, subsequent poor nidation, and early pregnancy wastage, when undertaking any in-depth assessment.[1]

Congenital uterine anomalies arise due to the disruption in the normal developmental process of the Müllerian ducts, which gives rise to the formation of the uterus, fallopian tubes, cervix, and proximal two-thirds of the vagina. The ovaries and distal one-third of the vagina originate from the primitive yolk sac and sinovaginal bud, respectively. Hence, patients with Müllerian duct anomalies (MDA) have normal external genitalia and ovarian function.

Most of the patients are asymptomatic or may present with dysmenorrhea and/or dyspareunia. There may be associated endometriosis and primary or secondary infertility. Patients who have conceived are more prone to miscarriages and ectopic gestation. Obstetrical complications include intrauterine growth restriction (IUGR), malpresentation, preterm labor, and increased rate of cesarean delivery. The above clinical presentations lead to the diagnosis of MDAs but imaging modalities help us in the confirmation of diagnosis and also with further management. Hysterosalpingography (HSG) along with 3D ultrasonography (USG) or magnetic resonance imaging (MRI) forms the preferred mode of imaging as the combination provides us with the details of the uterine cavity with tubal patency and external uterine contour.[2]

Accurate recognition of the anomaly subtype was recognized as very essential to be able to plan treatment accordingly and this led to the need for classifying MDAs. The most widely accepted is the classification proposed by the American Society for Reproductive Medicine (ASRM) which divides MDAs into seven different subtypes based on the anatomical variation. Correct identification of the anomaly followed by diagnostic with operative hysterolaparoscopy for correction of the anomaly may improve the reproductive potential of the patient.

The prevalence of associated renal anomalies with MDA is 30–50%, the most common one being unilateral renal agenesis. Other congenital malformations include anomalies of the axial skeletal system. Hence, a patient with MDA should also be screened for these anomalies.

With the advent of diagnostic and operative hysteroscopy in clinical practice, our approach to intrauterine abnormalities has undergone a radical change. This chapter addresses the diagnosis and management of congenital uterine abnormalities in a patient with infertility and reproductive wastage.

EMBRYOLOGY

The human uterus is of para-mesonephric origin, with any degree of failure of fusion of the Müllerian ducts or subsequent failure of resorption of the intervening tissue, resulting in a spectrum of clinical malformations. Incomplete Müllerian fusion results from partial or complete failure of the Müllerian ducts to fuse or canalize and leads to a variety of uterine and vaginal abnormalities—unicornuate uterus, arcuate uterus, septate uterus, bicornuate uterus, and didelphic uterus with or without a septate vagina.[3]

The first 8 weeks of the embryo is the ambisexual period of development in which both the Wolffian (mesonephric) and Müllerian (paramesonephric) ducts coexist. After this bipotent sexual phase, either the Wolffian or the Müllerian ducts persist while the other disappears up to 12th week of development. This process of sex determination of fetus is influenced mainly by Müllerian inhibiting substance (MIH) also known as the anti-Müllerian hormone (AMH) along with androgens and SRY protein. In the absence of the above factors, the fetus develops the uterus, fallopian tubes, and upper third of the vagina.[4]

The Wolffian ducts run on either side of the primitive gut as a longitudinal ridge covered by the coelomic epithelium. The Müllerian ducts run lateral to the Wolffian ducts but pass medially at its caudal end fusing to form a Y-shaped structure. By the 10th week of gestation, the Müllerian ducts fuse to form the fallopian tubes, uterus, and upper portion of the vagina. By the 22nd week of gestation, canalization to form the uterine cavity, cervical canal, and vagina is complete (Figs. 1 and 2).

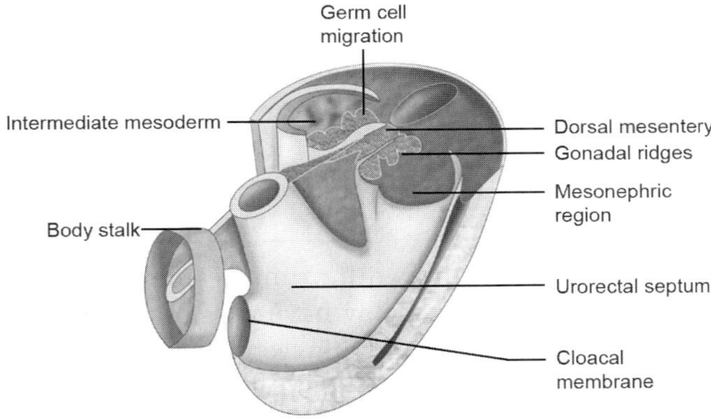

Fig. 1: The caudal half of the embryo (30–35 days).[3]

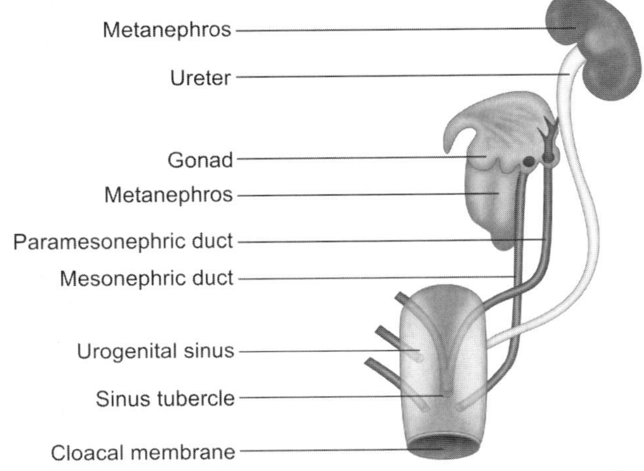

Fig. 2: The embryo with urogenital ducts (after 40 days).[3]

The following three phases lead to complete development of Müllerian ducts:

1. *Organogenesis*: Characterized by formation of both Müllerian ducts, failure of which results in uterine agenesis/hypoplasia or unicornuate uterus.
2. *Fusion*: Characterized by fusion of the ducts to form the uterus, failure of which results in bicornuate or didelphys uterus.
3. *Septal resorption*: Involves resorption of the central septum after ducts have been fused, failure of which results in septate or arcuate uterus.

Although the embryologic origin and mechanism of Müllerian abnormalities is understood, the cause is not. The role of genetic factors is suspected but unclear. Rare aggregates of incomplete uterine fusion have been reported in affected sisters, affected mother-daughter sets as also familial aggregates in which multiple members are affected.[5]

ETIOPATHOGENESIS

Various unknown factors affect either the organogenesis or fusion or resorption stages of embryological development resulting in congenital uterine anomalies.

The potential environmental factors are the endocrine disrupting chemicals, which are the natural and synthetic compounds found in the environment and these either simulate or antagonize the actions of endogenous hormones interfering with the normal functions of the endocrine system.

Differential expression of the *HOX* genes in the Müllerian duct governs the development of the uterus, fallopian tubes, and upper part of vagina. Exposure to various xenoestrogens alters *HOXA10* gene expression, disrupting the normal patterning of the Müllerian ducts leading to anomalies. The most common example to this is in utero exposure to diethylstilbestrol (DES) leading to T-shaped uterus.[6,7]

We also propose high maternal AMH may interfere with the normal development of the uterus leading to anomalies (Flowchart 1).

INCIDENCE

The overall incidence of uterine malformations in the general population is below 3%. This incidence is not significantly different in the infertile population (3.5%). Traditionally, uterine malformations did not seem to contribute directly to infertility nor interfere with conception in assisted reproduction. However, there is recent evidence of fertility compromise. It is now accepted that congenital uterine anomalies do contribute to delayed natural conception and are definitely associated with poor pregnancy outcomes

Flowchart 1: Endocrine disruptors influencing Müllerian development.

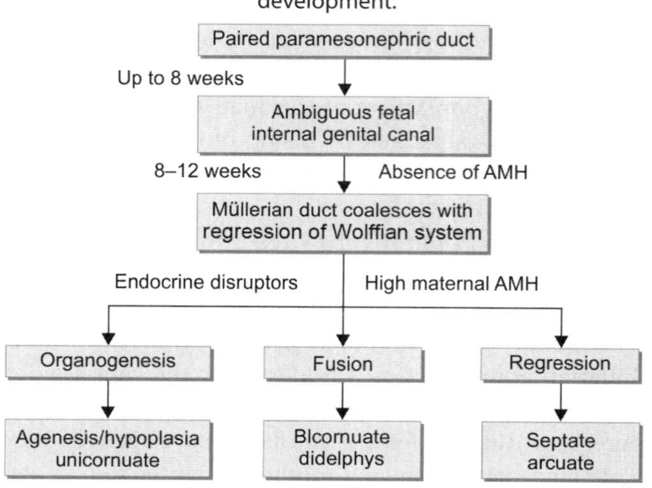

following conception. Hence, whenever diagnosed during infertility treatment, surgical correction may be considered and undertaken when warranted.

While the true incidence of uterine anomalies is difficult to ascertain as many of these conditions fail to present clinically, rates of incidence ranging from 0.1% to 2% have been reported in the general population, with significantly higher rates associated with infertility and reproductive wastage.[8]

A retrospective longitudinal study of 3,181 patients, which included fertile, infertile, and sterile patients, reported an overall frequency of uterine malformations as 4%. Infertile patients (6.3%) had a significantly higher incidence of Müllerian anomalies, in comparison with fertile (3.8%) and sterile (2.4%) women. Septate (33.6%) and arcuate (32.8%) uteri were the most common malformations observed.[9]

CLINICAL PRESENTATION

Patients with congenital uterine anomalies are generally asymptomatic but may present with amenorrhea, dysmenorrhea, or dyspareunia. Effect of these anomalies on reproduction includes infertility, ectopic pregnancy, recurrent pregnancy loss, IUGR, fetal malposition, and preterm delivery. These can be associated with decreased intraluminal volume, presence of medial wall or unfused uterine horn, inadequate vascularization, and greater uterine contractility and irritability.[10]

In a study of 176 patients with uterine malformations, Acien reported pregnancies resulting in a child surviving over 7 days in just 53% of women with malformations in contrast to 89% of women with a normal uterus. Uterine malformations were associated with a significantly higher spontaneous abortion rate (36%) and preterm delivery rate (18%) when compared with controls (8% and 6%, respectively). The poorest viability rates in this series were reported in the patients with septate (59%), arcuate (45%) and bicornuate uteri (40%).[11]

Patients with agenesis present with primary amenorrhea and dysmenorrhea. Unicornuate uterus may present with severe pelvic pain due to hematometra in cases associated with rudimentary, noncommunicating uterine horn with functional endometrium. Uterine septum is generally asymptomatic and only diagnosed during evaluation of women with recurrent pregnancy loss or infertility. It may present with pelvic pain if the menstrual flow is obstructed. Bicornuate or didelphys uterus mostly do not produce any symptoms. The reproductive outcome for patients with MDA is shown in Table 1.

Table 1: Reproductive outcome in patients with congenital uterine anomalies.[10]

Uterine anomaly	*Miscarriages (%)*	*Premature deliveries (%)*	*Fetus survival (%)*
Unicornuate	43.8	25	43.7
Bicornuate	40	–	62
Didelphys	35	19	60
Septate	Over 60	–	6–28

DIAGNOSIS

The patient presenting with primary amenorrhea or recurrent miscarriages may have associated uterine anomalies which need to be investigated further. The combination of various imaging modalities helps us to reach a final diagnosis.

Hysterosalpingography is the traditional method which helps in assessment of the cervical canal, uterine cavity, and fallopian tubes. It allows accurate evaluation of tubal patency and helps in diagnosing intrauterine conditions like septa and synechiae, but is limited in visualizing the external uterine contour. The specificity of HSG varies from 6% to 60% depending upon the type of anomaly present and the skill of the person performing the test (Figs. 3 and 4).

Sonohysterosalpingography is performed in the mid proliferative phase of the cycle (D6-D10 after the menstruation stops). Saline is injected through a catheter placed in the cervix and scanning is done to assess the distended cavity with passage of saline from the fallopian tubes. HyCoSy is the contrast hysterosalpingography in which positive contrast media (SonoVue) is used, and the fallopian tubes along with the uterine cavity are well delineated even on B mode scanning.[12]

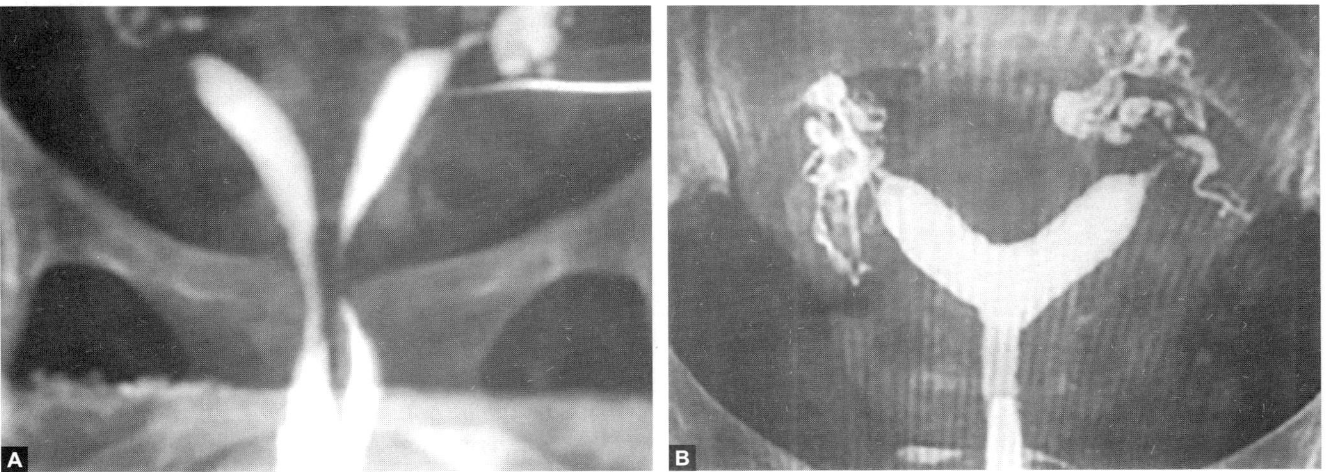

Figs. 3A and B: Hysterogram of septate uterus showing division of cavity to varying extent depending upon type of septum: (A) Complete septum extending down to cervical canal—AFS Class 5 i/CONUTA Class U2 b and (B) Partial septum extending different levels into the uterine cavity—AFS Class 5 ii/CONUTA Class U2 a. (AFS: American Fertility Society; CONUTA: CONgenital UTerine Anomalies)

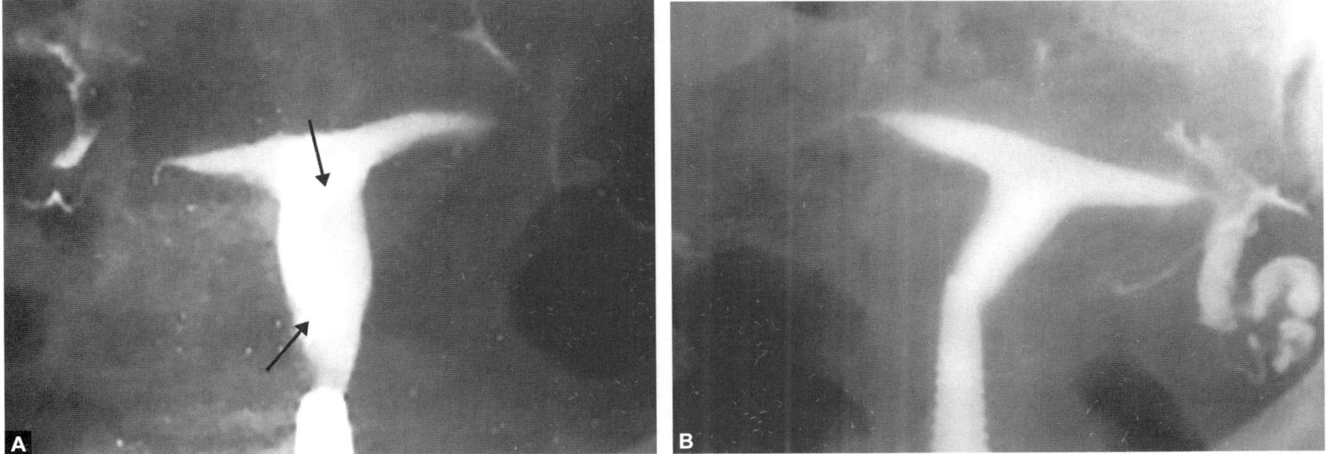

Figs. 4A and B: Hysterogram of DES exposed T-shaped uterus/dysmorphic uterus—AFS Class 7/CONUTA Class U1. (AFS: American Fertility Society; CONUTA: CONgenital UTerine Anomalies; DES: Diethylstilbestrol)

Ultrasonography is a quick, readily available, and economical method without radiation exposure, but external contour may be difficult to visualize in obese women or when there is overlying bowel gas. The specificity of USG ranges between 85% and 92% depending on the type of anomaly, patients body composition, and the skill of the radiologist. Transvaginal ultrasound gives a more detailed analysis of the cervical canal and the uterine cavity. Transvaginal 3D ultrasonography appears to be extremely accurate for the diagnosis and classification of congenital uterine anomalies, more than office hysteroscopy and MRI (Figs. 5 to 7). It may conveniently become the only mandatory step in the assessment of the uterine cavity in patients with a suspected septate or bicornuate uterus.[13]

However, currently, MRI is the best imaging modality as it lacks radiation and provides clear delineation of both the internal and external uterine anatomy (Fig. 8). The specificity of MRI is around 96–100% for diagnosing congenital uterine anomalies. Its use could be considered in cases in which findings on physical examination, HSG and USG remain equivocal, inpatients with vaginal agenesis, obstruction or transverse septum and in sexually inactive, premenarchal girls found to have a persistent adnexal mass.[14]

Hysterolaparoscopy is the most definitive method to diagnose uterine anomalies. Though invasive, it can be performed as a daycare procedure which allows for correction of the abnormality detected in the same sitting.

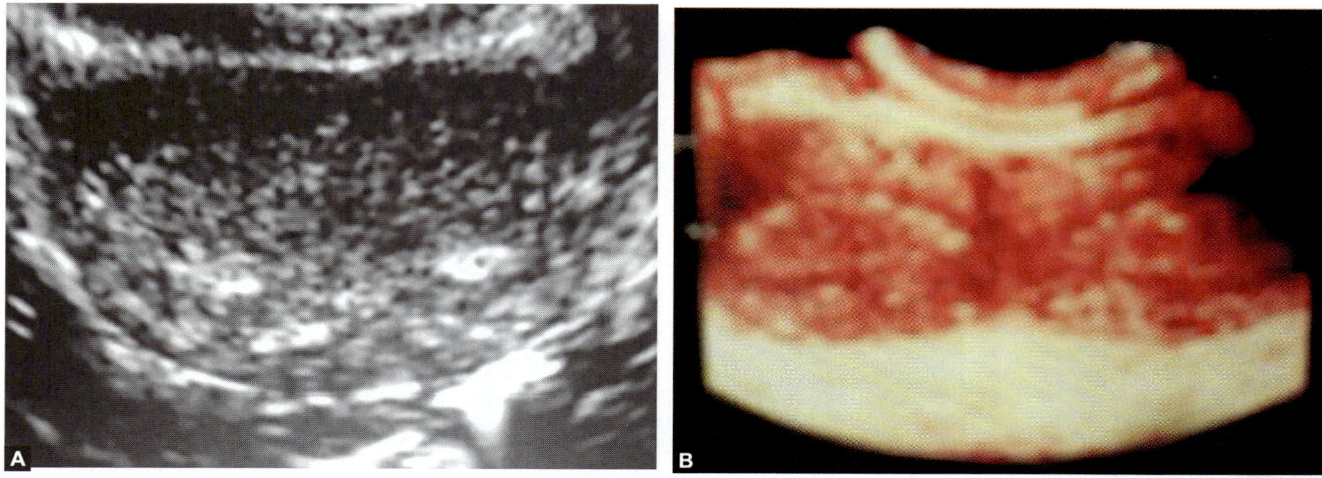

Figs. 5A and B: Ultrasound in transverse section of septate uterus showing division of cavity with an intact external contour differentiating this from a bicornuate uterus. (A) 2D ultrasound with two distinct cavities and (B) 3D ultrasound with two distinct cavities.

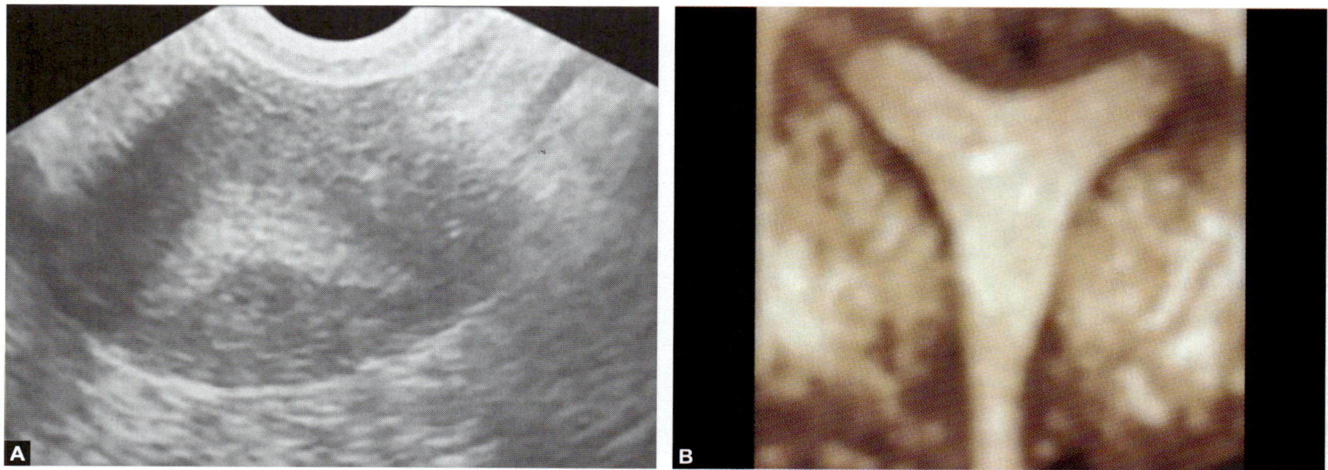

Figs. 6A and B: Ultrasound of arcuate septate uterus recognized as a distinct entity by the AFS classification but included as a variation of septate uterus in the CONUTA classification— AFS Class 6/CONUTA Class U2 a: (A) 2D ultrasound with a fundal prominence identified on angulating the TVS probe and (B) 3D ultrasound with a clear demonstration of cavity contours. (AFS: American Fertility Society; CONUTA: CONgenital UTerine Anomalies; TVS: Transvaginal sonography)

The superiority of a combined endoscopic examination over other diagnostic modalities regarding the reliability of diagnosis stands established and is the gold standard. It should be cautioned that hysteroscopic diagnosis of the intrauterine septum is not always easy, since the septum may be deviated to one side particularly following a previous pregnancy. In all cases where a tube-like uterine cavity with a single tubal ostium is seen on hysteroscopy a Müllerian abnormality should be suspected and in many cases a careful reinspection often reveals the lower edge of a septum. Simultaneous laparoscopy helps assess the external configuration of the uterus. Septate and subseptate uteri are invariably found to have a broad, flattened fundus with white streaks of fibrous tissue often seen in the midline.[15]

Many a times, the uterine anomalies are diagnosed during cesarean section when the uterus is exteriorized for suturing. These patients may experience discordant uterine contractions during labor.

CLASSIFICATION

Congenital uterine anomalies pose a challenge for therapeutic decision making in order to improve the reproductive potential. For efficient management of such patients, a clear diagnosis and effective categorization of these broad-spectrum anomalies is quite essential. Hence, arises the need for detailed classification of these anomalies for proper understanding and planning out the therapeutic options for their correction.

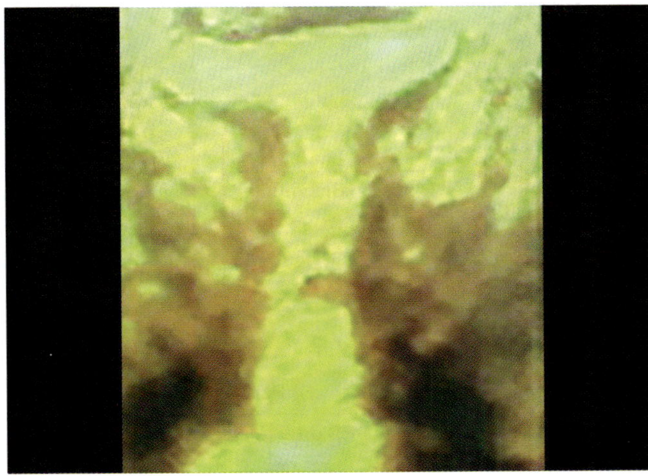

Fig. 7: Three-dimensional ultrasound of DES exposed T-shaped uterus/dysmorphic uterus—Reconstruction of cavity with shape identification comparable to hysterograms. (DES: diethylstilbestrol)

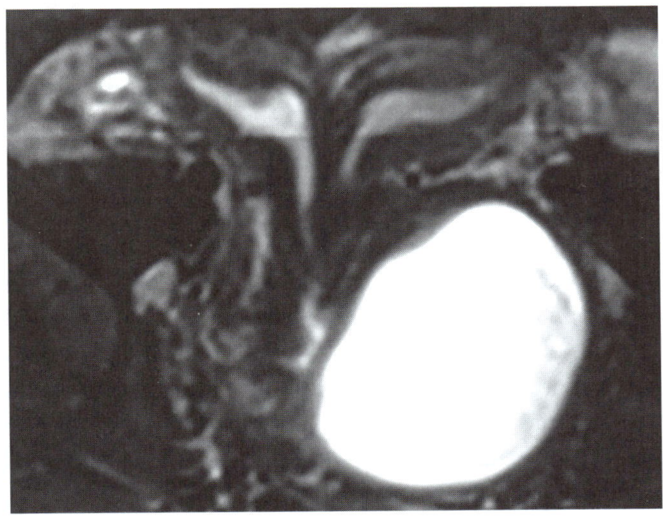

Fig. 8: Magnetic resonance imaging of septate uterus showing division of uterine cavity with complete septum extending down to cervical canal and vagina—AFS Class 5 i/CONUTA Class U2 b, V2. There is also a pyocolpos in a hemivagina. (AFS: American Fertility Society; CONUTA: CONgenital UTerine Anomalies)

In the beginning of the 19th century, Strassmann attempted to classify these anomalies and described septate and bicornuate uterus with some subgroups. However, based on the previous work of Buttram and Gibbons, the American Fertility Society (AFS) published the first classification in 1988[16] (Table 2). The AFS classification is based on anatomical origin and it is most successfully and widely adopted as the main classification till date[17] (Fig. 9). Later, Acien and Oppelt also proposed their classification

Table 2: American Fertility Society (AFS) classification.[16]

Class 1	Agenesis/Hypoplasia • Segmental • Complete
Class 2	Unicornuate • Noncommunicating with cavitary horn • Noncommunicating with noncavitary horn • Communicating with cavitary horn • No horn
Class 3	Didelphys
Class 4	Bicornuate • Complete • Partial
Class 5	Septate • Complete • Partial
Class 6	Arcuate
Class 7	DES-induced T-shaped uterus

(DES: Diethylstilbestrol)

based on embryological origin and VCUAM (vagina, cervix, uterus, adnexae, and associated malformations).

Recently, a more comprehensive classification has been established by the European Society of Human Reproduction and Embryology (ESHRE) and European Society for Gynaecological Endoscopy (ESGE) under the working name CONUTA (CONgenital UTerine Anomalies) (Table 3 and Fig. 10).[18,19]

Clinical Spectrum

Class I: Agenesis/Hypoplasia

The incidence of Müllerian agenesis is 1 in every 4,000–10,000 females. It is due to the early developmental failure of the Müllerian ducts (at around 5 weeks gestation) leading to agenesis or hypoplasia. There can be complete agenesis or sometimes a small amount of undifferentiated rudimentary tissue may be present. The most common form of complete agenesis is Mayer-Rokitansky-Kuster-Hauser syndrome. The patients present with primary amenorrhea and have normal sexual characteristics as the ovarian functions are preserved. These patients need a lot of psychological support to accept and deal with their pathology.

Class II: Unicornuate

The incidence of unicornuate uterus is 2.5–13% of uterine malformations. It occurs due to the complete or near complete arrest of the development of one of the Müllerian ducts. Patients with unicornuate uterus may present with dysmenorrhea, endometriosis, and hematometra.

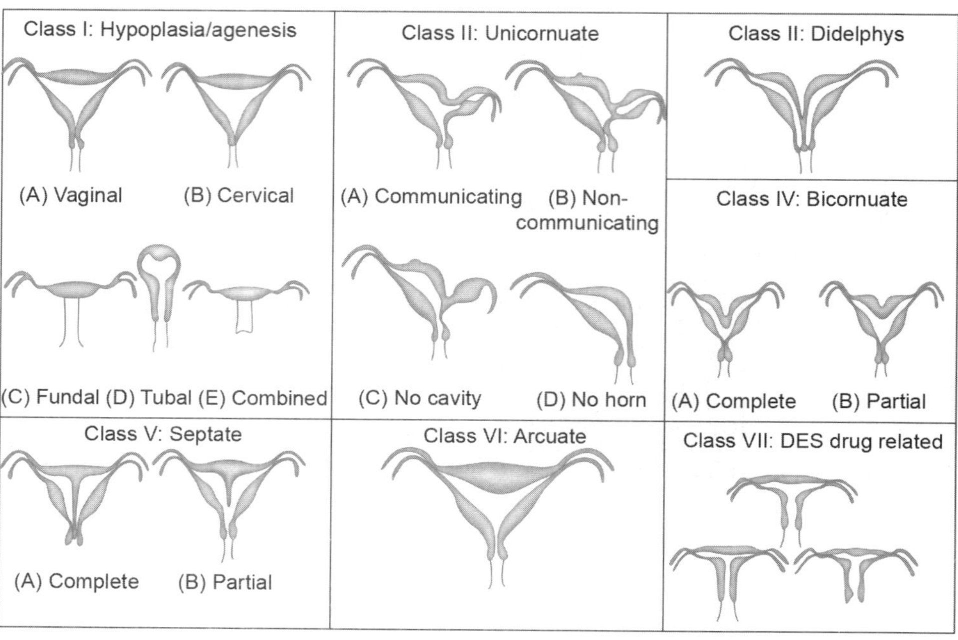

Fig. 9: American Fertility Society (AFS) classification.[16]

Table 3: European Society of Human Reproduction and Embryology (ESHRE) and European Society for Gynaecological Endoscopy (ESGE) CONUTA classification.[18]

Uterine anomaly		
	Main class	*Subclass*
U0	Normal uterus	
U1	Dysmorphic uterus	T shaped Infantilis Others
U2	Septate uterus	Partial Complete
U3	Bicorporeal uterus	Partial Complete Bicorporeal septate
U4	Hemi uterus	With rudimentary cavity (communicating or no horn), without rudimentary cavity (horn without cavity or no horn)
U5	Aplastic	With rudimentary cavity (bi or unilateral horn), without rudimentary cavity (bi or unilateral uterine remnants or aplasia)
U6	Unclassified	

Cervical/vaginal anomaly			
C0	Normal cervix	V0	Normal vagina
C1	Septate cervix	V1	Longitudinal nonobstructing vaginal septum
C2	Double normal cervix	V2	Longitudinal obstructing vaginal septum
C3	Unilateral cervical aplasia	V3	Transverse vaginal septum and/ or imperforate hymen
C4	Cervical aplasia	V4	Vaginal aplasia

(CONUTA: CONgenital UTerine Anomalies)

If conception occurs, there are increased chances of spontaneous abortion, ectopic gestation, malpresentation, IUGR, and preterm labor.

Class III: Didelphys

Uterus didelphys accounts for 11% of uterine malformations and it occurs due to the complete nonfusion of both the Müllerian ducts. The individual horns are fully developed and are of normal size with a deep fundal cleft with two cervices are present and a longitudinal or transverse vaginal septum may be present. Patients may be asymptomatic but have associated hematometra, hematometrocolpos, or hematosalpinx if obstruction is present.

Class IV: Bicornuate

The incidence of bicornuate uterus is 20% of uterine malformations and it is associated with increased rate of first trimester abortions. Partial nonfusion of the Müllerian ducts results in the formation of bicornuate uterus. The individual horns are smaller and are not fully developed as in didelphys uterus. The fundal cleft is more than 1 cm deep.

Bicornuate unicollis—central myometrium extends up to internal os.

Bicornuate bicollis—central myometrium extends up to external os.

The term live birth rate is approximately 60%, but there are increased chances of preterm delivery with malpresentation leading to increased rates of cesarean delivery.

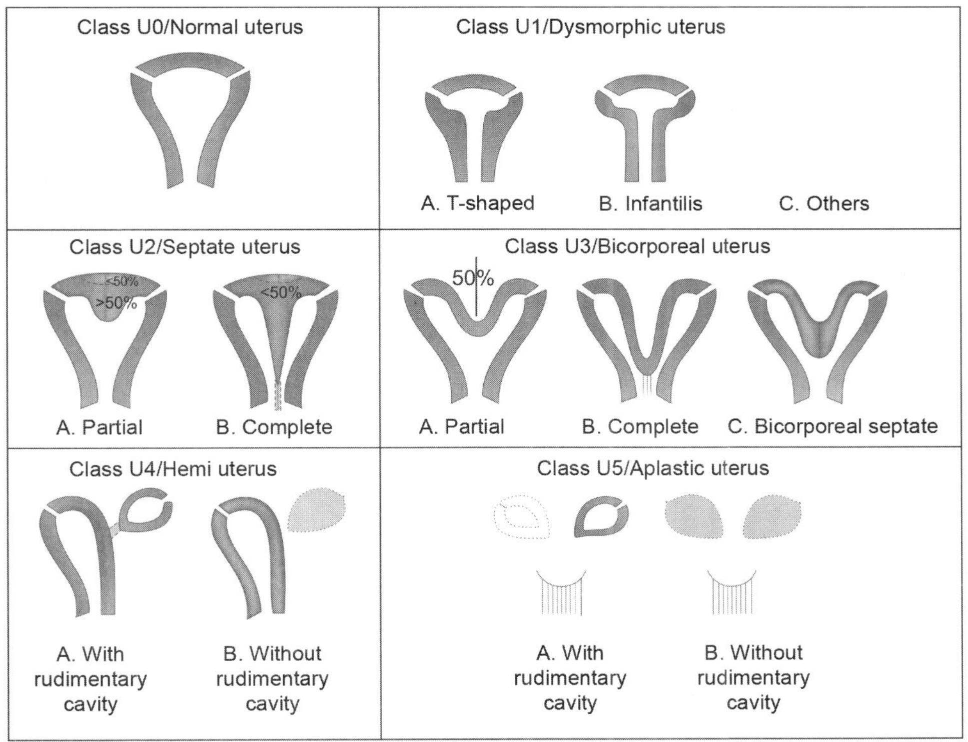

Fig. 10: European Society of Human Reproduction and Embryology (ESHRE) and European Society for Gynaecological Endoscopy (ESGE) CONUTA classification.[18] (CONUTA: CONgenital UTerine Anomalies)

Class V: Septate

The incidence of septate uterus is 33% of uterine malformations. Failure of resorption of the septum between the two Müllerian ducts results in a septate uterus. The septum can be muscular or fibrous or a combination of both. The uterus is partially or completely divided in two cavities. The fundal cleft is less than 1 mm deep with intercornual distance of less than 4 cm. The septate uterus has significant reproductive implications and is associated with poor obstetrical outcomes. The risk of miscarriage before 20 weeks is highest with the septate uterus.

Class VI: Arcuate

The incidence of arcuate uterus is 32.8% of uterine malformations. The near complete resorption of the uterovaginal septum results in the arcuate uterus leaving a mild indentation of the myometrium and endometrium at the fundus. Though generally considered asymptomatic, the arcuate uterus may be associated with an increased incidence of pregnancy wastage (25%) and preterm delivery (7.5%).

Class VII: DES Induced

The structural abnormalities associated with DES-include T-shaped uterus with smaller uterine cavities or a transverse septum. The primary pathology is the presence of constriction rings around the proximal uterine segment and a T-shaped uterine cavity with an arched base. These uteri are associated with increased incidence of miscarriages, ectopic gestation, and preterm delivery.

Management

Class I: Agenesis /Hypoplasia

With an absent uterus, surrogacy is the only option with in vitro fertilization of harvested ova from these patients.

Vaginal agenesis is rare and infrequently encountered and its association with a pelvic mass is even more uncommon. With vaginal agenesis, the uterus is usually absent or represented by rudimentary muscular buds (Mayer-Rokitansky-Kuster-Hauser syndrome). The classical treatment for vaginal agenesis has been vaginoplasty. When there is a functional uterus with vaginal agenesis, the proximal and distal vaginal mucosal ends can be joined and a few pregnancies have been reported following this procedure.

Class II: Unicornuate

There is no surgical therapy recommended for the unicornuate uterus without a rudimentary horn, unless an incompetent cervix is suspected. Reassurance and patience shown by the treating physician at times gives as good results as compared to surgical intervention, without the inherent morbidity of surgery.

When the unicornuate uterus has a noncommunicating cavitory rudimentary horn with a functional endometrial cavity, it is often associated with dysmenorrhea, hematometra, endometriosis, and ectopic pregnancy. In this situation excision of the rudimentary horn along with its oviduct should be considered since this eliminates a potential cause of persistent dysmenorrhea and the possible development of an ectopic pregnancy via transmigration from the contralateral adnexa. Laparoscopic excision of a noncommunicating rudimentary uterine horn was first reported in 1996 and has since become a feasible surgical option.[20]

Class III: Didelphys

This malformation is usually associated with premature labor. Because of the acceptable fetal salvage rate and the difficulty of a metroplasty, surgical therapy is rarely indicated or performed.

Class IV: Bicornuate

A bicornuate uterus is often considered an incidental finding. Patients usually have no difficulty becoming pregnant. They may present with premature labor and breech presentation leading to cesarean section. Approximately 60% of patients can expect to deliver a viable infant. While surgical correction for bicornuate uterus is seldom needed, for patients who have recurrent abortions or repeated preterm deliveries, the recommended therapy is the Strassman procedure, which has the advantage of not requiring excision of uterine tissue and thus not reducing the potential uterine space.

Class V: Septate

The traditional therapy for septate and subseptate uteri was abdominal metroplasty. Fortunately, this has been almost completely replaced by hysteroscopic resection of the uterine septum. With the accumulated experience with transcervical hysteroscopic metroplasty, transabdominal uterine unification of the symptomatic septate uterus is now an outmoded operation. Compared to hysteroscopy, the abdominal approach requires hospitalization, abdominal and uterine incisions, and a significant postoperative recovery period, including a wait of 3–6 months before conception can be attempted.

The effectiveness of hysteroscopic septectomy was established by March and Israel and confirmed by other researchers since. Pretreatment viable pregnancies were reported by them in just 5.0% and this improved dramatically to 85.7% posttreatment.[21]

Hysteroscopic approaches to septal resection use any one of the following modalities—resectoscope, flexible or semirigid scissors, neodymium-YAG laser or modified Metzenbaum scissors under portable fluoroscopy.[22,23] In a study by Cararach et al. of 81 cases that underwent a division of the septum, the post-treatment pregnancy success of 73% was uniformly distributed in the two groups—using the scissors or the resectoscope.[24] With different advantages provided by each technique, operator experience was the major consideration in technique selection.

Since hysteroscopy maintains myometrial integrity, any subsequent pregnancy can be delivered vaginally, unless cesarean section becomes indicated for purely obstetric reasons. In addition, because no tissue is removed, intrauterine volume should be greater after hysteroscopic incision than after transfundal metroplasty (Figs. 11 and 12).

Rare variations of septate uteri have been reported and require tailored surgical management. Perino et al. reported a case with dysmenorrhea and suspected unilateral adnexal tumescence for whom USG and endoscopy was performed. A diagnosis of a complete septate uterus with noncommunicating right hemicavity and hematometra, an exceptional type of Müllerian anomaly was made, for which hysteroscopic metroplasty was successfully performed.[25] Of course affected women may go through their entire obstetric career without being diagnosed of the uterine malformation. In fact, it may first get revealed at cesarean section done for an unrelated obstetric indication or at tubal sterilization.

Class VI: Arcuate

When an arcuate uterus is thought to be a cause of reproductive failure, this abnormality could occasionally have a clinical implication similar to septate uteri and hence could be treated on the same lines as a septate uterus.

Class VII: DES Induced

One of the earliest series of lateral metroplasty was reported in 1993 with hysteroscopic metroplasty using a semirigid scissor for nonfusion anomalies. The results were reassuring with live births reported in three out of five patients with recurrent pregnancy loss.[26]

For this condition, a plastic enlargement (metroplasty) is undertaken to widen the cavity by making careful incisions of the excess muscle tissue located on the uterus wall. The incisions are placed transversely at the fundus (similar to

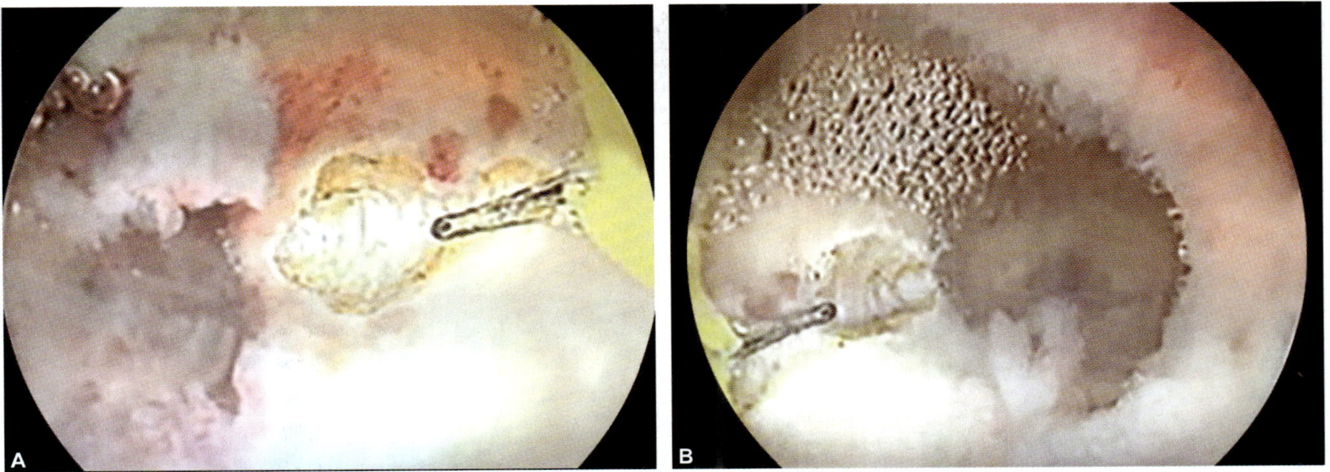

Figs. 11A and B: Hysteroscopic septal incision using a Collin's knife (HF resectoscope). (A) Transverse incision of the septum at the midpoint between the anterior and posterior uterine walls and (B) Monitor completion by visual and tactile check of the recessed cornu and till the electrode can easily move from side to side.

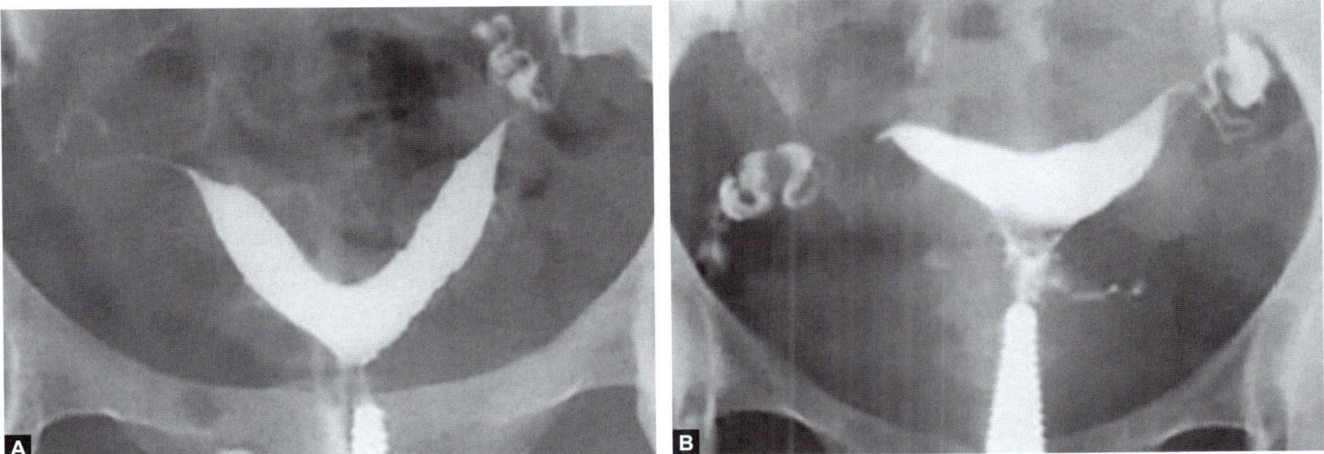

Figs. 12A and B: Preoperative hysterogram in a subseptate uterus with a postoperative hysterogram following a hysteroscopic septal incision using an HF resectoscope. (A) Preoperative hysterogram documenting a large septum and (A) Postoperative hysterogram documenting an adequate unified cavity.

hysteroscopic septal incision) and laterally, leading to the first author christening the procedure a lateral metroplasty for want of a better terminology.[27]

The procedure now consists of electrosurgical incision of the lateral walls of the uterine cavity with the help of a resectoscope using a Collins knife starting near the tubal ostia and extending proximally. Care must be taken to avoid incising the lateral wall in the region of the isthmus and internal os. The incision is done millimeter by millimeter till a normal uterine architecture is achieved and the underlying myometrium is visualized. The end point of the procedure is the visualization of both cornua satisfactorily on panoramic hysteroscopy (Figs. 13 and 14).

CONCLUSION

Uterine anomalies undoubtedly make women vulnerable to difficulty in conception and reproductive wastage. The septate uteri are the most significant followed by rarer abnormalities such as the T-shaped and the unicornuate uteri. There is now believed to be a marginalized role for reproductive implications of bicornuate uteri.

Fortunately, uterine abnormalities are one of the more successfully treatable forms of infertility and pregnancy wastage. Potential management options have progressed to a more conservative, less expensive and safer, even outpatient approach for patients, yielding results that are

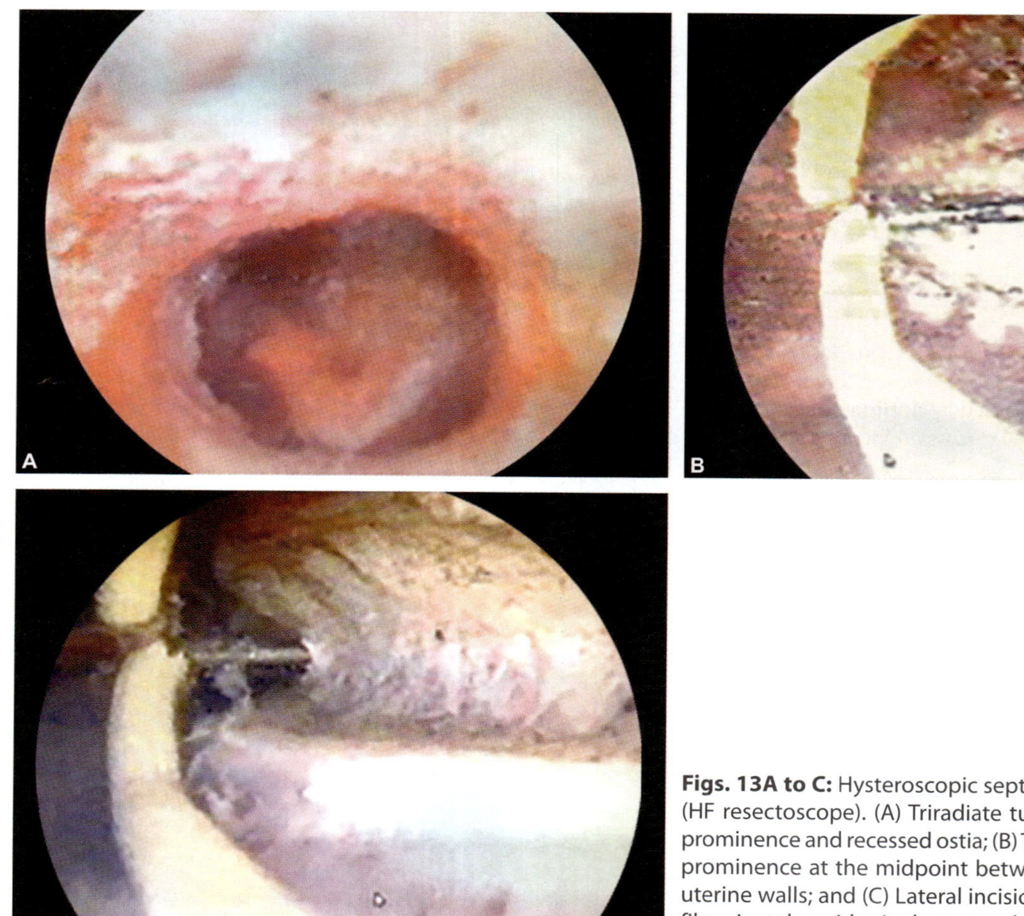

Figs. 13A to C: Hysteroscopic septal incision using a Collin's knife (HF resectoscope). (A) Triradiate tubular cavity often with fundal prominence and recessed ostia; (B) Transverse incision of the fundal prominence at the midpoint between the anterior and posterior uterine walls; and (C) Lateral incision of the constriction rings and fibrosis at the midpoint between the anterior and posterior uterine walls.

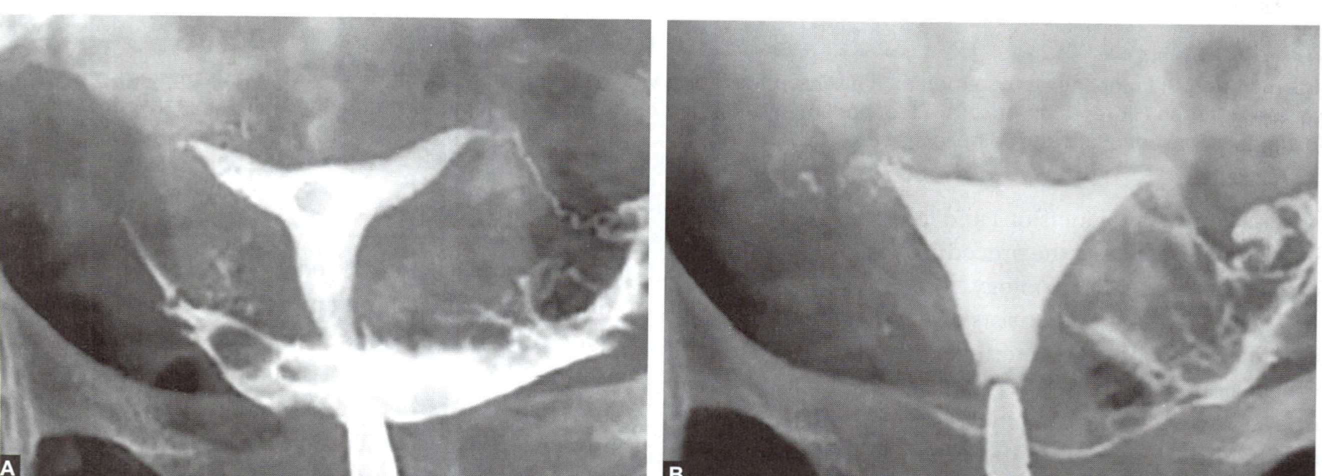

Figs. 14A and B: Preoperative hysterogram in a T-shaped uterus with a postoperative hysterogram following a hysteroscopic lateral incision using an HF resectoscope. Preoperative hysterogram documenting a triradiate cavity in a T-shaped uterus and Postoperative hysterogram documenting an adequate anatomically normal cavity.

as effective, if not more, as those achieved with the major operative procedures of the past. Of course there will always remain a group of patients who need only reassurance and no surgical intervention. With the significance of the uterine factor thus established, any neglect in evaluating the uterine cavity would be difficult to justify to our patients and ourselves.

REFERENCES

1. Sheriar NK. Management of congenital uterine abnormalities. In: Krishna UR, Shah DS, Salvi VA, Sheriar NK, Damania KR (Eds). Pregnancy at risk: a practical approach to high risk pregnancy & delivery (FOGSI). New Delhi: Jaypee Brothers Medical Publishers; 2010.
2. Behr SC, Courtier JL, Qayyum A. Imaging of Müllerian duct anomalies. Radiographics. 2012;32(6):E233-50.
3. Sheriar NK. Embryology and development of the female genital tract. In: Arulkumaran S, Chatterjee A, Pratap K (Eds). Essentials of gynecology. New Delhi: Jaypee Brothers Medical Publishers; 2011.
4. Chandler TM, Machan LS, Cooperberg MD, et al. Müllerian duct anomalies: from diagnosis to intervention. Br J Radiology. 2009;82:1034-42.
5. Verp MS, Simpson JL, Elias S, et al. Heritable aspects of uterine anomalies. Three familial aggregates with Müllerian fusion anomalies. Fertil Steril. 1983;40:80-5.
6. Taylor HS. Endocrine disruptors affect developmental programming of HOX gene expression. Fertil Steril. 2008;89(2):e57-8.
7. Zama AM, Uzumcu M. Epigenetic events of endocrine-disrupting chemicals on female reproduction: An ovarian perspective. Front Neuroendocrinol. 2010;31(4):420-39.
8. Diamond MP, DeCherney AH (Eds). Recurrent Pregnancy Loss. Infertility and Reproductive Medicine Clinics of North America. Philadelphia: WB Saunders; 1991.
9. Raga F, Bauset C, Remohi J, et al. Reproductive impact of congenital Müllerian anomalies. Hum Reprod. 1997;12(10):2277-81.
10. Ribeiro SC, Tormena RA, Peterson TV. Müllerian duct anomalies: review of current management. Sao Paulo Med J. 2009;127(2):92-6.
11. Acien P. Reproductive performance of women with uterine malformation. Human Reprod. 1993;8(1):122-7.
12. Panchal S, Nagori C. Imaging techniques for assessment of fallopian tube. J Human Reprod Sc. 2014;7(1):3-12.
13. Faivre E, Fernandez H, Deffieux X, et al. Accuracy of three-dimensional ultrasonography in differential diagnosis of septate and bicornuate uterus compared with office hysteroscopy and pelvic magnetic resonance imaging. J Minim Invasive Gynecol. 2012;19(1):101-6.
14. Chang YCG, Hricak H. Current status of MR imaging of the female pelvis. Crit Rev Diagn Imag. 1989;29:337-41.
15. Assaf A, Serour A, Elkady A, et al. Endoscopic management of the intrauterine PP septum. Int J Obstet Gynecol. 1990;32:43-51.
16. American Fertility Society. AFS classification of adnexal adhesions, distal tubal occlusion, tubal occlusions secondary to tubal ligation, tubal pregnancies, Müllerian anomalies and intrauterine adhesions. Fertil Steril. 1998;49:944-55.
17. Chandler TM, Machan LS, Cooperberg PL. Müllerian duct anomalies: from diagnosis to intervention. Br J Radiol. 2009;82:1034-42.
18. Grimbizis GF, Gordts S, Sardo AS. The ESHRE/ESGE consensus on the classification of female genital tract congenital anomalies. Human Reprod. 2013;2(8):2032-44.
19. Grimbizis GF, Campo R. Clinical approach for the classification of congenital uterine malformations. Gynecol Surg. 2012;9:119-29.
20. Kadir RA, Hart J, Nagele F, et al. Laparoscopic excision of a non-communicating rudimentary uterine horn. Br J Obstet Gynaecol. 1996;103(4):371-2.
21. March CM, Israel R. Hysteroscopic management of recurrent abortion caused by septate uterus. Am J Obstet Gynecol. 1987;156:834.
22. Hassiakos DK, Zourlas PA. Transcervical division of uterine septa. Obstet Gynecol Surv. 1990;45(3):165-73.
23. Valle JA, Lifchez AS, Moise JA. A simpler technique for reduction of uterine septum. Fertil Steril. 1991;56:1001-3.
24. Cararach M, Penella J, Ubeda A, et al. Hysteroscopic incision of the septate uterus: scissors versus resectoscope. Human Reprod. 1994;9(1):87.
25. Perino A, Chianchiano N, Simanaro C, et al. Endoscopic management of a case of complete septate uterus with unilateral haematometra. Human Reprod. 1995;10(8):2171-73.
26. Naegel TC, Malo JW. Hysteroscopic metroplasty inthe diethylstilbestrol-exposed uterus and similar nonfusion anomalies: effects on subsequent reproductive performance: a preliminary report. Fertil Steril. 1993;59:502-6.
27. Sheriar NK. Lateral hysteroscopic metroplasty. 42nd All India Congress of Obstetrics & Gynaecology, 27-30 December, 1998, Hyderabad.

CHAPTER

77

Intrauterine Pathologies: Evaluation and Treatment for Improving Assisted Reproductive Technology Outcomes

M Cerrillo, A Fabris, JM Puente, A Guillen, Juan A García-Velasco

INTRODUCTION

Correctly diagnosing an intrauterine pathology can determine the most suitable therapeutic strategy to be adopted. Although barely any evidence exists, a normal uterine cavity should be associated with better pregnancy rates, few obstetric complications and, consequently, with a better perinatal prognosis.

An ultrasound, which is sometimes combined with sonohysterography, is the first diagnostic step to evaluate the uterine factor prior to in vitro fertilization (IVF). Depending on the ultrasound findings, performing endoscopic techniques (hysteroscopy, laparoscopy) to achieve a diagnosis and to treat, may be needed.

When it comes to making ultrasound evaluations, it is important to adapt the examination to specific gynecological ultrasound requirements, and also to difficulties associated with certain pathologies, which are frequent in infertile patients (endometriosis, adenomyosis, myomas, scars or Müllerian malformations).

Both gynecological examination systematics and nomenclature to be used have been thoroughly studied, and there are well-defined criteria and recommendations supplied by several work groups (IOTA, IETA, MUSA, and IDEA) in ultrasound examinations for reproductive medicine.

DIAGNOSIS METHODS

2D-3D Ultrasonography

It is advisable to perform a complete and controlled evaluation of the female genital system. The examination begins by placing the probe in the vaginal fork. This allows us to obtain a transverse plane of the anal sphincter and, with it, a sagittal plane of the anal channel by rotating the probe 90°. As the probe is inserted into the vagina, we can evaluate the rectovaginal septum, the vagina and its cul-de-sacs. This is a very important step, particularly for those cases in which deep endometriosis or an adhesion syndrome is suspected.

Next, we evaluate the cervix and the uterus, firstly in the sagittal plane and secondly in the transverse plane. Then we gently move the probe from side to side to identify both adnexa. This evaluation must include any possible changes in the position of the adnexa in relation to the uterus, and if pain is noted during the examination.

Using the so-called shift signal or the uterine sliding sign is advisable to evaluate female genital system mobility. This sign was described in 1988 by Trimor-Tritsch,[1] and more recently by Hudelist[2] and Reid.[3] This simple test allows those patients with an adhesion syndrome of a different nature that affects Douglas cul-de-sacs to be identified. It consists in placing the ultrasound probe into the posterior vaginal cul-de-sac and applying pressure with it, while also applying suprapubic pressure on the uterus with the other hand. If we perceive that the vaginal wall and the posterior uterine wall shift in relation to the rectum, the signal is positive; if they shift together and appear to be adhered, the signal is negative.

This same signal can be applied if pressure is placed from the anterior vaginal cul-de-sac, combined with our hand (which is not normally necessary in most cases). In this case, we evaluate the mobility of the anterior vaginal and uterine walls in relation to the bladder wall.

The 3D Mode

Three-dimensional (3D) imaging in reproductive medicine is similar to imaging in general gynecology. The coronal plane is the most valuable when suspecting certain pathologies like anti-Müllerian malformations. While scanning ovaries with the help of 3D imaging the entire volume of the ovary can also be measured.

Adjusting the 3D Image

The most important adjustments are summarized as:

- The size and position of the volume "box", in order to adjust it to the organ that we must examine. It is important to encompass the whole uterus or ovary.
- Scanning angle: It is graduated in 5° intervals, as is size, and we must pay attention to include the whole volume at the smallest possible angle.

It is essential to avoid the patient from moving and making respiratory movements during the image acquisition process to prevent interference on the image.

Of all the 3D ultrasound modes available, the most important one is the multiplane mode because it allows us to view the uterine coronal plane.

Hysterosonography

Hysterosonography is a procedure where images are taken using a transvaginal probe while the uterine cavity is being distended using normal saline. The use of hysterosonography must be balanced against risks of a infectious disease in patients. It is necessary to pay attention to inflammatory pelvic disease, and to discard hydrosalpinx and endometriosis. Thus, antibiotic prophylaxis is advisable before proceeding with a hysterosonography (single dose of azithromycin or doxycycline).[4]

As for the technique itself, it is firstly important to perform an ultrasound examination to identify the cervix opposite the uterine fundus, and to evaluate the concomitant peritoneal tubo-ovarian pathology (hydrosalpinx, endometriosis, pelvic adhesions). Next, we carry out a speculoscopy to view and clean the cervix with 3% povidone iodine or chlorhexidine. An embryo transfer catheter or artificial insemination catheter or even a balloon catheter to avoid fluid reflux can be used. Then we remove the speculum and place the vaginal probe. We have to identify the catheter inside the uterine cavity so as to gradually insert 5–10 mL of an air bubble-free saline solution. Turbulence may occur if the solution is inserted too quickly, which makes the assessment of the cavity more difficult and could imply a higher degree of pain. Once the cavity is fully evaluated, we must aspirate the liquid that remains in the cavity under ultrasound control and remove the catheter by maintaining negative pressure with the syringe plunger. Using a balloon catheter prevents liquid from leaking and improves viewing, although insemination probes enable suitable viewing in most cases at a lower cost.

In those cases in which we also wish to view tubes (hysterosalpingosonography), a contrast can be used, or saline can be mixed with air. It is also worth having a reliable antireflux system.

Hysteroscopy

A hysteroscopy is a clinical procedure that allows the gynecologist to evaluate the uterine cavity with an endoscope, along with saline solution instillation. This procedure can be used for diagnosis purposes, to treat intrauterine pathologies, and also as a surgical method to eliminate certain uterine pathologies.

It is considered a simple outpatient minimally invasive technique, and is the gold standard technique to diagnose intracavity pathologies.

INTRAUTERINE PATHOLOGIES DIAGNOSIS

Myomas

The presence of myomas can affect fertility via several mechanisms. There appears to be a certain consensus[5] that those myomas which deform the uterine cavity should require treatment as they affect fertility. Apart from spontaneous fertility, we must assess the impact that a myoma can have on the success of ART and its relation with spontaneous abortion, prematurity, placenta previa, and postpartum hemorrhage, among others.[6] Therefore, we must make a detailed evaluation of the myomas' characteristics to help decide the appropriate management. The following parameters should be taken into consideration while doing fibroid mapping:

- Number, size (at least two diameters), type (subserous-pedicellata, intramural, submucous) and location of the myoma(s) in the uterus.
- If the fibroids make the access to the uterine cavity difficult, it is important to measure dimensions of the entire cavity. In IVF cases, always describe the distance from the cervix to where embryos must be deposited.
- Evaluate the uterine cavity. A 3D ultrasound is useful to obtain a coronal plane of the uterine cavity, and to know the extent to which the myoma affects it.
- If the cavity is affected by a submucous myoma, define the degree of the myoma's penetration into the cavity. This is useful as it correlates with the possibility of a hysteroscopic removal .[7,8]

- Finally, and this is valid especially for many myomas or doubtful cases, it is important to graphically document the examination, or to even store the ultrasound/video volume in order to jointly analyze the case with a specialist in reproduction and/or a surgeon, and to make a personalized decision in each case.

Myomas must be evaluated both on vaginal and abdominal ultrasound, because the abdominal ultrasound is better for patients with many or large-sized myomas as it offers better images than a vaginal ultrasound. It may also be the only option in such cases to be able to evaluate adnexa, and it also serves to study the relation between the myoma and surrounding organs. Abdominal evaluations can evaluate kidneys and rule out the presence of any associated hydronephrosis through extrinsic pressure from the urinary tract.

Polyps

Although very few randomized studies are available about the impact of polyps on fertility,[9] a general agreement exists on recommending their removal after observing endometrial polyps during an ultrasound examination since their removal is simple, and they may unfavorably affect fertility via several mechanisms.

An ultrasound evaluation is generally diagnostic; however, a sonohysterography can be used for more uncertain cases.

The polyp is generally viewed as a hyperechogenic image that contrasts with the hypoechogenic endometrium in the first phase of the cycle. The interphase between the two endometrial leaves is discontinued, with one vascular pedicle, or several, that feed it and can be easily identified by highdefinition power Doppler (Fig. 1). A description of the size, location, implantation site, polyp surface, and the vessels that feed it[10] are required. Nonetheless to avoid mistakes, we must pay attention to:

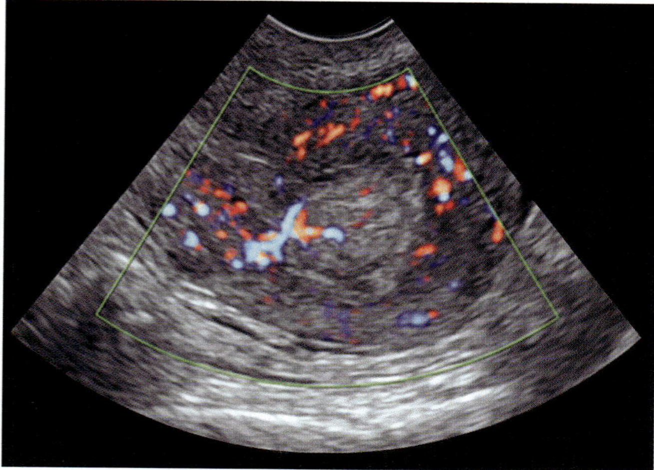

Fig. 1: Polyp.

- Performing the examination in the early follicular phase by delaying the scan a few days if necessary. The hyperechogenicity of a secretory endometrium can hide a polyp and, conversely, small folds in the endometrial mucous can simulate polyps.
- Optimizing equipment adjustments in both gray-scale (by reducing angle and depth) and color images by high-definition Doppler power, by slowing down speed to highlight the minor vessels that irrigate polyps, and to avoid artifacts, given their importance.

Adenomyosis

Adenomyosis is quite a frequent ultrasound finding in patients with endometriosis,[10,11] and with infertility in general,[12] although its association with infertility can be a matter of controversy.[11,13] Although some studies have associated it to a higher spontaneous abortion rate[14] along with a lower term pregnancy rate in ovum donation cycles. Perhaps its presence has been underestimated because it is not often considered. Yet despite its diagnosis being anatomopathological, ultrasounds have demonstrated good diagnostic accuracy that is almost comparable to MRI.[13-15] Therefore, the first step to diagnose adenomyosis is to suspect it in such patients. On ultrasound terms, it may present a nodular or fuzzy pattern, and its most common ultrasound findings include:

- The presence of hyperechogenic striations from the endometrium through the myometrium, along with other hypoechoic masses that correspond to smooth muscle hypertrophy and together form a heterogeneous pattern. This finding confers greater sensitivity (88%).[16]
- The uterus looks globular. There is an asymmetry of the myometrial walls, where the posterior wall is generally more affected (Fig. 2).
- The endometrium-myometrium interphase is lost, and small subendometrial cysts, formed by dilated glands, are present[17] (Fig. 3).
- In the nodular pattern, variable-sized nodules are present in the myometrium, with hyperechogenic limits and a hypoechoic content. This would be the most specific 2D scan finding (specificity of 98%, sensitivity of 78%).[18]
- Thickening of the endometrium-myometrium junction zone. The junction zone between the endometrium and myometrium comprises a portion of the myometrium, which is the richest portion in vessels, and is more

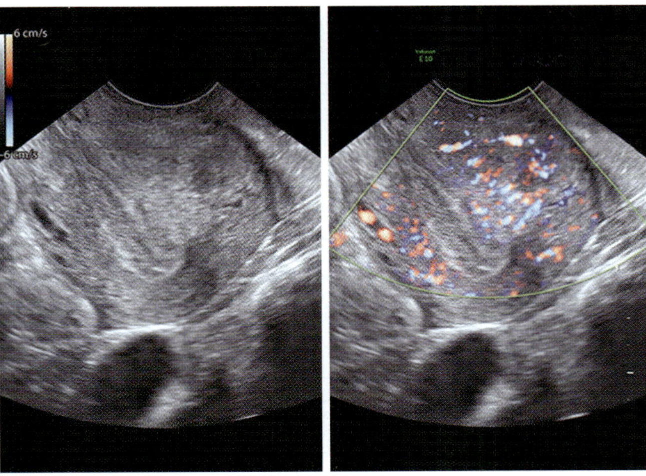

Fig. 2: Adenomyosis in posterior wall.

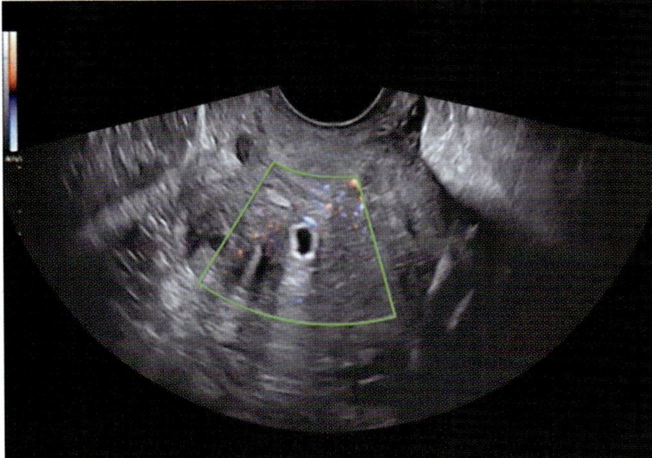

Fig. 3: Cyst of adenomyosis.

subject to changes in the ovarian cycle and pregnancy. Its thickness is around 4 mm,[19,20] and it is responsible for the uterine peristalsis in a nonpregnant uterus. This zone is invaded along with the decidua by the trophoblasts during the process of placentation.[21,22] The thickness of this zone increases in the presence of adenomyosis and is demonstrated clearly by the help of an MRI. Adenomyosis can also be seen in a 3D ultrasound as projections from the hyperechogenic endometrium into the hypoechogenic junction zone. The difference between the maximum and minimum thicknesses of the junction zone is more than 4 mm. Observing these endometrial projections is one of the most sensitive and specific 3D ultrasound findings (sensitivity of 88% in both, and a specificity of 85% and 82%, respectively).[22]

- Occasionally when the myometrial thickness considerably increases, it implies a reduced cavity size, which can be mild, moderate, or severe (cases

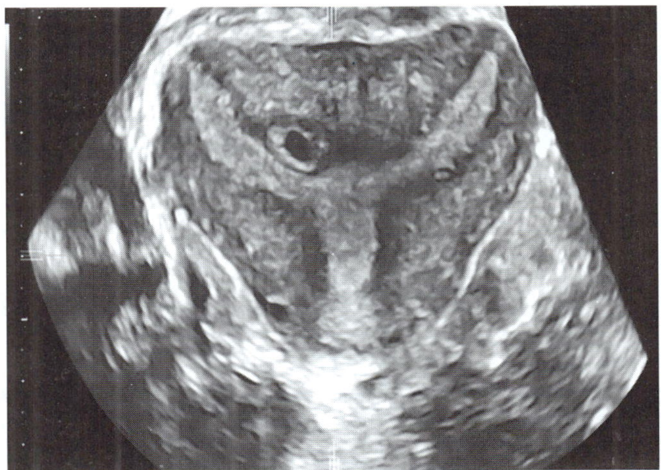

Fig. 4: T-shape secondary adenomyosis.

in which T-shaped cavities are seen) (Fig. 4). Recently our group published a series with a high prevalence of adenomyosis in infertile female patients with implantation failure, which was possibly due to patients' ever-increasing age.[23]

Müllerian Abnormalities

Congenital uterine abnormalities form a group of pathologies that result from alterations in the formation, merging, or reabsortion of the Müllerian ductus,[24] or through a combination of them. Depending on their type and severity, they can be associated with an adverse reproductive prognosis (implantation failure, early and/or late spontaneous abortions, preterm deliveries, fetal malpositions, etc.). Their incidence in the general population is not completely known, but a figure of 3–5% is assumed.[25,26] This figure rises to 8–13% in the infertile population. It is estimated a 13% of patients with a background of spontaneous abortion in the first trimester of pregnancy, and comes close to 25% if it corresponds to late spontaneous abortions.[27]

Many classifications for Müllerian duct abnormalities exist in literature. The 1998 *American Fertility Society* classification is still currently in use and establishes sevencategories (Fig. 5). Recently, a new more simplified system has been proposed by ESHRE (the European Society of Human Reproduction and Embryology), which divides them into six groups[28] (Fig. 6).

A diagnosis is made depending on the anomaly type by a combination of examinations, which include an palpation and speculoscopy, 2D and 3D ultrasounds, hysterosalpingography, hysteroscopy, laparoscopy, MRI, urography, etc., and also depending on each specific case. In this chapter, we will focus on the role of ultrasound. This is a fundamental test to diagnose a patient with a Müllerian malformation. Including a 3D ultrasound allows a coronal plane to be obtained, which is essential to classify different malformations, even though it is not necessary for them all. It is particularly useful to distinguish a bicorporal uterus (Fig. 7) from a septate uterus (Fig. 8), and it less expensive and simpler than MRI which is used in more complex malformations. T-shape uterus appears as a new Müllerian malformation (Fig. 9).

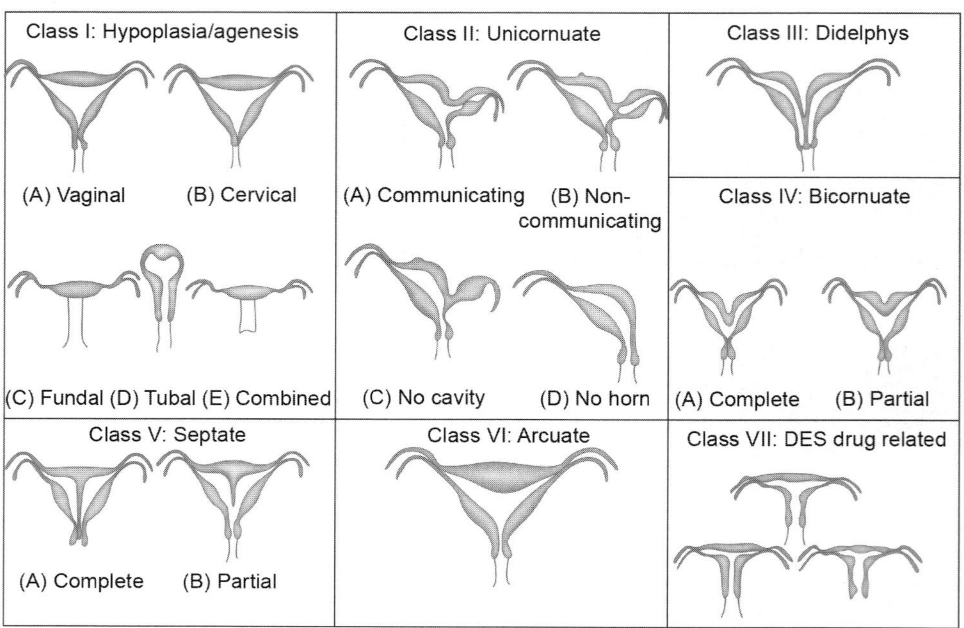

Fig. 5: American Fertility Society (AFS) classification.

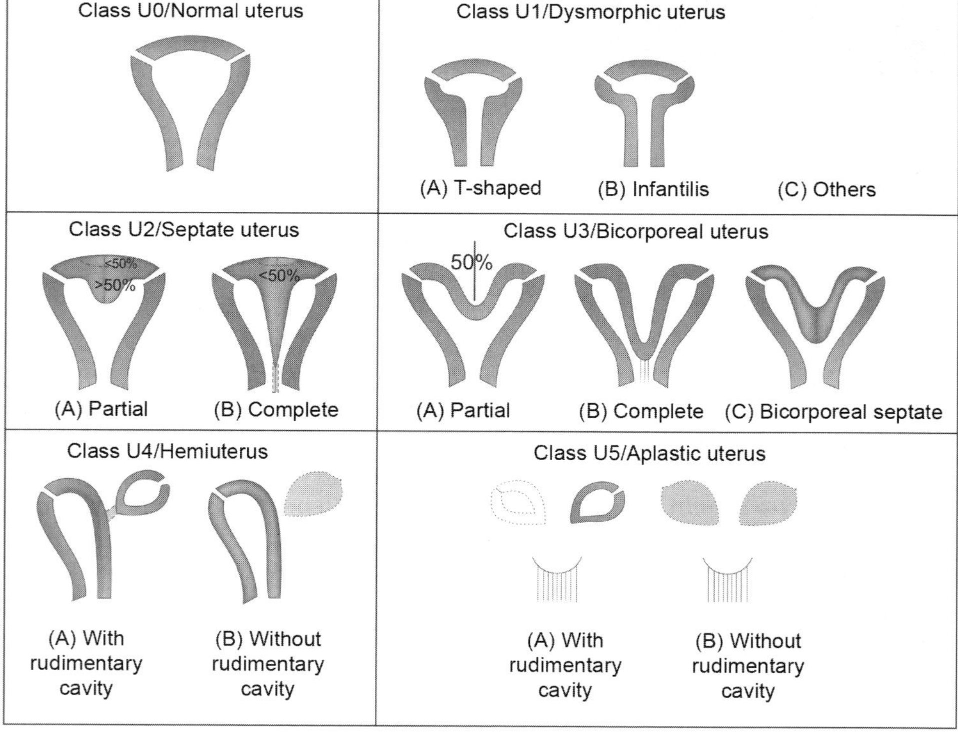

Fig. 6: European Society of Human Reproduction and Embryology-European Society of Gynecological Endoscopy (ESHRE-ESGE) classification.

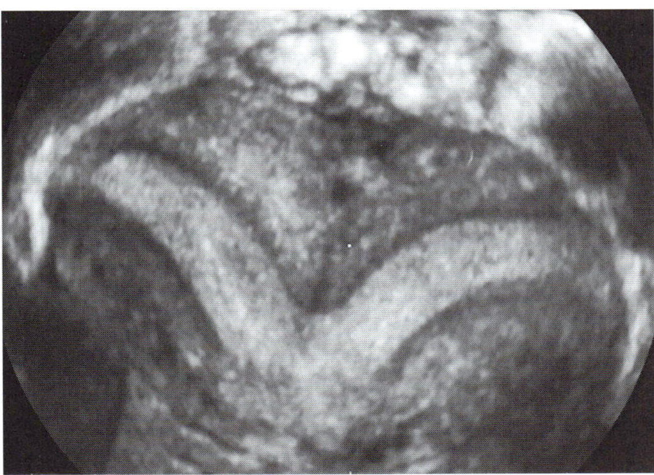

Fig. 7: Bicorporal uterus.

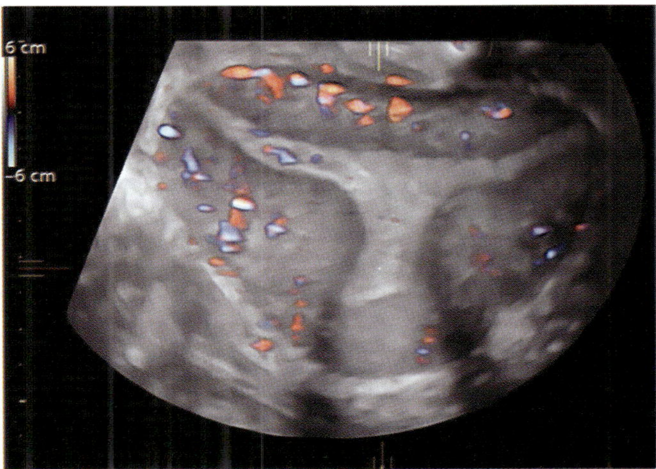

Fig. 9: T-shape uterus.

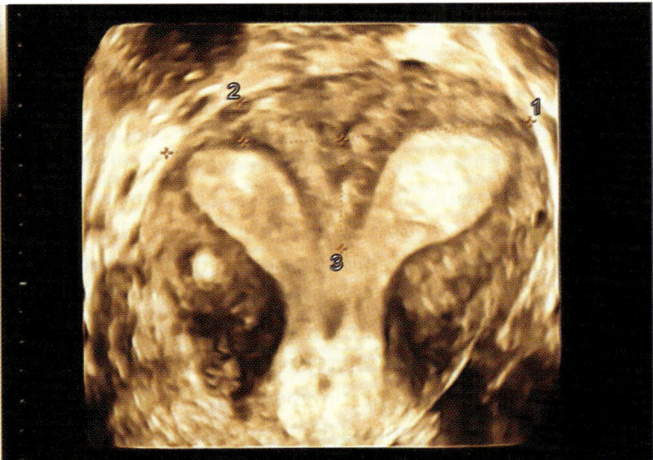

Fig. 8: Septum.

TREATING INTRAUTERINE PATHOLOGIES

Nowadays, treating exclusive intracavity pathologies is relatively easier thanks to the huge progress made in hysteroscopy in recent decades. Hysteroscopy is a clinical procedure that allows gynecologists to look inside a uterus with the help of an endoscope. Hysteroscopy can be performed for diagnostic purposes and also as a surgical procedure to treat intrauterine pathologies. It is considered a gold standard technique to diagnose polyps, myomas, or intracavitary pathology, and can be used as a surgical procedure to remove and treat them in most of the cases. In the majority of cases, outpatient minimally invasive hysteroscopic surgery, or surgery performed in an operating room under general anesthesia, allows lesions of any size to be removed.

Myomas

The myomas that can affect fertility are of the submucous or intramural types as they may distort the cavity. The mechanisms by which they can cause infertility are: chronic endometrial inflammation, abnormal vascularization, increased uterine contractility, or local endocrine alterations that can affect the transport of spermatozoa and implantation.[29]

Casini et al. in their randomized control trial have demonstrated a higher pregnancy rate after performing myomectomy in patients with submucous myomas, both with and without an intramural component, compared with expectant management (wait and see what happens).[30]

A hysteroscopy under general anesthesia or an epidural allows the cervical canal to be dilated and to remove submucous myomas of any size with a monopolar resectoscope. Modern loops and bipolar scissors enable an isotonic solution to be used, and avoid any excess absorption of hypotonic distension media through the vascularized myometrium, and the consequent compartment syndrome. In fibroids with intramural component, if we section the connective capsule of the myoma, it increases its intracavitary portion, thanks to the uterine contractions,[31] it simplifies the surgery and reduces the complications.

Myomas that measure less than 1.5 cm can be removed by office hysteroscopy, without anesthesia. It is advisable to firstly separate the capsule mechanically and then to remove the myoma by cutting it with a bipolar electrode in an isotonic distension medium. The OPPIuM technique, as previously described for hysteroscopy with anesthesia, consists in making an incision in the pseudocapsule of myomas with an intramural component so that with the next periods, uterine contractions increase the submucous portion of the myoma and the myomectomy will be simple.[32]

No evidence exists for the efficacy of medical intracavity treatments to reduce the formation of postmyomectomy intrauterine adhesions.[33]

In some cases of myomas with intramural components, a second hysteroscopy might be necessary to complete the myoma removal.

No cases of uterine rupture as the result of a hysteroscopic myomectomy have been described in the literature.[34]

The *intramural myomas* that distort the cavity can be removed during a laparotomy or laparoscopy, depending on their dimensions and the surgeon's choice. If cavity access is possible, 6 months have to pass before performing an embryo transfer.

Finally, therapy with Ulipristal acetate (a selective modulator of progesterone receptors) allows to reduce the size of uterine myomas and reduces the symptoms associated with medical treatment taken orally. Two 3-month treatment cycles are recommended for infertile women of reproductive age with many or large-sized myomas that affect the uterine cavity.[35]

Adenomyosis

The influence of adenomyosis on fertility is a controversial matter, but it is becoming a more frequently suspected and diagnosed pathology. As myomas, adenomyosis that result in a deformation of the cavity can affect the transport of spermatozoa and implantation.

A destroyed junction zone structure can affect normal uterine peristalsis. Women's endometria with adenomyosis seem to present metabolic and inflammatory alterations. It can present altered responses to estrogens and progesterone, and can occasionally not be adequately prepared for treatments.[36]

Adenomyosis can be treated medically or surgically.

Medical treatment: Gonadotropin-releasing hormone (GnRH) agonists have been used to lessen adenomyosis symptoms, such as pain and menorrhagia, but have not been studied in infertile women. However, a published case has reported that six of seven women became pregnant during the 24-month period following therapy.[37] Intrauterine or vaginal devices that administer Danazol doses have been used and a 41% pregnancy rate has been achieved in the months after therapy had ended.[38]

Surgical treatment: Laparoscopic techniques have been described for large laparatomic adenomyomas with an H incision technique that allowed uterine integrity and fertility to be preserved. However, the literature only includes retrospective studies or case studies, and does not recommend one technique rather than the other.[39-42]

Currently, hysteroscopy in reproduction is beginning to play a key role in correcting and improving uterine cavities affected by adenomyosis, but published data are lacking as very few series can be found.[43] Our group began to use it routinely when we encountered affected, T-shaped or small-sized cavities to widen them, and the results of the cycles performed later seem to be improved.

Studies with more scientific evidence are necessary before being able to recommend treating adenomyosis prior to ART, and to indicate the best treatment for the reproductive prognosis in adenomyosis affected patients.

Polyps

As mentioned earlier, very few randomized studies have been published on the repercussion of polyps on fertility,[44] and a general agreement exists on recommending their removal when found in an ultrasound. It is simple[44] and can unfavorably affect fertility via several mechanisms,[45] e.g. interfering with the transport of spermatozoa, embryo implantation, through inflammation or the altered production of factors relating to endometrial receptivity, like glycodelin.[45] If a polyp is detected in a fertility study prior to ovarian stimulation or to frozen embryo transfer, most centers perform a polypectomy.[46]

Although hysteroscopic polypectomy before performing intrauterine insemination (IUI) can increase the clinical pregnancy rate,[9,47,48] its efficiency in patients who undergo intracytoplasmic sperm injection (ICSI) or IVF has not been backed by randomized studies.

An in office polypectomy or under sedation allows us to directly visualize the lesions, their complete removal and the histological analysis of a lesion with very few complications.[45] Microscissors, a loop or a bipolar electrode (Gynecare Versapoint),[49,50] or a morcellator can be employed. Al Chami[48] in a recent review recommends outpatient hysteroscopic treatment, which offers a better cost-benefit ratio compared to procedures under sedation. Moreover, the fact that new instruments are now available for outpatient hysteroscopy allows polypectomies to be done with no limits as to the size, location, and number of polyps.[49]

If polyps are diagnosed during ovarian stimulation, various treatment options exist:

- Cancel the cycle and performing polypectomy
- Continue with stimulation and transfer fresh embryos

- Freeze oocytes or embryos, perform a polypectomy the day of the oocyte retrieval delaying and transfer to a different cycle.

Decisions depend on many factors, including the survival rate after vitrification in each laboratory. Lass et al. 1999 found no differences in the reproductive results of women who underwent a polypectomy as opposed to the finding of polyps of less than 2 cm during stimulation in which frozen embryo transfer was carried out *versus* the women in whom fresh embryos were transferred without removing the polyp. However, a high spontaneous abortion rate was observed in those patients who did not undergo polypectomy, but other studies have not reported different pregnancy rates in patients submitted to polypectomy.[9]

Another retrospective study by Tiras et al. (2012) discovered no benefit of performing polypectomy in polyps of less than 1.4 cm.[51]

As randomized studies are lacking, the doctor's preference, the efficiency of the vitrification program, and patients' reproductive history have to be assessed when a polyp is found during stimulation. Nowadays, and after all the vitrification progress made, our group only performs polypectomy and delays the transfers.

Synechiae

Uterine synechiae are mainly caused by damage to the endometrium while performing dilation and curettage (D&C) or by endometriosis. Presence of adhesions implies poor reproductive prognosis, characterized by infertility, spontaneous abortions, and preterm birth. Infertility can be caused by a mechanical obstacle that interferes with the transport of spermatozoa, or by lack of growth of endometrium, which does not allow the embryo to implant. This tends to be the first warning sign in reproductive medicine.

Synechiae can be removed by outpatient hysteroscopy or hysteroscopy done under sedation, but the risk of recurrence is high, and endometrial growth can still be poor post the procedure. No randomized studies exist about reproductive results after synechiolysis. Adhesiolysis with microscissors is preferable to minimize any thermal trauma caused by a bipolar electrode, and has shown the same results.[49]

In the last 10 years, efficacy of stem cell therapy has been investigated to treat women with Asherman's syndrome or an atrophic endometrium.[52] Promising results despite them being pilot studies[53] are available.

Müllerian Abnormalities

The new classification published by ESRHE-ESGE[28] allows us to better classify, which malformed uteri may benefit from a surgical treatment. As a meta-analysis has demonstrated,[27] many Müllerian malformations are at high risk of spontaneous abortion in the first and second trimesters, and of prematurity and fetal malpositions at the time of giving birth. Certain indications are clear, like a septate uterus, whose treatment would be septoplasty because it improves obstetric prognosis, as formerly demonstrated,[54,55]and hysteroscopy is not a complicated technique to perform. In complete septum, two or more hysteroscopies may be necessary to completely remove a septum (Figs. 10A to D).

The other indication would be a subtype C bicornuate uterus, which is a twin function-reabsorption defect. The septum resection in this case should be done with great care because the risk of perforation is high (Figs. 11A and B).

The third malformation for which surgery is beginning to be indicated in patients with infertility problems is the T-shaped uterus. This is quite a controversial matter, but infertility has been associated in many of these patients, of whom many have endometrial growth problems, or are associated with ectopic pregnancies or recurrent spontaneous abortions. One pilot study has demonstrated that performing an operation by hysteroscopic metroplasty on patients diagnosed with a T-shaped uterus on ultrasound substantially improves their prognosis and the possibility of having a live newborn child.[56] However, as it is a pilot study, larger series are needed to demonstrate these results. In our group, we tend to treat T-shaped uterus by metroplasty in patients with implantation failure, spontaneous abortions, or ectopic pregnancies, as shown in Figures 12A to C.

KEY POINTS

- Three-dimensional scan is the most effective, efficient, and noninvasive diagnostic method for the gynecologist to screen Müllerian malformations and intrauterine pathology.
- Hysteroscopy is the gold standard test to assess the intrauterine cavity, in minimally invasive way and at the same time allows us to treat lesions in the same sitting.
- Polyps do not usually affect reproductive outcomes when they are less than 1 cm, but because of the probability of growth under hormonal treatments in our group we usually remove them by hysteroscopic polypectomy.

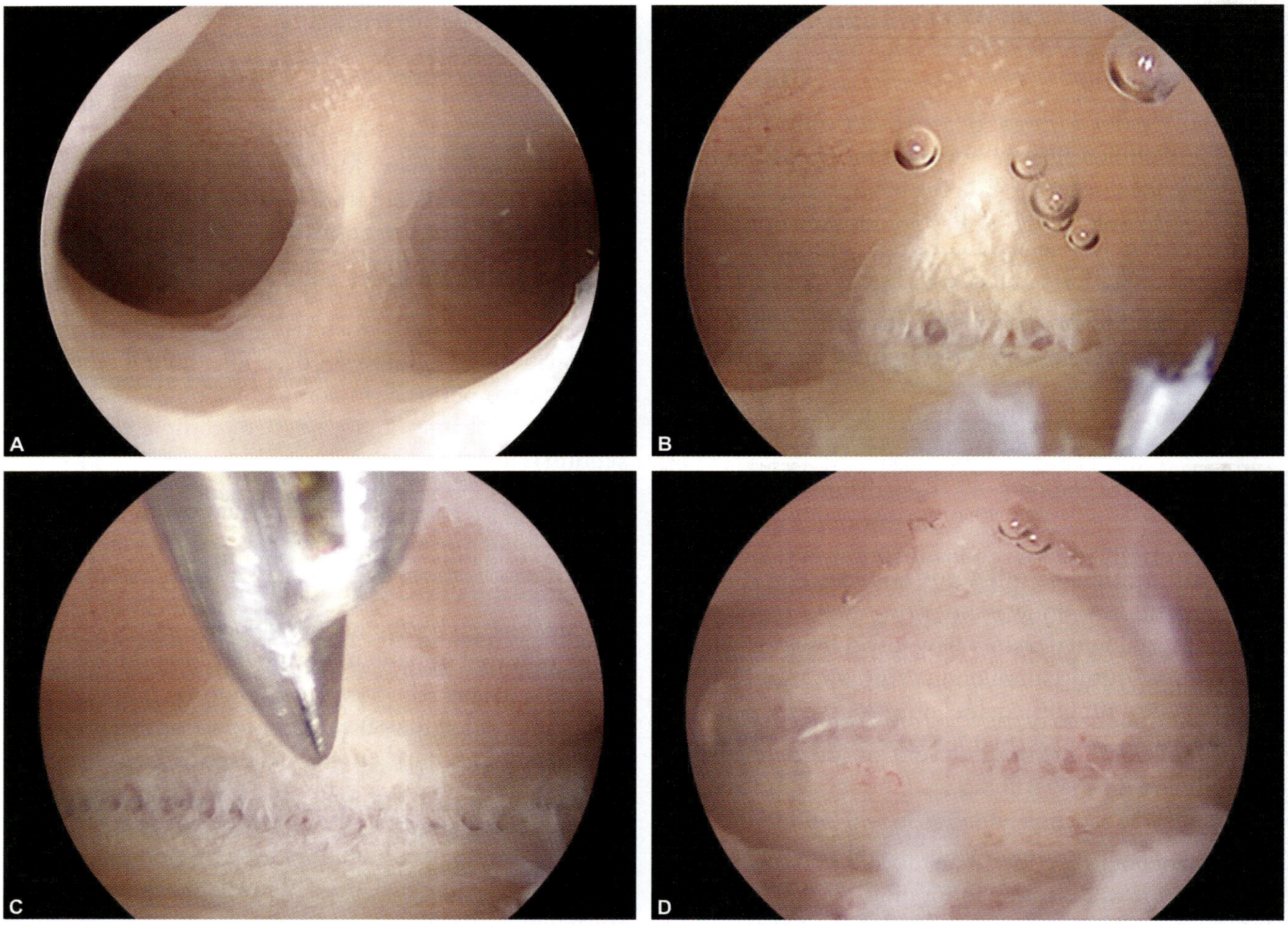

Figs. 10A to D: Septoplasty by hysteroscopy.

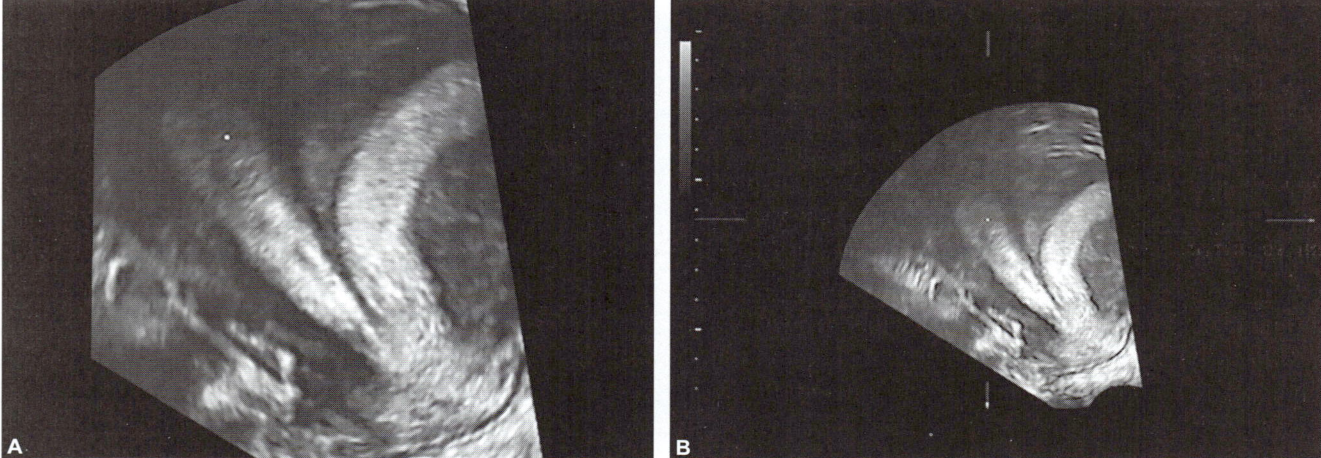

Figs. 11A and B: Bicorporal type 3 with part of septum.

- Submucosal myomas are a clear indication for hysteroscopic myomectomy.
- Adhesions should be removed by hysteroscopy.
- Müllerian malformations where hysteroscopic surgeries like septoplasty and metroplasty are indicated in order to improve the obstetric prognosis are septate uterus

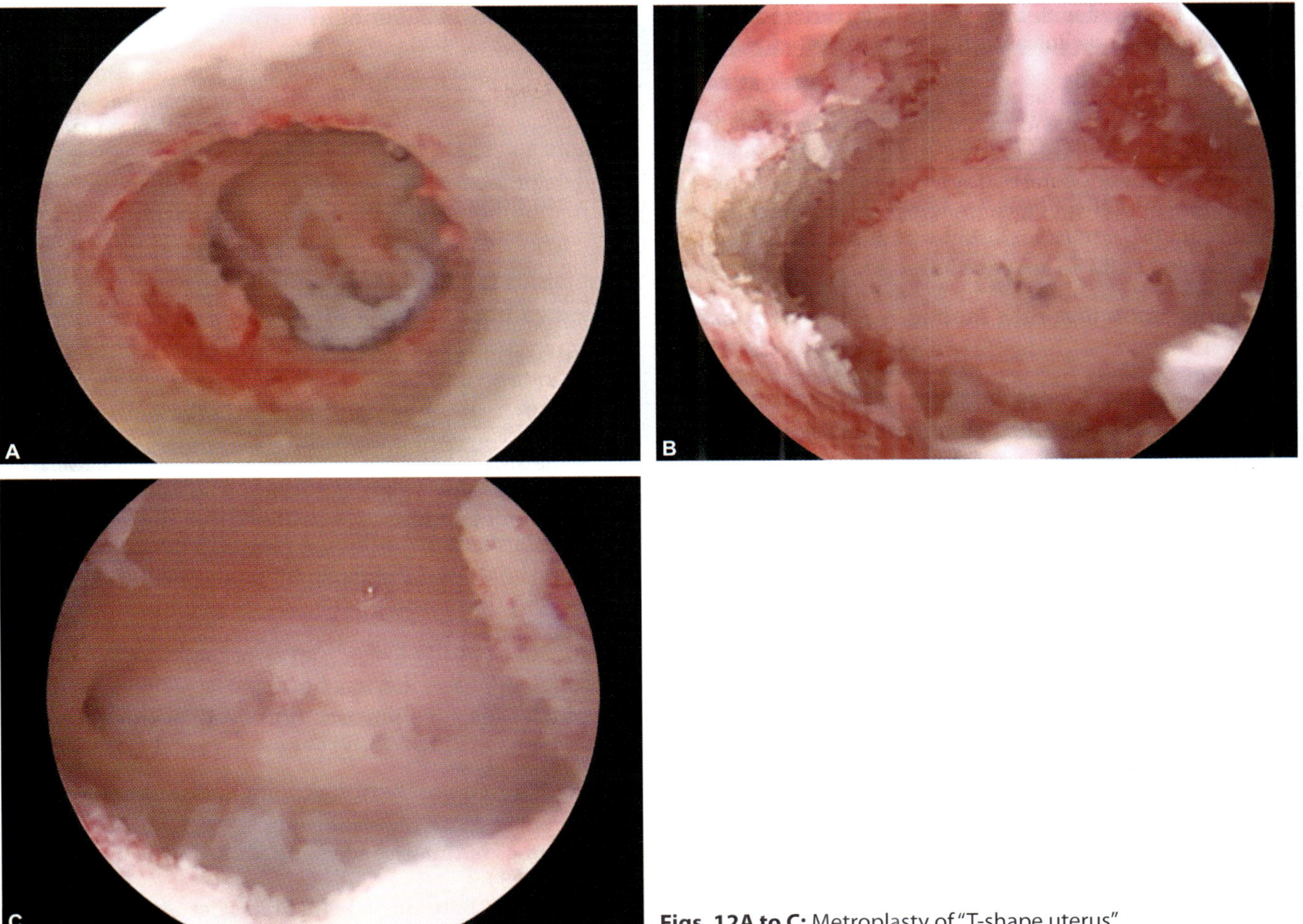

Figs. 12A to C: Metroplasty of "T-shape uterus".

and T-shaped uterus, especially if there is a history of implantation failure or recurrent miscarriages.

REFERENCES

1. Timor-Tritsch IE, Rottem S (Eds). Transvaginal sonography. New York: Elsevier; 1988.
2. Hudelist G, Fritzer N, Staettner S, et al. Uterine sliding sign: a simple sonographic predictor for presence of deep infiltrating endometriosis of the rectum. Ultrasound Obstet Gynecol. 2013;41:692-5.
3. Reid S, Condous G. Transvaginal sonographic sliding sign: accurate prediction of pouch of Douglas obliteration. Ultrasound Obstet Gynecol. 2013;41:605-7.
4. Saunders R, Shwayder J, Nakajima ST. Current methods of tubal patency assessment. Fertil Steril. 2011;95:2171-9.
5. Leone FP, Timmerman D, Bourne T, et al. Terms, definitions and measurements to describe the sonographic features of the endometrium and intrauterine lesions: a consensus opinion from the International Endometrial Tumor Analysis (IETA) group. Ultrasound Obstet Gynecol. 2010;35:103-12.
6. Galliano D, Bellver J, Díaz-GarcíaC, et al. ART and uterine pathology: how relevant is the maternal side for implantation? Hum Reprod Update. 2015;21(1):13-38.
7. Leone FP, Lanzani C, Ferrazzi E. Use of strict sonohysterographic methods for preoperative assessment of submucous myomas. Fertil Steril. 2003;79:998-1002.
8. Leone FP, Bignardi T, Marciante C, et al. Sonohysterography in the preoperative grading of submucous myomas: considerations on three-dimensional methodology. Ultrasound Obstet Gynecol. 2007;29:717-8.
9. Pérez-Medina T, Bajo-Arenas J, Salazar F, et al. Endometrial polyps and their implication in the pregnancy rates of patients undergoing intrauterine insemination: a prospective, randomized study. Hum Reprod. 2005;20:1632-5.
10. Fenzl V. Effect of different ultrasound contrast materials and temperatures on patient comfort during intrauterine and tubal assessment for infertility. Eur J Radiol. 2012;81(12):4143-5.
11. Kunz G, Beil D, Huppert P, et al. Adenomyosis in endometriosis prevalence and impact on fertility. Evidence from magnetic resonance imaging. Hum Reprod. 2005;20:2309-16.
12. Zacharia TT, O'Neill MJ. Prevalence and distribution of adnexal finding suggesting endometriosis in patients with MRI diagnosis of adenomyosis. Br J Radiol. 2006;79:303-7.
13. De Souza NM, Brosens JJ, Schwieso JE, et al. The potential value of magnetic resonance imaging in infertility. Clin Radiol. 1995;50:75-9.

14. Cakmak H, Taylor S. Implantation failure: molecular mechanisms and clinical treatment. Hum Reprod Update. 2011;17(2):242-53.
15. Martinez-conejero, Dueholm M, Lundorf E, et al. Magnetic resonance imaging and transvaginal ultrasonography for diagnosis of adenomyosis. Fertil Steril. 2001;76:588-94.
16. Bazot M, Cortez A, Darai E, et al. Ultrasonography compared with magnetic resonance imaging for the diagnosis of adenomyosis: correlation with histopathology. Hum Reprod. 2001;16:2427-33.
17. Dueholm M, Lundorf E. Transvaginal ultrasound or MRI for diagnosis of adenomyosis. Curr Opin Obstet Gynecol. 2007;19:505-12.
18. Exacoustos C, Brienza L, Rienza A, et al. Adenomyosis: three-dimensional sonographic findings of the junctional zone and correlation with histology. Ultrasound Obstet Gynecol. 2011;(37):471-9.
19. Hoad CL, Raine-Fenning NJ, Fulford J, et al. Uterine tissue development in healthy women during the normal menstrual cycle and investigations with magnetic resonance imaging. Am J Obstet Gynecol. 2005;192:648-54.
20. Hauth EA, Jaeger HJ, Libera H, et al. MR imaging of the uterus and cervix in healthy women: determination of normal values. Eur Radiol. 2007;17:734-42.
21. Abdallah Y, Naji O, Saso S, et al. Ultrasound assessment of the peri-implantation uterus: a review. Ultrasound Obstet Gynecol. 2012;39:612-9.
22. Brosens JJ, de Souza NM, Barker FG. Uterine junctional zone: function and disease. Lancet. 1995;346:558-60.
23. Puente JM, Fabris A, Patel J, et al. Adenomyosis in infertile women: prevalence and the role of 3D ultrasound as a marker of severity of the disease. Reprod Biol Endocrinol. 2016;14(1):60.
24. Moore KL, Persaud TVN, Torchia MG. The Urogenital System. Before We are Born: Essential of Embryology and Birth Defects, 7th edition. Philadelphia: Saunders/Elsevier; 2008. pp. 162-89.
25. Jayaprakasan K, Chan YY, Sur S, et al. Prevalence of uterine anomalies and their impact on early pregnancy in women conceiving after assisted reproduction treatment. Ultrasound Obstet Gynecol. 2011;37(6):727-32.
26. Raga F, Bonilla-Musoles F, Blanes J. Congenital Müllerian anomalies: diagnostic accuracy of three-dimensional ultrasound. Fertil Steril. 1996;64(3):523-8.
27. Chan YY, Jayaprakasan K, Tan A, et al. Reproductive outcomes in women with congenital uterine anomalies: a systematic review. Ultrasound Obstet Gynecol. 2011;38(4):371-82.
28. Grimbizis GF, Campo R. Clinical approach for the classification of congenital uterine malformations. Gynecol Surg. 2012;9(2):119-29.
29. Donnez J, Jadoul P. What are the implications of myomas on fertility? A need for a debate? Hum Reprod. 2002;17:1424-30.
30. Casini ML, Rossi F, Agostini R, et al. Effects of the position of fibroids on fertility. Gynecol Endocrinol. 2006;22:106-9.
31. Litta P, Vasile C, Merlin F, et al. A new technique of hysteroscopic myomectomy with enucleation in toto. J Am Assoc Gynecol Laparosc. 2003;10:263-70.
32. Cicinelli E, Mitsopoulos V, Fascilla FD, et al. The OPPIuM technique: office hysteroscopic technique for the preparation of partially intramural leiomyomas. Minerva Ginecol. 2016;68(3):328-33.
33. Bosteels J, Weyers S, Kasius J, et al. Anti-adhesion therapy following operative hysteroscopy for treatment of female subfertility. Cochrane Database Syst Rev. 2015;(11):CD011110.
34. Sentilhes L, Sergent F, Roman H, et al. Late complications of operative hysteroscopy: predicting patients at risk of uterine rupture during subsequent pregnancy. Eur J Obstet Gynecol Reprod Biol. 2005;120:134-8.
35. Donnez J, Donnez O, Dolmans MM. Safety of treatment of uterine fibroids with the selective progesterone receptor modulator, ulipristal acetate. Expert Opin Drug Saf. 2016;15:1679-86.
36. Harada T, Khine YM, Kaponis A, et al. The impact of adenomyosis on women's fertility. Obstet Gynecol Surv. 2016;71:557-68.
37. Maheshwari A, Gurunath S, Fatima F, et al. Adenomyosis and subfertility: a systematic review of prevalence, diagnosis, treatment and fertility outcomes. Hum Reprod Update. 2012;18:374-92.
38. Igarashi M, Abe Y, Fukuda M, et al. Novel conservative medical therapy for uterine adenomyosis with a danazol-loaded intrauterine device. Fertil Steril. 2000;74:412-3. No abstract available. Erratum in: Fertil Steril 2000;74:851.
39. Fujishita A, Masuzaki H, Khan KN, et al. Modified reduction surgery for adenomyosis. A preliminary report of the transverse H incision technique. Gynecol Obstet Invest. 2004;57:132-8.
40. Osada H, Silber S, Kakinuma T, et al. Surgical procedure to conserve the uterus for future pregnancy in patients suffering from massive adenomyosis. Reprod Biomed Online. 2011;22:94-9.
41. Saremi A, Bahrami H, Salehian P, et al. Treatment of adenomyomectomy in women with severe uterine adenomyosis using a novel technique. Reprod Biomed Online. 2014;28:753-60.
42. Kim MD, Kim NK, Kim HJ, et al. Pregnancy following uterine artery embolization with polyvinyl alcohol particles for patients with uterine fibroid or adenomyosis. Cardiovasc Intervent Radiol. 2005;28:611-5.
43. Zhang J, Shi W. Treatment of adenomyosis by hysteroscopy. J Mini Invasive Gynecol. 2015;22(6S):S123.
44. Jayaprakasan K, Polanski L, Sahu B, et al. Surgical intervention versus expectant management for endometrial polyps in subfertile women. Cochrane Database Syst Rev. 2014;30:CD009592
45. Jansen FW, Vredevoogd CB, van Ulzen K, et al. Complications of hysteroscopy: a prospective, multicenter study. Obstet Gynecol. 2000;96:266-70.
46. Richlin SS, Ramachandran S, Shanti A, et al. Glycodelin levels in uterine flushings and in plasma of patients with leiomyomas and polyps: implications for implantation. Hum Reprod. 2002;17:2742-7.
47. Bosteels J, Kasius J, Weyers S, et al. Hysteroscopy for treating subfertility associated with suspected major uterine cavity abnormalities. Cochrane Database Syst Rev. 2015;21:CD009461.
48. Al Chami A, Saridogan E. Endometrial polyps and subfertility. J Obstet Gynaecol India. 2017;67:9-14.

49. Bettocchi S, Achilarre MT, Ceci O, et al. Fertility-enhancing hysteroscopic surgery. Semin Reprod Med. 2011;29:75-82.
50. Litta P, Cosmi E, Saccardi C, et al. Outpatient operative polypectomy using a 5 mm-hysteroscope without anaesthesia and/or analgesia: advantages and limits. Eur J Obstet Gynecol Reprod Biol. 2008;139:210-4.
51. Tiras B, Korucuoglu U, Polat M, et al. Management of endometrial polyps diagnosed before or during ICSI cycles. Reprod Biomed Online. 2012;24:123-8.
52. Santamaria X, Cabanillas S, Cervelló I, et al. Autologous cell therapy with CD133+ bone marrow-derived stem cells for refractory Asherman's syndrome and endometrial atrophy: a pilot cohort study. Hum Reprod. 2016;31:1087-96.
53. Gargett CE, Schwab KE, Deane JA. Endometrial stem/progenitor cells: the first 10 years. Hum Reprod Update. 2016;22:137-63.
54. Esmaeilzadeh S, Delavar MA, Andarieh MG. Reproductive outcome following hysteroscopic treatment of uterine septum. Mater Sociomed. 2014;26(6):366-71.
55. Venetis CA, Papadopoulos SP, Campo R, et al. Clinical implications of congenital uterine anomalies: a meta-analysis of comparative studies. Reprod Biomed Online. 2014;29(6):665-83.
56. Di Spiezio Sardo A, Florio P, Nazzaro G, et al. Hysteroscopic outpatient metroplasty to expand dysmorphic uteri (HOME-DU technique): a pilot study. Reprod Biomed Online. 2015;30(2):166-74.

CHAPTER

78

Gynecological Cancers and Fertility: The Way Forward

Puneet Rana Arora, Aarthi Maini, Lovy Arora, Megha Malik Aneja

INTRODUCTION

Gynecological cancers are a collective term used for cancers involving the female reproductive system—ovaries, fallopian tubes, uterus, cervix, vagina, and vulva. Cancers of fallopian tube and vulva are relatively rare as compared to the other gynecological cancers.

More than 90% of cases of endometrial cancer occur in women above 50 years of age, with a median age at diagnosis of 63 years. Although it is primarily a disease of postmenopausal women, 25% are premenopausal and 3–5% are under age 40. The majority of endometrial cancers are diagnosed early (80% in stage I), with 5-year survival rates of over 95%. However, 5-year survival rates are much lower if there is regional spread or distant disease (68% and 17%, respectively).[1]

Every year in India, 122,844 women are diagnosed with cervical cancer.[1] It is the second most common cancer in women aged 15–44 years. India also has the highest age standardized incidence of cervical cancer in South Asia at 22.[1]

There are four types of ovarian cancer based on the cell type of origin— epithelial, germ cell, sex-cord stromal, and metastatic. The incidence of ovarian cancer depends on the type of the cancer.

Epithelial ovarian cancer derived from coelomic epithelium or mesothelium is the most common one with an incidence of 75–80% of all ovarian cancers. It predominantly occurs in the age group of 55–60 years but the age-specific incidence rises precipitously from 20 years to 80 years of age. The subtypes of epithelial ovarian cancer are—serous type accounting for 80%, endometroid 10%, clear cell 5%, mucinous type 5%, transitional and undifferentiated 1% each.[2]

Germ cell tumors derived from primordial germ cells have an incidence of 15% and usually occur in the age group below 25 years and the common types are dysgerminoma, teratoma, endodermal sinus tumor, embryonal carcinoma, choriocarcinoma, polyembryoma, and mixed germ cell tumor.[2]

Sex cord stromal tumors are derived from sex cords and ovarian stroma or mesenchyme, can occur in any age group, and account for 5–8% of all ovarian cancers. The subtypes are granulosa-stromal cell tumors, Sertoli-Leydig cell tumors, gynandroblastoma, sex cord stromal tumors (annular, unclassified), and steroid cell tumors.[2]

Borderline ovarian tumors are lesions of low malignant potential that tends to remain confined to the ovary for long periods, occur predominantly in premenopausal women between 30 years and 50 years, with the average age being 46 years.[2]

EFFECT OF GYNECOLOGICAL CANCERS AND THEIR TREATMENT ON FERTILITY

Cancer is a condition of oxidative stress and this itself can have a negative effect on fertility. Treatment of cancer in the form of chemotherapy, radiotherapy, and surgical interventions can also affect fertility.

Chemotherapy

Chemotherapeutic drugs act by interrupting vital cell processes and arresting the normal cellular proliferation cycle. They cause DNA abnormalities as well as oxidative damage in somatic and germ cells. Persistent unrepaired DNA double-strand breaks activate apoptotic death in oocytes.[2] Follicular depletion has been shown to be physiologically age dependent, the maximum rate of depletion occurring around the age of 38 years when the reserve is just about 10% the number present at menarche. The gonadotoxic effect is, thus, not just dependent on type and dosage of the cytotoxic drug employed but also on the age of the woman.[3]

The extent of damage to the ovary depends on the type and dose of chemotherapy, the radiotherapy dose, fractionation scheme and irradiation field and on the ovarian reserve before treatment.[3] The prepubertal ovary is less susceptible to damage by chemotherapeutic agents while older women have a lower ovarian reserve and hence are more susceptible to premature ovarian failure (POF).[4] Reduction in ovarian reserve occurs because of apoptosis of the growing follicles and activation of the resting follicle with subsequent apoptosis, leading to a burn-out effect. Fibrosis of stromal blood vessels adds to the ovarian damage. The clinical manifestation of this follicular loss ranges from complete amenorrhea to premature menopause and varying degree of infertility.

Different cytotoxic drugs have different effects on the ovarian tissue (Table 1). Ovarian markers like anti-Müllerian hormone (AMH), antral follicular count (AFC), and ovarian volume are decreased in patients receiving high dose compared to conventional dose of alkylating agents.[5]

Cyclophosphamide and cisplatin impact both, primordial and preantral/antral follicles, and both, mitotic and nonmitotic granulosa cells, whereas the antimetabolite cancer drug gemcitabine is detrimental only to preantral/antral follicles and mitotic nonluteinized granulose cells.[6]

Anthracycline antibiotics such as doxorubicin (DXR) induce oxidative stress.[2]

Antimetabolites like methotrexate and 5-fluorouracil do not seem to affect the ovary based on the limited current data available.[2] Methotrexate is commonly used to treat the ectopic pregnancy without any effect on subsequent fertility.

Table 1: Type of chemotherapy and their mechanism of action

Type of chemotherapy	*Effect on cells*
Alkylating agents	Not cell cycle-specific, highest risk of ovarian failure
Antimetabolites	Impact the cells of metabolically active ovarian follicles and are low risk for gonadal dysfunction
Platinum-based chemotherapy	Cause cell death by formation of chemical cross links in DNA thus interfering with DNA replication and transcription leading to cell death
Taxanes	Affect cell structure microtubules, which play an important role in cell function

Anti-Müllerian hormone levels rapidly decline to undetectable levels in most women during chemotherapy and generally persist at very low levels in most women after completion of treatment. Taxanes seem to have a negative impact on ovarian function, but data on ovarian reserve are scarce. AMH is a predictor of the occurrence of chemotherapy-related amenorrhea and is the most relevant hormonal marker of ovarian reserve.[7]

Biological targeted therapies (herceptin, tamoxifen, rituximab) are anticancer treatments that are derived from living organisms and are designed to interfere with specific molecules expressed by tumors (herceptin or tamoxifen), or act via the immune system (rituximab). Fertility risk data for these drugs are limited, but since they target specific cells, it is believed that the risk should be low. They are generally given as adjuvant therapy for 5 or more years after cancer treatment, and this delay by itself might pose a fertility risk[6] as fertility potential declines with increasing age of women.

Radiotherapy

Effective sterilizing dose (ESD) (Fig. 1) is one, which causes POF in 97.5% of patients and it decreases with increased age at treatment. The ESD at birth is 20.3 Gray (Gy), at 10 years 18.4 Gy, at 20 years 16.5 Gy, and after 30 years of age, application of 14.3 Gy is likely to render a woman irreversibly infertile and menopausal.[4] In adults, an exposure to total body irradiation (TBI) of 12 Gy is associated with significant uterine damage.[4] Patients receiving more than 15 Gy to the ovaries develop hormone failure.[4]

The damage due to a dose of 6 Gy to the ovaries of a woman under 30 years of age is usually reversible, but ultimately, it will bring menopause forwards.[4] Thus, not only fertility but also hormone production seems to be equally affected by radiotherapy.

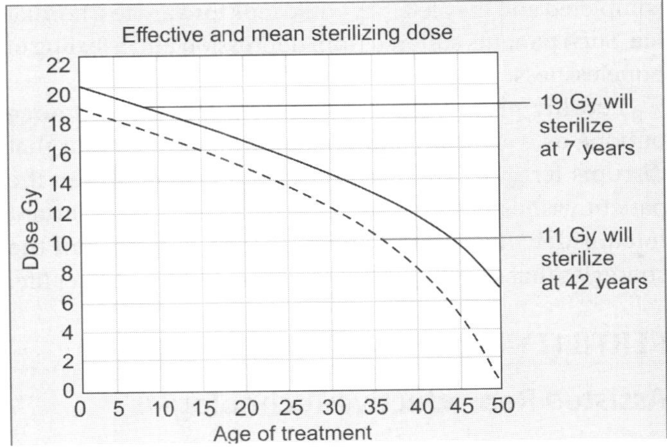

Fig. 1: Predicting age of ovarian failure after radiation to a field that includes the ovaries.[4]

Uterine irradiation will result in poor implantation.[8] This appears to be due to a number of factors including reduced uterine volume and blood flow which can lead to an increase in the risk of mid trimester losses, preterm labor, and intrauterine growth retardation. The vagina is relatively radio resistant; however, irradiation of this organ carries with it the risk of loss of lubrication and stenosis, which may result in physical impairments to fertility as well as major psychosexual issues.[9]

WHY SHOULD FERTILITY PRESERVATION BE CONSIDERED?

With significant advances in the early diagnosis of cancer and in its treatment, survival rates have highly improved and survivorship is being discussed more frequently. Cancer and its treatment can have some short- and long-term side effects. Cancer and quality of life with increased survivorship post-treatment is a big concern for some survivors. Effect on fertility is considered an important aspect of survivorship and studies suggest that women who did not have the chance to discuss about fertility or to preserve fertility prior to starting treatment for cancer were at higher risk of self-guilt and psychological issues.[10] It is imperative that fertility issues are discussed fully in the initial stages of cancer and when treatment is being planned. This gives the patient and everyone else concerned a chance to offer the patient the best options. If surgery is contemplated, a more conservative approach may be chosen by the patient. If chemotherapy and/or radiotherapy is planned, the help and advice of the fertility specialists may be sought well in time.

Many cancer survivors remain disappointed and unhappy about not having been counseled about the options for fertility preservation.[11] The regret was found to become more profound after the treatment was successfully completed and they felt they could look forward to a normal life. Such patients suffered from depression and a feeling of hopelessness.

Fertility preservation in cancer patients is a source of hope as well as an additional burden. Treatment that disrupts fertility can have a devastating effect when the patient wishes to start a family. Therefore, it is important to consider the effect of any proposed therapy and the strategies that exist to protect or restore fertility in later life.

FERTILITY PRESERVATION OPTIONS

Assisted Reproductive Technologies

For patients scheduled to undergo chemotherapy, radiotherapy, or bilateral oophorectomy, the loss of ovarian function will result in POF and permanent loss of fertility. Options available prior to these interventions are either to undergo embryo or oocyte cryopreservation.[12] Embryo cryopreservation is not suitable for children and unmarried women as it involves a male partner, unless sperm donation is acceptable. For embryo and oocyte cryopreservation, superovulation is required, which takes 12–14 days and in some cases where the treatment of cancer has to be started on an urgent basis, this is not feasible. Traditional stimulation protocols mandate start of superovulation with periods, whereas with better understanding of ovarian physiology, it is now known that there are multiple main follicle recruitment waves during the menstrual cycle and hence the concept of a narrow window of opportunity for follicle recruitment may not be accurate. Therefore, the current availability of gonadotropin-releasing hormone (GnRH) antagonists combined with the knowledge of multiple recruitment waves allows random-start controlled ovarian hyperstimulation (COH) in the late follicular or luteal phase of the menstrual cycle for embryo or oocyte cryopreservation.[13]

So far, in early stage gynecological cancers studies have been reassuring as to no increased risk of relapse with ovulation induction and subsequent pregnancies do not worsen oncological outcomes.[14]

To keep these risks to further minimum, advancements in assisted reproductive techniques have led to safer stimulation protocols. In hormone-sensitive tumors, strategies to keep estrogen levels low during COH have been used with success without compromising the outcomes of oocyte/embryo freezing. The use of aromatase-inhibitors in the ovarian stimulation protocols and of GnRH agonist as final injection to trigger ovulation is considered as safe to keep hormone's level down and to reduce the incidence of ovarian hyperstimulation syndrome (OHSS).[15]

Embryo cryopreservation is traditionally more common and has been studied extensively with regards to acceptability and safety. The American Society for Reproductive Medicine (ASRM) has recently reviewed the evidence on fertilization and pregnancy rates obtained after oocyte vitrification and warming. It has been noticed that results with frozen thawed oocytes are similar to those obtained when fresh oocytes are used in in vitro fertilization or intracytoplasmic sperm injection (IVF/ICSI) cycles and with no increase in the risk of chromosomal abnormalities, birth defects, or developmental alterations as compared to the general population.[16]Hence, cryopreservation of oocytes is an acceptable option particularly for single women aged 35 years or younger.[17] Success is also dependent on the availability of a quality controlled embryology laboratory.

Ovarian tissue cryopreservation is a promising strategy that offers the possibility to restore fertility by autotransplantation of ovarian tissue or in vitro culture and oocyte maturation.[16] It offers the advantages of enabling the storage of a large number of gametes and can be performed without the need for superovulation. It can be performed during any part of the cycle, without causing a delay in the oncological treatment, but requires laparoscopic removal of ovarian tissue for vitrification. The other advantage is the restoration of physiological ovarian function following replacement after completion of cancer treatment. It may be the only option for fertility preservation for prepubertal girls or young women with estrogen-sensitive cancers. However, it is assumed that autografting cryopreserved-thawed ovarian cortical tissue may pose a risk of reseeding the malignancy in some cancers.

Autotransplantation of ovarian tissue has yielded around 60 live births to date, including one from tissue that was cryopreserved in adolescence.[16] Ovarian tissue cryopreservation and subsequent transplantation, at present, is recommended only as an experimental protocol and to be used in carefully selected patients. It should not be offered to those who wish to delay pregnancy for social reasons, in benign conditions, or in situations where there is a potential risk of reintroducing malignancy.

Another novel approach for minimizing the gonadotoxic effect of chemotherapy is the use of GnRHa or oral contraceptives (OC) to stop the maturation of the dividing oocyte, leading to its involution and thus avoiding the noxious effect of chemotherapy on the dividing cell.[18] Possible mechanisms of action include reduction of the number of primordial follicles entering the differentiation stage, diminished ovarian perfusion and delivery of chemotherapy to the ovaries, and may be a direct effect with upregulation of an intragonadal anti-apoptotic molecule. There are still incidences of POF in patients who received GnRHa. There is absence of conclusive evidence regarding the safety and efficacy of GnRHa treatment.

Fertility Sparing Options: Surgical Aspect

Cervical Cancer

Fertility sparing option in early stage cervical cancer [stage Ia1 with or without lymphovascular space invasion (LVSI)] is conization with or without pelvic lymphadenectomy or simple/radical trachelectomy (robotic/laparoscopic/abdominal/vaginal) with pelvic lymphadenectomy. In patients for whom radiotherapy is advised postoperatively or as prime treatment, ovarian transposition (OT) should be considered and discussed. Ovarian transposition can reduce the risk of radiation exposure to the ovary by approximately 50–90%. Success of OT in maintaining ovarian function falls between 30% and 50%.[19]

Radical trachelectomy is a safe and feasible option for young women with early stage cervical cancer. But the size of the tumor is a limitation for this procedure. Tumor size larger than 2 cm is a high-risk factor for recurrence.[19] Hence, many young patients with early stage cervical cancer lose their opportunity for fertility preservation if their tumor is larger than 2 cm. Cervical cancer is a chemotherapy sensitive tumor and use of neoadjuvant chemotherapy is being considered to reducetum or size before trachelectomy. If neoadjuvant chemotherapy is used, it will mandate the discussion and use of fertility preservation options prior to using neoadjuvant chemotherapy.

Ovarian Cancer

The primary surgical treatment for stage I epithelial ovarian cancer is total abdominal hysterectomy, bilateral salpingo-oophorectomy, and surgical staging. For patients who undergo a thorough staging laparotomy and who have no evidence of spread beyond the ovary, abdominal hysterectomy and bilateral salpingo-oophorectomy are appropriate therapy. The uterus and the contralateral ovary can be preserved in women with stage IA, grade 1 to 2 disease who desire to preserve fertility. Patients who have a poorly differentiated disease or who have malignant cells, either in ascitic fluid or in peritoneal washings, must undergo complete surgical staging.

For advanced stage disease, if the patient is medically stable, cytoreductive surgery to remove as much of the tumor and its metastases as recommended. In cases of stage IIIc/IV disease, neoadjuvant chemotherapy may be given, followed by interval cytoreductive surgery after three cycles. Patients with high-grade, high-risk stage I epithelial ovarian cancer are given adjuvant chemotherapy. The type of chemotherapy depends on the patient's overall health and medical comorbidities. Treatment with carboplatin and paclitaxel for three to six cycles is used in these patients, whereas single agent carboplatin may be preferable for older women and patients with other medical comorbidities. Combination chemotherapy or intravenous carboplatin and paclitaxel or intraperitoneal cisplatin and paclitaxel (using the GOG 172 protocol) are the treatments of choice for patients with advanced disease. Whole abdominal radiation therapy is given as a treatment for recurrent or persistent disease.

Over the last 30 years, there has been a significant improvement in the 5-year survival rate for ovarian cancer. The overall survival rate, however, is still low at 46%.

Prognosis is closely related to the stage at diagnosis as determined by the staging system developed by FIGO.

The 5-year survival rate for epithelial ovarian carcinoma stage I–II is 55–90%; hence, fertility preservation options should be discussed and taken forward where clinically possible.

Endometrial Cancer

Endometrial cancer (EEC) is often diagnosed at endometrial biopsy or D&C in symptomatic women. Diagnosis is often followed by advanced imaging modalities and surgery to treat and stage the cancer.[20]

The standard treatment for endometrioid carcinoma includes staging laparotomy, total abdominal hysterectomy, and bilateral salpingo-oophorectomy with pelvic washing and lymph node sampling when appropriate. The 5-year survival rate after this approach is approximately 94%.[21]

The tissues removed at surgery are examined under a microscope to see how far the cancer has spread (the stage). For women with advanced cancer, or for those who are medically unfit for surgery, adjuvant treatments, such as radiation and/or chemotherapy may be recommended.

The reason for removal of adnexa is to prevent ovarian cancer and to rule out ovarian metastasis. If the woman has undergone fertility preservation options in the form of oocyte/embryo cryopreservation or ovarian tissue cryopreservation prior to surgery, future pregnancy will require surrogacy.

Preserving fertility can be considered in patients younger than 45 years with grade 1 EEC with myometrial invasion G50% and with no obvious ovarian or other extrauterine disease. Fertility sparing strategies should be offered to women with:[22]

- Grade 1 well-differentiated tumor
- Absence of lymphovascular space invasion (LVSI) on adequate curettage specimen
- No evidence of myometrial invasion on MRI
- No evidence of metastatic disease on CT imaging
- No evidence of a suspicious adnexal mass on CT or TVUS, and
- Strong and diffuse immunohistochemical expression of progesterone receptors on endometrial biopsy or curettage specimen.

Conservative management of endometrial carcinoma offers response rate of around 75%,[22] but recurrence rates can be 30–40%. Standard surgery with hysterectomy should be proposed to nonresponders. Maintenance treatment for a further 6 months can be considered in those who wish to delay pregnancy.[22,23]

Besides offering fertility preserving options in the form of fertility sparing surgeries, other options for preserving fertility in endometrial cancer are hormonal methods. Patients should be extensively counseled regarding potential risks as no scientifically proven optimal progestin regimen exists. Response to treatment may vary depending on tumor receptor status, ranging from 26% to 89% in estrogen and progesterone positive tumors but as low as 8–17% when these receptors are absent.[22] Conservative management of endometrial carcinoma is based on medical treatment with oral progestins mainly in the form of medroxyprogesterone acetate (MPA; 400–600 mg/day) or megestrol acetate (MA; 160–320 mg/day), and also levonogestral-releasing intrauterine device (LNG-IUD) with or without GnRH analogs. Other hormonal agents to consider after progestins include tamoxifen, fulvestrant, and aromatase inhibitors.

Selection of women suitable for such conservative treatment is a crucial part of management and should be done in discussion with gynecologist, oncologist, and fertility specialist. Importance of regular follow-up, evaluation for recurrence, obstetrical outcomes, and survival rates are vital parameters to be discussed when counseling these women. The stage of the tumor and histological grade of the tumor are important factors in predicting patients' outcome as it determines the mode of treatment which in turn significantly influences survival.

The initial stage should be confirmed by enhanced pelvic MRI to exclude overt myometrial invasion, as well as adnexal or pelvic nodes involvement. When inconclusive, laparoscopic exploration should be done before initiating conservative treatment.

Patient counseling needs to be emphasized that this is a nonstandard approach and they should be well prepared for close follow-up during and after the treatment. There is always a need for future hysterectomy in case of failure of the treatment and/or after pregnancies.

Pregnancy is not associated with an increased risk for endometrial cancer recurrence.[23] For patients achieving a complete response at 6 months, conception must be encouraged and these patients should be referred to a fertility clinic. After completion of childbearing (or after the age of potential pregnancy), standard treatment with hysterectomy and salpingo-oophorectomy is recommended.

RISK GROUPS FOR GYNECOLOGICAL CANCERS AND CONSIDERATION FOR FERTILITY COUNSELING

Advancements in the management of gynecological cancers have led to increased recognition of the risk factors associated with these cancers. Fertility-related counseling also should be an integral part when seeing such group of women.[24,25]

Obesity, nulliparity, polycystic ovarian syndrome associated with prolonged amenorrhea, early menarche, late menopause, and history of infertility itself are risk factors for endometrial cancer. Careful counseling of these women for timely planning of pregnancies is advised.[26]

Lynch syndrome or hereditary nonpolyposis colorectal cancer syndrome (HNPCC) is an autosomal dominant inherited disorder caused by germline mutations in DNA mismatch repair: MLH1, MSH2, MSH6, or PMS2 having up to a 40–60% lifetime risk of developing both endometrial and colorectal cancers.[27] Women with an HNPCC-associated mutation or with a family history of mutation or colon cancer should be annually screened beginning at age 35 due to the high risk of endometrial cancer and the potentially life-threatening nature of this disease. They should be encouraged to preserve their fertility or achieve conception by age of 35.[26,27]

Most epithelial ovarian cancer is sporadic, with familial or hereditary causes accounting for 5–10% of invasive epithelial ovarian cancer.[2] Hereditary ovarian cancers occur in women approximately 10 years younger than those with nonhereditary tumor. These kind of ovarian cancers are generally associated with mutations in the *BRCA1* gene, located on chromosome 17. A small proportion of inherited disease is associated with germline mutations in another gene, *BRCA2*, located on chromosome 13.

A mutation in the *BRCA1* or *BRCA2* gene is associated with an increased risk of developing ovarian cancer.[28] A woman with a *BRCA1* mutation has 54% lifetime risk of ovarian cancer and with a *BRCA2* mutation, it is 23%. If there is a history of two first degree relatives with premenopausal epithelial ovarian cancer, the risk of ovarian cancer is 35–40%, with one first degree relative and one second degree relative, the risk is increased 2–10-fold as compared to anyone without family history.

CONCLUSION

Addressing the fertility concerns of women diagnosed with gynecological cancer is important and requires a multi disciplinary approach in coordination with a fertility specialist. It is important to consider following aspects before offering any fertility preserving modality or option:

- Cancer prognosis, 5-year survival rate, and expected quality of life
- Fertility and obstetrical history and potential
- Availability and reliability of the FP technologies
- Surgical modalities and expertise
- Medical and laboratory modalities
- Detailed patient counseling with regards to success of surgery and probability of success of fertility preservation options if applied
- Psychosocial perspective
- Couple counseling
- Obtaining informed consent.

REFERENCES

1. WHO. GLOBOCAN 2012: Estimated cancer incidence, mortality and prevalence worldwide in 2012. Available from http://globocan.iarc.fr/Pages/fact_sheets_ population.aspx [Accessed Oct. 2017].
2. Berek JA. Berecks and Novoks Text Book of Gynaecology, 15th edition. USA: Lippincott Williams and Wilkins; 2011.
3. Meirow D, Biederman H, Anderson RA, et al. Toxicity of chemotherapy and radiation on female reproduction. Clin Obstet Gynecol. 2010;53:727-39.
4. Wallace WH, Thomson AB, Saran F, et al. Predicting age of ovarian failure after radiation to a field that includes the ovaries. Int J Radiat Oncol Biol Phys. 2005;62:738-44.
5. Thomas-Teinturier C, Allodji RS, Svetlova E, et al. Ovarian reserve after treatment with alkylating agents during childhood. Hum Reprod. 2015;30:1437-46.
6. Yuksel A, Bildik G, Senbabaoglu F, et al. The magnitude of gonadotoxicity of chemotherapy drugs on ovarian follicles and granulosa cells varies depending upon the category of the drugs and the type of granulosa cells. Hum Reprod. 2015;30:2926-35.
7. Fréour T, Barrière P, Masson D. Anti-Müllerian hormone levels and evolution in women of reproductive age with breast cancer treated with chemotherapy. Eur J Cancer. 2017;74:1-8.
8. Critchley HO, Wallace WH. Impact of cancer treatment on uterine function. J Natl Cancer Inst Monogr. 2005;34:64-8.
9. Liao L, Doyle J, Crouch NS, et al. Dilation as treatment for vaginal agenesis and hypoplasia: a pilot exploration of benefits and barriers as perceived by patients. J Obstet Gynaecol. 2006;26:144-8.
10. Tschudin S, Bitzer J. Psychological aspects of fertility preservation in men and women affected by cancer and other life-threatening diseases. Hum Reprod Update. 2009;15:587-97.
11. Rosen A, Rodriguez-Wallberg KA, Rosenzweig L. Psychosocial distress in young cancer survivors. Semin Oncol Nurs. 2009;25:268-77.
12. Zapardiel I, Cruz M, Diestro MD, et al. Assisted reproductive techniques after fertility-sparing treatments in gynaecological cancers. Hum Reprod Update. 2016;22:281-305.
13. Keskin U, Ercan CM, Yilmaz A, et al. Random-start controlled ovarian hyperstimulation with letrozole for fertility preservation in cancer patients: case series and review of literature. J Pak Med Assoc. 2014;64:830-2.
14. Fujimoto A, Ichinose M, Harada M, et al. The outcome of infertility treatment in patients undergoing assisted

reproductive technology after conservative therapy for endometrial cancer. J Assist Reprod Genet. 2014;31:1189-94.
15. Noyes N, Knopman JM, Long K, et al. Fertility considerations in the management of gynecologic malignancies. Gynecol Oncol. 2011;120:326-33.
16. Donnez J, Dolmans MM, Pellicer A, et al. Restoration of ovarian activity and pregnancy after transplantation of cryopreserved ovarian tissue: a review of 60 cases of reimplantation. Fertil Steril. 2013;99:1503-13.
17. Cobo A, Diaz C. Clinical application of oocyte vitrification: a systematic review and meta-analysis of randomized controlled trials. Fertil Steril. 2011; 96:277-85.
18. Blumenfeld Z, von Wolff M. GnRH-analogues and oral contraceptives for fertility preservation in women during chemotherapy. Hum Reprod Update. 2008;14:543-52.
19. Morice P, Juncker L, Rey A, et al. Ovarian transposition for patients with cervical carcinoma treated by radio-surgical combination. Fertil Steril. 2000;74:743-8.
20. Plante M, Renaud MC, François H, et al. Vaginal radical trachelectomy: an oncologically safe fertility preserving surgery. An updated series of 72 cases and review of the literature. Gynecologic Oncol. 2004;94:614-23.
21. Bakkum-Gamez JN, Gonzalez-Bosquet J, Laack NN, et al. Current issues in the management of endometrial cancer. Mayo Clin Proc. 2008;83:97-11.
22. Eskander RN, Randall LM, Berman ML, et al. Fertility preserving options in patients with gynecologic malignancies. Am J Obstet Gynecol. 2011;205:103-10.
23. Gallos ID, Yap J, Rajkhowa M, et al. Regression, relapse, and live birth rates with fertility-sparing therapy for endometrial cancer and atypical complex endometrial hyperplasia: a systematic review and metaanalysis. Am J Obstet Gynecol. 2012;207:266.e1-12.
24. Rodolakis A, Biliatis I, Morice P, et al. European Society of Gynecological Oncology Task Force for Fertility Preservation: Clinical Recommendations for Fertility-Sparing Management in Young Endometrial Cancer Patients. Int J Gynecol Cancer. 2015;25:1258-65.
25. Hahn HS, Yoon SG, Hong JS. Conservative treatment with progestin and pregnancy outcomes in endometrial cancer. Int J Gynecol Cancer. 2009;19: 1068-73.
26. Luo J, Beresford S, Chen C, etal. Association between diabetes, diabetestreatment and risk of developing endometrial cancer. Br J Cancer. 2014;111:1432-9.
27. Vasen HF, Blanco I, Aktan-Collan K, et al. Revised guidelines for the clinical management of Lynch syndrome (HNPCC): recommendations by a group of European experts. Gut. 2013;62:812-23.
28. Pan Z, Xie X. BRCA mutations in the manifestation and treatment of ovarian cancer. Oncotarget. 2017. In press.

Section 8

Miscellaneous

CHAPTER
79

Reproduction and Immunology

Diana Alecsandru, Juan Antonio Garcia Velasco

INTRODUCTION

Chromosome screening and fresh embryo transfer significantly increase in vitro fertilization (IVF) implantation and delivery rates, but we still lose euploid embryos.[1]

What happens to those embryos? Other factors, not just embryo aneuploidies, might contribute to implantation failure or miscarriage, such as endometrial factors, hydrosalpinges, infections, or immune maternal tolerance to pregnancy. The role of the immune system in recurrent miscarriage (RM) and recurrent implantation failure (RIF) is less known. As we know, maternal tolerance begins at the uterine level, and successful adaptation to the semiallogeneic fetus is more complicated than the initially suggested concept led us to believe.

Some reports[2] have presented an overview, for example, that peripheral blood natural killer (pbNK) and uterine natural killer (uNK) cells merge together with the simple "natural killer (NK) cells" marker as the "main immune cells at the maternal–fetal interface."[3] But pbNK cells and uNK cells are completely different types of immune cells. The number and functions of pbNK and uNK cells show wide variability depending on the patient's clinical condition, e.g. infections, autoimmunity or tumor, day of menstrual cycle, stress, time of day, exercise, etc. and is very difficult to quantify.

The fetal cells[4] that come into direct contact with the mother's immune system in the uterus are trophoblast cells, the layer that surrounds the blastocyst, and the mother's uterine immune system is dominated by uNK cells. CD56(bright)CD16$^-$ is the most abundant leukocyte population during the first trimester of human pregnancy.[5,6]

The key to the maternal–fetal tolerance process is the remodeling of the spiral arteries, with the destruction of the decidua by invading extravillous trophoblast (EVT) cells. The EVTs that invade the maternal decidua are of fetal origin, and express high levels of human leukocyte antigen-C (HLA-C) that is recognized by uNK KIRs (killer-cell immunoglobulin-like receptors). Maternal and paternal HLA-C allotypes are expressed at the same time and at high levels on the EVT cell surface.[7,8]

Placentation is regulated by interactions between maternal KIRs, expressed by uNKs, and fetal HLA-C molecules, expressed by EVTs. Insufficient invasion of the uterine lining by trophoblasts and vascular conversion in the decidua are thought to be the primary defect in disorders such as RM, preeclampsia, and fetal growth restriction (FGR).[7,9] This process is regulated by the interaction between maternal KIRs, expressed by the uNKs, and their ligand HLA-C, expressed by EVTs. Pregnancies are at increased risk of RM, preeclampsia, or FGR in mothers who are homozygous for KIR haplotype A (KIR AA), when the fetus has more *HLA-C2* genes than the mother and when additional fetal HLA-C2 alleles are of paternal origin. Thus, depending on the particular KIR–HLA-C interaction, is trophoblast cell invasion regulated. Thus, trophoblast cell invasion is regulated by the particular KIR-HLA-C interactions.[10,11]

SECTION

Maternal and fetal circulations do not mix, although a transient exchange of cells occurs, particularly during the trauma of delivery. Successful maternal adaptation to the semiallogeneic fetus occurs in the uterus at the site of placentation.[12] EVT cells express class I HLA-C and nonclassic HLA-G and HLA-E antigens, whereas class I antigens, HLA-A and HLA-B, and class II antigens are absent.[5,7,13] The villous trophoblast bathed in maternal blood is entirely HLA null. Nevertheless, HLA-E and HLA-G are oligomorphic, the HLA-C molecules expressed by EVT cells are polymorphic, and ligands for KIRs are expressed by uNK cells.[14] KIRs are the most variable receptors in uNKs, with diversity in gene number between individuals and allelic diversity at individual KIR loci.[15] Both polymorphic maternal KIRs and fetal HLA-C molecules are variable and specific to a particular pregnancy. In any pregnancy, the maternal KIR genotype could be AA (nonactivating KIRs), AB, or BB (one to ten activating KIRs). The HLA-C ligands for KIRs are divided into two groups: (1) HLA-C1, and (2) HLA-C2. Of these two, C2 is a stronger ligand than C1. KIR A haplotypes contain mainly genes for inhibitory KIR, and KIR B haplotypes have additional genes that encode activating KIR. Presence of activating KIR2DS1 (B haplotype)[16] confers protection from pregnancy disorders, and its absence (A haplotype) increases the risk of pregnancy complications. A similar protective effect has been recently described for another activating receptor, KIR2DS4, when carried together with KIR2DS1. Similarly to KIR2DS1, the triggering of KIR2DS4 to uNK cells leads to the secretion of granulocyte-macrophage colony-stimulating factor and other chemokines known to promote placental trophoblast invasion. Hiby et al.[10,11] showed that invading EVTs are the principal site of HLA-C expression in the decidua basalis, and that both maternal and paternal HLA-C allotypes are presented to KIRs. Insufficient invasion of the uterine lining by trophoblasts and vascular conversion in the decidua are thought to be the primary defect in disorders such as RM, preeclampsia, and FGR. This process is regulated by the interaction between maternal KIRs, expressed by the uNKs, and their ligand HLA-C, expressed by EVTs. Pregnancies are at increased risk of RM, preeclampsia, or FGR in mothers who are homozygous for KIR haplotype A (KIR AA), when the fetus has more HLA-C2 genes than the mother and when additional fetal HLA-C2 alleles are of paternal origin.[17] Protection from preeclampsia is likely mediated by activating KIR2DS1 (B haplotype), which also binds HLA-C2.

Hiby et al. and Faridi and Agrawal have reported differences in the outcomes of medically unassisted pregnancies, increased risk of RM, preeclampsia, and FGR, in mothers with KIR AA who carry a fetus with paternal HLA-C2. These findings suggest that placentation is deficient when a very strong inhibitory signal to uNK cells mediated by the KIR A haplotype gene exists. Hiby et al. performed larger cohort studies that analyzed both maternal and paternal genotypes along with a large control group. They demonstrated a clear difference between the KIR and HLA-C genotypes in patients with disorders such as RM, preeclampsia,[11] and FGR. Epidemiological studies have provided clear evidence that selection for human reproductive success has adapted to KIR and HLA-C genes and can be responsible for maintaining balanced polymorphisms between the HLA-C1 and HLA-C2 groups and the KIR A and B haplotypes.[18]

However, What Happens in ART?

Assisted pregnancies differ from medically unassisted pregnancies because the patients often receive more than one embryo per transfer; and donor oocytes, sperm, or embryos also are often used. After double-embryo transfer (DET), the expression of more than one paternal HLA-C per trophoblast cell is induced. In oocyte-donation cycles, which are increasingly demanded owing to advanced maternal age; oocyte-maternal HLA-C, which is genetically different from the mother's receptor, behaves as a paternal HLA-C. This implies that more nonself HLA antigens are presented to the maternal KIR per transfer compared with "normal" pregnancies. After DET in an oocyte-donation cycle, the expression of two nonself or "paternal" HLA-Cs in the EVTs per embryo is present in the decidua basalis. The presentation of trophoblast antigens (HLA-C) to uNK KIRs happens much more frequently than in natural pregnancies, because embryo transfer (ET) can be performed monthly in RIF patients. In human population, pregnancy disorders are predicted to reduce the frequency of KIR A, HLA-C2, or both; and this selection is thought to have originated during human evolution. An inverse correlation between frequencies of KIR AA and HLA-C2 has observed. Population with the highest KIR AA frequency (Japanese and Koreans) present the lowest HLA-C2 frequencies, whereas population with the lowest KIR AA frequency (aboriginal Australians and Asian Indians) have the highest HLA-C2 frequencies.[18,19] Natural selection seems to have driven an allele-level KIR A haplotype and HLA-C1 ligand to an unusually high frequency in Japanese and Koreans, because the detrimental KIR AA-HLA-C2 combination does not significantly affect pregnancy outcomes in those population. This correlation provides evidence that selection for human reproductive success has adapted to the KIR and HLA-C genes and can be responsible for maintaining balanced polymorphisms between the HLA-C1[20] and HLA-C2 groups and the A and B KIR haplotypes. However, this natural human evolution is not currently taken into account during assisted reproductive technology (ART). Furthermore, donor oocytes are often used in ART, and the literature describes higher maternal morbidity[21] (pregnancy-induced hypertension, 25% for preeclampsia,

FGR)[22] and preterm birth in oocyte donation pregnancies compared with ART pregnancies with own oocytes.[23] Although part of this increased frequency of complications may be due to the main indication for oocyte donation, which is advanced maternal age; recent age-matched data have confirmed this higher frequency of undesired events in young patients; and immunology maladaptation could be the reason.[24] Increased paternal HLA-C expression after DET could be associated with more pregnancy disorders than single embryo transfer (SET) in mothers with an inhibitory KIR haplotype (AA). A recent study has analyzed the pregnancy, miscarriage, and live birth rate (LBR) per cycle according to KIR haplotype, categorized by DET or SET.[25] A higher early miscarriage rate after DET when the patient's own oocytes were used occurred in those with KIR AA (22.8%), followed by those with KIR AB (16.7%), compared with mothers with KIR BB (11.1%; $p < 0.03$). A significantly decreased LBR per cycle after DET with the use of donated oocytes was observed in mothers with KIR AA (7.5%) compared with those with KIR AB (26.4%) and KIR BB (21.5%; $p < 0.006$). The lower LBR after DET in donor-oocyte cycles in KIR AA mothers may be due to an increased expression of nonself HLA-C (paternal and oocyte donor HLA-C). in this case four "paternal" HLA-Cs per trophoblast cell per DET are expressed. One paternal and one oocyte-donor HLA-C per trophoblast cell and embryo because oocyte-donor HLA-C behaves as "paternal" non-self HLA-C. Expressing four "paternal" HLA-Cs is more likely to find at least one paternal or oocyte-donor HLA-C2 (by allelic frequency) than in own oocytes and SET, and implantation or placentation failure is more likely to occur in KIR AA mothers.[25-27]

No other report has studied the impact of KIR-HLA-C on donor-oocyte cycles. The authors speculated that completing a normal pregnancy was possible only for mothers with the KIR AA haplotype who carried a baby with at least one nonself HLA-C1. Another recent study has reported that the proportion of pregnancies that ends in loss is significantly higher in KIR AA patients when a C2C2 euploid embryo is transferred than when C1C1 or C1C2 embryos are transferred (33% vs. 12.3% vs. 14.1%, respectively; $p < 0.01$).[28] These new findings show that maternal KIR haplotype and fetal HLA-C have an impact on LBR after IVF cycles, especially when donor oocytes and DET are used. Expressing four paternal HLA-Cs in EVT cells after DET with the use of donor oocytes is more likely to result in at least one nonself HLA-C2 (even with the HLA-C2 allelic frequency in a white population) than with the use of one's own oocytes after SET.[29] Therefore, selecting HLA-C1 among oocyte and/or sperm donors for patients who undergo oocyte donation and who express inhibitory KIR haplotypes can be more efficient and safer. The authors assume that it is a small sample and that it is the first report to observe differences in LBR according to oocyte donor HLA-C in KIR AA mothers with HLA-C2 partners. Apart from statistical significance, the association strength is noticeably high, which confers greater confidence to the findings. However, larger studies are needed and should be replicated by other groups before finally accepting and applying this theory to routine clinical practice. A new concept is emerging as evidence indicates important physiological roles for uNK cells in healthy placentation as well as for abnormal uNK cell function in pregnancy disorders. The combination of maternal KIR haplotype and parental/donor HLA-C could predict which couples could benefit from SET versus DET or from donor selection according to HLA-C to increase the LBR per cycle and would help to reduce the number of embryos transferred by facilitating the increase in elective SET. Therefore, selecting HLA-C1 among oocyte and/or sperm donors for patients who undergo oocyte donation ART and inhibitory KIR can be more efficient and safer, as epidemiologic studies have identified.[30,31]

REFERENCES

1. Scott RT Jr, Upham KM, Forman EJ, Hong KH, Scott KL, Taylor D, et al. Blastocyst biopsy with comprehensive chromosome screening and fresh embryo transfer significantly increases in vitro fertilization implantation and delivery rates: a randomized controlled trial. Fertil Steril 2013;100:697–703.
2. Tang AW, Alfirevic Z, Quenby S. Natural killer cells and pregnancy outcomes in women with recurrent miscarriage and infertility: a systematic review. Hum Reprod. 2011;26(8):1971-80.
3. Sacks G. Enough! Stop the arguments and get on with the science of natural killer cell testing. Hum Reprod. Jul;30(7):1526-31.
4. Horowitz A, Strauss-Albee DM, Leipold M, et al. Genetic and environmental determinants of human NK cell diversity revealed by mass cytometry. Sci Transl Med. 2013;5(208):208ra145.
5. Caligiuri MA. Human natural killer cells. Blood. 2008;112(3):461-9.
6. Cristiani CM, Palella E, Sottile R, et al. Human NK cell subsets in pregnancy and disease: toward a new biological complexity. Front Immunol. 2017;7:656.
7. King A, Hiby SE, Gardner L, Joseph S, Bowen JM, Verma S, et al. Recognition of trophoblast HLA class I molecules by decidual NK cell receptors—a review. Placenta 2000;21(Suppl A):S81–5.
8. Apps R, Murphy SP, Fernando R, Gardner L, Ahad T, Moffett A. Human leucocyte antigen (HLA) expression of primary trophoblast cells and placental cell lines, determined using single antigen beads to characterize allotype specificities of anti-HLA antibodies. Immunology 2009;127:26–39.
9. Koopman LA, Kopcow HD, Rybalov B, et al. Human decidual natural killer cells are a unique NK cell subset with immunomodulatory potential. J Exp Med. 2003;198(8):1201-12.
10. Hiby SE, Regan L, Lo W, Farrell L, Carrington M, Moffett A. Association of maternal killer-cell immunoglobulin-like

receptors and parental HLA-C genotypes with recurrent miscarriage. Hum Reprod. 2008 Apr;23(4):972-6.
11. Hiby SE, Walker JJ, O'Shaughnessy K M, Redman CW, Carrington M, Trowsdale J, et al. Combinations of maternal KIR and fetal HLA-C genes influence the risk of preeclampsia and reproductive success. J Exp Med. 2004 Oct 18;200(8):957-65.
12. Arck PC, Hecher K. Fetomaternal immune cross-talk and its consequences for maternal and offspring's health. Nat Med. 2013;19(5):548-56.
13. King A, Birkby C, Loke YW. Early human decidual cells exhibit NK activity against the K562 cell line but not against first trimester trophoblast. Cell Immunol. 1989;118(2):337-44.
14. Apps R, Murphy SP, Fernando R, et al. Human leucocyte antigen (HLA) expression of primary trophoblast cells and placental cell lines, determined using single antigen beads to characterize allotype specificities of anti-HLA antibodies. Immunology. 2009;127(1):26-39.
15. Uhrberg M, Valiante NM, Shum BP, et al. Human diversity in killer cell inhibitory receptor genes. Immunity. 1997;7(6):753-63.
16. Xiong S, Sharkey AM, Kennedy PR, et al. Maternal uterine NK cell-activating receptor KIR2DS1 enhances placentation. J Clin Invest. 2013;123(10):4264-72.
17. Winter CC, Gumperz JE, Parham P, Long EO, agtmann N. Direct binding and functional transfer of NK cell inhibitory receptors reveal novel patterns of HLA-C allotype recognition. J Immunol 1998;161:571–7.
18. Parham P, Moffett A. Variable NK cell receptors and their MHC class I ligands in immunity, reproduction and human evolution. Nat Rev Immunol. 2013;13(2):133-44.
19. Parham P. NK cells and trophoblasts: partners in pregnancy. J Exp Med. 2004;200(8):951-5.
20. Moffett A, Chazara O, Colucci F, et al. Variation of maternal KIR and fetal HLA-C genes in reproductive failure: too early for clinical intervention. Reprod Biomed Online. 2016;33(6):763-9.
21. Savasi VM, Mandia L, Laoreti A, et al. Maternal and fetal outcomes in oocyte donation pregnancies. Hum Reprod Update. 2016;22(5):620-33.
22. Levron Y, Dviri M, Segol I, et al. The 'immunologic theory' of preeclampsia revisited: a lesson from donor oocyte gestations. Am J Obstet Gynecol. 2014;211(4):383.e1-5.
23. Blazquez A, Garcia D, Rodriguez A, et al. Is oocyte donation a risk factor for preeclampsia? A systematic review and meta-analysis. J Assist Reprod Genet. 2016;33(7):855-63.
24. Masoudian P, Nasr A, de Nanassy J, et al. Oocyte donation pregnancies and the risk of preeclampsia or gestational hypertension: a systematic review and metaanalysis. Am J Obstet Gynecol. 2015;214(3):328-39.
25. Alecsandru D, Aparicio P, Aparicio M, et al. Maternal killer-cell immunoglobulin-like receptor (KIR) and fetal HLA-C compatibility in ART—oocyte donor influences live birth rate. ESHRE, 2016. [online] Available from http://www.madrid.org/cs/Satellite?blobcol=urldata&blobheader=application%2Fpdf&blobheadername1=Content-disposition&blobheadername2=cadena&blobheadervalue1=filename%3DInmunogenetica+Pre-eclampsia.pdf&blobheadervalue2=language%3Des%26site%3D Hospital12Octubre&blobkey=id&blobtable=MungoBlobs&blob where=1352923019463&ssbinary=true [Accessed January, 2019].
26. Alecsandru D, Garcia-Velasco JA. Immune testing and treatment: still an open debate. Hum Reprod. 2015;30(8):1994.
27. Alecsandru D, Garcia-Velasco JA. Immunology and human reproduction. Curr Opin Obstet Gynecol. 2015;27(3):231-4.
28. Morin SJ, Treff NR, Tao X, et al. Combination of uterine natural killer cell immunoglobulin receptor haplotype and trophoblastic HLA-C ligand influences the risk of pregnancy loss: a retrospective cohort analysis of direct embryo genotyping data from euploid transfers. Fertil Steril. 2017;107(3):677-83.e2.
29. Fertility and Sterility 2017.Why natural killer cells are not enough: a further understanding of killer immunoglobulin-like receptor and human leukocyte antigen Diana Alecsandru, M.D., Ph.D. and Juan A. García-Velasco, M.D., Ph.D.
30. Hiby SE, Apps R, Sharkey AM, Farrell LE, Gardner L, Mulder A, et al. Maternal activating KIRs protect against human reproductive failure mediated by fetal HLA-C2. J Clin Invest. Nov;120(11):4102-10.
31. Skjaerven R, Vatten LJ, Wilcox AJ, Ronning T, Irgens LM, Lie RT. Recurrence of pre-eclampsia across generations: exploring fetal and maternal genetic components in a population based cohort. BMJ 2005;331:877.

SUGGESTED READING

32. Alecsandru D, Garrido N, Vicario JL, et al. Maternal KIR haplotype influences live birth rate after double embryo transfer in IVF cycles in patients with recurrent miscarriages and implantation failure. Hum Reprod. 2014;29(12):2637-43.
33. Faridi RM, Agrawal S. Killer immunoglobulin-like receptors (KIRs) and HLA-C allorecognition patterns implicative of dominant activation of natural killer cells contribute to recurrent miscarriages. Hum Reprod. 2011;26(2):491-7.
34. Hiby SE, Apps R, Chazara O, et al. Maternal KIR in combination with paternal HLA-C2 regulate human birth weight. J Immunol. 2014;192(11):5069-73.
35. Hiby SE, Apps R, SharkeyAM, Farrell LE, Gardner L, Mulder A, et al.Maternal activating KIRs protect against human reproductive failure mediated by fetal HLA-C2. J Clin Invest 2010;120:4102–10.
36. Hiby SE, Ashrafian-Bonab M, Farrell L, et al. Distribution of killer cell immunoglobulin-like receptors (KIR) and their HLA-C ligands in two Iranian populations. Immunogenetics. 2010;62(2):65-73.
37. Hiby SE, Regan L, Lo W, Farrell L, Carrington M, Moffett A. Association of maternal killer-cell immunoglobulin-like receptors and parental HLA-C genotypes with recurrent miscarriage. Hum Reprod 2008;23:972–6.
38. Hiby SE, Walker JJ, O'Shaughnessy KM, et al. Combinations of maternal KIR and fetal HLA-C genes influence the risk of preeclampsia and reproductive success. J Exp Med. 2004;200(8):957-65.
39. Hiby SE, Walker JJ, O'Shaughnessy KM, Redman CW, Carrington M, Trowsdale J, et al. Combinations of maternal KIR and fetal HLA-C genes influence the risk of preeclampsia and reproductive success. J Exp Med 2004;200:957–65.

40. Jeve YB, Potdar N, Opoku A, et al. Three-arm age-matched retrospective cohort study of obstetric outcomes of donor oocyte pregnancies. Int J Gynaecol Obstet. 2016;133(2):156-8.
41. King A, Balendran N, Wooding P, et al. CD3-leukocytes present in the human uterus during early placentation: phenotypic and morphologic characterization of the CD56++ population. Dev Immunol. 1991;1(3):169-90.
42. King A, Hiby SE, Gardner L, et al. Recognition of trophoblast HLA class I molecules by decidual NK cell receptors—a review. Placenta. 2000;21(Suppl A):S81-5.
43. Moffett-King A. Natural killer cells and pregnancy. Nat Rev Immunol. 2002;2(9):656-63.
44. Moffett A, Colucci F. Co-evolution of NK receptors and HLA ligands in humans is driven by reproduction. Immunol Rev. 2015;267(1):283-97.
45. Moffett A, Colucci F. Uterine NK cells: active regulators at the maternal-fetal interface. J Clin Invest. 2014;124(5):1872-9.
46. Moffett A, Loke C. Immunology of placentation in eutherian mammals. Nat Rev Immunol. 2006;6(8):584-94.
47. Moffett A, Loke C. Implantation, embryo-maternal interactions, immunology and modulation of the uterine environment—a workshop report. Placenta. 2006;27(Suppl A):S54-5.
48. Moffett A, Shreeve N. First do no harm: uterine natural killer (NK) cells in assisted reproduction. Hum Reprod. 2015;30(7):1519-25.
49. Moffett A, Shreeve N. Reply: First do no harm: continuing the uterine NK cell debate. Hum Reprod. 2015;31(1):218-9.
50. Polanski LT, Barbosa MA, Martins WP, et al. Interventions to improve reproductive outcomes in women with elevated natural killer cells undergoing assisted reproduction techniques: a systematic review of literature. Hum Reprod. 2014;29(1):65-75.
51. Siewiera J, El Costa H, Tabiasco J, et al. Human cytomegalovirus infection elicits new decidual natural killer cell effector functions. PLoS Pathog. 2013;9(4):e1003257.
52. Skjaerven R, Vatten LJ, Wilcox AJ, et al. Recurrence of pre-eclampsia across generations: exploring fetal and maternal genetic components in a population based cohort. BMJ. 2005;331(7521):877.

CHAPTER

80

Unexplained Infertility

Aanchal Garg

INTRODUCTION

Worldwide around 12–15% couples suffer from the pain of not being able to conceive. About 15–30%[1] cases of infertility are unexplained where no definite cause can be determined. Such a diagnosis can be extremely frustrating for a couple as it fills them with the feelings of uncertainty. It is always reassuring to know that, if there is a certain problem, there may be a solution to overcome it, there is hope, but in the cases of unexplained infertility, the patient is left with doubts, hopelessness, and frustration as there is no definite cause of their infertility. Thankfully over the years there have been studies on unexplained infertility to help these patients with a working treatment plan.

The diagnosis of infertility is based on a time period in which a couple has a reasonable possibility of pregnancy. Once this does not occur, investigations are used to diagnose the obstacles to pregnancy. When diagnosed infertility is devoid of factors which can serve as barriers to conception then it can be termed unexplained infertility or subfertility.

Infertility is defined as 1 year of unwanted nonconception with unprotected intercourse in the fertile phase of the menstrual cycles.[1] The American Society for Reproductive Medicine (ASRM) has described "infertility as a disease, defined by the failure to achieve a successful pregnancy after 12 months or more of appropriately timed unprotected intercourse or therapeutic donor insemination. Earlier evaluation and treatment may be justified based on medical history and physical findings and is warranted after 6 months for women over 35 years of age."[2] The male and female factors are equally responsible for this global problem.

Unexplained infertility is one of the most fascinating challenges for reproductive medicine, which may involve undetected problems of ovarian reserve and male factor, or failure of implantation.[3] Even with the development of the investigative tools in reproductive medicine, infertility is still unexplained in around 25% of cases.[4] Unexplained infertility (also called subfertility) has been defined as the absence of a clear cause of infertility and no pregnancy after at least 12 cycles of unprotected intercourse or after 6 cycles of trying naturally in women above 35 years of age provided all the standard tests of tubal patency, ovulatory status, and semen analysis are normal.[5]

The prevalence of unexplained infertility (UI) is 6–30%. This difference is due to differences in the age of the female partner and the duration of infertility.[6] In women <35 years, it was 21% but in women >35 years it is 26%.[7] There is an increase in the prevalence with the chronological age of the female patient. It accounts for 40% of female infertility. The reported incidence is debatable as certain couples can be wrongly diagnosed with UI, such as couples with subtle causes—endometriosis, tubal infertility, diminished ovarian reserve, immunological causes, and endocrine causes, which may not be detected by special tests or the conception may be delayed by chance alone with the reduced fecundity potential of the couple.

The average monthly fecundity in humans is only 20%.[1] The mean number of cycles per year was assumed to be constant and set at 13. Women younger than 35 years have a fecundity rate of around 20%.[1,8] Fecundity rate decreases with age, from 20% at age 35 to almost 0% at age 45.[8] Every month of infertility reduces the chance of conception by 2% and for each year of females age above 30 years the conception rate is decreased by about 9%.

Couples with unexplained infertility might be reassured that even after 12 months of unsuccessful attempts, 50%

will conceive in the following 12 months, and another 12% in the year after.[9]

The prognosis mainly depends on the duration of infertility and the age of the female partner and previous pregnancy. When the duration is less than 2 years and age is less than 35 years prospects of conceiving are good with expectant management, but if the age is above 35 years and duration more than 3 years, the prognosis is bad and treatment should be taken earlier.[10]

ETIOLOGY AND PATHOPHYSIOLOGY

Despite scientific progress all these years, we have yet not been able to develop a perfect assessment method of the reproductive system of the male and the female partner. Specific tests to evaluate minute structure and function of certain parts of the reproductive tract have not been developed or are not routinely available. There can be numerous causes for not conceiving that may be associated with the minute steps in the process of ovulation, oocyte pick up by fallopian tube, tubal transport of the oocyte, sperm, and later the embryo and its interaction with tubal fluids and changes during transport meeting of sperm and oocyte, endometrial receptivity, and subsequent implantation.

ETIOLOGY OF MALE UNEXPLAINED INFERTILITY

Male factor infertility can be divided into two subgroups, idiopathic male infertility (IMI) and unexplained male infertility (UMI).[11] Both have normal physical examination and endocrine profile, but IMI has abnormal semen analyses, and UMI has a normal semen report.

Potential causes of UMI:

- Defective spermatogenesis
- Genetic—chromosomal abnormalities, mutations, compromised deoxyribonucleic acid (DNA) integrity
- Functional integrity of sperm-inability to negotiate the uterotubal junction
- Defective sperm fertilization potential poor zona pellucida binding, defects in capacitation, acrosome reaction
- Immunological—antisperm antibodies (ASAs)

The levels of sperm reactive oxygen species and DNA fragmentation due to oxidative damage were significantly higher in men with unexplained infertility, which affects the sperm motility and morphology and its fertilization potential.[12] Certain types of infertility could be caused by the inability of the sperm to correctly trigger the oocyte because of a faulty phospholipase C-zeta factor.[13,14]

Also according to Jodar et al. in male idiopathic infertility, the sperm lacked required sperm ribonucleic acid elements, which lead to reduced probability of a live birth compared with couples attempting to conceive by timed intercourse or intrauterine insemination (IUI).[15] In vitro fertilization (IVF)–embryo transfer (ET) or intracytoplasmic sperm injection (ICSI) can overcome this deficiency.

Overall male factor infertility is poorly defined, and the fertility prediction capacity of semen analysis result is less.[16]

ETIOLOGIES IN THE FEMALE

Causes can be at various levels of the system.

Ovarian

- Defective folliculogenesis and defective gametes leading to impaired fertilization;
- Genetic abnormalities—There may be genetically and functionally abnormal oocytes, especially in an aging patient;
- Ovulatory dysfunction—luteinized unruptured follicle, empty follicle, inadequate luteinization, incomplete maturation of follicle.

Tubal Dysfunction

- Defective oocyte pick up by fimbria
- Disturbed bidirectional gamete transportation
- Toxic tubal fluids due to endometriosis or due to other inflammatory causes
- Peritubal adhesions affecting the smooth transit of gametes.

Uterine Problems

- Endometrial implantation—failed implantation due to
    - Embryonic defects—chromosomal aneuploidy, thick zona
    - Altered endometrial receptivity
- Defective implantation leading to early embryonic losses
- Altered uterine peristalsis leading to impaired sperm transport.

Vaginal

- Raised pH—increased susceptibility to infections
- Altered vaginal flora leading to phagocytosis of sperms
- Lubricants toxic to sperm
- Abnormal liquefaction of semen

Cervix

Previous curettage, cervical conization, cauterization, cervical infections, chronic cervicitis.

Cervical mucus abnormalities:

- Genetic (cystic fibrosis), inflammatory conditions (chronic cervicitis or acute inflammation)
- Hormonal factors, clomiphene, nicotine, immunological (ASA).

Immunological factors—Antisperm, antiovarian, antiphospholipid antibodies, and anti-Chlamydia trachomatis antibodies have adverse effects on fertilization, implantation and lead to early embryonic losses.

Endocrinological factors—Affect ovulation, fertilization, luteal phase, implantation, and pregnancy rates (PRs).

Problems in thyroid function and hyperprolactinemia are familiar causes of infertility, but it is not certain whether thyrotropin [thyroid-stimulating hormone (TSH)] and prolactin levels within the normal range can lead to unexplained infertility. Women with UI have been seen to have higher TSH levels compared with a control population. It is debatable whether treatment of high-normal TSH levels decreases the time to conception in couples with UI. 26.9% women with UI had a TSH >2.5 mIU/L compared with controls (13.5%; $p < 0.05$).[17]

Oxidative stress and toxic effects of reactive oxygen species at ovarian, tubal, uterine, cervical, and peritoneal levels also have an adverse effect.

Environmental contaminants have endocrine disrupting potential. Cigarette smoke, bisphenol A, fluorinated compounds have toxic effects on gametogenesis. There is a 50% reduction in implantation in smokers and increased chances of pregnancy losses.

- The cervix has an important role of storing spermatozoa from where they go up the uterus at regular intervals, but we cannot assess the functional efficiency of the cervix through tests which may be reliable.[18]
- Even if the fallopian tubes are patent, their function may be compromised due to microscopic changes having an effect on the proper functioning of the tubal epithelium.[19] Bidirectional motility is important for sperm transport and embryo transport.
- No authentic test has been developed till date which can help us observe the functioning of the endometrium where implantation will take place. Embryo implantation is the most crucial step for conception.[20] It involves complex cellular and molecular interactions between the receptive endometrium and the embryo.[21] Disturbances in such biomarkers are seen in unexplained infertility. Beta 3 integrin and calcitonin have a role in endometrial receptivity. Decreased expression of these as seen in unexplained infertility may alter the window of implantation.[22]
- Serum kisspeptin, a neuropeptide, helps in regulating the hypothalamic-pituitary-gonadal axis and maturity of oocytes. Reduced Kimberley Process (KP) levels have been seen in unexplained infertility, and it was associated with reduced fertilization, defective egg maturation, thin endometrial lining, and blastocyst implantation failure. KP works as proinflammatory cytokine with tumor necrosis factor alpha and affects trophoblast cell invasion and implantation. Thus decreased implantation may be associated with decreased levels of cytokines and interleukins.[23]
- Leukemia inhibitory factor endometrial expression during the implantation window is decreased in patients with unexplained infertility.[24]

In reality, a number of fundamental steps of the fertility process cannot be precisely investigated.[25]

A better understanding of the mechanisms underlying UI could lead to less invasive and less expensive treatment strategies.

DIAGNOSIS AND EVALUATION

The Practice Committee of the American Society for Reproductive Medicine has published guidelines for a standard infertility evaluation.[5] These are as follows:

- Semen analysis (two properly performed semen analyses according to the strict criteria established in World Health Organization 2010 guidelines for the diagnosis of semen abnormalities).[26,27]
- Assessment of ovulation: Defects in ovulation are seen in around 30–40% of infertile women and in 15% of couples with infertility.[5]

  The various means of evaluation of ovulation include basal body temperature records, urinary luteinizing hormone (LH) ovulation prediction kits, and endometrial biopsy to assess for secretory endometrial development. Midluteal serum progesterone levels should be >3 ng/mL.[28] Endometrial biopsy is not recommended now as it has no relation with fertility status.[29]
- Assessment of tubal patency by hysterosalpingogram (HSG) or laparoscopy. The correlation of HSG with laparoscopic chromopertubation is about 80–90%.[30] Having said that, an HSG finding of patent fallopian tubes will not guarantee that ovum pick up will occur normally. It may be hampered due to adherent ovaries in the cul de sac with normal fallopian tubes as may be seen in endometriosis and after previous abdominal surgeries.

American Society for Reproductive Medicine recommends laparoscopy in women with unexplained infertility, those with signs and symptoms of endometriosis or in patients with suspected tubal adhesions but it can still miss tubal dysfunction or spasm or proximal occlusion.[31]

The diagnosis of UI is established after a standard evaluation fails to detect an abnormality. Unexplained infertility is a diagnosis of exclusion. These tests have been selected as they have definitive correlation with pregnancy.[5,9] It is estimated that a standard fertility evaluation will fail to identify an abnormality in approximately 15–30% of infertile couples.[9]

Controversy exists about the utility of endometrial biopsy, ovarian reserve (anti-Müllerian hormone, antral follicle count), and postcoital test (PCT). Earlier, the PCT was an integral part of the basic infertility evaluation. There has been a poor correlation between postcoital sperm motility and pregnancy outcome.[32] Its validity as a diagnostic test is further questioned due to poor reproducibility. Thus, it's outdated and has been abandoned.[25] In patients with normal results of standard tests, there still maybe undefined causes for infertility which have led to unexplained infertility.

In women above 40 years the cause of infertility may be reduced ovarian reserve, but since not many undergo the relevant diagnostic tests and these are also not included in the standard evaluation for UI, these women are misdiagnosed with UI. Problems in differentiating between real unexplained infertility (infertility due to undetectable causes) and age-related infertility increase markedly with a women's age. Older women should be referred earlier. It is recommended that after 35 years of age, infertility tests be advised before the conventional 1-year duration of pregnancy seeking.[31,33] The ASRM guidelines even suggest starting assessments after 6 months in this age-group.[33]

Starting tests earlier may have favorable clinical results if a clear barrier to fertility appears. For instance, if tubes are not patent, the woman will never conceive, and performing IVF earlier may improve the ultimate chance to become pregnant. If the fertility investigations fail to identify any cause of infertility or if they indicate subtle problems which cannot stop the process of natural conception the UI is diagnosed. It has been proposed that couples with mild male factor-infertility (total number of motile sperm between 3 million and 10 million), endometriosis stages I and II, only one patent tube, with cervical factor infertility, should be diagnosed with unexplained infertility.[34]

With age, fecundity decreases physiologically, and women with "age-related infertility" should not be considered having unexplained infertility. These two conditions, their treatment, and prognosis are entirely different and should not be put together in a similar group. It is very important to differentiate between age-related infertility in older women and unexplained infertility.[35]

Unexplained infertility is a diagnosis of exclusion and does not have a definite pathophysiologic basis. It may be a multifactorial disorder of reproduction. It is not possible to investigate all the etiologies despite an extensive evaluation as many causes are based on suspicion but have no definite diagnostic tests. Gleicher and Barad suggested substitution of the term "unexplained" by "undiagnosed".[36] It has been also addressed as subfertility as it is not a permanent disability, and with time, the patient may conceive spontaneously without treatment. However, one should not offer experimental tests or unnecessary additional tests as this can waste the crucial time for pregnancy without any positive effects.[37]

TREATMENT OPTIONS

The treatment of UI due to absence of a causative diagnosis is empirical as it is not meant for any particular defect, and thus several methods have been tried and used.[4] Therapeutic options for couples with unexplained infertility include empirical ovarian stimulation with or without IUI, IVF, and ICSI. Best approach to couples with unexplained infertility is individualized treatment based on resources, age, and duration of infertility. The treatment options for unexplained infertility comprise expectant observation with timed intercourse, clomiphene citrate (CC)/letrozole alone or with IUI, controlled ovarian hyperstimulation with IUI, and IVF/ICSI.

- Expectant management
- Controlled ovarian stimulation (Cos) and timed intercourse
- Only IUI
- Controlled ovarian stimulation + IUI
- In vitro fertilization/ICSI

It is very likely that the individual prognosis of the couple influences the effect of treatment. Taking into account the prognostic factors, may help in selecting the appropriate fertility treatment, tailored to the needs of the individual couple.[38] Notwithstanding its diverse pathogenesis, couples with unexplained infertility can still be given hope with working treatment plan.[4,31] ASRM recommendations propose a treatment line beginning with IUI and then proceeding to IVF.[4]

The National Institute for Health and Clinical Excellence (NICE) guidelines recommend advising an IVF cycle directly if patient has been trying with regular unprotected intercourse for more than 2 years.[31]

EXPECTANT MANAGEMENT

Spontaneous pregnancies have been seen in couples with UI. This possibility depends on the patient's age, duration of infertility, and history of previous pregnancy with the same spouse. It has a role in conditions with limited availability of resources or tests. The possibility of conception without treatment in couples with unexplained infertility is less than that of fertile couples but greater than zero.

We have to correctly diagnose and identify the couples that are eligible for tailored expectant management (TEM), i.e. calculating the chance of a natural conception within a year for couples with unexplained infertility with the prognostic model of Hunault.[39] The prognostic model takes four mandatory factors into account, female age (years), duration of infertility (years), type of infertility (primary/ secondary), and quality of semen (percentage progressive motile sperm).

Tailored expectant management[40] is recommended for at least 6–12 months for couples with a good prognosis (30% in 1 year) after finalizing the fertility workup. If TEM is advised by the professionals, the guideline recommends that the couple is educated on the most fertile period, optimal coital frequency, and healthy lifestyle factors to optimize the couples' chance of natural conception. NICE guideline, when referring to unexplained infertility, recommends expectant treatment for up to 2 years, and if it is not successful, then they propose proceeding to IVF, ruling out IUI as a possible interim treatment.[31] IUI was used with clomiphene in this, but when IUI is performed by stimulation with gonadotropins (Gns), it has a better success rate of about 25% over 3 cycles of treatment. Thus NICE 2013 guideline has been unacceptable to clinicians as it's not based on good evidence.

Expectant management was comparable in efficacy with treatments using clomiphene with IUI according to Deaton[41] and Wordsworth[42] or Gns with IUI in some studies by Steures et al.[43] It has comparable live birth rates (LBRs) as with the use of only IUI or only clomiphene.[44]

Thus expectant management has a crucial role where the resources are limited.

- Tubal flushing/perturbation has helped to increase the chance of pregnancy in unexplained infertility through a mechanical or immunological effect.[45]
- Spontaneous pregnancy has been achieved following HSG,[45] when oil-based media are used, there is a marked improvement in PR[46] (this may be due to the removal of tubal debris, lipiodol prevents peritoneal mast cell phagocytosis of sperm).
- It was proposed by Edelstom that clomiphene with perturbation and IUI could be the first option for treatment of UI.[47]

OVULATION INDUCTION

In patients with unexplained infertility, ovarian stimulation is beneficial even for ovulatory menstrual cycles, as it may overcome a subtle defect in ovulation not detected by routine testing. Moreover, it increases the chances of conception by increasing the number of oocytes available for fertilization and by increasing implantation by possible effects on endometrium.[48] Follicular recruitment and ovulation may be the rate-limiting step in conception in UI. CC and aromatase inhibitors, such as letrozole, are used for induction. When ovulation induction is coupled with IUI, it increases the number of gametes for fertilization and thus the chance of conception increases. It's also logical that when two effective treatments are combined, the results are better. Aromatase inhibitors, such as letrozole, have certain advantages over CC in that they lack antiestrogenic effect of clomiphene in late follicular phase and the effect on cervical mucus. Clomiphene and letrozole have advantages over Gns—lower incidence of multiple pregnancies, ovarian hyperstimulation syndrome (OHSS), low cost, oral administration, and less need for cycle monitoring.

Diamond et al.[49] concluded that ovarian stimulation with letrozole resulted in a significantly lower frequency of multiple gestations but also a lower frequency of live birth as compared with Gn but not as compared to clomiphene. Polyzos[50] enrolled five trials which supported the role of letrozole in UI. No significant difference was found, PRs were comparable with clomiphene in unexplained infertility, letrozole had a lower frequency of multiple gestation (as they are associated with monofollicular development in most cases) and lower chance of live birth as compared with Gn but not as compared with clomiphene. It was earlier off label but now again has been made available. Aromatase inhibitors have not been associated with a significantly increased risk of congenital anomalies.[51] CC has been in use for more than four decades, and its adverse effects are predictable, such as multiple pregnancy in 8–10% of cases and ovarian cysts in 5–10% are the most common.[52] Despite earlier studies inferring that CC was associated with increased ovarian cancer risk after 12 cycles of treatment use, more recent studies have observed no increased ovarian cancer risk related to the use of ovulation-inducing drugs.[53,54]

Anyways, prolonged treatment with oral drugs is not justified as none of the unexplained infertility trials offer evidence that ovulation stimulation is effective even after 6 cycles.

GONADOTROPINS

They have been used along with IUI and oral ovulation agents. Human menopausal Gn has higher clinical PR than clomiphene. In a number of cases of unexplained infertility, Gn stimulation and IUI may result in a doubling of the conception rate compared to oral agents, but at the cost of increase in multiple PRs of ≥30% also having higher order multiples.[49] PR with Gns is 25.5%, and with clomiphene, it is 8%. Disadvantages are the cost of treatment, patient inconvenience, OHSS, overresponse, and multiple pregnancies. In studies comparing Gn and IUI, results were in favor of IUI. The addition of IUI to empiric Gn therapy does improve fertility. The effect was confirmed in a trial among patients stimulated with Gns who were randomly allocated to receive IUI.[49] In yet another randomized clinical trial, IUI improved fertility in cycles; in which, CC was combined with Gns. Guzick et al.[55] conducted a study in 1999 where patients of unexplained infertility or male factor were randomized to IUI or ICI (intracervical insemination) with or without Gn stimulation showed that follicle-stimulating hormone (FSH) given with IUI produced higher PRs of 33% than only FSH (19%), with IUI alone it was (18%), and with ICI it was (10%). Per cycle PR was 2%, 4%, 5%, 9% for ICI, IUI, Gn with ICI, and Gn with IUI, respectively.[55] 20% multiple PR and OHSS was also seen.

Diamond et al. conducted the assessment of multiple intrauterine gestations from ovarian stimulation trial which had a cumulative PR of 35.5% with Gn/IUI and a multiple PR of 32% with triplets included.[56]

Gonadotropin therapy is more effective than CC or letrozole therapy, and when both are combined with IUI, their cumulative effect increases.

A recent systematic review by Gunn and Bates concluded that clomiphene is possibly more effective than letrozole, but Gns have a better response than both clomiphene and letrozole.[57]

INTRAUTERINE INSEMINATION

Intrauterine insemination is a widely used fertility treatment for couples with unexplained subfertility. It can be done during a natural cycle or following ovarian stimulation. It helps by increasing the number of motile and a greater number of normal formed sperms available to the oocytes. Timing it close to ovulation increases the probability of gamete interaction and can be performed in combination with natural ovulation timed with LH ovulation kit, ovulation induction using CC, letrozole, or Gns.

According to the Cochrane review,[58] IUI with ovulation induction increased the conception rate compared with IUI alone. A meta-analysis of 27 studies reported that the PR per cycle was 8% with Gn treatment alone and 18% when IUI was added to Gn stimulation.[59] Ovulation induction with Gns coupled with IUI markedly improved the possibility of pregnancy. Stimulated IUI is more cost-effective and less invasive than IVF and was proposed by Philips et al.[60] But stimulated IUI has the disadvantage of multiple follicular growth which may lead to cycle cancelation due to risk of multiple pregnancy which is the main concern with IUI [an update of a Cochrane review originally published in 2006 and updated in 2012].[58] The safety of IUI in combination with ovarian hyperstimulation is debated. Bhattacharya et al. due to this concern supported a more expectant management for 6 months.[61] If in IUI, we can control the number of follicles then we can reduce the multiple PRs without compromising the overall PR. In younger women, we can go for expectant management then stimulated IUI and later IVF. IUI can be done for 6 cycles in unexplained infertility. In ovulatory cycles, letrozole or clomiphene with IUI will result in conception rates only slightly more than a cycle monitoring and IUI. Use of clomiphene alone or IUI alone is unlikely to offer superior LBRs compared with expectant management as proposed by Bhattacharya et al.[61]

Stimulated IUI resulted in 10 times the multiple-birth rate with high-order multiple conceptions. But Cochrane review[58] and a randomized controlled trial from the Netherlands (2015)[62] proved that multiple PRs are the same or lower than in IVF. Here, the number of live births with 6 cycles of IUI (47%) was almost the same as 6 cycles of modified natural cycle IVF (43%) and 3 cycles of IVF with single ET (52%). For couples with unexplained or mild male infertility, IUI is the first line of treatment, associated with the lowest costs, and is neither invasive nor dangerous if performed correctly in properly selected patients.

Double IUI offers no clear benefit in the overall clinical PR in couples with unexplained infertility.[63] Side effects after IUI treatment are rarely seen. IUI with prepared spermatozoa does not change the frequency of ASAs.[64]

With ovarian stimulation and IUI combined, the couples conceive within the first 3–4 cycles of treatment, but there is a decrease in cycle fecundity later. Thus after 3–4 attempts of IUI and ovulation induction one must move to IVF.[65]

IN VITRO FERTILIZATION/ INTRACYTOPLASMIC SPERM INJECTION

In vitro fertilization is the most effective modality of treatment for unexplained infertility even though it's costly and an invasive procedure.[66] IVF is not only advised for treatment purpose but also to learn about the fertilization process in that given couple. Decreased fertilization and cleavage rates have been seen in IVF cycles done for unexplained infertility suggesting gamete defects in these couples. Total fertilization failure is seen in 20% couples and can recur in subsequent cycles.[67] ICSI can overcome fertilization defects, such as decreased or absent fertilization in unexplained infertility. A study conducted by Ruiz et al. concluded that ICSI avoids complete fertilization failure seen in 11.4% of patients of unexplained infertility when treated with routine IVF.[68] Thus ICSI should be offered to them. We cannot predict who can have fertilization failure, but after a failed cycle, ICSI is employed in the next. Drawbacks are that it is invasive, expensive, and associated with risks, such as multiple pregnancy and OHSS.

A failed conception can be due to various reasons, such as quality of gametes and their interaction development of embryo and its transportation and implantation and the development; ICSI can overcome all these.

The European Society for Human Reproduction and Embryology Multicentre Trial concluded that PRs per cycle were 15.2% in Gn only cycles, 27.4% in Gn and IUI cycles, and 25.7% in IVF cycles.[69]

According to Goverde et al., LBRs per cycle in the unexplained subgroup were 6.0% in IUI only cycles, 8.7% in Gn and IUI cycles, and 13.0% in IVF cycles.[70]

Two landmark National Institutes of Health trials were conducted to study the best course of treatment in women with unexplained infertility.

In 2010 the Fast Track and Standard Treatment (FASTT) Trial[71] was conducted in women less than 40 years. It compared the regular IUI management protocol in unexplained infertile couples. The conventional arm involved up to 3 cycles of clomiphene with IUI then 3 cycles with Gn (FSH) and IUI, followed by up to 6 cycles of IVF. The accelerated arm involved a fast tracked treatment protocol which did away with the FSH and IUI cycles. The results proved that the fast tracked approach to IVF lead to a lesser time to conception with pregnancies taking place in lesser number of cycles with cost-benefit, concluding that FSH with IUI had no extra advantage.[71] PRs were 8.5% with CC + IUI, 11.4% with Gn + IUI, and 38.6% with IVF. The conclusion derived was that the best protocol for such couples was directly proceeding to IVF after trial with CC + IUI. They first tried with CC + IUI since this would give the most fertile couples with a higher probability of multiple pregnancies to conceive before IVF is tried.[71]

A follow-up trial called the Forty and Over Treatment (FORT-T) Trial[72] was conducted for women between 38 years and 42 years old. They inferred that in older women 2 cycles of IVF will lead to a significantly greater conception and LBR as compared with two attempts with CC + IUI or FSH + IUI. Other European studies have proposed that starting with expectant approach saves cost without affecting much the time to or chances of pregnancy. Expectant management (EM) had the same conception results as IUI with COS proposing that 6-month expectant approach is advisable for these couples.[43] One cycle of IVF-elective single ET as first-line treatment has been advised in patients with unexplained or mild male subfertility by Gianaroli et al.[3] and found to be as good as three stimulated IUI cycles.

Thus above 40 years of age IVF is advised but a review[66] proposed that 2 cycles of Gn with IUI can be tried before going for IVF in some patients since IVF has its own complications, such as multiple pregnancy, ovarian hyperstimulation, and increased perinatal morbidity and mortality due to preterm and small-for-gestational-age births. In a report out of all the IVF/ICSI births, 34% were multiple, out of which 30% were twins and 3.2% were triplets or higher order births (2003 Assisted reproductive technology success rates. National summary and fertility clinic reports, 2003). Severe OHSS occurs in 2% of cycles (Table 1).[73]

Table 1: Studies comparing various treatment modalities in unexplained infertility.

Comparison between	*Inference in favor of*	*Study/Trial*
CC + TI vs. EM	CC + TI	Fisch et al.[74]
	No significant difference	Bhattacharya et al.[44]
CC + IUI vs. EM	No significant difference	Deaton et al.[41]
IUI (natural cycle vs. EM)	IUI but difference not significant	Bhattacharya et al.[44]
Gn + IUI vs. EM	No significant difference	Steures et al.[43]
CC + IUI vs. letroz + IUI	Letroz + IUI	Fouda et al.[75]
	CC but difference not significant	Diamond et al.[49]
Gn vs. IUI	IUI	Chung et al.,[76] Janko et al.,[77] Karlstrom et al.,[78] Melis et al.[79]

Contd...

Contd...

Gn (HMG) + IUI vs. CC + IUI	No significant difference No significant difference	Karlstrom et al.[78] Echocard et al.[80]
	No significant difference	Dankert et al.[81]
	No significant difference	Berker et al.[82]
	Gn + IUI	Diamond et al.[49]
Highly purified urinary Gn + IUI vs. CC + IUI	No significant difference	Balasch et al.[83]
Gn + IUI vs. letroz + IUI	No significant difference	Baysoy et al.[84]
	No significant difference	Gregoriou et al.[85]
	Gn + IUI	Diamond et al.[49]
Gn + IUI vs. IVF	No significant difference	Goverde et al.[70]
Gn + IUI vs. IUI natural cycle	No significant difference	Goverde et al.[70]
IVF vs. IUI natural cycle	No significant difference	Goverde et al.[70]
IVF vs. IVF + ICSI	No significant difference	Foong et al.[86]
IVF vs. Gn	IVF	Reindollar et al. (FASTT)[71]

(CC: clomiphene citrate; FASTT: fast track and standard treatment trial; Gn: gonadotropin; HMG: human menopausal gonadotropin; ICSI: intracytoplasmic sperm injection; IUI: intrauterine insemination; IVF: in vitro fertilization; TI: timed intercourse; EM: expectant management)

CONCLUSION

Around 25% of all couples worldwide seeking help for infertility may have normal findings on their clinical evaluation, making the unexplained infertility a more common provisional diagnosis. Our inability to find the causes of couples' infertility does not mean that there is no cause for the disorder. Research should be directed toward other probable causes of conception failure, such as parameters of quality of gametes, ovarian and testicular disorders, tubal transportation defects, uterine receptivity, implantation failures, and endometriosis. Individualized treatment should be offered to infertile couples with idiopathic causes. Factors, such as age, duration and history of infertility, treatments taken, costs, and risks, should be taken into consideration while selecting an appropriate treatment plan.

REFERENCES

1. Evers JL. Female subfertility. Lancet. 2002;360(9327):151-9.
2. The Practice Committee of the American Society for Reproductive Medicine. Definitions of infertility and recurrent pregnancy loss: a committee opinion. Fertil Steril. 2013;99(1):63.
3. Gianaroli L, Racowsky C, Geraedts J, et al. Best practices of ASRM and ESHRE: a journey through reproductive medicine. Hum Reprod. 2012;27(12):3365-79.
4. The Practice Committee of the American Society for Reproductive Medicine. Effectiveness and treatment for unexplained infertility. Fertil Steril. 2006;86(5 suppl):S111-4.
5. The Practice Committee of the American Society for Reproductive Medicine. Optimal evaluation of the infertile female. Fertil Steril. 2006;86(5 Suppl):S264-7.
6. Reza Sadeghi M. Unexplained infertility, the controversial matter in management of infertile couples. J Reprod Infertil. 2015;16(1):1-2.
7. Maheshwari A, Hamilton M, Bhattacharya S. Effect of female age on the diagnostic categories of infertility. Hum Reprod. 2008;23(3):538-42.
8. Leridon H. Can assisted reproductive technology compensate the decline in fertility with age? A model assessment. Hum Reprod. 2004;19:1548-53.
9. Gelbaya TA, Potdar N, Jeve YB, et al. Definition and epidemiology of unexplained infertility. Obstet Gynecol Surv. 2014;69(2):109-15.
10. Collins JA, Burrows EA, Wilan AR. The prognosis for live birth among untreated infertile couples. Fertil Steril. 1995;64:22-8.
11. Hamada A, Esteves SC, Nizza M, et al. Unexplained male infertility: diagnosis and management. Int Braz J Urol. 2012;38:576-94.
12. Agarwal A, Saleh RA, Bedaiwy MA. Role of reactive oxygen species in the pathophysiology of human reproduction. Fertil Steril. 2003;79:829-43.
13. Heytens E, Parrington J, Coward K. Reduced amounts and abnormal forms of phospholipase C zeta (PLCζ) in spermatozoa from infertile men. Hum Reprod. 2009;24(10):2417-28.
14. Kashir J, Jones C, Lee HC, et al. Loss of activity mutations in phospholipase C zeta (PLCζ) abolishes calcium oscillatory ability of human recombinant protein in mouse oocytes. Hum Reprod. 2011;26(12):3372-87.
15. Jodar M, Sendler E, Moskovtsev SI, et al. Absence of sperm RNA elements correlates with idiopathic male infertility. Sci Transl Med. 2015;7(295):295re6.
16. Wang C, Swerdloff RS. Limitations of semen analysis as a test of male fertility and anticipated needs from newer tests. Fertil Steril. 2014;102:1502-7.
17. Orouji Jokar T, Fourman L T, Lee H, et al. Higher TSH levels within the normal range are associated with unexplained infertility. J Clin Endocrinol Metab. 2018;103(2):632-9.

18. Martyn F, McAuliffe FM, Wingfield M. The role of the cervix in fertility: is it time for a reappraisal? Hum Reprod. 2014;29:2092-8.
19. Lyons RA, Saridogan E, Djahanbakhch O. The reproductive significance of human fallopian tube cilia. Hum Reprod Update. 2006;12:363-72.
20. Cakmak H, Taylor HS. Implantation failure: molecular mechanisms and clinical treatment. Hum Reprod Update. 2011;17:242-53.
21. Achache H, Revel A. Endometrial receptivity markers, the journey to successful embryo implantation. Hum Reprod Update. 2006;12(6):731-46.
22. Dorostghoal M, Ghaffari H, Shahbazian N, et al. Endometrial expression of B3 integrin, calcitonin and plexin-B1 in the window of implantation in women with unexplained infertility. Int J Reprod Biomed. 2017;15(1):33-40.
23. Mumtaz A, Khalid A, Jamil Z, et al. Kisspeptin: a potential factor for unexplained infertility and impaired embryo implantation. Int J Fertil Steril. 2017;11(2):99-104.
24. Margioula-Siarkou C, Prapas Y, Petousis S, et al. LIF endometrial expression is impaired in women with unexplained infertility while LIF-R expression in all infertility sub groups. Cytokine. 2017;96:166-72.
25. Practice Committee of the American Society for Reproductive Medicine. Diagnostic evaluation of the infertile female: a committee opinion. Fertil Steril. 2015;103(6):e44-50.
26. Kruger TF, Menkveld R, Stander FS, et al. Sperm morphologic features as prognostic factor in IVF. Fertil Steril. 1986;46:1118-23.
27. Cooper TG, Noonan E, von Eckardstein S, et al. World Health Organization reference values for human semen characteristics. Hum Reprod Update. 2010;16:231-45.
28. Crosignani PC, Collins J, Cooke ID, et al. Unexplained infertility (recommendations of ESHRE workshop). Hum Reprod. 1993;8:977-80.
29. Coutifaris C, Myers ER, Guzick DS, et al. Histological dating of timed endometrial biopsy tissue is not related to fertility status. Fertil Steril. 2004;82:1264-72.
30. Exacoustos C, Zupi E, Carusotti C, et al. Hysterosalpingo-contrast sonography compared with hysterosalpingography and laparoscopic dye pertubation to evaluate tubal patency. J Am Assoc Gynecol Laparosc. 2003;10:367-72.
31. NICE—National Institute for Health and Clinical Excellence; National Collaborating Centre for Women's and Children's Health. Fertility: assessment and treatment for people with fertility problems. London, UK: Royal College of Obstetricians & Gynaecologists; February 2013. p. 63. (Clinical guideline; No.156).
32. Collins JA, So Y, Wilson EH, et al. The postcoital test as a predictor of pregnancy among 355 infertile couples. Fertil Steril. 1984;41:703-8.
33. Practice Committee of the American Society for Reproductive Medicine. Diagnostic evaluation of the infertile female: a committee opinion. Fertil Steril. 2015;103(6):e44-50.
34. Kersten FA, Hermens RP, Braat DD, et al. Overtreatment in couples with unexplained infertility. Hum Reprod. 2015;30:71-80.
35. Somigliana E, Paffoni A, Busnelli A, et al. Age-related infertility and unexplained infertility: an intricate clinical dilemma. Hum Reprod. 2016;31(7):1390-6.
36. Gleicher N, Barad D. Unexplained infertility: does it really exist? Hum Reprod. 2006;21:1951-5.
37. Siristatidis C, Bhattacharya S. Unexplained infertility: does it really exist? Does it matter? Hum Reprod. 2007;22:2084-7.
38. Van den Boogaard NM, Hompes PG, Barnhart K, et al. The prognostic profile of subfertile couples and treatment outcome after expectant management, intrauterine insemination and in vitro fertilisation: a study protocol for the meta-analysis of individual patient data. BJOG. 2012;119(8):953-7.
39. Hunault CC, Habbema JDF, Eijkemans MJC, et al. Two new prediction rules for spontaneous pregnancy leading to live birth among subfertile couples, based on the synthesis of three previous models. Hum Reprod. 2004;19(9):2019-26.
40. Kersten FAM, Hermens RPGM, Braat DDM, et al. Tailored expectant management in couples with unexplained infertility does not influence their experiences with the quality of fertility care. Hum Reprod. 2016;31(1):108-16.
41. Deaton JL, Gibson M, Blackmer KM, et al. A randomised controlled trial of clomiphene citrate and intrauterine insemination in couples with unexplained infertility or surgically corrected endometriosis. Fertil Steril. 1990;54: 1083-8.
42. Wordsworth S, Buchanan J, Mollison J, et al. Clomiphene citrate and intrauterine insemination as first line treatments for unexplained infertility: are they cost effective? Hum Reprod. 2011;26:369-75.
43. Steures P, van der Steeg JW, Hompes PG, et al. Intrauterine insemination with controlled ovarian hyperstimulation versus expectant management for couples with unexplained subfertility and an intermediate prognosis: a randomized clinical trial. Lancet. 2006;368:216-21.
44. Bhattacharya S, Harrild K, Mollison J, et al. Clomiphene citrate or unstimulated intrauterine insemination compared with expectant management for unexplained infertility: pragmatic randomized controlled trial. Br Med J. 2008;337:a716.
45. Johnson N, Vandekerckhove P, Watson A, et al. Tubal flushing for subfertility. Cochrane Database Syst Rev. 2005;18:CD003718.
46. Watson A, Vandekerckhove P, Lilford R, et al. A meta-analysis of the therapeutic role of oil soluble contrast media at hysterosalpingography: a surprising result? Fertil Steril. 1994;61:470-7.
47. Edelstam G, Sjosten A, Bjuresten K, et al. A new rapid and effective method for treatment of unexplained infertility. Hum Reprod. 2008;23:852-6.
48. Collins JA. Superovulation in the treatment of unexplained infertility. Semin Reprod Endocrinol. 1990;8:165-73.
49. Diamond MP, Legro RS, Coutifaris C, et al. Letrozole, gonadotropin, or clomiphene for unexplained infertility. N Engl J Med. 2015;373:1230-40.
50. Polyzos NP, Tzioras S, Mauri D, et al. Treatment of unexplained infertility with aromatase inhibitors or clomiphene citrate. A systematic review and meta-analysis. Obstet Gynecol Surv. 2008;63:472-9.
51. Tatsumi T, Jwa SC, Kuwahara A, et al. No increased risk of major congenital anomalies or adverse pregnancy or neonatal outcomes following letrozole use in assisted reproductive technology. Hum Reprod. 2017;32(1):125-32.

52. Tarlatzis B, Grimbizis G. Future use of clomiphene in ovarian stimulation. Will clomiphene persist in the 21st century? Hum Reprod. 1998;13:2356-8.
53. Rossing MA, Tang MT, Flagg EW, et al. A case-control study of ovarian cancer in relation to infertility and the use of ovulation-inducing drugs. Am J Epidemiol. 2004;160:1070-8.
54. Brinton LA, Lamb EJ, Moghissi KS, et al. Ovarian cancer risk after the use of ovulation-stimulating drugs. Obstet Gynecol. 2004;103:1194-203.
55. Guzick DS, Carson SA, Coutifaris C, et al. The national cooperative reproductive medicine network. Efficacy of superovulation and intrauterine insemination in the treatment of infertility. N Engl J Med. 1999;340:177-83.
56. Diamond MP, Mitwally M, Casper R, et al. Estimating rates of multiple gestation pregnancies: sample size calculation from the assessment of multiple intrauterine gestations from ovarian stimulation (AMIGOS) trial. Contemp Clin Trials. 2011;32:902-8.
57. Gunn DD, Bates GW. Evidence-based approach to unexplained infertility: a systematic review. Fertil Steril. 2016;105(6):1566-74.
58. Veltman-Verhulst SM, Hughes E, et al. Intra-uterine insemination for unexplained subfertility. Cochrane Database Syst Rev. 2016;2:CD001838.
59. Guzick DS, Sullivan MW, Adamson GD, et al. Efficacy of treatment for unexplained infertility. Fertil Steril. 1998;70:207-13.
60. Philips Z, Barraza-Llorens M, Posnett J. Evaluation of the relative cost-effectiveness of treatments for infertility in the UK. Hum Reprod. 2000;15(1):95-106.
61. Bhattacharya S, Harrild K, Mollison J, et al. Clomifene citrate or unstimulated intrauterine insemination compared with expectant management for unexplained infertility: pragmatic randomised controlled trial. BMJ. 2008;337:a716.
62. Bensdorp AJ, Tjon-Kon-Fat RI, Bossuyt PMM, et al. Prevention of multiple pregnancies in couples with unexplained or mild male subfertility randomized controlled trial of in vitro fertilization with single embryo transfer or in vitro fertilization in modified natural cycle compared with intrauterine insemination with controlled ovarian hyperstimulation. BMJ. 2015;350:g7771.
63. Polyzos NP, Tzioras S, Mauri D, et al. Double versus single intrauterine insemination for unexplained infertility: a meta-analysis of randomized trials. Fertil Steril. 2010;94(4):1261-6.
64. Horvath PM, Beck M, Bohrer MK, et al. A prospective study on the lack of development of antisperm antibodies in women undergoing intrauterine insemination. Am J Obstet Gynecol. 1989;160:631-7.
65. Aboulghar M, Mansour RT, Serour G, et al. Controlled ovarian hyperstimulation and intrauterine insemination for treatment of unexplained infertility should be limited to a maximum of three trials. Fertil Steril. 2001;75:88-91.
66. Ray A, Shah A, Gudi A, et al. Unexplained infertility: an update and review of practice. Reprod Biomed Online. 2012;24:591-602.
67. Lipitz S, Rabinovici J, Ben-Shlomo I, et al. Complete failure of fertilization in couples with unexplained infertility: implications for subsequent in vitro fertilization cycles. Fertil Steril. 1993;59:348-52.
68. Ruiz A, Remohí J, Minguez Y, et al. The role of in vitro fertilization and intracytoplasmic sperm injection in couples with unexplained infertility after failed intrauterine insemination. Fertl Steril. 1997;68:171-3. Best practices of ASRM and ESHRE: a journey through reproductive medicine.
69. Crosignani PG, Walters DE, Soliani A. The ESHRE multicentre trial on the treatment of unexplained infertility: a preliminary report. European Society of Human Reproduction and Embryology. Hum Reprod. 1991;6:953-8.
70. Goverde AJ, McDonnell J, Vermeiden JP, et al. Intrauterine insemination or in-vitro fertilisation in idiopathic subfertility and male subfertility: a randomised trial and cost-effectiveness analysis. Lancet. 2000;355:13-8.
71. Reindollar RH, Regan MM, Neumann PJ, et al. A randomized clinical trial to evaluate optimal treatment for unexplained infertility: the Fast Track and Standard Treatment Trial (FASTT). Fertil Steril. 2010;94:888-99.
72. Goldman MB, Thornton KL, Ryley D, et al. A randomized clinical trial to determine optimal infertility treatment in older couples: the Forty and Over Treatment Trial (FORT-T). Fertil Steril. 2014;101(6):1574-81.
73. Van Voorhis BJ. Outcomes from assisted reproductive technology. Obstet Gynecol. 2006;107:183-200.
74. Fisch P, Casper RF, Brown SE, et al. Unexplained infertility: evaluation of treatment with clomiphene citrate and human chorionic gonadotropin. Fertil Steril. 1989;51:828-33.
75. Fouda UM, Sayed AM. Extended letrozole regimen versus clomiphene citrate for superovulation in patients with unexplained infertility undergoing intrauterine insemination: a randomized controlled trial. Reprod Biol Endocrinol. 2011;9:84.
76. Chung CC, Fleming R, Jamieson ME, et al. Randomised comparison of ovulation induction with and without intrauterine insemination in the treatment of unexplained infertility. Hum Reprod. 1995;10:3139-41.
77. Janko P, Hruzik P, Pruzinec J, et al. Induction of ovulation with or without intrauterine insemination in cases of unexplained sterility. Fertil Steril. 1998;70:S442.
78. Karlstrom PO, Bergh T, Lundkvist O. A prospective randomized trial of artificial insemination versus intercourse in cycles stimulated with human menopausal gonadotropin or clomiphene citrate. Fertil Steril. 1993;59:554-9.
79. Melis GB, Paoletti AM, Ajossa S, et al. Ovulation induction with gonadotropins as sole treatment in infertile couples with open tubes: a randomized prospective comparison between intrauterine insemination and timed vaginal intercourse. Fertil Steril. 1995;64:1088-93.
80. Echocard R, Mathieu C, Royere D, et al. A randomized prospective study comparing pregnancy rates after clomiphene citrate and human menopausal gonadotropin before intrauterine insemination. Fertil Steril. 2000;73:90-3.
81. Dankert T, Kremer JA, Cohlen BJ, et al. A randomized clinical trial of clomiphene citrate versus low dose recombinant FSH for ovarian hyperstimulation in intrauterine insemination cycles for unexplained and male subfertility. Hum Reprod. 2007;22:792-7.
82. Berker B, Kahraman K, Taskin S, et al. Recombinant FSH versus clomiphene citrate for ovarian stimulation in couples

with unexplained infertility and male subfertility undergoing intrauterine insemination: a randomized trial. Arch Gynecol Obstet. 2011;284:1561.
83. Balasch J, Ballesca JL, Pimentel C, et al. Late low dose pure FSH for ovarian stimulation in intrauterine insemination cycles. Hum Reprod. 1994;10:1863-6.
84. Baysoy A, Serdaroglu H, Jamal H, et al. Letrozole versus human menopausal gonadotropin in women undergoing intrauterine insemination. Reprod Biomed Online. 2006;13:208-12.
85. Gregoriou O, Vlahos NF, Konidaris S, et al. Randomized controlled trial comparing superovulation with letrozole versus recombinant FSH combined with intrauterine insemination for couples with unexplained infertility who had failed clomiphene citrate stimulation and intrauterine insemination. Fertil Steril. 2008;90(3):678-83.
86. Foong SC, Fleetham JA, O'Keane JA, et al. A prospective randomized trial of conventional in vitro fertilization versus intracytoplasmic sperm injection in unexplained infertility. J Assist Reprod Genet. 2006;23:137-40.

CHAPTER

81

Recurrent Implantation Failure

Guillermo Martínez-Canillas, Juan A García-Velasco

DEFINITION

The International Glossary on infertility and fertility care in the review of 2017 defines implantation as "the attachment and subsequent penetration by a zone-free blastocyst into the endometrium. This process starts 5–7 days after fertilization of the oocyte usually resulting in the formation of a gestational sac."[1] Based on this definition, we can understand the failure of implantation when there is no attachment or penetration due to a factor in the endometrium or poor quality of blastocyst.

To define recurrent implantation failure (RIF) is complicated. In fact, in the same glossary, which includes 283 terms, it is not defined.

In a systematic review, Polanski et al.[2] observed the enormous variability in the definition of the term RIF. Current descriptions incorporate the number of previously failed cycles and whether these were fresh or frozen, the number of embryos transferred and/or their respective quality, or a combination of these factors. The authors suggest that RIF should be defined as "the absence of implantation, itself defined by a negative serum HCG 14 days after oocyte collection, after two consecutive cycles of IVF, ICSI, or frozen embryo replacement, where the cumulative number of transferred embryos was no less than four for cleavage-stage embryos and no less than two for blastocysts, with all embryos being of good quality and of appropriate developmental stage." Moreover, the patients in oocyte donation programs failing to achieve pregnancy and meeting these criteria should also be treated as being affected by RIF.

Many authors also consider maternal age in the definition. A review by Coughlan et al.,[3] concluded defining RIF as "the failure to achieve a clinical pregnancy after transfer of at least four good-quality embryos in a minimum of three fresh or frozen cycles in a woman under the age of 40 years."

These definitions try to cover all the elements that make up a complex pathology, but they are still the opinion of authors. The truth is that a consensus of experts is needed to precisely define the term RIF in order to provide the best information to patients and offer a uniform treatment based on scientific evidence.

ETIOLOGY

Successful implantation is a complex process involving two main players: (1) the mother, as a host, and (2) the embryo. Problems originating from the host environment, such as abnormal uterine anatomy, nonreceptive endometrium, and the medical condition of the mother (such as endometriosis, undetected genetic defects, thrombophilia, uncontrolled diabetes, thyroid disease, and abnormal immunologic response), can adversely affect the implantation.[4] Similarly, this endometrial-embryo interaction may be hampered if the embryo is disordered. Compromised oocyte quality may be suspected when there is a poor response to ovarian stimulation associated with low antral follicle counts, high follicle-stimulating hormone, and low anti-Müllerian hormone, although is mainly age related.

The etiology is multifactorial; in advanced maternal age, the main cause is the increase in the incidence of aneuploidy in the embryo.[5] Other causes are endometrial alterations, such as congenital uterine abnormalities, hyperplasia, endometrial polyps, submucosal myomas, chronic endometritis, and uterine synechiae, which can

Flowchart 1: Diagnostic and treatment Algorithm for recurrent implantation failure

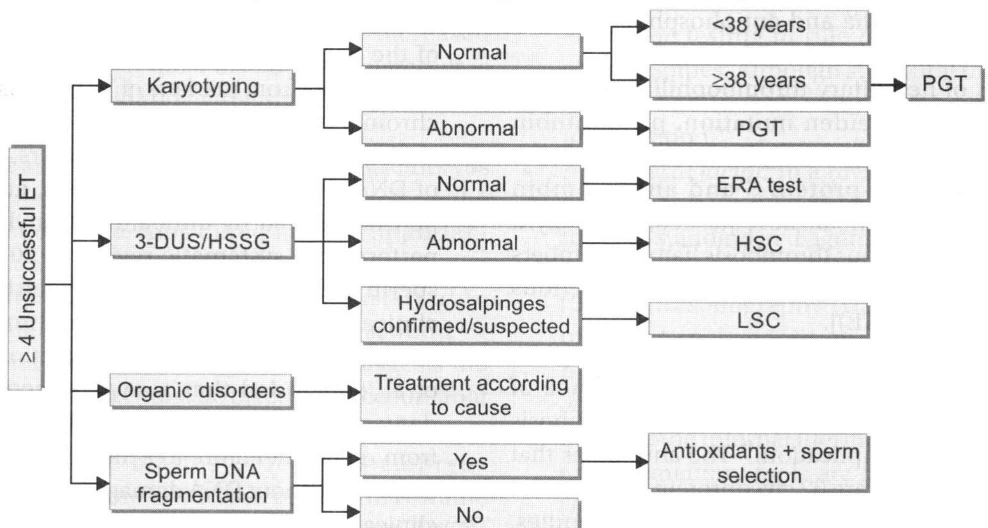

(ET: embryo transfer; 3-D US: three-dimensional ultrasound; HSSG: hysterosalpingosonography; PGT: preimplantation genetic testing; Hsc: hysteroscopy; Lsc: laparoscopy)

The application in clinical practice and its use have not been preceded by prospective and randomized studies. After randomized controlled trials and subsequent meta-analysis, the rates of newborns not only did not increase in patients undergoing PGT-A, they decreased significantly. In most of these studies, the embryo biopsy was performed in D3 and was examined with fluorescence in situ hybridization, a technique with limitations. The actual tendency is to perform the biopsy on D5 and a complete chromosomal screening using microarray comparative genomic hybridization (CGH) or next-generation sequencing (NGS).[5]

Performing the biopsy in the blastocyst stage and using complete chromosomal screening improves embryo selection and increases the PR/ET.[21] Embryo selection with PGT-A avoids failed cycles, reduces the time to pregnancy and the possibility of miscarriage. PGT-A should be considered an embryo selection technique, not a diagnostic technique. Further studies are required to confirm whether or not routine PGT-A using microarray CGH or NGS is beneficial in women with RIF.[3]

- *Endometrial receptivity*: Trials have shown that the ERA test is a reliable and reproducible method for determining the exact time of WOI that can be used with better results compared to the histological dating of endometrial receptivity.[20] The ERA test can be applied in clinical practice.[22] In patients with RIF, the endometrial receptivity evaluated with the ERA test and the ETs made according to the ERA data resulted in a PR of 62.8%. Simon et al.[23] investigated differences in implantation rate (IR), PR, ongoing pregnancy (OP) rates, and delivery among women undergoing transfer at the blastocyst stage in their first IVF/ICSI cycle randomized to fresh cycles (ET), deferred ET (DET), or personalized ET (pET) after endometrial receptivity analysis (ERA). They concluded that pET is associated with significant improvement in PR and trend toward increase IR and OP versus regular ET or DET. Personalization of the endometrial factor in the diagnostic workup of the infertile couple must be considered.
- *Anatomical factor*: Hysteroscopy may improve the outcome of women with RIF.[6] It is indicated to perform a therapeutic hysteroscopy, including uterine septum resection, removal of intrauterine adhesions, endometrial polypectomy or myomectomy, particularly the submucous type,[24] the possible contribution of intramural fibroids which are not distorting the uterine cavity to RIF is far from clear.
There is good evidence that the removal of hydrosalpinges, especially those visible by ultrasound, improves the implantation and live birth rates in women undergoing IVF.[25] When performing salpingectomy, it is recommended to use bipolar energy and incise as far away as possible from the ovary to avoid the interruption of the ovarian flow that leads to lower ovarian response in the future.
- *Thrombophilia*: In women with thrombophilia, anticoagulant treatment is prescribed with the aim to prevent VTE, according to evidence-based clinical guidelines.[26] In women with thrombophilia and RIF, it is presumed that the treatment prevents thrombosis in the

trophoblastic invasion (antithrombotic agents including aspirin and anticoagulants) and/or suppresses the immune system (immunological treatments), which is suggested to increase the chances of a successful result of pregnancy.

In the context of hereditary thrombophilia and RIF, anticoagulant therapy or immunosuppressive treatment with steroids is discussed. The evidence is not sufficient to recommend in clinical practice in women with RIF and hereditary thrombophilia anticoagulant therapy, unless in the context of research, or if indicated for VTE prevention.

On RPL, some authors reported improve reproductive results with human peripheral blood monocytes and aspirin in women with hereditary thrombophilia, but others did not find significant differences in the results with anticoagulant therapy in women with RPL and hereditary thrombophilia.[27]

For women who fulfill the laboratory criteria of Anti Phospholipid syndrome and a history of three or more pregnancy losses. It is suggested to administer low-dose aspirin (75–100 mg/day) before conception and a prophylactic dose of Low Molecular weight heparin from the date of a positive pregnancy test for Improved reproductive results.

- *Male factor*: Due to the association between increased sperm DNA fragmentation and unhealthy lifestyle, encourage the couple to live healthy habits, stop smoking, moderate alcohol consumption, healthy weight, and avoid excessive exercise. Oral antioxidant treatment has been shown to reduce the incidence of sperm DNA fragmentation,[28] but there are no clear data that improve outcomes. Moreover, it is possible to select spermatozoa with low levels of DNA damage from the ejaculated semen samples.[29]
- *Other*: If implantation does not occur despite repeated treatment attempts after approaching all therapeutic options, alternative treatment options should be considered. If the probable origin of the problem lies with the embryo, gamete donation should be recommended. If the problems are in the uterus, surrogacy should be discussed.

REFERENCES

1. Zegers-Hochschild F, Adamson GD, Dyer S, et al. The International Glossary on infertility and fertility care, 2017. Fertil Steril.2017;108(3):393-406.
2. Polanski LT, Baumgarten MN, Quenby S, et al. What exactly do we mean by 'recurrent implantation failure'? A systematic review and opinion. Reprod Biomed Online. 2014;28(4): 409-23.
3. Coughlan C, Ledger W, Wang Q, et al. Recurrent implantation failure: definition and management. Reprod Biomed Online. 2014;28:14-38.
4. Simon A, Laufer N. Repeated implantation failure: clinical approach. Fertil Steril. 2012;97:1039-43.
5. Kung A, Munne S, Bankowski B, et al. Validation of next generation sequencing for comprehensive chromosome screening of embryos. Reprod Biomed Online. 2015;31:760-9.
6. Demirol A, Gurgan T. Effect of treatment of intrauterine pathologies with office hysteroscopy in patients with recurrent IVF failure. Reprod Biomed Online. 2004;8:590-4.
7. Hashimoto T, Koizumi M, Doshida M, et al. Efficacy of the endometrial receptivity array for repeated implantation failure in Japan: a retrospective, two-centers study. Reprod Med Biol. 2017;16:290-6.
8. Penzias AS. Recurrent IVF failure: other factors. Fertil Steril. 2012;97:1033-8.
9. Harton GL, Munne S, Surrey M, et al. Diminished effect of maternal age on implantation after preimplantation genetic diagnosis with array comparative genomic hybridization. Fertil Steril. 2013;100:1695-703.
10. Ruiz-Alonso M, Galindo N, Pellicer A, et al. What a difference two days make: "personalized" embryo transfer (pET) paradigm: a case report and pilot study. Hum Reprod. 2014;29:1244-7.
11. Ziel A, Friedler S, Schachter M, et al. Increased frequency of female partner chromosomal abnormalities in patients with high-order implantation failure after in vitro fertilization. Fertil Steril. 2002;78:515-9.
12. Saravelos SH, Cocksedge KA, Li TC. Prevalence and diagnosis of congenital uterine anomalies in women with reproductive failure: a critical appraisal. Hum Reprod Update. 2008;14:415-29.
13. Strandell A, Lindhard A, Waldenstrom U, et al. Hydrosalpinx and IVF outcome: a prospective, randomized multicentre trial in Scandinavia on salpingectomy prior to IVF. Hum Reprod. 1999;14:2762-9.
14. El-Toukhy T, Campo R, Khalaf Y, et al. Hysteroscopy in recurrent in-vitro fertilisation failure (TROPHY): a multicentre, randomised controlled trial. Lancet. 2016;387(10038):2614-21.
15. Azem F, Many A, Ben Ami I, et al. Increased rates of thrombophilia in women with repeated IVF failures. Hum Reprod. 2004;19:368-70.
16. Miyakis S, Lockshin MD, Atsumi T, et al. International consensus statement on an update of the classification criteria for definite antiphospholipid syndrome (APS). J Thromb Haemost. 2006;4:295-306.
17. Hiby SE, Regan L, Lo W, et al. Association of maternal killer-cell immunoglobulin-like receptors and parental HLA-C genotypes with recurrent miscarriage. Hum Reprod. 2008;23:972-6.
18. Sharma R, Biedenharn KR, Fedor JM, et al. Lifestyle factors and reproductive health: taking control of your fertility. Reprod Biol Endocrinol. 2013;11:66.
19. Zhao J, Zhang Q, Wang Y, et al. Whether sperm deoxyribonucleic acid fragmentation has an effect on pregnancy and miscarriage after in vitro fertilization/intracytoplasmic sperm injection: a systematic review and meta-analysis. Fertil Steril. 2014;102:998-1005.
20. Diaz-Gimeno P, Horcajadas JA, Martinez-Conejero JA, et al. A genomic diagnostic tool for human endometrial

receptivity based on the transcriptomic signature. Fertil Steril. 2011;95(1):50-60.
21. Scott RT Jr, Upham KM, Forman EJ, et al. Blastocyst biopsy with comprehensive chromosome screening and fresh embryo transfer significantly increases in vitro fertilization implantation and delivery rates: a randomized controlled trial. Fertil Steril. 2013;100:697-703.
22. Diaz-Gimeno P, Ruiz-Alonso M, Blesa D, et al. The accuracy and reproducibility of the endometrial receptivity array is superior to histology as a diagnostic method for endometrial receptivity. Fertil Steril. 2013;99(2):508-17.
23. Simon C, Vladimirov I, Castillon-Cortes G, et al. Prospective, randomized study of the endometrial receptivity analysis (ERA) test in the infertility work-up to guide personalized embryo transfer versus fresh transfer or deferred embryo transfer. Fertil Steril. 2016;106(3):46-7.
24. Margalioth EJ, Ben-Chetrit A, Gal M, et al. Investigation and treatment of repeated implantation failure following IVF–ET. Hum Reprod. 2006;21:3036-43.
25. Practice Committee of American Society for Reproductive Medicine, Society of Reproductive Surgeons. Salpingectomy for hydrosalpinx prior to in vitro fertilization. Fertil Steril. 2008;90(5 Suppl):S66-8.
26. Bates SM, Greer IA, Middeldorp S, et al. VTE, thrombophilia, antithrombotic therapy, and pregnancy: antithrombotic therapy and prevention of thrombosis, 9th ed: American College of Chest Physicians Evidence-Based Clinical Practice Guidelines. Chest. 2012;141:e691S-736S.
27. Skeith L, Carrier M, Kaaja R, et al. A meta-analysis of low-molecular-weight heparin to prevent pregnancy loss in women with inherited thrombophilia. Blood. 2016;127:1650-5.
28. Greco E, Iacobelli M, Rienzi L, et al. Reduction of the incidence of sperm DNA fragmentation by oral antioxidant treatment. J Androl. 2005;26:349-53.
29. Sakkas D, Alvarez J. Sperm DNA fragmentation: mechanisms of origin, impact on reproductive outcome, and analysis. Fertil Steril. 2010;93:1027-36.

CHAPTER

82

Recurrent Pregnancy Loss

Azadeh Patel, Parnita Sardana, Manish Banker

INTRODUCTION

Pregnancy loss is a negative life event and it causes profound emotional impact on the couple. Implantation failure and recurrent pregnancy loss (RPL) represent a different point on a spectrum, which can be termed as reproductive failure as suggested by recent molecular studies.[1] The World Health Organization (WHO), Center for Disease Control and Prevention (CDC), and the National Center for Health Statistics all define miscarriage as pregnancy termination before 20 weeks of gestation or with the fetus born weighing less than 500 g. RPL is defined as two or more pregnancy losses and/or resolved and treated pregnancies of unknown location after 6 weeks.[2] The exact prevalence of RPL is difficult to estimate as the numerator (the patients who experience RPL) and the denominator (women at risk of RPL, women in fertile age, or all women who are trying for pregnancy) are difficult to obtain. But the prevalence of clinical RPL is between 0.8% and 1.4% and between 2% and 3% including biochemical pregnancies in general population.[3] RPL can be classified as primary or secondary. Primary RPL refers to RPL in a female with no previous viable pregnancies, whereas secondary RPL is when the woman had a previous pregnancy beyond 20 weeks of gestational age.

RISK FACTORS

The risk factors associated with RPL are:

- *Advanced maternal age*: Maternal age of more than 35 years is a risk factor for RPL. The risk of miscarriage increases significantly after the age of 30 years irrespective of previous obstetric history.[4] The risk of another pregnancy loss is double in women more than or equal to 35 years of age as compared to women of age less than 35 years.[5]
- *Previous obstetric history*: The risk ratio (RR) for live birth reduces by 10% after each nonvisualized pregnancy loss and by 20% after each clinical loss.[6] In cases of secondary unexplained RPL, the losses after the viable pregnancy are important and not the ones prior to that.[7]
- *Stress*: Stress is associated with RPL, but there is no evidence that stress is direct cause of RPL. Although several studies have confirmed an association between stress and RPL, heterogeneity in scales used and quality of the study were the main limitations.[8,9]
- Occupational or environmental exposure to heavy metals and lack of micronutrients are associated with RPL. Deficiencies of serum zinc, copper, and vitamin E levels are associated with RPL, and high levels of serum selenium, lead, and cadmium cause pregnancy loss in women with RPL.[10]
- Chronic endometritis is characterized by plasma cell infiltrate in the endometrium due to wide range of microorganisms. Treatment with antibiotics have shown to improve live birth rate.[11,12]

ETIOPATHOLOGY

Several factors have been associated with RPL like chromosomal abnormalities, uterine anomalies, hereditary and acquired thrombophilias, and endocrine factors, which are supported by various studies, whereas majority of the cases are unexplained. The causes and their management are discussed in detail in this chapter.

CYTOGENETIC ABNORMALITY

Cytogenetic abnormalities contribute around 2–5% of causes of RPL. The risk factors include high-maternal age (>35 years) and paternal karyotype abnormality, but majority of them are idiopathic. Sporadic cytogenetic abnormalities in the conceptus are diagnosed by analyzing the products of conception (POC). The abnormalities detected in fetus may show numerical chromosomal abnormalities (aneuploidy—trisomy or monosomy) or structural chromosomal abnormalities (balanced/unbalanced translocation, inversion, and deletion). The common causes of fetal aneuploidy are dispermy or failure of maternal meiotic disjunction resulting in diploid oocyte. Structural chromosomal abnormalities may arise de novo during gametogenesis or may be inherited from a parent carrying balanced translocation or inversion. When one of the parents is a carrier of a balanced structural chromosomal abnormality, it may result in either a child with a normal chromosome pattern or a child with balanced structural chromosomal abnormality or a conceptus with unbalanced structural chromosomal abnormality.[13] Balanced reciprocal/Robertsonian translocations are mainly associated with RPL.

Incidence

The risk of sporadic miscarriage between 6 weeks and 12 weeks of pregnancy in maternal age of less than 35 years is 9–12% and this markedly increases over the age of 35 years due to increased incidence of trisomic pregnancies. The risk of miscarriage after the age of 40 years is 50%. Also, the risk of aneuploidy in patients of RPL is lower than that of sporadic cases.[14]

Investigations

Karyotype of the POC and parents should be done in order to give prognostic information to the couple regarding subsequent pregnancy outcomes. Parental karyotype is carried out for all couples of RPL even though the frequency of finding an abnormality was found to be 1.9% in large retrospective cohort study (n = 20,432).[15,16] The methods commonly used are:

- Karyotyping by G-banding technique can assess the structural and numerical chromosomal rearrangements. Failure of tissue culture and inadequacy to distinguish between contaminated maternal tissue and normal euploid female fetus are its limitations.[17]
- *Fluorescence in situ hybridization (FISH)*: It is a molecular cytogenetic technique that uses fluorescent probes. It analyzes chromosome number 13, 18, 21, and sex chromosomes X and Y. Analysis of only certain and not all chromosomes is the limitation.
- *Array comparative genomic hybridization (aCGH)*: It is a better technique, as it avoids the limitations of karyotyping and FISH.[18,19] Although it can detect unbalanced translocations, but it cannot detect balanced chromosomal abnormalities such as reciprocal translocations and inversions, which can be detected by karyotyping by G-banding.
- *Next-generation sequencing (NGS)*: It is a newer technique and is not adequately studied for POC analysis, but has a good prospect in future.

Parental karyotyping may be more appropriate when unbalanced translocation is detected in products of conceptus.

Treatment

All couples should be offered genetic counseling whenever any fetal or parental chromosomal abnormality is detected. Genetic counseling offers a couple prognosis of future pregnancies with unbalanced chromosomal complement and opportunity for familial chromosomal studies. The likelihood of subsequent live birth depends on the number and the type of the chromosome(s) involved and the type of rearrangement. The cytogenetic abnormalities can be detected before implantation in embryos using newer technologies in IVF (in vitro fertilization) such as preimplantation genetic testing for aneuploidy (PGT-A) for screening the embryos for aneuploidies, preimplantation genetic testing-structural rearrangement (PGT-SR) for structural rearrangements, and preimplantation genetic diagnosis (PGD) for any known parental genetic abnormalities. Embryos are created in IVF cycle, which are then biopsied and screened for chromosomal anomalies which allow transfer of normal unaffected embryo(s) for implantation and thus it has been proposed as potential treatment in RPL. Earlier, most of the embryos were biopsied at day 3 using FISH, which looked at a specific number of chromosomes and at a very early stage with higher chances of mosaicism. Later on, array CGH and NGS have been introduced, which involve whole genome sequencing at blastocyst stage with higher accuracy. However, if the couple does not wish to opt for IVF then chorionic villus sampling and amniocentesis in pregnancy are other options. Change of either or both gamete may be required as last resort.

THROMBOPHILIAS

Thrombophilias are characterized by clinical tendency to thrombosis or molecular abnormality of hemostasis that predisposes to thromboembolic diseases. This tendency to form clots can arise from genetic factors or acquired changes in clotting mechanisms or interaction between genetic and acquired factors. There are two types of thrombophilias namely hereditary and acquired.

1. *Hereditary thrombophilias:* There are rare genetic conditions, which include factor V Leiden mutation, prothrombin mutation, protein C, protein S, antithrombin deficiency, methylenetetrahydrofolate reductase (MTHFR) mutation, and predispose patients to thromboembolic events. These causes should be evaluated in patients with family history or previous history of thromboembolic events. As there is no/very weak association between RPL and hereditary thrombophilias, routine screening is not recommended.
2. *Acquired thrombophilias*: Antiphospholipid syndrome (APS) was first defined as a syndrome in 1983 consisting of a triad of manifestation involving arterial and/or venous thrombosis, recurrent fetal loss, and accompanied by mild-to-moderate thrombocytopenia and elevated titers of antiphospholipid antibodies (APAs). APAs are a heterogeneous group of autoantibodies that bind to negatively charged phospholipids. The antibodies associated with thrombosis in APS are lupus anticoagulant, anticardiolipin antibodies IgG or IgM, beta-2-glycoprotein IgG or IgM (B2GPI). The antiphospholipids (aPL) are highly different from patient to patient and are specific for variety of cellular phospholipids and phospholipid-binding proteins.

Antiphospholipid syndrome is diagnosed by Miyakis criteria, which is an update of Sapporo criteria. The incidence of APS for RPL is 8–42%.[2]

International Consensus Classification Criteria for the Antiphospholipid Syndrome[20]

International Consensus Classification Criteria for the antiphospholipid syndrome are given in Table 1.

Table 1: International Consensus Classification Criteria for the antiphospholipid syndrome (APS).

APS is present, if one of the following clinical criteria and one of the laboratory criteria are met:	
Clinical criteria	*Laboratory criteria*
• Vascular thrombosis • Pregnancy morbidity: – One or more unexplained deaths of morphologically normal fetuses after the 10th week of gestation by ultrasound or direct examination of the fetus – One or more premature births of a morphologically normal neonate before the 34th week of gestation because of eclampsia or severe preeclampsia or recognized features of placental insufficiency – Three or more unexplained consecutive spontaneous abortions before the 10th week of gestation with maternal anatomic or hormonal abnormalities and paternal and maternal chromosomal causes excluded	• Lupus anticoagulant present in plasma on two or more occasions at least 12 weeks apart, or • Anticardiolipin antibody of IgG or IgM isotype in serum or plasma present in medium or high titer (>40 GPL or MPL or >99th percentile) on two or more occasions at least 12 weeks apart, or • Anti-beta-2-glycoprotein 1 antibody of IgG and/or IgM isotype in serum or plasma (in titer of >99th percentile) present on two or more occasions at least 12 weeks apart

(Ig: immunoglobulin)

Pathophysiology

The antiphospholipid antibodies have variety of effects like:

- Inhibition of villous cytotrophoblastic differentiation
- Inhibition of extravillous cytotrophoblastic invasion in decidua
- Induction of syncytiotrophoblast apoptosis
- Initiation of maternal inflammatory pathways on cytotrophoblast surface
- It induces thrombosis by decreasing prostacyclin production by endothelial cells and increasing thromboxane production by platelets and by decreasing protein C activation.

Treatment

After a pregnancy is diagnosed in patient with APS, management includes prevention of thrombosis and care of pregnancy. Pregnancy in women with diagnosed APS is at an increased risk of miscarriage and maternal complications (hypertension, preeclampsia, and thrombosis) during pregnancy and in puerperium. Close maternal and fetal monitoring with a multidisciplinary approach by a team comprising of an obstetrician, rheumatologist, hematologist, and a neonatologist should be done for timely intervention and prevention of complications. The treatment includes aspirin, heparin, glucocorticoids, and intravenous immunoglobulins (IVIG).

- *Aspirin*: It is an anti-inflammatory and antiplatelet drug. It has antithromboxane effect, hence it improves placental blood flow by decreasing thromboxane to prostacyclin ratio, inhibition of platelet aggregation, and thus in turn promotes implantation. Low-dose aspirin 75–100 mg per day is the recommended dose.
- *Heparin:* Unfractionated heparin (UFH) or low-molecular weight heparin (LMWH) is considered for prevention of thrombosis. It should be started before

pregnancy or as early as possible in first trimester or as soon as a live pregnancy is documented. It directly binds to APA and inhibits their activity causing APS. They also inhibit complement activation in formation of activation product (mainly C3a and C5a). Prophylactic dose (LMWH—enoxaparin 1 mg/kg/day) is given to patients with more than or equal to three early pregnancy losses (<10 weeks) with no history of arterial, venous, or small vessel thrombosis. Full dose (enoxaparin 1 mg/kg every 12 hourly) is given to patients who diagnosed with APS and having history of arterial, venous, or small vessel thrombosis and also to patients with pregnancy loss of more than 10 weeks with no history of thrombosis. LMWH is monitored with factor Xa levels. LMWH is preferred over UFH due to lower incidence of hemorrhage, osteoporosis, and heparin-induced thrombocytopenia.

The combination of heparin (UFH or LMWH) and low-dose aspirin is superior to aspirin alone in patients with RPL and APS.[21] As per the recent guidelines, women with APS should be started with low-dose aspirin (75–100 mg/day) before conception and a prophylactic dose of heparin should be started on the day of positive pregnancy test.[22]

Refractory Antiphospholipid Syndrome

Pregnancy losses continue in 20–30% of cases despite aspirin and heparin treatment. In these patients:

- Rule out fetal chromosomal abnormalities by POC karyotype.
- Optimal dose of heparin needs to be worked out and higher doses of heparin may be needed in case of abortion of a euploid embryo. Benefits should be weighed against the side effects.
- If there are other autoimmune phenomena then steroids (prednisolone) should be given to control the activity.
- Intravenous immunoglobulin should be given, if the pregnancy loss is due to any obstetric complications like preeclampsia and placental abruption.

INFECTIVE CAUSES

Mycoplasma, *Ureaplasma*, *Chlamydia trachomatis*, *Listeria monocytogenes*, and herpes simplex virus (HSV) are speculated to play a role in RPL. Certain infections like *Toxoplasma gondii*, Cytomegalovirus (CMV), rubella, HSV, *Listeria monocytogenes*, and Coxsackievirus are known to cause sporadic spontaneous pregnancy loss and very rarely in 0.5–5% of cases may cause RPL.[23] The mechanisms of pregnancy loss could be due to direct infection of the uterus, fetus or placenta, placental insufficiency, chronic endometritis or endocervicitis, and amnionitis. Routine infectious evaluation is not recommended, however, specific treatment for the cause, if diagnosed, should be given.

ENDOCRINE CAUSES

It is well known that the development and maintenance of pregnancy are dependent on numerous endocrinological events, which are responsible for successful growth and development of the fetus. It is estimated that approximately 8–12% of cases of RPL are caused by endocrine diseases.[24] RPL may be caused mainly by thyroid disorders, hyperprolactinemia, diabetes mellitus, polycystic ovary syndrome (PCOS), and inadequate progesterone production by corpus luteum.

Thyroid Disorder

The prevalence of thyroid dysfunction in general population is 2–3%. Thyroid disorders, especially hypothyroidism, have been linked with infertility and RPL. Thyroid hormone plays an important role in fetal neurocognitive development and is also involved in folliculogenesis, spermatogenesis, fertilization, and embryogenesis. T3 along with follicle-stimulating hormone (FSH) enhances granulosa cell proliferation and inhibits its apoptosis. It increases the expression of matrix metalloproteinases (MMP) namely MMP-2, MMP-3, fetal fibronectin in early placental extravillous trophoblasts.[25] Therefore, patients should be euthyroid before they plan for pregnancy and thyroid levels should be monitored strictly during pregnancy. The thyroid abnormalities associated with RPL are hyperthyroidism, overt hypothyroidism, subclinical hypothyroidism, and thyroid autoimmunity.

- *Hyperthyroidism*: Incidence of hyperthyroidism is approximately 0.1–0.4% of pregnancies.[26] Untreated overt hyperthyroidism may lead to increased risk of spontaneous miscarriage, preterm delivery, preeclampsia, congestive cardiac failure, fetal growth restriction, and increased perinatal morbidity and mortality.
  However, hyperthyroidism has not been reported as independent cause of RPL.
- *Hypothyroidism*: Causes of hypothyroidism can be Hashimoto's thyroiditis (chronic autoimmune thyroiditis), endemic iodine deficiency, thyroidectomy, and radioactive iodine therapy. Hypothyroidism can lead to miscarriage, preterm birth, low birth weight, and also has adverse effects on neurodevelopment of the fetus.

- *Thyroid autoimmunity*: The prevalence of autoimmune thyroid disorder is 10–15%.[27] Mechanism of thyroid antibodies causing RPL could be due to generalized activation of the immune system and an increased autoimmune reactivity against the fetoplacental unit. Women with RPL have a significant increase in Thl endometrial cell population, hypersecretion of interferon (IFN), and reduced secretion of interleukin-4 (IL-4) and IL-10. There are no clear recommendations as to whether euthyroid women with thyroid antibodies should be given thyroid replacement therapy.[28]

Investigation

Thyroid screening with thyroid-stimulating hormone (TSH) and antithyroid peroxidase (anti-TPO) antibodies is recommended in patients with RPL. If abnormal then free levels of T3 and T4 should be checked.

Treatment

Patients with overt hypothyroidism should be treated with levothyroxine. The aim is to maintain TSH levels below 2.5 mU/L in first trimester, 3 mU/L in second trimester, and 3.5 mU/L in third trimester. Treatment of subclinical hypothyroidism is controversial. The European Thyroid Association guidelines and American Thyroid Association Guidelines recommend treatment of subclinical hypothyroidism.[29] Two cohort studies contradict this and showed no difference in terms of live birth rates/miscarriage in patients with subclinical hypothyroidism.[30,31] There is a need for further investigating the role of potential treatment effects and risks of levothyroxine supplementation in patients with subclinical hypothyroidism. There is insufficient evidence to recommend levothyroxine in euthyroid patients with raised anti-TPO antibodies but should be prescribed to patients with raised TSH and anti-TPO antibodies.

Polycystic Ovarian Syndrome

Patients with PCOS have an increased rate of pregnancy loss, predominantly in first trimester. Factors responsible for RPL in PCOS patients could be hyperinsulinemia leading to increase in plasminogen activator inhibitor activity causing hypofibrinolysis and thus leading to miscarriage. Other factors could be obesity, luteinizing hormone (LH) hypersecretion, hyperandrogenism, and thrombophilias.[32] Insulin metabolism can be assessed by fasting glucose, fasting insulin, fasting glucose to insulin ratio, and glucose tolerance test. Routine assessment of PCOS, fasting glucose, and fasting insulin is not recommended. Although several studies have demonstrated the role of metformin in reducing RPL,[33] but due to lack of substantial studies, metformin is not recommended in patients with RPL.

Hyperprolactinemia

High-prolactin levels are associated with ovulatory dysfunction, impaired folliculogenesis and oocyte maturation and a short luteal phase, thus contributing to RPL. Prolactin testing is only recommended in the presence of clinical symptoms indicating hyperprolactinemia like oligomenorrhea, galactorrhea.[34] Treatment with bromocriptine should be considered, if hyperprolactinemia is diagnosed.

IMMUNOLOGICAL CAUSE

For a healthy pregnancy, a bidirectional communication takes place between the fetal trophoblastic cells and the endometrium, which is regulated by various maternal immune mediator cells, cytokines, chemokines, growth factors, and adhesion molecules. The proinflammatory cytokines regulate to establish endometrial receptivity and window of implantation; chemokines and adhesion molecules mediate blastocyst apposition and adhesion to the endometrium, and finally decidual immune cells mainly uterine natural killer cells (uNK cells), T-helper cells, and dendritic cells play a role for mediating and maintaining the immune tolerance and vascular remodeling with decidual development. Immune dysregulation has been proposed as a cause for fetal rejection and pregnancy loss. Therapies such as IVIG, intralipid therapy, paternal leukocyte immunization, third party donor cell immunizations, and trophoblastic infusions have been tried but are still not found to be beneficial.

Natural Killer Cells

The NK cells are detected in peripheral blood and endometrial tissue. Previously, studies have reported association between high prepregnancy peripheral blood NK cells and RPL,[35] but recent prospective studies reported no impact on RPL.[36-38] Several studies have tried to find an association between NK cells in endometrial biopsy and RPL. One case-control study reported that the CD56 bright NK cell subset was significantly lower in endometrial biopsies of women with RPL than controls,[39] whereas, other studies found that the frequency of CD56+ (or unspecified NK cells) cells was significantly higher in RPL than in controls.[40-42] In two case–control studies, no difference was found in NK cell subsets in the endometrium between women with RPL and controls.[43,44] So, NK cell testing in peripheral blood or endometrial tissue is not recommended as a routine.

Tumor Necrosis Factor-α

It is a marker for the degree of systemic inflammation. High levels are reported in patients of RPL. The plasma levels or in vitro production of many cytokines are influenced by polymorphisms in the cytokine genes, which have also been found in women with RPL. An association between transforming growth factor β-1 (TGF-β1) or tumor necrosis factor (TNF)-α gene polymorphisms and RPL has been reported.[45,46] Plasma cytokine concentrations may be completely different as compared to uterine concentrations. The measurement of cytokines in endometrial tissue, decidual tissue, or endometrial flushing is subject to technical difficulties.

Antinuclear Antibodies

They are antibodies against various components of the cell nuclei, frequently found in patients with autoimmune diseases. Although some studies have found an association between raised antinuclear antibody (ANA) and RPL,[47] a direct pathophysiological link between the presence of autoantibodies such as ANA in women with RPL and fetal death has not yet been documented.

Human Leukocyte Antigen-C and Killer-cell Immunoglobulin-like Receptors

During pregnancy, the developing fetal-placental unit is considered as semi-allograft, as allogeneic paternal human leukocyte antigens (HLAs) are presented to a mother's immune system. Maternal immune system should permit as well as restrict fetal cytotrophoblastic invasion for healthy implantation and maintenance of pregnancy. It is suggested that, in pregnancy, reactions of NK cells (cytotoxicity and cytokine production) are modified by interactions between specific receptors (killer immunoglobulin-like receptors or KIRs) on the NK cells and HLA-C or HLA-G, which are the only HLA genes expressed on the trophoblast. KIR can be activating or inhibitory and HLA has two allotypes C1 and C2. Combination of the woman carrying KIR genes that are mainly inhibitory and the man carrying C2 allotypes is more frequent among RPL than control couples.[48]

Human Leukocyte Antigen-G

The HLA-G polymorphisms have also been investigated in RPL, as they are suggested to modulate NK cell cytotoxicity and cytokine secretion at the fetomaternal interface. Low levels may be associated with homozygosity for HLA-G14-bp insertion in the HLA-G gene. Two meta-analyses concluded that the HLA-G14-bp insertion frequency was significantly increased in women with RPL [OR 1.27 (1.04–1.55) and 1.47 (1.13–1.91), respectively].[49,50] The association of RPL to HLA-G14-bp insertion may be secondary to a primary association to the HLA-DRB1*03 allele.[51]

ANATOMICAL CAUSES

Uterine anomalies have been associated with RPL. Till date, there has been a lack of clear understanding regarding causative mechanisms leading to pregnancy loss. Apart from pregnancy loss, uterine anomalies predispose women to infertility, abnormal fetal presentation, preterm labor, etc. Anatomical factors may be congenital or acquired. Congenital uterine defects are due to defects in development of Mullerian duct development.

Incidence

Congenital uterine anomalies are present in 5.5% (3.5–8.5%) in general population, 13.3% (8.9–20%) in patients with history of miscarriage and 24.5% (18.3–32.8%) in patients with miscarriage and infertility.[52] Septate uterus is most commonly associated with RPL.

Mechanism

The mechanism of RPL in congenital anomalies is that it mainly interferes with vasculature of endometrium leading to inadequate and abnormal placentation. Also, uterine anomalies may lead to reduced uterine cavity, uncoordinated uterine contractions leading to preterm births and preterm premature rupture of membranes (PPROM).

Diagnosis

All women with recurrent first-trimester miscarriage and all women with one or more second-trimester miscarriages should have a pelvic ultrasound to assess uterine anatomy. Suspected uterine anomalies may require further investigations to confirm the diagnosis using hysteroscopy, laparoscopy, or three-dimensional pelvic ultrasound. Uterine anomalies can be detected by:

- *Two-dimensional ultrasonography (USG)*: It provides information on anatomy of uterus and cervix. It involves low cost and is noninvasive but is highly dependent on experience of examiner.
- *Hysterosalpingography (HSG)*: It is simple, widely available, and easy to use diagnostic tool for evaluation of

uterus. Major disadvantage is its inability to differentiate uterine anomalies.

- *Hysterosalpingo-contrast sonography*: It is minimally invasive, simple, and low-cost test, which gives information about anatomy of uterus and cervix, but is grossly dependent on examiner's experience.
- *Three-dimensional USG*: It gives valuable information about anatomy of cervix and uterus, external contour of uterus, and adnexa. It provides precise information and objective measurements of uterine dimensions, and it is more reliable and has high sensitivity and specificity than 2D USG.
- *Magnetic resonance imaging (MRI)*: It is noninvasive technique with no radiation exposure. It gives detailed information of uterine contour, cavity, cervical canal, and adnexa. It is costly and requires training and experience.
- *Hysteroscopy*: It is minimally invasive procedure, which gives information about anatomy of uterus, ostia, cavity, cervix, and vagina and also allows correction in the same setting. It is unable to differentiate between septate and bicorporeal uterus.
- *Laparoscopy*: It is invasive technique, which provides valuable details about anatomy of uterus and adnexa when combined with hysteroscopy.

Management

Hysteroscopic metroplasty (resection of septum) should be considered for septate uterus. Significant decrease is reported in terms of pregnancy loss in patients who underwent metroplasty as compared to patients with no treatment.[53] It can be accomplished through resectoscope or scissors. No technique was found to be superior to the other.[54]

For hemiuterus, surgery is recommended only to remove the rudimentary horn, if present, so as to avoid risk of ectopic pregnancy. The surgical correction of a bicorporeal uterus can be performed by Strassman metroplasty operation, but it is not recommended. There is insufficient evidence in favor of metroplasty in women with bicorporeal uterus with double cervix (didelphic uterus) and hence it is not routinely recommended. Prophylactic cervical cerclage should be performed in patients with congenital uterine anomalies.

Acquired Intrauterine Malformations

Acquired uterine malformations contribute to either space-occupying causes (endometrial polyps or submucous fibroid) or space-restricting causes (intrauterine adhesions), which distort the endometrial cavity. Hysteroscopic correction is strongly recommended.

- *Endometrial polyps*: Although polyps do not have clear association with RPL, hysteroscopic removal can be considered for polyps more than 1 cm.[55]
- *Fibroids*: Submucosal fibroids deform the uterine cavity and the overlying endometrium is thin and inadequate for normal implantation and should be considered for myomectomy. Surgery for intramural fibroids not distorting the cavity is not recommended.
- *Intrauterine adhesions (Asherman's syndrome)*: Prior dilatation and curettage may be a predisposing factor for intrauterine adhesions.[56] Hysteroscopic adhesiolysis and prevention of recurrence are recommended in patients with RPL.
- *Cervical insufficiency*: It is the inability of the uterine cervix to retain a pregnancy in second trimester, in the absence of uterine contractions.[57] Congenitally, it may be associated with structural cervical weakness due to genetic disorders affecting collagen like Ehlers–Danlos syndrome, uterine anomalies, in utero diethylstilbestrol exposure or acquired due to cervical trauma, which may be from previous labor or delivery (spontaneous, forceps/vacuum, and cesarean) or rapid mechanical dilatation for gynecological procedure or may be as a result of treatment of cervical intraepithelial neoplasia (CIN). Cervical encerclage is associated with surgical risks and also has the risk of stimulating uterine contractions, therefore, it should be considered only in women who are likely to benefit.[58] Women with prior history of second-trimester loss should be offered serial cervical sonographic monitoring. Cochrane review found no benefit of prophylactic cervical cerclage in RPL.[59]

OTHERS

Vitamin D Deficiency

Vitamin D deficiency is highly prevalent in women of reproductive age group. Deficiency of vitamin D was associated with increased prevalence of antiphospholipid antibody, ANA, anti-single-stranded DNA (ssDNA), and antithyroid peroxidase antibody (TPOAb), and with higher peripheral blood CD19+B and CD56+NK cell levels and NK cytotoxicity.[60] Pregnancy causes a shift toward Th2 in T-cell immunity and vitamin D plays an important role in regulating immune response by promoting Th2 immune responses and suppressing Th1 responses. It has immune regulatory effects on NK cell cytotoxicity, cytokine secretion, and degranulation process. Lower expression of vitamin D receptor has been reported in women with RPL as compared to normal pregnant women.[61] Vitamin D deficiency is associated with maternal and fetal complications, therefore, prophylactic supplementation should be considered even though there is no conclusive evidence of vitamin D deficiency association with RPL.

Hyperhomocysteinemia

Elevated levels of homocysteine are a known risk factor for venous thromboembolism and adverse pregnancy outcome (RPL, preeclampsia, abruption, and neural tubal defects). Plasma homocysteine levels can be determined by several factors like levels of vitamin B6, B12, folate, MTHFR mutation, increased age, and hypothyroidism. Patients with hyperhomocysteinemia should be treated with high doses of folic acid, vitamin B6. Aspirin and LMWH should be started once pregnancy is detected.

Male Factor

Male factor is known to play a vital role in fertilization, human embryo development, its viability and placental proliferation. The role of the male partner of the couples with RPL still remains unclear as the majority has normal semen parameters. Men with very low-sperm counts (<1 million/mL) often have a higher incidence of chromosomal abnormalities or Y chromosomal microdeletion.[62] Sperm morphology, sperm function tests, sperm DNA fragmentation index (DFI), and sperm aneuploidy test are used for investigating the male factor associated with RPL.

Sperm morphology can be studied during routine semen analysis. Poor sperm motility has been found to have direct association with poor sperm capacitation ability and poor embryo development. This can be tested by various sperm function tests such as hypo-osmotic swelling test (HOST), nuclear chromatin decondensation test (NCDT), and acrosome status (AS) test.[63]

The DNA fragmentation occurs due to abnormal packaging of the sperm chromatin, which can be because of advanced paternal age or factors which increase oxidative stress like smoking, occupational exposure to toxins, exogenous heat, varicocele. Significant increase in miscarriage rates in men with high-DNA sperm damage has been reported as compared to those with low DNA sperm damage.[64] Y chromosome microdeletions were not found to be associated with RPL.[65] These tests should be offered in cases of unexplained RPL. The couples should be advised cessation of smoking, alcohol, excessive exercise as they may increase the chances of RPL. Antioxidants have not found to improve the chances of live birth. Magnetic activated cell sorting (MACS) can be used to separate the fragmented and the nonfragmented sperms after semen preparation in ART. Sperm donation can be used in severe cases. In cases of very high DFI, IVF with testicular sperms has better outcome than with sperms from the ejaculate.[66]

Sperm aneuploidy is defined as any deviation from the normal haploid state of sperms. The main causes of aneuploidy are nondisjunction, anaphase lag, and ineffective checkpoint control. Trisomy 13, 18, 21, X monosomy, and Klinefelter (XXY-XXXXY) are some aneuploidies, which are associated with sperm aneuploidy and are compatible with survival. FISH is used to detect sperm aneuploidy. Up to 40% of the men with RPL and normal semen parameters have abnormal aneuploidy with FISH.[67] IVF with preimplantation genetic screening (PGS) should be offered to these patients.

UNEXPLAINED RECURRENT PREGNANCY LOSS

Fifty to seventy-five percent of patients with RPL, where no definite cause can be found, are termed as unexplained RPL. The chance of successful pregnancy depends on maternal age and parity. The following treatments have been tried for such patients:

1. *Lymphocyte immunization therapy:* Women with RPL lack anti-paternal antibodies that protect the fetus against rejection and thus resultant antibodies after lymphocyte immunization therapy (LIT) was suggested to be beneficial, but the clinical impact of such antibodies is unclear.[68,69] LIT therapy has not been found to be beneficial for RPL.[70,71] This treatment raises safety concerns related to transfusion risks (HIV/hepatitis infection transmission, transfusion reactions), neonatal alloimmune thrombocytopenia, and production of red blood cells antibody, which may result in erythroblastosis fetalis. Hence, it is not recommended for treatment of unexplained RPL.
2. *Intravenous immunoglobulins:* Intravenous immunoglobulin is used in many autoimmune and inflammatory diseases, as it reduces symptoms through elimination of immune complexes, interaction with Fc receptors, elimination of activated complement factors, interference with antigen presentation, and neutralization of inflammatory cytokines. Role of IVIG in RPL has been studied and has not found to beneficial.[71,72] No serious adverse effects were noted except headache and skin rash.
3. *Prednisolone:* Glucocorticoids are used in treatment of most autoimmune diseases and have also been

tried in treatment of RPL with suspected immune etiology. Although several studies have demonstrated beneficial role of prednisolone in unexplained recurrent miscarriages but these studies had limitations of heterogeneity with different inclusion criteria, different regimens, and dose of steroids.[73,74] The adverse effects with prednisolone are gestational diabetes, hypertension, intrauterine growth restriction (IUGR), and preterm births.

4. *Anticoagulants:* Low-dose aspirin and heparin are beneficial in treatment of APLA and hereditary thrombophilias, but they have been increasingly used in treatment of patients with RPL without APLA. Cochrane review concluded that there was no significant benefit on live birth rates with anticoagulant therapy with placebo in patients with or without hereditary thrombophilias.[75] Later to this Cochrane, there were three randomized controlled trials (RCTs) published comparing heparin with placebo where two RCTs found no benefit with regards to live birth rate,[76,77] while the third study reported decrease in miscarriage rate with increase in live birth rates.[78]
5. *Progesterone:* A double-blind, placebo-controlled, RCT investigated vaginal progesterone to matched placebo and compared live birth rates in patients with unexplained RPL[79] and found no difference in terms of LBR in progesterone group (65.8%) compared to placebo group (63.3%), RR 1.04; 95% CI; 0.94–1.15. However, a meta-analysis of 10 trials reported lower risk of subsequent pregnancy loss in patients receiving progesterone (RR 0.72; 95% CI 0.53–0.97) and a higher LBR (RR 1.07; 95% CI; 1.02–1.15) when compared to those who did not.[80] Discrepancies of their results were explained by differences in the progesterone supplement and inclusion of seven trials published before 1990 when the quality standards were lower.
6. *Intralipid therapy:* Intravenous lipid emulsions (such as intralipid) are used for parenteral nutrition after surgery and in premature babies. Recently, they have been tried in unexplained RPL. One non-RCT trial compared intralipid versus IVIG in women with RPL and found that live birth rates were similar in both groups (92% and 88% respectively with p = 0.145).[81] Low-dose intralipid treatment is not associated with serious adverse effects but the higher doses are reported to cause acute kidney injury, cardiac arrest, acute lung injury, venous thromboembolism, fat embolism, fat overload syndrome, pancreatitis, allergic reactions, and increased susceptibility to infections.[82]
7. *Granulocyte colony-stimulating factor:* They are growth factors, which may help in promoting trophoblast growth and also have antiabortive effects. A RCT investigating the role of granulocyte colony-stimulating factor (G-CSF) in RPL found it to be beneficial as compared to no treatment (OR 5.1; 95% CI 1.5–18.4; p = 0.0061).[83] However, another RCT found no beneficial effect of G-CSF on implantation and pregnancy rates after IVF. Thus, due to lack of substantial evidence, it is not recommended in RPL.[84]

Though all these treatments have been proposed and researched, yet none of them have proven to have a definite role.

The experience of RPL is devastating, therefore, it is essential for the clinician to thoroughly evaluate the patient after two pregnancy losses. Full work-up should be done to rule out treatable causes like genetic causes, endocrine diseases, APS, and uterine anomalies. An individual's prognosis will depend on both the underlying causes of RPL and number of prior pregnancy losses. The treatment of the couple should be individualized and blanket therapy should be avoided. Regardless of the cause, patients should be counseled regarding good prognosis for the next pregnancy.

REFERENCES

1. Makrigiannakis A, Petsas G, Toth B, et al. Recent advances in understanding immunology of reproductive failure. J Reprod Immunol. 2011;90(1):96-104.
2. Practice Committee of the American Society for Reproductive Medicine. Evaluation and treatment of recurrent pregnancy loss: a committee opinion. Fertil Steril. 2012;98(5):1103-11.
3. Larsen EC, Christiansen OB, Kolte AM, et al. New insights into mechanisms behind miscarriage. BMC Med. 2013;11(1):154.
4. Bhattacharya S, Townend J, Bhattacharya S. Recurrent miscarriage: Are three miscarriages one too many? Analysis of a Scottish population-based database of 151,021 pregnancies. Eur J Obstet Gynecol Reprod Biol. 2010;150(1):24-7.
5. Lo W, Rai R, Hameed A, et al. The effect of body mass index on the outcome of pregnancy in women with recurrent miscarriage. J Family Community Med. 2012;19(3):167.
6. Kolte AM, Van Oppenraaij RH, Quenby S, et al.; ESHRE Special Interest Group Early Pregnancy. Non-visualized pregnancy losses are prognostically important for unexplained recurrent miscarriage. Hum Reprod. 2014;29(5):931-7.
7. Egerup P, Lindschou J, Gluud C, et al.; ImmuReM IPD Study Group. The effects of intravenous immunoglobulins in women with recurrent miscarriages: a systematic review of randomised trials with meta-analyses and trial sequential analyses including individual patient data. PloS One. 2015;10(10):e0141588.
8. Li W, Newell-Price J, Jones GL, et al. Relationship between psychological stress and recurrent miscarriage. Reprod Biomed Online. 2012;25(2):180-9.
9. Kolte AM, Olsen LR, Mikkelsen EM, et al. Depression and emotional stress is highly prevalent among women with recurrent pregnancy loss. Hum Reprod. 2015;30(4):777-82.

10. Ajayi OO, Charles-Davies MA, Arinola OG. Progesterone, selected heavy metals and micronutrients in pregnant Nigerian women with a history of recurrent spontaneous abortion. Afr Health Sci. 2012;12(2):153-9.
11. Cicinelli E, Matteo M, Tinelli R, et al. Chronic endometritis due to common bacteria is prevalent in women with recurrent miscarriage as confirmed by improved pregnancy outcome after antibiotic treatment. Reprod Sci. 2014;21(5):640-7.
12. McQueen DB, Bernardi LA, Stephenson MD. Chronic endometritis in women with recurrent early pregnancy loss and/or fetal demise. Fertil Steril. 2014;101(4):1026-30.
13. Goddijn M. Chromosome abnormalities in first-trimester pregnancy loss. Universiteit van Amsterdam (Host); 2003.
14. Ogasawara M, Aoki K, Okada S, et al. Embryonic karyotype of abortuses in relation to the number of previous miscarriages. Fertil Steril. 2000;73(2):300-4.
15. Franssen MT, Korevaar JC, van der Veen F, et al. Reproductive outcome after chromosome analysis in couples with two or more miscarriages: case-control study. BMJ. 2006;332(7544):759-63.
16. Barber JC, Cockwell AE, Grant E, et al. Is karyotyping couples experiencing recurrent miscarriage worth the cost? BJOG. 2010;117(7):885-8.
17. Robberecht C, Schuddinck V, Fryns JP, et al. Diagnosis of miscarriages by molecular karyotyping: benefits and pitfalls. Genet Med. 2009;11(9):646-56.
18. Kudesia R, Li M, Smith J, et al. Rescue karyotyping: a case series of array-based comparative genomic hybridization evaluation of archival conceptual tissue. Reprod Biol Endocrinol. 2014;12(1):19.
19. Mathur N, Triplett L, Stephenson MD. Miscarriage chromosome testing: utility of comparative genomic hybridization with reflex microsatellite analysis in preserved miscarriage tissue. Fertil Steril. 2014;101(5):1349-52.
20. Miyakis S, Lockshin MD, Atsumi T, et al. International consensus statement on an update of the classification criteria for definite antiphospholipid syndrome (APS). J Thromb Haemost. 2006;4(2):295-306.
21. Ziakas PD, Pavlou M, Voulgarelis M. Heparin treatment in antiphospholipid syndrome with recurrent pregnancy loss: a systematic review and meta-analysis. Obstet Gynecol. 2010;115(6):1256-62.
22. ESHRE Guideline Group on RPL, Bender Atik R, Christiansen OB, et al. ESHRE guideline: recurrent pregnancy loss. Hum Reprod. 2018;2(1):hoy004.
23. Ford HB, Schust DJ. Recurrent pregnancy loss: etiology, diagnosis, and therapy. Rev Obstet Gynecol. 2009;2(2):76-83.
24. Smith ML, Schust DJ. Endocrinology and recurrent early pregnancy loss. Semin Reprod Med. 2011;29(6):482-90.
25. Vissenberg R, Manders VD, Mastenbroek S, et al. Pathophysiological aspects of thyroid hormone disorders/thyroid peroxidase autoantibodies and reproduction. Hum Reprod Update. 2015;21(3):378-87.
26. Glinoer D. Thyroid hyperfunction during pregnancy. Thyroid. 1998;8(9):859-64.
27. Poppe K, Velkeniers B, Glinoer D. Thyroid disease and female reproduction. Clin Endocrinol. 2007;66(3):309-21.
28. Rushworth FH, Backos M, Rai RA, et al. Prospective pregnancy outcome in untreated recurrent miscarriers with thyroid autoantibodies. Hum Reprod. 2000;15(7):1637-9.
29. Lazarus J, Brown RS, Daumerie C, et al. 2014 European thyroid association guidelines for the management of subclinical hypothyroidism in pregnancy and in children. Eur Thyroid J. 2014;3(2):76-94.
30. Bernardi LA, Cohen RN, Stephenson MD. Impact of subclinical hypothyroidism in women with recurrent early pregnancy loss. Fertil Steril. 2013;100(5):1326-31.
31. van Dijk MM, Vissenberg R, Bisschop PH, et al. Is subclinical hypothyroidism associated with lower live birth rates in women who have experienced unexplained recurrent miscarriage? Reprod Biomed Online. 2016;33(6):745-51.
32. Kazerooni T, Ghaffarpasand F, Asadi N, et al. Correlation between thrombophilia and recurrent pregnancy loss in patients with polycystic ovary syndrome: a comparative study. J Chinese Med Assoc. 2013;76(5):282-8.
33. Al-Biate MA. Effect of metformin on early pregnancy loss in women with polycystic ovary syndrome. Taiwanese J Obstet Gynecol. 2015;54(3):266-9.
34. Li W, Ma N, Laird SM, et al. The relationship between serum prolactin concentration and pregnancy outcome in women with unexplained recurrent miscarriage. J Obstet Gynaecol. 2013;33(3):285-8.
35. Aoki K, Kajiura S, Matsumoto Y, et al. Preconceptional natural-killer-cell activity as a predictor of miscarriage. The Lancet. 1995;345(8961):1340-2.
36. Emmer PM, Veerhoek M, Nelen WL, et al. Natural killer cell reactivity and HLA-G in recurrent spontaneous abortion. Transplant Proc. 1999;31(4):1838-40.
37. Liang P, Mo M, Li GG, et al. Comprehensive analysis of peripheral blood lymphocytes in 76 women with recurrent miscarriage before and after lymphocyte immunotherapy. Am J Reprod Immunol. 2012;68(2):164-74.
38. Katano K, Suzuki S, Ozaki Y, et al. Peripheral natural killer cell activity as a predictor of recurrent pregnancy loss: a large cohort study. Fertil Steril. 2013;100(6):1629-34.
39. Lachapelle MH, Miron P, Hemmings R, et al. Endometrial T, B, and NK cells in patients with recurrent spontaneous abortion. Altered profile and pregnancy outcome. J Immunol. 1996;156(10):4027-34.
40. Clifford K, Flanagan AM, Regan L. Endometrial CD56+ natural killer cells in women with recurrent miscarriage: a histomorphometric study. Hum Reprod. 1999;14(11):2727-30.
41. Quenby S, Kalumbi C, Bates M, et al. Prednisolone reduces preconceptual endometrial natural killer cells in women with recurrent miscarriage. Fertil Steril. 2005;84(4):980-4.
42. Tuckerman E, Laird SM, Prakash A, et al. Prognostic value of the measurement of uterine natural killer cells in the endometrium of women with recurrent miscarriage. Hum Reprod. 2007;22(8):2208-13.
43. Michimata T, Ogasawara MS, Tsuda H, et al. Distributions of endometrial NK cells, B cells, T cells, and Th2/Tc2 cells fail to predict pregnancy outcome following recurrent abortion. Am J Reprod Immunol. 2002;47(4):196-202.
44. Shimada S, Kato EH, Morikawa M, et al. No difference in natural killer or natural killer T-cell population, but aberrant T-helper cell population in the endometrium of women with repeated miscarriage. Hum Reprod. 2004;19(4):1018-24.
45. Amani D, Dehaghani AS, Zolghadri J, et al. Lack of association between the TGF-β1 gene polymorphisms and recurrent

spontaneous abortion. J Reprod Immunol. 2005;68(1-2):91-103.
46. Zhang L, Wang L, Zhang X, et al. Sperm chromatin integrity may predict future fertility for unexplained recurrent spontaneous abortion patients. Int J Androl. 2012;35(5):752-7.
47. Cavalcante MB, Costa FD, Araujo Júnior E, et al. Risk factors associated with a new pregnancy loss and perinatal outcomes in cases of recurrent miscarriage treated with lymphocyte immunotherapy. Journal Matern Fetal Neonatal Med. 2015;28(9):1082-6.
48. Hiby SE, Regan L, Lo W, et al. Association of maternal killer-cell immunoglobulin-like receptors and parental HLA-C genotypes with recurrent miscarriage. Hum Reprod. 2008;23(4):972-6.
49. Fan W, Li S, Huang Z, et al. Relationship between HLA-G polymorphism and susceptibility to recurrent miscarriage: a meta-analysis of non-family-based studies. J Assist Reprod Genet. 2014;31(2):173-84.
50. Wang X, Jiang W, Zhang D. Association of 14-bp insertion/deletion polymorphism of HLA-G gene with unexplained recurrent spontaneous abortion: A meta-analysis. Tissue Antigens. 2013;81(2):108-15.
51. Hviid TV, Christiansen OB. Linkage disequilibrium between human leukocyte antigen (HLA) class II and HLA-G—possible implications for human reproduction and autoimmune disease. Human immunology. 2005;66(6): 688-99.
52. Chan YY, Jayaprakasan K, Tan A, et al. Reproductive outcomes in women with congenital uterine anomalies: a systematic review. Ultrasound Obstet Gynecol. 2011;38(4):371-82.
53. Venetis CA, Papadopoulos SP, Campo R, et al. Clinical implications of congenital uterine anomalies: a meta-analysis of comparative studies. Reprod Biomed Online. 2014;29(6):665-83.
54. Valle RF, Ekpo GE. Hysteroscopic metroplasty for the septate uterus: review and meta-analysis. J Minim Invasive Gynecol. 2013;20(1):22-42.
55. Lieng M, Istre O, Qvigstad E. Treatment of endometrial polyps: a systematic review. Acta Obstet Gynecol Scand. 2010;89(8):992-1002.
56. Hooker AB, Lemmers M, Thurkow AL, et al. Systematic review and meta-analysis of intrauterine adhesions after miscarriage: prevalence, risk factors and long-term reproductive outcome. Hum Reprod Update. 2014;20(2):262-78.
57. American College of Obstetricians and Gynecologists. ACOG practice bulletin No. 142: cerclage for the management of cervical insufficiency. Obstet Gynecol. 2014;123(2 Pt 1):372.
58. No GG. (2011). The investigation and treatment of couples with recurrent first-trimester and second-trimester miscarriage. [online] Available from https://www.rcog.org.uk/globalassets/documents/guidelines/gtg_17.pdf. [Accessed January, 2019].
59. Drakeley AJ, Roberts D, Alfirevic Z. Cervical stitch (cerclage) for preventing pregnancy loss in women. Cochrane Database Syst Rev. 2003(1):CD003253.
60. Ota K, Dambaeva S, Han AR, et al. Vitamin D deficiency may be a risk factor for recurrent pregnancy losses by increasing cellular immunity and autoimmunity. Hum Reprod. 2014;29(2):208-19.
61. Wang LQ, Yan XT, Yan CF, et al. Women with recurrent miscarriage have decreased expression of 25-hydroxyvitamin D3-1α-hydroxylase by the fetal-maternal interface. PloS One. 2016;11(12):e0165589.
62. Dewan S, Puscheck EE, Coulam CB, et al. Y-chromosome microdeletions and recurrent pregnancy loss. Fertil Steril. 2006;85(2):441-5.
63. Saxena P, Misro MM, Chaki SP, et al. Is abnormal sperm function an indicator among couples with recurrent pregnancy loss? Fertil Steril. 2008;90(5):1854-8.
64. Zhao J, Zhang Q, Wang Y, et al. Whether sperm deoxyribonucleic acid fragmentation has an effect on pregnancy and miscarriage after in vitro fertilization/intracytoplasmic sperm injection: a systematic review and meta-analysis. Fertil Steril. 2014;102(4):998-1005.
65. Pereza N, Crnjar K, Buretic-Tomljanovic A, et al. Y chromosome azoospermia factor region microdeletions are not associated with idiopathic recurrent spontaneous abortion in a Slovenian population: association study and literature review. Fertil Steril. 2013;99(6):1663-7.
66. Greco E, Romano S, Iacobelli M, et al. ICSI in cases of sperm DNA damage: beneficial effect of oral antioxidant treatment. Hum Reprod. 2005;20(9):2590-4.
67. Ramasamy R, Scovell JM, Kovac JR, et al. Fluorescence in situ hybridization detects increased sperm aneuploidy in men with recurrent pregnancy loss. Fertil Steril. 2015;103(4):906-9.
68. Mowbray JF, Liddell H, Underwood J, et al. Controlled trial of treatment of recurrent spontaneous abortion by immunisation with paternal cells. Lancet. 1985;325(8435):941-3.
69. Lashley EE, Meuleman T, Claas FH. Beneficial or harmful effect of antipaternal human leukocyte antibodies on pregnancy outcome? A systematic review and meta-analysis. Am J Reprod Immunol. 2013;70(2):87-103.
70. Wong LF, Porter TF, Scott JR. Immunotherapy for recurrent miscarriage. Cochrane Database Syst Rev. 2014;(10):CD000112.
71. Achilli C, Duran-Retamal M, Saab W, et al. The role of immunotherapy in in vitro fertilization and recurrent pregnancy loss: a systematic review and meta-analysis. Fertil Steril. 2018;110(6):1089-100.
72. Wang SW, Zhong SY, Lou LJ, et al. The effect of intravenous immunoglobulin passive immunotherapy on unexplained recurrent spontaneous abortion: a meta-analysis. Reprod Biomed Online. 2016;33(6):720-36.
73. Gomaa MF, Elkholy AG, El-Said MM, et al. Combined oral prednisolone and heparin versus heparin: the effect on peripheral NK cells and clinical outcome in patients with unexplained recurrent miscarriage. A double-blind placebo randomized controlled trial. Arch Gynecol Obstet. 2014;290(4):757-62.
74. Mekinian A, Cohen J, Alijotas-Reig J, et al. Unexplained recurrent miscarriage and recurrent implantation failure: is there a place for immunomodulation? Am J Reprod Immunol. 2016;76(1):8-28.
75. de Jong PG, Kaandorp S, Di Nisio M, et al. Aspirin and/or heparin for women with unexplained recurrent miscarriage with or without inherited thrombophilia. Cochrane Database Syst Rev. 2014;(7):CD004734.

76. Pasquier E, de Saint Martin L, Bohec C, et al. Enoxaparin for prevention of unexplained recurrent miscarriage: a multicenter randomized double-blind placebo-controlled trial. Blood. 2015;125(14):2200-5.
77. Schleussner E, Kamin G, Seliger G, et al. Low-molecular-weight heparin for women with unexplained recurrent pregnancy loss: a multicenter trial with a minimization randomization scheme. Ann Intern Med. 2015;162(9):601-9.
78. Shaaban OM, Abbas AM, Zahran KM, et al. Low-Molecular-Weight Heparin for the Treatment of Unexplained Recurrent Miscarriage with Negative Antiphospholipid Antibodies: A Randomized Controlled Trial. Clin Appl Thromb Hemost. 2017;23(6):567-72.
79. Coomarasamy A, Williams H, Truchanowicz E, et al. A randomized trial of progesterone in women with recurrent miscarriages. N Eng J Med. 2015;373(22):2141-8.
80. Saccone G, Schoen C, Franasiak JM, et al. Supplementation with progestogens in the first trimester of pregnancy to prevent miscarriage in women with unexplained recurrent miscarriage: a systematic review and meta-analysis of randomized, controlled trials. Fertil Steril. 2017;107(2):430-8.
81. Meng L, Lin J, Chen L, et al. Effectiveness and potential mechanisms of intralipid in treating unexplained recurrent spontaneous abortion. Arch Gynecol Obstet. 2016;294(1): 29-39.
82. Hayes BD, Gosselin S, Calello DP, et al.; Lipid Emulsion Workgroup. Systematic review of clinical adverse events reported after acute intravenous lipid emulsion administration. Clin Toxicol. 2016;54(5):365-404.
83. Scarpellini F, Sbracia M. Use of granulocyte colony-stimulating factor for the treatment of unexplained recurrent miscarriage: a randomised controlled trial. Hum Reprod. 2009;24(11):2703-8.
84. Barad DH, Yu Y, Kushnir VA, et al. A randomized clinical trial of endometrial perfusion with granulocyte colony-stimulating factor in in vitro fertilization cycles: impact on endometrial thickness and clinical pregnancy rates. Fertil Steril. 2014;101(3):710-5.

CHAPTER

83

Genetics of Fertility

Rajni Khajuria, Carmen Rubio Llues, Pere Mir Pardo

INTRODUCTION TO ROUTINE GENETIC TESTS IN FERTILITY

Infertility is a major human health problem worldwide. Known reasons for infertility are various, they can be endocrinological, uterine, genetics, etc., and some of them are still unclear or not clearly defined. Despite of all the known causes of infertility, in about 30% of the infertile patients, the cause of infertility remains unknown.[1] Genetics play an important role in fertility which will be described in the present chapter. Among the genetic factors that may be involved in infertility, it is worth to differentiate between cytogenetic factors and pure genetic factors. Within this classification, cytogenetic factors will be all the cases in which chromosomes are involved, while genetic factors will be specific gene defects, called mutations. Reproductive disorders are mostly associated with some cytogenetic abnormalities. Known genetic causes of infertility include chromosomal abnormalities, mitochondrial deoxyribonucleic acid (DNA) mutations, single gene variants, and phenotypes with multifactorial inheritance.[2]

CYTOGENETIC ASPECTS OF INFERTILITY

Couples with Abnormal Karyotype

The normal human chromosome complement consists of 23 pairs of chromosomes, in total 46 chromosomes (diploid), except for human gametes that contain 23 chromosomes. Chromosomal abnormality or aneuploidy is classified as a change in the number of chromosomes from the normal diploid chromosomal complement in somatic cells or haploid complement in gametes. Chromosomal abnormalities are the leading cause of infertility, pregnancy loss, and developmental disabilities.[3]

The chromosomal abnormalities observed in infertile couples are either numerical or structural. Numerical chromosome abnormalities involve either gain or loss of an entire chromosome [e.g. Turner's syndrome (45,X) or Klinefelter's syndrome (47,XXY)]; and structural chromosome abnormalities involve balanced reorganization of two segments from two chromosomes (e.g. translocation) or the reorganization of a segment of a chromosome (e.g. inversions), with the risk of unbalanced segregation during meiosis resulting in gametes with a gain or loss of a segment of a chromosome. The incidence of chromosomal abnormalities in live births is estimated to be around 90 per 10,000, including numerical as well as the structural chromosomal anomalies.[4]

Numerical Chromosomal Abnormalities

In humans, aneuploidy is surprisingly common occurring in around 4% of clinically recognized pregnancies. However, it is estimated that up to 60% of conceptions are aneuploid but are spontaneously aborted, often even before a pregnancy is clinically recognized.[5] Loss of a chromosome (monosomy) is much more fatal than gain of a chromosome (trisomy). Monosomy X is the only nonmosaic monosomic condition that is compatible with life[6] and is largely attributed to the phenomenon of X chromosome inactivation (lyonization).[7] Trisomies of chromosomes (13, 18, 21, X, and Y) can survive to term but it should be noted that while abnormalities for these chromosomes are compatible with live birth, the majority of them will be spontaneously aborted early on during development.[3]

Aneuploid and normal diploid cells can exist simultaneously in an individual leading to the phenomenon of mosaicism. Mosaicism involves two or more distinct cell lineages derived from a single zygote or fertilized egg. Mosaicism can involve either autosomes or sex chromosomes but most frequently involves sex chromosomes.[8] Mosaicism is seen in approximately 0.2% of fetus, mosaicism has been observed through prenatal genetic analysis, 1% of Down syndrome patients, 10% of Klinefelter's syndrome patients, and in more than 30% of patients with Turner's syndrome.[2]

Sex chromosomal abnormalities are more severe clinical anomalies than those associated with autosomal chromosomal imbalances, since they can survive to term, in contrast to autosomal aneuploidies for most chromosomes that end in miscarriage or pregnancy failure.[2,6] This difference can be attributed to the fact that one of the copies of X chromosome is inactivated in the cases where multiple copies are present. Sex chromosomal abnormalities are relatively common with an overall frequency of 1 in 500 live births. Some of them (as 47,XXX; 47,XXY; and 47,XYY) are relatively more common in newborns, but rare in spontaneous miscarriages.[9-11] The most common syndromes are described below:

Turner's syndrome (45,X): Turner's syndrome affects approximately 1 in 2,500–3,000 live born females and is characterized by either the loss of an entire X chromosome, loss of a portion of the X chromosome, or complex rearrangements affecting the X chromosome.[12] Loss of X chromosome is caused by nondisjunction of chromosomes during gametogenesis and, in the majority of the cases (80%), the X chromosome lost is of paternal origin.[13] Although 45,X is the karyotype typically seen in 50% of patients with Turner's syndrome, other sex chromosome anomalies, such as isochromosome Xq, ring X, deletion Xp, or an abnormal Y-chromosome, can also cause the syndrome,[8] and about 30% of Turner's patients are mosaic. Approximately 95–99% of 45,X conceptions fail to survive to term and account for about 18% of chromosomally abnormal spontaneous abortions. The incidence of 45,X is not directly associated with advanced maternal age (AMA).[14]

Klinefelter's syndrome (47,XXY): Klinefelter's syndrome is found in approximately 1 in 1,000 newborn males and is caused due to nondisjunction of the X chromosome during meiosis. The associated karyotype is 47,XXY, and about 50% of XXY are due to maternal meiotic (MI) errors, and the other 50% results from paternal first MI errors.[8] Klinefelter's 47,XXY males present gonadal defect, and they are generally sterile.[15] However, several numerical changes in sex chromosomes are involved with other types of Klinefelter mosaics (e.g. 45, X/47, XYY; 46, XY/47, XXY/48, XXXY).[2] At least 10% of Klinefelter patients are mosaic for sex chromosomes, and these patients may present more variable features and improved fertility, being most of them azoospermic and oligozoospermic males.[16]

47,XYY syndrome: The 47,XYY syndrome is found in approximately 1 in 1,000 male births and is the second most common sex chromosome abnormality after Klinefelter's syndrome (47,XXY).[9,17] Parental nondisjunction of Y-chromosome at meiosis II produces the 47,XYY karyotype in the affected offspring.[18] Parental nondisjunction during subsequent cell divisions after postzygotic mitosis can result in 46,XY/47,XYY mosaics.[11] Men with a 47,XYY karyotype are generally fertile, but increased incidence of chromosomally abnormal spermatozoa in the semen of men with 47,XYY syndrome has been observed.[18,19] Men with 47,XYY syndrome can have variable sperm parameters, ranging from normal to azoospermia.[11,17]

47,XXX syndrome (Triple-X syndrome): The frequency of 47,XXX is 1 in 1,000 females, and in 95% of cases, the extra X chromosome is maternal in origin. The 47,XXX karyotype is associated with AMA, and most of these cases are documented in women with premature ovarian failure[20] and also in women with premature ovarian aging.[21] Most of the 47,XXX females are fertile but have an early onset of menopause at about 30 years of age compared with the average of about 50 years old.[22]

Down's syndrome (Trisomy 21): Trisomy 21 is the most common chromosomal abnormality in newborns. Global incidence of Down's syndrome is 1 in 1,000 births.[23] Up to 95% of Down's syndrome cases are due to a single trisomy of chromosome 21, and about 80% of such cases result from errors in maternal meiosis I.[2] About 4% of Down's syndrome patients have an unbalanced Robertsonian translocation (ROB) involving chromosome 21. About half of these translocations occur de novo.[14,24] The risk of having a child with trisomy 21 increases with maternal age. At age 20, the chance is 1 in 1,441; at age 30, it is 1 in 959; at age 40, it is 1 in 84; and at age 50, it is 1 in 44.

Although the probability increases with maternal age, about 70% of children with Down's syndrome are born to women of 35 years of age and younger.[25] Affected females in rare cases can reproduce, however, most if not all of affected males are sterile.[14]

Edwards' syndrome (Trisomy 18): Trisomy 18 is the second most common autosomal trisomy syndrome in newborns. It has a frequency of ~1 in 6,000–8,000 live births, and its incidence increases with maternal age.[26,14] The phenotype results from full, mosaic, or partial trisomy 18q. Complete trisomy 18 is the most common form in about 94% of the cases, and mosaicism is reported in very few cases.[27] Most cases of trisomy 18 occur due to the de novo MI nondisjunction of the maternal meiosis phase II. Postnatal survival for these patients is poor and more than 90% die within the first 6 months. About 80% of these cases are reported to be females.[8] Many features characteristics of trisomy 18 have also been reported in patients with unbalanced translocations involving all or most of the long arm of chromosome 18 (18q). Although data is limited, the recurrence risk of trisomy 18 is approximately 1%.[26]

Patau's syndrome (Trisomy 13): Trisomy 13 is the least common of the major autosomal trisomies with an estimated incidence of 1 in 20,000 live births. There is a high fetal loss of 97% for trisomy 13 conceptions, and in the postnatal period, nearly all the Patau's syndrome patients die within 4 months. The incidence of trisomy 13 also increases with AMA.[28] The extra 13 chromosome usually results from maternal MI nondisjunction error. In about 20% of the Patau's syndrome cases, an unbalanced ROB involving chromosome 13 is present. Trisomy 13 mosaicism is rare and may be associated with less severe clinical anomalies and a longer survival.[14]

Structural Chromosome Abnormalities

Structural chromosome abnormalities are rearrangements of a portion of a chromosome and include translocations, inversions, deletions, and duplications.

A chromosome translocation is described as a rearrangement of genetic material involving two or more chromosomes and clinically is the most relevant structural abnormality. There are two types of chromosome translocations: ROB that implies an exchange of material involving only acrocentric chromosomes 13, 14, 15, 21, and 22; and reciprocal translocation (RCP) that is an exchange of material between any two chromosomes.[8] The karyotype of a balanced ROB shows only 45 chromosomes; in which, the translocated chromosome contains the two complete long arms of the two acrocentric chromosomes involved, while the short arms of the two translocated chromosomes are lost. Robertsonian translocations have an estimated incidence rate of 1/1,000 births, making this type of rearrangements the most common structural chromosomal abnormalities seen in the general population.[27,29] When the chromosomes pair during meiosis, the resulting gametes can be either chromosomally normal or aneuploid with an extra or missing q arm of any of the chromosomes involved in the translocation.[30] Translocations of chromosomes 13 and 14 are the most common to be observed in infertile males and constitute about 75% of all ROB.[31] It was proposed that the high prevalence of ROBs can be due to the similarities of the DNA sequences shared by the short arms of acrocentric chromosomes which confer susceptibility to chromosome rearrangement.[29]

Majority of ROB are found in adults with infertility and with history of previous miscarriage.[32] Meiotic studies of infertile couples carrying translocation between chromosome 13 and 14 and between chromosomes 14 and 21 have shown abnormal behavior of the rearranged autosomes in meiosis during spermatogenesis, causing infertility.[31,33] It is well known that balanced ROB carriers usually have normal phenotype but can have infertility problems associated with oligospermia in male adults, as well as miscarriages events or infertility in female adults. Although it is rare, a variety of abnormal phenotypes were described in some balanced ROB carriers.[34-36] The majority of heterologous ROBs are inherited from a carrier parent, and the minority of them occur de novo mainly in the stage of meiosis I of oogenesis, whereas almost all homologous ROBs occur de novo mitotically.[10,31]

Reciprocal translocations are the result of two way exchanges of chromosome material between two nonhomologous chromosomes. A break occurs in each arm of the chromosome and the portion of chromosome material distal to the breakpoints switch positions.[30] The portions exchanged are the translocated segments, and the rest of the chromosome including centromere is the centric segment. The resulting rearranged chromosome is called a derivative (der) chromosome. The breakpoint of a translocation is where the two chromosomes are joined. When there is no loss and no gain of exchanged material, such translocations are known as balanced RCP. Reciprocal translocation has an estimated incidence of 1 in 500 live births as per prenatal and newborn studies.[37]

Carriers of balanced RCP are usually normal but they have an increased risk for unbalanced offspring due to the presence of unbalanced gametes. The frequency of unbalanced gametes segregating during gametogenesis in an individual with a balanced translocation depends on the exact positioning of the translocation breakpoints. In general, viability is correlated with size of the unbalanced segment. Reciprocal translocation can either occur de novo or can be genetically transmitted from parental carriers.[30,38]

Chromosome inversions occur when two chromosome breaks occur in the same chromosome and the broken part of the chromosome joins in an inverted order with the intervening segment being rotated 180°. Like chromosome translocations, inversions can also cause infertility, spontaneous abortions, and birth defects.[2] In general, there is no loss or gain of genetic material in inversions, but difficulties arise during pairing of homologous chromosomes during meiosis. If a single crossover occurs in the inverted region of the paired chromosomes, offspring with chromosomal duplications and deficiencies can result from recombinant chromosomes.[30]

Inversion carriers are usually clinically normal but may have an increased risk for aneuploid offspring. When chromosomes pair during meiosis an inversion loop is formed when the inverted segment pairs with its normal homolog, and if an odd number of crossovers occur, unbalanced recombinant chromosomes are produced.[39] The formation of these loops can impact fertility due to the mechanics and time constraints associated with the formation of the inversion loop.[2] As with reciprocal chromosomal translocations, the relative frequency of normal or unbalanced gametes will depend on the chromosomes involved, the size of the region involved, and the likelihood of recombination events which can take place within the inverted segments.[3] The inversions that produce recombinant chromosomes are, in general, large inversions encompassing more than half of the chromosome length. In prenatal diagnosis cases, an overall risk of 10–15% has been estimated,[40] but it is clear that the risks are dependent on the individual inversion.

Inversions are classified in two types: paracentric and pericentric inversions. Paracentric inversions occur when both break points are in the same chromosome arm.[39] If a single crossover occurs within the inversion pairing loop, one half of the gametes are normal, one quarter are acentric (and they would be lost), and one quarter are dicentric (which could lead to a break between the centromeres and chromosome imbalance). Some investigators have suggested that paracentric inversions in man are generally harmless;[41] however, recombinant chromosomes have been observed in newborns, and the risk of viable recombinants has been estimated to be 3.8%.[42] Pericentric inversions occur when there is a breakage in each chromosome arm, and therefore, the centromere is included within the inversion. Pericentric inversions frequently produce a change in the relative arm lengths, and they can produce recombinants with duplication and deficiency of chromosome segments. The viability of these recombinant products is dependent upon the size of the unbalanced segments.[3] So far, pericentric inversion of chromosomes 1, 3, 5, 6, and 10 has been correlated to abnormal sperm production in infertile men.[30]

Marker chromosomes are additional chromosomes found in karyotypes that are not effectively recognized by typical cytogenetic methods. Carriers of marker chromosomes may be at risk of infertility because of MI arrest and instability.[33]

Risk Factors for Aneuploid Conceptions

Advanced Age

Natural fertility declines with the increasing of maternal age as the quality and number of oocytes decline with age.[43] All this is attributed to the age-related changes in the ovary and its function. It is reported that the number of aneuploidies in women's egg increases with advancing age primarily owing to MI nondisjunction errors associated with reduced recombination or crossing over prior to the MI division.[8] Prenatal and live birth risks for trisomy 21 are clearly associated with AMA. Along with trisomy 21, the other viable autosomal and sex chromosomal abnormalities, including trisomy 13, 18, XXX, and XXY, are also associated with AMA. Incidence of spontaneous abortion almost doubles among women in their late 30s, compared with women younger than 30. More than 50% of chromosomally abnormal spontaneous abortions are trisomic for various chromosomes and are more frequently associated with AMA.[43]

In contrast to women, there is no certain loss of fertility as men age. Male fertility may decline because of falling testosterone levels, but overall. men are capable of conceiving children well into their 90s. However, as men age, the quality of their gametes deteriorates, and as a result, the spermatozoa of aging males contain much more DNA damage than their younger counterparts, which leads to more segmental aneuploidies in sperm.[43]

Infertility

Karyotype analysis should be recommended as a diagnostic test when a couple is unable to conceive after 1 year of unprotected sexual intercourse. Karyotyping determines the critical regions on chromosomes which cause the chromosomal abnormalities. Knowledge of the critical regions in chromosomes is very useful in correlating the genotype and the phenotype.[44]

It is strongly recommended also during the diagnostic workup of infertile individuals, mainly in males with azoospermia, severe oligozoospermia, also in those cases, in which sperm parameters are within the normal ranges or only slightly abnormal and in infertile females presenting with primary ovarian dysfunction or primary/secondary amenorrhea.[45,46]

As previously showed in this chapter, most common types of karyotype abnormalities identified in males with infertility include sex chromosome abnormalities and ROBs. The frequency of somatic chromosome abnormalities in infertile men varies from 3% to 19% that is 3% in the cases of mild infertility and 19% in men with nonobstructive azoospermia (NOA).[47,48] In females, the higher frequency of abnormal karyotypes has been reported in patients experiencing primary amenorrhea, whose frequency vary between 20% and 31%.[6,49]

Many of the chromosome abnormalities especially related to the heterochromatin region, namely p+/q+ (for p arm and q arm, respectively), are frequently detected during routine cytogenetic analysis, being the most commons: 1qh, 9qh, and 16qh regions. Although inherited variants have been considered normal variants, which may or may not lead to infertility, chromosome heteromorphisms have been found to have a higher frequency relative to the normal population and have been regarded as abnormalities in some studies.[50-52]

Recurrent Pregnancy Loss

Spontaneous pregnancy loss can be due to several factors either maternal or fetal. The most common factor involved in spontaneous miscarriages is the presence of chromosome abnormalities in the embryo or the fetus, accounting for about 50% of all pregnancy losses before the 15th week of gestation.[53] The term recurrent pregnancy loss (RPL) is widely accepted as the loss of two or more pregnancies from the same partners and affects up to 5% of couples of reproductive age.[38] Common causes for RPL are immunological, endocrine, anatomic, or genetic factors, but about 50% of RPL cases still remain unexplained, or idiopathic. In this group of patients, fetal chromosomal abnormalities have been reported to be the most common cause of RPL, accounting for up to 55% of cases, thus leaving a remainder of 24.5% of truly unexplained RPLs.[54]

Many series of product of conception (POC) analysis through karyotype have confirmed that ~50% of all clinically recognized spontaneous miscarriages have a chromosome abnormality. Of these, ~9% have a 45,X constitution, 30% have trisomy, 10% are either triploid or tetraploid, and 2% have a structural rearrangement.[46]

Moreover, a large study that includes prenatal diagnosis in 46,939 women, confirmed the increased risk of karyotype abnormalities in the POCs in idiopathic RPL patients.[55] Mainly numerical chromosome abnormalities are present in those miscarriages, but also structural abnormalities. When an unbalanced structural abnormality is present in a miscarriage may well have caused the miscarriage and could result from chromosomal segregation errors during gametogenesis in a parent with a balanced rearrangement.[38] It is estimated that in 3% of RPL couples, one partner is carrier of a balanced structural chromosome abnormality.[56,57]

Therefore, while carriers of balanced translocations are normal, more than half of their gametes and embryos are chromosomally abnormal because chromosomal segregation is disrupted during meiosis. Thus it is prudent to recommend karyotyping for couples with RPL. If an abnormality is found, the couple should be referred to a clinical geneticist to decide on further family studies and to discuss the prognosis for a future pregnancy. The couple has an increased risk of having a future chromosomally abnormal pregnancy, hence not only prenatal diagnosis can be recommended,[38,56] but also their embryos can be tested by preimplantation genetic testing (PGT) for chromosome abnormalities before implantation and transfer to the uterus only chromosomally normal embryos, therefore reducing suffering in the couple and increasing the likelihood of having chromosomally normal offspring.[58]

The pattern of chromosomal abnormalities found in POCs from RPL couples is not substantially different from the pattern in spontaneous losses except for fewer Turner's syndromes in RPL. Trisomy is the leading anomaly (31%, most often chromosomes 15, 16, 22, and 21) (Fig. 1), followed by polyploidy (9%), Turner's syndrome (4%), and unbalanced translocations (2%).[59]

When a POC contains any unbalanced structural rearrangements, it is important to do chromosomal analysis of parent and determine whether a parent carries a balanced rearrangement which may put them at risk of having a further conceptus with additional and/or missing chromosome material.[9]

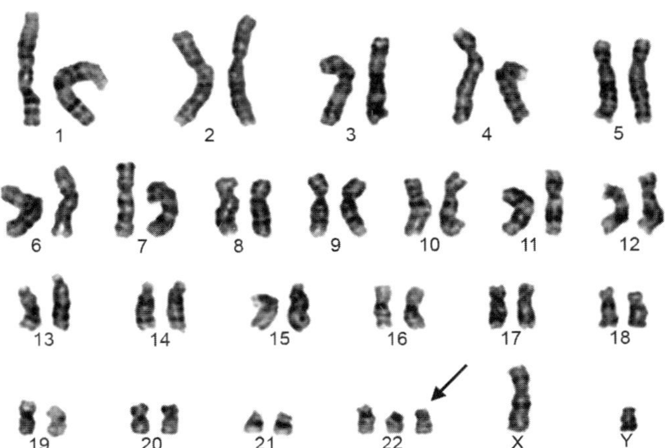

Fig. 1: Karyotype showing a trisomy for chromosome 22 (47,XY,+22) in a product of conception from a patient with RPL. (RPL: recurrent pregnancy loss)
Source: Inmaculada Campos Galindo, IGENOMIX, Spain.

GENETIC ASPECTS OF INFERTILITY

Genetic Aspects of Infertility in Males

The male factor (MF) is estimated to be responsible for up to 50% of the infertility cases, and in some of them, the infertility cause may remain unexplained.

For etiological cases, both genetic and nongenetic factors can be present. It has been estimated that genetic factors play a role in about 10% of the male infertility cases. Most important genetic factors comprise some chromosomal disorders, microdeletions of the Y-chromosome, and various single-gene disorders. Focusing on the management of infertile patients, the two genetic factors influencing more in clinical practice are Y-chromosome microdeletions and mutations in cystic fibrosis (CF) transmembrane conductance regulator (*CFTR*) gene.

Congenital bilateral absence of the vas deferens (CBAVD) due to CFTR mutations: Obstructive azoospermia (OA) due to CBAVD is an important genetic cause of male infertility. CBAVD occurs in all cases of CF with systemic manifestations. However, isolated CBAVD is recognized as a genital form of CF without any systemic manifestations.

Obstruction of the excretory ductal system can occur along ejaculatory ducts, vas deferens, or epididymis. History, physical examination, examination of semen, and radiologic studies can be used to identify the location of obstruction. Vasal obstruction may be caused by inguinal or pelvic surgery. Prior orchidopexy, hydrocelectomy, other scrotal surgery, or recurrent epididymitis may result in epididymal obstruction.[60] On physical examination, the absence of vas deferens is observed in patients with CBAVD, and dilated epididymis indicates possible obstruction.

About 25% of cases of OA and about 1–2% of cases of male infertility are caused by CBAVD.[61] In most cases, it is due to absence, dysfunction, or low level of CFTR protein. This disorder results in a broad range of clinical manifestations. The severe end of the phenotype is CF with pancreatic insufficiency and pulmonary dysfunction; at the other end, are relatively mild clinical manifestations, leading to a form of male infertility. Anatomically, CBAVD is a disorder characterized by bilateral regression of variable portions of epididymis, vas deferens and in about 80% of cases, absence of seminal vesicles.[62] The diagnosis of CBAVD relies on analysis of semen showing volume less than 1.5 mL, acidic power of hydrogen, absence of fructose and azoospermia. On physical examination, the palpation of spermatic cord reveals absence of the vas deferens. Confirmation can be obtained by transrectal ultrasound.

Given the fact that *CFTR* mutations are detected in men with CBAVD and, with a lower frequency, in men with congenital unilateral absence of the vas deferens, it appears that a normal amount of functional CFTR protein is required to ensure proper development of the vas deferens. However, the lack of *CFTR* mutations detected in CBAVD with renal abnormalities also suggests that the mesonephric duct plays an important role in the development of the vas deferens. Therefore, it can be hypothesized that the CFTR protein is required at some specific embryonic stage of the development of the vas deferens. Tizzano et al.[63] studied human fetuses from 10 weeks to 33 weeks gestation and found that low *CFTR* expression was present in the epithelium of the epididymis at all stages. The detection of *CFTR* messenger ribonucleic acid (RNA) in human fetuses suggests that *CFTR* acts as a chloride channel in the development of the reproductive tissues.[63] Recently, the relationship between *CFTR* mutations and the congenital absence of the uterus and vagina (CAUV), which affects 1 in 5,000 females, was examined upon the rationale that the embryological development of the Müllerian ducts directly depends on the prior normal development of the Wolffian ducts.[64] Samples from 25 patients with CAUV were tested for the 33 most common *CFTR* mutations, including the 5T allele. The data suggested that it is unlikely for *CFTR* mutations to cause CAUV in females.[64] Finding that *CFTR* mutations are associated with 80% of cases of CBAVD, a Wolffian duct anomaly, but are not associated with CAUV, a Müllerian duct anomaly provides further evidence on the timing of *CFTR* damage in CBAVD. The effects of the *CFTR* mutations on the Wolffian duct must occur after the ninth week of embryological development, at a time when the Wolffian and Müllerian ducts have completely separated and are developing independently.

The *CFTR* gene contains 27 exons encompassing, 180 kb of DNA on chromosome band 7q31.2. The CFTR protein is a glycosylated transmembrane protein that functions as a chloride channel. *CFTR* is expressed in epithelial cells of exocrine tissues, such as the lungs, pancreas, sweat glands, and vas deferens. Apart from its chloride channel function, *CFTR* also functions as a regulator of, and is regulated by, other proteins.[65] More than 1,500 CF-causing *CFTR* mutations have been identified. Mutations in *CFTR* gene are responsible of CF that is a single-gene disorder with autosomal recessive inheritance. This inheritance pattern implies that patients with classic CF carry severe mutations in both alleles. Patients with isolated CBAVD carry two changes in the *CFTR* gene; but at least one of these has to be a mild mutation/variant, otherwise classic CF would result.[66]

The most common mutation, F508del, reaches frequencies of about 70% in Northern European populations, while lower frequencies are observed in Southern European populations. In addition to F508del, other common mutations exist in most populations, each reaching frequencies of about 1–2%. Examples include the p.G542X, p.G551D, p.R553X, p.W1282X, and p.N1303K mutations. Finally, for a given population, ethnic-specific mutations that reach frequencies of about 1–2% might exist. For most populations, all these common mutations cover about 85–95% of all mutant *CFTR* genes. The remaining group of mutant *CFTR* genes in a particular population comprises rare mutations, some of them only found in a single family. In CBAVD patients having two mutant *CFTR* alleles, at least one will be a mild mutation. In CBAVD patients in which a mutation is found on both *CFTR* genes, about 88% carry one severe mutation on one *CFTR* gene and a mild mutation on the second *CFTR* gene, and about 12% carry mild mutations on both *CFTR* genes.[67] This is in contrast to CF patients, where about 88% of them carry severe mutations on both *CFTR* genes, and about 11% carry a severe mutation on one *CFTR* gene and a mild mutation on the other.[67,68]

The most frequent *CFTR* mutation conferring a mild phenotype found in CBAVD patients is the 5T polymorphism, which is one of the alleles found at the polymorphic locus in intron 8 of the *CFTR* gene. Possible alleles in this region are 5T, 7T, and 9T.[61,68] Frequency of the 5T polymorphism in Caucasians is about 21% in CBAVD patients, while it is only found on about 5% in control individuals. Frequency of the 5T polymorphism varies in different ethnic groups in CBAVD patients, ranging from 11% to 56%: 11% in Argentina,[69] 25% in India,[70] 31.4% in Iran,[71] 33.3% in France,[70] 44% in Israel,[72] 44.4% in Taiwan,[73] 56% in Egypt,[74] and 54.2% in India.[75]

When 5T allele is found in compound heterozygosity with a severe *CFTR* mutation, or even with another 5T allele, CBAVD might be observed. However, not all males who are compound heterozygous for a severe *CFTR* mutation and 5T develop CBAVD (e.g. some fathers of CF children).[76] The 5T polymorphism was therefore classified as a disease mutation with partial penetrance.[77] Different alleles in this locus can be found depending on the number of thymine-guanine (TG) repeats in the contiguous region of *CFTR* gene. The 5T polymorphism can be found in combination with a TG11, TG12, or TG13 allele (11, 12, or 13 TG repeats, respectively). In CBAVD patients, the milder TG11-5T allele is seldom found, while TG12-5T is the most frequently found genotype in CBAVD. The TG13-5T allele is rarer but is also found in CBAVD patients. TG13-5T might even result in some cases in pancreatic sufficient CF, possibly because of additional polymorphisms that affect *CFTR*, such as V470.[78,79]

Molecular studies in the cases of CBAVD have important clinical implications. Infertile males with CBAVD can have children by assisted reproductive techniques (ART), such as in vitro fertilization (IVF) and intracytoplasmic sperm injection (ISCI). Many of these patients have mutations in *CFTR* gene. If the other partner is a carrier of *CF* gene, the offspring may inherit the mutant gene from both the parents and suffer from CF. Therefore, genetic testing and counseling needs to be offered to all couples undergoing IVF or ICSI procedure to avoid having children with CF disease.

The genetic counselor should determine whether there is a family history of CF and determine the couple's ethnicity. The genetic aspect of CBAVD is more complex than in CF, since genetic analysis is able to prove but not to exclude the diagnosis of a genital form of CF,[80] and the risk of CF or CBAVD in the offspring may be unpredictable when rare mutations are identified in the male or the female.[81] For accurate genetic counseling, the screening of the most common mutations in a particular ethnic group is very useful for a cost-effective and rapid screening protocol for the partner to determine the carrier status for CF. However, the couple should be informed that routine screening tests cannot detect all mutations within the gene. Therefore, a negative mutation screen reduces, but does not eliminate, the risk of being a carrier, only a full sequencing of the *CFTR* will detect all the possible mutations.[82]

Y-Chromosome Microdeletions and Male Infertility

The Y-chromosome is an obvious area of interest in the study of MF infertility because it contains many of the genes that are critical for spermatogenesis and the development of male gonads. The variations present on the Y-chromosome and the occurrence of deletions of large segments of the chromosome involving multiple genes make it difficult to determine the exact cause of certain infertile phenotypes.[83] Furthermore, the same phenotype may be produced by several different deletions or mutations. This fact complicates efforts to distinctively correlate mutations with infertile phenotypes. Y-chromosome microdeletions are a frequent cause of infertility in males. A microdeletion is defined as a chromosomal deletion that spans several genes but is not large enough to be detected using conventional cytogenetic methods.[84] Routine karyotyping will not identify these microdeletions; they must be detected through specific DNA analysis.

Y-chromosome microdeletions have been studied in infertile males, and its frequency varies widely among different studies (ranging from 0.9% to 55.5%), but these studies have been performed in many countries including different study groups. Y-chromosome microdeletions have been identified in about 10–12% of men with severe sperm abnormalities but with normal karyotype.[85] In fact, several studies showed that the prevalence of microdeletions in azoospermic men was in a range from 10% to 15%.[75,86,87] In another study performed in oligozoospermic men, the prevalence of microdeletions was 5–10%.[86] It is essential to consider these deletions when discussing ART because microdeletions are always passed on to the male offspring,[88,89] and fertilization and pregnancy rates (PRs) are not affected by microdeletions on the azoospermia factor (AZF) c region when using ICSI.[89]

Regarding the type of microdeletions in infertile male, most frequently they occur on the long arm of the Y-chromosome, Yq, and deletions in this region are specifically related to failure of spermatogenesis.[90,91] A particular area of interest on Yq is the AZF region, which contains genes involved in the growth and development of sperm. The AZF region contains three subregions found in Yq11: AZFa, AZFb, and AZFc (Fig. 2).[92] The most common aberrations that occur in the AZF region are multiple gene deletions in the AZFb and AZFc areas,[75,93] which can produce a wide range of infertile phenotypes.[92]

The two main genes located in AZFa region are *USP9Y* and *DBY* (also called *DDX3Y*) (Fig. 2).[93] Deletions in the AZFa region that remove both of these genes cause Sertoli cell-only syndrome, a condition characterized by the presence of complete Sertoli cells in the testes but a lack of spermatozoa in the ejaculate.[75,92,94] *DBY*, the major gene located in the AZFa region, has a probable role in infertility because it is localized in the testis and is involved in the development of premeiotic germ cells (Table 1).[92]

A study of the transcriptional activity of several AZF region genes found that men with Sertoli cell-only syndrome had reduced levels of *DBY* transcripts but other genes examined were transcribed normally.[95] This finding suggests that *DBY* may play an important role in spermatogenesis. The *USP9Y* gene is also involved in spermatogenesis.[96] Different studies suggest that shortening or deletion of the *USP9Y* gene causes azoospermia,[97] oligozoospermia,[98] or oligoasthenozoospermia.[90] However, it seems that this gene may only be involved in the efficiency of spermatogenesis because it can be passed on to offspring (Table 1).

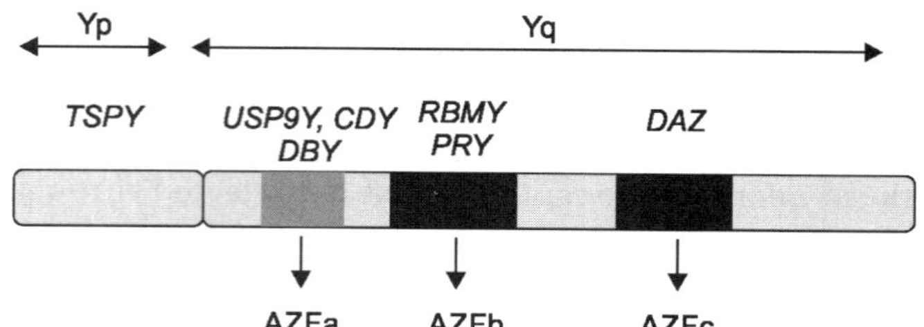

Fig. 2: Image of Y-chromosome displaying AZF regions and its genes associated with infertility. (AZF: azoospermia factor)

Deletions of the AZFb region cause arrest of spermatogenesis at the primary spermatocyte stage,[92] indicating that the region is essential for fertility.[94] The main gene in the AZFb region is *RBMY*, and there are six copies of the gene located on the Y-chromosome (Fig. 2).[91] *RBMY1* codes for an RNA-binding protein,[99] which is a testis-specific splicing factor expressed in the nuclei of spermatogonia, spermatocytes, and round spermatids (Table 1).[92] In the study by Lavery et al.,[99a] *RBMY1* expression was reduced in azoospermic men.

A family of *PRY* genes is also found in the AZFb region (Fig. 2) of the Y-chromosome. The *PRY* genes are involved in the regulation of apoptosis, an essential process that removes abnormal sperm from the population of spermatozoa.[92] In the cases in which all the genes in the AZFb region except *RBMY* and *PRY* are deleted, patients present hypospermatogenesis.[100] However, if both the *RBMY* and *PRY* genes are removed, spermatogenesis is completely arrested,[75,101] indicating that both are the major genes involved in infertility in the AZFb region (Fig. 2).

Deletions in the AZFc region produce a wide range of phenotypes, many of which are associated with low sperm concentration due to reduced spermatogenesis.[92]

Table 1: Genes on Y-chromosome with suspected involvement in male factor infertility.[92,94,116,117]

Gene	*Location*	*Reasons for investigation*
USP9Y	AZFa	Involved in efficiency of spermatogenesis; deletion or shortening may case azoospermia, oligozoospermia, or oligoasthenozoospermia
DBY	AZFa	Involved in premeiotic germ cell development
RBMY	AZFb	RNA-binding protein/testis-specific slicing factor; reduced expression in azoospermic men
PRY	AZFb	Regulation of apoptosis
DAZ	AZFc	Regulation of translation, meiosis, and germ cell population; codes for RNA-binding proteins; reduced expression in azoospermic men; partial deletion related to oligozoospermia
CDY	Yq	Involved in histone replacement
TSPY	Yq	Regulates timing of spermatogenesis; greater copy number in infertile patients

(AZF: azoospermia factor; RNA: ribonucleic acid)

AZFc deletions cause approximately 12% of NOA and 6% of severe oligozoospermia.[75,102] In many cases, men can still achieve fertilization with the assistance of ART.[92] Studies demonstrate that only the AZFa and AZFb regions are needed to initiate spermatogenesis but that without the AZFc region, spermatogenesis will not be completely normal.[103] Complete deletions of the AZFc region may occur in two different ways: either as a result of a previous deletion within the AZFc or spontaneously from a normal AZFc region.

A deletion of the AZFc region may also predispose men to Y-chromosome loss, leading to sexual reversal. Several studies have found this deletion to be a kind of premutation for 45,X0[104] and for the mosaic phenotype 45,X/46,XY.[105] The AZFc region is prone to many smaller subdeletions that are thought to be caused by intrachromosomal recombinations.[106] These partial deletions produce a wide array of phenotypes, ranging from normospermic to azoospermic, due to many factors, including the interaction of the environment and the genetic background of the region involved in the microdeletion.

Genetic studies of different ethnic groups produce diverse results because of the variations in their genomes that have evolved over generations to cope with environmental pressures specific to their region.[107] Therefore studies of the partial deletions of the AZFc region have produced conflicting results that relate to the genetic background of the groups studied. The complex interaction of genes and environment makes it difficult to replicate the results of studies and definitively associate subdeletions with infertile phenotypes.[93] The three most frequent subdeletions on the AZFc region of the Y-chromosome are gr/gr, b1/b3, and g1/g3 (b2/b3). The gr/gr subdeletion, which removes half of the content in the AZFc region, illustrates the complicating effects of ethnic background on gene function. Several studies have identified the deletion as a risk factor for the loss of spermatogenesis, while others failed to find a correlation.[108] Furthermore, a study of the Han Chinese population discovered that a duplication of the gr/gr region was also detrimental to fertility, contributing to further uncertainty about the role that this region may play in determining a man's fertility status.[109]

The AZFc region also contains genes involved in spermatogenesis. The *DAZ* gene has four copies on the Y-chromosome (Fig. 2).[110] *DAZ* genes are thought to serve a variety of roles throughout the spermatogenic process because they are expressed in all stages of germ cell development.[83] They regulate translation, code for germ cell-specific RNA-binding proteins,[111] and are involved in the control of meiosis and maintenance of the primordial germ cell population.[83] Deletions of the *DAZ* genes can cause a spectrum of phenotypes ranging from oligozoospermia to azoospermia.[112] In addition, *DAZ* gene expression was reduced in azoospermic patients,[99a] and partial deletions of *DAZ* genes seem to be related to oligozoospermia.[113] It is critical that azoospermic and severely oligozoospermic men be tested for microdeletions both for accurate diagnosis and genetic counseling before performing ART.[114,115] However, the lack of association between testicular phenotype and genotype in affected men forces clinicians to employ inefficient and costly methods, such as polymerase chain reaction (PCR), to determine diagnosis. The Y-chromosome contains 300 sequence tagged sites (STS), which correspond to the AZF regions and could be exploited for easier characterization of microdeletions.[86]

Another gene involved in spermatogenesis and located on Yq is *CDY*, the chromodomain protein Y-linked gene (Fig. 2). It is expressed exclusively in the testis and is involved in facilitating the replacement of histones in spermatogenesis. It also grants the proteins that regulate transcription easier access to the postmeiotic sperm DNA through the acetylation of histones (Table 1).[92] The *CDY* gene seems to have diverged functionally from its autosomal homolog (CDYL, located on chromosome 6) during evolution and then subsequently migrated to the Y-chromosome.

This fact makes it an interesting gene to study and demonstrates that there may be a tendency for genes with spermatogenic function to consolidate on the Y-chromosome.[92] The *TSPY* gene is located on the short arm of the Y-chromosome, Yp, and it also has copies on the long arm of the chromosome (Fig. 2).[95] The gene is expressed in the testis, and its protein has been identified in spermatogonia.[116] The *TSPY* gene may regulate the timing of spermatogenesis by signaling spermatogonia to enter meiosis.[94] A study of copy number variation of the *TSPY* gene found that more copies were found in infertile patients.[117] This finding warrants further investigation of *TSPY* to characterize its role in infertility. Table 1 is a visual representation of the information presented above to serve as an easy reference for the reader.

Microdeletions of Y-chromosome are a common genetic cause of male infertility, and screening for these microdeletions in azoospermic or severely oligospermic men is standard practice.[118] A positive test provides a firm diagnosis of the man's problem, which, for couples with longstanding infertility, can help to resolve stress, blame, or feelings of guilt. Second, knowledge of the type of Yq deletions may assist the clinician in determining the best ART treatment. For example, a Yq microdeletion involving the AZFa or AZFb regions carry poor prospect of sperm retrieval, even with testicular biopsy. In several cases, treatment with donor sperm would be preferred. Third, if sperm from males carrying microdeletions of Y-chromosome are used in ISCI, there is risk that their male offspring may be infertile.[90]

However, the high diversity of results observed in studies analyzing Y-chromosome microdeletions may be due to the small sample size in most of the studies, variable inclusion criteria for patients, and the number of genetic markers analyzed as well. Although almost 80 markers have been shown to be deleted in various studies, in practice only, a limited number of markers can be analyzed, therefore the European Academy of Andrology recommends the study of Y-chromosome microdeletions in infertile male, but only the analysis of six genetic markers (called STS, sequence-tagged sites), which are expected to detect of over 90% of the deletions in the AZF loci.[119a,119b]

Genetic Aspects of Infertility in Females

Some genetic causes of infertility in females are related with RPL, while others are mainly related with repetitive implantation failure (RIF) cases. Among the genetic factors involved in RPL, hereditary or acquired hypercoagulation disorders promoting thrombosis, collectively termed "thrombophilias," form the molecular basis for the majority of unexplained pregnancy loss.[120] Normal pregnancies are characterized by a hypercoagulability state that predisposes to thrombosis.[121] Hereditary thrombophilic defects in combination with these physiological changes may increase the risk of pregnancy loss.[122] An overview of inherited genetic defects found in the majority (70%) of thrombophilic patients is shown in Table 2. Two of them, factor V Leiden (FVL) mutation (c.1696G > A) and the prothrombin (PTm) mutation (20210G > A), account together for more than half of all cases with inherited thrombophilia.

Factor V Leiden

Factor V Leiden mutation (c.1691G > A) results in an amino acid replacement at one of the three contact residues where activated protein C (APC) would normally cleave and inactivate procoagulant factor Va. As a result, activated FVL becomes partially resistant to the anticoagulant action of APC and is inactivated at an approximately tenfold slower rate than normal, thereby resulting in increased thrombin generation and a prothrombotic state.

Factor V Leiden is the most common inherited cause of thrombophilia, being present in heterozygous form in about 12–20% of patients with venous thrombosis and in 40–50% of those with recurrent venous thrombosis. The mutation is very common in the Caucasian population, where about 3–7% of individuals from North Europe are heterozygous. FVL heterozygosity has been shown to be associated with a three- to seven-fold increase of venous thrombosis risk, while homozygotes have a 50- to 100-fold increased risk.[124-126] An elevated thrombosis risk may be due to a combined defect of FVL mutation plus another risk factor.[126-128] In a meta-analysis published by Rey et al.,[123] FVL was found to be associated with early and late recurrent fetal loss [odds ratio (OR) 2.01, 95% confidence interval (CI) 1.13–3.58] and with late nonrecurrent fetal loss (OR 7.83, 95% CI 2.83–21.67) (Table 2). Upon the exclusion of women with other pathologies that could explain fetal loss, the association between FVL and recurrent abortions increased. While protein S deficiency was related to non-RPL occurring after 22 weeks of gestation, APC resistance not due to FVL was associated with recurrent early pregnancy loss.

Factor II/Prothrombin Mutation

The PTm mutation results in greater synthesis of PTm protein.[129] Its overall prevalence in Europe is approximately 2%, the highest prevalence has been observed in Southern

Table 2: Known hereditary thrombophilia risk factors.[123]

	Prevalence in the white population (%)			
Thrombophilic defect	*Incident VTE*	*Recurrent VTE*	*Normal population*	*Relative thrombotic risk*
Antithrombin deficiency	1–2	2–5	0.02–0.04	5
Protein C deficiency	2–5	5–10	0.2–0.5	6–10
Protein S deficiency	1–3	5–10	0.1–1	2
Factor V Leiden	20	40–50	3–7	3–7 (heterozygotes)
				5–100 (homozygotes)
Prothrombin G20210A	3–8	15–20	1–3	2–8 (heterozygotes)

(VTE: venous thromboembolism)

Europe (approximately 3%) and the lowest in the northern parts of the continent (approximately 1.7%). Heterozygous carriers have a two- to eight-fold increased risk for venous thrombosis.[130] Very few cases of homozygosity for this mutation have been described.[131] Although the severity of the phenotype and the concurrent thrombosis risk would be expected to be higher in the homozygous state, a broad clinical spectrum with striking heterogeneity has emerged in a very small case number.[132] The meta-analysis of Rey et al.[123] shows a significant association between PTm carriers and recurrent abortion before 13 weeks of pregnancy (OR 2.56, 95% CI 1.04–6.29) as well as with nonrecurrent fetal loss after 20 weeks (*see* Table 2). Individuals carrying both an FVL and a PTm mutation have a 20-fold increased risk for venous thrombosis, which is higher than for heterozygous carriers of FVL or PTm alone.

Methylenetetrahydrofolate Reductase Gene

An elevated plasma homocysteine level (hyperhomocysteinemia) has been suggested to represent another factor predisposing to thrombosis. A quite common variant in the methylenetetrahydrofolate reductase (*MTHFR*) gene, c.677C > T, may cause increased levels of plasma homocysteine. This variant shows reduced activity and increased thermolability of the protein. Approximately 12% of the Caucasian population is homozygous for the mutation that would cause typical manifestation of moderate hyperhomocysteinemia when folate levels are at the lower end of the normal range.[133]

A second common polymorphism in the *MTHFR* gene, c.1298A > C, has been described by van der Put et al.[134] The prevalence of homozygotes for this variant in the white population is approximately 10%, and 23% of people are compound heterozygotes for both c.677C > T and c.1298A >C.[133] It has been described that compound heterozygosity for both mutations, but not homozygosity for c.1298A > C, is associated with increased homocysteine plasma levels.[133]

A meta-analysis has been performed on 31 publications in the literature regarding the association between inherited thrombophilia and pregnancy loss.[123] In addition to estimating the actual strength of association between inherited thrombophilia and fetal loss, this meta-analysis also served to clarify whether the associations vary by the timing or definition of fetal loss.

The initial observation that homozygosity for *MTHFR* c.677C > T could be related to pregnancy loss,[135,136] supported by more recent studies,[137,138] could not be confirmed, neither in another sample[139] nor by the mentioned meta-analysis.[124] However, when additional thrombophilic factors were considered, *MTHFR* c.677C > T seemed to significantly increase the risk of pregnancy wastage.[121,140,141] The *MTHFR* c.1298A > C variant alone showed no significant association with RPL, but a good correlation was confirmed in the presence of other prothrombotic mutations.[137,138] Hyperhomocysteinemia is a risk factor for placenta-mediated diseases, such as preeclampsia and placenta abruption as well as for fetal neural tube defects.[136,139] However, it does not appear that homozygosity for *MTHFR* c.667C > T, the genetic abnormality most commonly associated with hyperhomocysteinemia, is linked to an increased risk of venous thromboembolism (VTE) in pregnant women. As clinical events in homozygotes are likely to reflect the interaction of the genotype with a relative deficiency of vitamins, such as B12 and folic acid, the absence of an association of this genotype with gestational VTE may reflect pregnancy-related physiologic reduction in homocysteine levels and/ or the effects of folic acid supplements that are now taken widely by women in pregnancy for the prevention of neural tube defects. According to the guidelines of the Italian Society for Haemostasis and Thrombosis, evidence of association between pregnancy complications and MTHFR polymorphisms is not sufficient. Therefore the use of folic acid is suggested for the whole pregnancy in women with mild hyperhomocysteinemia.[142]

Taking into account the literature published so far, DNA analysis of both FVL and PTm mutations is recommended in patients with a personal or family history of thrombosis.[143,144] However, other hereditary deficiencies of anticoagulant proteins as antithrombin, protein C, and protein S are heterogeneous in nature and can be caused by many different genetic lesions.[145] Although they have been the target of intense clinical research, taken together, they account for less than 10% of patients with thrombophilia.[146]

Preimplantation Genetic Testing

Preimplantation genetic testing is an early analysis to obtain genetic information from cultured embryos, leading to the selection of normal embryos to be transferred. The first use of PGT was to discard affected embryos in carriers of single-gene disorders.[147] Techniques have changed since those years and clinical indications for the use of PGT have increased. Nowadays, PGT is used to discard affected embryos in carriers of monogenic disorders and to discard embryos having structural chromosome abnormalities in couples having known abnormal karyotype. In addition, a variant of PGT is applied to the screening of numerical chromosome abnormalities in couples with normal karyotype, but with infertility problems, and it is called PGT for aneuploidy (PGT-A) or PGS.

Preimplantation Genetic Testing for Aneuploidy

Preimplantation genetic testing for aneuploidy is offered in many IVF centers to improve IVF outcome of certain groups of patients. Current clinical indications for PGT-A are AMA, recurrent miscarriage (RM), RIF, and severe MF (SMF) infertility.

Initially PGT-A was done using a technique called fluorescence in situ hybridization (FISH) for the screening of only a selected panel of chromosomes (in most of the cases ranging from 5 to 12).[148,149] However, there was controversy regarding the benefits of PGT-A. Some randomized controlled trials with FISH-based PGT-A showed no improvement in live birth rates after IVF and presented even lower live birth rates for women with AMA,[150,151] whereas other studies showed improvement in live birth rates.[152] Despite, the controversy, what these studies pointed out was the need to have methods which can comprehensively screen all 23 pairs of chromosomes in human embryos for appropriate evaluation.

With advancements in reproductive technologies, many methodologies were incorporated for PGT-A to asses all 23 pairs of chromosomes, these include CGH (comparative genetic hybridization) arrays, SNP (single-nucleotide polymorphism) arrays, NGS (next-generation sequencing), and quantitative PCR. Among these methods, array CGH (aCGH) was the first technology to be widely used and has been validated by testing cells of a known genotype.[153] Three pilot randomized controlled trials (RCTs) that tested trophectoderm (TE) biopsy and aCGH on patients with a good prognosis for live birth showed significant improvements in ongoing PRs and have changed the view of the PGT-A field,[154-156] and aCGH became a gold standard test to be offered to the patient with good prognosis. However, owing to the ability of the new technologies to better discriminate the copy number for each chromosome, the possibility of identifying the presence of embryonic mosaicism has also increased, and now it is possible to consider the potential impact of embryo mosaicism on diagnosis accuracy and whether mosaic embryos should be used for transfer or not.[157]

Several studies have used mixture of cell lines to estimate the sensitivity and specificity of these novel methods (aCGH and NGS) for detecting mosaicism in TE biopsy, estimating levels of detection to be 40–50% for aneuploid cells with the use of aCGH and 20% with the use of NGS.[158-161] The results of a TE biopsy may not be representative of the entire embryo, the unbiopsied TE cells, or the ICM.[157] Some studies have attempted to determine how frequently a TE biopsy correctly represents the embryo mosaicism. Analysis of two to three biopsies in the same embryo showed concordance rates as high as 95–100%.[158,162] In addition, these studies also analyzed the ICM of the same embryos to estimate the discordance frequencies between cell lineages. The TE and ICM showed discordant mosaicism rates of 3–4%. Therefore, TE biopsy is a good method to accurately diagnose blastocyst mosaicism.[157]

Next-generation sequencing offers more potential advantages including reduced cost, reduced time, higher resolution and improved detection of partial or segmental aneuploidies, and the detection of mosaicism as compared to all other methods.[163-166] It has been demonstrated by recent RCTs that PGT-A based on NGS is equally concordant (99.5%) to PGT-based on aCGH in the detection of chromosomal aneuploidy after TE biopsy. Clinical pregnancy and implantation rates (IRs) using aCGH (63.8%) and NGS (62%) after the transfer of euploid blastocyst transfer were also similar.[166] The sensitivity and specificity of NGS for the detection of aneuploid chromosome number are 100% and 99.98%, respectively.[167]

Advanced Maternal Age

Chromosome aneuploidies are common in preimplantation human embryos, and it is a fact that aneuploidy rates are higher in embryos from AMA women,[168] probably due to age-related MI recombination defects.[169] The increase of aneuploidies with maternal age results in higher aneuploidy rates in the offspring involving chromosomes 13, 18, 21, X, and Y; and increasing spontaneous abortions, reducing in fact ongoing IRs.[170,171]

There has been a huge controversy about the usefulness of PGT-A in AMA patients, but all the studies showing detrimental results after the application of PGT-A were done using FISH technique. Even with FISH technique for nine chromosomes (13, 15, 16, 17, 18, 21, 22, X, and Y), some improvement in clinical outcome of certain AMA patients was observed using day 3 embryo biopsies for PGT-A and subsequent day 5 embryo transfer in fresh cycle when compared to a similar control group of AMA patients but without PGT-A treatment.[172] And in AMA patients, the improvement in pregnancy and IRs is higher after the application of aCGH technology for PGT-A.[152] A recent RCT by Rubio et al. demonstrates the superiority of PGT-A in achieving live birth at the first attempt, both per transfer and per cycle. The results were possible despite a significant decrease in the percentage of cycles reaching ET in PGT-A versus control patients (69.0% vs. 90.5%) due to significantly fewer miscarriages in the PGT-A group versus control (2.7% vs. 39.0%).[173] The study proposed that the clinicians must choose between a higher number of ETs with a greater risk of miscarriage; or decreased number of ETs with chromosomally normal embryos, reducing the chance of miscarriage and potential live births with chromosomal abnormalities. From the patients' perspective, this question has a straightforward response.[173]

Recurrent Pregnancy Loss

It has been shown previously in this chapter that RPL can be caused by several factors, and the presence of any chromosomal abnormality in the fetus accounts for about 50% of those cases. Added to the studies showing the presence of chromosomal abnormalities in pregnancies of RPL patients, there is evidence demonstrating that RPL couples have an increased number of chromosomally abnormal embryos (ranging from 50% to 80%).[58,174]

The initial studies published using PGT-A in RPL patients were done using FISH technique for a limited number of chromosomes to select chromosomally normal embryos for transfer. In a study[58] using FISH for chromosomes 13, 15, 16, 18, 21, 22, X, and Y demonstrated that reproductive outcome was improved by PGT-A. Moreover, this study demonstrated that, after PGT-A, significantly higher IRs were obtained in couples who previously suffered aneuploid miscarriages. Second, similar embryo aneuploidy rate, PR, and IR were recorded in couples with RPL after fertility treatments as in those with previous spontaneous pregnancies.

Third, there were no miscarriages after PGT-A in couples in which the FISH assay first showed that the male partner's sperm was abnormal. Finally, lower IRs are observed in couples with more than or equal to five previous miscarriages, which is associated with a lower incidence of chromosomally abnormal embryos. Authors concluded that PGT-A should be recommended when RPL is associated with chromosomopathy in up to five previous miscarriages, and when there is a high incidence of chromosomal abnormalities in sperm.[58] Moreover, there is increasing evidence supporting the use of PGT-A even in idiopathic RPL patients.[175]

A case series report by Hodes-Wertz et al. used aCGH technology on 287 IVF cycles from couples with unexplained RPL, defined as two or more losses. They used PGT-A both on cleavage-stage biopsy (193 cycles) and blastocyst biopsy (94 cycles) and compared the miscarriage rate from these IVF-PGT-A cycles with the expected miscarriage rate determined as reported in the United States to the Society of Assisted Reproduction Technology. The overall aneuploidy rate for all analyzed embryos was 64.8%. The aneuploidy rate was 68.8% for cleavage-stage embryos and 53% for blastocyst embryos. The overall clinical PR per embryo transfer was 55.2%, with a significantly higher PR for blastocyst biopsy compared with cleavage-stage biopsy (63.6% vs. 50.4%, $p < 0.001$).[176] The results of this study by Hodes-Wertz look promising for the new technology; however, the data require careful interpretation as the conclusions drawn are limited to certain groups.[177]

Repetitive Implantation Failure

Couples who had failed three or more IVF attempts or who had failed an IVF treatment after cumulative transfer of more than 10 good quality embryos are considered RIF. There are several causes that can result in implantation failure: endocrinological, uterine, immunological, and embryonic factors. Although not all the RIF cases are due to embryonic defects, there are reports of higher chromosomal abnormalities in their embryos, compared to control groups.[178]

There is no agreement in the PGT-A studies in RIF patients using FISH technique, as different chromosomes were analyzed (from 5 to 9), and study designs were also different: different inclusion criteria, stimulation protocols, and day of embryo transfer. However, some of them could show that PGT-A seems to be beneficial at least in younger RIF patients[179] and in those patients having good embryo morphology in which blastocyst transfer is possible.[178]

However, the use of aCGH technique in RIF patients has improved the benefit of PGT-A for those patients. In a study that applied PGT-A using aCGH in day 3 embryo biopsies and subsequent day 5 embryo transfer in the same cycle, very promising ongoing PR and IR were obtained.[152] Another study that applied day 5 embryo biopsy showed similar clinical PR and IR in RIF patient with PGT-A and non-RIF patients with PGT-A (68.3% and 70.5%) and concluded that the combined use of aCGH and single blastocyst transfer can provide an efficient tool for improving IVF clinical outcomes in RIF patients without increasing the number of transferred embryos and the risk of unwished multiple pregnancies.[180]

Severe Male Factor

Males having impaired sperm parameters can be considered SMF. However, the most commonly included in PGT-A programs are: severe oligozoospermia (≤5 millions of spermatozoa/mL), azoospermia, teratozoospermia, increased incidence of chromosome abnormalities in spermatozoa, abnormal male meiosis and, also patients after undergoing chemotherapy.

Preimplantation genetic testing for aneuploidy studies in SMF patients have shown higher incidence of chromosome abnormalities in embryos from infertile men with altered sperm parameters. In azoospermic patients, higher rates of mosaic embryos and chromosomally abnormal embryos have been reported, most frequently for sex chromosomes.[181,182] This increase was more remarkable in embryos from NOA patients.[183] We found significantly higher incidence of abnormal embryos in severe oligozoospermic patients (≤5 millions of spermatozoa/mL); in patients with OA and in NOA patients compared to a control group of fertile couples undergoing PGT-M (PGT for monogenic diseases) due to sex-linked diseases.[171,184] Nonobstructive azoospermia patients showed the highest aneuploidy and mosaicism rates, as reported in other studies. Pregnancy and implantation rates in these patients after a PGT-A cycle were as high as in the control group of patients without infertility problems. In teratozoospermic patients, it is harder to elucidate which morphological dysmorphism could imply a higher rate of embryo aneuploidy. It has been observed a correlation between sperm aneuploidy rates and sperm head anomalies[185] with higher incidence of abnormal embryos in patients with macrocefalic spermatozoa.[186,187] In the study of Kahraman et al., PGT-A was performed, and the results were compared with ICSI cycles without PGT-A, obtaining better IRs and a significant reduction of miscarriage rates.[186]

An increased incidence of aneuploid sperm has been reported for all the above-mentioned indications, mainly in patients with $\leq 5 \times 10^6$ sperm/mL, in OA, and in NOA patients.[163,165] In most of these patients, an increase in sex chromosomes aneuploidy is observed on sperm that can be translated into an increase of aneuploidy in preimplantation embryos. Couples with higher incidence of chromosome abnormalities on sperm have lower fertilization rates and higher percentages of chromosomally abnormal embryos than controls. In normal karyotype patients with increased disomy for sex chromosomes, we observed increased percentages of aneuploid embryos for all the chromosomes analyzed, not only for sex chromosomes, whereas in those with increases in diploid spermatozoa, there was a higher production of triploid embryos.[188] For these reasons, these patients should be informed of their genetic risks. Several strategies could be offered to the couple, such as PGT-A, prenatal testing, or sperm donation.

Men with altered karyotype for sex chromosomes (47,XXY; 47,XYY; and mosaics 46,XY/47,XXY) can have abnormal spermatogenesis, although frequently they do not have fertility problems. In 29 PGT-A cycles performed in 47,XXY men, higher incidence of abnormal embryos was reported than in a control group, mostly for sex chromosomes aneuploidy, but also in chromosomes 18 and 21, and haploid embryos. In a group of 47,XYY patients, those with abnormal FISH on sperm showed increases of diploidy and sex chromosomes disomy. The chromosomal abnormalities of their spermatozoa seem to be reflected in their embryos, showing high incidence of triploid embryos and aneuploid embryos for chromosomes 13, 16, and sex chromosomes, respectively.[188]

A recent RCT published in SMF patients using aCGH in day 3 embryo biopsies and subsequent day 5 embryo transfer in fresh cycle showed a clear improvement in ongoing PR and IR in this patient group compared to a similar control group of SMF patients but without PGT-A treatment.[189] A recent study on Indian patients using aCGH in day 3 biopsies in different poor prognosis patients including patients AMA, RIF, RM, and MF showed that the best clinical results after PGT-A are observed in MF couples (PR 60.0% and IR 42.9%) than in any other group.[190] Another retrospective cohort study by Coates et al. performed aCGH on TE biopsies and reported that SMF was associated with a significant increase of sex chromosome abnormalities in blastocysts compared with subjects with normozoospermia and highlighted that SMF infertility as a possible referral category for PGT-A.[191]

Preimplantation Genetic Testing for Monogenic Diseases

Genetic disorders are the leading cause of infant death in the United States, accounting for approximately 20% of annual infant mortality.[192] For patients at risk of having offspring with a type of genetic disorders called single-gene disorder or monogenic disease, either prenatal genetic diagnosis (PND) or PGT-M can be offered to avoid the birth of affected offspring for the analyzed condition.

Preimplantation genetic testing for monogenic diseases is applied to diagnose embryos at high risk of suffering a specific monogenic disease. It is possible to distinguish between genetically normal or abnormal embryos using molecular analysis techniques, mainly PCR in its diverse methods. Embryos carrying the specific mutation or the disease's linked haplotype can be discarded, and only genetically normal embryos for the condition analyzed will be candidates to be transferred.

Polymerase chain reaction is the most common technique applied to PGT-M, and two main approaches are followed: (1) to perform a whole genome amplification of the embryo biopsy and then several simplex PCR for each of the genetic markers as well as the mutation/s and (2) to develop individualized protocols for each couple by multiplex-PCR assays with linked polymorphic markers.[147]

The number of inherited disorders diagnosed by PGT-M has grown progressively due to new strategies for single-cell analysis. There is a worldwide experience for PGT-M being applied in more than 300 different conditions. Independently of the analyzed condition, the aim in all the cases is to avoid the transmission of a severe hereditary disease to the offspring. Moreover, an increasing number of new genetic diseases are reported worldwide in a yearly basis by the European Society for Human Reproduction and Embryology Preimplantation Genetic Diagnosis Consortium.[193,194]

However, PGT-M needs a previous step of genetic counseling to evaluate the family history of the disease, and it is mandatory to follow the law, as it can be different in different countries. Before patients undergo PGT-M, the genetic cause of the disorder has to be identified. In some cases, patients already have a genetic study showing the mutation because they have a previous family history of the disease. However, a mutation may appear de novo, that is a new mutation present in a patient which was not present in his parents, this mainly happens in cases of a dominant pattern of inheritance of the disease; present symptoms in the patients and therefore they further have possibility of being at risk of having affected offspring for this condition.[195]

Recent technological advances in the reproductive medicine field have made genetic carrier screening test possible and affordable for everyone. These tests provide the screening of hundreds of recessive genetic disorders simultaneously in one test.[192] Moreover, these tests can be applied to patients not having any family history of a particular genetic disease; therefore, they can be used as preconceptional screening tests. Finally, in those cases; in which, the test shows the presence of any mutation, the couple should be tested too, and if both members of the couple shared the same mutations, then, PGT-M should be offered to these couples to avoid the birth of affected offspring for the tested condition.

In the developed countries, there is an increasing number of patients who prefer PGT-M over PND because of the less risky procedure. The use of PGT-M implies a costlier and longer treatment than PND, and it also requires ART. However, PND implies a risk of fetal loss that can vary from 0.5% to 1%, and in cases, in which the fetus is genetically abnormal, the medical termination of the pregnancy may imply some risk to the mother, both physical and emotional.[34] Therefore, both PND and PGT-M have to be recommended to these couples along with the proper genetic counseling, informing all the advantages and disadvantages of both options so that patients can make the right decision.

Concurrent Preimplantation Genetic Testing

The field of clinical genetics is evolving so fast along with the evolution of newer reproductive technologies. The techniques, such as PGT, is providing help to the families to reduce the transmission of monogenic diseases (PGT-M) and also chromosomal aneuploidies (PGT-A). However, as we know that prevalence of aneuploidies is high in the embryos, particularly in AMA patients, so the embryos which are found to be free of disease mutation remain at high risk of implantation failure or pregnancy loss due to aneuploidy. So, there is a need of simultaneous detection of disease mutation and chromosomal aneuploidies in the same sample (known as concurrent PGT), to achieve a higher IR and reduce the miscarriage rate. Concurrent PGT is becoming popular nowadays although has not become standard. A recent retrospective cohort study explored the value of concurrent screening, and they compared two groups including patients who underwent PGT-M with or without aneuploidy screening and demonstrated that only 25.6% of embryos were both negative for PGT-M and PGT-A despite young mean age (32.4 ± 5.9 years) of the patients. This study demonstrated higher IR (75% vs. 53.3%) and lower miscarriage rate (20% vs. 40%) suggesting that PGT-A when performed concurrently with PGT-M provides valuable information for embryo selection and improves clinical outcome.[196] The screening for chromosomal aneuploidies revealed that 50.6% of blastocysts diagnosed free of genetic disease or balanced were aneuploid, therefore avoiding the transfer of blastocysts potentially resulting in implantation failures, miscarriages, or in some cases, in health affected live births.[197]

Noninvasive Preimplantation Genetic Testing

The selection of the best embryo based on the morphology and normal genetic content is crucial for improving patients' chance of achieving a live birth with the use of IVF. As described above too, PGT nowadays is frequently being used to select embryos that is unaffected by a monogenic disease (PGT-M) or by chromosomal abnormalities (PGT-A). Preimplantation genetic testing, however, relies on the invasive biopsy of a single cell or a few cells from the developing embryo, which has to be performed by highly trained and experienced individuals, and the potential effect of this biopsy procedure on future development of an embryo or fetus has not been fully established.[198] Therefore, there is a need for a technique which should not be invasive for the embryos to assess the genetic and chromosomal defects in the embryos.

Recently some studies reported the presence of cell-free nuclear DNA (cfDNA) in blastocoelic fluid (BF) and in spent embryo culture medium (SEM).[199,200] Palini et al. found that cfDNA was present in approximately 90% of investigated BF samples, and several genes were also characterized using the same DNA for real-time PCR.[199] Study by Wu et al. verified that the cfDNA present in SEM can be successfully amplified for the diagnosis of human alpha thalassemia, demonstrating that this medium, which is typically discarded by IVF centers after blastocyst transfer or vitrification, may represent a potential sources of genetic material for noninvasive PGT.[200] Recent studies have documented the ability to detect and sequence cfDNA in SEM with the use of techniques, such as aCGH, SNP sequencing, and NGS.[200-206] Xu et al. reported high concordance of the results obtained by the noninvasive technique and from the biopsy for detection of chromosomal aneuploidy (sensitivity: 88% and specificity: 84%, respectively),[202] and another recent study showed that the full chromosome concordance rate between biopsied cells and SEM was 64.52%, and it increased to 90.00% for diploid blastocyst samples.[204] Recent study demonstrated that cfDNA can be successfully sequenced at the cleavage and blastocyst stages, showing concordance of 65% and 70% between day 5 cfDNA and TE biopsies.[205] Study by Vera-Rodriguez et al. demonstrated significantly higher quantity of cfDNA in SEM cocultured with embryos versus control media samples. The presence of cfDNA in the SEM enabled a chromosomal diagnosis, although results differed from those of TE biopsy analysis in most cases (67%) and reported a high percentage of maternal DNA in the SEM. This study highlighted the need of first developing either in vitro or in silico methods for reducing maternal contamination before this new noninvasive technique can be used for diagnosing human embryos.[206] Another recent study demonstrated that the aneuploidy information generated by the noninvasive technique was not entirely identical to the information obtained from the biopsied TE or the remaining embryo and highlighted that as the origins of the DNA extracted from the different sample types were not the same, the significance and interpretation of each result would have its own meaning, so should be interpreted carefully.[203]

The noninvasive technique has more advantages over the currently used embryo biopsy method. Most importantly, it is less harmful to the embryo, and there would be little concern of potential damage to the developing embryo. Release of the BF would not cause any damage to the embryo as this is being routinely used in the frozen embryo IVF technique. Possible contamination of the sample is also reduced to the minimum due to much less manipulation of the embryo in the procedure.[203]

Although results have been encouraging, the differences in sensitivity and specificity shown by different studies challenge more proper evaluation and explanation to assess the validity of this technique. This also warrants that this technique is not yet ready for clinical application and needs further optimization using more validated studies on different sequencing and bioinformatics platforms before its clinical implementation.

REFERENCES

1. Poongothai J, Gopenath TS, Manonayaki S. Genetics of human male infertility. Singapore Med J. 2009;50:336-47.
2. Shah K, Sivapalan G, Gibbons N, et al. The genetic basis of infertility. Reproduction. 2003;126:13-25.
3. Harton GL, Tempest HG. Chromosomal disorders and male infertility. Asian J Androl. 2012;14:32-9.
4. Mueller RF, Young ID (Eds). Emery's elements of medical genetics, 11th edition. Edinburgh, UK: Churchill Livingstone; 2001. pp. 249.
5. Hassold T, Hunt PA, Sherman S. Trisomy in humans: incidence, origin and etiology. Curr Opin Genet Dev. 1993;3:398-403.
6. Anglani F, Baccichetti C, Artifoni L, et al. Frequency of abnormal karyotypes in relation to the ascertained method in females referred for suspected sex chromosome abnormality. Clin Genet. 1984;25:242-7.
7. Lyon MF. Possible mechanisms of X chromosome inactivation. Nat New Biol. 1971;232:229-32.
8. Gardner RJ, Sutherland GR. Chromosome abnormalities and genetic counselling. 2nd edition. Oxford, UK: Oxford University Press; 1996.
9. Jacobs PA, Melville M, Ratcliffe S, et al. A cytogenetic survey of 11,680 newborn infants. Ann Hum Genet. 1974;37:359-76.
10. Nielsen J, Wohlert M. Chromosome abnormalities found among 34,910 newborn children: results from a 13-year incidence study in Arhus, Denmark. Hum Genet. 1991;87:81-3.
11. Kim IW, Khadilkar AC, Ko EY, et al. 47,XYY syndrome and male infertility. Rev Urol. 2013;15:188-96.
12. Gonzalez L, Witchel SF. The patient with Turner syndrome: puberty and medical management concerns. Fertil Steril. 2012;98:780-6.
13. Suri M, Kabra M, Jain U, et al. A clinical and cytogenetic study of Turner syndrome. Indian Pediatr. 1995;32:433-42.
14. Witters G, Van Robays J, Willekes C, et al. Trisomy 13, 18, 21, triploidy and Turner syndrome: the 5T's. Look at the hands. Facts Views Vis Obgyn. 2011;3:15-21.
15. Rives N, Joly G, Machy A, et al. Assessment of sex chromosome aneuploidy in sperm nuclei from 47,XXY and 46,XY/47,XXY males: comparison with fertile and infertile males with normal karyotype. Mol Hum Reprod. 2000;6:107-12.

16. Skakkebaek N, Zenthen E, Nielsen J, et al. Abnormal spermatogenesis in XYY males: a report on 4 cases ascertainment through a population study. Fertil Steril. 1973;24:390-5.
17. Morel F, Roux C, Bresson JL. Sex chromosome aneuploidies in sperm of 47,XYY men. Arch Androl. 1999;43:27-36.
18. Lim AS, Fong Y, Yu SL. Analysis of the sex chromosome constitution of sperm in men with a 47,XYY mosaic karyotype by fluorescence in situ hybridization. Fertil Steril. 1999;72:121-3.
19. Wong EC, Ferguson KA, Chow V, et al. Sperm aneuploidy and meiotic sex chromosome configurations in an infertile XYY male. Hum Reprod. 2008;23:374-8.
20. Otter M, Constance TR, Schrander S, et al. Triple X syndrome: a review of the literature. Eur J Hum Genet. 2010;18:265-71.
21. Kodandapani S, Pai MV, Nambiar J, et al. Premature ovarian aging in primary infertility: triple X syndrome. J Hum Reprod Sci. 2011;4:153-4.
22. May KM, Jacobs PA, Lee M, et al. The parental origin of the extra X chromosome in 47,XXX females. Am J Hum Genet. 1990;46:754-76.
23. Weijerman ME, de Winter JP. Clinical practice. The care of children with Down syndrome. Eur J Pediatr. 2010;169: 1445-52.
24. Blouin JL, Binkert F. Antonarakis SE. Biparental inheritance of chromosome 21 polymorphic markers indicates that some Robertsonian translocations t(21;21) occur postzygotically. Am J Med Genet. 1994;49:363-8.
25. Morris JK, Mutton DE, Alberman E. Revised estimates of the maternal age specific live birth prevalence of Down's syndrome. J Med Screen. 2002;9:2-6.
26. Cereda A, Carey JC. The trisomy 18 syndrome. Orphanet J Rare Dis. 2012;7:81.
27. Hamerton JL, Canning N, Ray M, et al. A cytogenetic survey of 14,069 newborn infants. I. Incidence of chromosome abnormalities. Clin Genet. 1975;8:223-43.
28. Nybo Andersen AM, Wohlfahrt J, Christens P, et al. Maternal age and fetal loss: population based register linkage study. BMJ. 2000;320:1708-12.
29. Kim SR, Shaffer LG. Robertsonian translocations: mechanisms of formation, aneuploidy, and uniparental disomy and diagnostic considerations. Genet Test. 2002;6:163-8.
30. Martin RH. Cytogenetic determinants of male fertility. Hum Reprod Update. 2008;14:379-90.
31. Therman E, Susman B, Denniston C. The nonrandom participation of human acrocentric chromosomes in Robertsonian translocations. Ann Hum Genet. 1989;53:49-65.
32. Tharapel AT, Tharapel SA, Bannerman RM. Recurrent pregnancy losses and parental chromosome abnormalities: a review. Br J Obstet Gynaecol. 1985; 92:899-914.
33. Chandley AC. Infertility and chromsomal abnormality. In: Clark JR (Ed). Oxford reviews of reproductive biology, vol. 6. Oxford: Oxford University Press; 1984. pp. 1-46.
34. Berend SA, Bejjani BA, McCaskill C, et al. Identification of uniparental disomy in phenotypically abnormal carriers of isochromosomes or Robertsonian translocations. Am J Med Genet. 2002;111:362-5.
35. Choi BH, Kim UH, Lee KS, et al. Various endocrine disorders in children with t(13;14)(q10; q10) Robertsonian translocation. Ann Pediatr Endocrinol Metab. 2013;18:111-5.
36. Warburton D. De novo balanced chromosome rearrangements and extra marker chromosomes identified at prenatal diagnosis: clinical significance and distribution of breakpoints. Am J Hum Genet. 1991;49:995-1013.
37. Nigam A, Ahmad A, Batra S. Absent endometrium due to balanced translocation [t(4;20)] presenting as primary amenorrhea. J Hum Reprod Sci. 2014;7:63-5.
38. Stephenson MD, Awartani KA, Robinson WP. Cytogenetic analysis of miscarriages from couples with recurrent miscarriage: a case-control study. Hum Reprod. 2002;17: 446-51.
39. Madan K, Seabright M, Lindenbaum RH, et al. Paracentric inversions in man. J Med Genet. 1984;21:407-12.
40. Daniel A, Hook E, Wulf G. Risks of unbalanced progeny at amniocentesis to carriers of chromosome rearrangements: data from United States and Canadian laboratories. Am J Med Genet. 1989;33:14-53.
41. Madan K. Paracentric inversions: a review. Hum Genet. 1995;96:503-15.
42. Pettenati M, Rao P, Phelan M, et al. Paracentric inversion in humans: a review of 446 paracentric inversions with presentation of 120 new cases. Am J Med Genet. 1995;55: 171-87.
43. Aitken RJ. Age, the environment and our reproductive future: bonking baby boomers and the future of sex. Reproduction. 2013;147:S1-11.
44. Laxmi KV, Babu SJ, Dayakar S, et al. Cytogenetic investigation of patients with primary amenorrhea. Indian J Hum Genet. 2012;18:112-6.
45. Foresta C, Ferlin A, Gianaroli L, et al. Guidelines for the appropriate use of genetic tests in infertile couples. Eur J Hum Genet. 2002;10:303-12.
46. ESHRE Capri Workshop Group. Genetic aspects of female reproduction. Hum Reprod Update. 2008;14:293-307.
47. Lissitsina J, Mikelsaar R, Punab M. Cytogenetic analyses in infertile men. Arch Androl. 2006;52:91-5.
48. Ferlin A, Arredi B, Foresta C. Genetic causes of male infertility. Reprod Toxicol. 2006;22:133-41.
49. Opitz O, Zoll B, Hansmann I, et al. Cytogenetic investigation of 103 patients with primary or secondary amenorrhea. Hum Genet. 1982;65:46-7.
50. Nakamura Y, Kitamura M, Nishimura K, et al. Chromosomal variants among 1790 infertile men. Int J Urol. 2001;8:49-52.
51. Yakin K, Balaban B, Urman B. Is there a possible correlation between chromosomal variants and spermatogenesis? Int J Urol. 2005;12:984-9.
52. Madon PF, Athalye AS, Parikh FR. Polymorphic variants on chromosomes probably play a significant role in infertility. Reprod Biomed Online. 2005;11:726-32.
53. Warren JE, Silver RM. Genetics of pregnancy loss. Clin Obstet Gynecol. 2008;51:84-95.
54. Sugiura-Ogasawara M, Ozaki Y, Katano K, et al. Abnormal embryonic karyotype is the most frequent cause of recurrent miscarriage. Hum Reprod. 2012;27:2297-303.
55. Bianco K, Caughey AB, Shaffer BL, et al. History of miscarriage and increased incidence of fetal aneuploidy in subsequent pregnancy. Obstet Gynecol. 2006;107:1098-102.
56. Franssen MT, Korevaar JC, van der Veen F, et al. Reproductive outcome after chromosome analysis in couples with two or

more miscarriages: index [corrected]-control study. BMJ. 2006;332:759-63.

57. Stephenson MD, Sierra S. Reproductive outcomes in recurrent pregnancy loss associated with a parental carrier of a structural chromosome rearrangement. Hum Reprod. 2006;21:1076-82.
58. Rubio C, Buendía P, Rodrigo L, et al. Prognostic factors for preimplantation genetic screening in repeated pregnancy loss. Reprod BioMed Online. 2009;18:687-93.
59. Carr DH. Chromosome studies in spontaneous abortions. Obstet Gynaecol. 1965;26:308-26.
60. Brugh V, Matscke M, Lipshultz L. Male factor infertility. Endocrinol Metab Clin North Am. 2003;32:689-707.
61. Chillón M, Casals T, Mercier B, et al. Mutations in the cystic fibrosis gene in patients with congenital absence of the vas deferens. N Engl J Med. 1995;332:1475-80.
62. Patrizio P, Leonord DG. Mutation of cystic fibrosis gene and congenital bilateral absence of vas deferens. In: McElreavey K (Ed). The genetic basis of male infertility. Berlin: Springer-Verlag; 2000. pp. 175-86.
63. Tizzano EF, Chitayat D, Buchwald M. Cell-specific localization of CFTR mRNA shows developmentally regulated expression m human fetal tissues. Hum Mol Genet. 1993;2:219-24.
64. Timmreck LS, Gray MR, Handelin B, et al. Analysis of cystic fibrosis transmembrane conductance regulator gene mutations in patients with 512 congenital absence of the uterus and vagina. Am J Med Genet. 2003;120:72-6.
65. Egan M, Flotte T, Afione S, et al. Defective regulation of outwardly rectifying Cl2 channels by protein kinase A corrected by insertion of CFTR. Nature. 1992;358:581-4.
66. Xu WM, Shi QX, Chen WY, et al. Cystic fibrosis transmembrane conductance regulator is vital to sperm fertilizing capacity and male fertility. Proc Natl Acad Sci USA. 2007;104:9816-21.
67. Claustres M, Guittard C, Bozon D, et al. Spectrum of CFTR mutations in cystic fibrosis and in congenital absence of the vas deferens in France. Hum Mutat. 2000;16:143-56.
68. Sachdeva K, Saxena R, Majumdar A, et al. Mutation studies in the CFTR gene in Asian Indian subjects with congenital bilateral absence of vas deferens: report of two novel mutations and four novel variants. Genet Test Mol Biomarkers. 2011;15(5):307-12.
69. Levy E, Guranados P, Rave V, et al. Mutation in CFTR gene and clinical correlation in Argentine patients with congenital bilateral absence of vas deferens. Medicine. 2004;64:213-8.
70. Sharma N, Acharya N, Singh SK, et al. Heterogeneous spectrum of CFTR gene mutation in Indian patient with congenital bilateral absence of vas deferens. Hum Reprod. 2009;24:1229-36.
71. Radpour R, Gilani S, Gourabi H, et al. Molecular analysis of IVS8-T splice variant 5T and M470V exon 10 missence polymorphism in Iranian males with congenital bilateral absence of vas deferens. Mol Hum Reprod. 2006;12:469-73.
72. Rave-Harel N, Kerem E, Nissim-Rafinia M, et al. The molecular basis of partial penetrance of splicing mutations in cystic fibrosis. Am J Hum Genet. 1997;60:87-94.
73. Wong LJ, Alper OM, Hsu E, et al. The necessity of complete CFTR mutational analysis of an infertile couple before in vitro fertilization. Fertil Steril. 2004;82:947-49.
74. Lissen W, Mahmoud KZ, Elgindi E. Molecular analysis of cystic fibrosis gene reveal a high frequency of intron 8 splice variant 5T in Egyptian male with congenital bilateral absence of vas deferens. Mol Hum Reprod. 1999;5:10-3.
75. Sachdeva K, Saxena R, Majumdar A, et al. Use of ethnicity-specific sequence tag site markers for Y-chromosome microdeletion studies. Genet Test Mol Biomarkers. 2011;15:451-9.
76. Chu CS, Trapnell BC, Curristin S, et al. Genetic basis of variable exon 9 skipping in cystic fibrosis transmembrane conductance regulator mRNA. Nat Genet. 1993;3:151-6.
77. Cuppens H, Lin W, Jaspers M, et al. Polyvariant mutant cystic fibrosis transmembrane conductance regulator genes. The polymorphic (Tg)m locus explains the partial penetrance of the T5 polymorphism as a disease mutation. J Clin Invest. 1998;10:487-96.
78. Welsh MJ, Smith AE. Cystic fibrosis. Sci Am. 1995;273:52-9.
79. Wilschanski M, Zielenski J, Markiewicz D, et al. Correlation of sweat chloride concentration with classes of the cystic fibrosis transmembrane conductance regulator gene mutations. J Pediatr. 1995;127:705-10.
80. Augarten A, Yahav Y, Kerem BS, et al. Congenital bilateral absence of vas deferens in the absence of cystic fibrosis. Lancet. 1994;344:1473-4.
81. Blau H, Freud E, Mussaffi H. Urogenital abnormalities in male children with cystic fibrosis. Arch Dis Child. 2002;87:135-8.
82. Loukas YL, Thodi G, Molou E, et al. Clinical diagnostic next-generation sequencing: the case of CFTR carrier screening. Scand J Clin Lab Invest. 2015;75:374-81.
83. Reynolds N, Cooke HJ. Role of the DAZ genes in male fertility. Reprod Biomed Online. 2005;10:72-80.
84. Schlegel PN. Causes of azoospermia and their management. Reprod Fertil Dev. 2004;16:561-72.
85. Katagiri Y, Neri QV, Takeuchi T, et al. Y-chromosome assessment and its implications for the development of ICSI children. Reprod Biomed Online. 2004;8:307-18.
86. Foresta C, Moro E, Ferlin A. Y-chromosome microdeletions and alterations of spermatogenesis. Endocr Rev. 2001;22:226-39.
87. Dohle GR, Halley DJ, Van Hemel JO, et al. Genetic risk factors in infertile men with severe oligozoospermia and azoospermia. Hum Reprod. 2002;17:13-6.
88. De Vries JW, Repping S, Oates R, et al. Absence of deleted in azoospermia (DAZ) genes in spermatozoa of infertile men with somatic DAZ deletions. Fertil Steril. 2001;75:476-9.
89. Peterlin B, Kunej T, Sinkovec J, et al. Screening for Y-chromosome microdeletions in 226 Slovenian subfertile men. Hum Reprod. 2002;17:17-24.
90. Krauz C, Forti G. Clinical aspects of male infertility. In: McElreavey K (Ed). The genetic basis of male infertility. Berlin: Springer-Verlag; 2000. pp. 1-21.
91. Skaletsky H, Kuroda-Kawaguchi T, Minx PJ, et al. The male-specific region of the human Y-chromosome is a mosaic of discrete sequence classes. Nature. 2003;423:825-37.
92. Vogt PH. Azoospermia factor (AZF) in Yq11: towards a molecular understanding of its function for human male fertility and spermatogenesis. Reprod Biomed Online. 2005;10:81-93.

93. Ferlin A, Raicu F, Gatta V, et al. Male infertility: role of genetic background. Reprod Biomed Online. 2007;14:734-45.
94. Nuti F, Krausz C. Gene polymorphisms/mutations relevant to abnormal spermatogenesis. Reprod Biomed Online. 2008;16:504-13.
95. Lardone MC, Parodi DA, Ebensperger M, et al. AZFc partial deletions in Chilean men with severe spermatogenic failure. Fertil Steril. 2007;88:1318-26.
96. Tyler-Smith C. An evolutionary perspective on Y-chromosomal variation and male infertility. Int J Androl. 2008;31:376-82.
97. Galan JJ, Guarducci E, Nuti F, et al. Molecular analysis of estrogen receptor alpha gene AGATA haplotype and SNP12 in European populations: potential protective effect for cryptorchidism and lack of association with male infertility. Hum Reprod. 2007;22:444-9.
98. Brown GM, Furlog RA, Sargent CA, et al. Deletion of the DFFRY gene in patients with the AZFa genotype and of the murine homologue (Dffry) in XO Sxrb mice correlated with an early failure of spermatogenesis and infertility. Hum Mol Genet. 1998;7:97-107.
99. Elliott DJ. The role of potential splicing factors including RBMY, RBMX, hnRNPG-T and STAR proteins in spermatogenesis. Int J Androl. 2004;27:328-34.
99a. Lavery R, Glennon M, Houghton J, et al. Investigation of DAZ and RBMY1 gene expression in human testis by quantitative real-time PCR. Arch Androl. 2007;53:71-3.
100. Ferlin A, Moro E, Rossi A, et al. The human Y-chromosome's azoospermia factor b (AZFb) region: sequence, structure, and deletion analysis in infertile men. J Med Genet. 2003;40:18-24.
101. Vogt PH. Human chromosome deletions in Yq11, AZF candidate genes and male infertility: history and update. Mol Hum Reprod. 1998;4:739-44.
102. Kuroda-Kawaguchi T, Skaletsky H, Brown LG, et al. The AZFc region of the Y-chromosome features massive palindromes and uniform recurrent deletions in infertile men. Nat Genet. 2001;29:279-86.
103. Georgiou I, Syrrou M, Pardalidis N, et al. Genetic and epigenetic risks of intracytoplasmic sperm injection method. Asian J Androl. 2006;8:643-73.
104. Siffroi JP, Le Bourhis C, Krausz C, et al. Sex chromosome mosaicism in males carrying Y-chromosome long arm deletions. Hum Reprod. 2000;15:2559-62.
105. Patsalis PC, Sismani C, Quintana-Murci L, et al. Effects of transmission of Y-chromosome AZFc deletions. Lancet. 2002;360:1222-4.
106. Ferlin A, Moro E, Rossi A, et al. The human Y-chromosome's azoospermia factor b (AZFb) region: sequence, structure, and deletion analysis in infertile men. J Med Genet. 2003;40: 18-24.
107. Bateson P, Barker D, Clutton-Brock T, et al. Developmental plasticity and human health. Nature. 2004;430:419-21.
108. Zhang F, Lu C, Li Z, et al. Partial deletions are associated with an increased risk of complete deletion in AZFc: a new insight into the role of partial AZFc deletions in male infertility. J Med Genet. 2007;44:437-44.
109. Lin YW, Hsu LC, Kuo PL, et al. Partial duplication at AZFc on the Y-chromosome is a risk factor for impaired spermatogenesis in Han Chinese in Taiwan. Hum Mutat. 2007;28:486-94.
110. Ferlin A, Moro E, Garolla A, et al. Human male infertility and Y chromosome deletions: role of the AZF-candidate genes DAZ, RBM and DFFRY. Hum Reprod. 1999;14:1710-6.
111. Yen HW, Jakimiuk AJ, Munir I, et al. Selective alterations in insulin receptor substrates-1, -2 and -4 in theca but not granulosa cells from polycystic ovaries. Mol Hum Reprod. 2004;10:473-9.
112. Reijo R, Lee TY, Salo P, et al. Diverse spermatogenic defects in humans caused by Y-chromosome deletions encompassing a novel RNA-binding protein gene. Nat Genet. 1995;10:383-93.
113. Writzl K, Zorn B, Peterlin B. Copy number of DAZ genes in infertile men. Fertil Steril. 2005;84:1522-5.
114. Cram DS, Ma K, Bhasin S, et al. Y-chromosome analysis of infertile men and their sons conceived through intracytoplasmic sperm injection: vertical transmission of deletions and rarity of de novo deletions. Fertil Steril. 2000;74:909-15.
115. Sadeghi-Nejad H, Farrokhi F. Genetics of azoospermia: current knowledge, clinical implications, and future directions. Part II. Y-chromosome microdeletions. Urol J. 2007;4:192-206.
116. Schnieders F, Dörk T, Arnemann J, et al. Testis-specific protein, Y-encoded (TSPY) expression in testicular tissues. Hum Mol Genet. 1996;5:1801-7.
117. Vodicka R, Vrtel R, Dusek L, et al. TSPY gene copy number as a potential new risk factor for male infertility. Reprod Biomed Online. 2007;14:579-87.
118. Vogt PH, Affara N, Davey P, et al. Report of the third international workshop on Y chromosome mapping 1997. Heidelberg, Germany, April 13-16, 1997. Cytogenet Cell Genet. 1997;79:1-20.
119a. Simoni M, Bakeker E, Eurling MC, et al. Laboratory guidelines for molecular diagnosis of Y chromosomal microdeletions. Int J Androl. 1999;22:292-9.
119b. Simoni M, Gromoll J, Hoppner W, et al. Mutational analysis of the follicle-stimulating hormone (FSH) receptor in normal and infertile men: identification and characterization of two discrete FSH receptor isoforms. J Clin Endocrinol Metab. 1999;84:751-5.
120. Kupferminc MJ, Eldor A, Steinman N, et al. Increased frequency of genetic thrombophilia in women with complications of pregnancy. N Engl J Med. 1999;340:50-2.
121. Sanson BJ, Simioni P, Tormene D, et al. The incidence of venous thromboembolism in asymptomatic carriers of a deficiency of antithrombin, protein C, or protein S: a prospective cohort study. Blood. 1999;94:3702-6.
122. Kupferminc MJ. Thrombophilia and pregnancy. Reprod Biol Endocrinol. 2003;1:111.
123. Rey E, Kahn SR, David M, et al. Thrombophilic disorders and fetal loss: a meta-analysis. Lancet. 2003;361:901-8.
124. Griffin JH, Evatt B, Wideman C, et al. Anticoagulant protein C pathway defective in majority of thrombophilic patients. Blood. 1993;82:1989-93.
125. Koster T, Rosendaal FR, de Ronde H, et al. Venous thrombosis due to poor anticoagulant response to activated protein C: Leiden Thrombophilia Study. Lancet. 1993;342:1503-6.

126. Ridker PM, Hennekens CH, Selhub J, et al. Interrelation of hyperhomocyst(e)inemia, factor V Leiden, and risk of future venous thromboembolism. Circulation. 1997;95:1777-82.
127. Cattaneo M, Tsai MY, Bucciarelli P, et al. A common mutation in the methylenetetrahydrofolate reductase gene (C677T) increases the risk for deep-vein thrombosis in patients with mutant factor V (factor V: Q506). Arterioscler Thromb Vasc Biol. 1997;17:1662-6.
128. Eldibany MM, Caprini JA. Hyperhomocysteinemia and thrombosis: an overview. Arch Pathol Lab Med. 2007;131:872-84.
129. Gehring NH, Frede U, Neu-Yilik G, et al. Increased efficiency of mRNA 3′ end formation: a new genetic mechanism contributing to hereditary thrombophilia. Nat Genet. 2001;28:389-92.
130. Poort SR, Rosendaal FR, Reitsma PH, et al. A common genetic variation in the 3′-untranslated region of the prothrombin gene is associated with elevated plasma prothrombin levels and an increase in venous thrombosis. Blood. 1996;88:3698-703.
131. Rosendaal FR, Doggen CJ, Zivelin A, et al. Geographic distribution of the 20210 G to A prothrombin variant. Thromb Haemost. 1998;79:706-8.
132. Bosler D, Mattson J, Crisan D. Phenotypic heterogeneity in patients with homozygous prothrombin 20210AA genotype. J Mol Diagn. 2006;4:420-5.
133. Hanson NQ, Aras O, Yang F, et al. C677T and A1298C polymorphisms of the methylenetetrahydrofolate reductase gene: incidence and effect of combined genotypes on plasma fasting and post-methionine load homocysteine in vascular disease. Clin Chem. 2001;47:661-6.
134. Van der Put NM, Gabreëls F, Stevens EM, et al. A second common mutation in the methylenetetrahydrofolate reductase gene: an additional risk factor for neural-tube defects? Am J Hum Genet. 1998;62(5):1044-51.
135. Nelen WL, Blom HJ, Steegers EA, et al. Hyperhomocysteinemia and recurrent early pregnancy loss: a meta-analysis. Fertil Steril. 2000;74:1196-9.
136. Van der Molen EF, Arends GE, Nelen WL, et al. A common mutation in the 5,10-methylenetetrahydrofolate reductase gene as a new risk factor for placental vasculopathy. Am J Obstet Gynecol. 2000;182:1258-63.
137. Goodman CS, Coulam CB, Jeyendran RS, et al. Which thrombophilic gene mutations are risk factors for recurrent pregnancy loss? Am J Reprod Immunol. 2006;56:230-6.
138. Subrt I, Ulvova-Gallova Z, Bibkova K, et al. Recurrent pregnancy loss and frequency of eight antiphospholipid antibodies and genetic thrombophilic factors in Czech women. Am J Reprod Immunol. 2008;59:193-200.
139. Foka ZJ, Lambropoulos AF, Saravelos H, et al. Factor V Leiden and prothrombin G20210A mutations, but not methylenetetrahydrofolate reductase C677T, are associated with recurrent miscarriages. Hum Reprod. 2000;15:458-62.
140. Coulam CB, Jeyendran RS, Fishel LA, et al. Multiple thrombophilic gene mutations rather than specific gene mutations are risk factors for recurrent miscarriage. Am J Reprod Immunol. 2006;55:360-8.
141. Tranquilli AL, Giannubilo SR, Dell'Uomo B, et al. Adverse pregnancy outcomes are associated with multiple maternal thrombophilic factors. Eur J Obstet Gynecol Reprod Biol. 2004;117:144-7.
142. Lussana F, Dentali F, Abbate R, et al. Screening for thrombophilia and antithrombotic prophylaxis in pregnancy: guidelines of the Italian Society for Haemostasis and Thrombosis (SISET). Thromb Res. 2009;124:e19-25.
143. McGlennen RC, Key NS. Clinical and laboratory management of the prothrombin G20210A mutation. Arch Pathol Lab Med. 2002;126:1319-25.
144. Press RD, Bauer KA, Kujovich JL, et al. Clinical utility of factor V Leiden (R506Q) testing for the diagnosis and management of thromboembolic disorders. Arch Pathol Lab Med. 2002;126(11):1304-18.
145. Seligsohn U, Lubetsky A. Genetic susceptibility to venous thrombosis. N Engl J Med. 2001;344:1222-31.
146. Florell SR, Rodgers GM. Utilization of testing for activated protein C resistance in a reference laboratory. Am J Clin Pathol. 1996;106:248-52.
147. Verlinsky Y, Pergament E, Strom C. The preimplantation genetic diagnosis of genetic diseases. J In Vitro Fert Embryo Transf. 1990;7(1):1-5.
148. Colls P, Escudero T, Cekleniak N, et al. Increased efficiency of preimplantation genetic diagnosis for infertility using "no result rescue." Fertil Steril. 2007;88(1):53-61.
149. Mir P, Rodrigo L, Mateu E, et al. Improving FISH diagnosis for preimplantation genetic aneuploidy screening. Hum Reprod. 2010;25:1812-7.
150. Mastenbroek S, Twisk M, van Echten-Arends J, et al. In vitro fertilization with preimplantation genetic screening. N Engl J Med. 2007; 357(1):9-17.
151. Mastenbroek S, Twisk M, van der Veen F, et al. Preimplantation genetic screening: a systematic review and meta-analysis of RCTs. Hum Reprod Update. 2011; 17(4):454-66.
152. Rubio C, Rodrigo L, Mir P, et al. Use of array comparative genomic hybridization (array-CGH) for embryo assessment: clinical results. Fertil Steril. 2013;99:1044-8.
153. Wells D, Alfarawati S, Fragouli E. Use of comprehensive chromosomal screening for embryo assessment: microarrays and CGH. Mol Hum Reprod. 2008;14(12):703-10.
154. Yang Z, Liu J, Collins GS, et al. Selection of single blastocysts for fresh transfer via standard morphology assessment alone and with array CGH for good prognosis IVF patients: results from a randomized pilot study. Mol Cytogenet. 2012;5(1):24.
155. Forman EJ, Li X, Ferry KM, et al. Oocyte vitrification does not increase the risk of embryonic aneuploidy or diminish the implantation potential of blastocysts created after intracytoplasmic sperm injection: a novel, paired randomized controlled trial using DNA fingerprinting. Fertil Steril. 2012;98:644-9.
156. Scott RT Jr, Upham KM, Forman EJ, et al. Blastocyst biopsy with comprehensive chromosome screening and fresh embryo transfer significantly increases in vitro fertilization implantation and delivery rates: a randomized controlled trial. Fertil Steril. 2013;100(3): 697-703.
157. Vera-Rodriguez M, Rubio C. Assessing the true incidence of mosaicism in preimplantation embryos. Fertil Steril. 2017;107(5):1107-12.
158. Capalbo A, Wright G, Elliott T, et al. FISH reanalysis of inner cell mass and trophectoderm samples of previously

array-CGH screened blastocysts shows high accuracy of diagnosis and no major diagnostic impact of mosaicism at the blastocyst stage. Hum Reprod. 2013;28:2298-307.
159. Maxwell SM, Colls P, Hodes-Wertz B, et al. Why do euploid embryos miscarry? A case-control study comparing the rate of aneuploidy within presumed euploid embryos that resulted in miscarriage or live birth using next-generation sequencing. Fertil Steril. 2016;106(6):1414-9.e5.
160. Goodrich D, Tao X, Bohrer C, et al. A randomized and blinded comparison of qPCR and NGS-based detection of aneuploidy in a cell line mixture model of blastocyst biopsy mosaicism. J Assist Reprod Genet. 2016;33:1473-80.
161. Ruttanajit T, Chanchamroen S, Cram DS, et al. Detection and quantitation of chromosomal mosaicism in human blastocysts using copy number variation sequencing. Prenat Diagn. 2016;36:154-62.
162. Johnson DS, Cinnioglu C, Ross R, et al. Comprehensive analysis of karyotypic mosaicism between trophectoderm and inner cell mass. Mol Hum Reprod. 2010;16:944-9.
163. Handyside AH. 24-Chromosome copy number analysis: a comparison of available technologies. Fertil Steril. 2013;100:595-602.
164. Gardner DK, Meseguer M, Rubio C, et al. Diagnosis of human preimplantation embryo viability. Hum Reprod Update. 2015;21(6):727-47.
165. Yin X, Tan K, Vajta G, et al. Massively parallel sequencing for chromosomal abnormality testing in trophectoderm cells of human blastocysts. Biol Reprod. 2013;88(3):69.
166. Fiorentino F, Bono S, Biricik A, et al. Application of next-generation sequencing technology for comprehensive aneuploidy screening of blastocysts in clinical preimplantation genetic screening cycles. Hum Reprod. 2014;29(12):2802-13.
167. Fiorentino F, Biricik A, Bono S, et al. Development and validation of a next-generation sequencing-based protocol for 24-chromosome aneuploidy screening of embryos. Fertil Steril. 2014;101(5):1375-82.
168. Hassold T, Chen N, Funkhouser J, et al. A cytogenetic study of 1000 spontaneous abortions. Ann Hum Genet. 1980;44(Pt 2):151-78.
169. Lamb NE, Freeman SB, Savage-Austin A, et al. Susceptible chiasmate configurations of chromosome 21 predispose to non-disjunction in both maternal meiosis I and meiosis II. Nat Genet. 1996;14(4):400-5.
170. Munne S, Sandalinas M, Escudero T, et al. Improved implantation after preimplantation genetic diagnosis of aneuploidy. Reprod Biomed Online. 2003;7(1):91-7.
171. Rubio C, Rodrigo L, Perez-Cano I, et al. FISH screening of aneuploidies in preimplantation embryos to improve IVF outcome. Reprod Biomed Online. 2005;11(4):497-506.
172. Milán M, Cobo AC, Rodrigo L, et al. Redefining advanced maternal age as an indication for preimplantation genetic screening. Reprod Biomed Online. 2010;21(5):649-57.
173. Rubio C, Bellver J, Rodrigo L, et al. In vitro fertilization with preimplantation genetic diagnosis for aneuploidies in advanced maternal age: a randomized, controlled study. Fertil Steril. 2017;107(5):1122-9.
174. Garrisi JG, Colls P, Ferry KM, et al. Effect of infertility, maternal age, and number of previous miscarriages on the outcome of preimplantation genetic diagnosis for idiopathic recurrent pregnancy loss. Fertil Steril. 2009;92:288-95.
175. Mir P, Al-Asmar N, Rodrigo L, et al. Debate: should preimplantation genetic screening be performed in recurrent pregnancy loss? Yes. In: Carp H(Ed). Recurrent pregnancy loss: causes, controversies, and treatment, 2nd edition. 2015. ISBN 9781482216141.
176. Hodes-Wertz B, Grio J, Ghadir S, et al. Idiopathic recurrent miscarriage is caused mostly by aneuploid embryos. Fertil Steril. 2012;98:675-80.
177. Shahine L, Lathi R. Recurrent pregnancy loss: evaluation and treatment. Obstet Gynecol Clin North Am. 2015;42(1):117-34.
178. Pehlivan T, Rubio C, Rodrigo L, et al. Impact of preimplantation genetic diagnosis on IVF outcome in implantation failure patients. Reprod Biomed Online. 2003;6(2):232-7.
179. Caglar GS, Asimakopoulos B, Nikolettos N, et al. Preimplantation genetic diagnosis for aneuploidy screening in repeated implantation failure. Reprod Biomed Online. 2005;10(3):381-8.
180. Greco E, Bono S, Ruberti A, et al. Comparative genomic hybridization selection of blastocysts for repeated implantation failure treatment: a pilot study. BioMed Res Int. 2014;2014:457913.
181. Gianaroli L, Magli MC, Ferraretti AP, et al. Preimplantation diagnosis after assisted reproduction techniques for genetically-determined male infertility. J Endocrinol Invest. 2000;23(10):711-6.
182. Rodrigo L, Rubio C, Mateu E, et al. Analysis of chromosomal abnormalities in testicular and epididymal spermatozoa from azoospermic ICSI patients by fluorescence in-situ hybridization. Hum Reprod. 2004;19(1):118-23.
183. Silber S, Escudero T, Lenahan K, et al. Chromosomal abnormalities in embryos derived from testicular sperm extraction. Fertil Steril. 2003;79(1):30-8.
184. Rubio C, Gil-Salom M, Simon C, et al. Incidence of sperm chromosomal abnormalities in a risk population: relationship with sperm quality and ICSI outcome. Hum Reprod. 2001;16(10):2084-92.
185. Cinar C, Yazici C, Ergunsu S, et al. Genetic diagnosis in infertile men with numerical and constitutional sperm abnormalities. Genet Test. 2008;12(2):195-202.
186. Kahraman S, Sertyel S, Findikli N, et al. Effect of PGD on implantation and ongoing pregnancy rates in cases with predominantly macrocephalic spermatozoa. Reprod Biomed Online. 2004;9(1):79-85.
187. Mateu E, Rodrigo L, Prados N, et al. High incidence of chromosomal abnormalities in large-headed and multiple-tailed spermatozoa. J Androl. 2006;27(1):6-10.
188. Rodrigo L, Peinado V, Mateu E, et al. Diploid and sex chromosome aneuploid sperm: do they behave similarly in preimplantation embryos? Fertil Steril. 2010;94(4):1380-6.
189. Rubio C, Castillón G, Rodrigo L, et al. Improvement of clinical outcome in severe male factor infertility with embryo selection based on array-CGH: a randomized controlled trial. Fertil Steril. 2014;102(Suppl 3):e24-5.
190. Kotdawala A, Patel D, Herrero J, et al. Aneuploidy screening by array comparative genomic hybridization improves success rates of in vitro fertilization: a multicenter Indian study. J Hum Reprod Sci. 2016;9(4):223-9.

191. Coates A, Hesla JS, Hurliman A, et al. Use of suboptimal sperm increases the risk of aneuploidy of the sex chromosomes in preimplantation blastocyst embryos. Fertil Steril. 2015;104:866-72.
192. Nazareth SB, Lazarin GA, Goldberg JD. Changing trends in carrier screening for genetic disease in the United States. Prenat Diagn. 2015;35(10):931-5.
193. Verlinsky Y, Cohen J, Munne S, et al. Over a decade of experience with preimplantation genetic diagnosis: a multicenter report. Fertil Steril. 2004;82(2):292-4.
194. De Rycke M, Belva F, Goossens V, et al. ESHRE PGD Consortium data collection XIII: cycles from January to December 2010 with pregnancy follow-up to October 2011. Hum Reprod. 2015;30(8):1763-89.
195. Rechitsky S, Pomerantseva E, Pakhalchuk T, et al. First systematic experience of preimplantation genetic diagnosis for de-novo mutations. Reprod Biomed Online. 2011;22(4):350-61.
196. Goldman KN, Nazem T, Berkeley A, et al. Preimplantation genetic diagnosis (PGD) for monogenic disorders: the value of concurrent aneuploidy screening. J Genet Couns. 2016;25(6):1327-37.
197. Minasi MG, Fiorentino F, Ruberti A, et al. Genetic diseases and aneuploidies can be detected with a single blastocyst biopsy: a successful clinical approach. Hum Reprod. 2017;32(8):1770-7.
198. Labonte ML. An analysis of US fertility centre educational materials suggests that informed consent for preimplantation genetic diagnosis may be inadequate. J Med Ethics. 2012;38(8):479-84.
199. Palini S, Galluzzi L, De Stefani S, et al. Genomic DNA in human blastocoele fluid. Reprod Biomed Online. 2013;26(6):603-10.
200. Wu H, Ding C, Shen X, et al. Medium-based noninvasive preimplantation genetic diagnosis for human α-thalassemias-SEA. Medicine. 2015;94(12):e669.
201. Shamonki MI, Jin H, Haimowitz Z, et al. Proof of concept: preimplantation genetic screening without embryo biopsy through analysis of cell-free DNA in spent embryo culture media. Fertil Steril. 2016;106:1312-8.
202. Xu J, Fang R, Chen L, et al. Noninvasive chromosome screening of human embryos by genome sequencing of embryo culture medium for in vitro fertilization. Proc Natl Acad Sci USA. 2016;113:11907-12.
203. Li P, Song Z, Yao Y, et al. Preimplantation genetic screening with spent culture medium/blastocoel fluid for in vitro fertilization. Sci Rep. 2018;8(1):9275.
204. Liu W, Liu J, Du H, et al. Non-invasive pre-implantation aneuploidy screening and diagnosis of beta thalassemia IVSII654 mutation using spent embryo culture medium. Ann Med. 2017;49(4):319-28.
205. Ho JR, Arrach N, Rhodes-Long K, et al. Pushing the limits of detection: investigation of cell-free DNA for aneuploidy screening in embryos. Fertil Steril. 2018;110(3):467-75.e2.
206. Vera-Rodriguez M, Diez-Juan A, Jimenez-Almazan J, et al. Origin and composition of cell-free DNA in spent medium from human embryo culture during preimplantation development. Hum Reprod. 2018;33:745-56.

CHAPTER

84

Troubleshooting in the In Vitro Fertilization Laboratory

Nicolás Prados

TROUBLESHOOTING IN AN IN VITRO FERTILIZATION PROGRAM

The in vitro fertilization (IVF) laboratory is one of the main parts of an assisted reproduction center. An IVF program is a complex and multidisciplinary activity where professionals from different fields come together to try to help an infertile couple.

The IVF program does not offer a product but a medical service. The patients want a healthy baby at home. As pregnancy is not guaranteed, in some cases the treatment fails in spite of the couple's emotional and financial investment. Although this may seem at first to make more difficult, the application of the traditional industrial and engineering concepts of quality to IVF, these concepts are equally applicable. More so, they are fundamental for achieving a successful and stable IVF program.[1-4]

Another aspect to take into account is the complexity of an IVF treatment. Many procedures are not completely standardized between different laboratories and depend on manual work. Furthermore, the treatment is irreversible, and we cannot undo a failed treatment. If one of the many steps in an IVF treatment is suboptimal and it has affected the quality of the gametes or the embryos, there is nothing we can do to improve this quality. This is another factor why we need a strong quality management program in an IVF center. In a manufacturing center, not everything affects the product. A worker who is taking longer to screw part of a product may cause delays, but it is not affecting the quality of the final product. An embryologist who is taking longer in scoring embryos may cause delays, but more importantly will affect the quality of the embryos and the increase the probability of failure of the cycle.

There is another destabilizing factor in an IVF program that we cannot avoid. The main factor that affects the treatment result is the patient characteristics. Age, male and female characteristics, their genomes, diets, body mass index, or their response to the medication among other factors are going to affect the quality of gametes and the embryos we get from them. This variability makes even more difficult from the IVF indicators analysis.

The quality management program of an IVF program tries to answer some simple questions in an organized and registered way:[3]

- Are the patients getting their babies? [quality control (QC)]
- Are we working properly? [quality assurance (QA)]
- Can we improve? (risk management)
- What has gone wrong? (troubleshooting)
- Are we good enough? (benchmarking).

This is a very rough sketch of the different parts of a quality management program that highlights to sides of the same coin. Corrective actions to solve problems we find (troubleshooting) and preventive actions to avoid possible problems (risk management). There is no perfect organization. Accidents, mistakes, and wear happen. One of the objectives in quality management is to avoid risks and minimize their effects. It may seem a paradox that the more efficient the quality program is, more valuable is an error. Errors and noncompliances are one source of the sources for continuous improvement in the real world.

Troubleshooting can be frustrating in IVF as we do not have always all the indicators (or robust enough indicators) to point us the origin of the problem.

There are different flowcharts available for troubleshooting, but they basically have six parts:[3]

1. Problem activation
2. Data collection
3. Problem definition
4. Roots identification
5. Prioritization of corrective actions
6. Corrective actions execution
7. Outcome monitorization.

Problem Activation and Monitoring Key Performance Indicators

We start a troubleshooting process after a standard operating procedure (SOP) noncompliance, an accident, a negligence, or an indicator alarm. The objective is to avoid further repetition of these events that may impair the quality of our service (lower pregnancy rates, higher costs, or patient's discontent).

We cannot follow-up on all the possible indicators of an IVF program. Hence we focus on those areas which reflect most on our results and procedures, usually our QC indicators. Once we select these key performance indicators (KPIs), we must select a threshold or an algorithm that triggers an alarm. Some basic statistics must be applied.[5] First, most indicators are proportions whose descriptive statistics are easy to understand and apply. In second place, these alarms are diagnostic binary tests. As such, parameters as sensitivity and specificity of the alarms are of relevance. These relate to the frequency of fall positives and negatives for our KPI.

Data Collection and Problem Definition

If we have an accident (incubator not working, accident with a petri dish), we must gather more information (frequency of the event, details of the event, and effect on the procedure of the patient, etc. If we have an alarm in monitoring KPI, we may have enough data for a confirmation analysis. But this is not always the case. We must be sure that a problem is really happening as making unfounded corrective actions after false-positive alarms will just increase the instability of the program. Changes in the SOPs are introduced that will make us believe that they are true improvements. The two main factors that trigger these false alarms with KPIs are—(1) low numbers and (2) patient variability.

When we get a KPI for a period of time, there is a level of uncertainty with it.[5] We do not use directly the value of the indicator but its interval of confidence (IC). If the IC does not overlap to our alarm value, we have a true alarm. The range of the IC is inversely proportional to the number of cases (retrievals, transfers, and transferred embryos, etc.), we are using calculate it. We must also arbitrary establish an alpha error. This value is usually 90%, 95%, or 99%. In IVF programs, it is usually fixed in 95% although in the industry, it is fixed in 99%. This is a compromise between false-positive and negative alarms due to the low number we usually manage in the programs.

We can have a statistically significant alarm due to patient variability. We may have during a period of time a higher number of older patients or low responders, any other bad prognosis characteristic or a combination of them. If this change is not detected and we act modifying our SOPs, again we get misled by the apparent improvement of the KPI when the characteristics of the patients become stable.

We can also face an ineffective positive troubleshooting where we try to find the reasons for an exceptional significant KPI which has been really caused by chance or a change in the prognosis of the group of patients affected.

So, to confirm our problem we must make sure that the problem is real. We can look for trends or wait for confirmation. In both cases, we are increasing the numbers of the analysis. There are different tools to detect these variations with six-sigma analysis on Shewhart graphs or mobile averages with cumulative sum control chart or exponentially weighted moving average (EWMA) graphs.[5,6] To avoid the variation in patients' characteristics, we can make control analysis groups (e.g. patients with good prognosis or patients with at least eight oocytes).

Once we are dealing with what we think is a true alarm, we must gather all the data that may be related to the initial problem. We are trying to locate and outline the exact problem. We gather the data through different indicators. We can classify the indicators as:

- *Program indicators or QC indicators*: They measure the results of the program: pregnancies, multiple pregnancies, or live births. They are usually KPIs of the program. These indicators tell us if the IVF program is achieving our standards but if they fail, they do not specify at all where the problem is[4]
- *Laboratory indicators (QC/QA)*: They are general indicators related to the global efficiency of an area of the program. Laboratory indicators are related to embryo scoring or embryo quality, multinuclearity, cleavage rate, blastocyst rate, or transfer cancellation rate. They may point to an issue in the laboratory, but they do not clarify which laboratory process is faulty. Some of them can be used as the QC indicators of the department. Implantation rate is a proxy pregnancy rate designed to normalize the number of embryos transferred. We can consider it a program indicator not a laboratory indicator. Clinical, administrative, or

nursing indicators should also be managed in the quality management program. Clinical indicators should include patient characteristics to check variations in their profile

- *Process indicators (QA)*: These are more interesting during troubleshooting. They are affected only by the performance of a SOP and can single out problems specific to it. Unfortunately, they are the most difficult to define per SOP. Process indicators are sperm mobility after capacitation, post-intracytoplasmic sperm injection (ICSI) degeneration rate, or survival rates after embryo warming.
- *Performance indicators (QA)*: These indicators are the backbone of a good quality management program. They include the control of equipment parameters (temperature, CO_2, and pH, etc.), compliance with maintenance of the equipment and traceability of embryologists, patients, and batches of consumables among many others
- *Efficiency indicators (QA)*: These indicators are related to nontechnical issues of the procedures. They include, for example, number of procedures per embryologist, time from retrieval to ICSI, time per oocyte during ICSI, consumable cost per cycle, number of nonused dishes discarded per procedure, and QC indicators per procedure performed by a specific embryologist or doctor.

The two first types of indicators help us to trigger a troubleshooting analysis. The last three points help us to define what is exactly the problem. If, e.g. our pregnancy rate per retrieval has lowered, we must start gathering information. First to check if it is a laboratory or a clinical issue. Maybe embryo quality is worse or may be the stimulation cancellation rate has changed.

Then we start zooming into specific areas to see if we can narrow the problem. This is where procedure, performance, and efficiency indicators are helpful. Maybe we have junior staff that has not been properly trained doing ICSI or transfers. Maybe time to ICSI is shortening or taking to long. Only if we have the possibility to access all these indicators we may detect where the problem is localized. For this, a comprehensive database is needed in order to not become overwhelmed with the amount of information to transcript.

Ideally, the initial trigger (lower pregnancies rate per retrieval) can be defined in a specific problem (junior embryologists need more training in vitrification). As an IVF program has a high number of steps, many times we do not find the exact problem. This is where a strong QA program is helpful. If all the procedures, performance, and efficiency indicators are correct, caution is demanded in case we are dealing with a false alarm.

Roots Identification and Prioritization of Corrective Actions

Once we have identified a specific problem (e.g. it is associated with a change in media manufacturer), we must make an exercise of examining every detail related and decide whether it is relevant. This is a very important exercise, very similar to risk management and requires checking not only the compliance of the procedures but the reason why every step is performed in order to detect deviations in a specific accident or a period of time with a low KPI. In our example, it would be a mistake to just change back to the previous media. We may detect media handling problems, incubator CO_2 or pH mismanagement, and patient allocations to incubators or refrigerator issues that may have been concealed while using the previous media. If this is not corrected, even with the first media, the problem will rise at some point when it gets worse.

After this identification, we will end with a list of possible causes for the problem. We must prioritize them depending on the impact we assume and their feasibility. If we suspect that we have a problem because we are using an old domestic refrigerator to keep our media and it may be freezing our media, our first solution would be to buy a new professional refrigerator with forced-air cooling. But maybe we cannot acquire it right away. We can make previously a temperature mapping of the actual refrigerator and localize the areas where no freezing occurs.

Corrective Actions Execution and Outcome Monitorization

Sometimes, the correction is self-evident (a masked faulty equipment). Other times, we develop a hypothesis to explain the problem. In this case, we are not correcting the problem as much as testing this hypothesis. We must make a small test or retrospectively check the evolution of the indicator. If the problem is not corrected, we must ask ourselves if the change should be applied in our SOPs.

If our outcome returns to its normal values, we can close our troubleshooting analysis. If not, other corrective actions should be taken into account.

TROUBLESHOOTING VERSUS RISK ASSESSMENT: TWO SIDES OF THE MIRROR

Troubleshooting is a reactive procedure (*a posteriori*). We can describe risk assessment as a hypothetical troubleshooting. It is a preventive tool (*a priori*). We can assess the SOP of a procedure and ask ourselves in detail what could go wrong. We start a very similar analysis where we measure the probability of occurrence and the impact of the different issues and we make a root analysis of its causes. This way, we adapt and make improvements on our SOPs. The sum of all these minor changes will impact positively in our outcomes.

A particular way of doing risk assessment is checking the performance and efficiency indicators of a particular process. The more time we focus on these indicators, the easiest is the troubleshooting. This micro-troubleshooting becomes a way to prevent or lower the impact of accidents or deviations on our main KPIs. If we have a faulty incubator that does not regulate correctly the CO_2 and we wait for our pregnancy rates to lower before checking with a calibrated CO_2 meter of the incubator or the (pH of the media), it may take weeks to react since the start of the problem. Daily CO_2 checks or weekly pH checks can limit the number of affected patients in a way that it does not affect our QC KPIs.

Risk management is a friendlier and more useful tool than troubleshooting. Troubleshooting is a forensic QC where we must be a detective trying to find a culprit. In risk management, we are monitoring the process and preventing the effects of deviations.

MAIN AREAS OF TROUBLESHOOTING IN THE IVF LABORATORY

We can define an IVF laboratory in many ways. It is a cell culture-transplant-auxiliary laboratory. Gamete and embryos are processed, cultured, manipulated, generated, stored, and transferred to patients. This chapter cannot but summarize briefly some of the aspects to review when troubleshooting problem in the laboratory. The monography by Kay Elder and collaborators reviews with more detail of all these issues.[7]

There are four parameters that affect the culture of embryos:

1. Asepsis
2. Temperature
3. CO_2 and pH
4. Defined environment (osmolarity and toxic components).

There are three levels of encompassing areas in the laboratory regarding these parameters:

1. *Embryo culture (the incubator)*: Most of the time, the embryos are cultured inside the incubator. This is the main piece of equipment in the laboratory and their design and number must be correctly decided.
   Microorganisms contamination is easily detected and analyzed. Contamination is related to poor aseptic techniques in the manipulation of the samples or the sterile media and consumables, defective cabinets, or manufacturer issues.

The temperature and pH of the environment of the gametes and embryos are provided by the media and the incubators. Temperature is a physical parameter efficiently controlled by most equipment. The pH of the media is reached with a bicarbonate/CO_2 buffer where the incubator controls the %CO_2 in the chamber with the injection of 100% CO_2 or a premixed gas. Some issues we may detect:

- *Too many openings of the incubator door*: Absence of working incubators or too few incubators may cause to have more than one patient per incubator chamber
- Faulty equipment (of the incubator or the calibrating meters we use)
- *Problems with CO_2 supply to the incubators:* In the case of pH, adjustment of the level of CO_2 with the media or the altitude of the laboratory.
- Dishes not equilibrate for enough time.

Embryos are cultured in a defined media. Though different manufacturers have their own proprietary formulations, they are all quite similar with an osmolarity between 260 and 290 mOsm/L. It is very rare to lower this level. On the contrary, it is extremely easy to increase the level. Over 300 mOsm/L, embryos may start to impair. Some reasons to this increase could be:

- Use of dry incubators (no humidity) and no oil overlay. Even if the droplets of media are covered, evaporation is present
- Improper preparation of culture dishes when the media is exposed too long to ambient air without being covered
- Improper handling of the media bottles.

The composition of the media can also be altered if the bottles are frozen causing precipitations or changes in the protein and amino acids concentration.

Also related to the chemical environment that affects the embryo is the presence of volatile organic compounds (VOCs). These can be present in the media from many different sources as for example:

- Nonoutgassed plasticware
- Quality of the gas cylinders that provide the CO_2 and the N_2 to the incubators (or the premixed gas). If the supplier is not reliable or the quality of the available gas is not sufficient, VOC filters should be attached to the gas inlet.

2. *Embryo manipulation*: At some points, gametes and embryos are manipulated outside the incubators. During this time, the parameters may change.
   - *Faulty equipment*: Heated surfaces and stages may be too hot or too cold
   - *Slow procedures*: The equipment is not designed to maintain the conditions the same as in an incubator. Too many oocytes during ICSI or junior embryologists may be taking too long
   - *Insufficient mineral oil*: A very thin overlay may not affect the osmolarity inside a humidified incubator but in the dry ambient of the laboratory, the media may evaporate
   - There are glass hoods or working incubators that can minimize the loss of the CO_2 dissolved in the media.

   Cryopreservation is a particular process in the laboratory with its own possible steps to analyze during troubleshooting. Not only the procedure must be reviewed, but also the storage in the cryobanks and the supply of the liquid nitrogen
3. *Laboratory environment*: Incubators and flow cabinets are used inside a space usually designed as a clean room where a team of embryologists work. Different issues in the laboratory can affect the embryo environment and impair their implantation potential.

Design and services: The design of the laboratory may be also a cause for problems in the laboratory.

- Construction elements may outgas VOCs
- Absence of generators and uninterruptible power supplies
- Poorly distribution of equipment may cause accidents or long movement of embryos around the laboratory
- Doors without windows and slippery floors also may cause accidents.

Air quality can affect the asepsis, the temperature, or the chemical environment of our embryos. Faulty filters and ducts can be a source of fungal spores. Stations under a strong air inlet may cool too quickly the ICSI dishes. Weak air conditioning units that cannot cool external high temperatures may make the laboratory reach 30°C which make most incubators stop heating. This also may happen when air conditioning is turned off when the laboratory work is finished. Embryologist can pollute the air with VOCs with their cosmetics or perfumes. If airlocks are not properly used and designed, VOCs form the clinic (air fresheners, cleaning products) that will enter the laboratory. Also, external contingencies (fire, street painting, and construction works) can also affect the air quality of the laboratory.

Staff: Their number and training of embryologists can affect the embryos. This is very relevant in organizations with no continuous training and review of results and techniques. Other staff must also be trained. Operating room staff may change temperature parameters of heating blocks and incubators. Unsupervised cleaning staff in the laboratory may alter or unplug equipment.

Organization and quality management: Closing the laboratory on weekends or suboptimal timing of the procedures because of nonscientific reasons can affect the outcomes. Poorly written, absent, or nonreviewed SOPs are also an important cause of alarms.

OTHER ASPECTS

An IVF laboratory is part of a medical process where we are transplanting embryos generated in the laboratory from previously obtained gametes. Traceability of the samples and the consumables are mandatory. Transferring embryos from another couple or using out of date drugs, media, or consumables are risks that should be proactively avoided and part of a rigorous risk management assessment. Troubleshooting is usually straightforward in these cases and always shows a poor-quality management program.

As an IVF quality program becomes improves with time correcting and improving the different procedures and processes, troubleshooting becomes a rarer event. There is always a risk of an accident or an equipment malfunction, but a strong risk assessment analysis and a preventive use of performance and efficiency indicators should minimize these events.

REFERENCES

1. Gardner DK, Reed L, Linck D, et al. Quality control in human in vitro fertilization. Semin Reprod Med. 2005;23(4):319-24.
2. Alper MM. Experience with ISO quality control in assisted reproductive technology. Fertil Steril. 2013;100(6):1503-8.
3. Mortimer ST, Mortimer D. Quality and Risk Management in the IVF Laboratory, 2nd edition. Cambridge: Cambridge University Press; 2015.
4. Carson BE, Alper MM, Keck C. Quality Management Systems for Assisted Reproductive Technology. New York: CRC Press; 2016.
5. Montgomery DC. Statistical Quality Control: A Modern Introduction, 7th edition. United States: John Wiley & Sons; 2012.
6. Dessolle L, Biau DJ, de Larouziere V, et al. Learning curve of vitrification assessed by cumulative summation test for learning curve (LC-CUSUM). Fertil Steril. 2009;92(3):943-5.
7. Elder K, Van den Bergh M, Woodward B. Troubleshooting and Problem-Solving in the IVF Laboratory. Cambridge: Cambridge University Press; 2015.

CHAPTER

85

Third-party Reproduction

Gautam Nand Allahbadia, Akanksha Allahbadia Gupta

SUMMARY

Third-party reproduction is any human reproduction in which DNA or gestation is provided by a third party or donor other than the one or two parents who will raise the resulting child. This goes beyond the traditional father–mother model, and the third party's involvement is limited to the reproductive process and does not extend into the raising of the child. Third-party reproduction is used by couples unable to reproduce where they would otherwise be unable to do so, by same-sex couples, and by men and women without a partner. Where donor gametes are provided by a donor, the donor will be a biological parent of the resulting child, but in third-party reproduction, he or she will not be the rearing parent. Third-party reproduction can be segregated into several categories, some of which may be combined:

- *Sperm donation*: A donor provides sperm in order to father a child for a third-party female
- *Oocyte donation*: A donor provides ova to a woman or couple in order for the egg to be fertilized and implanted in the recipient woman
- *Spindle transfer*: A third party's mitochondrial DNA is transferred to the future mother's ovum. This is used to prevent mitochondrial disease
- *Embryo donation*:
  - With embryos which were originally created for a genetic mother's assisted pregnancy. Once the genetic mother has completed her own treatment, she may donate unused embryos for use by a third party
  - Or where embryos are specifically created for donation using donor eggs and donor sperm
  - Embryo adoption: Embryos created during a donor's assisted pregnancy are adopted to be implanted in a third-party recipient.
- *Surrogacy*: An embryo is gestated in a third party's uterus (gestational surrogacy) or a woman is inseminated in order to gestate a child for a third party (traditional surrogacy).

INTRODUCTION

Pregnancy is typically initiated by artificial insemination in the case of sperm donation and by embryo transfer after in vitro fertilization (IVF) in the case of egg donation, embryo donation, and surrogacy. Thus a child can have a genetic and social (nongenetic, nonbiological) father, and a genetic, gestational, and social (nonbiological) mother, and any combinations thereof. Theoretically a child thus could have five parents. Human response to new developments regarding birth, death, marriage, and divorce is largely shaped by religious beliefs. When assisted reproduction was introduced into medical practice in the last quarter of the 20th century, it was fiercely attacked by some religious groups and highly welcomed by others. Today, assisted reproduction is accepted in nearly all its forms by Judaism, Hinduism, and Buddhism, although most Orthodox Jews refuse third party involvement.[1] On the contrary assisted reproduction is totally unacceptable to Roman Catholicism, while Protestants, Anglicans, Coptic Christians, and Sunni Muslims accept most of its forms, which do not involve gamete or embryo donation. Orthodox Christians are less strict than Catholic Christians but still refuse third party involvement. Interestingly, in contrast to Sunni Islam, Shi'a Islam accepts gamete donation and has made provisions to institutionalize it. Chinese culture is strongly influenced by Confucianism, which accepts all forms of assisted reproduction that do not involve third parties. Other communities follow the law of the land, which is usually dictated by the religious group(s) that make(s) the majority of that specific community.[1]

SPERM DONATION

Sperm donation is an increasingly common method of assisted reproduction. In the debate on sperm donation, the right to privacy—construed as a right that refers to the limits of the realm of information to which others have access—plays a pivotal role with regard to two questions. The first question is whether the sperm donor's right to privacy implies his right to retain his anonymity; the second is whether the gamete recipients' right to privacy entitles them to withhold information about the circumstances of their conception from their donor-conceived offspring. There are no regulations in the majority of countries worldwide regarding the exchange of important genetic information that has become available after the birth of a child conceived with donor gametes. This may lead to difficult situations such as when the gamete donor is found to suffer from a genetic cancer-predisposition disorder. Genetic information about the donor that becomes available later may be of great importance to donor offspring. Genetic information uncovered in the donor child may likewise be of importance to legal offspring of the gamete donor.

Schieb et al.[2] reported findings from 10 years of requests from adults eligible to obtain their open-identity sperm donor's information. Just above 35% of eligible donor insemination (DI) adults requested their donor's identity. Adults ranged from 18 to 27 years, requesting at median age 18 years. More women than men requested. Proportionally fewer adults requested when they had heterosexual-couple parents, and proportionally more when they had one rather than two parents. In interviews, the common theme was wanting to know more about the donor, especially about shared characteristics. Most adults planned to contact their donor. More than 94% of adults had donors who were open to contact; adults expressed modest expectations about this contact. In 2001, the first adults became eligible to obtain their open-identity sperm donor's information. Ten years of identity requests at one program indicates that information about one's donor is important to a significant proportion of these DI adults. Most requested their donor's identity soon after becoming eligible, suggesting some urgency to wanting the information. Interview data highlighted the role of donor information in helping adults better understand themselves and their ancestry.[2] Findings hold important implications for practice and policy.

How do female-partnered mothers in Lesbian relationships deal with the third-party involved in their reproductive arrangement? The aim of an Italian study by Lingiardi et al.[3] is to identify the meaning-making of the sperm donor, exploring different patterns between genetic and nongenetic mothers, as well as between open-identity and anonymous donation. Semi-structured interviews were conducted with 24 Italian female-partnered mothers, who at the time of data collection had at least one donor-conceived child. Interpretative phenomenological analysis was performed to identify emergent themes. None of the mothers considered the donor as the father of their child. Three patterns of thoughts and feelings recurred—"donor as an entity", "donor as a medical process", "donor as a person".[3] Genetic and nongenetic mothers constructed shared meanings regarding the donor. Mothers who opted for anonymous donors were more likely to describe the donor as an entity and as a medical process compared with mothers who opted for open-identity donors.

Hu et al.[4] investigated the pregnancy outcomes of assisted reproductive technology (ART) with cryopreserved donor sperm and the safety of the offspring thus conceived. The Human Sperm Bank of CITIC Xiangya Hospital provided cryopreserved donor semen to 31 reproductive centers in China between January 2006 and December 2012, with which 50247 ART cycles were accomplished. Authors compared the rates of birth defects and spontaneous abortion of intracervical insemination (ICI), intrauterine insemination (IUI), IVF, and intracytoplasmic sperm injection (ICSI). A total of 39,047 ART cycles were performed by artificial insemination with cryopreserved donor sperm, including 36,674 cycles of ICI and 2,372 cycles of IUI. Among the 8,612 clinical pregnancies achieved by ICI, there were 917 cases of spontaneous abortion (at <28 gestational weeks) (10.6%) and 6,133 live births, with 43 cases of birth defect (0.70%). Of the 547 clinical pregnancies achieved by IUI, there were 41 cases of spontaneous abortion (7.5%) and 426 live births, with two cases of birth defects (0.47%). Totally, 11,200 cycles of IVF and ICSI were accomplished with cryopreserved donor sperm. Of the 5,860 clinical pregnancies achieved by IVF, there were 456 cases of spontaneous abortion (7.8%) and 5,089 live births, with 55 cases of birth defects (1.08%). Among the 350 clinical pregnancies achieved by ICSI, there were 30 cases of spontaneous abortion (8.6%) and 229 live births, with three cases of birth defects (1.31%). The birth defect rate of ART with cryopreserved donor sperm was significantly lower than that published by the Chinese Ministry of Health

(0.86% vs. 1.53%, p <0.01). The study concluded that the safety of the offspring conceived by ART with cryopreserved donor sperm is at par with the normal population.[4]

The aim of a recent Spanish study is to estimate the weight of each relevant factor in such unions of inadvertent consanguinity and to determine a "reasonable" limit for the number of children per donor, matching the probability of inadvertent consanguinity arising from the use of sperm donor in assisted reproduction with that of such a union arising from false paternity.[5] In this study, the authors applied to Spanish data a mathematical model of consanguineous unions, taking into account the following factors—maximum number of live births per donor, fertility rate, average number of births per donor in a pregnancy, donor success rate, matings per phenotype, number of newborns per year, and number of donors needed in the population per year and births by false paternity. In Spain, the number of inadvertent unions between descendants of the same donor in Spain has been estimated at 0.4/year (one every two and a half years), although this frequency decreases as the reference population increases.

On the other hand, the frequency of unions between family members due to false paternity has been estimated at 6.1/year. Thus, only 6% of such unions are due to the use of donor sperm. A total of 25 children per sperm donor are needed to align the probability of inadvertent consanguinity arising from the use of assisted reproduction with that due to false paternity. Therefore, the authors consider this number to be the maximum "reasonable" number of children born per donor in Spain.[5]

An international working group was established with the aim of making recommendations on the number of offspring for a sperm donor that should be allowable in cases of international use of his sperm.[6] Considerations from genetic, psychosocial, operational, and ethical points of view were debated. For these considerations, it was assumed that current developments in genetic testing and internet possibilities mean that, now, all donors are potentially identifiable by their offspring, so no distinction was made between anonymous and nonanonymous donation. Genetic considerations did not lead to restrictive limits (indicating that up to 200 offspring or more per donor may be acceptable except in isolated social-minority situations). Psychosocial considerations on the other hand led to proposals of rather restrictive limits (10 families per donor or less). Operational and ethical considerations did not lead to more or less concrete limits per donor, but seemed to lie in-between those resulting from the aforementioned ways of viewing the issue. In the end, no unifying agreed figure could be reached; however the consensus was that the number should never exceed 100 families.[6]

Zarek et al.[7] compared the pregnancy outcomes in the setting of a single versus double-donor sperm IUI treatment cycle. There were 2,486 double and 673 single-donor sperm IUI cycles. Two groups were similar for age, body mass index, and the number of prior cycles. The clinical pregnancy rates were similar between the two groups (single: 16.4% vs. double: 13.6%). In univariate regression analysis, age, total motile sperm, and diminished ovarian reserve (DOR) were associated with pregnancy. Generalized estimating equation models accounting for repeated measures, age, DOR, and total motile sperm and the interactions of these factors demonstrated that single and double IUI had similar odds of pregnancy [odds ratio (OR) 1.12; 95% confidence interval (CI), 0.96–1.44]. Pregnancy rates remained similar between the two groups in matched comparison and other subgroup analyses. The study concluded that single and double-donor IUI cycles had similar clinical pregnancy rates. This large data set did not demonstrate a benefit to routine double IUI in donor sperm cycles.[7]

A systematic review and meta-analysis were performed to evaluate whether women who conceive with donor sperm have an increased risk of preeclampsia compared with those who use their partner's sperm.[8] Studies that compared women who were impregnated by donor and partner sperm were included. The main outcomes assessed were preeclampsia and gestational hypertension rates. Altogether, 10,898 women (2,342 pregnancies by donor sperm versus 8,556 by the partner's sperm) were included from seven observational studies. Conception using donor sperm was associated with an increased risk of preeclampsia (OR 1.63, 95% CI 1.36–1.95) compared with using a partner's sperm. No difference was observed in the risk of gestational hypertension (OR 0.94, 95% CI 0.43–2.03). In conclusion, pregnancies achieved by donor sperm significantly increase the risk of preeclampsia, although the underlying mechanisms remain unclear.[8]

OOCYTE DONATION

Although oocyte donation is widely practiced, few interventions in this field are evidence based. The objective of a study by Weissman et al.[9] was to describe the current practices for evaluation and treatment of oocyte donors and recipients worldwide. Through an IVF-focused website, an internet-based survey was addressed to physicians in IVF units worldwide. A total of 161 units responded, reflecting 14,890 annual oocyte donation cycles. The majority (83.3%) of centers perform genetic testing for oocyte donors, and in 94.6% of cycles, donors are below 35 years old. Anonymous donors are most commonly used (91.3%) and 95.8% are fresh donations. In 51.4% of donor cycles, the gonadotropin-releasing hormone (GnRH) antagonist protocol is used, and in 29.8% of these cycles, a GnRH agonist is prescribed for the ovulatory trigger. Recipient pituitary suppression is used in 76.7% of cycles, and oral estrogen (86.4%) and vaginal progesterone (73.8%) are the preferred routes of administration for endometrial preparation. In the majority (51.5%) of cycles, a minimum endometrial thickness of more than or equal to 7 mm is required. This study reflects a relative lack of homogeneity in management of oocyte donors and recipients and highlights the need for developing a consensus in the practice of oocyte donation based upon evidence-based medicine.[9]

The fetus is a semi-allograft for the maternal host in natural pregnancy, but the fetus is a complete allograft after oocyte donation (OD), and there is greater antigenic dissimilarity with the mother. Thus, OD pregnancy is a good model for understanding how the fetus is protected by the maternal immune system. Recent clinical data have revealed a higher risk of miscarriage, gestational hypertension, preterm birth (PTB), and low birth weight (LBW) with OD pregnancy. There is also a higher incidence of chorionic deciduitis, dense fibrinoid deposits in the chorionic basal plate, inflammatory lesions in the chorionic plate, and C4d deposition on syncytiotrophoblasts in OD pregnancy.[10] Impaired accumulation of T cells, regulatory T (Treg) cells, natural killer (NK) cells, and monocytes in the decidua basalis and poor remodeling of spiral arteries are observed in OD pregnancy irrespective of whether preeclampsia occurs. Oocyte donation seems to be independently associated with a higher rate of pregnancy-induced hypertension and preeclampsia. An explanatory hypothesis is that an immunological maladaptation causes placenta-mediated disorders in oocyte donation pregnancies.[11] The risks are even higher in twin pregnancies. Oocyte donation also seems to be associated with lower fetal birth-weight.[11] However, after adjusting for obstetric complications, most studies report less pronounced differences in birth-weight or no dissimilarities. The incidence of cesarean section is increased without clear clinical indications. Pregnancies achieved by oocyte donation confer a threefold increase in the likelihood of developing PE than those achieved by IVF with own oocytes.[12] Physicians should be aware of this risk in order to both counsel patients and monitor pregnancies accordingly.

Oocyte donation represents a unique in vivo experimental model in the human that permits the study of endometrial development under controlled variable conditions. Early studies have shown that adequate endometrial preparation can be achieved by sequential E and P only. The successful implementation of the simplified approach to oocyte donation demonstrated that satisfactory endometrial receptivity is not dependent on incremental administration of E and P and similarly can be achieved by fixed dosages of these steroids. Moreover, numerous clinical oocyte donation studies have shown that both physiologic and supraphysiologic levels of E and P have resulted in good endometrial development and pregnancy rates, underlining the relative insensitivity of the endometrium to extreme hormonal conditions. In addition, it has been clarified that the endometrium is tolerant of some manipulations during the follicular phase. Contrary to morphological studies that demonstrated preservation of endometrial preparation after luteal E depletion, preliminary evidence suggests that the functional capacity of the endometrium could be affected adversely. In contrast to early oocyte donation studies, which indicated a correlation between morphologic integrity and functional capacity of the endometrium, some evidence presented by Younis et al.[13] demonstrated that adequate endometrial morphology does not always imply normal endometrial receptivity.

The Ethics Committee Opinion of the American Society for Reproductive Medicine (2016) stated that financial compensation of women donating oocytes for infertility therapy or for research is justified on ethical grounds and should acknowledge the time, inconvenience, and discomfort associated with screening, ovarian stimulation, and oocyte retrieval, and not vary according to the planned use of the oocytes, the number or quality of oocytes retrieved, the number or outcome of prior donation cycles, or the donor's ethnic or other personal characteristics.[14]

Oocyte donations have increased with improvements in oocyte cryopreservation procedures in recent years. Women with medical conditions that require chemotherapy or radiotherapy have begun to opt for oocyte cryopreservation prior to their treatment or to enroll in an oocyte donation program. Alternatively, some women apply for "third-party" oocyte donation programs for nonmedical reasons such as delayed childbearing. Although society seems to accept oocyte donations for medical reasons, it appears that there are still some moral issues surrounding nonmedical oocyte donations.

Mascarenhas et al.[15] performed a systematic review and meta-analysis of the known literature to assess whether the perinatal outcomes are different after oocyte donation compared to autologous oocyte (AO) IVF pregnancies. A systematic literature search was done for studies published in English from 1980 to 2016. Studies comparing perinatal outcomes of pregnancies following fresh or frozen OD and AO IVF were included. Meta-analysis was performed using the Rev Man 5.3 software (Cochrane Collaboration) for the perinatal outcomes of PTB (<37 weeks), early PTB (<32 weeks), LBW (<2,500 g), very LBW (<1,500 g), and small for gestational age (SGA) (<10th centile). There is an increased risk of PTB following fresh embryo transfer in OD pregnancies than in AO IVF pregnancies (OR 1.45, 95% CI 1.20–1.77). If the PTB risk is assumed to be to 9% for pregnancies following AO IVF, then OD pregnancies will have a PTB risk between 10.8% and 15.9%. Similarly, the risk of LBW is higher after fresh embryo transfer in OD pregnancies than AO IVF pregnancies (OR 1.34, 95% CI 1.12–1.60). If the assumed LBW risk is 9% for AO IVF pregnancies, then OD pregnancies have a LBW risk between 10.1% and 14.4%. There is an increased risk of early PTB (OR 2.14, 95% CI 1.40–3.25) and very LBW (OR 1.51, 95% CI 1.17–1.95) in a fresh embryo transfer after OD as compared to AO IVF pregnancies. There appears to be a higher risk of adverse perinatal outcomes following fresh OD compared to AO IVF pregnancies.[15]

Bortoletto et al.[16] set up a cross-sectional study to determine whether the general public supports intergenerational oocyte donation. Characteristics of respondents who supported (strongly agree and agree) various oocyte donation practices were compared with participants who did not support them (disagree and strongly disagree) using log binomial regression to calculate risk ratios (RRs) and 95% CIs of support (95% CIs). Models were adjusted for age, gender, and religion to yield adjusted risk ratios (aRR). A total of 1,915 people responded to the web-based survey; 53% were female, and 24% were racial/ethnic minorities. 85% had prior knowledge of oocyte donation, and 74% felt that a woman should be able to donate oocytes to a family member. The desire to help a family member was the most commonly perceived motivation for donors (79%). Christian-Catholics compared with Christian-non-Catholics (aRR 0.91, 95% CI 0.86–0.98), African Americans compared with non-Hispanic Caucasians (aRR 0.86, 95% CI 0.76–0.97), and Republicans compared with Democrats (RR 0.93, 95% CI 0.88–0.98) were less likely to support intergenerational oocyte donation. Respondents with three or more biological children (RR 1.06, 95% CI 1.00–1.11) compared with those with no children were less likely to support this practice. 8% of participants disapproved of donation to any family member. The most common reason for disapproval was the potential negative impact on the child (53%). The study summarized that a majority of Americans support the practice of intergenerational oocyte donation; however, support varies according to demographic characteristics.[16]

Egg donation is a common fertility treatment in female cancer survivors with reproductive wish and iatrogenic ovarian failure. Marklund et al.[17] examined whether women previously treated for cancer have a higher risk of pregnancy complications after egg donation treatments when compared to women without cancer history. In this prospective cohort treated during 2003–2015 at a single center, 31 women with previous history of cancer achieved 25 deliveries and 212 women without cancer history achieved 244 deliveries. All egg donor treatments were performed with a strict policy of single embryo transfer (SET) to reduce pregnancy and perinatal complications. Women without previous history of cancer were used as the reference group in the regression models. Women with a history of cancer presented with a significantly increased risk of pregnancy complications, including PTB [adjusted OR (aOR) 5.54, 95% CI 2.01–15.31] and preeclampsia (aOR 2.79, 95% CI 1.07–7.34), compared to women without cancer history. The findings of this study suggest that the risks of PTB and preeclampsia in women with prior cancers who become pregnant by egg donor treatment significantly exceed those of women without cancer history undergoing similar treatments. As pregnancies using donor eggs are already acknowledged of higher risk for hypertensive pathologies, this study alerts toward characterization of specific increased risks in women who are cancer survivors to provide adapted pregnancy monitoring.[17]

The aim of a recent study[18] was to evaluate whether pregnancies resulting from oocyte donation have a higher risk of preeclampsia compared with pregnancies after IVF using AOs. Propensity score matching on maternal age and parity was carried out on a one to one basis, and a total of 144 singleton pregnancies resulting in delivery beyond 22 gestational weeks, achieved by oocyte donation, were compared with 144 pregnancies achieved through IVF and ICSI with the use of AOs. All pregnancies were achieved after fresh embryo transfer. Obstetric and neonatal outcomes were compared for each pregnancy. Singleton pregnancies after oocyte donation were associated with a significantly higher risk for preeclampsia (OR 2.4, CI 1.02–5.8; $p = 0.046$), as well as for pregnancy-induced hypertension (OR 5.3, CI 1.1–25.2; $p = 0.036$), and cesarean delivery (OR 2.3, CI 1.4–3.7; $p = 0.001$) compared with pregnancies using AOs.[18]

Utilization of cryopreserved instead of fresh donor oocytes has rapidly increased in recent years. Whether treatment outcomes are comparable has, however, remained controversial. More than 24% of initiated oocyte donation cycles in the USA during 2013–2014 involved previously cryopreserved oocytes.[19] The use of cryopreserved-donated oocytes may simplify logistics and lower costs per treatment cycle. Whether cryopreserved donor oocytes also lower costs per live birth is still undetermined as they result in lower live birth rates in comparison to fresh donor oocyte cycles. National data regarding the safety of donated oocytes, including miscarriage rates and neonatal health outcomes, are lacking. Currently available data on cryopreserved-donated oocytes are incomplete and, therefore, still insufficient to claim equivalency between fresh and cryopreserved donor oocytes. Until sufficient data are available, patients should be advised about advantages and disadvantages of both methods of oocyte donation, and the use of cryopreserved oocytes should be considered only with caution and appropriate informed consent.[19]

With the introduction of oocyte vitrification, a special form of intergenerational intrafamilial medically assisted reproduction has now become feasible—fertility preservation for mother-to-daughter oocyte donation (FPMDD).[20] For girls diagnosed with premature ovarian insufficiency (POI), banking of their mothers' oocytes can preserve the option of having genetically related offspring. Since policy documents on IMAR do not discuss specific concerns raised by FPMDD, clinicians can feel at a loss for guidance with regard to handling these requests. Through a comparison of FPMDD with reproductive practices in which similar concerns were raised, proportionality of cryopreservation for self-use and pressure to use the oocytes in fertility preservation in minors, the authors argued that FPMDD can be acceptable under specific conditions.[20]

Guesdon et al.[21] compared maternal, obstetric, and neonatal outcomes between women who underwent oocyte donation at or after age 50 years and from 45 through 49 years. The rate of multiple-gestation pregnancies was similar in both groups (35% in the older and 37.7% in the younger group). They observed no significant difference globally between the two groups for outcomes, except for the mean duration of postpartum hospitalization, which was significantly longer among the older women (mean ± SD, 9.5 ± 7.4 days vs. 6.8 ± 4.4 days). The rates of isolated pregnancy-related hypertension and of fetal growth restriction in singleton pregnancies were statistically higher in the older than in the younger group (19.2% vs. 5.5%, and 30.7% vs. 14.3%, respectively). Complication rates with twin pregnancies were similar between groups and very high compared with singleton pregnancies. Complication rates were similar among women aged 50 years and older and those aged 45–49 years. Nonetheless, given the high rate of complication in both groups, especially among twin pregnancies, SET needs to be encouraged for oocyte donations after age 45 years.[21]

Pregnancies resulting through oocyte donation have been associated with increased risk for adverse outcomes for the mother, such as gestational hypertensive disorders. However, little is known about possible neonatal complications of such pregnancies. The purpose of Elenis et al. study[22] was to evaluate the neonatal health outcomes among singleton pregnancies in a population of relatively young and healthy oocyte recipients in Sweden, taking into account the medical indication leading to treatment. This cohort study involved 76 women conceiving with donated oocytes, 149 age-matched nulliparous women conceiving spontaneously and 63 women conceiving after nondonor IVF. Participants were recruited during 2005–2008 and followed up until delivery. Data on neonatal outcomes were retrieved from the National Birth Medical Register and the medical records of oocyte recipients from seven Swedish University Hospitals with IVF clinics. Infants conceived through oocyte donation had higher odds for premature delivery [OR 2.36, 95% CI (1.02–5.45)], for being small for gestational age [OR 4.23, 95% CI (1.03–17.42)] and having Apgar score below 7 at 5 minutes [OR 10.57, 95% CI (1.21–92.20)] compared to spontaneously conceived infants. Similar trends were observed when comparing infants conceived through oocyte donation to those conceived by traditional IVF. Furthermore, donor oocyte infants had a lower mean birth-weight and length compared to AO neonates ($p = 0.013$); however, no differences were noted among infants born at term. Neonatal outcomes were more favorable among women with DOR compared to those with other indications for oocyte donation. Infants conceived after oocyte donation in Sweden have higher odds of being born prematurely and having lower mean birth-weight in comparison to nondonor infants.[22]

Turner syndrome (TS) is a chromosomal defect with partial or total absence of the X chromosome. Deligeoroglou et al.[23] reported a series with patients suffering from TS and trying to conceive who underwent IVF (ICSI) with donor oocytes in order to get pregnant. Three out of four patients managed to conceive and bring pregnancy to completion. It was shown that patients diagnosed in childhood or adolescence with TS have the possibility to undergo hormone replacement therapy (HRT) and thus, secondary sexual characteristics as well as uterus of almost normal size can develop. Assisted reproduction techniques, predominantly with donated oocytes, could give these patients the possibility to have children.[23]

During the last decade oocyte donation has been highly successful for treating women previously thought to be hopelessly infertile. The pregnancy rate after oocyte donation is among the highest reported for any fertility-enhancing procedure. Most investigators have noted an increased rate of obstetric complications in these pregnancies. In particular, pregnancy-induced hypertension appears to occur more often than expected, and the cesarean section rate is high. However, the majority of oocyte recipients experience a favorable pregnancy and perinatal outcome. When perinatal complications occur they are usually related to multiple gestation. The high frequency of multiple pregnancies after oocyte donation, as well as in all other fields of assisted reproduction, deserves attention, and efforts to avoid multifetal gestation must be made. There are only a few studies on postnatal growth and development of young children born after oocyte donation. The health of these children appears to be within normal ranges. The psychological consequences of the treatment on the child require further investigation. Thus far, studies have shown normal socioemotional development in the child and a warm relationship between the parents and the child in oocyte donation families.

Physicians should obtain a complete medical evaluation before deciding to attempt transfer of embryos to any woman over age 50. Embryo transfer should be strongly discouraged or denied to any woman over age 50 with underlying issues that could increase or further obstetrical risks and discouraged in women over age 55 without such issues.[24]

Barad et al.[25] evaluated pregnancy and live birth rates in donor oocyte-recipient cycles after the first embryo transfer with day 5/6 embryos. Statistical models, adjusted for patient and donor ages, number of embryos transferred, race, infertility diagnosis, and cycle year were created to compare live birth rates in 392 preimplantation genetic screening (PGS) and 20,616 control cycles. Overall, pregnancy and live birth rates were significantly lower in PGS cycles than in control cycles. The authors concluded that PGS, as practiced in donor oocyte-recipient cycles over the past 9 years, has not been associated with improved odds of live birth or reduction in miscarriage rates.

EMBRYO DONATION/EMBRYO ADOPTION

Embryo donation is where extra embryos from a successful IVF of a couple are given to other couples or women for transfer with the goal of producing a successful pregnancy. Embryos for embryo donation may also be created specifically for embryo transfer using donor eggs and sperm, or in some cases donor eggs and donor sperm. It may thus be seen as a combination of sperm donation and egg donation, since what is donated is a combination of these. Such embryos may also be donated to a "commissioning" woman or a "commissioning" couple and gestated by a surrogate where, e.g. the "commissioning" woman or the female partner (FP) of the "commissioning" couple is infertile and is unable to bring a pregnancy to full term on medical grounds, or is unwilling for social, medical or other reasons, to do so.

The number of women receiving IVF cycles with both oocyte and sperm donation [double donation (DD)] has grown globally in the last decade. The aim of a retrospective study by Blázquez et al.,[26] which included 1139 DD cycles, was to describe the characteristics of patients receiving DD and the outcomes of this assisted reproductive treatment. A cluster analysis identified couple "status" as the main variable in dividing patients into categories. Three such status groups were identified for further analysis: (1) single women (SW) that is women without a partner either male or female; (2) women with a male partner (MP); (3) women with a female partner. SW were significantly older (43.9) than patients with a MP (40.4) and a FP (41.3). Women with a MP or FP comprised fewer patients with no previous ART cycles (18.4% and 25.7%, respectively) compared to SW (43.5%). The proportion of patients without children before treatment was significantly different between SW (94.7%) and women with a MP (87.2%). There were no differences in clinical outcomes among the three groups studied. Biochemical pregnancy rate was 58.2% in SW, 58.4% in women with a MP, and 64.9% in women with a FP. For the same groups, clinical pregnancy rates were 50.2%, 49.4%, and 55.4%, while "take-home baby" rates were 36.6%, 38.9%, and 40.3%. Multiple birth and caesarean section rates were not different among the groups, with twinning rates 21.1%, 30.4%, and 36% and cesarean section rates 25.6%, 24%, and 26.4% for SW, women with MP and women with FP, respectively.[26]

Egg sharing in female couples can be used to allow dual participation of female couples in the pregnancy process.[27] The oocyte donor-partner provides the eggs and the recipient partner provides the uterine environment for gestation. Yeshua et al. published descriptive data of their experience in female couples to establish a better understanding of utilization of co-in vitro fertilization (Co-IVF) for social and medical reasons.[27] Female couples (n = 21) who participated in Co-IVF cycles were analyzed. Over time, 16/21 (76%) of couples achieved at least one pregnancy, 9 (42%) couples delivered, and there are another 5 (23%) ongoing pregnancies. This analysis presents descriptive data and sheds realistic expectations for Co-IVF couples.[27] Co-IVF cycles can result in a shared experience with regard to the process of creating a family, while preserving a female couple's desire for dual partner participation in the gestational process.

SURROGACY

A first mention about surrogacy was discovered on a 4,000-year-old clay tablet of marriage contract belonging to the Assyrian period exhibited at Istanbul Archeology Museum in Turkey.[28] Surrogacy is an assisted reproduction-based approach in which the intended parents assign the gestation and birth to another woman called the surrogate mother. In a "conventional surrogacy", a surrogate agrees to be inseminated with the sperm of the male partner of the "commissioning" couple, or with the sperm of one of the male partners in a same-sex relationship, or with sperm provided by a sperm donor. The surrogate is inseminated, conceives, and hands over the baby at the completion of the pregnancy. In conventional or traditional surrogacy, the egg which is fertilized is therefore that of the surrogate. In a "gestational surrogacy", a surrogate agrees to the implantation in her of an embryo which may be created either by using an egg provided by another woman who may be part of a "commissioning" couple, or she may be a single woman. Alternatively, an egg provided by a donor may be used to create the embryo. The embryo implanted in the surrogate may be fertilized using sperm from the male partner of the "commissioning couple", or by using sperm provided by a sperm donor.

The drivers of surrogacy refer largely to infertility, medical conditions, same-sex couples' parenting, and cases of diversity regarding sexual identity and orientation. Surrogacy consists of a valid option for a variety of conditions or circumstances ranging from medical to social reasons.

Anonymized data were obtained from the Human Fertilization and Embryology Authority to determine whether gestational surrogacy influences perinatal outcomes compared with pregnancies after autologous IVF.[29] A total of 103,160 singleton live births, including 244 after gestational surrogacy, 87,571 after autologous fresh IVF and ICSI, and 15,345 after autologous frozen embryo transfers were analyzed. Perinatal outcomes of PTB, LBW, and high birth weight (HBW) were compared. No difference was found in the risk of PTB and LBW after gestational surrogacy compared with autologous fresh IVF-ICSI—PTB (adjusted OR 0.90, 95% CI 0.56–1.42), LBW (adjusted OR 0.90, 95% CI 0.57–1.43) and gestational surrogacy compared with autologous frozen embryo transfers—PTB (adjusted OR 0.96, 95% CI 0.58–1.60), LBW (adjusted OR 1.16, 95% CI 0.69–1.96). The incidence of HBW was significantly higher after gestational surrogacy compared with fresh IVF-ICSI (adjusted OR 1.94, 95% CI 1.38–2.75); no difference was found in HBW between gestational surrogacy and autologous frozen embryo transfers.[29]

Söderström-Anttila et al.[30] examined a variety of main outcomes for the surrogate mothers, children, and intended mothers, including obstetric outcome, relationship between surrogate mother and intended couple, surrogate's experiences after relinquishing the child, PTB, LBW, birth defects, perinatal mortality, child psychological development, parent-child relationship, and disclosure to the child. PubMed, Cochrane, and Embase databases up to February 2015 were searched. The search returned 1795 articles of which 55 met the inclusion criteria. The medical outcome for the children was satisfactory and comparable to previous results for children conceived after fresh IVF and oocyte donation. The rate of multiple pregnancies was 2.6–75.0%. PTB rate in singletons varied between 0% and 11.5% and LBW occurred in between 0% and 11.1% of cases. At the age of 10 years there were no major psychological differences between children born after surrogacy and children born after other types of ART or after natural conception. The obstetric outcomes for the surrogate mothers were mainly reported from case series. Hypertensive disorders in pregnancy were reported in between 3.2% and 10% of cases and placenta previa/placental abruption in 4.9%. Cases with hysterectomies have also been reported. Most surrogate mothers scored within the normal range on personality tests. Most psychosocial variables were satisfactory, although difficulties related to handing over the child did occur. The psychological well-being of children whose mother had been a surrogate mother between 5 years and 15 years earlier was found to be good. No major differences in psychological state were found between intended mothers, mothers, who conceived after other types of ART and mothers whose pregnancies were the result of natural conception.[30]

Woo et al.[31] studied the perinatal outcomes between singleton live births achieved with the use of commissioned versus spontaneously conceived embryos carried by the same gestational surrogate. They identified 124 gestational surrogates who achieved a total of 494 pregnancies. Pregnancy outcomes for surrogate and spontaneous pregnancies were significantly different ($p < 0.001$), with surrogate pregnancies more likely to result in twin pregnancies—33% versus 1%. Miscarriage and ectopic rates were similar. Of these pregnancies, there were 352 singleton live births: 103 achieved from commissioned embryos and 249 conceived spontaneously. Surrogate births had lower mean gestational age at delivery (38.8 ± 2.1 vs. 39.7 ± 1.4), higher rates of PTB (10.7% vs. 3.1%), and higher rates of LBW (7.8% vs. 2.4%). Neonates from surrogacy had birth weights that were, on average, 105 g lower. Surrogate births had significantly higher obstetrical complications, including gestational diabetes, hypertension, use of amniocentesis, placenta previa, antibiotic requirement during labor, and cesarean section. Neonates born from commissioned embryos and carried by gestational surrogates have increased adverse perinatal outcomes, including PTB, LBW, hypertension, maternal gestational diabetes, and placenta previa, compared with singletons conceived spontaneously and carried by the same woman.[31] Woo et al. data suggest that assisted reproductive procedures may potentially affect embryo quality and that its negative impact cannot be overcome even with a proven healthy uterine environment.[31]

Preimplantation genetic screening is a component of IVF entailing selection of an embryo for transfer on the basis of chromosomal normalcy. If PGS were integrated with SET in a surrogacy setting, this approach could improve pregnancy rates, minimize miscarriage risk, and limit multiple gestations.[32] Even without PGS, pregnancy rates for IVF surrogacy cases are generally satisfactory, especially when treatment utilizes embryos derived from young oocytes and transferred to a healthy surrogate. However, there could be a more general role for PGS in surrogacy, since background aneuploidy in embryos remains a major factor driving implantation failure and miscarriage for all infertility patients.

WHAT IS NEW IN THIRD PARTY REPRODUCTION?

A recent study aimed to describe a novel strategy that increases the accuracy and reliability of PGD in patients using sperm donation by preselecting the donor whose haplotype does not overlap the carrier's one.[33] A panel of 4–9 informative polymorphic markers, flanking the mutation in carriers of autosomal dominant/X-linked disorders, was tested in DNA of sperm donors before PGD. Whenever the lengths of donors' repeats overlapped those of the women, additional donors' DNA samples were analyzed. The donor that demonstrated the minimal overlapping with the patient was selected for IVF. In 8 out of 17 carriers the markers of the initially chosen donors overlapped the patients' alleles and 2–8 additional sperm donors for each patient were haplotyped. The selection of additional sperm donors increased the number of informative markers and reduced misdiagnosis risk from 6.00% ± 7.48 to 0.48% ± 0.68. The PGD results were confirmed and no misdiagnosis was detected.

This study demonstrated that preselecting a sperm donor whose haplotype has minimal overlapping with the female's haplotype, is critical for reducing the misdiagnosis risk and ensuring a reliable PGD.[33] This strategy may contribute to prevent the transmission of affected IVF-PGD embryos using a simple and economical procedure.

CONCLUSION

Third-party IVF use and efficacy have increased over the past decade, now comprising more than 20% of the total IVF birth cohort. In women who are above 40 years old, third-party IVF has become the dominant treatment.[34]

The rise of the Internet Age has brought a host of sweeping changes to the landscape of third-party reproduction. What began as a dyadic relationship between doctor and patient has evolved into a more complex system in which patients are able to access information online from a variety of external sources.[35] Patients often seek to play a more active role in their third-party reproductive care, and the internet allows them to do so. Further, demand for both medical and psychosocial information about donors and donor-conceived siblings, available online through patient forums and genetic registries, has altered the perception of gamete donation from a one-time event to an ongoing relationship.[35]

The proliferation of medically assisted reproduction for the treatment of infertility has brought benefit to many individuals around the world. But infertility and its treatment continue to be a cause of suffering, and over the past decade, there has been a steady growth in a new global market of inter-country medically assisted reproduction (IMAR) involving "third-party" individuals acting as surrogate mothers and gamete donors in reproductive collaborations for the benefit of other individuals and couples who wish to have children. At the same time there is evidence of a double standard of care for third-party women involved in IMAR, violations of human rights of children and women, and extreme abuses that are tantamount to reproductive trafficking.[36] A recent report of an interdisciplinary working group of experts who convened in Israel to discuss the complex issues of IMAR describes documented practices that are harmful, suggests principles of good practice based on an ethic of care, and calls for action at the international, national, and professional levels to establish a human rights based system of international governance for IMAR based on three regulatory models—public health monitoring, inter-country adoption, and trafficking in human beings, organs, and tissues.[36]

REFERENCES

1. Sallam HN, Sallam NH. Religious aspects of assisted reproduction. Facts Views Vis Obgyn. 2016;8(1):33-48.
2. Scheib JE, Ruby A, Benward J. Who requests their sperm donor's identity? The first ten years of information

releases to adults with open-identity donors. Fertil Steril. 2017;107(2):483-93.
3. Lingiardi V, Carone N, Morelli M, et al. It's a bit too much fathering this seed: the meaning-making of the sperm donor in Italian lesbian mother families. Reprod Biomed Online. 2016;33(3):412-24.
4. Hu J, Xing L, Wu HL, et al. Safety of the offspring conceived by assisted reproductive technology with cryopreserved donor sperm. Zhonghua Nan Ke Xue. 2016;22(6):525-9.
5. Sánchez-Castelló IM, Gonzalvo MC, Clavero A, et al. Maximum number of children per sperm donor based on false paternity rate. J Assist Reprod Genet. 2017;34(3):345-8.
6. Janssens PM, Thorn P, Castilla JA, et al. Evolving minimum standards in responsible international sperm donor offspring quota. Reprod Biomed Online. 2015;30(6):568-80.
7. Zarek SM, Hill MJ, Richter KS, et al. Single-donor and double-donor sperm intrauterine insemination cycles: does double intrauterine insemination increase clinical pregnancy rates? Fertil Steril. 2014;102(3):739-43.
8. González-Comadran M, Urresta Avila J, Saavedra Tascón A, et al. The impact of donor inseminate ion on the risk of preeclampsia: a systematic review and meta-analysis. Eur J Obstet Gynecol Reprod Biol. 2014;182:160-6.
9. Weissman A, Leong M, Sauer MV, et al. Characterizing the practice of oocyte donation: a web-based international survey. Reprod Biomed Online. 2014;28(4):443-50.
10. Saito S, Nakabayashi Y, Nakashima A, et al. A new era in reproductive medicine: consequences of third-party oocyte donation for maternal and fetal health. Semin Immunopathol. 2016;38(6):687-97.
11. Savasi VM, Mandia L, Laoreti A, et al. Maternal and fetal outcomes in oocyte donation pregnancies. Hum Reprod Update. 2016;22(5):620-33.
12. Blázquez A, García D, Rodríguez A, et al. Is oocyte donation a risk factor for preeclampsia? A systematic review and meta-analysis. J Assist Reprod Genet. 2016;33(7):855-63.
13. Younis JS, Simon A, Laufer N. Endometrial preparation: lessons from oocyte donation. Fertil Steril. 1996;66(6):873-84.
14. Ethics Committee of the American Society for Reproductive Medicine. Electronic address: ASRM@asrm.org(1); Ethics Committee of the American Society for Reproductive Medicine. Financial compensation of oocyte donors: an Ethics Committee opinion. Fertil Steril. 2016;106(7):e15-e19.
15. Mascarenhas M, Sunkara SK, Antonisamy B, et al. Higher risk of preterm birth and low birth weight following oocyte donation: A systematic review and meta-analysis. Eur J Obstet Gynecol Reprod Biol. 2017;218:60-7.
16. Bortoletto P, Farland LV, Ginsburg ES, et al. Public support for intergenerational oocyte donation in the United States. Fertil Steril. 2018;109(2):343-8.e1.
17. Marklund A, Nasiell J, Berger AS, et al. Pregnancy Achieved Using Donor Eggs in Cancer Survivors with Treatment-Induced Ovarian Failure: Obstetric and Perinatal Outcome. J Womens Health (Larchmt). 2018;27(7):939-45.
18. Tarlatzi TB, Imbert R, Mercadal AB, et al. Does oocyte donation compared with autologous oocyte IVF pregnancies have a higher risk of preeclampsia? Reprod Biomed Online. 2017;34(1):11-8.
19. Kushnir VA, Gleicher N. Fresh versus cryopreserved oocyte donation. Curr Opin Endocrinol Diabetes Obes. 2016;23(6):451-7.
20. Balkenende EM, Dondorp W, Ploem MC, et al. A mother's gift of life: exploring the concerns and ethical aspects of fertility preservation for mother-to-daughter oocyte donation. Hum Reprod. 2017;32(1):2-6.
21. Guesdon E, Vincent-Rohfritsch A, Bydlowski S, et al. Oocyte donation recipients of very advanced age: perinatal complications for singletons and twins. Fertil Steril. 2017;107(1):89-96.
22. Elenis E, Sydsjö G, Skalkidou A, et al. Neonatal outcomes in pregnancies resulting from oocyte donation: a cohort study in Sweden. BMC Pediatr. 2016;16(1):170.
23. Deligeoroglou E, Stergioti E, Dimopoulos KD, et al. Pregnancy outcome after oocyte donation in patients with Turner's syndrome: Clinical experience and management. J Obstet Gynaecol. 2016;36(4):504-7.
24. Ethics Committee of the American Society for Reproductive Medicine. Oocyte or embryo donation to women of advanced age: a committee opinion. Fertil Steril. 2013;100(2):337-40.
25. Barad DH, Darmon SK, Kushnir VA, et al. Impact of preimplantation genetic screening on donor oocyte-recipient cycles in the United States. Am J Obstet Gynecol. 2017;217(5):576.e1-576.e8.
26. Blázquez A, Vassena R, Rodríguez A, et al. Characteristics and clinical outcomes of patients undergoing fertility treatment by double gamete donation. Hum Fertil (Camb). 2016;19(3):180-5.
27. Yeshua A, Lee JA, Witkin G, et al. Female Couples Undergoing IVF with Partner Eggs (Co-IVF): Pathways to Parenthood. LGBT Health. 2015;2(2):135-9.
28. Turp AB, Guler I, Bozkurt N, et al. Infertility and surrogacy first mentioned on a 4000-year-old Assyrian clay tablet of marriage contract in Turkey. Gynecol Endocrinol. 2018;34: 25-27.
29. Sunkara SK, Antonisamy B, Selliah HY, et al. Perinatal outcomes after gestational surrogacy versus autologous IVF: analysis of national data. Reprod Biomed Online. 2017;35(6):708-14.
30. Söderström-Anttila V, Wennerholm UB, Loft A, et al. Surrogacy: outcomes for surrogate mothers, children and the resulting families-a systematic review. Hum Reprod Update. 2016;22(2):260-76.
31. Woo I, Hindoyan R, Landay M, et al. Perinatal outcomes after natural conception versus in vitro fertilization (IVF) in gestational surrogates: a model to evaluate IVF treatment versus maternal effects. Fertil Steril. 2017;108(6):993-8.
32. Sills ES, Anderson RE, McCaffrey M, et al. Gestational surrogacy and the role of routine embryo screening: Current challenges and future directions for preimplantation genetic testing. Birth Defects Res C Embryo Today. 2016;108:98-102.
33. Malcov M, Gold V, Peleg S, et al. Improving preimplantation genetic diagnosis (PGD) reliability by selection of sperm donor with the most informative haplotype. Reprod Biol Endocrinol. 2017;15(1):31.
34. Kushnir VA, Darmon SK, Shapiro AJ, et al. Utilization of third-party in vitro fertilization in the United States. Am J Obstet Gynecol. 2017;216(3):266.e1-266.e10.
35. Woodward JT. Third-party reproduction in the Internet Age: the new, patient-centered landscape. Fertil Steril. 2015;104(3):525-30.
36. Shalev C, Moreno A, Eyal H, et al. Ethics and regulation of inter-country medically assisted reproduction: a call for action. Isr J Health Policy Res. 2016;5:59.

CHAPTER 86

Fertility Preservation

Devika Gunasheela, N Ashwini

INTRODUCTION

The survival rates of young people with cancer have increased substantially due to fast-growing innovations in cancer treatment. Most frequently diagnosed cancers in adults aged 25–49 years include breast, colorectal and cervical cancer, and malignant melanoma (Cancer Research United Kingdom, 2009). About 90% of 5-year survival rates are now reported in young people for many malignancies. The diagnosis and treatment of cancer often poses a threat to fertility.

The primary objective in the minds of most oncologists is to cure the system of killer illness. As the overall survival rates of young cancer patients treated with radiation or chemotherapeutic agents are 65%, the prevalence of longtime survivors in young adult population has been estimated to be 1 in 1,000.[1]

Awareness needs to grow in the medical community regarding the evolving methods of fertility preservation. The ability to have biological children is of great importance to many people. A detailed counseling should be done with all patients afflicted with cancer who still have a good reproductive potential regarding the effects of chemotherapy or radiotherapy on fertility. Maximum attempts should be made to preserve gonadal function of young men and women treated with cancer drug therapy.

ONCOLOGY THERAPY ON FERTILITY—THE IMPACT

Radiotherapy

The extent of damage caused by radiotherapy depends on the type and dose of radiation and dose per fraction. Radiotherapy results in ionization of cellular atoms and molecules leading to the destruction of double and single deoxyribonucleic acid structures within the cell structure. A chain of events causes disruption of the cell cycle leading to apoptosis of the cells.

Impact on Males

Immature sperm cells are very sensitive to low doses of radiation. The application of greater than 6 Gy to the testes will result in irreversible azoospermia. Reversible sterility occurs at levels of 3.5 Gy, and the testis will recover over 18–24 months. The Leydig cells[2] are more resistant to chemotherapeutic agents. Hence, testosterone production and the development of secondary sexual characteristics are preserved even when the spermatogenesis has failed completely.[3] Extent of Leydig cell damage is directly related to the dose of cytotoxic agents and inversely to the age of the patient.[1] Libido and erection will usually remain normal in the male, and it is sterility that is the main concern. However, it is not unusual for patients who have had pelvic irradiation to suffer from erectile dysfunction as a long-term complication as a result of radiation-induced vascular disease leading to reduced blood flow in the pelvic and penile vessels.[4]

Impact on Females

The mature cells take the onslaught of the effect of radiotherapy, while the immature resting cells escape in the female gonads. In females the follicular function and sex steroid functions are interdependent where damage of either results in failure of both functions.[1]

Recent results suggest that the dose necessary to destroy 50% of primordial follicles (lethal dose 50) would be 2 Gy.[5] Factors influencing the degree of ovarian impairment include the volume treated, total irradiation dose, fractionation schedule, and age at the time of treatment.[6-9] The effective sterilizing dose (ESD) decreases with increasing age at treatment (ESD—dose of fractionated radiotherapy at which premature ovarian failure occurs immediately after treatment in 97.5% of the patients).

There is an increased incidence of infertility, fetal loss, and intrauterine growth restriction in young girls who have been irradiated in prepubertal age, which is attributed to reduced elasticity of the myometrial tissue, and decreased endometrial receptivity due to uterine vascular damage.[2,10]

Irradiation of vagina carries with it the risk of loss of lubrication and stenosis, which may result in physical impairments to fertility as well as major psychosexual issues.[11]

Chemotherapy

Almost every chemotherapeutic agent used for cancer has a degree of gonadotoxicity. Factors governing this are as follows:[12]

- Radical chemotherapy generally has more profound effects on fertility than adjuvant chemotherapy
- Increasing complexities of regimes are more likely to have impacts upon fertility than single agents[13-15]
- Increasing doses are likely to have more profound effects on fertility than lower doses
- Different agents have a markedly different impact upon fertility with some chemotherapeutic agents sparing fertility, whilst others are extremely toxic in this regard
- In the female, in particular, age has a profound effect on chemotherapy toxicity[16]
- The testis in the male is exquisitely sensitive to chemotherapy, while in the female, it is variable in terms of the tolerance to chemotherapy agents.

Chemotherapy and the Testis

The testis is more sensitive to chemotherapy than the ovary.[17,18] The germinal epithelium is extremely sensitive when compared to the Leydig cells. Hence, gonadal toxicity of the testis affects spermatogenesis more than it does testosterone production. The prepubertal testis is less susceptible than postpubertal testis[19] when exposed to cytotoxic drugs.

Chemotherapy and the Ovary

Postpuberty, the primordial follicles contain single oocytes arrested in the prophase of the first meiotic division and are highly sensitive to cytotoxic drugs, leading to cellular death.[20] Follicular depletion is physiologically age dependent, the maximum rate of depletion occurring around the age of 38 years when the reserve is just about 10% of the number present at menarche.[21] The cytotoxic effects are dependent on the types of cytotoxic drugs, the dosage of the drugs, and also the age of the women.

The estimated risks of premature ovarian failure (listed from highest to lowest) and, consequently, loss of future fertility potential in a patient of reproductive age are represented in Tables 1 and 2.

STRATEGIES FOR FERTILITY PRESERVATION

In Males

Sperm banking remains the choice of fertility preservation for males capable of producing a semen sample. Young males will only start producing sperm cells suitable for cryopreservation around the age of 12–13 years.[22] If the testicular volume is less than 10 mL, it is very

Table 1: Risk to fertility with different modalities of radiotherapy and chemotherapy.

Risk	*Treatment*[17]
High >80%	1. High-dose external beam radiation to the ovaries: a. Adult women ≥6 Gy b. Postpubertal girls ≥10 Gy c. Prepubertal girls ≥15 Gy (Gy—Gray: absorbed dose of radiation) 2. Bone marrow transplant or stem cell transplant alkylating agent chemotherapy (cyclophosphamide, busulfan, or melphalan) in preparation for transplant 3. Breast cancer combination chemotherapy in women over 40 years: a. Chemotherapy with alkylating agents which are cyclophosphamide, busulfan or melphalan, and methotrexate, fluorouracil, doxorubicin or epirubicin
Intermediate~30–70%	1. Breast cancer or severe autoimmune disease chemotherapy in women 30–39 years: a. Alkylating chemotherapy (cyclophosphamide, busulfan, melphalan, or chlorambucil) 2. Breast cancer combination chemotherapy in women over 40 years: a. Alkylating agent chemotherapy (cyclophosphamide, busulfan, or melphalan) plus doxorubicin

Contd...

Contd...

Low <20%	1. Breast cancer or severe autoimmune disease chemotherapy in women less than 30 years: a. Alkylating agent chemotherapy (cyclophosphamide, busulfan, melphalan, or chlorambucil) 2. Breast cancer combination: chemotherapy in women less than 40 years: a. Alkylating agent chemotherapy (cyclophosphamide, busulfan, or melphalan) plus doxorubicin 3. Cancer chemotherapy for: a. Leukemia (ALL, AML) b. Non-Hodgkin lymphoma

(ALL: acute lymphocytic leukemia; AML: acute myeloid leukemia)

Table 2: Risk levels for infertility promoted by various chemotherapeutic agents.

Risk level	*Risk due to nature or risks caused by nature of treatment of malignancy*
High	Alkylating agents
Medium	Cyclophosphamide, ifosfamide, chlormethine, busulfan, melphalan, chlorambucil, carmustine, lomustine, mechlorethamine, procarbazine
Low <20%	Cisplatin, carboplatin, doxorubicin vincristine, methotrexate, dactinomycin, bleomycin, mercaptopurine, vinca alkaloids (vinblastine), fluorouracil
Risk exists unknown	Nitrosources and antimetabolites
Unknown risk	Cytosine arabinoside, taxanes, oxaliplatin, monoclonal antibodies (trastuzumab, bevacizumab, cetuximab), tyrosine kinase inhibitors (erlotinib, imatinib)

Taken with kind permission from Ronit Abir. Cancer in Female Adolescents.[30] Elad Feigin, Ronit Abir, Fertility Preservation in Female Adolescents with Malignancies. © 2008 Nova Science Publishers, Inc.

unlikely that the patient will demonstrate any significant spermatogenesis. Electroejaculation[23] or epididymal or testicular sperm extraction[24] may be done when young males are unable to ejaculate.

Testicular biopsy, followed by the cryopreservation of spermatogonia, may be performed in prepubertal boys where spermatogenesis has not yet commenced. Disadvantages of testicular biopsy include psychological trauma to young boys and anxiety in parents.[25]

Semen samples can be stored indefinitely in liquid nitrogen.

Cryopreservation fee is about $350 with an additional cost of approximately $100/specimen. Semen samples are frozen for free in Gunasheela IVF Center for a period of 10 years.

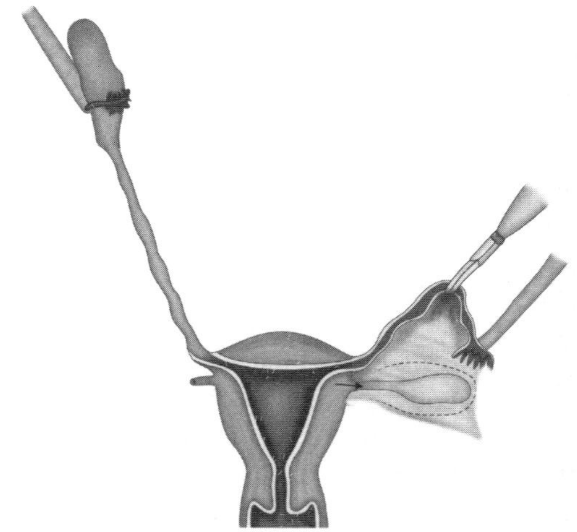

Fig. 1: Laparoscopic lateral ovarian transposition.

Obstacles to Cryopreservation

- Failure to collect sample(s)
- Stress of having the semen frozen may not be worth the possible benefits
- Patient may not be able to fit the process into a busy treatment schedule.

Use of Frozen Semen Sample

- Artificial insemination
- In vitro fertilization (IVF)
- Intracytoplasmic sperm insemination (ICSI).

In Females

Laparoscopic Ovarian Suspension before Irradiation[26]

Pelvic irradiation may be indicated in some women with genitourinary or low intestinal tumors which results in the loss of ovarian function.

Ovarian transposition to an extra pelvic site out of the field of radiation has been advocated in an attempt to protect the ovaries from radiation. Ovarian transposition is done by laparotomy either as a part of surgical staging or as a separate procedure[27-34] (Fig. 1).

Preservation of ovarian function occurs in 83% of the patients after lateral ovarian transposition prior to pelvic irradiation.[30] Lateral transposition is more effective than medial transposition of the ovaries behind the uterus. The upper and lower poles of the ovaries can be marked with hemoclips (Fig. 1) which help to verify that they are out of the radiation portals on radiation verification films.[34] Good blood supply to both ovaries should be confirmed at the end of the procedure.

Ovaries can otherwise be exteriorized under the skin through an opening in the flank. This approach is not used widely and has been associated with ovarian cyst formation.[33] Injury and torsion of the ovarian blood vessels are known complications of ovarian transposition.[30]

The ovaries frequently migrate back into the pelvic irradiation fields, especially when there is a long delay between oophoropexy and the onset of irradiation therapy.[35] It is therefore suggested that oophoropexy must be done immediately before starting pelvic irradiation.

Ovarian Suppressor Agents

A 68% increase in the rate of preserved ovarian function is noted with the use of a gonadotrophin-releasing hormone (GnRH) agonist (GnRHa) during chemotherapy compared with women not receiving a GnRHa.[36]

The mechanisms of action by means of which of GnRH analogs preserve ovarian function, even though not fully understood, may include the interruption of follicle-stimulating hormone (FSH) secretion, a decrease in utero-ovarian perfusion, the activation of GnRH receptors, the upregulation of intragonadal antiapoptotic molecules, or the protection of undifferentiated germline stem cells.[37]

It should be noted that GnRHa cannot provide protection from ovarian damage caused by irradiation. Some alkylating agents can destroy the resting primordial follicles on which GnRHa has no effect at all.

The study by Elgindy et al.[38] concluded that GnRH treatment has minimal benefit when used during chemotherapy for breast cancer. Prolonged GnRHa use is accompanied by undesired adverse effects (hot flushes, vaginal dryness, mood swings, and osteoporosis). These side effects have to be borne by the patients along with the additional side effects of chemotherapy.

The PROMISE-GIM6 (Prevention of Menopause Induced by Chemotherapy: A Study in Early Breast Cancer Patients—Gruppo Italiano Mammella 6) study[38] showed that the administration of the GnRH analog triptorelin, before and during chemotherapy, led to a 17% absolute reduction in the occurrence of early menopause in premenopausal patients with breast cancer undergoing adjuvant or neoadjuvant chemotherapy. Early menopause occurred in 25.9% of the patients treated with chemotherapy alone and 8.9% of those treated with chemotherapy plus triptorelin.

The use of GnRH analogs may be justified in specific cancers alone rather than its generalized application.

Cryopreservation of Embryos, Oocytes, and Ovarian Tissue

Embryo Storage

For an adult woman who is married or in a stable relationship, embryo storage as a means of fertility preservation is the best option. Embryo storage involves stimulating the ovaries using gonadotrophins to produce mature eggs, which are then aspirated and injected with the partner's sperm. This technique is called intracytoplasmic sperm injection (ICSI). A success rate of approximately 40% per cycle (age dependent) can be achieved with ICSI. The limitations would include:

- The deficiency of time that is there between the detection of the cancer and the start of the treatment
- Only a limited number of embryos would be available for transfer at a later date
- In some tumors, such as breast cancer, with an estrogen receptor positive status, the use of gonadotrophins results in elevated estrogen levels which is of concern. The risks of such techniques in terms of tumor progression or relapse in hormone-dependent cancers are still unclear.

Oktay et al.[39] reported 600 women with breast cancer, who underwent ovarian stimulation with either tamoxifen or letrozole in combination with a low dose of FSH. It was seen that a combination of low-dose letrozole with FSH resulted in a higher embryo yield and lower peak estradiol levels.[39]

The unpredictability of the number of good embryos that one gets in IVF in any one cycle makes it undependable method of preserving reproductive potential. Second, embryo storage demands that there should be a stable male partner for the individual concerned. In the absence of a stable male partner, one has no alternative but to arrange for the cryopreservation of oocytes either by slow cooling or by vitrification.

Oocyte Storage

Cryopreservation of oocytes is, especially, suited for adults and for older teenagers without a current partner. The technique involves ovarian stimulation, oocyte pickup, and freezing of oocytes. Oocyte cryopreservation is technically more difficult than embryo cryopreservation. Stored oocytes can later be thawed, and ICSI techniques can be used when a stable partner is available and pregnancy is desired. Oocytes from isolated antral follicles of the size of

2–3 mm can also be aspirated, maturated in vitro, and then cryopreserved.

Freezing of oocytes has become highly successful after the advent of vitrification (rapid freezing method). Pregnancy rates are in the range of 32–65% per embryo transfer, and live birth rates of over 50% have been reported[40] in certain centers world over.

Ovarian Tissue Storage

The cortical tissue of the ovary contains the maximal number of ovarian follicles, which can be peeled off the medullary stromal tissue. This tissue can then be teased into several strips of 8–10 mm^2 and cryopreserved for future use. The frozen cortical tissue can be later thawed when the patient is declared disease free and can be transplanted into the patient's ovary or other sites. This technique can be used for young adults and adolescent children. It unfortunately involves a laparoscopy to undertake a biopsy of an ovary or to remove the whole ovary for preservation. It is an invasive procedure under general anesthesia and carries a mortality rate of 1 in 12,000.

Silber et al.[41] reported that oocytes obtained from ultrafast-frozen ovarian tissue produced the same success rates as fresh tissue, claiming that vitrification of thin cortical ovarian tissue containing follicles of various stages of growth had the same kind of viability as that in the fresh oocytes. They also found that 91.9% of the fresh oocytes and 88.9% of the vitrified and thawed oocytes were viable, whereas among the cohort of oocytes tested after slow freezing and thawing, only 56% were viable.

Safety Concerns and Alternative Treatments

Ovarian tissue transplantation is not recommended for patients with blood-borne malignancies, malignancies that metastasize to the ovary or for those with an inherent predisposition to ovarian cancer due to the uncertainties about transmission of disease. However, ovarian tissue transplantation in women with cancers that have a negligible risk of ovarian involvement may be considered for future autotransplantation.

Patients should be explained regarding the surgical and anesthetic risks involved with the ovarian transplantation procedure. In the event of death of the donor, there should be no ambiguity regarding the disposition of ovarian tissue.

Ethical Issues

Fertility preservation raises several ethical issues which include the discussion of danger or the safety of fertility preservation in the setting of available techniques, cultural issues, the consent process,[42,43] and the dilemma of counseling a young candidate who has not yet reached adulthood to make decisions, regarding his or her reproductive health.

The cancer patient or their guardians must interact with not only the oncologists but also the fertility specialists and the andrology/embryology laboratories where the biological material of cancer sufferers is going to be preserved. Treatment for cancer may not allow the luxury of time for necessary consultations and decision-making.

Decision-making is not very complicated in sperm banking as it is in ovarian tissue banking.

The patient must also be aware that the technique does not guarantee either the birth of a child or its well-being. The technology of cryopreservation of gametes and embryos is not a part of the care for cancer; but it runs parallel to the main treatment, which may be accepted or rejected depending on patient's philosophy of life. She may opt adoption or a gamete donation; in which case, one must agree that it may not reduce the joy of parenting.

With the exception of a few heritable cancer syndromes, a history of cancer or its treatment does not seem to increase the rate of congenital abnormalities or cancer in the offspring.[44] Some types of cancer, such as leukemia and lymphoma, have greater tendency to metastasize to the ovary or testes. The potential risk of development of a metastatic tumor in the reproductive tract must be disclosed to the patient and the family before proceeding.[45]

There are no guidelines formulated in India regarding freezing of the gametes or ovarian tissue of cancer-afflicted patients for their own use at a later date when they are deemed to be cured of the disease.

American Society of Clinical Oncology

Recommendations[46]

American Society of Clinical Oncology convened an expert panel to conduct a systematic review of 233 studies published between 1987 and 2005 to develop recommendation. The panel concluded that oncologists should address the possibility of infertility and options for fertility preservation with all patients who are to be treated in their reproductive years, and that these discussion and resultant referrals to reproductive endocrinologists should occur as soon as possible during treatment planning.

GUNASHEELA INSTITUTE OF RESEARCH IN CANCER AND FERTILITY (CHARITABLE TRUST)

Gunasheela Institute of Research in Cancer and Fertility found its inception in 2010 with a noble purpose of helping patients suffering from various cancers in the reproductive age-group to preserve fertility despite their ongoing cancer therapies.

Patients referred for fertility preservation are evaluated, given thorough counseling on the impact of cancer therapies on fertility and the importance of fertility preservation prior to cancer therapy.

This program is an ongoing social initiative by Gunasheela Institute of Research in Cancer and Fertility, and fertility preservation has been offered and continued as a charitable program from 2010 till date for all male and female patients.

Statistics of Fertility Preservation Program in Gunasheela Institute of Research in Cancer and Fertility

Male Patients

A total of 285 male patients have undergone fertility preservation from December 2010 to April 2018 in Gunasheela Institute of Research in Cancer and Fertility. Patients belong to the age-group of 15–40 years with 62% of patients belonging to the age-group of 21–30 years.

Distribution of cancers is as follows:
- Testicular tumors: 115 patients
- Hodgkin's and non-Hodgkin's lymphoma: 77 patients
- Others (bone, colon, blood): 93 patients.

Female Patients

A total of 31 female patients have undergone fertility preservation from December 2010 to August 2017 in Gunasheela Institute of Research in Cancer and Fertility.

Distribution of various cancers among female patients include:
- *Breast cancer:* 16 patients
- *Ovarian malignancy:* 7 patients
- *Rectum/colon cancer:* 3 patients
- *Spindle cell cancer:* 2 patients
- *Lymph node malignancy:* 3 patients.

Fertility preservation strategy distribution among female patients:
- *Cortical tissue cryopreservation:* 12 patients
- *Oocyte vitrification:* 12 patients
- *Embryo freezing:* 10 patients.

Fertility Preservation in Noncancer Conditions

Fertility preservation can be considered in certain noncancer conditions, which affect the reproductive system.

Indications

- Genital tuberculosis and sexually transmitted diseases causing reduced ovarian reserve
- Autoimmune conditions, such as rheumatoid arthritis, systemic lupus erythematosus, where the patients are required to be on immunosuppressive therapy
- Young adults with severe endometriosis causing rapid decline in ovarian reserve
- *Social freezing*: When the woman concerned wishes to postpone pregnancy and childbirth, perhaps for career reasons or because she does not currently have a partner, fertility preservation can be considered.

Techniques

Ovarian tissue and unfertilized oocytes can be preserved if the woman is single. If the woman is in a stable relationship, fertilized oocytes in the form of zygotes or embryos can be placed in storage.

Efficacy and Safety of Oocyte Cryopreservation and Storage

With the age-related decrease in the ovarian reserves, the number of oocytes that can be harvested goes down. Hence, cryopreservation should be ideally carried out before the woman reaches the age of 35. Risks of hemorrhage and/or injury during follicular aspiration and severe hyperstimulation syndrome should be carefully considered while using reproductive medicine techniques without a medical indication.

The risks associated with fertility preservation for nonmedical reasons must always be described in detail during the counseling process.

Potential Advantages and Disadvantages of Social Freezing

Advantages

- As childbirth is postponed to a later time, it gives the patient the opportunity to fulfill her need of motherhood when she deems that the time is right
- The cryopreserved oocytes may increase the likelihood of conception in fertility-reducing diseases, such as premature ovarian failure or endometriosis
- There is a lower risk of chromosomal malformations, such as Down syndrome, as the eggs used to achieve conception were harvested when the woman was younger.

Disadvantages

- Only limited number of embryos or oocytes is available to achieve a pregnancy
- High costs for every stimulation, oocyte retrieval, and cryopreservation procedure; for each year of storage; and for subsequent IVF of the oocytes and embryo transfer
- Increased risk of multiple pregnancy
- Elevated risk of complications, such as preeclampsia and gestational diabetes in women >40 years of age
- Lack of clarity with regard to the danger of epigenetic changes and other malformation risks due to the necessary IVF procedure.

The perspective for obstetricians

Single pregnancy at 50 is associated with a sixfold risk of gestational diabetes (6%) and a fourfold chance of mild (14.4%) or severe (9%) preeclampsia. It should be considered that IVF is associated with a higher rate of multiple pregnancies because usually more than one embryo is transferred leading to a higher risk of complications during pregnancy and thus greater risk to the children.

REFERENCES

1. Waring A, Wallace W. Subfertility following treatment for childhood cancer. Hosp Med. 2000;61:550-7.
2. Janson PO. Possibilities of fertility preservation in children and young adults undergoing treatment for malignancy. Acta Obstet Gynecol Scand. 2000;79:240-3.
3. Petersen PM, Daugaard G, Rørth M, et al. Endocrine function in patients treated for carcinoma in situ in the testis with irradiation. Acta Pathol Microbiol Immunol Scand. 2003;111(1):93-9.
4. Basavaraju SR, Easterly CE. Pathophysiological effects of radiation on atherosclerosis development and progression, and the incidence of cardiovascular complications. Med Phys. 2002;29(10):2391-403.
5. Wallace W, Thomson A, Kelsey T. The radiosensitivity of the human oocyte. Hum Reprod. 2003;18:117-21.
6. Lushbaugh CC, Casarett GW. The effects of gonadal irradiation in clinical radiation therapy: a review. Cancer. 1976;37:1111-25.
7. Green DM. Fertility and pregnancy outcome after treatment for cancer in childhood or adolescence. Oncologist. 1997;2:171-9.
8. Meirow D, Nugent D. The effects of radiotherapy and chemotherapy on female reproduction. Hum Reprod Update. 2001;7:535-43.
9. Wallace W, Thomson A, Saran F, et al. Predicting age of ovarian failure after radiation to a field that includes the ovaries. Int J Radiat Oncol Biol Phys. 2005;62:738-44.
10. Green DM, Hall B, Zevon MA. Pregnancy outcome after treatment for acute lymphoblastic leukemia during childhood or adolescence. Cancer. 1989;64:2335-9.
11. Liao L, Doyle J, Crouch NS, et al. Dilation as treatment for vaginal agenesis and hypoplasia: a pilot exploration of benefits and barriers as perceived by patients. J Obstet Gynaecol. 2006;26(2):144-8.
12. Howell S, Shalet S. Gonadal damage from chemotherapy and radiotherapy. Endocrinol Metab Clin North Am. 1998;27(4):927-43.
13. Meirow D. Reproduction post-chemotherapy in young cancer patients. Mol Cell Endocrinol. 2000;169:123-31.
14. Viviani S, Santoro A, Ragni G, et al. Gonadal toxicity after combination chemotherapy for Hodgkin's disease. Comparative results of MOPP vs ABVD. Eur J Cancer Clin Oncol. 1985;21:601-5.
15. Papdakis V, Valchopapadopoulou E, Van Syckle K, et al. Gonadal function following therapy for childhood Hodgkin's disease. Med Pediatr Oncol. 1999;32:366-72.
16. Byrne J, Fears TR, Gail MH. Spontaneous recovery of chemotherapy-induced primary ovarian failure: implication for management. Clin Endocrinol. 1997;46:217-9.
17. Thomson A, Critchley H, Kelnar C, et al. Late reproductive sequelae following treatment of childhood cancer and options for fertility preservation. Best Pract Res Clin Endocrinol Metab. 2002;16:311-34.
18. Bahadur G, Ralph D. Gonadal tissue cryopreservation in boys with paediatric cancers. Hum Reprod. 1999;14:11-17.
19. Rivkees SA, Crawford JD. The relationship of gonadal activity and chemotherapy-induced gonadal damage. J Am Med Assoc. 1988;259(14):2123-5.
20. Warne GL, Fairley KF, Hobbs JB, et al. Cyclophosphamide induced ovarian failure. N Engl J Med. 1973;289(22):1159-62.
21. Richardson SJ, Senikas V, Nelson JF. Follicular depletion during the menopausal transition: evidence for accelerated loss and ultimate exhaustion. J Clin Endocrinol Metab. 1987;65(6):1231-7.
22. Aslam I, Fishel S, Moore H, et al. Fertility preservation of boys undergoing anti-cancer therapy: a review of the existing situation and prospects for the future. Hum Reprod. 2000;15(10):2154-9.
23. Rosenlund B, Sjoblom P, Tornblom M, et al. In-vitro fertilization and intracytoplasmic sperm injection in the treatment of infertility after testicular cancer. Hum Reprod. 1998;13(2):414-8.
24. Schwarzer JU, Fiedler K, Hertwig IV, et al. Sperm retrieval procedures and intracytoplasmatic spermatozoa injection with epididymal and testicular sperms. Urol Int. 2003;70(2):119-23.
25. Hovatta O. Cryopreservation of testicular tissue. Mol Cell Endocrinol. 2000;169:113-5.
26. Togas Tulandi MD, Sundus Al-Took MD. Laparoscopic ovarian suspension before irradiation. Fertil Steril. 1998;70:381-3.
27. Ray GR, Trueblood HW, Enright LP, et al. Oophoropexy (a means of preserving ovarian function following pelvic megavoltage radiotherapy for Hodgkin's disease). Radiology. 1970;96:175-80.
28. Nahhas WA, Nisce LZ, D'Angio GL, et al. Lateral ovarian transposition. Obstet Gynecol. 1971;38:785-8.
29. Belinson JL, Doherty M. A new technique for ovarian transposition. Surg Gynaecol Obstet. 1984;159:157-60.

30. Husseinzadeh N, Nahhas WA, Velkley DE, et al. The preservation of ovarian function in young women undergoing pelvic radiation therapy. Gynecol Oncol. 1984;18:373-9.
31. Gabriel DA, Bernard SA, Lambert J, et al. Oophoropexy and the management of Hodgkin's disease. Arch Surg. 1986;121:1083-5.
32. Thomas PRM, Winstanly D, Peckham MJ, et al. Reproductive and endocrine function in patients with Hodgkin's disease (effects of oophoropexy and irradiation). Br J Cancer. 1976;33:226-31.
33. Kovacev M. Exteriorization of ovaries under the skin of young women operated upon for cancer of the cervix. Am J Obstet Gynecol. 1968;101:756-9.
34. Leporrier M, von Theobald P, Roffe JL, et al. A new technique to protect ovarian function before pelvic irradiation. Cancer. 1987;60:2201-4.
35. Farber LA, Ames JW, Rush S, et al. Laparoscopic ovarian transposition to preserve ovarian function before pelvic radiation and chemotherapy in a young patient with rectal cancer. Med Gen Med. 2005;7(1):66.
36. Williams RS, Little RD, Mendenhall NP. Laparoscopic oophoropexy and ovarian function in the treatment of Hodgkin disease. Cancer. 1999;86(10):2138-42.
37. Clowse MEB, Behera MA, Anders CK, et al. Ovarian preservation by GnRH agonists during chemotherapy: a meta-analysis. J Womens Health. 2009;18:311-9.
38. Elgindy EA, El-Haieg DO, Khorshid OM, et al. Gonadotrophin suppression to prevent chemotherapy induced ovarian damage: a randomized controlled trial. Obstet Gynaecol. 2013;121:178-86.
39. Oktay K, Buyuk E, Linertella N, et al. Fertility preservation in Breast Cancer patients: A prospective controlled comparison of ovarian stimulation with Tamoxifen and Letrozole for embryo cryopreservation. J Clin Oncol. 2005;23:4347-53.
40. Homburg R, van der Veen F, Silber SJ. Oocyte vitrification—women's emancipation set in stone. Fertil Steril. 2009;91:1319-20.
41. Silber S. Ovarian transplantation: new technique gives greatly improved results in this delicate operation. In: 25th annual conference of the European Society of Human Reproduction and Embryology. Amsterdam, The Netherlands; 2009. Abstract no: O-037.
42. Grundy R, Gosden RG, Hewitt M, et al. Personal practice: fertility preservation for children treated for cancer (1): scientific advances and research dilemmas. Arch Dis Child. 2001;84(4):355-9.
43. Grundy R, Larcher V, Gosden RG, et al. Fertility preservation for children treated for cancer (2): ethics of consent for gamete storage and experimentation. Arch Dis Child. 2001;84(4):360-2.
44. Hawkins MM, Draper GJ, Smith RA. Cancer among 1,348 offspring of survivors of childhood cancer. Int J Cancer. 1989;43(6):975-8.
45. Kim SS, Radford J, Harris M, et al. Ovarian tissue harvested from lymphoma patients to preserve fertility may be safe for autotransplantation. Hum Reprod. 2001;16(10):2056-60.
46. Lee SJ, Schover LR, Partridge AH, et al. American Society of Clinical Oncology. American Society of Clinical Oncology recommendations on fertility preservation in cancer patients. J Clin Oncol. 2006;24(18):2917-31.

SUGGESTED READING

1. Del Mastro L, Boni L, Michelotti A, et al. Effect of the gonadotropin-releasing hormone analogue Triptorelin on the occurrence of chemotherapy-induced early meno-pause in premenopausal women with breast cancer-a randomized trial. JAMA. 2011;306:269-76.

CHAPTER

87

Role of a Counselor in ART Treatment

Diana Divya Crasta

INTRODUCTION

Bearing a child is an important goal of everyone's life. The concept of bearing children is been routed deeply into the mind of people ever since they are born.

Infertility is one of the most not spoken, yet one of the common concerns of mankind. It affects the feeling of "no child" and creates lots of stress and anxiety among the couple and family. Infertility also comes with huge stigma and discrimination primarily for the women in Indian scenario. It has been observed that the people who come for infertility treatment require lot of motivation and support in taking decision and manage their own issues, which may be hampering them in taking the right decision for themselves.

INFERTILITY COUNSELING

What is infertility counseling?

Infertility counseling aims at providing psychological support to the patients and their family members during their treatment. This involves identifying the concerns or problem that the patient is going through because of not having children or may be past experience of stigma and discrimination, which resulted in various psychological conditions. In other words, counseling is required for the patients while taking treatment depending on the situation, treatment, or concerns they are experiencing at that point of time.

Infertility can impact a person's life and it may create a problem to lead a normal life. Some of the emotional impacts of infertility are:

- *Anger*: The fact that the couple is not able to have a child like some of their friends makes them feel angry as well as jealous. The anger and jealousy feeling harm their emotional and mental health and this will result in physical problems
- *Loss*: The patient may experience the feeling of loss. They may feel that the dreams or desire they had to have a child are not met with and their life has no meaning
- *Denial*: Most of the people do not want to accept that they have a problem in conceiving a child naturally. This will make them to wait for some miracle to happen and leaves them childless for quite a long time
- *Shame*: People will feel shame and experience stigma due to the infertility problems. Some time, society makes them feel ashamed for being childless
- *Blame*: Blaming themselves or each other for not able to conceive is a common factor. This feeling also results in being "incomplete" and creates guilt among the patient. The other factor is blaming the spouse. In most of the cases, it is the woman who takes blame for not able to conceive. This also results in husband planning for another marriage.

At the same time, people who are facing infertility do not talk or share the problems or concerns they face. Some of the common reasons are:

- Social stigma related to infertility
- For Indian couples, infertility is more of social issue than a biological issue. At the same time, it is very emotional subject
- Family members do not encourage such discussions and it is been always hushed
- Fear of being judgmental
- Fear about people's comments or the opinion created
- Fear of social gatherings
- Feeling of embracement.

All these aspects impact a person emotionally and they are left with no answer nor do they know whom and where to approach. When people come to visit fertility center for treatment, they bring lot of unsolved or unspoken pains. During these situations, the role of the counselor is very crucial. They need to recognize and address the "current" or "felt need" of the patient. Hence, it is important to have a psychological counseling for such patients.

Addressing Psychological Needs of People Going for Treatment

Keeping the family, social, and environmental factors, the role of the counselor is very essential for people taking infertility treatment. The need for psychological counseling majorly can be divided in three stages of the treatment that are before, during, and after the treatment.

Before Treatment

People respond differently to the infertility problems they face and everyone has their own way of dealing with it. People may accept infertility or they may blame themselves or each other, blame their fate, etc. when patient decides to visit the fertility center, he/she comes with lots of hope. This hope also includes lot of fear, confusion, stress, or anxiety. In other words, people hope for the best but the fear of failure always there.

Some of the important factors/points that the patient may feel before treatment are:

- *Clinical factors*: These include everything about the treatment. Starting from understanding the treatment to success rate and the different things involved in the treatment
- *Personal factors*: The personal factors like selection of the right clinic, ethical practices, working on the unspoken pains, dealing with the spouse/family and working on own self, keeping themselves positive from the friends and social media, etc. All these factors are present in each one's life, they affect the psychological well being and is an import factor in their mental health. The psychological counselor is required to understand these factors and many other while counseling the patients.

These are very common concerns that each and every patient experiences before or during the treatment. It becomes very important to identify the emotional stress they are going through.

Role of the counselor before the treatment:

- *Identify the concerns or needs*: Counselor with his/her empathetic skills explores the underlying reasons, which are bothering the patients. This may include multiple sessions with the patient, i.e. one to one, one to couple, or one to group before starting the treatment. It is important for the counselor to help the patient in reducing the stress and anxiety related to treatment
- *Working with the changes*: The psychological counselor helps the patient to deal with the emotional changes that may occur during the treatment. This may include the relationship between the couple, family, or social changes. The counselor deals with the sensitive issues while dealing with the changes. In the counseling sessions, therapeutic interventions will help in dealing with the changes that may occur and help in attaining the quality of life
- *Accepting the advised treatment*: One of the important concerns that the patient may experience is of accepting the treatment advised. Patients may have myths and misconceptions regarding assisted reproductive technology (ART) treatment. The role of the counselor is to counsel the need and reason for the kind of treatment advised, legal implications involved and thus helps them to take a decision by providing awareness, supportive counseling, and implication counseling.

During the Treatment

Once the patient decides to start the treatment, the role of the counselors also inflates. The counselor is required to keep a close look on the different things that may happen during the treatment. Not all patients will be able to give positive results. The consultant may have to change the treatment, based on the response or developments after initiating the treatment. Therefore, it is important for a counselor to consider the following stages during the treatment.

Stages to be considered:

- *Day of the stimulation*: The 1st day of the stimulation can be a combination of various emotions and feelings for the patient—the feeling of anxiety, stress, fear or happiness, and thinking about the future. Counseling on the 1st day of the stimulation means helping the patient to be calm and positive. Couple counseling is very important when the patient starts treatment
- *Day of follicle scan*: This is the day when the consultants decide to continue or stop the stimulation based on the response. It will be a heart-breaking moment for the patient, if the stimulation gets canceled. This may also result in changes in the kind of treatment offered further. The counselor is required to understand the importance of this stage and support the patient to cope up with the changes and prepare them.

- *Day of ovum pick-up (OPU)*: The day of OPU is the day where the patient is looking forward for good quality and good number of eggs. It is important for the counselor to meet the patient before the pick-up and work toward reducing felt emotions of the patient. Counseling post pick-up is also important, as the patient and her family member are looking forward for the details. However, it is important for the counselor to understand the different aspects of OPU day and counsel the patient accordingly. Some of the situations that may arise post-OPU are:
  - No oocytes
  - Less number of oocytes or not good quality oocytes and resulting in a cancelled cycle post egg retrieval.

  The counselor should be aware of the emotions and feelings associated with post-OPU. Having an understanding will help them in working with the patients based on the situations. It is important to remember and consider that each and every patient has a different way of seeing and handling things. At the same time, working in collaboration and coordination with the clinical team is essential in this situation.
- *Day of embryo transfer*: Another important day for the patients, where their hopes are focused. The counselor is required to meet them before and after the transfer to make sure that the patients are calm and stress free. It is important to understand the emotions patient is experiencing and counsel them accordingly. Similarly, patient may want to meet the clinical team to give instructions post-transfer. However, the patient may go through the following situation and thus there will not be any embryos transfer.
  - No embryos formed, resulted in no embryos for transfer
  - Total number of embryos and embryos grade.

  Not having embryos for transfer creates and brings lots of emotional disturbance and the patient may go through emotional breakdown. Counseling the patients post the embryo status is very important to help them to cope up with their situation and prepare them for the next treatment plan.

Role of the counselor during the treatment:

- *Counseling based on the stage*: The counselor is required to understand the stages of the treatment and the kind of the emotions associated with the same. Good awareness of the stage and being sensitive and empathetic will help in doing the right counseling at the right time
- *Focus on both gender*: Counseling and preparing the men is as important as counseling the women. The counselor should understand that the men also go through lots of unspoken emotional problems and they also need emotional support. At the same time, women may experience more stress and anxiety due to the medication. Therefore, couple counseling is very important during the treatment
- *Dealing with the changes*: The changes in treatment during the treatment period may be unexpected or patients may not have prepared for the same. The psychological counselor will understand the emotions involved during this phase and help the patients to cope up with the changes
- *Counseling on the day of the procedure*: Relaxation of body and mind is a key during the procedure. By meeting the patient before and after the procedure, the counselor will make it easy for the patient. Deep breathing exercises and relaxation techniques before the procedure are helpful. At the same time, answering all the quarries post the procedures (mostly clinical team) makes them relax as well
- *Helping the patients to stay calm and positive*: It is important to stay positive during the treatment for both husband and wife. Positive mind and body help to bring positivity in life. However, being anxious during this period is normal. The regular counseling sessions when the patient is on treatment will help the patent during the treatment. The counselor can plan the counseling sessions based on the need and situation.

After the Treatment

One of the stressful and anxious periods for the patient is the waiting period for result. This means that the patients require emotional support to stay positive and need to keep themselves occupied in different activities. The major stage or factor post-treatment is the result. The stages in post treatment are:

- *Waiting period*: Postembryos transfer till the result, the patient may experience anxiety due to result. Even though the doctors ask them to have a normal life, the patients may find it difficult to lead one. However, knowing the situation the psychological counselors help the patients to handle their anxiety
- *Day of the result*: This is one of the most awaited days and most difficult days. Handling the patient postnegative results should be the high priority for the clinical as well as for the counseling team
- *Dealing with miscarriages/abortions/ectopic*: This can happen at any stage of the pregnancy and this is another important factor, which requires to be handled well.

Role of the counselor post-treatment:

- *Waiting period*: It is important to counsel the patients about how to handle the waiting period. The counselor can encourage them to take up different activity/follow dreams, etc. depending on their interest level. Couple counseling may be very effective during the waiting period. Calling the (telephonic conversation) patient during the waiting period will be more effective also, because the counselor will get the better clarity on patient's mind set and they can counsel accordingly
- *Counseling postnegative results*: Dealing with the negative result is the most important role of a counselor. Understanding the emotions that the patient is going through should be the priority in patients with a negative pregnancy test, coming back for counselling. The counseling sessions and rapport established before and during the treatment will help in dealing postresults. There are two aspects here:
  1. Patients with frozen embryos
  2. Patients without frozen embryos.

The counseling will defer based on the patients with or without frozen embryos. However, it is important to check if the patient is able to handle the negative result. This can be checked only by having a counseling session with the patient. The counseling session should be the combination of clinical and psychological and thus helps the patient to cope up with the negative result. It is good to have a couple counseling during clinical counseling; however, the psychological counseling can be individual or couple or both. Depending on the coping skills of the patient, the counselor can perform therapies.

The key aspects during the negative β-hCG counseling are:

- Check the acceptance level postresult
- Look for the situations around the negative result and look for the "current felt need" of the patient
- *The matters bothering the patient much and the blocks (emotional or physical) created due to the negative result*: This can be clinical, personal, family, society, etc.
- Once the counselor understands the patient, the counselor can work on managing the loss, stress, depression, or any feeling expressed by the patient
- *Counseling postmiscarriages/abortions/ectopic*: Like the negative β-hCG counseling, it is important to counsel the patient postmiscarriage/abortions/ectopic pregnancy. Counselor should check the next treatment plan advised before counseling the patient.

Counseling during the Third-party Reproduction

This is when one or the couple is not able to produce good-quality oocytes or sperms and is looking for third party or donor. When third-party reproduction is been advised, the couple requires support in accepting and also understanding its implications.

Third-party reproduction has three major categories; they are:

1. *Sperm donation*: When a man is not able to produce sperm naturally or through a surgical procedure then the donor sperm is advised for the couple.
   Psychological factors associated with the sperm donation:
   - The man who advised to go for sperm donation may feel that he is incomplete and the emotions are associated with the male ego
   - Feeling of guilt that he is not able to give a child of his own and not able to continue the family legacy
   - Acceptance of the child born of different genes
   - Concern about matching and identifying the right donor
   - Feelings of frustration, anger, isolation, depression, sadness, hopelessness, helplessness, suicidal ideation etc. are the common feelings that the man may go though.
2. *Oocytes donation*: There are clinical reasons when woman is advised to go for oocytes donation. The IVF center identifies healthy and eligible donor as per Indian Council of Medical Research (ICMR) guidelines for oocytes donation.
   Psychological factors associated with the oocytes donation:
   - Getting pregnant and having a baby is fundamental life event for women in Indian society. There is no other major life goal for them apart from becoming a mother and taking of the child and family
   - Women are being blamed or held responsible for infertility—this means if a woman is not able to have her own then she is not complete
   - Family pressure, societal pressure, and more than this a woman herself feels guilty for not able to give a child of her own to the family
   - Fear of losing husband or abandoning her for not able to have a child of their own. In a few cases, it may be irrespective of who is having clinical reasons
   - Accepting a child born from donor gametes
   - Living in the fear of life being out of control, so as the relationships and social life.
3. *Embryo donation*: There could be clinical or financial reasons for a couple to opt for donor embryo made from donor egg and donor sperm.
   Psychological factors associated with the embryo donation:
   - Couple advised to go for embryo donation goes through mixed feelings regarding taking the treatment

   - The dilemma between embryo donation versus adoption
   - Acceptance of the gametes
   - Concern about the selecting the right match for the couple
   - Feeling of guilt, frustration, loss, and desire to have a child are the major factors in the couple.

Role of the counselor: The counselor plays an important role based on the treatment advised to the patient. The role of the counselor is been explained in detail below:

- *Awareness*: It is important for the counselor to create awareness about the donor program that is been carried out at the IVF clinics. The selection of the donor, identification, matching the donor, clinical aspects that are taken care of, confidentiality, etc. needs to explain well in advance. The awareness helps the patient to evaluate the details and decide based on that. Basically, the recipient will get to know that the agency or the IVF center finalizes the healthy (with mind and body) donor. Transparency and ethical practice are the top most priority in cases of donor gametes
- *Acceptance*: Accepting donor gametes is not as easy as it is seen. It is a matter of lifelong commitment for the recipient. The recipient may have questions about what kind of donor been selected, their health, ethnicity, level of matching, etc. Understanding the mind set or concerns shared by the recipient will help the counselor to counsel them accordingly. The important point to counsel is not only accepting the donor gametes but also nurturing the child born through this treatment without any bias
- *Implication*: It is important to counsel the recipients on the implications of donor gametes. This means that the recipient is aware and prepared for the child, which is not completely born from their genes. But environment, upbringing, and nurturing play an important role in shaping the personality of an individual. Considering each person is unique in their own way and being nonjudgmental is an important consideration
- *Dealing with the family*: It is completely left on the couple to decide whom they would like to or how much they would like to share regarding their treatment, especially when donor gametes been advised. The counselor can share the pros and cons related to the same, which help the recipients to decide what suits best for them. However, the counselor should remember that it is absolutely fine, if the couple does not want to share about the same to their family members.

Types of Counseling

Based on the need and situation at any stage of the treatment cycle, the counselor will decide to have session through one to one, one to couple, or one to group. Depending on the treatment situation discussed in the previous section, the counseling can be divided into the following methods:

- *Individual counseling*: Individual counseling is a kind of counseling, which helps the patient to get the focused counseling sessions. This is very useful when the patient has concerns about him-/herself or in situations where he/she is not able to come out of it and that block him/her in taking the right decision regarding treatment. Some of the examples are patients who have experienced multiple negative cycles and are not able to cope up with it or to those who are not able to accept that they need donor gametes or situations where they are victims of stigma and discrimination, etc. These situations cause stress, depression, or in a few cases suicidal ideation, thus overall affects the patients emotionally and physically. Individual counseling can be a combination of counseling and therapy, depending on the patient and his/her condition
- *Couple counseling*: Fertility treatment is a journey of the couple; both of them go through physical and emotional changes. However, in a few situations, the couple may disagree for treatment or they may go through marital issues, which are common. But it is important for them to accept each other and decide about the treatment. Relationship plays very important role at any stage of life. Couple counseling facilitates in keeping the couple positive, support each other, work on the differences (if any), accept the strength and weakness, improve communication with each other and thus helps them during the journey of parenthood. Overall couple counseling provides better way of accepting the treatment and to start a new journey as parents. The counselor can use counseling and therapeutic sessions for the same
- *Family counseling*: Having a child in Indian context is not only a decision of the couple but also a decision of the close family members. Similarly, during the fertility treatment, the family members are involved or interested in understanding about the treatment and then influence the decision-making process. In this situation, it is very essential for the counselor to counsel the family members as well. Also, remember what and how much to counsel or what kind of information to be given. For example in a few cases, the couple may not

want the center to talk/inform about the donor gametes to the family members. Counseling session should be planned based on the need, situation, and level of involvement of the family members.

Support Group Meetings

Infertility or fertility treatment brings a lot of psychosomatic situations for a patient. Not sharing about infertility makes them feel lonely and isolated many a time. In these cases, support group meetings could be the better options for patients to interact, listen to others on how they coped up, managed, or faced different situations in life because of infertility.

Support group meetings are those gatherings or get-togethers where the group of people with the similar problem and/or patients with a positive outcome come together and provide help and companionship to one another. Support group meeting brings together those people with the similar issues or problems and connects them, it makes the people to understand that they are not alone, it helps them to ventilate and helps in bringing the positivity.

CONCLUSION

The role of psychological counselor is very important for patients who are planning or have decided to take fertility treatment. Counselor brings changes in the life of a patient through his/her empathetic listening, allowing ventilating the feelings, being nonjudgmental, counseling at the right time, making the patient feel important, encouraging, supporting, and more importantly responding to their emotional needs. Taking treatment is not just to have a baby, but it is a responsibility and commitment. A good and positive family produces a healthy and positive child. Getting the right information and going for right treatment with all positive mind and body give a happy family.

SUGGESTED READING

1. Ahuja M, Counseling in Infertility : Practice Guideline. South Asian Federation of Obstetrics and Gynecology, 2009;1(2): 38-43. (published by Jaypee Journals)
2. Appleton TC, Baron J, Bitzer, et al. "Guidelines for Counselling in Infertility" Human Reproduction (Oxford, Englan), 2001 Jun;16(6):1301-4.
3. Covington SN, Burns LH. Infertility Counseling: A Comprehensive Handbook for Clinicians. London: Cambridge University Press; 2006.
4. Gameiro S, Boivin J, Dancet E, et al.; ESHRE guideline: Routine Psychosocial Care in Infertility and Medically Assisted Reproduction-A Guide for Fertility Staff. Hum Reprod. 2015;30(11):2476-85.
5. Indian Council of Medical Research National Academy of Medical Sciences (India), New Delhi. (2005). National Guidelines for Accreditation, Supervision and Regulation of ART Clinics in India. [online] Available from https://www.icmr.nic.in/sites/default/files/guidelines/Guidline_content.pdf [Accessed January, 2019].
6. Peterson B, Boivin J, Norré J, et al. An introduction to infertility counseling: a guide for mental health and medical professionals. J Assist Reprod Genet. 2012;29(3):243-8.

CHAPTER

88

Deriving Happiness through Adoption

Avinash Kumar

Adoption is a beautiful experience providing us with a unique opportunity to look beyond our own need or desire (to adopt) and connect with another human being with selfless love and compassion. However, owing to its stereotyped projection in films and fiction, many people in India do not consider it as a default choice for initiating one's family, or continue to harbor myths when a need arises them to adopt a child.

There are 60 million destitute children in India and about 30 million families affected by infertility. Yet the country clocks fewer than 20,000 parents registered for adoption and an even fewer 4,000 adoptions per year. Contrast this with the United States, a country with almost one fourth the population of India, which registers more than 200,000 adoptions per year. The challenge lies with gross misconceptions prevalent in the society around adoption.

Such beliefs have been perpetrated for generations that adoption is kind of last resort for middle-aged couple who fails to conceive a biological child of their own. As and when they are *pushed* to such a need (of adopting), there exists a pool of infants from amongst which the couple can choose the most adorable, healthy, and handsome baby. Further, the child has to be adopted when infant, so that it is unaware of the fact of adoption, and this truth need not be told to the child ever, for it will break the bond—and the heart. For the same reason, the fact of adoption has to be hush-hushed within the family, neighbors, and workplace, because it somewhere reflects upon the couple inability to reproduce. In this whole saga of overemphasizing the (lack of) ability to reproduce, the need of the parent and the choice of a child—the core constituency that makes adoption possible—is completely ignored and suffers (Fig. 1).

Children are the first casualty when parents decide to give them up for adoption. Children struggle to survive in the most critical hours after its birth, for want of love and care that they need and rightly deserve. Children face challenges yet again in getting a reentry into a family with parents judging them for their looks, abilities, age, complexion, cast, and religion. Children are robbed of support and accommodations that could help them realize their potential, and children live in humiliation carrying the label of "being adopted" for the rest of their lives. All because adoption is looked through the lens of a parent's need and its redemption so much so that our laws too have reinforced this doctrine of need. Need of the parent!

It is time we began looking at adoption from the child's perspective and began the "Number of Reimagining Adoption" section.

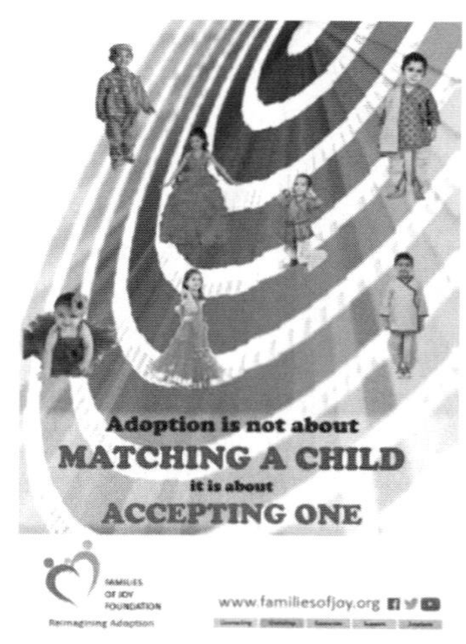

Fig. 1

NUMBER OF REIMAGINING ADOPTION

Unlike law, religion, science, taxation, relations, marriage, careers, and whole lot of domains prescribed at school and college education, adoption has completely escaped the attention of our educators. It is not part of any curriculum, there are no festivals dedicated to it, it is not enshrined in any political party's manifesto, and there is hardly any family or public conversations around it. Whatever little people understand of adoption is largely fed through Bollywood and fiction in melodramatic overtones. Their portrayal of adoption is oblivious of the legalities and contemptuous of transparency that it deserves. Little wonder that even those people who are presented with an opportunity to experience adoption whether for themselves or for their kith and kin—react with sympathy, disagreement, bewilderment, shock, and disbelief.

Adoption sounds like a serious, gloomy, and secret affair so long as we drive the discussions from a parent's need. A need that is unfulfilled. A need that raises expectations. A need that defies reality. But the moment we place the child at the center of the dialog, the whole discourse gets filled with positivity, enthusiasm, and child-like energy, for a child's presence brings hope. When a child blossoms, the family blossoms. Even the darkest fears of how a child may react when told about adoption are easily addressed not by how we tell the child about its adoption—but how we think and talk of adoption—in the first place. The child merely reflects our own comfort and ease with the subject. And this comfort can come only through an objective assimilation of facts associated with adoption, not from Bollywood (Fig. 2).

That calls for putting adoption into our curriculum by the educators, developing inspiring content by the filmmakers, embracing positive adoption language (PAL) by the community, undertaking research in adoption by the scholars, offering tax incentives for adoptions by the Government, announcing child-centric policies by the regulators, declaring adoption-friendly policies by the employers, and rendering professional services by the lawyers, doctors, counselors, and therapists engaged in the adoption cycle. Together as a community, we need to build a positive identity in adoption for the child.

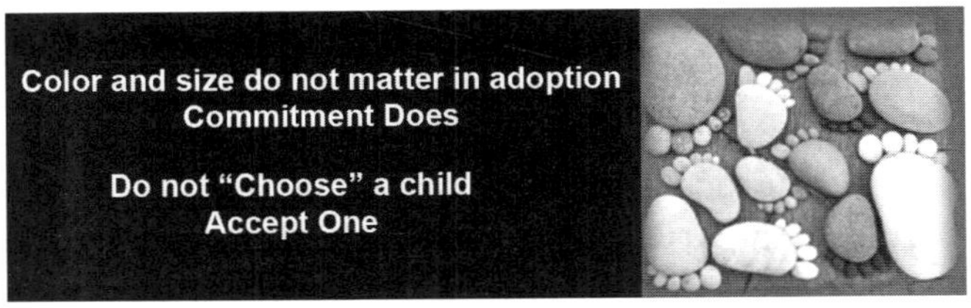

Color and size do not matter in adoption
Commitment Does

Do not "Choose" a child
Accept One

Fig. 2

ADOPTION IS NOT PLAN B

The first principle of adoption lies in accepting it with 100% of your commitment.

Each one of us is gifted uniquely. Some can sing, dance, play cricket, negotiate a business deal, swim, give a lecture, fight in military, etc. Reproducing a child is just another facet. Ability or inability to do either cannot be a judgment on one's life and personality. Moreover, there is a trigger for every decision that we take in life. Some decisions are consciously taken by us, while a few others are decided for us. The need to adopt may also come packaged in various options. That need is not important. The fact that you have decided to adopt IS. And that decision has to bear your 100% commitment. It is immaterial what transpired before adoption became relevant for you. Today we have all sorts of parents wanting to adopt a child—those affected by infertility, those who are single (mother or father), and those who want to add a sibling to their existing children through adoption. Those who only want to build their families through adoption. Those who hope to make up for the loss of a child. No one driver is more important than the other. No one driver is worth spending a thought. What matters is—how to make most of adoption.

ADOPTION NEEDS PREPARATION

Having a need to adopt does not automatically qualify a parent to adopt a child. Parents may not be ready to adopt—howsoever desperate they may be. Even those parents who voluntarily decide to adopt need to prepare for adoption. Here are just few of the aspects related to adoption where parents need to upgrade their skills, refine their language, align their thoughts, and level their expectations:

- Understanding the legal process
- Learning PAL
- Engaging the extended family
- Managing preferences and waiting in adoption
- Accepting the first child referred in adoption
- Settling the child in the family
- Empowering the child through support, accommodations, custom care, and *love*
- Telling the child about adoption.

You should be flexible to throw away some of the hardened stereotypes. For example, be open to adopt a child above 2 years of age. Apart from a much shorter wait time, the health of the child has stabilized by the age of 2 years, and you are likely to run into fewer surprises.

Or, refrain from "choosing a child" or waiting to see all the three referrals. Approach a counselor if you are facing challenge in accepting the first child referred to you.

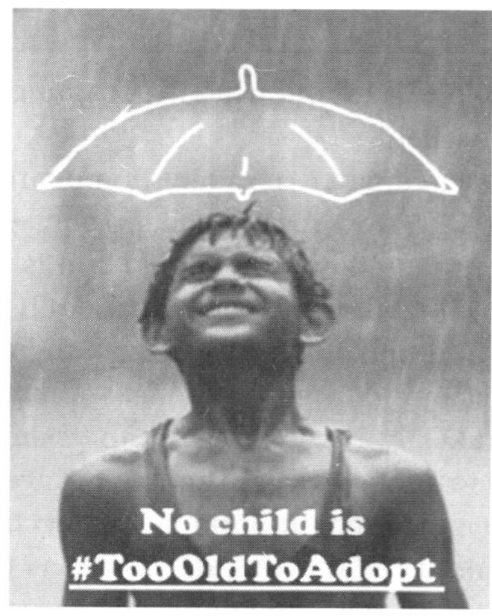

Fig. 3

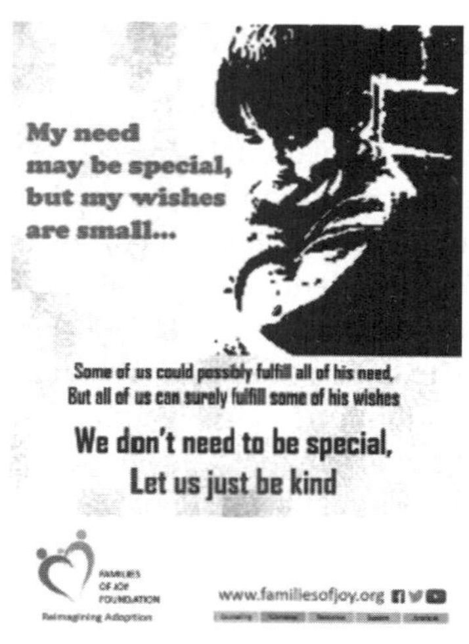

Fig. 4

Make it a habit to view the profiles under the "Number of Immediate Placement Category" and "Number of Special Needs Category" to locate a child you can support. There is *zero wait* time in either categories, and you will be amazed at how you discover the child destined to come to you.

A professionally qualified counselor can guide you in preadoption and postadoption phases (Fig. 3).

CHECK YOUR READINESS

A parent is ready for adoption once it starts looking at adoption from the child's perspective, beyond their own need, biases, or myths. The parent has to be comfortable with the idea of adoption, engage their kith and kin, believe in telling the child about adoption, and to position adoption as a happy event to the child. This requires setting aside the notions developed through hearsay or casual conversations, some of those include:

- Adoption is for childless couples only—there are several parents who are adopting children in addition of or even without requiring to have their biological kids. Adopting a child does not mean that you should not or cannot have your biological children
- Older children do not bond well—80% of the parents registered for adoption in India opt for an infant or youngest possible child owing to this misconception. Older children are more responsible, have a more stable health, and bond better with age-appropriate parents
- Child should be matched with the parent—nothing could be more racial, discriminatory, and illogical than the ill-conceived concept of matching a child with the parent. Unfortunately, even the government regulations provide for and use the term "matching-of-a-child". A child will develop its own personality, and it is naïve to seek comfort in similar looks of the child. This also leads to debate upon adopting a child from local agencies so that the child matches the appearance of the parents. Several parents add months to their wait in adoption opting for nearby regions to adopt from, even as there may be no children available for adoption in certain areas
- Don't tell the child about adoption—a child has to be told about its adoption because it is very much part of their identity, resolves several situations that may arise out of medical necessity, and reflects upon the parents comfort and commitment in the first place. It is important to tell the child about adoption, first of all, and in a positive context, even before you tell the child that it was adopted
- Children should not be placed with single parents—the marital status of parent is irrelevant. There are millions of "couples" who could adopt a child but may not be simply interested in adoption. On the contrary, there are thousands of people who may make an excellent parent (Fig. 4).

NOT ALL ADOPTIONS ARE LEGAL—NOT ALL LEGAL ADOPTIONS ARE SAFE!

For parents who may be emotionally drained by the time they decide to adopt a child, it may be difficult to overcome the temptation of Bollywood-styled adoptions—where in you visit an agency, choose a child, and start singing lullabies 3 days later. Nothing could be farther from truth.

Adoption today in India requires online registration with Central Adoption Resource Authority (CARA), a proper due diligence process, and a long wait as per your preferences indicated at the time of registration. Anyone promising you an instant adoption is bound to be an unethical agent, to be avoided at all cost.

Save an exception. Hindus in India can still adopt under the Hindu Adoption and Maintenance Act (1956) or HAMA as it is popularly known. Except that, HAMA was never meant for large-scale adoptions between anonymous parties. Apart from the fact that one can technically and legally adopt a child from any source claiming to offer a Hindu child from a Hindu parent, in matter of days—there are huge risks of child trafficking, adoption of child of fragile health, blackmailing, and money trail for adoptions under HAMA. The HAMA does not even require a court order to legalize the adoption—but does not safeguard the child's interest in absence of one. Only adopt through online registrations with CARA.

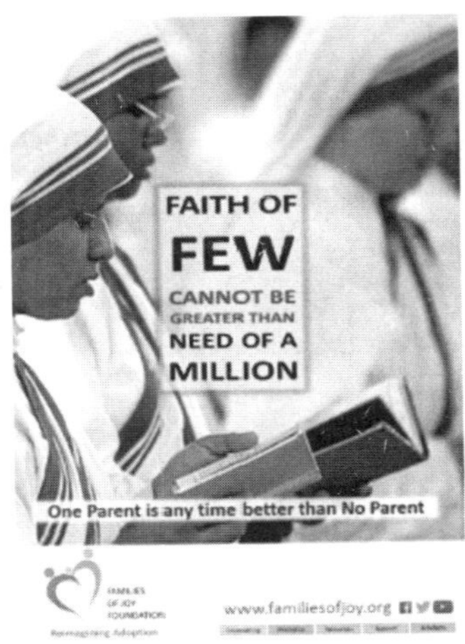

Fig. 5

THE PROCESS WITH CENTRAL ADOPTION RESOURCE AUTHORITY IS TRANSPARENT AND EQUITABLE

Parents desirous to adopt a child need to register with the CARA on their website www.cara.nic.in where the entire process is online. They don't need to visit any agency to search for a child. They need to upload required documentation and indicate their preferences at the time of registration. Once the registration is accepted, a home study is conducted by the nearest adoption agency that qualifies the parents for their eligibility to adopt a child. Once the home study is approved and uploaded, parents are awarded the seniority, and they receive a referral of the child, as per availability of children according to their preferences. Parents are referred a maximum of three profiles. Each profile is offered one at a time—60 days apart.

Upon receiving a referral, parents have choice to confirm the profile within 48 hours or let it pass (waiting for another). In the event of not accepting a child after confirming its profile (within 20 days of confirming the profile), or not confirming any of the three profiles, the parents are relegated to the bottom of the waitlist. They remain eligible for next referral as per the new seniority, as long as their home study is valid in the system. The home study is valid for 3 years. If the parents do not adopt a child in this 3-year period, they need to get their home study done once again.

Your seniority is determined solely by your date of registration. So if you are fairly certain of your decision to adopt, do not lose any further time in registering online. There are about 100 parents registering everyday on an average. However, your wait time depends upon your relative seniority within the group of parents who have the same choices as yours in terms of gender, age, and chosen states of adoption. Choose your preferences carefully to reduce avoidable wait (Fig. 5).

At present, there are roughly 18,000 parents registered for adoption with CARA and just under 2,000 children. More than half of these children have a special need, leaving just about 400 children below 2 years of age, legally free for adoption in the CARA system. This has resulted in a wait for about 15–18 months for getting your first referral. The wait time varies and could be shorter for different preferences according to age, gender, and state of the child. Most parents fall into the trap of adopting under HAMA to avoid this wait, but it is simply not worth it. Seek counseling to validate your preferences, explore options on tweaking your preferences, and how to manage this wait time.

Parents pay a total sum of 48,000 for all expenses, including the home study, legal fees, and other services rendered by the adoption agency. Once the child is adopted, the adoption agency files for an adoption order in the court, on behalf of the parents. The agency also arranges for the birth certificate in their name.

COUNSELING IS MUST

Even if you are aware of the overall process, it is a good idea to seek counseling in adoption. CARA itself offers counseling, there are nongovernmental organizations (NGOs) and adoption support groups who can also offer counseling. Counseling not only advises you in choosing the right preferences, it prepares you for adoption, helps you overcome the feeling of loss, connects you with the child, networks you with other families in adoption, trains you in PAL, and offers postadoption support. Genuine advice can help you decide which category to adopt from, e.g. immediate placement category, special need group,

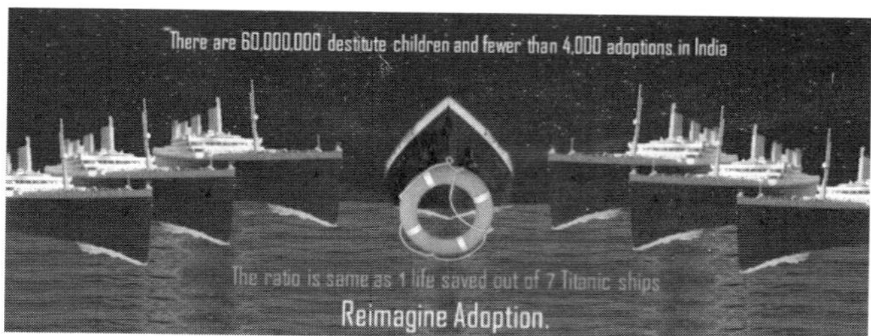

Fig. 6

older children, from anywhere in India, or from a given set of states.

Do not be restrained with a layman presumption of these categories. There are opportunities within each and only a good counselor can advise the option best suited for you—as each parent is different and capable of supporting a different kind of child. Consequently, you may be able to save a few months of your wait by opting a child who is more suitable for you—not necessarily for others. A good counselor can also point you to authentic resources in adoption, such as books, videos, families, lawyers, doctors, etc. and engage you in events associated with adoption (Fig. 6).

ACCEPTING THE FIRST CHILD YOU SEE IS ESSENTIAL

Most parents carry a mindset of seeing a few children before they make up their mind or "choose" a child. Waiting to see another child may be futile as the earlier profile may seem best to you, which you cannot revert to. Moreover, there is little comparison that is possible across children. So do not elongate your wait and delay the happy times in seeking multiple profiles. Adoption is not about "matching" a child. It is about accepting one.

You are bound to experience multitude of emotions as you meet "your" child. The child may appear different from the photo in the CARA profile. This is normal. Most children tend to appear weak and will pick up health once in family care. The child could have been sleeping, shy, hesitant, or hyperactive. If need be, plan for a couple of days and give yourself some time to understand child's behavior.

There are several benefits of accepting the first child that is referred to you as follows:

- Just as in a birth in the family where we accept the child wholeheartedly, irrespective of the color, weight, height, shape of the child, accepting the first child referred to us, helps us retain our innocence, commitment, and dedication to the child. We are not judging but accepting the child

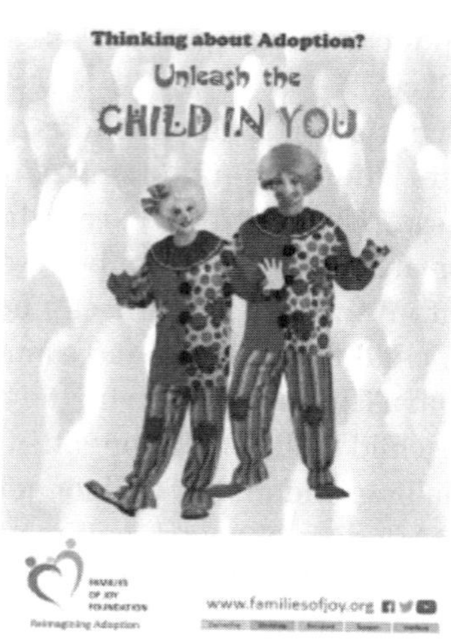

Fig. 7

- Given the ever-changing situation around availability of children and parents' commitments (there have been instances where people had to suddenly travel abroad, after they received their first referral, which they declined—or some constraint in the family requiring them to delay adoption, etc.), it is best to begin our beautiful journey on parenting—than delay the happiness coming our way
- Complete honesty, truthfulness, and commitment are the bedrock of relationships in adoption. As you share the story of adoption with your child, he/she will feel more confident when you tell that you accepted him/her as the first child you saw—than if you shared that you did not accept him/her as the first child that you saw
- Reserving and not accepting even the first child—puts you down at the bottom of the waitlist, and you lose your other two chances also. Not even reserving the first child, for fear of losing your seniority—but to keep your option open to "see" another child—is not even giving a fair chance to the child. For all you know, you are giving away the happiness rightfully destined for you (Fig. 7)!

REFRAIN FROM CONDUCTING ADDITIONAL MEDICAL TESTS

At times, parents have the doubt on how much to rely on the child's Medical Examination Report (MER) prepared by the agency. They want to know if they can conduct their own tests. Take care not to stress the child in this activity. In most cases, talking to the agency will assure you if their MER is reliable or not. Their body language, eye contact, quality of documentation will give you additional inputs for you to trust their due diligence.

Each child that is referred to you has been medically examined, and the medical reports are available along with the referral. These reports are valid for 6 months. Do not be tempted to conduct extramedical tests, unless really called for. Remember, a child loses up to 5% of its blood every time a new set of parents conducts its tests (blood test is the most basic requirement, in addition to other tests) and needs 2 weeks to recuperate the loss. Repeated tests by parents, sometimes week after week, cause extreme pain, trauma, and setback to the child's development. Even a perfectly healthy child may become sick with repeated exposure to tests, radiation, diagnostics, and strain.

Parenthood comes with lot of uncertainties. Follow you basic instincts. When in doubt, always keep the child's interest above everything else—and the best shall happen to you.

TELLING ABOUT ADOPTION

Contrary to what you see in films, it is absolute necessary to share the fact of adoption with your child. Not just because it may create challenges later, but primarily because it is your child's right to be aware of its identity, it helps your child to discover its true potential and relate to its own personality and physicality. One must remember that even if you do not tell, most likely the child will discover on its own, or through someone else about the fact of adoption, and that will create a huge trust deficit in you. Further, it will reinforce the stereotype that there must be something wrong in "adoption"—which is so very untrue. You will also come across several instances where you will need to share the fact of adoption, especially with the pediatrician as you cannot conceal that the child was not a natural delivery to you (Fig. 8).

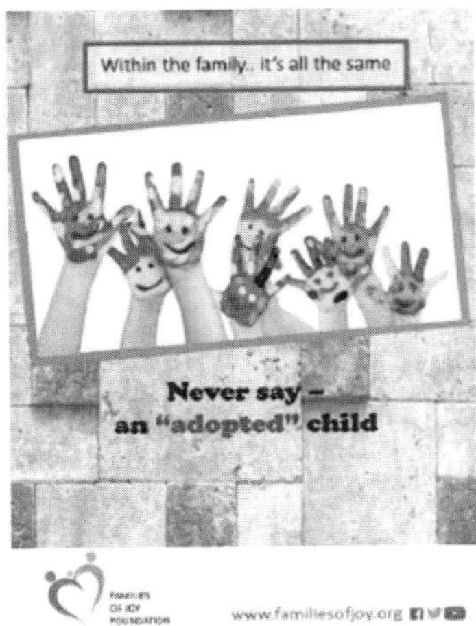

Fig. 8

What is most important that even before you share the fact of adoption, you refer to adoption as a happy event? So that as and when the child is made aware of the fact of its own adoption, it relates to it as a positive experience, rather than an undesirable experience.

ACCEPTING SOME GOSPEL TRUTHS

There are certain truths that you need to accept as a parent-in-adoption, in order to experience joy and bliss through adoption.

- *That* your child indeed has birth parents. Refer to them with respect, especially during growing up years of the child. This is required for a positive self-esteem of the child
- *That* your child will have a different personality that yours. Allow your child to realize his/her true potential and accept the child with its uniqueness. Given the space, your child will outperform your expectations, in a field of his/her competence
- *That* the child may develop some challenges postadoption, through growing years or later in life. Do not thrust your wishes—moral, academic, or emotional—on your child. Your child may live in the shadow of being different from you. Allow the child to take pride in the difference, rather than feeling ashamed or defensive about it
- *That* the child may continue to feel a void and an urge to search for its roots. Enable the child and support him/her in her quest for an identity. You have no reason to feel insecure.

EMBRACING POSITIVE ADOPTION LANGUAGE

What we think of adoption gets reflected in the words we choose, to describe of it. It is very common to come across phrases, such as "She is our adopted child/Do you know his real parents?/I would not like to adopt an older child/How can you adopt an illegitimate child?" Such expressions gain popularity due to their unabated use in films and fiction. Over a period of time, we get conditioned and immune to the insensitivity inherent in such phrases. We cannot even imagine the harm caused by reckless use of such terms. Such irresponsible lingo severely dents the self-confidence of a child who may already be grappling with her identity and seeking an approval as an adoptee in mainstream society.

Think again—there are far nicer and humane ways of communicating what we may actually need to, rather than using words that have coined to sell a drama of a novel. The beauty of using the PAL is that it shifts the focus from qualifying people in adoption or judging them to communication of the underlying fact.

You need to make a conscious effort to refer to it with a positive overtone. Labeling the child as an "adopted" child, comparing it with "real" children, and referring to adoption as "Plan B" are a result of conditioning over hundreds of years and stereotypes established by Bollywood and fiction. Make no big deal about adoption. Share your values, beliefs, and underlying message of humanity and love through adoption. Make your child feel comfortable with adoption and do not shy from correcting, educating, or sensitizing the uninitiated folks when accosted with uncomfortable situations. Prepare your children to expect these situations and train them to deal with such occasions through PAL. Make sure adoption is perceived as a positive identity by you, the child, and all those in your ecosystem (Fig. 9).

Life is a journey. Each one of us is blessed uniquely. Adoption may be the opportunity to rediscover ourselves, our hidden potentials, and our ability to love and connect with another soul bonded with love. Have faith in those

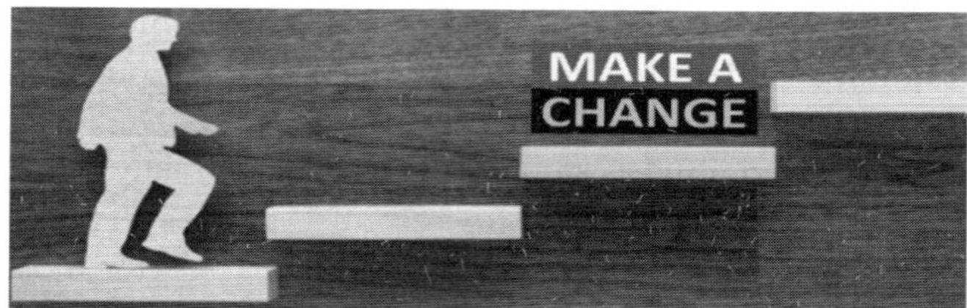

Fig. 9

core human principles, and when in doubt, always keep the child's interest above everything else. The best shall happen to you.

WISH YOU GOOD LUCK!

The author is a member of CARA Steering Committee, author, counselor, and a parent-in-adoption. He is the founder of the Families of Joy Foundation—an NGO espousing the cause of adoption and engaging with all the stakeholders in adoption. For more information, log on to www.familiesofjoy.org.

CHAPTER

89

Cross-border Reproductive Care

Pilar Alamá, José Remohí

INTRODUCTION

Infertility, or the inability to conceive, is a condition affecting an increasing number of people over the world. In recent years, this phenomenon has spread across both the Western countries and the developing countries (although with different characteristics), thus developing the features of a pandemic. For this reason the World Health Organization (WHO) acknowledged that infertility should be considered a disease to all intents and purposes, as it diminishes the health and well-being of the individuals who suffers from.[1] According to WHO data in 2010, it is estimated that 48.5 million couples worldwide were infertile.[2]

In more than 80% of countries, assisted reproductive technology (ART) was regulated by legislation, guidelines, or a combination of both. ART legislation depends on a variety of factors, such as social structure, political choices, ethical issues, and religious beliefs. There are huge variations noted when the regulatory legislations adopted by different countries to govern infertility treatment.[3]

A recent publication conducted a systematic review of published national and regional ART registry data to assess how has changed in clinical practice between 2004 and 2013 in Australia and New Zealand, Canada, Continental Europe, the United Kingdom (UK), Japan, Latin America, and the United States (US). The data reflect that about 7 million of ART cycles were performed utilizing both fresh and previously cryopreserved embryos from autologous oocytes.[4] It is estimated about 30% of ART cycles involving egg donation treatment. Therefore it could be possible that in this study period about 10 million of ART cycles have been performed.

DEFINITION OF CROSS-BORDER REPRODUCTIVE CARE

Cross-border reproductive care (CBRC) has been in the news for several years now. Health professionals prefer the term "CBRC" to the more derogatory "medical tourism" or "reproductive tourism" often used by the press. The word tourism implies choice, pleasure, and relaxation, very far from the physical and emotional challenges of fertility treatment. CBRC has been proposed by several societies. CBRC emphasizes that most patients who cross borders in search of reproductive treatment do this because they must and not by choice or for leisure as one would for a holiday.[5]

INCIDENCE OF CROSS-BORDER REPRODUCTIVE CARE

The full extent of CBRC in Europe is not precisely known because many national treatment registries do not record the patient's country of origin, only the treatment cycle. However, based on surveys performed over the past 10 years, it has been estimated that around 5% of all fertility care in Europe involves cross-border patients. It means that each year between 11,000 and 14,000 patients (24,000–30,000 cycles) in Europe travel outside of their country of residence to seek infertility-related CBRC.[6]

Spain and Belgium appear to be the most frequently visited European countries for treatment. Spain is the most active country in Europe with around 116,000 cycles performed in 2014 due to its efficient services (minimal waiting time) and plentiful donor gametes. Data from the Spanish national registry for in vitro fertilization (IVF) (2014) show that 10% of all fertility treatments in Spain were in foreign residents, most of them for egg donation treatment (66%). Patients come mostly from Italy, France, the Netherlands, and Germany.[7]

The United States remains a worldwide destination. A recent study performed by the Centers for Disease Control in the US found that almost 4% of all US cycles in 2013 were in non-US residents. According to a recent study published in 2017, the largest groups of incoming patients were from Canada (23.9%), México (14.2%), UK (10.2%), Japan (9.6%), and the People's Republic of China (6.5%).[8,9] In those cases where American and Canadian patients seek treatment outside, they tend to go to India/Asia and Europe. Traffic was highest in specialized procedures, such as egg donation, surrogacy, and preimplantation genetic testing.[10]

In Asia, India and Thailand are the main destinations for international assisted reproductive care, although Singapore, Malaysia, and South Korea are increasingly important as destinations, especially for regional patients. There are no accurate figures available of the numbers of people traveling for assisted reproductive services in these places, but it is estimated that approximately 400,000 foreign patients travel to Thailand each year for medical treatment.[11]

The volume of CBRC activity is difficult to estimate accurately, but according to the European Society of Human Reproduction and Embryology (ESHRE) and US data from a survey, it is estimated that approximately 5% of all fertility treatments involve cross-border travel.[12]

THE REASONS FOR CROSS-BORDER REPRODUCTIVE CARE

Most patients who cross borders in search of reproductive treatment do this because they must and not by choice or for leisure as one would for a holiday.[6]

There are several explanations for this trend among patients:

1. *Travel to avoid legal restrictions at home*:
   i. Legal regulation of ART worldwide occurs on a country-by-country basis. Logically jurisdictions with restrictive laws are more likely to serve as departure countries, while nations with few or no legal restrictions are supported as destination countries. The act of seeking fertility care outside of one's country of residence to avoid application of prevailing law is sometimes referred to as "circumvention tourism"[13]
   ii. Assisted reproductive technology regulation that motivates CBRC falls into two broad categories:
      a. Restrictions on *who* can access fertility care. Laws addressing "who" typically restrict access based on patient demographics. Restrictions on patient age (older), marital status (single), and sexual orientation (gays) are enclosed in law in some countries, sending these patients across national borders
      b. Restrictions on *what* fertility care can be accessed. Prohibitions on ART services, including preimplantation genetic diagnosis (PGD), sex selection, compensated gamete donation, and compensated gestational surrogacy. It is argued that bans on certain treatments express a country's core values, but dilemma arises when patients who return after receiving not allowed treatments face no legal, medical, or social consequences, likely contributing to continued travel to avoid restrictive laws in a patient's home jurisdiction. At the same time, there is little or no support to punish patients who participate in the evasion of the law in search of biological paternity, nor is there a generalized defense to penalize doctors who help patients in their search to access CBRC, although laws in some countries consider such behavior illegal. The International Federation of Fertility Societies[14] lists a range of clinical practices which carry differing regulations in various jurisdictions. These include definitions of eligibility for treatment; number of embryos transferred; cryopreservation; the availability of posthumous insemination, sperm, and egg donation; the micromanipulation of sperm (intracytoplasmic sperm injection) and embryos (assisted hatching and cytoplasmic transfer); requirements regarding anonymity of donors, PGD, and IVF surrogacy (particularly restrictions on commercial surrogacy).
2. *Travel to seeking of a better quality care abroad*:
   i. A patient's ability to access fertility care in their country of residence depends on the amount or ART services, the quality of care offered, the treatments options available, and the waiting time to access to ART treatments
   ii. Travel is also more prevalent from countries where the supply of donor gametes and gestational services is low. Both, the restrict payments to gamete donors and the gestational carriers and national policies that require disclosure of donor identity are the main reasons to travel for ART
   iii. Patients' desire to access higher quality care also figures prominently in CBRC. Most of the

patients who travel abroad for care have received treatment in their home country, often for several years. Treatment failures, along with a perception that clinics abroad employ more highly trained personnel, utilize more up-to-date equipment, and offer more specialized services, incentivize experienced ART patients to seek treatment abroad

iv. Patients travel to avoid long wait times at home, a reality in countries that include infertility care as part of their national health service.

3. *Travel to reduce the cost of fertility care*:

   i. The high cost of ART is a well-described barrier to its use. Because fertility treatment can be very expensive, it is utilized by only a fraction of those in need of care. Global price variations are published, with the average price of an IVF cycle highest in the US and significantly lower in countries, such as India.[15] In the past, medical travel was associated with travel to wealthy nations for specialized health care, but now it has expanded to include travel by wealthy patients to the developing countries, promoting an opportunity for the developing countries to generate investment capital[11]

   ii. The impact of ART on patients differs across the world; patients in the countries that fund care as part of a national health service are impacted the least, while those in non-reimbursement countries are impacted the most. Disparities in the fees paid to gamete donors and gestational carriers also incentivize travel. Surveys of patients who travel to access third-party reproductive services indicate that cost is a significant factor in their decision to leave home.[6,7]

4. *Travel for privacy and cultural comfort*:

   i. The physical, psychological, emotional, and financial burdens that infertility can engender lead some patients to seek treatment abroad. Often these patients will patronize a country in which they have extended family or possess a degree of cultural familiarity. For example, the most popular destination for Japanese infertile couples is the US due to familial ties and/or large population of Japanese-Americans as potential gamete donors. A desire for privacy as well as increasingly easy access to international travel is cited by patients.[16]

Although some authors have tried to differentiate the reasons for patient travel by country, where the patients are asked, most patients mentioned a combination of factors leading them to seek cross-border treatment.[6,17]

ADVANTAGES OF CROSS-BORDER REPRODUCTIVE CARE

Fertility travel can potentially benefit patients and their partners, offspring, ART providers, gamete donors and gestational carriers, and local populations in destination countries. Potential benefits to CBRC are the following:

- *Improving access to care*: Increase in worldwide utilization of ART is a benefit to patients and their partners, especially those whose treatment produces a successful outcome. On a more philosophical level, arguably access to CBRC is a benefit to the offspring who would not have been born without the foreign treatment. Improved access to donor gametes and gestational services is also an overall benefit of CBRC. Third-party participants, particularly oocyte donors, play an increasing important role in ART. In countries with legislation limiting payment for oocyte donation, utilization of donor oocytes is very low (e.g. 3% of all UK cycles compared with 12% in the US).[18] Improving access to donor oocytes improves success rates, thus benefiting those who travel to procure donor gametes. In a publication based on the health-care providers experience in CBRC, they adapted their service to foreign patients: providing all appointments one day, providing interpreters, adapting treatment, collaboration with the doctors in the home country, and providing consent forms in appropriate languages[19]
- *Avoiding discrimination*: Traveling to avoid application of restrictive laws in place in a home jurisdiction allows patients to escape discrimination based on demographic characteristics that are unrelated to medical suitability for treatment. In a field sometimes criticized for catering to white, middle- and upper-income individuals, increasing diversity among the patient population by removing discriminatory barriers and lowering costs is a benefit to the individual patients as well to the medical practice[5]
- *Reducing the costs of care*: The internet emerges as a major source of information for patients traveling or planning CBRC, followed by the council of their own doctor in countries, such as Germany, Italy, UK, or Sweden. Patients could feel motivated to choose a country or a clinic depending on the price of the ART treatment. Patients benefit from the lower cost of care. Lower costs can improve outcomes by increasing the number of cycles a patient can afford to undergo[7]
- *Cross-border care can benefit ART providers*, health professionals, gamete donors, gestational carriers, and providers of general tourism services in destination

countries. Increased demand for fertility services can enhance access to both ART and general medical care for local populations. These improvements can benefit local populations in the form of increased ART services or convertible medical infrastructure

- *Protecting privacy*: Some patients will benefit from the privacy that CBRC provides. Couples or individuals who fight with infertility may wish to escape the scrutiny that even well-intentioned family and friends can apply. Receiving treatment without having to report daily progress and eventual outcomes can be a relief for some patients. For others, accessing treatment in a country of origin with a familiar language and cultural sensibility can also enhance the ART experience.

DISADVANTAGES OF CROSS-BORDER REPRODUCTIVE CARE

- *Absence of international standards of care*: The most important worry for traveling patients is the protection of their health and safety. In the ART context, health and safety concerns can focus on the transmission of infectious diseases to patients or genetic disorders to offspring. In the absence of international policies and norms dictating quality control measures, patients are disadvantaged in their ability to discover and assess the standard of care in any given foreign jurisdiction
- *Impact in quality of live (QoL) and psychosocial aspects*: Infertility and ARTs have a known impact on the psychosocial well-being of patients, mainly in terms of loss of control, stigmatization, negative emotional responses, such as anxiety and depression and QoL impairments.[20] The decision to undergo reproductive care abroad might add further emotional and practical complexity to treatment.[21] One of the reasons for this is linked to the fact that patients usually choose to CBRC after failed attempts in their countries, and this is usually associated with increased anxiety during treatments. Although several clinics offer simplified treatments for CBRC patients, the interference of medical procedures with professional and personal routines is worsened by traveling abroad, which impacts QoL, and the couples also need to adjust to a new cultural and medical care context[5]
- *Language, information, and legal barriers*: Patients may be harmed by lack of access to understandable information about their treatment options. In many instances, patients do not speak the native language in the destination country. Reduced quality of care and language barriers can combine to victimize patients once they arrive in the destination country. Additional harms include the possibility of changing or evolving legal schemes in destination jurisdictions. The timing and effective dates of such legal changes could put at risk an individual or couple's anticipated or ongoing reproductive plan, possibly resulting in the inability to remove a newborn from the subject country. Intended parents who contract a gestational carrier in a destination country for the purposes of safeguarding citizenship for their child in the place of birth can also experience legal difficulties upon return to their country of domicile. The increasing complexity surrounding the legal status of CBRC offspring cautions patients and their partners to give serious attention to matters, such as legal parentage, immigration, and citizenship
- *Policy responses to CBRC*: CBRC has emerged for a lot of reasons as an area of concern, generating corresponding debate about how various stakeholders should respond to this phenomenon.
  - Those advocating the prohibition of CBRC. Few authors advocate this approach. This option could theoretically operate, such as restricting the movements of citizens for the purpose of CBRC, allowing people to have treatment in their home country only and applying penalties for "offenders". Their suggestions were should be illegal for doctors to refer patients to countries, who have different forms of regulation of ART treatments. Some authors argue that such a move has the potential for the violation of individual privacy and freedom[22]
  - Those promoting harmonization of relevant regulation across borders. Some authors suggest that harmonization is not feasible because it would require culturally and politically diverse nation states to accept universal ethical principles or moral truths[23]
  - Those endorsing the operation of CBRC under certain conditions or with specific safeguards (or "harm minimization"). This third argument has received most discussions in the literature to date and would appear to reflect current dominant thinking on interventions in CBRC. The development of an international code of practice for professionals and/or a system of international clinic accreditation which allows patients (and presumably donors and surrogates) to identify affiliated clinics with agreed quality standards has been proposed. Others have called for additional international protection for children conceived via CBRC and for donors and surrogates.[24]

- *Harm to offspring*: The quality of ART care can impact offspring health, particularly in the context of multiple pregnancy. The morbidity and mortality associated with high-order multiple pregnancy are well described and have prompted some countries to limit the number of embryos transferred in any single IVF cycle. Patients who travel are at increased risk for multiple pregnancy. In addition, offspring who are the result of gamete donation abroad may have less access to information about their genetic origins than donor-conceived children produced by domestic arrangements. While access to and information about gamete donors are highly variable, offspring attempting to locate their gamete donors abroad would likely face greater hurdles[25]
- *Harm to donors and gestational carriers*: Concern about the exploitation of gamete donors and gestational carriers in destination countries occupies much of the critique of CBRC.[26] This critique presumes that patients seeking third-party reproduction will be wealthier and more politically powerful than women who act as donors or gestational carriers. In countries where the status of women is already problematically low, building a market for reproductive services can fuel the view that a woman's value is limited to her physical characteristics and childbearing capacity. While payments to donors and gestational carriers can temporarily raise their economic status, some argue that such practices permanently harm women by reducing them to commodities available for exploitation[12]
- *Harm to equity in low-income countries*: A primary concern is that the development of the foreign patient trade in health services will have a detrimental effect upon the public health systems of these countries, by encouraging the further development of inequitable, two-tiered health systems, where elite, technologically sophisticated hospitals, catering to wealthy foreign clients, stand beside poorly resourced public hospitals. Negative effects generated by the development of the international trade in health services in low-income countries include a local brain drain of skilled medical staff from the public health system into private, elite hospitals, affecting access for the local population.[11]

ETHICAL CONSIDERATIONS

Patients who travel for ART begin this journey in their home country, often by consulting several sources for information, including physicians. If a potential ART traveler has a pre-existing relationship with a provider in a departure country, several legal and ethical dilemmas can be anticipated.[27]

- *For departure-country physicians*:
  - A fundamental principle of medical ethics is to respect patients by treating them as autonomous individuals. It enhances patient autonomy in providing an equal opportunity of treatment to all, even if that autonomy may imply national law evasion and variable costs. Physicians have a duty to provide patients with information necessary to understand their diagnosis and treatment options, as well as the risks and benefits of accepting treatment. If a patient asks a physician about options for care abroad, the provider has an ethical duty to not misrepresent his or her knowledge about those options. A physician with experiential or secondary knowledge about CBRC, including specific information about clinical options abroad, may disclose such information to inquiring patients. A physician has a duty to disclose any conflicts of interest, such as financial interests in an overseas ART program
  - Duty to disclose risks and benefits of CBRC: Informed consent requires physician disclosure of the risks and benefits of suggested treatment. The physician is free to share opinions about the merits of CBRC and should be clear about whether the information is given as a recommendation or merely as guidance
  - Duty to resume care of a patient who receives CBRC treatment: A patient who returns from abroad may have little or no documentation explaining the care she received. Lack of medical records can pose significant challenges for treating physicians, raising concerns about whether to treat or continue treatment of returning patients. Where no such duty exists, physicians are free to accept or decline patients into their practice. The physician–patient relationship is largely a voluntary one, which both parties may choose to enter or not, so long as their conduct is nondiscriminatory.
- *For destination-country physicians*:
  - Providers who treat traveling patients are held to whatever standards of care govern medical care in their jurisdiction, including informed consent.

The first step to providing guidance for fertility clinics in Europe has been pioneered by the ESHRE Task Force on CBRC. The ESHRE has developed a good practice guide (GPG) for practitioners, which takes into account the patients themselves, their future child, and the interests of third-party collaborators, such as gamete donors and surrogates.[28] This GPG provides guidance for centers and physicians treating foreign patients. The operational principles to be considered include the following:

- Equity in CBRC for patients and donors: Equity implies that similar protocols and fees are applied and that the same information, counseling, and psychological support are provided for foreign as for national patients. Donors should receive similar care to patients and local donors
- Quality, safety, and evidence-based care in cross-border treatment includes the following:
  - Patients should receive clear information about necessary investigations and their cost, about waiting list times and the expected time they will have to spend outside their country
  - Communication and collaboration between the clinical team in the home country and the team abroad
  - It is essential to propose a stimulation cycle that minimizes the health risk for the oocyte donors
  - It is necessary to establish national registers of gametes donors
  - In surrogacy treatment, single-embryo transfer is the only acceptable option
  - The decline in the number of multiple births can be regulated only with a reduction of the number of embryos transferred
  - Follow-up of ART children, whether conceived after treatment at home or abroad, should be encouraged
  - Collaboration between doctors: If a home practitioner refers the patient to a specific clinic, the practitioner shares a responsibility for the general standards used in that center
  - Counseling and psychological support should be available in a language understood by the patients.

CONCLUSION

Cross-border reproductive care is a growing reality in ART. The main factors that incentivize patients to travel abroad for fertility care—access, cost, regulation, and privacy—are poised to remain features of the global reproductive health market. Physicians who treat ART patients from abroad have a duty to deliver the same quality of care required for all domestic patients. Referral to qualified experts, including legal and mental health professionals, should be considered and is encouraged when appropriate. As the practice and delivery of reproductive medicine becomes more internationalized, physicians are well served to understand the extent and limits of their medical, ethical, and legal duties to traveling ART patients.

REFERENCES

1. Gianaroli L, Ferraretti AP, Magli MC, et al. Current regulatory arrangements for assisted conception treatment in European countries. Eur J Obstet Gynecol Reprod Biol. 2016;207:211-3.
2. Mascarenhas MN Flaxman SR, Boerma T, et al. National, regional, and global trends in infertility prevalence since 1990: a systematic analysis of 277 health surveys. PLoS Med. 2012;9(12):e1001356.
3. IFFS. IFFS Surveillance 2016. Global Reprod Health. 2016;1(e1):1-143.
4. Kushnir, VA. Systematic review of worldwide trends in assisted reproductive technology 2004-2013. Reprod Biol Endocrinol. 2017;15(1):1-9.
5. Ferraretti AP, Pennings G. Cross-border reproductive care: a phenomenon expressing the controversial aspects of reproductive technologies. Reprod Biomed Online. 2010;20(2):261-6.
6. Shenfield F, de Mouzon J, Pennings G, et al. Cross border reproductive care in six European countries. Hum Reprod. 2010;25(6):1361-8.
7. Hudson N, Culley L, Blyth E, et al. Cross-border reproductive care: a review of the literature. Reprod Biomed Online. 2011;22(7):673-85.
8. Hughes EG, Dejean D. Cross-border fertility services in North America: a survey of Canadian and American providers. Fertil Steril. 2010;94(1):e16-9.
9. Levine A, Boulet SL, Berry RM, et al. Assessing the use of assisted reproductive technology in the United States by non–United States residents. Fertil Steril. 2017;108(5):815-21.
10. Hughes EG, Sawyer A, DeJean D, et al. Cross-border reproductive care in North America: a pilot study testing a prospective data collection program for in vitro fertilization clinics in Canada and the United States. Fertil Steril. 2016;105(3):786-90.
11. Whittaker A. Cross-border assisted reproduction care in Asia: implications for access, equity and regulations. Reprod Health Matters. 2011;19(37):107-16.
12. Daar J, Benward J, Collins LR, et al. Cross-border reproductive care: an Ethics Committee opinion. Fertil Steril. 2016;106(7):1627-33.
13. Cohen IG. Circumvention tourism. Cornell Law Rev. 2012;97(6):1309-98.
14. Jones Jr HW, Cooke I, Kempers R, et al. International Federation of Fertility Societies Surveillance 2010. Fertil Steril. 2010. [online] Available from http://www.iffs-reproduction.org/documents/IFFS_Surveillance_2010.pdf
15. Dyer SJ, Patel M. The economic impact of infertility on women in developing countries—a systematic review. Facts Views Vis Obgyn. 2012;4:102-9.
16. Hibino Y, Shimazono Y, Kambayashi Y, et al. Attitudes towards cross-border reproductive care among infertile Japanese patients. Environ Health Prev Med. 2013;18(6):477-84.
17. Inhorn MC, Shrivastav P. Globalization and reproductive tourism in the United Arab Emirates. Asia Pac J Public Health. 2010;22(3 Suppl):68S-74S.

18. Calhaz-Jorge CD. Assisted reproductive technology in Europe, 2013: results generated from European registers by ESHRE. Human Reprod. 2017;32(10):1957-73.
19. Pennings G, Autin C, Decleer W, et al. Cross-border reproductive care in Belgium. Hum Reprod. 2009;24:3108-18.
20. Gameiro S, van den Belt-Dusebout AW, Smeenk JM, et al. Women's adjustment trajectories during IVF and impact on mental health 11-17 years later. Hum Reprod. 2016;31(8):1788-98.
21. Blyth E. Fertility patients' experiences of cross-border reproductive care. Fertil Steril. 2010;94(1):e11-5.
22. Mertes H, Pennings G. Ethical aspects of the use of stem cell derived gametes for reproduction. Health Care Anal. 2010;18(3):267-8.
23. Pennings G. Legal harmonization and reproductive tourism in Europe. Hum Reprod. 2004;19(12):2689-9.
24. Cohen J. Procreative tourism and reproductive freedom. Reprod Biomed Online. 2006;13:145-6.
25. McKelvey A, David AL, Shenfield F, et al. The impact of cross-border reproductive care or 'fertility tourism' on NHS maternity services. BJOG. 2009;116:1520-3.
26. Whittaker A, Speier A. "Cycling overseas": care, commodification, and stratification in cross-border reproductive travel. Med Anthropol. 2010;29:363-83.
27. Van Hoof W, Pennings G, De Sutter P. Cross-border reproductive care for law evasion: should physicians be allowed to help infertility patients evade the law of their own country? Eur J Obstet Gynecol Reprod. 2016;202:101-5.
28. Shenfield FP. ESHREs good practice guide for cross-border reproductive care for centers and practitioners. Hum Reprod. 2011;26(7):1625-7.

CHAPTER

90

Medicolegal Issues in Assisted Reproductive Technology

Taswin Kaur, Kamini A Rao

INTRODUCTION

The birth of Louise Brown in 1978 revolutionized modern medicine and surgery, especially in the field of assisted reproductive technology (ART). Breathtaking breakthroughs in reproductive medicine have occurred in the recent years since the birth of the world's first ART baby. In the past four decades, we have leaped over from creating an embryo in vitro to almost creating a human in the laboratory! The atomic bomb which can be used as a germ warfare!

The volcanic explosion of this technology has not only given hopes and smiles to millions of infertile couples, but this double-edged sword has also opened its doors to a myriad of legal, ethical, and social challenges or controversies.

In vitro fertilization (IVF) is the most common form of ART. The ART has resulted in a tectonic shift in the way physicians and the general population perceives infertility and ethics. Long gone are those days where doctors were looked upon as saints or as a step lower, if not equivalent than the creator himself. The recent explosion and propagation by the media have made doctors stand in the limelight for any blame game in a hospital setting. With the increasing accessibility, publicity, and advancement of assisted reproductive methods, there are numerous gray areas, especially in the legal aspects that a medical practitioner can be held responsible for.

It is impossible to describe in this chapter of all the laws of reproductive medicine and the medicolegal issues that can arise in all the countries of the world, especially since the rules, regulations, and legislations regarding reproductive medicine are different in between countries. Hence, this chapter aims at providing an overview of the medicolegal aspects in reproductive medicine based on the current laws of the land, especially in India (Table 1).

Table 1: Gray areas for medicolegal problems.

Consent and documentation	*Wrong insemination*	*Confidentiality*
Adultery	Divorce	Consummation of marriage
Legitimacy	Posthumous insemination	HIV transmission
Confidentiality	Donor gametes—sperms, oocytes	Surrogate mother
Embryo transferred—number	Single parents/gay/lesbians	Storage of embryos
Fate of gametes	Research	Cloning

(HIV: human immunodeficiency virus)

CONSENT AND DOCUMENTATION

The concept of consent comes from the ethical issue of respect of individual integrity, autonomy, and self-determination. Every individual has a right to determine what should be done to his body. In the court of law, a legally valid consent for a procedure or treatment is one, i.e.

- *Given by the person himself*, if above 12 years of age [Section 88 IPC (Indian Penal Code)], conscious, and mentally sound or given by the parent, guardian, or close relative, if the patient is less than 12 years of age or is insane or is unconscious. In such circumstances consent given by parent, guardian, or close relative is known as "substitute or proxy consent"

- *Informed expressed written consent*
- *Given before* actually doing the *procedure*
- Given in the present of *two witnesses*
- Given freely, voluntarily, and directly
- Given without fear, fraud, or force
- *Signed by the doctor, patient (or guardian), and witnesses*
- Should be written in patient's own handwriting.

It is important to ensure that the consent includes the nature of the diagnosis, the nature of the planned treatment, foreseeable risks of the treatment, prognosis if the treatment is not carried out, and if any alternative therapies are available.

A blanket consent is one that is taken on a printed form that covers almost everything the doctor or hospital might do to a patient without mentioning anything specifically. Blanket consents are usually legally inadequate for any procedure that has risks or multiple alternatives.

In an infertility clinic, consent taking is very essential, and consent from both the partners—husband and wife—is mandatory prior to treatment. It is very crucial to counsel, document, and to take necessary consents, especially when donor gametes or when a surrogate mother is involved in part of the treatment to avoid unforeseen legal complications. The use of gametes of the partner without their consent amounts to forgery.

The couple should be made to understand that there is no guarantee on the success of the ART procedure. This is important as many patients, especially in the developing countries like India, assume that they will walk home with a baby in their arms once they step into an infertility clinic.

In India the ART Bill 2010 by the Ministry of Health and Family Welfare, Government of India and the Indian Council of Medical Research has laid down guidelines to be followed by the ART clinics and banks.[1]

According to the ART Bill 2010 as quoted as follows, it is the duty of the ART clinic to obtain a written consent:

- No clinic shall perform any treatment or procedure of ART without a written consent of all the parties (couple/donors/surrogate mothers) seeking treatment or procedure at all stages
- No ART clinic shall freeze human embryos without the consent and specific instructions from parties seeking treatment on what is to be done with the gametes/embryos in the case of death or incapacity of any one party
- No ART clinic shall use any human reproductive material to create an embryo or to use an in vitro embryo for any purpose without the specific consent in writing of all the parties to whom the treatment relates
- The consent of any of the parties obtained under this section may be withdrawn at any time before the embryos or the gametes are transferred to the concerned woman's uterus.

Specific consent forms have been provided in the ART Bill 2010, and it is advisable to adhere to these formats (Table 2; Fig. 1).

Apart from necessary consent taking, documentation at each and every step is essential. It is important to document the couples visits, complaints, medication given, options offered to the couple.

It is mandatory that all ART clinics maintain detailed records legibly written or computerized, including of all donor sperms/oocytes used surrogate mothers. Records should be maintained for at least 10 years and upon the expiry of which the ART clinic shall transfer the records to

Table 2: Consent forms as given in ART Bill 2010.

Form	*Use*
Form D	Consent form signed by the couple for IVF/ICSI
Form E	Consent for artificial insemination or intrauterine insemination by husband's semen/sperms
Form F	Consent for artificial insemination or intrauterine insemination with donor semen
Form G	Consent for freezing of embryos
Form H	Consent for the surgical extraction of sperm
Form I	Consent for oocyte retrieval/embryo transfer
Form J	Agreement for surrogacy
Form K	Consent form for the donor of oocytes
Form L	Consent form for the donor of sperm

(ART: assisted reproductive technology; IVF: in vitro fertilization; ICSI: intracytoplasmic sperm injection)

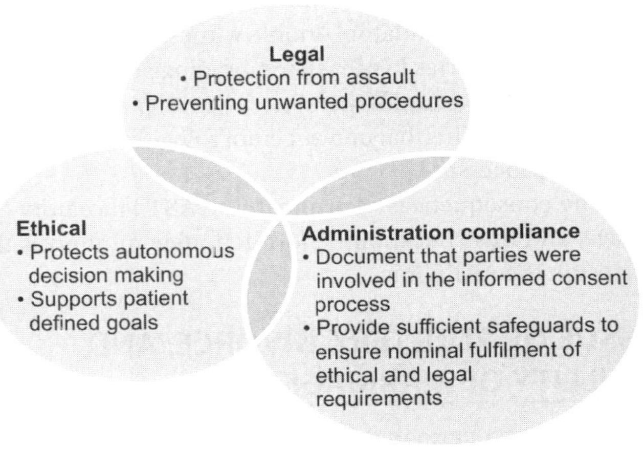

Fig. 1: Venn diagram showing the multiple overlapping purposes of informed consent.[2]

a central database which is to be set up. However, if an ART clinic closes before the expiry of the 10-year period, the clinic or the bank should immediately transfer the records to a central database.

WRONG INSEMINATION

Infertility is synonymous as the disease of the 21st century. ART clinics are mushrooming worldwide, and none of them seem less occupied. With the increase in demand, chances of errors also dwindle. Wrong insemination of gametes—sperms, oocytes, or embryos—is a crime! At no cost, at no event of time, this should happen.

Several measures can be employed to assure that mistake of wrong insemination is avoided. Each couple or patient is provided with at least three identification methods—name, date of birth, and personal identification number. At every point of treatment or procedure, this identification should be verified.

The Human Fertilization and Embryology Authority in the United Kingdom has made it mandatory that double witnessing should be carried out at predefined checkpoints in the IVF laboratory to minimize mix-ups. Manual double witnessing method is often practiced in an ART laboratory where the identification check is done by two separate individuals before proceeding with the procedure. This method is done on the basis that if the "operator" makes an error, it will be caught by other "witness".

Manual double checking has been related to many problems such as attentional blindness, independent redundancy, and ambiguous accountability. Hence, recently, an electronic witnessing system using radiofrequency identification technology—RI-Witness™, has been developed to track samples at predefined procedural steps in IVF laboratories across the world.[3] This system is used to prevent mix-ups and is an automated solution for the mandatory double witnessing. This system has inbuilt defenses to prevent embryologist working from more than one couple's gametes at a time, and it has an inbuilt checkpoints that prevent embryologist from omitting key step processes.

The consequences of errors in the ART laboratory are grave, and this checkpoint effort definitely minimizes the errors in the ART clinic.

ISSUE OF ADULTERY, DIVORCE, AND NULLITY OF MARRIAGE

The Indian scenario in this issue is quite bleak as there are no laws on artificial insemination applicable in the entire country. The Delhi Artificial Insemination (Human) Act, 1995 is applicable only in Delhi and is the only statutory act prevailing in India. This is unlike the United Kingdom where laws regarding artificial reproduction are clearly defined under the Human Fertilization and Embryology Act, 2008.

According to the Indian law under Section 497 IPC, an ART procedure when used for a married woman with the consent of her husband does not amount to adultery on the part of the wife or the donor.[4,5] This offense requires sexual intercourse as a necessary ingredient for the charge of adultery. Adultery can only be committed in the absence of the husband's consent. However, donor inseminations without the consent of the husband can be a ground for judicial separation or a ground for divorce under the Hindu Marriage Act, 1955, provided the husband is sterile or impotent. The use of donor gametes should be done with caution and precautions as there is no space for "oops" or "sorry" if any mistakes were to occur. A doctor can be held liable if inseminations are done without the consent—of the husband, wife, or even donor.

Conception of the wife by artificial reproductive techniques does not amount to consummation of the marriage. A marriage is said to be consummated when the parties have a sexual intercourse—with full or at least partial penetration after its solemnization.

The separation of a family—the husband and the wife—should be avoided as far as possible for the believe that a two-parent family would be always better for the child than a single parent one; and the child's interest must be prioritized outweighing all other interests.

A mere artificial insemination is not a ground for nullity of marriage or divorce since sterility is not a ground. However, if artificial insemination is due to impotence of the husband, it may be a ground for divorce.

POSTHUMOUS INSEMINATION

According to the Indian Evidence Act, 1872, a child is considered to be a legitimate child if the child is born within 280 days after dissolution of a marriage—by death or a divorce. We have come a far way beyond history in this science and technology era, perhaps it is wise to reconsider and reframe this century-old law where a child is illegitimate if he or she is not born within the 280-day time frame. With scientific advancements, couples are freezing their gametes for future use.[6] A child born to a woman artificially inseminated with stored sperms of her deceased husband, provided there is a detailed written consent from him while freezing the sperms to hand the sperms for use to his partner, the child born is still considered a legitimate child. Study has shown that use of posthumous sperms results in developmentally normal children.[7]

LEGITIMACY

A child born after ART treatment is presumed to be the legitimate child of the couple born within wedlock provided the necessary consents were obtained prior to the procedure. The couple shall have all the rights of parentage, and the child shall have the rights of support and inheritance. The donors or gametes—sperms and oocytes—shall remain anonymous and will not hold any legitimacy nor parental rights. All parental rights are also relinquished from the surrogate mother. As per the ART Bill 2010, a child born in the following situations is considered to be a legitimate child of the couple:

- Through the use of ART procedures, after the consent of both spouses
- Unmarried couple through the use of ART but with the consent of both parties
- Single woman or single man—the child will be a legitimate child of that individual
- Couple—married or unmarried separates or gets divorced, after they had consented for the ART procedure but before birth of the child
- Woman is artificially inseminated with the stored sperm of her dead husband.

HUMAN IMMUNODEFICIENCY VIRUS TRANSMISSION

Couples should be made aware that during their course of treatment, especially with donor gametes, human immunodeficiency virus (HIV) transmission cannot be completely prevented. All donors are screened for transmissible diseases, especially HIV, hepatitis B, and hepatitis C. Semen donor samples are usually quarantined and cryopreserved for 6 months and rescreened for HIV, hepatitis B, and hepatitis C again after the window period to rule out the possibility of the disease being in the dormant stage. It is of utmost importance to inform the partner if one of them on routine testing is found to be seropositive. Universal precautions should be maintained at all times in the laboratory.

EMBRYO TRANSFERRED

Multiple pregnancies are viewed as a complication of ART. Therefore under optimal conditions, wherever possible, elective transfer of a single embryo is preferred. This is in concordance with the American Society for Reproductive Medicine 2017 guidelines on the number of embryos to be transferred in an IVF-intracytoplasmic sperm injection cycle. At no point of time, more than three embryos should be transferred into the uterus. Under exceptional circumstances, the transfer of more than three embryos may be considered.[1]

- Elderly women (>37 years)
- Poor implantation (>three previous failures)
- Advanced endometriosis
- Poor embryo quality.

The reason and justification of transferring additional embryos should be clearly documented in the patient's records (Table 3).

Table 3: Recommendations for the limit to the number of embryos to transfer.

	Age years			
Prognosis	*<35*	*35–37*	*38–40*	*41–42*
Cleavage-stage embryos[a]				
Eupolid	1	1	1	1
Other favorable[b]	1	1	≤3	≤4
All others	≤2	≤3	≤4	≤5
Blastocysts[a]				
Euploid	1	1	1	1
Other favorable[b]	1	1	≤2	≤3
All others	≤3	≤2	≤3	≤3

[a]See text for more complete explanations.
[b]Other favorable = Any ONE of these criteria—Fresh cycle: expectation of 1 or more high-quality embryos available for cryopreservation, or previous live birth after an IVF cycle, FET cycle: availability of vitrified day 5 or day-6 blastocysts, euploid embryos, 1st FET cycle, or previous live birth after an IVF cycle.
Please note: Justification for transferring additional embryos beyond recommended limits should be clearly documented in the patient's medical record.
ASRM. Limits on number of embryos to transfer. Fertil Steril 2017
Adapted from ASRM Committee Opinion 2017.[8]

PROVIDING ASSISTED REPRODUCTIVE TECHNOLOGY TO SINGLE PARENTS/GAY/ LESBIAN

India, a country, where roots of traditions and culture are very strong, has somehow not been very open to gays, lesbians, or even single parents on having a child. This parenthood concept is also believed to be the spark of many medicolegal issues. The ART Bill clearly states that ART—IVF or surrogacy should be offered to a couple who has been married for a minimum period of 2 years.

STORAGE OF EMBRYOS AND FATE OF THE GAMETES

Usually in an ART cycle, controlled ovarian stimulation is preferred to maximize the number of oocytes-embryos obtained during the stimulation cycle. Excess embryos are invariably stored for future use. According to the Human

Fertilization and Embryology Act, the United Kingdom, 1990, a 5-year storage period is accepted for embryos.[9] If the couple wishes to dispose, donate, or use their embryos for research purpose, a written consent should be taken mentioning the same. However, storing an increasing number of embryos raises many concerns regarding disputes regarding ownership as well as disposition of the embryos. The embryo storage period is different worldwide. Some countries, such as Portugal, allow storage for 3 years, 5 years in Norway, Egypt, and India; 10 years in Australia and Taiwan. It is possibly longer in countries such as the United Kingdom (55 years) and unlimited in Canada and Finland.[10,11] The unused gametes or embryos may be discarded, allowed to perish, or used for further research in reproductive medicine. However, more often than not, they are usually preserved for further future use. Donating embryos for research is a noble initiative which should be encouraged. There should not be a sale or transaction for the use of these embryos in research.

DONOR GAMETES

Late marriages, decreased fertility potential, postponement of child bearing further accelerate the infertility muddle. Many couples therefore opt for donor gametes to bear a legitimate offspring. There is much controversy worldwide regarding the use of donor gametes or the transfer of embryos into surrogate mothers.

- *Donor gametes*: In India as accordance to the ART Bill 2010, guidelines have been laid, respectively, for oocyte and sperm donors (Table 4)

Table 4: Guidelines for gamete donation.

	Donor sperms	*Donor oocytes*
Age (years)	21–45	18–35
Maximum donation in a lifetime	75 times	6 times (minimum 3-month interval between each oocyte retrieval)
Quarantine period	At least 6 months	–
	One semen sample to be used only once one recipient	All unused oocytes can be cryopreserved
Sharing of gametes	No mixing of two semen sample	Can be shared between 2 recipients (provided each have ≥7 oocytes)
Storage	Not more than 5 years	
Information of the donor	Confidential—no name/address/ personal details to be shared	Confidential—no name/address/ personal details to be shared

- *Surrogate mother*: Lending a womb has always been a controversial issue. Much litigation have aroused, women have been misused. In lines with the ART Bill 2010, surrogate mothers should be between 21 and 35 years of age, and she shall not act as a surrogate for more than five successful live births, including her own children. Much controversy is sparked regarding the use of surrogate mothers. Lending a womb is associated with a vast scope of litigations.

SEX SELECTION

In a female feticide rampant country, a male child is considered a blessing, while the female offspring is considered a curse. Socioeconomic status holds no bar when couples and their families wish for a male child. Female fetuses are killed and aborted. The issue of selection has long been an issue in India and has always been associated with a lot of controversy and conspiracy. In India, sex selection is against the law.

CONCLUSION

Assisted reproduction technology is a Pandora's Box which has doors that are yet to be opened. It is an atom bomb that can be used as a germ warfare if not used with care. In the 21st century where doctors are the main targets of litigations, it is wise to look at both the sides of the coin before making a decision or treatment. Above all practices, a good consent and neat documentation shall always be the cornerstone that speaks up in the court of law.

As said by Plato a long time ago, "Good people do not need laws to tell them to act responsibly and bad people will find ways around them".

REFERENCES

1. Ministry of Health and Family Welfare Government of India. The assisted reproductive technologies (regulation) rules—2010. New Delhi: Indian Council of Medical Research; 2018.
2. Hall DE, Prochazka AV, Fink AS. Informed consent for clinical treatment. Can Med Assoc J. 2012;184(5):533-40.
3. Brunetti X, Bird S, Rogers S, et al. OP-2 identifying human error in the ivf laboratory using electronic witnessing. Reprod Biomed Online. 2012;24:S1.
4. Deore V. (2018). Adultery—Section 497 IPC. [online] Available from http://www.legalserviceindia.com/article/l291-Adultery.html [Accessed February 2018].
5. Govt. of India. (2018). Law Commission of India, Ministry of Law & Justice. [online] Available from http://www.lawcommissionofindia.nic.in/ [Accessed February 2018].

6. Benshushan A, Schenker J. The right to an heir in the era of assisted reproduction. Hum Reprod. 1998;13(5):1407-10.
7. Robson SJ, Campbell S, McDonald J, et al. Pregnancy and childhood health and developmental outcomes with the use of posthumous human sperm. Hum Reprod. 2015;30(10):2259-62.
8. Penzias A, Bendikson K, Butts S, et al. Guidance on the limits to the number of embryos to transfer: a committee opinion. Fertil Steril. 2017;107(4):901-3.
9. Pereira M, Samorinha C, Alves E, et al. Patients' views on the embryo storage time limits. Reprod Biomed Online. 2015;31(2):232-8.
10. Ory SJ, Devroey P, Banker M, et al. IFFS surveillance 2013. International Federation of Fertility Societies; 2013.
11. The Human Fertilization and Embryology (statutory storage period for embryos and gametes) regulations. No. 1582. [online] Available from http://www.legislation.gov.uk/uksi/2009/1582/made

CHAPTER

91

Ethics and Reproduction

Antonio Pellicer, Mauro Cozzolino

INTRODUCTION

Ethics is a branch of philosophy that studies the rational foundations that allow us to assign a deontological status to human behavior, according to an ideal behavioral model to distinguish good, just, or legitimate from unjust, illicit, improper, or bad behaviors. Ethics is based on some fundamental principles:

- *Principle of autonomy:* It is the obligation to observe individual's own values and free will
- *Principle of beneficence:* It is the obligation to do well
- *Principle of nonmaleficence:* Respecting the integrity of human beings, even more regarding technical and scientific advances
- *Principle of justice:* It is the equitable division of charges and benefits, avoiding discrimination on the access to health-care resources.

Role of gynecologists and obstetricians: To ensure equal access to health services for women, regardless of age, race, marital, socio-economical, or religious status and recognizing sexual and reproductive rights, which are fundamental human rights.

Professionals providing medically assisted reproduction must take into consideration the welfare of the future child. This is the main distinction between the normative framework of medically assisted reproduction and that of traditional genetic counseling, emphasizing nondirectiveness.[1] The introduction of assisted reproduction technology (ART) has generated ethical debates within the scientific field. ART has solved numerous infertility problems, yet religious ethics question, if it is acceptable to generate embryos outside the mother's uterus. However, from an ethical point of view, the principles of beneficence and nonbeneficence make it possible. ART has introduced new treatments, such as third-party reproduction, which go beyond treating sterile couples. It has also opened the field to the application of genetics with preimplantation genetic diagnosis (PGD) and preimplantation genetic testing for aneuploidy (PGT-A) in the cases of sterility, preserving fertility in the cases of cancer, benign diseases, such as endometriosis, or as a social matter. Further debates will be created with the advent of genome editing and stem cells. Due to space constraints, this chapter will not cover the issues concerning ethics and ART, but with the daily issues faced in our profession such as

- Multiple pregnancy
- Screening of donor gametes
- Selection of sex for nonmedical reasons
- Fertility treatments in human immunodeficiency virus (HIV)-positive patients
- Aspects of welfare of child born with ART
- Preimplantation genetic diagnosis and its application in the field of human leukocyte antigen (HLA)
- Preservation of fertility for social cause, cancer, and scientific research
- The equity in ART
- The rights of gay, lesbian, transsexual, and single couples
- The posthumous ART and the surrogacy.

SAFETY IN ASSISTED REPRODUCTION TECHNOLOGY

Welfare of the Child in Medically Assisted Reproduction

Numerous factors may have implications for the welfare of the child, which are as follows:

- Medical conditions of the would-be parent(s), including transmittable, genetic, and infectious disorders (HIV, hepatitis B and C). Other conditions are serious physical disabilities, which impede functioning and/or reduce life expectancy, and substance abuse

- Psychosocial factors, such as child abuse, violence in the family, addiction, mental retardation, psychiatric disorders, poverty, widowhood, or single women.

There are three different standards. The strictest one, "maximal welfare," states that no medical assistance should be provided when the life conditions of the future child will not be optimal.[2] "Minimum threshold" states that medical assistance to reproduction is unacceptable only if the life quality of the future child is so low, it would had been better not to have been born. "Reasonable welfare," the intermediate standard, states that assistance is acceptable if the future person will have the abilities and opportunities to achieve the goals that make a human life valuable.[2] ART must always try to follow "reasonable welfare," although it is not always possible. In this context, the physicians are divided between two ethical positions, their obligation of care, including responsibility to the would-be parents and the welfare of the future child. However, physicians cannot be expected to behave as detectives, so they should be allowed to accept certain patients' declarations as true. Physicians should not contact outsiders, as the obligation to verify only exists when there is a well-grounded reason to not trusting neither the information given by the would-be parent nor the patients' parenting capacity. If a certain condition is too risky, the physician may decide to collaborate only if the risk for the future child can be diminished. If the physician is uncertain about the evaluation of any medical or nonmedical (psychological, relational, or social) aspect of the patient's situation, the decision must be taken after consulting experts from other relevant disciplines, such as psychology, psychiatry, counseling, genetics, and pediatrics. At IVIRMA, our physicians always have the possibility to provide the patients psychological assistance or genetic counseling, in situations where the child's welfare cannot be assured.

Ethics of Medically Assisted Fertility Treatment for HIV-positive Men and Women

The improvement of HIV treatments has led to the increase of life expectancy and quality of those infected, who were often advised to avoid procreation but have now reconsidered this possibility. The question of treating HIV-positive persons generates conflict between two ethical principles: respect for the autonomy of the patient regarding their reproduction and that of beneficence, as expressed in the concern for the child's welfare.[3] We respect these two principles by offering our couples the possibility to be parents without discrimination, and ensuring the future child's right to health. Information enhances patients' autonomy, so there is a need for valuable information for the public on matters, such as risk of transmission or progress of the disease and treatment. In the case of HIV, two groups need to be distinguished—fertile and infertile couples. The rationale for intervention in the former is to avoid harming the uninfected spouse and, indirectly, the future offspring. Since these couples can procreate, the contribution of the physician is directed, mainly, at risk reduction, which is not only part of the physician's obligation but relevant to the ethical decision-making process. Hence, why using insemination with washed sperm in fertile couples where the male partner is HIV-positive and insemination when the female partner is HIV-positive are considered good practice. When the woman is pregnant and infected, she should accept treatment with antiretroviral agents, agree to a cesarean, if necessary, and to bottle feeding. When the couple also suffers from infertility, the aim is contributing to the conception and reducing horizontal risk. The physician assumes special responsibility for the future offspring by offering treatment, as conception would not be possible without medical intervention. We should take the short- and long-term consequences and outlook of the disease for the parents and offspring into account, to determine the acceptability of any risk. There is no reason to exclude these couples from the considerations applied to all of those seeking infertility treatment. In fact, the additional disease transmission risk for the child regarding HIV infection is not excessively high at present, compared to the risk accepted for older women, people with chromosomal abnormalities, multiple pregnancies, or to the base rate risk of congenital abnormalities in the general population.

Multiple Pregnancies: Prevention or Reduction

Multiple pregnancies are the result of either ovulation induction or transfer of several embryos in in vitro fertilization (IVF) and generate social, psychological, and medical issues for the offspring and parents—such as obstetric complications[4] or the risk of depression. These problems increase when children are physically or mentally disabled, and when higher order multiples are involved.[5] The attitude toward the effects of multiple pregnancies toward the newly created family is a test case for the moral quality of medically assisted reproduction.[6] Regarding the number of embryos transferred, some physicians consider restrictions on the patients' wishes as paternalism, which is viewed as unacceptable. Moreover, studies show that infertility patients do not consider twins and triples as an undesirable result. Regarding the number of embryos to be transferred, it is limited by how many IVF cycles parents can afford and by the causal and intentional contribution of the physician, who is professionally responsible. The patients that accept a single-embryo transfer (SET) have a good prognosis.[7] The physician's refusal to replace more embryos than what is considered acceptable is seen as paternalistic, yet it should be considered an exercise of responsibility for the welfare of the future offspring, based on the "do no harm" principle. The ignorance of the professional duty to avoid harm is difficult to accept when the continuing rate of multiples is found in the competition between centers.[8] However, avoidance of multiple pregnancies should not be an absolute rule, as the task is to balance low pregnancy rates and the risk increase of multiple pregnancies. In IVIRMA, we advise patients with good prognosis to choose SET. Our patients trust our professionalism, so their decisions regarding SET depend on the information given by the physicians and the auxiliary personnel. We always explain our patients the risks involved in multiple pregnancy in the first visit. Many of our patients, then, choose SET. Similar cumulative live birth rates can be obtained by sequential SET compared to double-embryo transfer (DET).[9-11] These discussions must take place weeks before the embryo transfer. Patients are more receptive to an SET policy when they see the clinic's commitment to achieve both, a high pregnancy rate and an optimal maternal and neonatal outcome. Couples are inclined to have twins. In one study, 30% of the infertility patients listed a twin, triplet, or quadruplet pregnancy as their most desired outcome. This is due to the lack of counseling, the limited knowledge about medical complications from twin pregnancies, nulliparity, and other factors.[12] After our physicians have carefully explained all the process and its risks to the patients, they tend to prefer the idea of a DET. Physicians and health professionals should always follow the highest standards of good clinical practice. At IVIRMA clinics, we consider patient autonomy to be an important bioethical principle. Moreover, we also highlight the importance of nonmaleficence principle "do no harm" and the right of conscientious practice for physicians. Although we respect patient autonomy, the physician always must abide by the ethical and moral responsibilities.

EMBRYO SELECTION

Preimplantation Genetic Diagnosis

Reproductive autonomy regards people's liberty right to decide whether to have children or not and to decide about the health of their future children.[13] At the heart of the latter is the parent's freedom to avoid the conception or birth of affected children, to which PGD is a morally sound method to use and people's preferences for this should be respected, at least in principle.[14] Professionals involved in medically assisted reproduction should avoid serious risks to the future child.[15] Furthermore, even if a risk is not, a priori, unacceptable, professionals should try reducing it, as it may have harmful psychosocial, medical/genetic, or mixed consequences for the child.[16] Situations where PGD is applied are as follows:

- Preimplantation genetic diagnosis for lower penetrance mutations and for disorders that have a highly variable expression
- Preimplantation genetic diagnosis to avoid the conception of healthy carriers who are at high risk of having affected children themselves
- Preimplantation genetic diagnosis for risk reduction (if the risk of transmitting a disorder cannot be completely eliminated)
- Transferring (possibly) affected embryos after failed PGD or when no "healthy" embryos (e.g. embryos unaffected with the disorder tested for) are available for transfer.

In traditional genetic counseling, especially in prenatal diagnosis, it is accepted that professionals should not try imposing their own views upon pregnant women, hence the use of nondirective counseling, aimed at supporting people's autonomous reproductive choice.[17] However, this normative framework cannot be simply extrapolated to medically assisted reproduction in general, and PGD, as professionals involved have a co-responsibility for the welfare of the future children conceived. Hence why most PGD centers accept the policy to never transfer an affected embryo and abstain from transferring an embryo after failed PGD—even if no other "healthy" embryos are available. This policy fits the principle to avoid serious harm to future children. Yet, despite being justified, there are an increasing number of exceptions to the traditional policy. The first variable relates to the severity of the disorder. In many cases the severity is evident, so a transfer would be fully unacceptable—not only when the embryo is proven to be affected but also after a PGD failure, as the risk that the embryo is affected will be in the range of 25–50%. Unquestionably, if the couple is fertile, they may then decide to engage in natural reproduction, which may be ethically problematic. However, this freedom is not a reason for professionals to disregard their own professional responsibility to abstain from assistance in reproduction in case of risk of serious harm. Nonetheless, situations may vary. Sometimes, a transfer of a possibly severely affected embryo does not result in the birth of a child affected with the particular disorder, due to natural selection in utero. Moreover, a flexible use of the proportionality criterion regarding indications for PGD may allow for other exceptions to the rule to never transfer an affected embryo or an embryo at high risk. Transferring an embryo carrying a less serious disorder, such as male infertility, may be well acceptable if there are no other embryos available for those infertile applicants who will engage in IVF/intracytoplasmic sperm injection. PGD/sex selection for indirect medical reasons, aiming at the avoidance of transgenerational transmission, may be morally justified—preconception sex selection would be useful. On another note, screening of numerical chromosome abnormalities is now under the terms of the PGT-A. At IVIRMA, this is used in patients with recurrent pregnancy loss, women above 38 years old and in the cases of semen alterations. In these patients, the use of PGT-A is essential. However, despite the principle of autonomy of the patients, it is necessary to inform them that in these situations the risk of genetic abnormal embryo is very high, and so is the rate of miscarriages.

The Application of Preimplantation Genetic Diagnosis for Human Leukocyte Antigen Typing of Embryos

Planning having a child with the intention to use it as a "donor" of hematopoietic stem cells for a sibling has been done for years with the means available each time. Before the possibility of prenatal HLA typing, parents would have another child hoping that it would be a match.[18] The dilemma for the parents is balancing the interests of both children. Moreover, the acceptability of this balance can be argued by referring to the notion of hypothetical consent: the future sibling on whose behalf the donation is made will agree with it when he/she becomes autonomous. For the sick child the benefits are obvious, since transplantation of stem cells from cord blood is the only treatment offering the chance of cure. The collaboration of the physician in these projects is justified, as this practice is morally acceptable. The team involved has the responsibility to provide full information, genetic and implication counseling to the future parents. It is also acceptable using PGD for the creation of an HLA-matched sibling to cure a sick child suffering from a serious nongenetic disease. Given the low chances of success of the procedure, it may be inappropriate to recommend the technique in the cases of advanced maternal age and/or poor ovarian reserve. The team may also conclude that the technique is not advisable if the chance of delivering an HLA-matched child given the specific circumstances is estimated as very low; parents should be urged to think about the disposition of the remaining healthy embryos that are not HLA compatible.[19] In these cases the options should be freezing for future reproduction by themselves, donation for research, or disposal. Donation to other couples is not advisable until sufficient information about the health of children after embryo biopsy is available. The creation of a donor child for harvesting nonregenerative organs is extremely difficult to justify in view of the risks involved. Creating a child to obtain an organ for a sibling is not acceptable, as solid organ donation by children or incompetent adults is not morally acceptable either, due to the more than minimal risk for the donor. Only empirical research will corroborate or refute the concerns about the psychological and social consequences for the donor sibling. It is therefore advisable to collate a register of such donations for this purpose. Given the relevance of parental motives for the moral evaluation, their intentions regarding the upbringing of the future child and their coping capacity should be discussed by a psychologist before the start of the treatment.

Sex Selection for Nonmedical Reasons

An overview of all 36 countries with laws or policies regarding sex selection, including 25 European countries,[20] with Israel as a qualified exception, shows that none of these allow sex selection for nonmedical reasons. Article 14 of the Convention on Human Rights and Biomedicine (Council of Europe) states that "the use of techniques of medically assisted procreation shall not be allowed for choosing a future child's sex, except where serious hereditary sex-related disease is to be avoided." It is suspected that sexist motives will be at work in most, if not all, cases of sex selection for nonmedical reasons, a deeply problematic practice from a moral point of view. "Sexism" refers to the discriminatory belief that one sex is better than the other and to the stereotyped views about gender role behavior.[21] This would also apply to sex selection aimed at having a "balanced family," not necessarily based on the supremacy of one sex, yet sexist in expressing and reinforcing preconceived gender role expectations. It has been suggested that sex selection by parent with stereotyped gender role expectations may negatively affect the welfare of their children. Sex selection in countries with a culturally mediated gender preference may reinforce societal patterns of inequality between the sexes.[22] There are concerns that the marketing of sex selection will reify sex differences and reinforce gender stereotypes in seemingly nonsexist western societies. If sex selection is motivated by a concern for reproductive health, there is no reason for questioning its acceptability. For prospective parents unable to cope in a responsible way with technology failure, IVF/PGT-A would be the better chosen methods in this respect. Although a reliable sex selection technology, PGT-A is burdensome, costly, and may raise ethical concerns related to the use of embryos. IVF/PGT-A material and immaterial costs make them only available for parents at risk of transmitting a serious genetic disease, excluding their use for parental sex preference. However, doctors performing PGT-A are questioned to be legally allowed to do so in countries with legislation banning sex selection. Despite not being against the letter of the law, additional sex selection (not involving any extra procedures or use of techniques) may still violate its spirit. Leaving the embryos' selection for transfer to a professional who is not aware of the couple's preferences may be a solution. Sex selection for nonmedical reasons through prenatal diagnosis, followed by abortion in the case of a fetus of the "wrong" sex, is widely regarded as morally problematic. This is the most used method in countries where sex selection has led to a distorted sex ratio. Forbid the use of prenatal diagnosis and abortion for sex selection (beyond medical reasons) had the adverse effect of making safe medical abortion less available for women who need such procedures.

FERTILITY PRESERVATION

Ethical Considerations for the Cryopreservation of Gametes and Reproductive Tissues for Self-use

The autonomy of males and females should be respected, as both should be able to take measures to preserve his or her fertility, whether threatened by disease or voluntary chosen interventions or life-plan considerations. The moral and legal recognition of autonomy is achieved by obtaining the informed consent of the patient, although obtaining this differs from adults to children, based on their decision-making capacity. Two considerations may complicate the decision-making of the parents: the imperative character of the offer and the principle of parental responsibility.[23] Due to the phenomenon of anticipated decision regret preserving gametes or tissues may take on an imperative character in decision-making, people are led by anticipation of the negative feelings of finding out later that they made the wrong decision. Second, some people may think that it is their duty as parents to take up every possibility to promote the child's future well-being, despite the possible complications of the intervention.[23] The reproductive tissues and gametes should only be stored until it is acceptable to be used, taking the welfare of the child, which is unlikely to be met when both parents are of a highly advanced age, and the risks to the pregnant mother into account. For stored embryos the storage period previously proposed may be extended to more than 10 years.[23]

Ethical Aspects of Social Freezing

The main argument against freezing oocytes by healthy women is the absence of a medical reason, which seems straightforward but very difficult to specify. The term "medical" has several functions in the debate, as it demarcates justified from unjustified interventions: "A medical indication appears rather as a practical normative construct in which medical and social justifications are woven together" but also indicates which interventions should be reimbursed by the health insurance system.[24] This is an essential element in the debate on oocyte freezing, since several IVF cycles may cost thousands of euros. Authors agree that approximately 25 good-quality oocytes should be stored to have a chance of success. Since most women who want to cryopreserve their oocytes for reasons of age are over 35, they will need 3–4 IVF cycles. Only people with sufficient financial resources will access the treatment, as no support from the public health system is offered. However, the meaning of the term in this debate is to keep open the possibility of having a genetically related child. Freezing eggs is labeled a mere preference since the woman has the option of becoming pregnant, so the freezing would be mainly based on social reasons. The IVI-RMA clinic in Valencia has been the first clinic worldwide to close an agreement with the Valencian *Club de Primeras Marcas*. This club puts together the best brands in the autonomous community of Valencia. A similar agreement has been made for brands, such as Google, Facebook, and Apple in the United States. This agreement allows companies to offer advantageous arrangements for the preservation of the fertility of its workers. We believe in giving the opportunity to motherhood whenever it is deemed appropriate, putting the interests of our patients first. It could be argued that women should not wait for the ideal situation, as financial resources or the family context may never be the preferred ones. Nonetheless, some concerns are considered essential, such as finding a stable and loving partner to raise a child with, something that cannot be planned. It seems ironic that women are now being blamed for wanting an appropriate environment for their future child.

Fertility Preservation for People with Cancer

A relatively new field of assisted reproductive technology deals with prevention of "oncofertility." The fertility of people with cancer can be threatened by the disease itself, radiotherapy or chemotherapy received to survive. Fertility preservation is not the best for the patient, as its measures often hold many risks. Sperm cryopreservation is the main exception. Oocyte vitrification is an efficient option for elective fertility preservation.[25] When ovarian stimulation is needed, either to cryopreserve oocytes or embryos, there will be a treatment delay of 2–3 weeks when one stimulation cycle is performed, or longer if several are carried out. Risks involve surgical complications, ovarian hyperstimulation syndrome, diminished ovarian reserve (when an entire ovary is removed), and possible reintroduction of malignant cells. Ovarian cortex autotransplantation can be a valid alternative to ovarian stimulation, with a 30% pregnancy rate after autotransplantation.[26] Moreover, fertility preservation can also be giving false hope to the patients, as some interventions may prove to be useless. Except for the use of cryopreserved sperm, the success rates of establishing a pregnancy are rather low. Either of these arguments seems convincing enough to abandon fertility preservation, based on the reasonable welfare standard, for all people with cancer. Although genetic components are at play in many types of cancer, sometimes it is the inheritance of an affected gene that results in an increased predisposition to develop the disease. According to the American Society of Reproductive Medicine, people with cancer have a higher risk than the general population that disease will recur and may be fatal, but this increase is not prohibitively high. Also in this case, the situation can be re-evaluated at the time of embryo transfer. Physician's reluctance to transfer embryos may be warranted if a woman has not recovered from the disease after radiotherapy or chemotherapy. However, excluding all people with cancer from taking fertility-preserving measures would be out of proportion. In countries struggling to provide their citizens with basic health care, it is, indeed, unrealistic to expect funding for sperm and oocyte cryopreservation, as well as ovarian and testicular tissue cryopreservation. Yet it seems logical that countries with generous policies for public funding of infertility treatments also cover measures to prevent future infertility. At IVIRMA, we are convinced that preservation should not only be indicated in cases of cancer but also to young women who suffer from endometriosis, those patients with bilateral unoperated endometriomas and those who had excision of unilateral endometriomas and have required surgery for a contralateral recurrence. However, pilot studies aimed at assessing the feasibility and potential benefits of fertility preservation procedures in women with endometriosis are prior to its introduction in routine clinical practice. If fertility preservation is useful for women as a whole, it would be highly suitable for women with endometriosis.

ISSUE PROVIDING SERVICES

Surrogacy

Problematic indications include serious health risks for the intended mother, difficulties in becoming pregnant (relative indication), and the absence of the uterus regardless of etiology (absolute indication). Surrogacy is an acceptable procedure, if made altruistically, to help a couple for which it is impossible, or medically contraindicated, to carry a pregnancy.[27] Several arguments against payment for surrogacy include insulting human dignity, instrumentalization of the human body, potential exploitation of vulnerable women and women's coercion.[27] Hence why only altruistic surrogacy is accepted. However, medical expenses incurred during the pregnancy and pregnancy-related complications, related expenses and the loss of actual income, not covered by the national health service, private insurance, or national social security system, should be reimbursed. Restrictions on both parties' autonomy are voluntarily accepted, and only in the case of the commissioning parents' death before birth would the surrogate have the first choice of keeping the child or giving it up for adoption. The surrogate simultaneously accepts restrictions on her autonomy when accepting to conceive and deliver a child on behalf of another couple voluntarily.[27] She is expected to behave responsibly and to conform to the original agreement with the future parents regarding prenatal screening and testing, which includes to consider terminating a pregnancy in the case of severe malformation of the fetus. The surrogate should behave reasonably by taking all the precautions advised in modern prenatal care (vitamins, no smoking, moderate alcohol use, etc.). Terminating a pregnancy can be justified for medical reasons, although it is impossible to prevent the surrogate from terminating the pregnancy or to force termination upon her, given the principle of respect for her autonomy and bodily integrity. However, she has the *prima facie* moral obligation to continue the pregnancy. Following the principle of autonomy, the surrogate cannot be forced to accept advice of the obstetric team, but she is obliged to accept the advice that ensures the best outcome for the child and for herself.[27] The IVIRMA clinic in Lisbon is the first in our clinics to allow surrogacy, Portugal is currently one of the countries in Europe that allows surrogacy. The current law in Portugal allows surrogacy in women who cannot use their uterus or who do not have one. The physician is responsible to assess the surrogacy in the cases of uterine diseases that make pregnancy impossible. Following medical indication, surrogacy is indicated in the cases of

- Absence of uterus
- Lack of functionality of the uterus
- Other clinical conditions that justify its use: This third group is astonishingly vague and broad, but, as in all cases of surrogacy, it needs to be previously approved by the National Council of Reproductive Medicine (CNPMA, in Portuguese). After having received the documents listed above, the CNPMA has 60 days to decide about the request. In case its decision is positive, the process is then sent to the Physicians Association. This entity has another 60 days to send a decision back to the CNPMA. The lack of response is assumed as an acceptance. After that, the CNPMA has 60 more days to inform the couple/carrier about the final decision.

There are certain conditions that need to be accepted and followed. First, the couple must choose the carrier on their own. The carrier is not allowed to accept any economic compensation, apart from the expenses generated by the treatment, pregnancy, and delivery. Second, one of the gametes must come from one of the members of the couple; the carrier cannot be the donor of the oocytes, even in the cases of oocyte donation. Third, for the contract to be valid, delivery must obviously take place in Portugal. Moreover, authorities have specified that couples/carriers from abroad can undergo the whole process in Portugal. Lastly, surrogacy is forbidden in homosexual couples, as well as in those cases where the uterus is not the issue.

Posthumous

Posthumous reproduction can be generally separated into distinct categories: fertilization and pregnancy take place after the death of one of the partners, but fertilization and cryopreservation of embryos take place before, or fertilization and pregnancy take place before the death of one of the partners, yet birth happens after it. Posthumous reproductive treatment may generate a conflict between two ethical principles—respect for the autonomy of people to decide about reproduction and of beneficence as expressed in the concern for the welfare of the child.[28] There are three possible situations. First, the gametes or embryos are solely put at the disposal of the surviving partner. The family of the deceased has no say in this matter, and the surviving partner has no legal or moral obligation to use the gametes or embryos for reproduction. A minimum waiting period of a year is obligatory to prevent hasty and ill-considered decisions. Psychological evaluation is essential in the assessment of this point, which should also stimulate the would-be parent to consider the social implications of the procedure, especially on the welfare of the future child. Second, the partner can only use the gametes or embryos for his/her own reproduction.[28] If he/she does not want to use them, they cannot be donated for the reproduction of others. The only options left are donation for scientific research or disposal. The main question is whether the wish, or acceptance, of parenthood after one's death is rational, although casuistry suggests that knowing that their wish may be realized after their death increases the quality of their lives. Third, the gametes or embryos must be destroyed (possibly preceded by research) when both partners die. Third parties cannot continue a parental project in which they had no part during the life of the intentional parents. Posthumous reproduction is highly controversial, due to the absence of empirical data on the psychosocial development of children born after this procedure, and to differences in appreciation of the parental project. If posthumous reproduction is applied in that context, the following steps are recommended:

- Writing a consent, before dying, on the use of the gametes or embryos
- Counseling of the surviving partner during the decision-making
- A minimum waiting period of 1 year after the death before the treatment starts.

Medically-assisted Reproduction in Singles, Lesbian and Gay Couples, and Transsexual People

Reproduction is an essential element of the autonomy of an individual. The acknowledgment of reproductive needs and interests of homosexual people, combined with the notion of equal citizenship, has increased the support for the view that lesbians and gays share the same right to reproduce as others. Recent studies show that many transsexuals, likewise, desire to have children.[29] From a human rights perspective, there are critics who would deny that particular groups have the right to reproduce. However, there are concerns regarding medical and/or psychosocial risks for the parties involved in nonstandard cases (especially children) and for society.[30] The debate is on psychosocial risks of growing up in a nonnuclear familial environment for the future child. Regarding the mother-headed families (single women, lesbian couples), critics fear that the absence of a father will have detrimental psychological development effects for the child. The sparse studies on single women opting for donor insemination to become a mother mostly report that they are psychologically healthy and can rely on a supportive family and social network; individuals raised in such families function well up into entering adult life if compared with children raised in heterosexual families. It is concluded that the quality of the family relationships matters more than the way in which the family is formed. There are far less data about the implications for the development and welfare of the child growing up with gay couples. It is far more difficult for gay men to convince people of the acceptability of their wish to parent and of their parental competency. It is often simply assumed that children need a mother to develop normally. However, the empirical literature available suggests that children are not adversely affected or harmed by being raised by homosexual fathers.[30,31] Many transsexuals have children, but the majority were born before their parents' transition. Preliminary findings suggest that children adapt, so their parents' transsexualism does not adversely impact them. However, children conceived by transsexual people after their gender identity shift need no adaptation to a new parental identity, which make things easier. A 12-year follow-up exploratory study of 42 children raised by transmen and their heterosexual wives after donor insemination suggests that those children are normal and happy.[32]

Equity of Access to Assisted Reproductive Technology

The question arises as to whether assistance to reproduction should be included in basic health care and eligible for reimbursement. The wish to reproduce encompasses people suffering from infertility and people needing infertility techniques to prevent the birth of a child with a specific genetic disorder, so people with the latter may need IVF combined with PGD. The pivotal point in the discussion is whether the desire for a child should be considered a fundamental need or a personal wish. The view, adopted by European Society of Human Reproduction and Embryology, argues that infertility may be a serious handicap that prevents people from realizing an important life goal.[33] However, funding of infertility treatment is not sufficient to eliminate inequity completely. In countries with mandatory insurance coverage or full reimbursement by the public system, groups with low income and low education make less use of health-care provisions. In societies with limited resources, minimal effectiveness is needed before treatment is reimbursed. Funding is extremely difficult to justify if the chance of success is close to zero. There are two sides in this debate—some people argue that everyone should have at least one chance, however small, to a child, although some others argue access should not only be given to patients with a high change of getting pregnant.[33] Nevertheless, some people say that the available resources should be distributed efficiently, implying that those with the highest chance of success should have priority. Almost all the countries that fund medically assisted reproduction have fixed a maximum number of cycles or interventions that will be reimbursed.

The Right of the Donor to Information About Children Conceived from his or her Gametes

The claims for a right to some type of information about the offspring conceived by donors through their donations are based on the following information:

- Medical information about the donor offspring can be fundamental to the donors' and their own children's health
- Basic information is a minimal reward for the altruistic behavior of the donors
- General information about the donor offspring should be given to ease their potential concern and sense of responsibility for the offspring
- Basic information can provide an important enrichment of the donors' identities
- The open-identity system creates a "new" type of donor that desires contact with their offspring.

There are three reasons why donors could claim an equal right to medical information about the offspring. The first reason is their own well-being: if the donor offspring develops a genetic disease and the donor is informed, he/she can be tested for the disease.[34] At best, adequate measures can then be taken to prevent it. The second reason deals with the donors' reproduction, as they could make informed reproductive decisions about whether they should have children of their own and about the need for prenatal or preimplantation diagnosis.[34] Finally, this information could also benefit the donors' own children, as they could seek treatment if needed or make informed reproductive decisions in the future.[34] Donors are seen as altruistic helpers who do the recipients a favor. The question arises on whether donors deserve to be rewarded for the donation, on top of the social recognition they may receive, particularly for the physical burden oocyte donors endure. Our society is highly sensitive to the needs and well-being of children, so it is not surprising that this concern heightens when it involves children who carry your genes. Anonymous feedback on the general well-being of the donor offspring could be given to donors, through a rating scale that covers various welfare issues; it could be updated every 5–10 years. This information should only be passed on to those donors who ask for it, and the possibility of bad news should be made clear. Granting donors general information about the offspring conceived by their donations could be a way to reassure them about the children's well-being. At IVIRMA, informing our donors about the success of the donation in terms of pregnancy and live births is not a problem. We believe that it is essential to undergo an altruistic process; the donor knows that her/his action has helped a couple become parents. Donors tend to ask if the donation was successful, and if the child who has been born from their donations enjoys good health. For us, denying this information is not acceptable.

REFERENCES

1. Pennings G, de Wert G. Evolving ethics in medically assisted reproduction. Hum Reprod Update. 2003;9(4):397-404.
2. Pennings G, de Wert G, Shenfield F, et al. ESHRE Task Force on Ethics and Law 13: the welfare of the child in medically assisted reproduction. Hum Reprod. 2007;22(10):2585-8.
3. Shenfield F, Pennings G, Cohen J, et al. Taskforce 8: ethics of medically assisted fertility treatment for HIV positive men and women. Hum Reprod. 2004;19(11):2454-6.
4. Olivennes F. Avoiding multiple pregnancies in ART. Double trouble: yes a twin pregnancy is an adverse outcome. Hum Reprod. 2000;15(8):1663-5.
5. Elster N. Less is more: the risks of multiple births. The Institute for Science, Law, and Technology Working Group on Reproductive Technology. Fertil Steril. 2000;74(4):617-23.
6. Pennings G. Avoiding multiple pregnancies in ART: multiple pregnancies: a test case for the moral quality of medically assisted reproduction. Hum Reprod. 2000;15(12):2466-9.
7. Practice Committee of the American Society for Reproductive Medicine; Practice Committee of the Society for Assisted Reproductive Technology. Guidance on the limits to the number of embryos to transfer: a committee opinion. Fertil Steril. 2017;107:901-3.
8. Templeton A. Avoiding multiple pregnancies in ART: replace as many embryos as you like-one at a time. Hum Reprod. 2000;15(8):1662.
9. Sazonova A, Kallen K, Thurin-Kjellberg A, et al. Neonatal and maternal outcomes comparing women undergoing two in vitro fertilization (IVF) singleton pregnancies and women undergoing one IVF twin pregnancy. Fertil Steril. 2013;99:731-7.
10. McLernon DJ, Harrild K, Bergh C, et al. Clinical effectiveness of elective single versus double embryo transfer: meta-analysis of individual patient data from randomised trials. BMJ. 2010;341:c6945.
11. Mancuso AC, Boulet SL, Duran E, et al. Elective single embryo transfer in women less than age 38 years reduces multiple birth rates, but not live birth rates, in United States fertility clinics. Fertil Steril. 2016;106:1107-14.
12. Ryan GL, Zhang SH, Dokras A, et al. The desire of infertile patients for multiple births. Fertil Steril. 2004;81:500-4.
13. Harper JC, Harton G. The use of arrays in preimplantation genetic diagnosis and screening. Fertil Steril. 2010;94(4):1173-7.
14. Harper JC, Sengupta SB. Preimplantation genetic diagnosis: state of the art 2011. Hum Genet. 2012;131(2):175-86.
15. De Wert G, Dondorp W, Shenfield F, et al. ESHRE Task Force on Ethics and Law 22: preimplantation genetic diagnosis. Hum Reprod. 2014;29(8):1610-7.
16. de Wert G. Preimplantation genetic diagnosis: the ethics of intermediate cases. Hum Reprod. 2005;20(12):3261-6.
17. Hens K, Dondorp W, Handyside AH, et al. Dynamics and ethics of comprehensive preimplantation genetic testing: a review of the challenges. Hum Reprod Update. 2013;19(4):366-75.
18. Burgio GR, Locatelli F. Transplant of bone marrow and cord blood hematopoietic stem cells in pediatric practice, revisited according to the fundamental principles of bioethics. Bone Marrow Transplant. 1997;19(12):1163-8.
19. Shenfield F, Pennings G, Cohen J, et al. Taskforce 9: the application of preimplantation genetic diagnosis for human leukocyte antigen typing of embryos. Hum Reprod. 2005;20(4):845-7.
20. Darnovsky M. Voluntary isn't working. Recent events show need for regulation of assisted reproduction. Mod Healthc. 2009;39(15):24.
21. Dondorp W, De Wert G, Pennings G, et al. ESHRE Task Force on Ethics and Law 20: sex selection for non-medical reasons. Hum Reprod. 2013;28(6):1448-54.
22. FIGO Committee for the Ethical Aspects of Human Reproduction and Women's Health. Ethical guidelines on sex selection for non-medical purposes. FIGO Committee for the Ethical Aspects of Human Reproduction and Women's Health. Int J Gynaecol Obstet. 2006;92(3):329-30.
23. ESHRE Task Force on Ethics and Law. Taskforce 7: ethical considerations for the cryopreservation of gametes and reproductive tissues for self use. Hum Reprod. 2004;19(2):460-2.
24. Pennings G. Ethical aspects of social freezing. Gynecol Obstet Fertil. 2013;41(9):521-3.
25. Cobo A, García-Velasco JA, Coello A, et al. Oocyte vitrification as an efficient option for elective fertility preservation. Fertil Steril. 2016;105(3):755-64.e8.
26. Jadoul P, Guilmain A, Squifflet J, et al. Efficacy of ovarian tissue cryopreservation for fertility preservation: lessons learned from 545 cases. Hum Reprod. 2017;32(5):1046-54.
27. Shenfield F, Pennings G, Cohen J, et al. ESHRE Task Force on Ethics and Law 10: surrogacy. Hum Reprod. 2005;20(10):2705-7.
28. Pennings G, de Wert G, Shenfield F, et al. ESHRE Task Force on Ethics and Law 11: posthumous assisted reproduction. Hum Reprod. 2006;21(12):3050-3.
29. Wierckx K, Van Caenegem E, Pennings G, et al. Reproductive wish in transsexual men. Hum Reprod. 2012;27(2):483-7.
30. De Wert G, Dondorp W, Shenfield F, et al. ESHRE Task Force on Ethics and Law 23: medically assisted reproduction in singles, lesbian and gay couples, and transsexual people. Hum Reprod. 2014;29(9):1859-65.
31. Golombok S, Mellish L, Jennings S, et al. Adoptive gay father families: parent-child relationships and children's psychological adjustment. Child Dev. 2014;85(2):456-68.
32. Chiland C, Clouet A-M, Golse B, et al. A new type of family: transmen as fathers thanks to donor sperm insemination. A 12-year follow-up exploratory study of their children. Neuropsychiatr Enfance Adolesc. 2013;61(6):365-70.
33. Pennings G, de Wert G, Shenfield F, et al. ESHRE Task Force on Ethics and Law 14: equity of access to assisted reproductive technology. Hum Reprod. 2008;23(4):772-4.
34. Raes I, Ravelingien A, Pennings G. The right of the donor to information about children conceived from his or her gametes. Hum Reprod. 2013;28(3):560-5.

Index

Page numbers followed by *f* refer to figure, *fc* refer to flowchart, and *t* refer to table.

B

D

E

F

G

K

L

M

N

O

P

Q

R

U

V

W

X

Y

Z